Robert Carachi · Jay L. Grosfeld · Amir F. Azmy

The Surgery of Childhood Tumors

Robert Carachi · Jay L. Grosfeld · Amir F. Azmy (Eds.)

The Surgery of Childhood Tumors

Second Corrected and Enlarged Edition

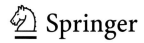

Springer

Robert Carachi, MD, PhD, FRCS
Professor of Surgical Paediatrics
at the University of Glasgow and Honorary Consultant
Paediatric Surgeon at the Royal Hospital for Sick Children
NHS Greater Glasgow and Clyde, Women & Children's Directorate, Yorkhill
Glasgow G3 SSJ, Scotland
UK

Jay L. Grosfeld, MD, FACS, FAAP, FRCS
Lafayette Page Professor and Chairman, Emeritus
Department of Surgery
Indiana University School of Medicine
Indianapolis, IN 46202
USA

Amir F. Azmy, MB, ChB, DS, FRCS
Consultant Paediatric Surgeon Department of Surgical Paediatrics
Royal Hospital for Sick Children, Yorkhill
Glasgow G3 SSJ, Scotland
UK

The first edition was published by Arnold, London, © 1999 (ISBN 0-340-69269-3)

ISBN 978-3-540-29733-8   e-ISBN 978-3-540-29734-5

DOI 10.1007/978-3-540-29734-5

Library of Congress Control Number: 2007932198

Cover design: Frido Steinen-Broo, eStudio, Calamar, Spain

Printed on acid-free paper

9 8 7 6 5 4 3 2 1

springer.com

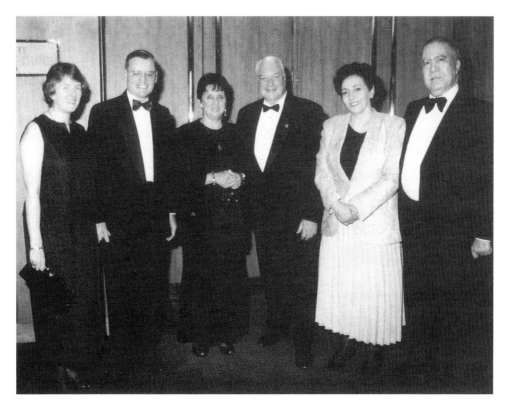

This photograph was taken in Glasgow (March, 1998) when Professor Jay Grosfeld was awarded the Honorary Fellowship of The Royal College of Physicians and Surgeons of Glasgow. The three editors in the picture with their wives are, from left to right, Robert and Annette Carachi, Jay and Margie Grosfeld, Amir and Fatima Azmy.

*This volume is dedicated to our wives,
our children, and our grandchildren.*

Foreword

Surgery was at one time the only modality of treatment which was capable of curing children unfortunate enough to develop cancer. Then along came radiotherapy, chemotherapy, and now even immunotherapy; however, surgery still retains an important place and in some instances good surgery is a prerequisite for cure.

In Europe and the UK, as in the US, much of the early treatment for children with solid tumors was led by and often given by surgeons. We now, however, have multidisciplinary teams with each member having a key role to play.

Survival for childhood cancer has improved dramatically over the last 50 years and although we continue to make progress the rate of improvement has inevitably slowed down. In developed countries the major scope for improvement still lies in the organization of care. Ensuring that the pathway to diagnosis is as short as possible and ends at the team that can deliver best modern treatment, preferably in a clinical trial setting, has to be a goal for all countries. One of the biggest hurdles, however, remains getting on to that diagnostic journey in the first place and there remains a great deal to be done in education of both parents and primary care physicians to take lumps and bumps seriously. Even within Europe there are marked disparities in outcome in spite of similar treatments. Social factors and access to and compliance with care must also be considered.

The role of the surgeon is important in the direct management of children with cancer but they also play a huge supportive role. The advent of central venous lines to facilitate access for chemotherapy has revolutionized the giving of treatment. Insertion of these lines is a skilled procedure and needs to be done in a timely fashion. The oncology team surgeon usually plays this vital role.

I am delighted to see the second edition of this important book. The editors have done an excellent job in drawing together a real team of experts. This book will facilitate the education of young surgeons, keen to join the pediatric oncology team, and provide refreshment and stimulation for those already in the field.

Professor Sir Alan W. Craft

Foreword

In managing a child thought to have a malignant tumor, the day starts in the operating room, literally and figuratively. The surgeon is the key figure, whether in taking a biopsy or undertaking a major extirpation. Much depends on how that procedure is done, starting with the incision. Is it correctly placed – whether for a biopsy or a radical procedure – or will it make for problems in subsequent management? Even at this perhaps simplest of levels, it is obvious that the surgeon from the beginning plays a pivotal role in ensuring success in pediatric oncology. A trans-scrotal biopsy of a subsequently proven testicular or paratesticular malignant tumor complicates matters. How best to deal with the unnecessarily contaminated hemi-scrotal sac?

It is also inherent in the example given that modern management of the child with cancer entails working as a member of a coordinated, multimodal team. Long gone are the days when any specialist could embark on a solo course of action. The pediatric radiation therapist and chemotherapist along with the surgeon make up that team, each depending on the skill and expertise of the other.

Modern multimodal care in pediatric oncology has led to the rapid rise in survival rates of the various malignant entities to the present astonishing levels. Effective anticancer drugs have been credited with much of that progress – and rightly so. That has, however, also led in recent decades to an unfortunate undervaluation of the part surgeons have played and continue to play in contributing to that success. The surgeon's role too often is being taken for granted. It must be more appreciated and understood that the day does indeed start in the operating room. I feel this perhaps more keenly because I had the privilege of working as an intern under two great pioneering pediatric surgeons: Drs. William E. Ladd and Robert E. Gross. They were the Fathers of Pediatric Surgery in the USA, and were responsible for major steps forward in the management of children with cancer. Their surgical skills were remarkable, and made a deep impression, of course, as did their willingness to look beyond accepted techniques and methods. They were ready to explore the new and promising; Dr. Ladd, for instance trying and then advocating the transperitoneal approach to Wilms' tumors. Dr. Gross did so for routine postoperative radiation therapy for that neoplasm, thus forging the first link in the chain of interdisciplinary care. Even more memorable and important was their systematic, careful method for moving forward. Their innovations were not capricious. They came about only after careful thought, observation, and even laboratory experimentation when appropriate. Their textbooks were models of building on the logical conclusions. From the organization of those books, I first began to understand the meaning of the "scientific method."

Despite the fact that some of the best survival rates in the world resulted from what they were doing, the chemotherapist was quickly added to the radiotherapist to form the modern multimodal team. Great credit is due Drs. Ladd, Gross, and other surgeons like them, in so quickly embracing a pattern of care that was completely new, and helping to pave the path to progress.

But the day for the multimodal team nonetheless starts with the surgeon, who ideally should be a member of an experienced, interdisciplinary unit. If not, and such a well-staffed and competent pediatric cancer center is available locally, the child should be referred there. This is so because childhood cancers are very different from those that occur in the adult. Few surgeons accumulate sufficient personal experience to feel confident in undertaking the care of a child with a malignant tumor. To help them understand the intricacies of the pediatric surgical oncology, the editors have brought together in these pages the experience and expertise of an international array of surgeons and other authorities. The Table of Contents shows the wide range topics covered. They start with basic considerations such as the epidemiology of childhood tumors. The roles of associated specialties are then discussed along with a review of specific tumor types. Supportive and palliative care – extremely important topics sometimes neglected in "how to" books – are not neglected. Chapter 29 adds information concerning how best to interact with parents' groups and other psychosocial support associations. Such groups are making their voices heard more and more, and it is appropriate and proper that they should. The surgeon must be ready to meet with such associations, to discuss their problems and to answer their questions. The second edition of this book thus brings detailed and up-to-date informing concerning what needs to be done not only before surgery, but also at the operating table and thereafter. It does more than that: It provides a blue print of how the surgeon can best fit within the modern practice of pediatric oncology.

Emeritus Professor J. Giulio D'Angio

Preface

The first edition of The Surgery of Childhood Tumors was published in 1999. The purpose of the book was to produce a comprehensive illustrated reference book on the management of childhood solid tumors focusing on those neoplasms of specific interest to pediatric surgeons. It was also intended for use by pediatricians, pediatric and adult medical oncologists, general and pediatric urologists, orthopedic surgeons, otolaryngologists and neurosurgeons. Each chapter was written by an authority in that field of pediatric oncology. Authors were selected from Europe, the United States, and Asia. Most were members of the major cancer study groups worldwide. This book was well received and the editors believed that a second edition was due because of the new important knowledge that has become available in the last few years. There have been new developments in epidemiology, tumor biology, molecular genetics of cancer, concepts of risk in relation to pediatric surgical pathology, diagnostic imaging techniques, radiation and chemotherapy. In particular, there are new surgical concepts in the evolution of minimally invasive surgery in the diagnosis and management of surgical oncology as well as the problem of vascular access provided by the surgeon and the interventionalist. Novel methods of treatment in cancer patients have advanced with the increased knowledge of the molecular biology of the cancer cell. As a consequence, the 2nd edition has had to include chapters on new therapies and technologies and up-to-date literature reviews. We trust that the readers will find these changes valuable.

We have retained our main aim in the 1st edition to have the book well illustrated with clinical images as well as detailed operative techniques and up-to-date references. The book consists of three sections:

Part A consists of eight chapters dealing with epidemiology of childhood cancer, tumor biology, and environmental carcinogens, the genetics of cancer including inherited syndromes and counseling, tumor markers and results of tumor screening programs, tumor imaging, the general pathologic principles of childhood solid tumors, and information regarding chemotherapy, radiation therapy, and immunotherapy in pediatric cancer.

Part B consists of seven chapters concerning tumors encountered in the neonatal period, and the contemporary management of Wilms' tumor and other renal neoplasms, neuroblastoma and other adrenal lesions, malignant hepatic tumors, germ cell tumors, soft tissue sarcomas, and Hodgkin's and non-Hodgkin's lymphoma.

Part C deals with some tumors managed by the specialist surgeons and other members of the cancer team and consists of fourteen chapters including chapters about malignant bone tumors, and head and neck tumors with extensive coverage of medullary thyroid cancer and multiple endocrine neoplasia syndromes. The chapter on brain tumors has been altered to include orbital and periorbital tumors. The other chapters in this section cover thoracic tumors (lung, chest wall, and mediastinum), other rare tumors observed in children, and unique aspects of reconstructive surgery following extensive procedures (limb salvage, chest wall replacement, etc.). Surgical and other complications of cancer treatment, patient and family support and counseling at diagnosis and during early postoperative care in potential survivors, palliative and terminal care, and bereavement, as well as the late effects of cancer treatment in long-term survivors are also covered in detail. This chapter also includes an extensive review on fertility in children treated for cancer. Four other new chapters have been included on minimal invasive surgery, new treatments and new strategies, central venous access and pain management. There is occasional overlap in some chapters when dealing with tumors in anatomical regions, and this was intentionally left in place and cross-referenced.

The editors wish to thank all the contributing 47 authors for taking valuable time from their busy schedules to participate in the development of this text and for submitting their manuscripts in a timely manner.

Robert Carachi
Jay L. Grosfeld
Amir F. Azmy

Acknowledgements

We are grateful to Professor Dr. Giulio D'Angio and Sir Alan Craft for writing the Foreword to this 2nd edition of 'The Surgery of Childhood Tumors'. We would also like to thank our secretaries Kay Byrne (Glasgow) for the tremendous amount of work in corresponding with the authors of all the chapters and collating all the material to hand over to the publishers as well as Karen Jaeger (Indianapolis) for her help in preparing the manuscripts during the production of this text. Our gratitude goes to Gabriele Schröder, Editorial Director and Stephanie Benko, Desk Editor Clinical Medicine of Springer Verlag for their help and support in the production of this book.

Finally we would like to thank our wives and children for their continuing support and understanding while we were editing this book.

Robert Carachi
Jay L. Grosfeld
Amir F. Azmy

Contents

List of Contributors

Mr. Basith Amjad
Department of Surgical Paediatrics
Royal Hospital for Sick Children, Yorkhill
Glasgow G3 8SJ, Scotland
UK

Professor Richard J. Andrassy
Chairman, Department of Surgery
University of Texas Medical Center
6431 Fannin, MSB 4-020
Houston, TX 77020
USA

Emeritus Professor J. Giulio D'Angio
University of Pennsylvania Medical Center
2 Donner Building
3400 Spruce Street
Philadelphia, PA 19104-4283
USA

Dr. G. Suren Arul
Consultant Paediatric Surgeon
Department of Surgery
Birmingham Children's Hospital
Steelhouse Lane
Birmingham B4 6NH
UK

Professor Richard G. Azizkhan
Children's Hospital of Cincinnati
3333 Burnet Avenue MLC 301 8
Cincinnati, OH 45239-3039
USA

Mr. Amir F. Azmy
Department of Surgical Paediatrics
Royal Hospital for Sick Children, Yorkhill
Glasgow G3 8SJ, Scotland
UK

Professor Edward M. Barksdale
Children's Hospital of Pittsburgh
Department of Pediatric Surgery
3705 Fifth Avenue, Suite 4A-485
Pittsburgh, PA 15213-2583
USA

Dr. Louise E. Bath
Department of Paediatric Oncology
Royal Hospital for Sick Children
9 Sciennes Road
Edinburgh EH9 1LF, Scotland
UK

Professor Deborah F. Billmire
Riley Children's Hospital
702 Barnhill Drive, Suite 2500
Indianapolis, IN 46202
USA

Miss Elspeth Livingston Brewis
2 Grosvenor Crescent
Glasgow G12 9AE, Scotland
UK

Mr. Stephen V. Cannon
London Bone and Soft Tissue Service
Royal Orthopaedic Hospital
Stanmore
Middlesex, HA7 4LP
UK

Professor Robert Carachi
Department of Surgical Paediatrics
Royal Hospital for Sick Children, Yorkhill
Glasgow G3 8SJ, Scotland
UK

Mr. Paul D. Chumas
Consultant Paediatric Neurosurgeon
The General Infirmary
Leeds, LS1 3EX
West Yorkshire
UK

Professor J. Michael Connor
Duncan Guthrie Institute of Medical Genetics
Royal Hospital for Sick Children, Yorkhill
Glasgow G3 8SJ, Scotland
UK

Dr. Fiona Cowie
Consultant Clinical Oncologist
Beatson Oncology Centre
Western Infirmary
Durnbarton Road
Glasgow G1 1 6NT, Scotland
UK

Professor Sir Alan W. Craft
Sir James Spence Institute
Royal Victoria Infirmary
Newcastle upon Tyne NE1 4LP
UK

Dr. John Currie
Consultant Anaesthetist
Royal Hospital for Sick Children, Yorkhill
Glasgow G3 8SJ, Scotland
UK

Associate Professor Andrew M. Davidoff
St. Jude Children's Research Hospital
332 N. Lauderdale-Mail Stop 133
Memphis, TN 38105-2794
USA

Dr. Diana L. Diesen
Duke University Medical Center
Division of Pediatric Surgery
Box 3815
Durham, NC 17710
USA

Professor Jay L. Grosfeld
Riley Children's Hospital
702 Barnhill Drive, Suite 2500
Indianapolis, IN 46202
USA

Mr. Constantinos A. Hajivassiliou
Consultant Paediatric Surgeon
Royal Hospital for Sick Children, Yorkhill
Glasgow G3 8SJ, Scotland
UK

Professor Hugo A. Heij
Head of Pediatric
Surgical Centre Amsterdam
University Hospital Vrije Universiteit
De Boelelaan 11 17
P.O. Box 7057
107 MB Amsterdam
The Netherlands

Dr. Melanie Hiorns
Great Ormond Street Hospital for Children NHS Trust
Great Ormond Street
London WC1N 3JH
UK

Professor George W. Holcomb
Children's Mercy Hospital
240 1 Gillham Road
Kansas City, MO 64108
USA

Dr. Allan G. Howatson
Consultant Pathologist
Royal Hospital for Sick Children, Yorkhill
Glasgow G3 8SJ, Scotland
UK

Professor Christopher J. Kelnar
Department of Paediatric Oncology
Royal Hospital for Sick Children
9 Sciennes Road
Edinburgh EH9 1LF, Scotland
UK

Mr. Charles Keys
Department of Surgical Paediatrics
Royal Hospital for Sick Children, Yorkhill
Glasgow G3 8SJ, Scotland
UK

Professor Jean-Martin Laberge
Montreal Children's Hospital
2300 Tupper Street C-1 137
Montreal, Quebec
H3H 1P3
Canada

Professor Michael P. LaQuaglia
Memorial Sloan-Kettering Cancer Center
Dept. of Pediatric Surgery
1275 York Avenue, Room C1 17
New York, NY 10021
USA

Dr. Dermot Murphy
Consultant Pediatric Oncologist
Schiehallion Unit
Royal Hospital for Sick Children, Yorkhill
Glasgow G3 8SJ, Scotland
UK

Mrs. Marianne C. Naafs-Wilstra
Director VOKK
Scgiywstede 2d
343 1 JB Nieuwegein
The Netherlands

Emeritus Professor Jean-Bernard Otte
Cliniques Saint-Luc
Avenue Hippocrate
B- 1200 Brussels
Belgium

Dr. Susan V. Picton
Consultant Paediatric Oncologist
Department of Paediatric Oncology
Children's Day Hospital
St James' Hospital
Beckett Street
Leeds LS9 7TF
UK

Dr. Michelle Reece-Mills
Department of Paediatric Oncology
Royal Hospital for Sick Children
9 Sciennes Road
Edinburgh EH9 1LF, Scotland
UK

Professor Frederick J. Rescorla
Riley Children's Hospital
702 Barnhill Drive, Suite 2500
Indianapolis, IN 46202
USA

Dr. Milind Ronghe
Consultant Pediatric Oncologist
Schiehallion Unit
Royal Hospital for Sick Children, Yorkhill
Glasgow G3 8SJ, Scotland
UK

Dr. Daniel N. Rutigliano
Memorial Sloan Kettering Cancer Center
Dept. of Surgery, Division of Pediatric Surgery
1275 York Avenue, Room H1315
New York, NY 10021
USA

Professor Robert C. Shamberger
Children's Hospital Boston
Department of Surgery
300 Longwood Avenue
Boston, MA 02115
USA

Dr. Michael A. Skinner
Duke University Medical Center
Division of Pediatric Surgery
Box 3815
Durham, NC 17710
USA

Mr. Richard D. Spicer
Consultant Paediatric Surgeon
Royal Hospital for Sick Children
St. Michaels Hill
Bristol BS2 8BJ
UK

Mr. Charles A. Stiller
Research Officer
CCRG
57 Woodstock Road
Oxford 0x2 6HJ
UK

Dr. Wendy Su
UCI Medical Center
101 The City Drive
Building 55, Room 110
Orange, CA 92828
USA

Mr. Edward S. Tobias
Duncan Guthrie Institute of Medical Genetics
Royal Hospital for Sick Children, Yorkhill
Glasgow G3 8SJ, Scotland
UK

Professor Benno M. Ure
Director, Kinderchirurgische Klinik
Medizinische Hochschule
30623 Hannover
Germany

Mr. Gregor Walker
Consultant Pediatric Surgeon
Department of Surgical Paediatrics
Royal Hospital for Sick Children, Yorkhill
Glasgow G3 8SJ, Scotland
UK

Dr. Hamish B. Wallace
Consultant Oncologist
Royal Hospital for Sick Children
9 Sciennes Road
Edinburgh EH9 1LF, Scotland
UK

Dr. Harry Willshaw
Consultant Ophthalmologist
Birmingham Children's Hospital NHS Trust
Steelhouse Lane
Birmingham B4 6NH
UK

Glossary of Terms

Alleles
Alternative forms of a gene or DNA sequence occuring at the same locus an homologous chromosomes.

Aneuploid
Chromosome number that is not an exact multiple of the haploid set – for example, 2n – 1 or 2n × 1.

Clone
All cells arising by mitotic division from a single original cell and having the same genetic constitution.

Diploid
Normal state of human somatic cells, containing two haploid sets of chromosomes (2n).

DNA polymerase
Enzyme concerned with synthesis of double-stranded DNA from single-stranded DNA.

Haploid
Normal state of gametes, containing one set of chromosomes (n).

Heritability
The contribution of genetic as opposed to environmental factors to phenotypic variance.

Hybridization
Process by which single strands of DNA with homologous sequence bind together.

Oncogene
Gene with potential to cause cancer.

Polymerase chain reaction (PCR)
Method of amplification of specific DNA sequences by repeated cycles of DNA synthesis to permit rapid analysis of DNA restriction fragments subsequently.

Polyploid
Chromosome numbers representing multiples of the haploid set greater than diploid – for example 3n.

Probe
Labeled DNA fragment used to detect complementary sequences in DNA sample.

Southern blotting
Process of transferring DNA fragments from agarose gel to nitrocellulose filter or nylon membrane.

Translocation
Transfer of chromosomel material between two non-homologous chromosomes.

Triploid
Cells containing three haploid sets of chromosomes (3n).

Deletion
A deletion occurs when a section of a chromosome either terminal or intestitial is lost.

Proto-oncogene
First recognized as viral oncongenes (*v-onc*) carried by RNA viruses. Subsequent ones found in the human genome are called cellular oncogenes *(c-onc)*. More than 60 such proto-oncognes have been described. Their normal function is the control of cell growth and differentiation. Mutation results in appropriate expression leading to neoplasia.

Northern blotting
Blotting for analysis from RNA detects gene expression.

FISH
Fluorescent in situ hybridization. DNA probe labeled with fluorochrome and hybridized direct with a metaphase chromose spread. A fluorescent signal produced by the hybridization to the relevant chromosome is visualized using a fluorescent microscope.

Abbreviations

Organizations

CCG	Children's Cancer Group
CCLG	Children's Cancer and Leukemia Group
CESS	German Cooperative Ewing's Sarcoma Study
CLGB	Cancer and Leukemia Group B
CWS	German Cooperative Sarcoma Group
EC	European Community
ENSG	European Neuroblastoma Study Group
IACR	International Association of Cancer Registries
IARC	International Agency for Research and Cancer
ICDO	International Classification of Disease for Oncology
INSS	International Neuroblastoma Staging System
IRS	Intergroup Rhabdomyosarcoma Study Group
NCI	National Cancer Institute (USA)
NWTS	National Wilms' Tumor Study
POG	Pediatric Oncology Group (USA)
SEER (Program)	Surveillance, Epidemiology and End-Results Program
SIOP	International Society of Pediatric Oncology (Society Internationale Oncologie Pediatrique)
SWOG	Southwest Oncology Group
UKW	United Kingdom Wilms' Tumor Trials
WHO	World Health Organization

Common Abbreviations Used in the Text

ABMT	Autologous Bone Marrow Transplant
ACTH	Adrenocorticotropic Hormone
ADEPT	Antibody Directed Enzyme Prodrug Therapy
AFP	Alpha-Fetoprotein
AIDS	Acquired Immunodeficiency Syndrome
ALL	Acute Lymphoblastic Leukemia
ALL	Acute Lymphocytic Leukemia
AML	Acute Myelogenous Leukemia
ANLL	Acute Nonlymphoblastic Leukemia
APUD	Amine Precursor Uptake and Decarboxylation
ARDS	Adult Respiratory Distress Syndrome
ASR	Age Standardized Rate
ASRM	Age Standardized Mortality Rate
bFGF	Basic Fibroblast Growth Factor
BMRTC	Bone Metastasing Renal Tumor of Childhood
CFS	Congenital Fibrosarcoma
CK	Creatine Kinase
CMN	Congenital Mesoblastic Nephroma
CMV	Cytomegalovirus
CNS	Central Nervous System
COMT	Catechol-O-Methyltransferase
CPDN	Cystically Partially Differentiated Nephroblastoma
CT	Computed Tomography
CUM	Cumulated Incidence Rate
DDC	DOPA Decarboxylase
DGH	dopamine β-hydroxylase
DNET	Dysembryoplastic Neuroepithelial Tumor
DOPA	3, 4-Dihydroxyphenylalanine
EBV	Epstein-Barr virus
EMG	Exomphalos, Macroglossia and Gigantism Syndrome
FAP	Familial Adenomatous Polyposis
FISH	Fluorescent In Situ Hybridization
FNA	Fine Needle Aspiration
FRC	Functional Residual Capacity
FSH	Follicle Stimulating Hormone
5-FU	5-Fluorouracil
FVC	Forced Vital Capacity
G-CSF	Granulocyte Colony Stimulating Factor
GCT	Germ Cell Tumors
GLC	Gas Liquid Chromatography
GM	Granulocyte Macrophage
HAL	Hepatic Artery Ligation
HCG	Human Chorionic Gonadotropin

HIV	Human Immunodeficiency Virus
HMMA	Hydroxymethoxymandellic Acid
HPLC	High Performance Liquid Chromatography
HSV	Herpes Simplex Virus
HVA	Homovanillic Acid
IGF	Insulin-Like Growth Factor
IR	Incidence Rate
ITP	Idiopathic Thrombocytopenic Purpura
LCH	Lens Culinaris Hemagglutinin
LDH	Lactic Dehydrogenase
LH	Luteinizing Hormone
LT	Linear Trend
Mab	Monoclonal Antibodies
MAO	Monoamine Oxidase
MDP	Methylene Diphosphonate
MDR	Multiple Drug Resistance
MEN	Multiple Endocrine Neoplasia
Mesna	2-Mercaptoethane Sulfate
MFH	Malignant Fibrous Histiocytoma
MIBG	Meta-Iodo-Benzylguanidine
MKI	Mitosis/Karryorrhexis Index
6-MP	6-Mercaptopurine
MPNST	Malignant Peripheral Nerve Sheath Tumors
MR	Mortality Rate
MRA	Magnetic Resonance Angiography
MRP	Multiple Drug Resistance Associated Protein Gene
MTC	Medullary Thyroid Carcinoma
NGF	Nerve Growth Factor
NHL	Non-Hodgkin's Lymphoma
NPY	Neuropeptide Y
NRSTS	Non-Rhabdomyosarcoma Soft Tissue Sarcomas
NSE	Neuron-Specific Enolase
OMIM	On-line Mendelian Inheritance in Man
OPSI	Overwhelming Post-Splenectomy Infection
PAS	Periodic Acid-Schiff
PCA	Patient-Controlled Analgesia
PCNA	Proliferating Cell Nuclear Antigen
PCR	Polymerase Chain Reaction
PEFR	Peak Expiratory Flow Rate
PEI	Percutaneous Ethanol Injection
PNET	Primitive Neuroectodermal Tumor
PNMT	Phenylethanolamine-N-Methyl-transferase
RMS	Rhabdomyosarcoma
SIR	Standardized Incidence Rate
SMN	Second Malignant Neoplasms
SMR	Standardized Mortality Rate
SPECT	Single Photon Emission Computed Tomography
TBI	Total Body Irradiation

TGF	Transforming Growth Factor
TLC	Total Lung Capacity
RMN	Third Malignant Neoplasms
TNM	Tumor-Node-Metastasis
TRK	Tyrosine Kinase Receptor
TS	Tuberous Sclerosis
TSH	Thyroid-Stimulating Hormone
VIP	Vasoactive Intestinal Polypeptide
VLA	Vanillactic Acid
VMA	Vanillylmandelic Acid
WAGR	Wilms' Tumor, Aniridia, Genitourinary Abnormalities (or Gonadoblastoma), Abnormalities and Mental Retardation

Acronyms of Drug Combinations

ABVD	Adriamyciri (Doxorubicin) Bleomycin, Vinblastine, Dacarbazine
Adria-VAC	Adriamycin (Doxorubicin), Vincristine, Actinomycin-D, Cyclophosphamide
BEP	Bleomycin, Etoposide, Cisplatin
BiCNU	Carmustine (Bischloroethyl-N-Nitro-surea)
CADO	Cyclophosphamide, Adriamyciri (Doxorubicin)
CCNU	Lomustine (Chloroethyl-N-Cyclohexyl-N-Nitrosurea)
Ch1VPP	Chlorambucil, Vinblastine, Procarbazine, Prednisone
COMP	Cyclophosphomide, Vincristine (Oncovin) Methotrexate, Prednisone
IVA	Ifosfamide, Vincristine, Adriamycin (Doxorubicin)
JEB	Carboplatin, Etoposide, Bleom Cin
MOPP	Mustine, Vincristine (Oncovin) Procarbazine, Prednisolone
OPEC	Vincristine (Oncovin) Cisplatin or
OJEC	Etoposide, Carboplatin
PEI	Cisplatin, Etoposide, Ifosfamide
PVB	Cisplatin, Vinblastine, Bleomycin
PLADO	Cisplatin, Adriamyciri (Doxorubicin)
VA	Vincristine, Actinomycin-D
VAC	Vincristine, Actinomycin-D, Cyclophosphamide
VAdriaC	Vincristine, Adriamyciri (Doxorubicin), Cyclophosphamide
VIA	Vincristine, Ifosfamide, Actinomycin-D
VIE	Vincristine, Ifosfamide, Etoposide

Part A

Epidemiology of Childhood Tumors

1

Charles A. Stiller

Contents

1.1 Classification

Traditionally, descriptive data on cancers occurring in people of all ages combined have been presented with the diagnoses categorized according to the International Classification of Diseases (ICD), in which cancers other than leukemias, lymphomas, Kaposi's sarcoma, cutaneous melanoma, and mesothelioma are classified purely on the basis of primary site. The malignant solid tumors of children are histologically very diverse and a substantial proportion consists of characteristic entities that are rarely seen in adults. Therefore, it is appropriate to group childhood cancers in a way which more fully takes morphology into account, and standard classifications have been devised with the categories defined according to the codes for topography and morphology in the International Classification of Diseases for Oncology (ICD-O) [4, 25, 59]. The current scheme is the International Classification of Childhood Cancer, Third Edition (ICCC-3), based on the third edition of ICD-O [59]. ICCC-3 contains 12 main diagnostic groups:

I   Leukemias, myeloproliferative diseases, and myelodysplastic diseases

II   Lymphomas and reticuloendothelial neoplasms

III   CNS and miscellaneous intracranial and intraspinal neoplasms

IV   Neuroblastoma and other peripheral nervous cell tumors

V   Retinoblastoma

VI   Renal tumors

VII   Hepatic tumors

VIII   Malignant bone tumors

IX   Soft tissue and other extraosseous sarcomas

X   Germ cell tumors, trophoblastic tumors, and neoplasms of gonads

XI   Other malignant epithelial neoplasms and malignant melanomas

XII   Other and unspecified malignant neoplasms

All of the groups except retinoblastoma are split into subgroups, and the most heterogeneous subgroups are in turn split into divisions. Most groups contain only malignant neoplasms, but groups III and X also include nonmalignant intracranial and intraspinal tumors since they are usually recorded by cancer registries.

Successive classifications have been designed to have as much continuity as possible with their predecessors, while recognizing advances in understanding of tumor pathology and biology. Although the nomenclature of many groups and subgroups has changed since the previous version of the classification, their contents are largely the same.

1.2 Incidence

The annual incidence of cancer in children under 15 years of age is usually between 100 and 160 per million. There is a risk of 1 in 650 to 1 in 400 that a child will be affected during the first 15 years following birth. Table 1.1 shows annual incidence rates per million children in Great Britain for the decade 1991–2000 [61]. The total incidence, just under 140 per million, was slightly lower than in many industrialized countries, but the relative frequencies of the different groups and subgroups were fairly typical. In Table 1.1, the ICCC-3 subgroups for Burkitt lymphoma and other non-Hodgkin lymphoma (NHL) have been combined because they are usually considered together clinically, and data for some other subgroups and divisions are not shown separately because of small numbers.

Table 1.1 Registration rates for cancers diagnosed at age 0–14 years in Great Britain, 1991–2000. Source: National Registry of Childhood Tumors [61]

ICCC-3 categories	Total registrations	Annual rates per million children for age group (years)				Age standardized rates per million (world standard population)		
		0	1–4	5–9	10–14	Boys	Girls	Children
I-XII. All cancers	14,659	187.9	185.9	108.3	110.8	150.5	127.4	139.2
I. Leukemias	4,695	38.3	78.2	34.4	24.8	50.1	40.7	45.5
(a) Lymphoid leukemias	3,715	18.0	66.7	28.3	17.0	39.9	32.1	36.1
(b) Acute myeloid leukemias	693	13.5	7.9	4.4	5.8	7.1	6.1	6.6
(c) Chronic myeloproliferative diseases	63	-	0.3	0.5	1.1	0.6	0.5	0.6
(d) Myelodysplastic syndrome and other myeloproliferative	173	4.9	2.7	1.0	0.6	1.9	1.5	1.7
(e) Other and unspecified	51	2.0	0.6	0.2	0.3	0.5	0.5	0.5
II. Lymphomas, etc.	1424	1.1	7.9	12.9	20.1	17.0	13.9	12.5
(a) Hodgkin lymphoma	584	-	1.3	4.2	11.1	6.5	3.4	5.0
(b, c) Non-Hodgkin lymphomas	815	0.8	6.4	8.5	8.8	10.2	4.3	7.3
(d, e) Other and unspecified	25	0.3	0.2	0.2	0.3	0.3	0.1	0.2
III. CNS, intracranial, intraspinal	3,605	35.2	36.0	35.4	28.3	34.7	32.3	33.5
(a) Ependymomas & choroid plexus tumors	352	6.9	5.5	2.2	1.7	4.0	2.9	3.5
1. Ependymomas	261	1.8	4.2	1.9	1.6	2.7	2.2	2.5
2. Choroid plexus tumors	91	5.0	1.4	0.3	0.1	1.3	0.6	1.0
(b) Astrocytomas	1,551	10.4	15.1	15.8	13.0	13.3	15.4	14.3
(c) Intracranial & intraspinal embryonal tumors	697	9.0	8.1	7.2	3.7	7.8	5.4	6.6
1. Medulloblastomas	509	4.1	5.4	6.0	2.9	5.9	3.6	4.8
2. Primitive neuroectodermal tumor	161	3.8	2.3	1.1	0.7	1.7	1.5	1.6
4. Atypical teratoid/ rhabdoid tumor	24	1.1	0.3	0.1	0.1	0.2	0.2	0.2
(d) Other gliomas	380	2.0	3.2	4.5	3.0	3.5	3.5	3.5
(e) Other specified	452	3.9	2.8	4.3	5.2	4.5	3.7	4.1
2. Craniopharyngioma	201	0.7	1.2	2.3	2.2	2.0	1.6	1.8
4. Neuronal, neuronal-glial	142	2.4	0.8	1.4	1.4	1.4	1.2	1.3
5. Meningiomas	48	0.1	0.3	0.4	0.7	0.5	0.3	0.4
(f) Unspecified	173	3.1	1.4	1.4	1.7	1.7	1.6	1.6
IV. Neuroblastoma etc	897	36.0	17.5	3.0	0.6	10.3	8.4	9.3
(a) Neuroblastoma & ganglioneuroblastoma	886	36.0	17.3	2.9	0.5	10.2	8.3	9.2
(b) Other peripheral nervous cell	11	-	0.1	0.1	0.1	0.1	0.1	0.1

Table 1.1 *(Continued)* Registration rates for cancers diagnosed at age 0–14 years in Great Britain, 1991–2000. Source: National Registry of Childhood Tumors [61]

ICCC-3 categories	Total registrations	Annual rates per million children for age group (years)				Age standardized rates per million (world standard population)		
		0	1–4	5–9	10–14	Boys	Girls	Children
V. Retinoblastoma	430	25.4	7.9	0.5	0.1	4.5	4.6	4.6
VI. Renal tumors	811	15.9	17.4	3.9	1.3	8.3	8.3	8.3
(a) Nephroblastoma & other nonepithelial	787	15.6	17.3	3.8	0.9	8.0	8.1	8.1
1. Nephroblastoma (Wilms tumor)	732	13.2	16.4	3.6	0.8	7.2	7.8	7.5
2. Rhabdoid	24	2.0	0.3	-	-	0.4	0.2	0.3
3. Sarcomas	24	0.3	0.6	0.1	-	0.4	0.1	0.3
4. Peripheral neuroectodermal tumor	7	0.1	-	0.1	0.1	0.1	0.1	0.1
(b) Renal carcinoma	19	-	0.1	0.1	0.4	0.2	0.2	0.2
(c) Unspecified	5	0.3	-	0.1	-	0.1	0.0	0.1
VII. Hepatic tumors	138	5.9	2.2	0.3	0.6	1.7	1.1	1.4
(a) Hepatoblastoma	112	5.9	2.1	0.1	0.1	1.5	0.9	1.2
(b) Hepatic carcinoma	25	-	0.1	0.2	0.4	0.2	0.2	0.2
(c) Unspecified	1	-	0.0	-	-	0.0	-	0.0
VIII. Malignant bone tumors	563	0.7	0.9	4.1	10.8	4.7	4.9	4.8
(a) Osteosarcoma	307	-	0.2	2.4	6.1	2.4	2.7	2.6
(c) Ewing sarcoma family	217	0.1	0.7	1.6	4.0	2.0	1.8	1.9
(b, d, e) Other & unspecified	39	0.6	0.0	0.1	0.8	0.3	0.4	0.3
IX. Soft tissue & extraosseous sarcomas	1028	14.7	11.1	8.1	8.6	10.6	8.7	9.7
(a) Rhabdomyosarcoma	547	6.6	8.5	4.6	2.3	6.3	4.3	5.3
(b) Fibrosarcoma etc	80	2.2	0.3	0.5	1.1	0.6	0.9	0.7
(c) Kaposi's sarcoma	5	-	-	0.1	0.1	0.0	0.1	0.0
(d) Other specified	340	4.5	2.0	2.5	4.5	3.2	3.0	3.1
1, 2. Ewing sarcoma family	122	1.4	1.1	0.9	1.3	1.0	1.2	1.1
7. Synovial sarcoma	56	-	0.1	0.4	1.2	0.6	0.4	0.5
(e) Unspecified	56	1.4	0.3	0.4	0.7	0.5	0.5	0.5
X. Germ cell, trophoblastic & gonadal	486	11.2	4.2	2.2	5.7	4.2	4.9	4.5
(a) Intracranial & intraspinal germ cell	165	2.0	0.6	1.1	2.6	1.7	1.2	1.5
(b) Other malignant extragonadal	107	6.3	1.8	0.1	0.2	0.7	1.6	1.1
(c) Malignant gonadal germ cell	204	3.1	1.8	0.9	2.7	1.8	2.0	1.9
(d, e) Other & unspecified gonadal	10	0.1	-	0.1	0.2	0.1	0.1	0.1

Table 1.1 *(Continued)* Registration rates for cancers diagnosed at age 0–14 years in Great Britain, 1991–2000. Source: National Registry of Childhood Tumors [61]

ICCC-3 categories	Total registrations	Annual rates per million children for age group (years)				Age standardized rates per million (world standard population)		
		0	1–4	5–9	10–14	Boys	Girls	Children
XI. Other malignant epithelial & melanoma	483	1.4	1.6	2.9	9.1	3.7	4.7	4.2
(a) Adrenocortical carcinoma	24	0.3	0.5	0.1	0.1	0.2	0.3	0.2
(b) Thyroid carcinoma	71	-	0.2	0.5	1.4	0.4	0.8	0.6
(c) Nasopharyngeal carcinoma	24	-	-	0.1	0.6	0.3	0.1	0.2
(d) Malignant melanoma	154	1.0	0.7	1.1	2.5	1.1	1.6	1.4
(e) Skin carcinoma	82	0.1	0.2	0.5	1.6	0.7	0.7	0.7
(f) Other & unspecified carcinomas	128	-	0.1	0.6	2.9	1.0	1.2	1.1
XII. Other & unspecified	99	2.1	1.1	0.5	0.9	0.8	1.1	0.9
(a) Other specified	17	0.3	0.3	0.0	0.2	0.2	0.2	0.2
(b) Unspecified	82	1.8	0.8	0.5	0.7	0.7	0.9	0.8

Leukemia formed the most frequent diagnostic group, about one third of the total incidence. The lymphoid subgroup, which in childhood consists almost entirely of precursor cell acute lymphoblastic leukemia (ALL), accounted for about 80% of leukemias and one quarter of all childhood cancers; nearly all the remaining leukemias were acute myeloid (AML). The most numerous solid neoplasms were CNS and other intracranial and intraspinal tumors, accounting for just under a quarter of total cancer incidence. The next most frequent diagnostic groups were, in descending order of incidence, lymphomas, soft tissue sarcomas, neuroblastoma and other peripheral nervous cell tumors, and renal tumors, each accounting for 6–9% of the total. The remaining groups together accounted for 15%. Overall, incidence in the first 5 years of life was about 1.7 times that at 5–14 years of age. Boys were affected 1.2 times as often as girls. There were, however, pronounced differences in age distribution and sex ratio between different types of childhood cancer. The principal embryonal tumors, namely those of the CNS (including medulloblastoma and other primitive neuroectodermal tumors), neuroblastoma, retinoblastoma, nephroblastoma (Wilms tumor) and hepatoblastoma, all had their highest incidence in early childhood, and about 40% of the cumulative incidence of retinoblastoma and hepatoblastoma were observed in the first year of life. Contrastingly, incidence of some diagnostic categories increased with age, and more than two thirds of the cumulative childhood incidence of Hodgkin lymphoma and osteosarcoma occurred at age 10–14 years. Incidence was higher among boys than girls in most diagnostic categories and NHL had a male:female ratio of more than 2:1, but for a few cancers, notably germ cell tumors of certain sites, thyroid carcinoma and malignant melanoma, there was a marked excess of girls.

Table 1.2 shows the distribution by morphology of childhood cancers in selected anatomical sites, based on the same data as Table 1.1. The proportions of lymphomas in some sites are probably underestimates, as some cases coded to less specific or multiple sites may in fact have arisen in one of the sites listed. While most cancers of most sites in adults are carcinomas, the pattern in childhood is strikingly different. Tumors of the head and neck included substantial numbers of lymphomas and sarcomas. Lymphomas predominated among cancers of the gastro-intestinal tract. Most cancers of the liver, kidney, and eye were characteristic childhood embryonal tumors. Cancers of the ovary were nearly all germ cell tumors. The majority of testicular cancers were germ cell tumors, but there were also substantial numbers of paratesticular rhabdomyosarcomas. Rhabdomyosarcoma was the most common type of childhood cancer in other genito-urinary sites of both sexes.

In addition to the diseases included in ICCC-3, children can also develop many types of nonmalignant

Table 1.2 Histological types of cancers of selected primary sites diagnosed at age 0–14 years in Great Britain, 1991–2000. Source: National Registry of Childhood Tumors

Primary site (ICD-O-3)	Type	Number of registrations
Major salivary glands (C07–08)	Total	46
	Lymphoma	8 (17%)
	Rhabdomyosarcoma	4 (9%)
	Other sarcoma	2 (4%)
	Germ-cell tumor	1 (2%)
	Carcinoma	30 (65%)
	Unspecified	1 (2%)
Other mouth (C00–06)	Total	38
	Lymphoma	4 (11%)
	Rhabdomyosarcoma	14 (37%)
	Other sarcoma	10 (26%)
	Carcinoma	9 (24%)
	Unspecified	1 (3%)
Tonsil (C09)	Total	35
	Lymphoma	34 (97%)
	Rhabdomyosarcoma	1 (3%)
Nasopharynx (C11)	Total	97
	Lymphoma	27 (28%)
	Rhabdomyosarcoma	44 (45%)
	Other sarcoma	2 (2%)
	Carcinoma	24 (25%)
Other upper aerodigestive (C10, 12–14, 30–32)	Total	68
	Lymphoma	8 (12%)
	Neuroblastoma	2 (3%)
	Esthesioneuroblastoma	5 (7%)
	Rhabdomyosarcoma	38 (56%)
	Other sarcoma	7 (10%)
	Germ cell	3 (4%)
	Carcinoma	2 (3%)
	Unspecified	3 (4%)
Stomach (C16)	Total	11
	Lymphoma	4 (36%)
	Sarcoma	2 (18%)
	Germ cell	2 (18%)
	Carcinoma	1 (9%)
	Unspecified	2 (18%)
Small intestine (C17)	Total	51
	Lymphoma	45 (88%)
	Carcinoma	4 (8%)
	GIST	2 (4%)
Colon, rectum (C18–19)	Total	53
	Lymphoma	39 (74%)
	Carcinoma	12 (23%)
	Unspecified	2 (4%)
Liver (C22)	Total	171
	Lymphoma	6 (4%)
	Hepatoblastoma	112 (65%)
	Carcinoma	25 (15%)
	Sarcoma	22 (13%)
	Germ cell	5 (3%)
	Unspecified	1 (1%)
Pancreas (C25)	Total	9
	Lymphoma	2 (22%)
	Sarcoma	1 (11%)
	Carcinoma	2 (22%)
	Pancreatoblastoma	4 (44%)

Table 1.2 *(Continued)* Histological types of cancers of selected primary sites diagnosed at age 0–14 years in Great Britain, 1991–2000. Source: National Registry of Childhood Tumors

Primary site (ICD-O–3)	Type	Number of registrations
Lung (C34)	Total	28
	NHL	6 (21%)
	Sarcoma	3 (11%)
	Carcinoid/bronchial adenoma	8 (29%)
	Other carcinoma	2 (7%)
	Pleuropulmonary blastoma	7 (25%)
	Unspecified	2 (7%)
Ovary (C56)	Total	126
	Lymphoma	6 (5%)
	Neuroblastoma	1 (1%)
	Germ cell	112 (89%)
	Carcinoma	6 (5%)
	Mesothelioma	1 (1%)
Other female reproductive (C52–55,57)	Total	37
	Rhabdomyosarcoma	19 (51%)
	Other sarcoma	1 (3%)
	Germ cell	12 (32%)
	Carcinoma	5 (14%)
Prostate (C61)	Total	18
	Rhabdomyosarcoma	18 (100%)
Male genital (C62–63)	Total	160
	Lymphoma	6 (4%)
	Neuroblastoma	2 (1%)
	Rhabdomyosarcoma	55 (34%)
	Other sarcoma	2 (1%)
	Germ cell	92 (58%)
	Carcinoma	1 (1%)
	Unspecified	2 (1%)
Kidney (C64)	Total	829
	Lymphoma	5 (1%)
	Neuroblastoma	12 (1%)
	Nephroblastoma (Wilms)	728 (88%)
	Rhabdoid	24 (3%)
	Clear cell sarcoma	24 (3%)
	pPNET	7 (1%)
	Other sarcoma	4 (<0.5%)
	Germ cell	1 (<0.5%)
	Carcinoma	19 (2%)
	Unspecified	5 (1%)
Bladder (C67)	Total	47
	Lymphoma	1 (2%)
	Rhabdomyosarcoma	36 (77%)
	Other sarcoma	3 (6%)
	Carcinoma	6 (13%)
	Unspecified	1 (2%)
Orbit (C69.6)	Total	57
	Chloroma	2 (4%)
	Lymphoma	3 (5%)
	Rhabdomyosarcoma	47 (82%)
	Other sarcoma	4 (7%)
	Unspecified	1 (2%)
Other eye (C69.0–69.5, 69.7–69.9)	Total	443
	Lymphoma	1 (<0.5%)
	Astrocytoma	2 (<0.5%)
	Medulloepithelioma	1 (<0.5%)
	Retinoblastoma	430 (97%)
	Melanoma	8 (2%)
	Unspecified	1 (<0.5%)

neoplasm. They are not generally notified to cancer registries, hence estimates of their incidence are difficult to obtain. A few categories, however, have been routinely ascertained by some specialist population-based registries, namely the Manchester Children's Tumour Registry (MCTR) and West Midlands Regional Children's Tumour Registry (MWRCTR), both in England, and the German Childhood Cancer Registry (GCCR). The incidence of Langerhans cell histiocytosis (LCH) has been reported as around 6 per million in the GCCR [12] and 2–3 per million in the MCTR [3]. Mesoblastic nephroma accounted for 3% of all renal tumors in the MCTR, 4% in the GCCR, and 6% in the WMRCTR [2, 12, 33], indicating an annual incidence of about 0.4 per million. In the MCTR 61% of all extracranial germ cell tumors were nonmalignant [32]; they represented 48% of germ cell tumors in the testes, 60% in the ovaries and 69% in other sites. In the WMRCTR, all 49 extracranial germ cell tumors diagnosed in the first 3 months of life were benign teratomas, though four did recur as malignant tumors [45]; benign teratomas represented 29% of all registered neoplasms in this age group, making them more numerous than neuroblastomas. Adrenocortical adenoma accounted for 29% of adrenocortical tumors in the MCTR [14], implying an annual incidence of about 0.1 per million. It is not always possible to distinguish morphologically between benign and malignant adrenocortical tumors, however they should perhaps be regarded as lying on a continuum of clinical behavior [51]. Carcinoid tumors of the appendix had an annual incidence of 1.1 per million children in the WMRCTR [44].

There are pronounced variations in the occurrence of different types of childhood cancer between ethnic groups and world regions. ALL is less common among less affluent populations, including not only those of developing countries but also African-Americans in the USA. The deficit is largely due to the attenuation or even the absence of the early childhood peak that has been characteristic of western industrialized countries since the mid-twentieth century. Lymphomas, on the other hand, tend to be more frequent in less developed countries, the most extreme example being the very high incidence of Burkitt lymphoma in a broad band across equatorial Africa and also in Papua New Guinea.

Increases in the incidence of various childhood cancers have been recorded in many countries during past decades [20, 49]. Mostly the changes have been quite small, often of the order of 1% per year [20]. There have, however, been a few examples of much larger increases. Where population screening for neuroblastoma in infancy was offered either as a service or in the context of a scientific study, there was a dramatic increase in incidence resulting from detection of additional cases that would otherwise never have presented clinically [17, 54, 72]. The very large increase in childhood Kaposi's sarcoma in some sub-Saharan African countries is linked to the AIDS epidemic, probably through immunosuppression consequent on HIV infection allowing HHV8 viral load to increase uncontrollably [46]. The equally spectacular rise in thyroid cancer among children in regions most severely contaminated with radioactive fallout from Chernobyl was certainly due in part to radiation exposure, though intensive screening also contributed [71].

Recent increases in the incidence of ALL among young children in former socialist countries of central and eastern Europe, resulting in the more marked early childhood peak that has been characteristic of western countries for decades, seem likely to reflect improved socioeconomic conditions [18, 58]. An increase in the incidence of CNS tumors, especially low-grade gliomas, in the USA in the mid-1980s was attributed to improved detection with the introduction of magnetic resonance imaging (MRI) [56]. While an increase in low-grade gliomas in Sweden could also have resulted from improved detection [16, 57], it has been argued that increases in childhood CNS tumors in north-west England and in Denmark represent a true increase in risk [37, 47]. It is difficult to apportion the relative contributions of improved detection and diagnosis, improved registration and genuine increases in risk to the rather small increases in incidence of most other childhood cancers.

1.3 Etiology

Despite intensive research over several decades, very little is known about the causes of most childhood cancers. Some of the most well-established risk factors are genetic in nature. An increasingly long list of hereditary syndromes, mostly associated with identified single gene defects, carry a raised risk of specific childhood cancers [64, 67]. Germline mutations or deletions of RB1 give rise to heritable retinoblastoma. Children with neurofibromatosis 1 have an increased risk of gliomas, soft-tissue sarcomas, and juvenile myelomonocytic leukemia. Germline mutations of TP53 carry a raised risk of various cancers including soft tissue sarcoma, osteosarcoma, adrenocortical carcinoma, brain tumors, and leukemia, as well as premenopausal breast cancer; Li-Fraumeni syndrome is the resulting aggregation of specific combinations of these cancers within a family. An especially wide range of genetic disorders, both heritable and sporadic, is associated with Wilms tumor, including Beckwith-Wiedemann, Denys-Drash, WAGR, and Simpson-Golabi-Behmel syndromes [55]. Constitutional chromosomal abnormalities are implicated in about 1% of all childhood cancers [65]. The most important is Down syndrome, which carries a greatly raised risk of leukemia and almost certainly an increased risk of germ cell tumors, though the total excess of cancer is reduced by an apparent protective effect against several other types of solid tumors [15]. Risks associated with other, usually isolated, congenital abnormalities will be discussed towards the end of this section.

In 1991 it was estimated that genetic conditions were responsible for about 3% of all childhood cancer [42]. That figure will now be higher, not least because the 1991 estimate did not include Li-Fraumeni syndrome, but the proportion attributable to known genetic disorders is probably still under 5% in most populations. The main exception must be North African populations with high frequencies of the recessive DNA repair disorder xeroderma pigmentosum (XP), which carries a 1000-fold increased risk of skin cancer among children and adolescents [24]. In a series of 900 childhood cancers other than leukemia from the National Cancer Institute in Tunisia, 8% were skin carcinomas associated with XP [39].

An enormous number of exogenous or environmental exposures have been investigated as possible risk factors for childhood cancer [30, 63]. The only ones to which more than a handful of cases can be attributed worldwide are ionising radiation and certain infectious agents.

The relationship between in utero radiation exposure from obstetric x-rays and subsequent cancer in the child was established almost half a century ago [60]. At that time as many as 1 in 20 cases of childhood cancer may have been attributable to obstetric irradiation but the proportion nowadays must be much lower since ultrasound has largely supplanted x-rays. The use of x-rays to treat certain benign conditions produced an increased risk of cancer but this practice is also obsolete and therefore responsible for virtually no new cases of childhood cancer. Radiotherapy treatment for childhood cancer is itself carcinogenic but the numbers of subsequent malignancies occurring within childhood are relatively small. Large numbers of thyroid carcinomas occurred among children in the areas of Ukraine, Belarus, and Russia most heavily exposed to radioactive iodine as a result of the Chernobyl nuclear power station explosion in 1986, but there is little evidence of increased risk in less severely contaminated regions [7]. It is plausible that some childhood cancers are caused by naturally occurring gamma rays and radon, but there is limited consistency between studies and the numbers of attributable cases must be small [9, 22, 26, 69].

Ultraviolet (UV) radiation from the sun causes malignant melanoma and skin carcinomas, mainly in adults. The excess of skin cancers in children with XP results from UV exposure of a highly susceptible group. The possibility of carcinogenic effects of electromagnetic fields arising from electric power cables has caused public concern for two decades. A moderately raised risk of leukemia has consistently been found for the highest exposure levels experienced by fewer than 1 in 20 children in industrialized countries, but the reasons for this are unclear [1, 21, 38].

Several specific infections are known to increase the risk of cancer. Among children worldwide, the types of cancer with the largest numbers of cases attributable to infectious agents are Burkitt lymphoma, Hodgkin lymphoma, and nasopharyngeal carcinoma (all associated with Epstein-Barr virus, with malaria as a cofactor for Burkitt lymphoma in the region of highest incidence), hepatocellular carcinoma (hepatitis B), and Kaposi's sarcoma (HHV8) [46]. The incidence of childhood hepatocellular carcinoma fell dramatically in Taiwan following the introduction of universal vaccination against hepatitis B [27], and a similar decrease would also be expected in other countries of hitherto high incidence as they introduce immunization.

Many epidemiological studies support the suggestion that infection is involved in the etiology of some childhood leukemias [36]. Most of these studies are relevant to either or both of two hypotheses. Kinlen's hypothesis that leukemia is a rare response to a specific, but unidentified infection is supported by the finding of increased incidence in many situations of population mixing which could have led to impaired herd immunity [6, 23]. Greaves's hypothesis that common ALL can arise as an abnormal response to infectious challenge, especially in children with weaker immunity, is supported by studies showing a protective effect of breast feeding and early daycare attendance [6, 13, 34].

Some medical treatments are undoubtedly carcinogenic. The excess risk from radiotherapy has already been mentioned. Some chemotherapeutic drugs used to treat cancer produce an increased risk of subsequent cancers but relatively few of these occur in childhood. Daughters of women who took diethylstilboestrol (DES) in pregnancy had an increased risk of clear cell carcinoma of the vagina or cervix but most of these tumors occurred in early adulthood and DES ceased to be used more than 30 years ago. Despite considerable public concern generated by a positive finding in one early study, there is no consistent evidence that intramuscular vitamin K given neonatally to prevent hemorrhagic disease of the newborn is a risk factor for childhood cancer [10, 52]. Many studies have found associations between exposure to other medical treatments in utero or postnatally and various childhood cancers but there has been little consistency between reports. With the increasing use of assisted reproductive technology (ART), there has been a succession of anecdotal reports of cancer in children born following

ART. Follow-up of cohorts of children born after ART has so far failed to reveal any significant increase in the risk of cancer [28, 48], but the expected numbers of cancers are still relatively small and follow-up is as yet short for children born after some types of ART.

A wide range of other exogenous exposures to the child, to the mother antenatally, or to the father pre-conceptionally, have been suggested as contributing to the etiology of childhood cancer. Mostly the evidence comes from a small number of studies or is inconsistent between studies [29]. There are two exposures for which the evidence seems relatively strong, though it is still short of conclusive and further research is needed to clarify the nature of any etiological relationship. A possible role for benzene in relation to leukemia has not only been found in several childhood studies but is also supported by its acceptance as a risk factor for AML in adults [6, 29]. Maternal consumption of cured meats during pregnancy has been repeatedly linked to increased risk of a brain tumor in the child [29], perhaps as a result of increased exposure of the fetus to N-nitrosamides [8].

Malformations and other physical characteristics associated with certain childhood cancers could be markers for underlying genetic or environmental causes. In a large population-based study, more than 4% of children with malignant solid tumors also had a congenital anomaly, in many cases not as part of any recognized syndrome [41]. Such an occurrence could result from an unknown genetic defect or, as seems more likely, for example, in the association of inguinal hernia with Ewing sarcoma, have a common environmental cause [70].

1.4 Survival

Table 1.3 shows actuarial 5-year survival rates for children in Great Britain with cancer diagnosed during 1996–2000 [61]. More than three quarters of children survived for 5 years, and the survival rate comfortably exceeded 80% for several important diagnostic groups. Five-year survival rates above 75% are seen in many other industrialized countries [49, 53]. Survival tended to be lower in less affluent countries of Eastern Europe [53], and lower still in developing countries [40]. The prognosis for many childhood cancers has improved dramatically over past decades. In Great Britain, 5-year survival of children diagnosed in 1971–1975 was 39%, compared with 77% for those diagnosed a quarter century later [61]. This means that the risk of death within 5 years from diagnosis has been reduced by 63%. Figures 1.1–1.3 show that survival for all major diagnostic groups increased in Europe between 1978–1982 and 1993–1997, though the timing of the largest increases varied between di-

Table 1.3 Five-year survival of children in Great Britain with cancer diagnosed during 1996–2000. Source: National Registry of Childhood Tumors [61]

	Five-year survival (%)
All cancers	77
Leukemia	79
ALL	83
AML	65
Lymphomas	86
Hodgkin	94
Non-Hodgkin (incl. Burkitt)	81
CNS tumors	71
Ependymoma	69
Astrocytoma	81
Embryonal	55
Other glioma	43
Craniopharyngioma	99
Neuroblastoma	59
Retinoblastoma	96
Renal tumors	88
Nephroblastoma (Wilms tumor)	91
Hepatic tumors	66
Hepatoblastoma	79
Bone tumors	64
Osteosarcoma	62
Ewing sarcoma family	63
Soft tissue sarcoma	66
Rhabdomyosarcoma	68
Germ cell and gonadal	87
CNS germ cell	81
Other extragonadal germ cell	79
Gonadal germ cell	96
Other epithelial and melanoma	87
Thyroid carcinoma	100
Malignant melanoma	85

agnostic groups [31]. Broadly similar trends have been observed in the USA [49].

The results quoted here are derived from cancer registry data and estimate survival rates at the population level. Survival data can also be found in countless publications from clinical trials and single or multi-institutional case series. Very often the results appear better than those from population-based data, but they could well be unrepresentative of all cases in the population because of selective exclusion of those with a poor prognosis or not offered most effective treat-

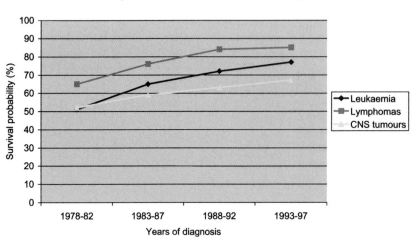

Fig. 1.1 Five-year survival of children in Europe with leukemias, lymphomas and CNS tumors diagnosed 1978–1997. Source: Automated Childhood Cancer Information System [31]

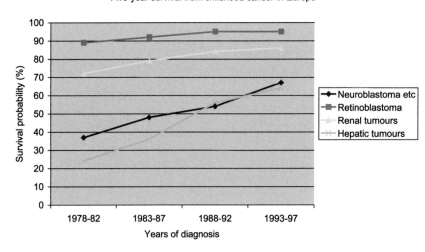

Fig. 1.2 Five-year survival of children in Europe with sympathetic nervous system tumors (neuroblastoma etc.), retinoblastoma, renal tumors and hepatic tumors diagnosed 1978–1997. Source: Automated Childhood Cancer Information System [31]

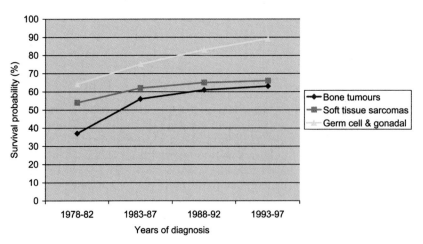

Fig. 1.3 Five-year survival of children in Europe with bone tumors, soft tissue sarcomas, and germ cell and gonadal tumors diagnosed 1978–1997. Source: Automated Childhood Cancer Information System [31]

ment. Increases in survival have, nevertheless, occurred concurrently with the development of pediatric oncology clinical trials groups and increased referral to specialist treatment centers in many countries. Several studies have found that survival was higher for children who were treated at large or specialist centres or entered in clinical trials [62, 66].

Improved survival has resulted in increasing numbers of long-term survivors of childhood cancer. The risk of a second primary malignancy within 25 years of the original childhood cancer diagnosis is about 4% [19, 43]. Many other aspects of the health of long-term survivors and their offspring are the subject of several large epidemiological studies [5, 50, 68].

1.5 Mortality

Population mortality rates from childhood cancer in western countries have fallen dramatically since the mid-20th century, in line with the moderate increase in incidence and very marked improvements in outcome. Table 1.4 shows estimated age-standardized mortality rates for childhood cancer by world region in 2002 [11]. In wealthy industrialized countries, mortality was typically around 25–30 per million. It was considerably higher in Eastern Europe, reflecting the lower survival rates still obtained in that region. Results for other world regions are harder to interpret because of incompleteness and inaccuracy in the data for many countries [35]. Overall, and for cancers other than those of the brain and nervous system, mortality rates tended to be highest in developing countries, reflecting their generally lower survival rates. Mortality from cancers of the brain and nervous system showed a different pattern with low rates in developing countries outside the Americas and Western Asia; since survival is lower in these countries, the lower mortality must be a result of under-recording and lower incidence.

Table 1.4 Estimated age-standardized mortality rates per million for cancer at age 0–14 years, 2002, by world region. Source: GLOBOCAN 2002 [11]

	Total		Leukemia		Lymphoma		Brain/nervous system		Other	
	Boys	Girls	Boys	Girls	Boys	Girls	Boys	Girls	Boys	Girls
North Africa	72.8	52.7	20.6	12.2	17.1	9.1	6.8	4.0	28.3	27.4
Sub-Saharan Africa	74.2	52.5	11.1	6.6	23.2	13.7	3.3	3.6	36.6	28.6
USA/Canada	26.5	23.2	8.6	7.1	1.4	0.8	7.5	7.1	9.0	8.2
Central America	60.6	52.2	31.9	28.2	6.2	3.0	8.2	7.1	14.3	13.9
South America	63.5	51.9	26.8	21.4	6.9	3.6	11.7	9.5	18.1	17.4
Western Asia	72.7	58.2	29.4	22.1	14.3	9.6	12.7	9.4	16.3	17.1
India	36.2	23.2	15.0	9.8	4.6	1.5	5.4	3.0	11.2	8.9
Other South Asia	55.5	36.5	16.9	13.3	9.6	3.1	7.1	4.9	21.9	15.2
China	52.3	38.9	32.2	23.0	3.4	1.7	7.8	7.9	8.9	6.3
Japan	27.6	18.5	11.5	8.2	1.5	1.1	5.1	3.5	9.5	5.7
South East Asia	68.7	54.7	33.0	25.5	8.8	4.9	8.3	7.4	18.6	16.9
Nordic Countries	27.1	24.5	7.9	7.5	2.8	0.0	8.4	7.9	8.0	9.1
British Isles	33.8	25.4	11.6	10.4	1.1	1.0	10.7	7.7	10.4	6.3
Former USSR in Europe	57.3	47.9	18.5	14.8	6.2	2.7	13.7	12.1	18.9	18.3
Other Eastern Europe	50.5	40.0	15.5	11.3	4.6	2.2	14.0	12.8	16.4	13.7
Western Europe	30.9	22.1	9.9	6.3	1.3	0.9	9.9	6.5	9.8	8.4
Southern Europe	34.7	30.4	12.3	10.3	2.6	1.9	9.8	6.9	10.0	11.3
Australia/New Zealand	37.0	26.7	12.2	10.1	1.8	1.1	12.4	6.0	10.6	9.5

References

1. Ahlbom A, Day N, Feychting M, et al. (2000) A pooled analysis of magnetic fields and childhood leukaemia. Br J Cancer 83:692–698

2. Barrantes JC, Muir KR, Toyn CE, et al. (1993) Thirty-year population-based review of childhood renal tumours with an assessment of prognostic features including tumour DNA characteristics. Med Pediatr Oncol 21:24–30

3. Birch JM, United Kingdom—Manchester children's tumour registry 1954–1970 and 1971–1983. In: Parkin DM, et al., eds. (1988) International Incidence of Childhood Cancer. IARC, Lyon

4. Birch JM, Marsden HB (1987) A classification scheme for childhood cancer. Int J Cancer 40:620–624

5. Boice JD, Tawn EJ, Winther JF, et al. (2003) Genetic effects of radiotherapy for childhood cancer. Health Phys 85:65–80

6. Buffler PA, Kwan ML, Reynolds P, et al. (2005) Environmental and genetic risk factors for childhood leukemia: Appraising the evidence. Cancer Invest 23:60–75

7. Cardis E, Krewski D, Boniol M, et al. (2006) Estimates of the cancer burden in Europe from radioactive fallout from the Chernobyl accident. Int J Cancer 119:1224–1235

8. Dietrich M, Block G, Pogoda JM, et al. (2005) A review: Dietary and endogenously formed N-nitroso compounds and risk of childhood brain tumors. Cancer Causes Control 16:619–635

9. Evrard A-S, Hémon D, Billon S, et al. (2006) Childhood leukemia incidence and exposure to indoor radon, terrestrial and cosmic gamma radiation. Health Phys 90:569–579

10. Fear NT, Roman E, Ansell P, et al. (2003) Vitamin K and childhood cancer: A report from the United Kingdom Childhood Cancer Study. Br J Cancer 89:1228–1231

11. Ferlay J, Bray F, Pisani P, et al. (2004) GLOBOCAN 2002: Cancer Incidence, Mortality and Prevalence Worldwide, IARC Cancerbase No. 5, version 2.0. IARC Press, Lyon

12. German Childhood Cancer Registry (2004) Jahresbericht Annual Report 2004 (1980–2003), German Childhood Cancer Registry, Mainz

13. Greaves M (2006) Infection, immune responses and the aetiology of childhood leukaemia. Nat Rev Cancer 6:193–203

14. Hartley AL, Birch JM, Marsden HB, et al. (1987) Adrenal cortical tumours: Epidemiological and familial aspects. Arch Dis Child 62:683–689

15. Hasle H (2001) Pattern of malignant disorders in individuals with Down's syndrome. Lancet Oncol 2:429–436

16. Hjalmars U, Kulldorff M, Wahlquist Y, et al. (1999) Increased incidence rates but no space-time clustering of childhood astrocytoma in Sweden, 1973–1992. Cancer 85:2077–2090

17. Honjo S, Doran HE, Stiller CA, et al. (2003) Neuroblastoma trends in Osaka, Japan, and Great Britain 1970–1994, in relation to screening. Int J Cancer 103:538–543

18. Hrusák O, Trka J, Zuna J, et al. (2002) Acute lymphoblastic leukemia incidence during socioeconomic transition: selective increase in children from 1 to 4 years. Leukemia 16:720–725

19. Jenkinson HC, Hawkins MM, Stiller CA, et al. (2004) Long-term population-based risks of second malignant neoplasms after childhood cancer in Britain. Br J Cancer 91:1905–1910

20. Kaatsch P, Steliarova-Foucher E, Crocetti E, et al. (2006) Time trends of cancer incidence in European children (1978–1997): Report from the Automated Childhood Cancer Information System project. Eur J Cancer 42:1961–1971

21. Kabuto M, Nitta H, Yamamoto S, et al. (2006) Childhood leukemia and magnetic fields in Japan: A case-control study of childhood leukemia and residential power-frequency magnetic fields in Japan. Int J Cancer 119:643–650

22. Kendall GM, Smith TJ (2005) Doses from radon and its decay products to children. J Radiol Prot 25:241–256

23. Kinlen L (2004) Infections and immune factors in cancer: The role of epidemiology. Oncogene 23:6341–6348

24. Kraemer KH, Lee M-M, Andrews AD, et al. (1994) The role of sunlight and DNA repair in melanoma and nonmelanoma skin cancer. The xeroderma pigmentosum paradigm. Arch Dermatol 130:1018–1021

25. Kramárová E, Stiller CA (1996) The international classification of childhood cancer. Int J Cancer 68:759–765

26. Laurier D, Valenty M, Tirmarche M (2001) Radon exposure and the risk of leukemia: A review of epidemiological studies. Health Phys 81:272–288

27. Lee C-L, Hsieh K-S, Ko Y-C (2003) Trends in the incidence of hepatocellular carcinoma in boys and girls in Taiwan after large-scale hepatitis B vaccination. Cancer Epidemiol Biomarkers Prev 12:57–59

28. Lightfoot T, Bunch K, Ansell P, et al. (2005) Ovulation induction, assisted conception and childhood cancer. Eur J Cancer 41:715–724

29. Linet MS, Wacholder S, Zahm SH (2005) Interpreting epidemiologic research: Lessons from studies of childhood cancer. Pediatrics 112:218–232

30. Little J (1999) Epidemiology of Childhood Cancer, IARC, Lyon

31. Magnani C, Pastore G, Coebergh JWW, et al. (2006) Trends in survival after childhood cancer in Europe, 1978–1997: Report from the Automated Childhood Cancer Information System project (ACCIS). Eur J Cancer 42:1981–2005

32. Marsden HB, Birch JM, Swindell R (1981) Germ cell tumours of childhood: A review of 137 cases. J Clin Pathol 34:879–883

33. Marsden HB, Newton WA (1986) New look at mesoblastic nephroma. J Clin Pathol 39:508–513

34. Martin RM, Gunnell D, Owen CG, et al. (2005) Breast-feeding and childhood cancer: A systematic review with metaanalysis. Int J Cancer 117:1020–1031

35. Mathers CD, Fat DM, Inoue M, et al. (2005) Counting the dead and what they died from: An assessment of the global status of cause of death data. Bull World Health Organ 83:171–177

36. McNally RJQ, Eden TOB (2004) An infectious aetiology for childhood acute leukaemia: A review of the evidence. Br J Haematol 127:243–263

37. McNally RJQ, Kelsey AM, Cairns DP, et al. (2001) Temporal increases in the incidence of childhood solid tumors seen in Northwest England (1954–1998) are likely to be real. Cancer 92:1967–1976

38. Mezei G, Kheifets L (2006) Selection bias and its implications for case-control studies: A case study of magnetic field exposure and childhood leukaemia. Int J Epidemiol 35:397–406

39. Mourali N, Tunisia—Institut Salah-Azaiz, 1969–1982. In: Parkin DM, Stiller CA, Draper GJ, et al., (eds) (1988) International Incidence of Childhood Cancer (IARC Scientific Publications No. 87). International Agency for Research on Cancer, Lyon

40. Nandakumar A, Anantha N, Appaji L, et al. (1996) Descriptive epidemiology of childhood cancers in Bangalore, India. Cancer Causes Control 7:405–410

41. Narod SA, Hawkins MM, Robertson CM, et al. (1997) Congenital anomalies and childhood cancer in Great Britain. Am J Hum Genet 60:474–485

42. Narod SA, Stiller C, Lenoir GM (1991) An estimate of the heritable fraction of childhood cancer. Br J Cancer 63:993–999

43. Olsen JH, Garwicz S, Hertz H, et al. (1993) Second malignant neoplasms after cancer in childhood or adolescence. BMJ 307:1030–1036

44. Parkes SE, Muir KR, Al Sheyyab M, et al. (1993) Carcinoid tumours of the appendix in children 1957–1986: incidence, treatment and outcome. Br J Surg 80:502–504

45. Parkes SE, Muir KR, Southern L, et al. (1994) Neonatal tumours: A thirty-year population-based study. Med Pediatr Oncol 22:309–317

46. Parkin DM (2006) The global health burden of infection-associated cancers in the year 2002. Int J Cancer 118:3030–3044

47. Raaschou-Nielsen O, Sørensen M, Carstensen H, et al. (2006) Increasing incidence of childhood tumours of the central nervous system in Denmark, 1980–1996. Br J Cancer 95:416–422

48. Raimondi S, Pedotti P, Taioli E (2005) Meta-analysis of cancer incidence in children born after assisted reproductive technologies. Br J Cancer 93:1053–1056

49. Ries LAG, Harkins D, Krapcho M, et al. (2006) SEER Cancer Statistics Review, 1975–2003, National Cancer Institute Bethesda, MD

50. Robison LL, Green DM, Hudson M, et al. (2005) Long-term outcomes of adult survivors of childhood cancer. Results from the Childhood Cancer Survivor Study. Cancer 104:2557–2564

51. Rodriguez-Galindo C, Figueiredo BC, Zambetti GP, et al. (2005) Biology, clinical characteristics, and management of adrenocortical tumors in children. Pediatr Blood Cancer 45:265–273

52. Roman E, Fear NT, Ansell P, et al. (2002) Vitamin K and childhood cancer: Analysis of individual patient data from six case-control studies. Br J Cancer 86:63–69

53. Sankila R, Martos Jiménez MC, Miljus D, et al. (2006) Geographical comparison of cancer survival in European children (1988–1997): Report from the Automated Childhood Cancer Information System project. Eur J Cancer 42:1972–1980

54. Schilling FH, Spix C, Berthold F, et al. (2002) Neuroblastoma screening at one year of age. N Eng J Med 346:1047–1053

55. Scott RH, Stiller CA, Walker L, et al. (2006) Syndromes and constitutional chromosomal abnormalities associated with Wilms tumour. J Med Genet 43:705–715

56. Smith MA, Freidlin B, Gloeckler Ries LA, et al. (1998) Trends in reported incidence of primary malignant brain tumors in children in the United States. J Natl Cancer Inst 90:1269–1277

57. Smith MA, Freidlin B, Ries LAG, et al. (2000) Increased incidence rates but no space-time clustering of childhood astrocytoma in Sweden, 1973–1992: A population-based study of pediatric brain tumors (corres). Cancer 88:1492–1493

58. Steliarova-Foucher E, Stiller C, Kaatsch P, et al. (2004) Geographical patterns and time trends of cancer incidence and survival among children and adolescents in Europe since the 1970s (the ACCIS project): An epidemiological study. Lancet 364:2097–2105

59. Steliarova-Foucher E, Stiller C, Lacour B, et al. (2005) International classification of childhood cancer, third edition. Cancer 103:1457–1467

60. Stewart A, Webb J, Hewitt D (1958) A survey of childhood malignancies. Br Med J 30:1495–1508

61. Stiller C (2007) Childhood cancer in Britain: Incidence, Survival, Mortality. Oxford University Press, Oxford

62. Stiller CA (1994) Centralised treatment, entry to trials and survival. Br J Cancer 70:352–362

63. Stiller CA, Aetiology and Epidemiology. In: Pinkerton CR, Plowman PN, Pieters R, (eds) (2004) Paediatric Oncology. Arnold, London

64. Stiller CA (2004) Epidemiology and genetics of childhood cancer. Oncogene 23:6429–6444

65. Stiller CA (2006) Constitutional chromosomal abnormalities and childhood cancer. Ital J Pediatr 31:347–353

66. Stiller CA, Passmore SJ, Kroll ME, et al. (2006) Patterns of care and survival for patients aged under 40 years with bone sarcoma in Britain, 1980–1994. Br J Cancer 94:22–29

67. Strahm B, Malkin D (2006) Hereditary cancer predisposition in children: Genetic basis and clinical implications. Int J Cancer 119:2001–2006

68. Taylor A, Hawkins M, Griffiths A, et al. (2004) Long-term follow-up of survivors of childhood cancer in the UK. Pediatr Blood Cancer 42:161–168

69. UK Childhood Cancer Study Investigators (2002) The United Kingdom Childhood Cancer Study of exposure to domestic sources of ionising radiation: 2: gamma radiation. Br J Cancer 86:1727–1731

70. Valery PC, Holly EA, Sleigh AC, et al. (2005) Hernias and Ewing's sarcoma family of tumours: A pooled analysis and meta-analysis. Lancet Oncol 6:485–490

71. Williams D (2002) Cancer after nuclear fallout: Lessons from the Chernobyl accident. Nature Rev Cancer 2:543–549

72. Woods WG, Tuchman M, Robison LL, et al. (1996) A population-based study of the usefulness of screening for neuroblastoma. Lancet 348:1682–1687

Tumor Biology and Environmental Carcinogenesis

2

Andrew M. Davidoff

Contents

2.1 Introduction

During normal development and renewal, cells evolve to perform highly specialized functions to meet the physiologic needs of the organism. Development and renewal involve tightly regulated processes that include continued cell proliferation, differentiation into specialized cell types, and programmed cell death (apoptosis). An intricate system of checks and balances ensures proper control over these physiologic processes. The genetic composition (genotype) of a cell determines which pathway(s) will be followed and exerting that control. The environment also plays a crucial role in influencing cell fate. Cells use complex signal transduction pathways to sense and respond to neighboring cells and their extracellular milieu. In addition, however, environmental factors may have a direct impact on cell phenotype and fate by causing DNA damage that permanently alters the host genome. Cancer is a genetic disease whose progression is driven by a series of accumulating genetic changes influenced by hereditary factors and the somatic environment. These genetic changes result in individual cells acquiring a phenotype that provides those cells with a survival advantage over surrounding normal cells. Our understanding of the processes that occur in malignant cell transformation is increasing with many discoveries in cancer cell biology having been made using childhood tumors as models.

2.2 Cell Fate

2.2.1 Stem Cells

The development and maintenance of the tissues that comprise an organism are processes driven by stem cells. These are cells with the potential for both self-renewal and terminal differentiation into one or more cell types. They, therefore, play a critical role in normal tissue turnover and repair. The fate of most of these stem cells is generally one of terminal differentiation and either quiescence or apoptosis. However, a small percentage of stem cells maintain their pleuripotent capacity. It is becoming increasingly recognized that these same stem cells that are essential for maintaining an organism are also central to the development of malignancy and therapy resistance [116]. Cancer stem cells, like normal stem cells, possess remarkable proliferative and self-renewal capacities, while the larger portion of partially differentiated tumor cells possess quite limited reproductive potential.

2.2.2 Programmed Cell Death

Multicellular organisms have developed a highly organized and carefully regulated mechanism of cell death in order to maintain cellular homeostasis. Normal development and morphogenesis are often associated with the production of excess cells, which are removed by the genetically programmed process called apoptosis. Apoptosis is a highly regulated event which can be effected by either death receptor-mediated or mitochondrial pathways by activating specific signaling molecules. Both pathways converge onto a group of effector caspases, leading to morphologic and biochemical changes characteristic of apoptosis. Cells undergoing apoptosis have distinct morphologic features (plasma membrane blebbing, reduced volume, nuclear condensation), and their DNA is subjected to endonucleolytic cleavage.

Receptor-mediated apoptosis is initiated by the interaction of "death ligands" such as tumor necrosis factor alpha (TNFα), Fas, and TNF-related apoptosis-inducing ligand (TRAIL) with their respective receptors. This interaction is followed by aggregation of the receptors and recruitment of adaptor proteins to the plasma membrane, which activate caspases [79]. Caspases are a large family of proteases that function in both the initiation of apoptosis in response to proapoptotic signals and in the subsequent effector pathway that disassembles the cell. Thus, apoptosis limits cellular expansion and counters cell proliferation. Because cell survival signals may also be activated through pathways mediated by nuclear factor-kappa B (NF-KB), the fate of a cell is determined by the balance between death signals and survival signals [57]. Other signals arising from cellular stress (e.g., DNA damage, hypoxia, oncogene activation) may also effect cell cycle arrest or apoptosis.

An alternative to cell death mediated by receptor-ligand binding is cellular senescence, which is initiated when chromosomes reach a critical length. Eukaryotic chromosomes have DNA strands of unequal length, and their ends – telomeres – are characterized by species-specific nucleotide repeat sequences. Telomeres stabilize the ends of chromosomes, which are otherwise sites of significant instability [106]. Over time and with each successive cycle of replication, chromosomes are shortened by failure to complete replication of their telomeres. Thus, telomere shortening acts as a biologic clock, limiting the lifespan of a cell. Germ cells, however, avoid telomere shortening by using telomerase, an enzyme capable of adding telomeric sequences to the ends of chromosomes. This enzyme is normally inactivated early in the growth and development of an organism. Persistent activation or the reactivation of telomerase in somatic cells appears to contribute to the immortality of transformed cells.

2.2.3 Malignant Transformation

Alteration or inactivation of any of the components of normal cell regulatory pathways may lead to the dysregulated growth that characterizes neoplastic cells. Malignant transformation may be characterized by cellular dedifferentiation or failure to differentiate, cellular invasiveness and metastatic capacity, or decreased drug sensitivity. Tumorigenesis reflects the accumulation of excess cells that results from increased cell proliferation and decreased apoptosis or senescence. Cancer cells do not replicate more rapidly than normal cells, but they show diminished responsiveness to regulatory signals. Positive growth signals are generated by proto-oncogenes, so named because their dysregulated expression or activity can promote malignant transformation. These proto-oncogenes may encode growth factors or their receptors, intracellular signaling molecules, and nuclear transcription factors (Table 2.1). Conversely, tumor suppressor genes, as their name implies, control or restrict cell growth and proliferation. Their inactivation, through various mechanisms, permits the dysregulated growth of cancer cells. Also important are the genes that regulate cell death. Their inactivation leads to resistance to apoptosis and allows accumulation of additional genetic aberrations.

Cancer cells carry DNA that has point mutations, viral insertions, or chromosomal or gene amplifications, deletions, or rearrangements. Each of these aberrations can alter the context and process of normal cellular growth and differentiation. Although genomic instability is an inherent property of the evolutionary process and normal development, it is through genomic instability that the malignant transformation of a cell may arise. This inherent instability may be altered by inheritance or exposure to destabilizing factors in the environment. Point mutations may terminate protein translation, alter protein function, or change the regulatory target sequences that control gene expression. Chromosomal alterations create new genetic contexts within the genome and lead to the formation of novel proteins or to the dysregulation of genes displaced by aberrant events.

Genetic abnormalities associated with cancer may be detected in every cell in the body or only in the tumor cells. Constitutional or germline abnormalities are either inherited or occur de novo in the germ cells (sperm or oocyte). Interestingly, despite the presence of a genetic abnormality that might affect growth regulatory pathways in all cells, people are generally predisposed to only certain tumor types. This selectivity highlights the observation that gene function contributes to growth or development only within a particular milieu or physiologic context. Specific tumors occur earlier and are more often bilateral (in paired organs)

Table 2.1 Proto-oncogenes and tumor suppressor genes in pediatric malignancies

Oncogene family	Proto-oncogene	Chromosome location	Tumors
Growth factors and receptors	erb B2	17q21	Glioblastoma
	trk	9q22	Neuroblastoma
Protein kinase	src	7p11	Rhabdomyosarcoma, Osteosarcoma, Ewing sarcoma
Signal transducers	H-ras	11p15.1	Neuroblastoma
Transcription factors	c-myc	18q24	Burkitt lymphoma
	N-myc	2p24	Neuroblastoma
Syndrome	**Tumor suppressor gene**	**Chromosome location**	**Tumors**
Familial polyposis coli	APC	5q21	Intestinal polyposis, colorectal cancer
Familial retinoblastoma	RB	13q24	Retinoblastoma, osteosarcoma
WAGR*	WT1	11p13	Wilms tumor
Denys-Drash**	WT1	11p13	Wilms tumor
Beckwith-Wiedemann***	WT2 (?)	11p15	Wilms tumor, hepatoblastoma, adrenal tumor
Li-Fraumeni	p53	17q13	Multiple
Neurofibromatosis type 1	NF1	17q11.2	Sarcomas, breast cancer
Neurofibromatosis type 2	NF2	22q12	Neurofibroma, neurofibrosarcoma, brain tumor
Von Hippel-Lindau	VHL	3p25-26	Renal cell cancer, pheochromocytoma, retinal angioma, hemangioblastoma

*WAGR: Wilms tumor, aniridia, genitourinary abnormalities, and mental retardation
**Denys-Drash: Wilms tumor, pseudohermaphroditism, mesangeal sclerosis, renal failure
***Beckwith-Wiedemann: multiple tumors, hemihypertrophy, macroglossia, hyperinsulinism
Reprinted with permission from Davidoff, AM and Krasin MJ (2006) Principles of pediatric oncology/genetics of cancer.
In: Grosfeld JL, (ed): Pediatric surgery, 6th edn. 2006.

when they result from germline mutations than when they result from sporadic or somatic alterations. Such is often the case in two pediatric malignancies, Wilms tumor and retinoblastoma. These observations led Alfred Knudson to propose a "two-hit" model of carcinogenesis in which the first genetic defect, already present in the germ line, must be complemented by an additional spontaneous mutation before a tumor can arise [54]. In sporadic cancer, cellular transformation occurs only when two (or more) spontaneous mutations take place in the same cell. The critical features of the Knudson model – the small number of mutations required for malignant transformation, the possible inheritance of a first mutation, and the gradual disappearance of transformable target cells with increasing age – provide a conceptual framework for mutational theories of the genetics of most childhood tumors. In this scheme familial tumors will present earlier than sporadic tumors of the same histologic type; inheri-

tance of a tumorigenic mutation will also predispose to multiple tumor occurrences.

Much more common, however, are somatically acquired chromosomal aberrations, which are confined to the malignant cells. These aberrations affect growth factors and their receptors, signal transducers, and transcription factors. The general types of chromosomal alterations associated with malignant transformation are shown in Fig. 2.1. Although a low level of chromosomal instability exists in a normal population of cells, neoplastic transformation occurs only if these alterations affect a growth-regulating pathway and confer a growth advantage.

2.2.3.1 DNA Content

Normal human cells contain two copies of each of 23 chromosomes; a normal "diploid" cell therefore has

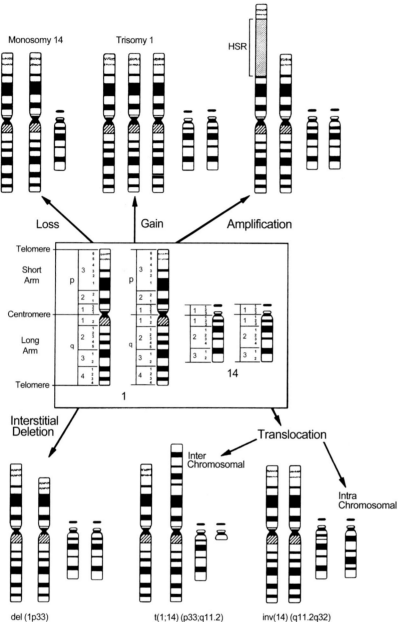

Fig. 2.1 The spectrum of gross chromosomal aberrations using chromosomes 1 and 14 as examples. Reprinted with permission from [69].

46 chromosomes. Although cellular DNA content, or ploidy, is accurately determined by karyotypic analysis, it can be estimated by the much simpler method of flow cytometric analysis. Diploid cells have a DNA index of 1.0, whereas near-triploid cells have a DNA index ranging from 1.26 to 1.76. The majority (55%) of primary neuroblastoma cells are triploid or near triploid, for example, having between 58 and 80 chromosomes, whereas the remainder are near diploid (35–57 chromosomes) or near tetraploid (81–103 chromosomes) [49]. Neuroblastomas consisting of near-diploid or near-tetraploid cells usually have structural ge-

netic abnormalities (e.g., chromosome 1p deletion and amplification of the *MYCN* oncogene), whereas those consisting of near-triploid cells are characterized by three almost complete haploid sets of chromosomes with few structural abnormalities [12]. Importantly, patients with near-triploid tumors typically have favorable clinical and biologic prognostic factors and excellent survival rates compared with those who have near-diploid or near-tetraploid tumors [67].

2.2.3.2 Chromosomal Translocations

Many pediatric cancers, specifically hematologic malignancies and soft-tissue neoplasms, have recurrent, nonrandom abnormalities in chromosomal structure, typically chromosomal translocations (Table 2.2). The most common result of a nonrandom translocation is the fusion of two distinct genes from different chromosomes. The genes are typically fused within the reading frame and express a functional, chimeric protein product that has transcription factor or protein kinase activity. These fusion proteins contribute to tumorigenesis by activating genes or proteins involved in cell proliferation. For example, in Ewing sarcoma the consequence of the t(11;22)(q24;q12) translocation is a fusion of *EWS,* a transcription factor gene on chromosome 22, and *FLI-1,* a gene encoding a member of the ETS family of transcription factors on chromosome 11 [72]. The resultant chimeric protein, which contains the DNA-binding region of FLI-1 and the transcription activation region of EWS, has greater transcriptional activity than does EWS alone [73]. The EWS:FLI-1 fusion transcript is detectable in approximately 90% of Ewing sarcomas. At least four other EWS fusions have been identified in Ewing sarcoma; fusion of EWS with ERG (another ETS family member) accounts for an additional 5% of cases [109]. Alveolar rhabdomyosarcomas have characteristic translocations between the long arm of chromosome 2 (75% of cases) or the short arm of chromosome 1 (10% of cases) and the long arm of chromosome 13. These translocations result in the fusion of *PAX3* (at 2q35) or *PAX7* (at 1p36) with *FKHR,* a gene encoding a member of the forkhead family of transcription factors [41]. The *EWS:FLI-1* and *PAX7:FKHR* fusions appear to confer a better prognosis for patients with Ewing sarcoma and alveolar rhabdomyosarcoma, respectively [5, 28]. Translocations that generate chimeric proteins with increased transcriptional activity also characterize desmoplastic small round cell tumor [61], myxoid liposarcoma [94], extraskeletal myxoid chondrosarcoma [21], malignant melanoma of soft parts

Table 2.2 Common, recurrent translocations in soft tissue tumors

Tumor	Genetic abnormality	Fusion transcript
Ewing sarcoma/Primitive neuroectodermal tumor	t(11;22)(q24;q12)	*FLI1-EWS*
	t(21;22)(q22;q12)	*ERG-EWS*
	t(7;22)(p22;q12)	*ETV1-EWS*
	t(17;22)(q12;q12)	*E1AF-EWS*
	t(2;22)(q33;q12)	*FEV-EWS*
Desmoplastic small round cell tumor	t(11;22)(p13;q12)	*WT1-EWS*
	t(11;22)(q24;q12)	*FLI1-EWS*
Synovial sarcoma	t(X;18)(p11.23;q11)	*SSX1-SYT*
	t(X;18)(p11.21;q11)	*SSX2-SYT*
Alveolar rhabdomyosarcoma	t(2;13)(q35;q14)	*PAX3-FKHR*
	t(1;13)(p36;q14)	*PAX7-FKHR*
Malignant melanoma of soft part (clear cell sarcoma)	t(12;22)(q13;q12)	*ATF1-EWS*
Myxoid liposarcoma	t(12;16)(q13;p11)	*CHOP-TLS(FUS)*
	t(12;22)(q13;q12)	*CHOP-EWS*
Extraskeletal myxoid chondrosarcoma	t(9;22)(q22;q12)	*CHN-EWS*
Dermatofibrosarcoma protuberans and Giant cell fibroblastoma	t(17;22)(q22;q13)	*COL1A1-PDGFB*
Congenital fibrosarcoma and Mesoblastic nephroma	t(12;15)(p13;q25)	*ETV6-NTRK3*
Lipoblastoma	t(3;8)(q12;q11.2)	?
	t(7;8)(q31;q13)	?

Reprinted with permission from Davidoff AM, Hill DA (2001) Molecular genetic aspects of solid tumors in childhood. Semin Pediatr Surg 10:106–118.

[122], synovial sarcoma [22], congenital fibrosarcoma [114], cellular mesoblastic nephroma [97], and dermatofibrosarcoma protuberans [81].

2.2.3.3 Proto-Oncogene Activation

Proto-oncogenes are commonly activated in transformed cells by point mutations or gene amplification. The classic example of proto-oncogene activation by a point mutation involves the cellular proto-oncogene *RAS* RAS-family proteins are associated with the inner, cytoplasmic surface of the plasma membrane and function as intermediates in signal transduction pathways that regulate cell proliferation. Point mutations in *RAS* result in constitutive activation of the RAS protein and, therefore, the continuous activation of the RAS signal transduction pathway. Activation of RAS appears to be involved in the pathogenesis of a small percentage of pediatric malignancies, including leukemia and a variety of solid tumors [20].

Gene amplification (i.e., selective replication of DNA sequences) enables a tumor cell to increase expression of crucial genes whose products are ordinarily tightly controlled. The amplified DNA sequences, or amplicons, may be maintained episomally (i.e., extrachromosomally) as double minutes – paired chromatin bodies lacking a centromere – or as intrachromosomal, homogeneously staining regions. In about one third of neuroblastomas, for example, the transcription factor and proto-oncogene *MYCN* is amplified. *MYCN* encodes a 64-kDa nuclear phosphoprotein (MycN) that forms a transcriptional complex by associating with other nuclear proteins expressed in the developing nervous system and other tissues [55]. Increased expression of MycN increases the rates of DNA synthesis and cell proliferation and shortens the G1 phase of the cell cycle [69]. The *MYCN* copy number in neuroblastoma cells can be amplified 5- to 500-fold and is usually consistent among primary and metastatic sites and at different times during tumor evolution and treatment [11]. This consistency suggests that *MYCN* amplification is an early event in the pathogenesis of neuroblastoma. Because gene amplification is usually associated with advanced stages of disease, rapid tumor progression, and poor outcome, it is a powerful prognostic indicator [13, 104]. The cell surface receptor gene *ERBB2* is another proto-oncogene commonly overexpressed, due to gene amplification, an event that occurs in breast cancer, osteosarcoma, and Wilms tumor [90].

Comparative genomic hybridization studies have shown that a gain of genetic material on the long arm of chromosome 17 (17q) is perhaps the most common genetic abnormality in neuroblastomas: such gain occurs in approximately 75% of primary tumors [113]and is strongly associated with other known prognostic factors, but may be a powerful independent predictor of adverse outcome [10]. Gain of 17q most often results from an unbalanced translocation of this region to other chromosomal sites, most frequently 1p or 11q. The term "unbalanced" indicates that extra copies of 17q are present in addition to the normal chromosome 17. Although it is unclear what the crucial gene(s) are on 17q and how extra copies of 17q contribute to the malignant phenotype of neuroblastoma, the existence of 17q amplification in neuroblastoma suggests the presence of a proto-oncogene on 17q.

2.2.3.4 Inactivation of Tumor Suppressor Genes

Tumor suppressor genes, or antioncogenes, provide negative control of cell proliferation. Loss of function of the proteins encoded by these genes, through deletion or mutational inactivation of the gene, liberates the cell from growth constraints and contributes to malignant transformation. The cumulative effect of genetic lesions that activate proto-oncogenes or inactivate tumor suppressor genes is a breakdown in the balance between cell proliferation and cell loss due to differentiation or apoptosis. Such imbalance results in clonal overgrowth of a specific cell lineage. The first tumor suppressor gene to be recognized was the retinoblastoma susceptibility gene, *RB*. This gene encodes a nuclear phosphoprotein that acts as a "gatekeeper" of the cell cycle. RB normally permits cell cycle progression through G1 phase when it is phosphorylated but prevents cell division when it is unphosphorylated. Inactivating deletions or point mutations of *RB* cause the protein to lose its regulatory capacity. The nuclear phosphoprotein, p53, has also become recognized as an important tumor suppressor gene, perhaps the most commonly altered gene in all human cancers. Inactivating mutations of the p53 gene also cause the p53 protein to lose its ability to regulate the cell cycle. The p53 gene is frequently inactivated in solid tumors of childhood, including osteosarcoma, rhabdomyosarcoma, brain tumors, anaplastic Wilms tumor, and a subset of chemotherapy-resistant neuroblastoma [4, 51, 58]. In addition, heritable cancer-associated changes in the p53 tumor suppressor gene occur in families with Li-Fraumeni syndrome, an autosomal dominant predisposition for rhabdomyosarcoma, other soft tissue and bone sarcomas, premenopausal breast cancer, brain tumors, and adrenocortical carcinomas [70]. Other tumor suppressor genes inactivated in pediatric malignancies include Wilms tumor 1 (*WT1*), neurofibromatosis type 1 (*NF1),* and von Hippel-Lindau (*VHL).*

Other tumor suppressor genes are presumed to exist but have not been definitively identified. For example, early karyotype analyses of neuroblastoma-derived cell lines found frequent deletion of the short arm of chromosome 1 [14]. Deletion of genetic material in tumors suggests the presence (and subsequent loss) of a tumor suppressor gene, but no individual tumor suppressor gene has been identified on chromosome 1p. Functional confirmation of the presence of a 1p tumor suppressor gene comes from the demonstration that transfection of chromosome 1p into a neuroblastoma cell line results in morphologic changes of differentiation and ultimately cell senescence [3]. Approximately 20–35% of primary neuroblastomas exhibit 1p deletion, as determined by fluorescent in situ hybridization (FISH), and the smallest common region of loss is located within region 1p36 [40]. Deletion of 1p is also common in Wilms tumor [42].

2.3 Metastasis

Metastasis is the spread of cancer cells from a primary tumor to distant sites and is the hallmark of malignancy. The development of tumor metastases is the main cause of treatment failure and a significant contributing factor to morbidity and mortality resulting from cancer. Although the dissemination of tumor cells through the circulation is probably a frequent occurrence, the establishment of metastatic disease is a very inefficient process. It requires several events, including the entry of the neoplastic cells into the blood or lymphatic system, the survival of those cells in the circulation, avoidance of immune surveillance, invasion of foreign (heterotopic) tissues, and the establishment of a blood supply to permit expansion of the tumor at the distant site. Simple, dysregulated cell growth is not sufficient for tumor invasion and metastasis. Many tumors progress through distinct stages that can be identified by histopathologic examination, including hyperplasia, dysplasia, carcinoma in situ, invasive cancer, and disseminated cancer. Genetic analysis of these different stages of tumor progression suggests that uncontrolled growth results from progressive alterations in cellular oncogenes and inactivation of tumor suppressor genes, but these genetic changes driving tumorigenicity are clearly distinct from those that determine the metastatic phenotype.

Histologically, invasive carcinoma is characterized by a lack of basement membrane around an expanding mass of tumor cells. Matrix proteolysis appears to be a key part of the mechanism of invasion by tumor cells, which must be able to move through connective tissue barriers, such as the basement membrane, to spread from their site of origin. The proteases involved in this process include the matrix metalloproteinases and their inhibitors, tissue inhibitors of matrix metalloproteinases. The local environment of the target organ may profoundly influence the growth potential of extravasated tumor cells [34]. The various cell-surface receptors that mediate interactions between tumor cells and between tumor cells and the extracellular matrix include cadherins, integrins (transmembrane proteins formed by the noncovalent association of a and b subunits), and CD44, a transmembrane glycoprotein involved in cell adhesion to hyaluronan [112]. Tumor cells must decrease their adhesiveness to escape from the primary tumor, but at later stages in metastasis, the same tumor cells need to increase their adhesiveness during arrest and intravasation to distant sites.

2.4 Angiogenesis

Angiogenesis is the biologic process of new blood vessel formation. This complex, invasive process involves multiple steps including proteolytic degradation of the extracellular matrix surrounding existing blood vessels, chemotactic migration and proliferation of endothelial cells, the organization of these endothelial cells into tubules, the establishment of a lumen that serves as a conduit between the circulation and an expanding mass of tumor cells, and functional maturation of the newly formed blood vessel [39, 96]. Angiogenesis involves the coordinated activity of a wide variety of molecules including growth factors, extracellular matrix proteins, adhesion receptors, and proteolytic enzymes. Under physiologic conditions the vascular endothelium is quiescent and has a very low rate of cell division, such that only 0.01% of endothelial cells are dividing [39, 45, 96]. However, in response to hormonal cues or hypoxic or ischemic conditions, the endothelial cells can be activated to migrate, proliferate rapidly, and create tubules with lumens.

Angiogenesis occurs as part of such normal physiologic activities as wound healing, inflammation, the female reproductive cycle, and embryonic development. In these processes, angiogenesis is tightly and predictably regulated. However, angiogenesis can also be involved in the progression of several pathologic processes in which there is a loss of regulatory control that results in persistent growth of new blood vessels. Such unabated neovascularization occurs in rheumatoid arthritis, inflammatory bowel disease, hemangiomas of childhood, ocular neovascularization, and the growth and spread of tumors [38].

Compelling data implicate the requirement for tumor-associated neovascularization in tumor growth, invasion, and metastasis [8, 36, 37, 91]. A tumor in the prevascular phase (i.e., before new blood vessels have developed) can grow to only a limited size, approximately 2–3 mm^3. At this point the rapid cell proliferation is balanced by equally rapid cell death by apoptosis resulting in a nonexpanding tumor mass. The switch to an angiogenic phenotype with tumor neo-vascularization results in a decrease in the rate of tumor cell apoptosis, thereby shifting the balance to cell proliferation and tumor growth [47, 66]. This decrease in apoptosis occurs, in part, because the increased perfusion resulting from neovascularization permits improved nutrient and metabolite exchange. In addition, the proliferating endothelium may supply, in a paracrine manner, a variety of factors that promote tumor growth, such as insulin-like growth factors I and II (IGF-I, IGF-II) [44].

In experimental models, increased tumor vascularization correlates with increased tumor growth, whereas restriction of neovascularization limits tumor growth. Clinically, the onset of neovascularization in many human tumors is temporally associated with increased tumor growth [111], and high levels of angiogenic factors are commonly detected in blood and urine from patients with advanced malignancies [80]. In addition, the number and density of new microvessels within primary tumors have been shown to correlate with the likelihood of metastasis as well as the overall prognosis for patients with a wide variety of neoplasms, including pediatric tumors such as neuroblastoma and Wilms tumor [1, 74].

It has become increasingly evident that the regulation of tumor angiogenesis is complex: new blood vessel formation occurs as the result of competing pro- and antiangiogenic signals originating in multiple tissues [19]. Specific genetic events in certain cancers, such as altered expression of the p53 tumor suppressor gene [26, 121] or the human EGFR gene [63, 89, 119], not only affect the cell cycle but also play a role in angiogenesis by modulating key signals (e.g., upregulating the expression of vascular endothelial growth factor [VEGF], or downregulating the expression of the endogenous angiogenesis inhibitor thrombospondin 1).

Metastasis also appears to be dependent on angiogenesis [35, 65]. This dependence is probably due to several factors. First, new blood vessels in the primary tumor provide increased opportunities for the shedding of tumor cells into the circulation. Also, disruption of the basement membrane by proteases released by the proliferating endothelial cells may contribute to the metastatic potential of a tumor [15, 98]. Finally, successful growth of metastatic cells in foreign target organs depends on the stimulation and formation of new blood vessels, perhaps even when cells metastasize to the bone marrow.

2.5 Environmental Carcinogenesis

As stated previously, tumorigenesis is a complex process in which the progressive acquisition of combina-tions of critical genetic alterations shifts normal cells into uncontrolled growth and clonal expansion. These alterations in the genome can either be inherited or acquired, the latter being a result of the influence of the environment on the host genome or factors intrinsic to a dividing cell. The most significant host factor relates to the normal, albeit low, rate of inaccurate DNA replication that goes uncorrected by normal host mechanisms. Living organisms have been selected for their ability to accurately replicate their genomes, although not with absolute precision. This ensures stability while permitting the dynamic of genetic change essential to environmental adaptation and consequent evolution. Variability in the local environment may make such mistakes more or less likely. This rate of accumulating alterations in the genome can also be significantly increased when there are defects in the normal genetic corrective mechanisms, or when there is increased host cell genomic instability. Critical for tumorigenesis, however, in addition to the initial occurrence of DNA damage, is the persistence of the DNA alterations and their eventual transmission to clonal descendants of the originally affected cell. Two conditions need to be fulfilled for persistence and inheritance of DNA damage: (1) The DNA repair systems of the cell fail to remove or correct the damage and (2) the residual lesion should not only be compatible with continued cell viability and proliferative capacity but also should confer a survival advantage.

The first line of cellular defense against DNA damage is the recognition of the damage and the implementation of a variety of molecular mechanisms which have evolved to effect repair. An important class of genetic lesions are mismatches which result in non-complementary DNA sequence over a short region. Unrepaired mismatches generate point mutations at the next round of cell division and the synthesis of mutant or truncated proteins. Removal of these mismatches and restoration of normal complementary base-pairing is the responsibility of mismatch repair enzymes. Other DNA lesions require different sorts of repair. DNA strands can be broken, generating a spectrum of lesions from point mutations to large-scale chromosomal aberrations. Several mechanisms exist for strand break repair including the process of homologous recombination. The DNA repair processes are intimately linked to cell cycle control in proliferating cells, with several check points existing at which DNA-damaged cells are blocked until the repair processes have been completed. One example is the p53 tumor suppressor gene and its role in cell cycle arrest. DNA damage by a variety of extrinsic agents leads to cellular accumulation of the p53 protein, largely by stabilization of the protein, and the resultant blocking of the damaged cell at the G1 checkpoint. Successful repair of DNA damage leads to a reduction in p53 levels and release from the G1 block. However, incomplete or unsuccessful repair continues to generate the p53 blocking signal. Long-term-G1 blocking then invokes a cell death pathway, usually apoptosis, to eliminate unrepairable mutant cells. Thus p53 plays a critical role as the "guardian of the genome" to prevent the onset of genetic instability [62].

2.5.1 Epidemiology

The opportunity to practice prevention of cancer depends on the existence of potentially avoidable factors and their recognition so that appropriate action can be taken. The impact or causal role of environmental factors on the development of human malignancies was first recognized by noting unexpectedly high cancer incidences in certain occupational groups. Fabia and Thuy first suggested that a father's occupation might increase the risk of a child developing cancer [32]. The ability of certain chemicals was then documented in various animal models of carcinogenesis. In addition, population-based studies confirmed histology and anatomic site-specific cancer rates among geographically distinct populations. Changes in cancer frequency among migrating ethnic groups, high cancer rates associated with specific occupations and most notably the risk of cancer associated with such activities as smoking and tobacco use have confirmed that environmental and lifestyle exposures contribute to human cancer risk. In addition, it has become recognized that certain people carry hereditary susceptibility genes that increase risk for developing cancer with particular environmental exposures. Environmental agents may cause mutations which are distinct or different from the predominant mutational type resulting from intrinsic mutagenesis or from the action of other environmental agents. This gives rise to the possibility of "molecular fingerprinting" by which environmental agents might be identified by the characteristic mutational type they have caused in the oncogenes or tumor suppressor genes of a tumor suspected of having environmental causation. One example is the characteristic mutations in the p53 gene associated with aflatoxin-mediated hepatocellular carcinoma [48].

The critical corollary to the identification of these factors is that exposure or lifestyle modification may be able to decrease the incidence of cancer development. Epidemiology, broadly defined, is the study of disease occurrence in different population groups in order to help identify causative risk factors and to plan appropriate preventive strategies. Epidemiology may also provide clues to etiology and pathogenesis.

Strong evidence exists that a substantial proportion of adult cancers are environmentally influenced, with tobacco, alcohol, and diet being among the most

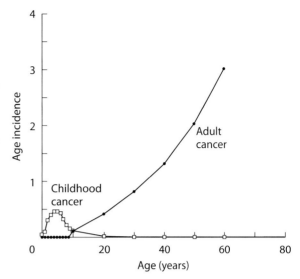

Fig. 2.2 Schematic illustration of the differing age-incidence patterns of adult and childhood cancer (not to scale). (This is Figure 2.4 from the prior edition of this textbook.)

important factors [2]. It is much less obvious that environmental factors play an important role in the development of childhood cancer. However, there are fundamental differences between oncogenesis in children and adults that influence the impact of environmental exposures on carcinogenesis. Most adult tumors are of epithelial origin, such as in the gastrointestinal or respiratory tracts, surfaces that are directly exposed to carcinogens, whereas most pediatric tumors are of mesenchymal origin in tissues or sites with minimal contact with the environment. In addition, during embryogenesis, fetal tissues are normally undergoing rapid cell division with high rates of proliferation, much like cancer cells, and then ultimately undergo differentiation or apoptosis. Additionally, adult cancers, despite variations between pathologic types, usually conform to a pattern in which the incidence increases with age, reflecting an accumulation of multiple mutations with time. Childhood cancers, in distinction to those in adults, typically have an incidence that initially increases with age, reaches a peak, and then falls (Fig. 2.2), suggesting that other epigenetic factors, other than simply an accumulation of genetic mutations, contribute to the development of malignancies in children. Finally, the cumulative effects of carcinogens such as irradiation and other environmental exposures often are not apparent for many years and, therefore, are less likely to have a direct impact on the development of pediatric malignancies. Thus, few environmental factors have been identified as being associated with pediatric oncogenesis. Nevertheless, some environmental factors have been associated with the evolution of pediatric tumors and are discussed below.

2.5.2 Potential Causative Agents

2.5.2.1 Radiation

Ionizing radiation is tumorigenic and is capable of causing or contributing to the development of a wide variety of malignancies. It causes a variety of heritable DNA lesions, from point mutations to chromosomal deletions or rearrangements, induces transformation to a malignant state in cells in culture and causes a range of types of cancer in experimental animals in a dose-dependent fashion. The developing fetus is particularly sensitive to the effects of ionizing irradiation, which increases the risk of childhood cancer by approximately 6%/Gy exposure [30]. For postnatal irradiation the risk is about half of that for the fetus [95]. The radiation being delivered to children as part of diagnostic imaging studies, particularly CT scans, is currently being closely scrutinized as its potential role in the subsequent development of cancer is becoming increasingly appreciated [31]. It should be noted, however, that most of the cancers to which childhood irradiation makes a contribution will appear in adulthood, as radiation-induced cancer generally has a very long latency period [77]. Non-ionizing radiation such as ultraviolet light and electromagnetic fields may also contribute to the development of cancer, although, again, the association of skin cancer with UV exposure, for example, is well known but typically results in a heightened incidence in adult years. The epidemiologic evidence that electromagnetic radiation leads to cancer is conflicting [60], and the data regarding the effects of high-voltage transmission lines, electrical appliances, and video display screens do not seem to support a causal role for these factors.

2.5.2.2 Chemical Agents

There are many chemical agents which have DNA-damaging capacity and therefore tumorigenic potential, but few for which there is any clear evidence of significant involvement in the causation of childhood cancer. Several chemical factors have been suggested as relevant to childhood cancer, including pesticides, vitamin K administration, passive cigarette smoke, and maternal use of "recreational" drugs. An uncommon but very striking factor is the well-known risk of the hormone diethylstilbestrol, which used to be administered in pregnancy in some cases where miscarriage was anticipated. This resulted in a 0.1% risk of the development of clear cell adenocarcinomas of the cervix or vagina in female offspring [78]. There have been some reports of other childhood cancers, particularly neuroblastoma, associated with induced ovulation, although the evidence is not overwhelming [71].

2.5.2.3 Viruses

The role played by several viruses in human malignancies has been well established, most notably Epstein-Barr virus (EBV) and its association with Burkitt lymphoma, whereby immortalization of B cells by EBV has been suggested to be the initial event in multistep carcinogenesis [53]. EBV also appears to have a causal role in the development of nasopharyngeal carcinoma and some cases of Hodgkin lymphoma [43]. Cancer also occurs with increased frequency in children with human immunodeficiency virus (HIV) infection. The most common types are lymphomas and leukemias, although solid tumors including leiomyosarcoma and Kaposi sarcoma also occur with an increased incidence [92, 108]. However, neither the specific clinical, immunological, and viral risk factors for malignancy in these patients, nor the pathogenesis of HIV-related pediatric malignancies have been clearly elucidated.

2.5.2.4 Parental Occupation and Exposure to Noxious Agents

Parental occupation and exposures have been linked to an increased risk of a variety of childhood cancers [24, 101]. Transgenerational effects may be due to direct germ cell mutation, transport of carcinogens in the semen or epigenetic alterations of gene expression [87]. Paternal exposure to solvents such as benzene, xylene, toluene, and carbon tetrachloride have been implicated in the pathogenesis of hematologic malignancies and brain tumors as have paints and pesticides [82]. Increased risk of childhood cancers such as leukemia, Ewing sarcoma germ cell tumor, and Wilms tumor have been associated with certain paternal occupations including auto mechanic and welder, and to exposure at work to motor vehicle exhaust fumes, pesticides, petroleum, and ether [46, 105, 107]. Although increased risk of some childhood cancers in association with potential carcinogen exposure is suggested by multiple studies, methodological limitations common to many studies restrict conclusions; these include exposure classification, small sample size, and potential biases in control selection

2.5.2.5 Iatrogenic Factors

Because the survival rates for childhood cancers have improved to more than 80%, the proportion of childhood cancer survivors within the general population increases every year. Survivors are at risk for multiple late sequelae of therapy, including the development of a secondary malignancy. A significant factor contributing to this risk, in addition to the genetic predisposition of the patient, is the type of therapy received [6]. For example, an increased risk of subsequent leukemia is well-documented after exposure to epipodophyllotoxins and alkylating agents [93]. Similarly, the risk of carcinomas of the breast and thyroid, particularly after childhood Hodgkin lymphoma, has been extensively reported, and is related, in part to exposure to ionizing radiation as part of the treatment of the initial cancer [7]. Other examples include therapy-related brain tumors after cranial irradiation, osteosarcoma after irradiation for retinoblastoma and tumors, such as thyroid cancer, arising as a complication of low-dose irradiation given in the past as treatment for tinea capitis and acne, which often occurs in adulthood but may occur late in the teenage years.

2.5.3 Tumor Types

2.5.3.1 Neuroblastoma

Several case-control studies have examined the relationship between maternal and paternal occupation and exposure, and the risk of neuroblastoma in offspring [18, 75, 110, 117]. Two studies found an association with fathers employed in electronics-related occupations including electricians and welders (odds ratio = 11.7, 95% confidence interval 1.4–98.5) [110]. Another study found increased risks in electrical, farming and gardening, and painting occupations [85]. A variety of other paternal occupations and industries have been shown to have an increased risk of having a child with neuroblastoma [18, 117]. Paternal exposures to hydrocarbons such as diesel fuel, lacquer thinner, and turpentine were associated with an increased incidence of neuroblastoma as were exposures to wood dust and solders [29]. Pesticide use in both home and garden were modestly associated with neuroblastoma [27]. Certain maternal occupations have also been found to have an association with an increased risk [18, 110, 117].

Several epidemiologic and case series have suggested a relationship between the use of certain medications just prior to and during pregnancy and neuroblastoma, specifically hormone use and fertility drugs [56, 76, 103], although others studies have not confirmed such an association [25]. One study by Schuz,

et al. observed a positive association with the use of oral contraceptives or other sex hormones during pregnancy (particularly with male offspring), a shorter gestational duration, lower birth weight, and maternal alcohol consumption during pregnancy [102]. Other drugs have been implicated, although the data have not always been consistent among different studies. Similarly, the results for smoking, alcohol use, and the use of hair dye in some studies are suggestive but not conclusive [52, 56, 103], while other studies find no association [120]. Maternal use of illicit or recreational drug around pregnancy has been associated with an increased risk of neuroblastoma in offspring (odds ratio = 1.82, 95% confidence interval 1.13–3.00), particularly the use of marijuana in the first trimester of pregnancy [9]. Other studies have suggested an association between maternal hair dye use and elevated risk of childhood cancer including neuroblastoma (OR = 1.6, 95%CI = 1.2–2.0). Vitamin use during pregnancy might reduce the incidence of neuroblastoma, consistent with findings for other childhood cancers [86]. Also, children with neuroblastoma were less likely to have been breast-fed than control children (CR = 0.6, 95% CI = 0.5–0.9) with the decreased association between breast-feeding and neuroblastoma increasing with increasing duration of breast-feeding.

2.5.3.2 Wilms Tumor

The first suggestion that paternal occupational exposures might be of importance in the etiology of Wilms tumors came from Kantor, et al. [50]. From a comparison of birth certificates for 149 Connecticut tumor registry cases with 149 matched controls, they estimated relative risks of 2.4 for hydrocarbon-related occupations and 3.7 for those with a potential for lead exposure. This was later supported by Wilkins and Sinks, although their results did not reach statistical significance for the association [118]. Others have attempted to confirm this finding [17, 59, 99]. Although suggestive associations have been found in some studies for machinists, mechanics, and welders the numbers are small and the patterns are inconsistent. Olshan, et al. found no consistent pattern of increased risk for paternal exposure to hydrocarbons and lead but did find that certain paternal occupations did have an elevated odds ratio of Wilms tumor including vehicle mechanics, auto body repairmen, and welders [83]. Offspring of fathers who were auto mechanics had a four- to seven-fold increased risk of Wilms tumor. Other early studies have suggested possible associations with maternal smoking, coffee/tea drinking, and exposure to synthetic progestins during pregnancy and the use of hair coloring products [17, 64, 82]. However, these studies are subject to several methodologic limitations including misclassification of exposure, selection bias, and small sample size, and later studies have, in general, failed to confirm most of the previously reported maternal risk factors for Wilms tumor [84]. Breast feeding was associated with a reduced risk of Wilms tumor (odds ratio = 0.7, 95% confidence interval = 0.5–0.9).

2.5.3.3 Liver Tumors

Environmental factors have also been implicated in hepatoblastoma. An association with certain occupational exposures in fathers of children with hepatoblastoma, including excess exposures to metals such as in welding and soldering fumes (odds ratio 8.0), petroleum products, and paints (odds ratio 3.7), has been observed [16]. Prenatal exposure to acetaminophen in combination with petroleum products has also been noted in association with hepatoblastoma [100]. There is a striking association of hepatoblastoma with prematurity, with the relative risk increasing with decreasing birth weight [33]. However, the etiology behind this association is currently unknown. An increased incidence of liver tumors is also seen in association with fetal alcohol syndrome, exposure to hepatitis B and aflatoxin, and prolonged parenteral nutrition in infancy [88]. The most striking association, however, is in children with metabolic diseases such as tyrosinemia. In children with these disorders, the tissues are exposed to high, continuous levels of endogenous carcinogens, and are at such high risk for the development of malignancies such as hepatocellular carcinoma early in life, that early organ transplantation is recommended [23, 115].

2.6 Summary

The potential role of environmental exposures in the etiology of childhood cancer remains uncertain. The relatively few epidemiologic studies that have been conducted have been limited by a number of confounding factors, including sample size, exposure misclassification and selection bias. Nevertheless, sufficient suggestive data exist to warrant further evaluation into the role of environmental exposures in pediatric oncogenesis. The goal being, of course, to identify factors that can be eliminated or avoided in order to decrease the risk for developing a malignancy.

References

1. Abramson LP, Grundy PE, Rademaker AW, et al. (2003) Increased microvascular density predicts relapse in Wilms' tumor. J Pediatr Surg 38:325–330
2. Ames BN, Gold LS, Willett WC (1995) The causes and prevention of cancer. Proc Natl Acad Sci USA 92:5258–5265
3. Bader SA, Fasching C, Brodeur GM, et al. (1991) Dissociation of suppression of tumorigenicity and differentiation in vitro effected by transfer of single human chromosomes into human neuroblastoma cells. Cell Growth Differ 2:245–255
4. Bardeesy N, Falkoff D, Petruzzi MJ, et al. (1994) Anaplastic Wilms' tumour, a subtype displaying poor prognosis, harbours p53 gene mutations. Nat Genet 7:91–97
5. Barr FG (1999) The role of chimeric paired box transcription factors in the pathogenesis of pediatric rhabdomyosarcoma. Cancer Res 59:1711s–1715s
6. Bassal M, Mertens AC, Taylor L, et al. (2006) Risk of selected subsequent carcinomas in survivors of childhood cancer: A report from the Childhood Cancer Survivor Study. J Clin Oncol 24:476–483
7. Bhatia S, Robison LL, Oberlin O, et al. (1996) Breast cancer and other second neoplasms after childhood Hodgkin's disease. N Engl J Med 334:745–751
8. Bicknell R, Harris AL (1996) Mechanisms and therapeutic implications of angiogenesis. Curr Opin Oncol 8:60–65
9. Bluhm EC, Daniels J, Pollock BH, et al. (2006) Maternal use of recreational drugs and neuroblastoma in offspring: A report from the Children's Oncology Group (United States). Cancer Causes Control 17:663–669
10. Bown N, Cotterill S, Lastowska M, et al. (1999) Gain of chromosome arm 17q and adverse outcome in patients with neuroblastoma. N Engl J Med 340:1954–1961
11. Brodeur GM, Hayes FA, Green AA, et al. (1987) Consistent N-myc copy number in simultaneous or consecutive neuroblastoma samples from sixty individual patients. Cancer Res 47:4248–4253
12. Brodeur GM, Maris JM, Yamashiro DJ, et al. (1997) Biology and genetics of human neuroblastomas. J Pediatr Hematol Oncol 19:93–101
13. Brodeur GM, Seeger RC, Schwab M, et al. (1984) Amplification of N-myc in untreated human neuroblastomas correlates with advanced disease stage. Science 224:1121–1124
14. Brodeur GM, Sekhon G, Goldstein MN (1977) Chromosomal aberrations in human neuroblastomas. Cancer 40:2256–2263
15. Brooks PC, Silletti S, von Schalscha TL, et al. (1998) Disruption of angiogenesis by PEX, a noncatalytic metalloproteinase fragment with integrin binding activity. Cell 92:391–400
16. Buckley JD, Sather H, Ruccione K, et al. (1989) A case-control study of risk factors for hepatoblastoma. A report from the Childrens Cancer Study Group. Cancer 64:1169–1176
17. Bunin GR, Nass CC, Kramer S, et al. (1989) Parental occupation and Wilms' tumor: Results of a case-control study. Cancer Res 49:725–729
18. Bunin GR, Ward E, Kramer S, et al. (1990) Neuroblastoma and parental occupation. Am J Epidemiol 131:776–780

19. Carmeliet P, Jain RK (2000) Angiogenesis in cancer and other diseases. Nature 407:249–257

20. Chen Y, Takita J, Hiwatari M, et al. (2006) Mutations of the PTPN11 and RAS genes in rhabdomyosarcoma and pediatric hematological malignancies. Genes Chromosomes Cancer 45:583–591

21. Clark J, Benjamin H, Gill S, et al. (1996) Fusion of the EWS gene to CHN, a member of the steroid/thyroid receptor gene superfamily, in a human myxoid chondrosarcoma. Oncogene 12:229–235

22. Clark J, Rocques PJ, Crew AJ, et al. (1994) Identification of novel genes, SYT and SSX, involved in the t(X;18)(p11.2;q11.2) translocation found in human synovial sarcoma. Nat Genet 7:502–508

23. Coire CI, Qizilbash AH, Castelli MF (1987) Hepatic adenomata in type Ia glycogen storage disease. Arch Pathol Lab Med 111:166–169

24. Colt JS, Blair A (1998) Parental occupational exposures and risk of childhood cancer. Environ Health Perspect 106(Suppl 3):909–925

25. Cook MN, Olshan AF, Guess HA, et al. (2004) Maternal medication use and neuroblastoma in offspring. Am J Epidemiol 159:721–731

26. Dameron KM, Volpert OV, Tainsky MA, et al. (1994) Control of angiogenesis in fibroblasts by p53 regulation of thrombospondin-1. Science 265:1582–1584

27. Daniels JL, Olshan AF, Savitz DA (1997) Pesticides and childhood cancers. Environ Health Perspect 105:1068–1077

28. de Alava E, Kawai A, Healey JH, et al. (1998) EWS-FLI1 fusion transcript structure is an independent determinant of prognosis in Ewing's sarcoma. J Clin Oncol 16:1248–1255

29. De Roos AJ, Olshan AF, Teschke K, et al. (2001) Parental occupational exposures to chemicals and incidence of neuroblastoma in offspring. Am J Epidemiol 154:106–114

30. Doll R, Wakeford R (1997) Risk of childhood cancer from fetal irradiation. Br J Radiol 70:130–139

31. Donnelly LF, Emery KH, Brody AS, et al. (2001) Minimizing radiation dose for pediatric body applications of single-detector helical CT: Strategies at a large Children's Hospital. AJR Am J Roentgenol 176:303–306

32. Fabia J, Thuy TD (1974) Occupation of father at time of birth of children dying of malignant diseases. Br J Prev Soc Med 28:98–100

33. Feusner J, Buckley J, Robison L, et al. (1998) Prematurity and hepatoblastoma: More than just an association? J Pediatr 133:585–586

34. Fidler IJ (2002) The organ microenvironment and cancer metastasis. Differentiation 70:498–505

35. Fidler IJ, Ellis LM (1994) The implications of angiogenesis for the biology and therapy of cancer metastasis. Cell 79:185–188

36. Folkman J (1990) What is the evidence that tumors are angiogenesis dependent? J Natl Cancer Inst 82:4–6

37. Folkman J (1992) The role of angiogenesis in tumor growth. Semin Cancer Biol 3:65–71

38. Folkman J (1995) Clinical applications of research on angiogenesis. N Engl J Med 333:1757–1763

39. Folkman J, D'Amore PA (1996) Blood vessel formation: What is its molecular basis? Cell 87:1153–1155

40. Fong CT, Dracopoli NC, White PS, et al. (1989) Loss of heterozygosity for the short arm of chromosome 1 in human neuroblastomas: Correlation with N-myc amplification. Proc Natl Acad Sci USA 86:3753–3757

41. Galili N, Davis RJ, Fredericks WJ, et al. (1993) Fusion of a fork head domain gene to PAX3 in the solid tumour alveolar rhabdomyosarcoma. Nat Genet 5:230–235

42. Grundy P, Coppes MJ, Haber D (1995) Molecular genetics of Wilms tumor. Hematol Oncol Clin North Am 9:1201–1215

43. Gutensohn N, Cole P (1981) Childhood social environment and Hodgkin's disease. N Engl J Med 304:135–140

44. Hamada J, Cavanaugh PG, Lotan O, et al. (1992) Separable growth and migration factors for large-cell lymphoma cells secreted by microvascular endothelial cells derived from target organs for metastasis. Br J Cancer 66:349–354

45. Hobson B, Denekamp J (1984) Endothelial proliferation in tumours and normal tissues: Continuous labelling studies. Br J Cancer 49:405–413

46. Holly EA, Aston DA, Ahn DK, et al. (1992) Ewing's bone sarcoma, paternal occupational exposure, and other factors. Am J Epidemiol 135:122–129

47. Holmgren L, O'Reilly MS, Folkman J (1995) Dormancy of micrometastases: Balanced proliferation and apoptosis in the presence of angiogenesis suppression. Nat Med 1:149–153

48. Hsu IC, Metcalf RA, Sun T, et al. (1991) Mutational hotspot in the p53 gene in human hepatocellular carcinomas. Nature 350:427–428

49. Kaneko Y, Kanda N, Maseki N, et al. (1987) Different karyotypic patterns in early and advanced stage neuroblastomas. Cancer Res 47:311–318

50. Kantor AF, Curnen MG, Meigs JW, et al. (1979) Occupations of fathers of patients with Wilms tumour. J Epidemiol Community Health 33:253–256

51. Keshelava N, Zuo JJ, Waidyaratne NS, et al. (2000) p53 mutations and loss of p53 function confer multidrug resistance in neuroblastoma. Med Pediatr Oncol 35:563–568

52. Kinney H, Faix R, Brazy J (1980) The fetal alcohol syndrome and neuroblastoma. Pediatrics 66:130–132

53. Klein G, Klein E (1985) Evolution of tumours and the impact of molecular oncology. Nature 315:190–195

54. Knudson AG Jr (1971) Mutation and cancer: Statistical study of retinoblastoma. Proc Natl Acad Sci USA 68:820–823

55. Kohl NE, Kanda N, Schreck RR, et al. (1983) Transposition and amplification of oncogene-related sequences in human neuroblastomas. Cell 35:359–367

56. Kramer S, Ward E, Meadows AT, et al. (1987) Medical and drug risk factors associated with neuroblastoma: A case-control study. J Natl Cancer Inst 78:797–804

57. Kucharczak J, Simmons MJ, Fan Y, et al. (2003) To be, or not to be: NF-kappaB is the answer – Role of Rel/NF-kappaB in the regulation of apoptosis. Oncogene 22:8961–8982

58. Kusafuka T, Fukuzawa M, Oue T, et al. (1997) Mutation analysis of p53 gene in childhood malignant solid tumors. J Pediatr Surg 32:1175–1180

59. Kwa SL, Fine LJ (1980) The association between parental occupation and childhood malignancy. J Occup Med 22:792–794

60. Lacy-Hulbert A, Wilkins RC, Hesketh TR, et al. (1995) Cancer risk and electromagnetic fields. Nature 375:23

61. Ladanyi M, Gerald W (1994) Fusion of the EWS and WT1 genes in the desmoplastic small round cell tumor. Cancer Res 54:2837–2840

62. Lane DP (1992) Cancer - P53, Guardian of the Genome. Nature 358:15–16

63. Laughner E, Taghavi P, Chiles K, et al. (2001) HER2 (neu) signaling increases the rate of hypoxia-inducible factor 1alpha (HIF-1alpha) synthesis: Novel mechanism for HIF-1-mediated vascular endothelial growth factor expression. Mol Cell Biol 21:3995–4004

64. LeMasters GK, Bove KE: Genetic/environmental significance of multifocal modular renal blastema. Am J Pediatr Hematol Oncol 2:1980:81–87

65. Liotta LA, Steeg PS, Stetler-Stevenson WG (1991) Cancer metastasis and angiogenesis: An imbalance of positive and negative regulation. Cell 64:327–336

66. Liotta LA, Steeg PS, Stetler-Stevenson WG (1991) Cancer metastasis and angiogenesis: An imbalance of positive and negative regulation. Cell 64:327–336

67. Look AT, Hayes FA, Nitschke R, et al. (1984) Cellular DNA content as a predictor of response to chemotherapy in infants with unresectable neuroblastoma. N Engl J Med 311:231–235

68. Look AT, Kirsch IR (1997) Molecular basis of childhood cancer. In: Pizzo PA, Poplack DG (eds) Principles and practices of pediatric oncology. Lippincott, Philadelphia, pp 38–53

69. Lutz W, Stohr M, Schurmann J, et al. (1996) Conditional expression of N-myc in human neuroblastoma cells increases expression of alpha-prothymosin and ornithine decarboxylase and accelerates progression into S-phase early after mitogenic stimulation of quiescent cells. Oncogene 13:803–812

70. Malkin D, Li FP, Strong LC, et al. (1990) Germ line p53 mutations in a familial syndrome of breast cancer, sarcomas, and other neoplasms. Science 250:1233–1238

71. Mandel M, Toren A, Rechavi G, et al. (1994) Hormonal treatment in pregnancy: A possible risk factor for neuroblastoma. Med Pediatr Oncol 23:133–135

72. May WA, Gishizky ML, Lessnick SL, et al. (1993) Ewing sarcoma 11;22 translocation produces a chimeric transcription factor that requires the DNA-binding domain encoded by FLI1 for transformation. Proc Natl Acad Sci USA 90:5752–5756

73. May WA, Lessnick SL, Braun BS, et al. (1993) The Ewing's sarcoma EWS/FLI-1 fusion gene encodes a more potent transcriptional activator and is a more powerful transforming gene than FLI-1. Mol Cell Biol 13:7393–7398

74. Meitar D, Crawford SE, Rademaker AW, et al. (1996) Tumor angiogenesis correlates with metastatic disease, N-myc amplification, and poor outcome in human neuroblastoma. J Clin Oncol 14:405–414

75. Michaelis J, Haaf HG, Zollner J, et al. (1996) Case control study of neuroblastoma in West Germany after the Chernobyl accident. Klin Padiatr 208:172–178

76. Michalek AM, Buck GM, Nasca PC, et al. (1996) Gravid health status, medication use, and risk of neuroblastoma. Am J Epidemiol 143:996–1001

77. Miller R (1986) Radiogenic cancer after prenatal or childhood exposure. In: Boice JD Jr, Upton AC, Albert RE, Burns FJ (eds) Radiation carcinogenesis. Elsevier, New York, pp 379–386

78. Mittendorf R (1995) Teratogen update: Carcinogenesis and teratogenesis associated with exposure to diethylstilbestrol (DES) in utero. Teratology 51:435–445

79. Nagata S (1997) Apoptosis by death factor. Cell 88:355–365

80. Nguyen M, Watanabe H, Budson AE, et al. (1993) Elevated levels of the angiogenic peptide basic fibroblast growth factor in urine of bladder cancer patients. J Natl Cancer Inst 85:241–242

81. O'Brien KP, Seroussi E, Dal Cin P, et al. (1998) Various regions within the alpha-helical domain of the COL1A1 gene are fused to the second exon of the PDGFB gene in dermatofibrosarcomas and giant-cell fibroblastomas. Genes Chromosomes Cancer 23:187–193

82. O'Leary LM, Hicks AM, Peters JM, et al. (1991) Parental occupational exposures and risk of childhood cancer: A review. Am J Ind Med 20:17–35

83. Olshan AF, Breslow NE, Daling JR, et al. (1990) Wilms' tumor and paternal occupation. Cancer Res 50:3212–3217

84. Olshan AF, Breslow NE, Falletta JM, et al. (1993) Risk factors for Wilms tumor. Report from the National Wilms Tumor Study. Cancer 72:938–944

85. Olshan AF, De Roos AJ, Teschke K, et al. (1999) Neuroblastoma and parental occupation. Cancer Causes Control 10:539–549

86. Olshan AF, Smith JC, Bondy ML, et al. (2002) Maternal vitamin use and reduced risk of neuroblastoma. Epidemiology 13:575–580

87. Olshan AF, van Wijngaarden E (2003) Paternal occupation and childhood cancer. Adv Exp Med Biol 518:147–161

88. Patterson K, Kapur SP, Chandra RS (1985) Hepatocellular carcinoma in a noncirrhotic infant after prolonged parenteral nutrition. J Pediatr 106:797–800

89. Petit AM, Rak J, Hung MC, et al. (1997) Neutralizing antibodies against epidermal growth factor and ErbB-2/neu receptor tyrosine kinases down-regulate vascular endothelial growth factor production by tumor cells in vitro and in vivo: Angiogenic implications for signal transduction therapy of solid tumors. Am J Pathol 151:1523–1530

90. Pinthus JH, Fridman E, Dekel B, et al. (2004) ErbB2 is a tumor associated antigen and a suitable therapeutic target in Wilms tumor. J Urol 172:1644–1648

91. Pluda JM (1997) Tumor-associated angiogenesis: Mechanisms, clinical implications, and therapeutic strategies. Semin Oncol 24:203–218

92. Pollock BH, Jenson HB, Leach CT, et al. (2003) Risk factors for pediatric human immunodeficiency virus-related malignancy. JAMA 289:2393–2399

93. Pui CH, Ribeiro RC, Hancock ML, et al. (1991) Acute myeloid leukemia in children treated with epipodophyllotoxins for acute lymphoblastic leukemia. N Engl J Med 325:1682–1687

94. Rabbitts TH, Forster A, Larson R, et al. (1993) Fusion of the dominant negative transcription regulator CHOP with a novel gene FUS by translocation t(12;16) in malignant liposarcoma. Nat Genet 4:175–180

95. Richardson RB (1990) Past and revised risk estimates for cancer induced by irradiation and their influence on dose limits. Br J Radiol 63:235–245

96. Risau W (1997) Mechanisms of angiogenesis. Nature 386:671–674

97. Rubin BP, Chen CJ, Morgan TW, et al. (1998) Congenital mesoblastic nephroma t(12;15) is associated with ETV6-NTRK3 gene fusion: Cytogenetic and molecular relationship to congenital (infantile) fibrosarcoma. Am J Pathol 153:1451–1458

98. Ruegg C, Yilmaz A, Bieler G, et al. (1998) Evidence for the involvement of endothelial cell integrin alphaVbeta3 in the disruption of the tumor vasculature induced by TNF and IFN-gamma. Nat Med 4:408–414

99. Sanders B (1981) Occupations of fathers of children dying from neoplasms. J Epidemiol Community Health 35:245–250

100. Satge D, Sasco AJ, Little J (1998) Antenatal therapeutic drug exposure and fetal/neonatal tumours: Review of 89 cases. Paediatr Perinat Epidemiol 12:84–117

101. Savitz DA, Chen JH (1990) Parental occupation and childhood cancer: Review of epidemiologic studies. Environ Health Perspect 88:325–337

102. Schuz J, Kaletsch U, Meinert R, et al. (2001) Risk factors for neuroblastoma at different stages of disease. Results from a population-based case-control study in Germany. J Clin Epidemiol 54:702–709

103. Schwartzbaum JA (1992) Influence of the mother's prenatal drug consumption on risk of neuroblastoma in the child. Am J Epidemiol 135:1358–1367

104. Seeger RC, Brodeur GM, Sather H, et al. (1985) Association of multiple copies of the N-myc oncogene with rapid progression of neuroblastomas. N Engl J Med 313:1111–1116

105. Sharpe CR, Franco EL, de Camargo B, et al. (1995) Parental exposures to pesticides and risk of Wilms' tumor in Brazil. Am J Epidemiol 141:210–217

106. Sharpless NE, DePinho RA (2004) Telomeres, stem cells, senescence, and cancer. J Clin Invest 113:160–168

107. Shu XO, Nesbit ME, Buckley JD, et al. (1995) An exploratory analysis of risk factors for childhood malignant germ-cell tumors: Report from the Childrens Cancer Group (Canada, United States). Cancer Causes Control 6:187–198

108. Sinfield RL, Molyneux EM, Banda K, et al. (2006) Spectrum and presentation of pediatric malignancies in the HIV era: Experience from Blantyre, Malawi, 1998–2003. Pediatr Blood Cancer (epub ahead of print)

109. Sorensen PH, Lessnick SL, Lopez-Terrada D, et al. (1994) A second Ewing's sarcoma translocation, t(21;22), fuses the EWS gene to another ETS-family transcription factor, ERG. Nat Genet 6:146–151

110. Spitz MR, Johnson CC (1985) Neuroblastoma and paternal occupation. A case-control analysis. Am J Epidemiol 121:924–929

111. Srivastava A, Laidler P, Davies RP, et al. (1988) The prognostic significance of tumor vascularity in intermediate-thickness (0.76–4.0 mm thick) skin melanoma. A quantitative histologic study. Am J Pathol 133:419–423

112. Toole BP (1990) Hyaluronan and its binding proteins, the hyaladherins. Curr Opin Cell Biol 2:839–844

113. Vandesompele J, Van Roy N, Van Gele M, et al. (1998) Genetic heterogeneity of neuroblastoma studied by comparative genomic hybridization. Genes Chromosomes Cancer 23:141–152

114. Wai DH, Knezevich SR, Lucas T, et al. (2000) The ETV6-NTRK3 gene fusion encodes a chimeric protein tyrosine kinase that transforms NIH3T3 cells. Oncogene 19:906–915

115. Weinberg AG, Mize CE, Worthen HG (1976) The occurrence of hepatoma in the chronic form of hereditary tyrosinemia. J Pediatr 88:434–438

116. Weissman IL (2000) Stem cells: Units of development, units of regeneration, and units in evolution. Cell 100:157–168

117. Wilkins JR (1990) Paternal occupational exposure to electromagnetic fields and neuroblastoma in offspring. Am J Epidemiol 131:990–1007

118. Wilkins JR, III, Sinks TH Jr (1984) Paternal occupation and Wilms' tumour in offspring. J Epidemiol Community Health 38:7–11

119. Xiong S, Grijalva R, Zhang L, et al. (2001) Up-regulation of vascular endothelial growth factor in breast cancer cells by the heregulin-beta1-activated p38 signaling pathway enhances endothelial cell migration. Cancer Res 61:1727–1732

120. Yang Q, Olshan AF, Bondy ML, et al. (2000) Parental smoking and alcohol consumption and risk of neuroblastoma. Cancer Epidemiol Biomarkers Prev 9:967–972

121. Zhang L, Yu D, Hu M, et al. (2000) Wild-type p53 suppresses angiogenesis in human leiomyosarcoma and synovial sarcoma by transcriptional suppression of vascular endothelial growth factor expression. Cancer Res 60:3655–3661

122. Zucman J, Delattre O, Desmaze C, et al. (1993) EWS and ATF-1 gene fusion induced by t(12;22) translocation in malignant melanoma of soft parts. Nat Genet 4:341–345

Genetic Counseling for Childhood Tumors and Inherited Cancer-Predisposing Syndromes

Edward S. Tobias, J. Michael Connor

3

Contents

3.1 General Principles of Cancer Genetics

Chromosomal changes are common in all types of malignancy and are helpful for identification of the underlying pathogenesis and for prognostic assessment. These chromosomal changes usually occur after birth and are thus acquired rather than inherited. The cells at birth usually have normal chromosome constitutions (46, XY or 46, XX) and a variety of acquired changes are seen (Figs. 3.1–3.5) including loss or gain of chromosomes (in part or whole) and chromosome rearrangements. Loss of chromosomal material means that genes on the partner chromosome are unmatched and such loss of heterozygosity has been an important clue to the location of tumor suppressor genes. For example, cytogenetic analysis in neuroblastomas commonly reveals loss of the distal short arm of chromosome 1 and this area is believed to hold as yet uncloned tumor suppressor gene(s) for this tumor type. Table 3.1 lists examples of regions which show loss of heterozygosity (by cytogenetic or molecular analysis) with the associated childhood tumor types and names of the tumor suppressor genes where these have been cloned. These genes in Table 3.1 are all on the autosomes (chromosomes 1–22 inclusive) and as these autosomes are paired there are normally two copies of each tumor suppressor gene in each cell. Both copies

Table 3.1 Examples of tumor suppressor genes known to be involved in childhood tumors

Chromosomal location	Tumor type(s)	Cloned tumor suppressor gene(s)
1p	MutYH- or MYH-associated polyposis	*MutYH or MYH*
3p	Retinal angiomas, phaeochromocytomas	*VHL*
5q	Familial polyposis	*APC*
7p	SPNET	*PMS2*
8q	Exostoses	*EXT1*
9q	BCC, medulloblastoma, Gorlin syndrome	*PTCH*
11p	Nephroblastoma	*WT1, WT2, CDKN1C*
11p	Exostoses	*EXT2*
13q	Retinoblastoma, osteosarcoma	*RB1*
17p	Adrenocortical carcinoma, Li-Fraumeni syndrome	*TP53*
17q	Neurofibroma, CNS tumors	*NF1*

p, short arm; q, long arm of a chromosome; BCC, basal cell carcinoma; SPNET, supratentorial primitive neuroectodermal tumor. Human gene symbols are shown in italic capitals.

Table 3.2 Examples of proto-oncogenes implicated in human malignancy

Proto-oncogene	Molecular abnormality	Disorder
RET	Point mutation	Medullary thyroid cancer and MEN2
MYC	Translocation 8q24	Burkitt's lymphoma
ABL1	Translocation 9q34	Chronic myeloid leukemia
MOS	Translocation 8q22	Acute myeloid leukemia
MYC	Amplification	Carcinoma of breast, lung, cervix, esophagus
MYCN	Amplification	Neuroblastoma, small cell carcinoma of lung
KRAS2	Point mutation	Carcinoma of colon, lung and pancreas; melanoma
HRAS	Point mutation	Carcinomas of genitourinary tract, thyroid

Reproduced in part from Ref. 60 with permission from Macmillan Magazines Ltd., Basingtoke, UK.

need to be inactivated for a tumor to occur or progress. In sporadic tumors two separate mutations are required to inactivate each normal gene. These mutations may be unexplained or induced by mutagenic agents. In contrast, in many familial forms of pediatric cancer only one of the tumor suppressor genes is active at birth as the partner gene is inherited in an inactive form from a parent. The parent thus carries one normal and one underactive copy of this tumor suppressor gene and on average one half of the children will inherit the underactive gene and be predisposed to cancer (i.e., inherited as an autosomal dominant trait). As only a single mutation step is required to inactivate the remaining gene, tumors tend to occur at an earlier age in the familial forms than their sporadic counterparts and are more commonly multifocal or bilateral in paired organs. In some tumors the somatic inactivation of a single remaining copy of a tumor suppressor gene occurs by an epigenetic event (rather than by a mutation) whereby methylation of cytosine bases in the promoter region of the gene causes transcriptional repression or silencing.

Chromosome rearrangements can also provide important clues to the other main class of genes which are involved in tumor occurrence and progression: the oncogenes (Table 3.2). For example (Fig. 3.1), Ewing's sarcoma is commonly associated with a specific translocation between chromosomes 11 and 22 (with breakpoints on the long arm of 11 at band q24 and the long arm of 22 at band q12). This translocation results

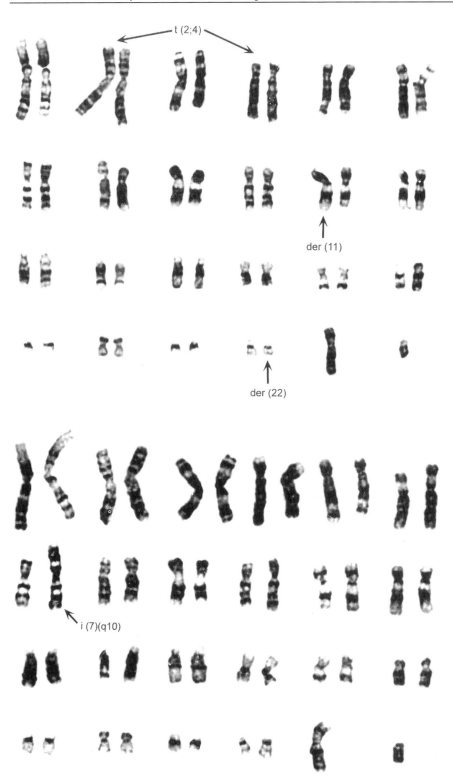

t (2;4)

der (11)

der (22)

Fig. 3.1 G-banded karyotype of a cell from a patient with Ewing's sarcoma showing the characteristic translocation between chromosomes 11 and 22 [t(11;22)(q24;q12)]. This translocation is found in 90% of cases of Ewing's sarcoma. The cells from this patient also carried an apparently balanced translocation between chromosomes 2 and 4 [t(2;4)(p23;p14)].

i (7)(q10)

Fig. 3.2 G-banded karyotype from a patient with Wilms' tumor showing an isochromosome for the long arm of chromosome 7. This results in monosomy for the short arm of chromosome 7 and trisomy for the long arm.

in a novel fused gene (*EWS* with either *ETS* or *FUS)* whose product is believed to cause the tumor [1, 2]. This and other oncogenes usually produce their effect via an altered gene product rather than loss of activ-ity as for the tumor suppressor genes. Oncogenes may also be involved in tumor progression by amplification (a selective increase in the number of copies of a specific gene) to produce an increased level of the

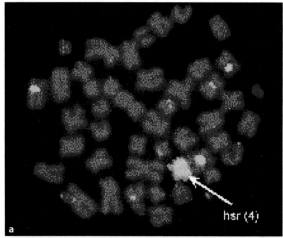

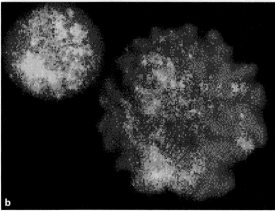

Fig. 3.3 a, b a Metaphase cell from a patient with neuro-blastoma showing a homogeneously staining region (hsr) on chromosome 4. Hybridization with a probe for *MYCN* shows the hsr to be comprised of amplified sequences of the *MYCN* gene. b Fluorescence in situ hybridization of *MYCN* in a case of neuroblastoma exhibiting double minute chromosomes. This figure contains both a metaphase spread and an interphase nucleus; however, both show the presence of multiple copies of the double minutes.

normal protein product. For example, amplification of *MYCN* on chromosome 2 occurs in some neuroblastomas and is associated with a worse prognosis (Figs. 3.3a, b).

The effects of these chromosomal changes can also be influenced by the parental origin of the chromosome. For example, in patients with neuroblastoma but without *MYCN* amplification, the associated 1p deletion is almost always maternal in origin [3]. In contrast, familial mutations in the succinate dehydrogenase D, *SDHD*, gene appear to predispose to phaeochromocytomas and paragangliomas only when inherited from the father [4]. These observations reflect genomic imprinting – a process in which defined parts of particular chromosomes are only active if inherited from the mother or father, but not both.

Thus the occurrence and progression of tumors is influenced by a variety of genetic changes. Retinoblastoma appears to be an exceptional tumor in that it occurs with inactivation of the tumor suppressor gene *RB1* alone whereas most tumors involve multiple genetic changes. This accumulation of changes varies between tumor types and the exact pattern varies even for a particular tumor type. In general, early changes are viewed as key steps in the pathogenesis and in some instances the cumulative pattern or particular changes can be useful in assessment of prognosis.

3.2 Genetic Counseling Aspects of Childhood Cancer

Epithelial cancers in infancy and childhood (i.e., lung, breast and gastrointestinal cancer) are extremely rare. Tumors in childhood are generally of mesodermal origin and may be subdivided into leukemias (35%), brain tumors (20%) and solid tumors (45%). The solid tumors and brain tumors are of most relevance to the pediatric surgeon and hence this chapter will focus on the genetic aspects of the more common types of these tumors and their associated inherited syndromes.

3.2.1 General Principles of Genetic Counseling

Genetic counseling is the communication of information and advice about inherited conditions [5, 6]. A standard medical history and examination is required for the affected person and in addition the family pedigree needs to be constructed. Figure 3.6 illustrates the pedigree from a family with a child with Wilms' tumor. Squares symbolize males, and circles females. All members of the same generation are placed on the same horizontal level and brothers and sisters are ordered with the eldest to the left. In this family the affected boy (shown shaded) has a normal older brother and a younger sister and no other relatives are or were affected. If other relatives had related tumors then it would be necessary to either see them in the clinic or confirm the details from their records. For certain tumor syndromes it might also be necessary to examine apparently normal parents and other relatives for minor features of the condition. Alternatively, if a specific mutation is identified in the proband, genetic testing for this mutation can subsequently be offered to the relatives where appropriate. It should be noted that if neither parent of a proband with an autosomal dominantly inherited syndrome has the condition or the causative mutation, the risk to siblings of the proband

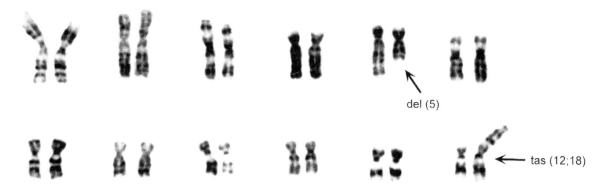

Fig. 3.4 G-banded karyotype from a patient with a giant cell tumor showing an interstitial deletion of chromosome 5 [del (5) (q15q33)] and also a telomeric association between chromosomes 12 and 18 [tas(12; 18)p13;q23)].

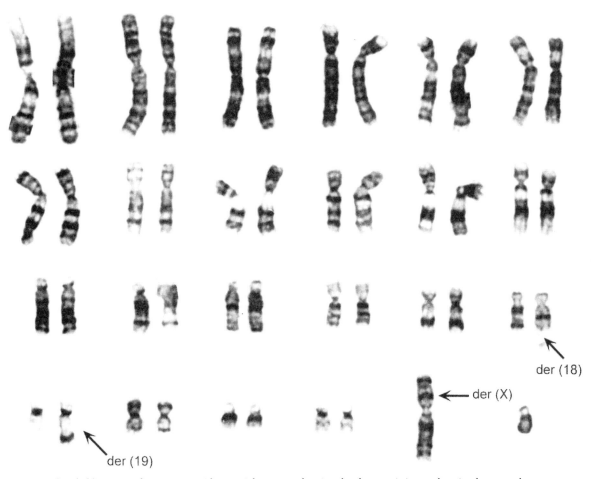

Fig. 3.5 G-banded karyotype from patient with synovial sarcoma showing the characteristic translocation between chromosomes 18 and X [t(X;18)(p11;q11)]. This karyotype also has a derivative chromosome 19 from a translocation between chromosomes 17 and 19 [der (19)t(17;19)(q21;q13)].

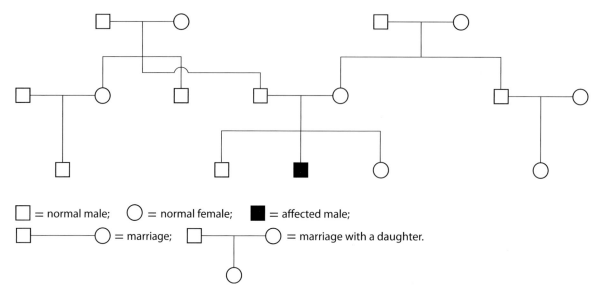

Fig. 3.6 Pedigree of a family with a child who has Wilms' tumor.

may be very low but not zero. The residual recurrence risk is due to the possibility of gonadal mosaicism whereby a proportion of gonadal cells in a parent may contain the mutation without it being present constitutionally in that individual.

The key is to establish the precise diagnosis before attempting to provide genetic counseling. This may involve further tests or literature searches or opinions from colleagues in the regional clinical or cancer genetics services. Once the diagnosis is secure adequate time in an appropriate setting needs to be allowed for discussion of the facts. Ideally both parents should be seen and few couples can be adequately counseled in under 30 minutes. A crowded clinic or the corner of a hospital ward are inappropriate and the information is unlikely to be retained if given too soon after the initial shock of a serious diagnosis. Counseling needs to include all aspects of the condition and the depth of explanation should be matched to the educational background of the couple. Pictures of chromosomes can be helpful in explaining modes of inheritance and we routinely send the parents a summary letter of the salient points after the session. Most couples can be counseled in a single session with the option to return if new questions arise or for recall if relevant new research advances occur. Parents may feel responsible for the condition of their child. These fears need to be aired and allayed. In inherited tumors and syndromes there is an additional need to minimize feelings of guilt and stigmatization.

3.2.2 Genetic Counseling for Specific Tumor Types

In this section general counseling information is provided for the more common tumor types of relevance to the pediatric surgeon and further information is available in the specific references provided or in textbooks of general cancer genetics [7].

3.2.2.1 Ependymoma

Most ependymomas are sporadic with a low recurrence risk but one exceptional family has been described where sisters and a maternal male cousin were affected [8]. Another has been reported in which two siblings had cervical spinal cord ependymoma and another had schwannoma, with evidence for the possible involvement of a tumor suppressor gene on chromosome 22 in familial ependymoma [9]. Ependymomas can occur as part of the spectrum of neurofibromatosis type 2.

3.2.2.2 Ewing's Sarcoma

Ewing's sarcoma is usually a sporadic event and has not so far been reported in a parent and child. Furthermore, the tumor does not appear to occur as part of specific familial cancer syndromes.

3.2.2.3 Gliomas

Genetic conditions associated with a predisposition to glioma include Gorlin's syndrome, Li-Fraumeni syndrome, Maffucci's syndrome, neurofibromatosis type 1, neurofibromatosis type 2, tuberous sclerosis and Turcot's syndrome. Familial glioma not associated with these conditions occurs but is rare [10].

3.2.2.4 Gonadoblastoma

The majority of gonadoblastomas develop in 46, XY individuals with gonadal dysgenesis. Gonadal dysgenesis has a variety of causes and recurrence risk will depend upon the precise diagnosis.

3.2.2.5 Hepatoblastoma

Congenital abnormalities are common in children with hepatoblastoma and have been reported in up to a third of cases. The abnormalities include hemihypertrophy, polycystic kidney disease and abnormalities of the urogenital system. Hepatoblastoma is a recognized complication of several overgrowth syndromes including congenital hemihypertrophy, Beckwith-Wiedemann syndrome, Sotos syndrome and Bannayan-Riley-Ruvalcaba syndrome. Hepatoblastoma may also rarely occur in children with familial adenomatous polyposis coli [11]. Congenital hypertrophy of the retinal pigment epithelium has been observed with the latter association. In the absence of these associated syndromes a low recurrence risk is appropriate as familial cases appear to be rare [12, 13]. For further information concerning hepatoblastoma see Chap. 12.

3.2.2.6 Lymphoma

A variety of genetic immunodeficiency disorders predispose to malignant lymphoma. They include ataxia-telangiectasia, Chédiak-Higashi syndrome, common variable immunodeficiency, hyper IgM syndrome, severe combined immunodeficiency, Wiskott-Aldrich syndrome and X-linked lymphoproliferative syndrome (Duncan disease). Non-Hodgkin's lymphoma is about six times as frequent as Hodgkin's disease in these patients with primary immunodeficiencies. In the absence of an underlying primary immunodeficiency there is a sevenfold increased risk for siblings of a young (<45 years) patient with Hodgkin's disease. The low incidence means, however, that the actual risk to siblings is still low [14]. Part of this familial risk might relate to shared environment but part appears to relate to the HLA locus which might operate by pre-

disposing to a particular infection or by producing an aberrant response to a particular infectious agent. In addition, a non-HLA genetic factor (a susceptibility gene on chromosome 4 in particular) is now also believed to play a causative role [15]. For more in depth information concerning lymphoma see Chap. 15.

3.2.2.7 Medulloblastoma and Primitive Neuroectodermal Tumor (PNET)

Familial medulloblastomas are uncommon but have been reported in twins and siblings [16]. Genetic disorders associated with medulloblastoma include ataxia-telangiectasia, blue rubber bleb nevus syndrome, familial adenomatous polyposis, Gorlin's syndrome and von Hippel-Lindau syndrome. A childhood medulloblastoma (or primitive neuroectodermal tumor) of the desmoplastic subtype at the age of less than 2 years is highly suggestive of Gorlin's syndrome [17]. Childhood PNETs can also occur in patients with inherited *TP53* mutations (Li-Fraumeni syndrome) [18].

Histologically similar to the medulloblastoma is another embryonal CNS tumor, supratentorial primitive neuroectodermal tumor (SPNET). This tumor is however more aggressive, has a poorer prognosis and is most likely derived from primitive neuroepithelial cells. It is now recognized that SPNET can occur together with café-au-lait skin pigmentation (similar to that occurring in neurofibromatosis type 1) in patients who have inherited mutations in both copies of the *PMS2* DNA mismatch repair gene [18]. Such patients are also now believed to possess an increased risk of leukemias, lymphomas, astrocytomas, glioblastomas, and in early adult life, colorectal neoplasia [19]. Homozygous *PMS2* syndrome is an important cause of pediatric malignancy among a population in the UK that originated from south Asia and its risk of recurrence in siblings is 25% [19].

3.2.2.8 Nephroblastoma (Wilms' Tumor)

Most cases of nephroblastoma are sporadic with a low recurrence risk but multiple families with familial Wilms' tumor have been described. Familial Wilms' tumor, which accounts for less than 1% of affected patients, is inherited as an autosomal dominant trait (OMIM 194070) with incomplete penetrance (i.e., not all gene carriers develop the tumor). Bilateral tumors are more likely to be familial. Sporadic (and, more rarely, familial) Wilms' tumor can be caused by mutations in the *WT1* gene at chromosome 11p13, although mutations in other genes can also predispose to the condition. In up to 5% of cases, Wilms' tumor occurs as a recognized complication of Beckwith-Wi-

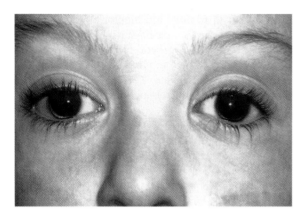

Fig. 3.7 A child with bilateral aniridia.

edemann syndrome, Denys-Drash syndrome, hemi-hypertrophy, Perlman's syndrome, sporadic aniridia and WAGR syndrome (*Wilms'* tumor, *a*niridia, genitourinary abnormalities or *g*onadoblastoma and mental *r*etardation) (Fig. 3.7). Wilms' tumor is described in depth in Chap 10.

3.2.2.9 Neuroblastoma

Most cases of neuroblastoma are sporadic and familial cases (in which predisposition to neuroblastoma is inherited as an autosomal dominant trait, OMIM 256700) account for less than 1% of the total. The mean age at diagnosis in familial cases is 9 months compared with 30 months in nonfamilial cases and familial tumors are frequently multiple [20]. Neuroblastoma is occasionally a feature of neurofibromatosis type 1, Hirschsprung disease, Beckwith-Wiedemann syndrome and congenital hemihypertrophy. More information concerning neuroblastoma is noted in Chap. 11.

3.2.2.10 Osteogenic Sarcoma

Most osteosarcomas are sporadic but affected sibs have been described. Osteosarcoma may occur in patients with inherited retinoblastoma, Li-Fraumeni syndrome, multiple exostoses and Rothmund-Thomson syndrome.

3.2.2.11 Retinoblastoma

Retinoblastoma may be sporadic (60%) or inherited as an autosomal dominant trait caused by mutations in the *RB1* tumor suppressor gene on chromosome 13 (OMIM 180200). Sporadic cases are always unilat-

eral and have a later age of onset than the inherited form. Around 15% of patients with unilateral retinoblastoma have an inherited mutation. In the inherited form, the penetrance is high with a risk of developing retinoblastoma of approximately 90%, and bilateral tumors occur in 30%. Mutation carriers are also at an increased risk for later osteogenic sarcoma. Retinoblastoma is described in depth in Chap. 18.

3.2.2.12 Rhabdomyosarcoma

Most rhabdomyosarcomas are sporadic with a low recurrence risk for other relatives. Associated syndromes include Beckwith-Wiedemann syndrome, Li-Fraumeni syndrome, neurofibromatosis type 1 and WAGR syndrome.

3.2.2.13 Teratoma

Most teratomas develop in the sacrococcygeal area and these tend to be benign. There may be associated malformations of the sacrum, vertebrae and gastrointestinal or urogenital tracts. Most are sporadic with a low recurrence risk but familial teratoma with an autosomal dominant mode of inheritance has been described. The hallmark of this condition is the presence of partial sacral agenesis with intact first sacral vertebrae. Other common features are a presacral mass and an anorectal malformation (forming, with the sacral bone defect, the Currarino triad) and urogenital malformations [21] (Fig. 3.8 a, b). Gene tracking in affected families supported a localization of this gene to the long arm of chromosome 7 [22] and mutations have now been found in the *HLXB9* gene in most familial cases of Currarino triad and in some apparently sporadic cases [23].

After the first few years of life, most teratomas are gonadal. Ovarian teratomas (dermoid cysts) originate through failure of extrusion of the second polar body or refusion of it with the ovum (i.e., self-fertilization). They are usually sporadic with low recurrence risks but occasional families have been described where the condition appears to be inherited [24]. In comparison with sporadic dermoid cysts the familial cases tended to be of earlier onset and were often (10–25%) bilateral. For further information concerning teratoma see Chap. 13.

3.3 Inherited Cancer-Predisposing Syndromes

Over 200 syndromes have been described in which cancer occurs as a recognized complication. Many of these syndromes are inherited and detailed continu-

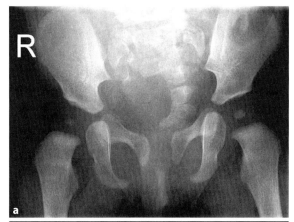

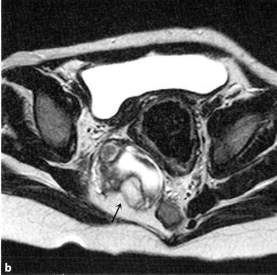

Fig. 3.8 a, b **a** Pelvic anteroposterior radiograph showing a left hemisacrum with a sickle-shaped defect distal to S2 vertebrae. (Figure 1 from Currarino triad: Characteristic appearances on magnetic resonance imaging and plain radiography, Low G, Irwin GJ, Haddock G, Maroo SV (2006) Australasian Radiology 50:249–251.) **b** Axial T2-weighted turbo spin-echo sequence showing the pre-sacral mass (*arrow*). The mass is of mixed composition with elements of fluid and fat signal. (Figure 2 from Currarino triad: Characteristic appearances on magnetic resonance imaging and plain radiography, Low G, Irwin GJ, Haddock G, Maroo SV (2006) Australasian Radiology 50:249–251.)

ously updated information is available for each in Online Mendelian Inheritance in Man (OMIM). The web site for OMIM is www.ncbi.nlm.nih.gov/omim. In OMIM each condition has a unique number and these are provided for each entry in this section. Some of these conditions can be caused by mutations in more than one gene and these have two or more OMIM numbers. This chapter focuses on the main features of the more common syndromes which are associated with childhood tumors. For more detailed information

including further references, and for rarer syndromes or syndromes mainly associated with adult tumors see OMIM.

3.3.1 Bannayan-Zonana Syndrome (Bannayan-Riley-Ruvalcaba Syndrome or Macrocephaly, Multiple Lipomas and Hemangiomata, OMIM 153480)

This rare condition is inherited as an autosomal dominant trait and is characterized by macrocephaly, pseudopapilledema, hamartomatous intestinal polyps, café-au-lait spots on the penis, a lipid storage myopathy, Hashimoto's thyroiditis and lipomas [25]. The lipomas and hemangiomas may be aggressive in growth and the intestinal hamartomas may have the potential to become malignant. Mutations in the *PTEN* gene are found in the blood of 50–60% of patients with this syndrome and in 80% of patients with the related Cowden syndrome (with associated adult cancer risks for breast, follicular thyroid and endometrial cancers) [26]. As a precaution, it is suggested that all *PTEN* mutation carriers should undergo physical screening for tumors from the age of 18 years [26, 27].

3.3.2 Beckwith-Wiedemann Syndrome (EMG Syndrome, OMIM 130650)

The cardinal features in the neonate are exomphalos, macroglossia and gigantism and the alternative name is an acronym of these features (EMG). Other features include earlobe grooves or posterior helical ear pits, visceromegaly (liver, kidney and spleen), cryptorchidism and neonatal hypoglycemia.

The majority of cases appear to be sporadic with a low recurrence risk but autosomal dominant inheritance with very variable expression is evident in 10–15% of cases. The principal cause of Beckwith-Wiedemann syndrome is the deregulation of imprinted growth-regulatory genes within a region on the short arm of chromosome 11 at 11p15. Loss of activity of cyclin-dependent kinase inhibitor 1c (*CDKN1C*) appears to underlie the condition in at least some familial cases [28]. This gene is located at 11p15 and normally only the maternally inherited copy is active. This copy can be inactivated by a variety of point mutations or by chromosomal changes which lead to a paternally derived duplication of chromosome 11p or uniparental disomy for chromosome 11 (where both copies of chromosome 11 are derived from the father). In one of the families described by Hatada, et al. [28] the mother of an affected child carried the same mutation in *CDKN1C* as her child but was clinically unaffected, as this mutation had been inherited from her father and was thus imprinted. This mother had a 1 in 2 recurrence risk for each subsequent pregnancy. Molecular analysis should help to confirm that sporadic cases are truly new mutations with a low recurrence risk.

Patients with Beckwith-Wiedemann syndrome have an increased risk of Wilms' tumor, neuroblastoma, adrenal carcinoma, rhabdomyosarcoma and hepatoblastoma and this risk is enhanced in the patients who have hemihypertrophy. Overall, 12.5% of children with Beckwith-Wiedemann syndrome have hemihypertrophy and this figure rises to 49% in those with tumors. The increased risk of tumors relates largely to the first 8 years of life and the estimated combined risk approximates to 7.5%.

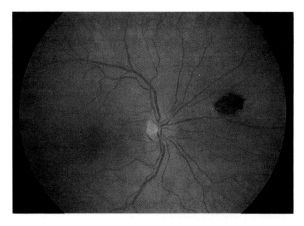

Fig. 3.9 Congenital hypertrophy of the retinal pigment epithelium (*CHRPE*) in familial adenomatous polyposis.

3.3.3 Blue Rubber Bleb Nevus Syndrome (Bean Syndrome, OMIM 112200)

This condition may be sporadic or be inherited as an autosomal dominant trait. Multiple hemangiomas occur especially on the trunk and upper limbs and mucous membranes. Intestinal and pulmonary angiomas may occur and may bleed. Patients appear to be at increased risk of cerebellar medulloblastoma.

3.3.4 Denys-Drash Syndrome (Wilms' Tumor and Pseudohermaphroditism, OMIM 194080)

This rare disorder is due to a variety of point mutations in the Wilms' tumor gene (*WT1*) and is characterized by male pseudohermaphroditism, Wilms' tumor and a progressive renal failure due to mesangial sclerosis [29]. Over 90% of patients with Denys-Drash syndrome possess constitutional heterozygous mutations in the *WT1* gene [30]. Wilms' tumor in patients with the syndrome presents early (mean 18 months) and is usually bilateral. Gonadoblastoma or diaphragmatic hernia may also occur. Children who survive will be at high risk of having affected offspring (on average 1 in 2 will be affected) but for normal parents and other relatives of an affected child the recurrence risk will be very low.

3.3.5 Familial Adenomatous Polyposis Coli (APC, OMIM 175100)

This condition is inherited as an autosomal dominant trait and is caused by a variety of mutations in the *APC* tumor suppressor gene on chromosome 5q. The most consistent feature is childhood onset of multiple intestinal polyps which have a high risk of malignant degeneration in adulthood. Other less consis-

tent features are retinal pigmented spots (congenital hypertrophy of the retinal pigment epithelium) (Fig. 3.9), facial bone osteomas, desmoid tumors and epidermoid or sebaceous cysts. In addition to gastrointestinal malignancy, patients are at increased risk of gliomas.

3.3.6 Gorlin's Syndrome (Nevoid Basal Cell Carcinoma Syndrome, OMIM 109400)

This condition is inherited as an autosomal dominant trait and is caused by a variety of mutations in the *PTCH* gene on chromosome 9q [31]. About 20–30% of patients possess de novo mutations rather than having inherited a mutation from a parent. The main features are multiple basal cell carcinomas of the skin and palmar and plantar pits. By 30 years of age 90% of patients will have skin lesions but only 15% manifest before puberty. Nondermatological features include hypertelorism with a broad nasal bridge, frontal and parietal bossing, a prominent chin, jaw odontogenic keratocysts, cleft lip and palate, fusion defects of the cervical spine, rib abnormalities and calcification of the falx cerebri [32]. There is an increase in the incidence of nondermatological tumors including squamous cell carcinoma and fibrosarcoma in jaw cysts, nasopharyngeal carcinoma, medulloblastoma, meningioma, craniopharyngioma, cardiac fibroma and ovarian fibroma. In fact, about 5% of individuals with Gorlin's syndrome develop the childhood brain malignancy medulloblastoma (or primitive neuroectodermal tumor [PNET]). This tends to be of desmoplastic histology [17] and to have a favorable prognosis. The peak incidence of medulloblastoma in Gorlin's syndrome is about 2 years of age compared to 7 years in its sporadic form [17].

3.3.7 Li-Fraumeni Syndrome (OMIM 151623)

This condition is inherited as an autosomal dominant trait and is characterized by a predisposition to breast cancer, brain tumors, sarcomas, leukemia and adrenocortical carcinoma in children and young adults. Additional tumors which appear to occur with increased frequency include pancreatic, prostatic, lung and laryngeal carcinomata and malignant melanoma. Of affected patients, almost 50% develop cancer by 30 years of age and 90% by 70 years of age. Multiple primaries may occur and recurrent cancers often arise in the radiotherapy field, suggesting a susceptibility to radiation carcinogenesis. In the majority of families the cause is an inherited inactivating mutation in one copy of *TP53* on chromosome 17p [33]. This gene encodes a protein that plays a pivotal role in both DNA repair and programmed cell death (apoptosis). A deletion in the *TP53* gene is responsible for around 10% of these mutations [34]. Unusually for a tumor suppressor gene, a single mutated copy of the *TP53* gene can occasionally give rise to cancer development without the inactivation of the other allele. This phenomenon is most likely to be due to a "dominant negative" effect of some mutations whereby the mutation prevents the normal efficient assembly of the protein into functional tetramers [34]. It relates especially to those mutations located within the central core (DNA-binding) domain of the gene [35]. Interestingly, missense (amino acid substitution) mutations located within this domain are reported to be associated with a higher risk of breast and brain cancer while those located outside the DNA-binding domain are more commonly associated with adrenocortical carcinoma [34]. In Li-Fraumeni syndrome families possessing normal *TP53* genes, heterozygous germline mutations have, rarely, been found in another gene, the *CHK2* gene (Barlow, et al., 2004) but this and several other candidate genes (including *MDM2*, *PTEN*, *CDKN2A*, *BCL10*, *CHK1*, *TP63* and *BAX*) have now been excluded as important causes of the syndrome [34–36]. At present, it remains unclear whether mutations in any other genes predispose to Li-Fraumeni syndrome.

3.3.8 McCune-Albright Syndrome (Polyostotic Fibrous Dysplasia, OMIM 174800)

This sporadic syndrome is usually caused by mosaicism for an activating mutation in the *GNAS1* gene, which encodes the alpha subunit of the stimulatory signal transduction protein, Gs. The syndrome is characterized by polyostotic fibrous dysplasia, café-au-lait pigmented skin patches and endocrinological abnormalities including precocious puberty, thyrotoxicosis,

pituitary gigantism and Cushing's syndrome. Osteosarcomatous transformation in areas of fibrous dysplasia has been described as a complication of this condition [37]. The timing of occurrence of the somatic mutation during embryonic development appears to determine the extent of disease, with earlier occurrence resulting in McCune-Albright syndrome and later occurrence resulting in more focal disease such as just a thyroid or pituitary adenoma. Transmission of mutations from parent to child has almost never been observed and the inheritance of such mutations is presumed to be incompatible with embryonic survival [38].

3.3.9 Maffucci's Syndrome (Osteochondromatosis, Multiple Enchondromatosis, Ollier Disease, OMIM 166000)

This is usually a sporadic condition in which osteochondromatosis (mostly enchondromas) and hemangiomas occur. The enchondromas may result in pathological fractures or deformity. Patients are predisposed to malignancy including chondrosarcoma most commonly, but also fibrosarcoma, angiosarcoma, osteosarcoma, teratomas, ovarian granulosa cell tumors and gliomas [39]. The condition in some cases may result from mutations in the PTH/PTHRP type I receptor (*PTHR1*) gene [40] but such cases are likely to represent a minority, with other unidentified causative genes being responsible for the majority [41].

3.3.10 Multiple Exostoses (Diaphyseal Aclasis, Multiple Osteochondromatosis, OMIM 133700, 133701, 600209)

This condition is inherited as an autosomal dominant trait and is caused by a variety of mutations in one of three genes: *EXT1*, a tumor suppressor gene on the long arm of chromosome 8; *EXT2*, a tumor suppressor gene on the short arm of chromosome 11; and a third as yet uncloned gene on chromosome 19 [42]. Clinically the families with mutations in the different genes appear to be indistinguishable. Affected patients develop cartilaginous excrescences near the ends of the diaphyses of the bones of the extremities, which later undergo ossification. They may result in local deformity or nerve compression and patients may show disproportionate short stature in severe cases. Sarcomatous degeneration of an exostosis occurs in 0.5–2% of patients and should be suspected when growth of an exostosis occurs after puberty. Each affected person has a high risk of passing the condition to his or her offspring (on average 1 in 2 will be affected). Gene carriers invariably show exostoses by puberty but these may not be prominent, especially in females, and it is important to radiograph the long bones before concluding that an apparently unaffected person at risk has received the normal gene and hence has a negligible risk for their family [43]. Multiple exostoses may also form part of the Langer-Giedion syndrome (microdeletion of chromosome 8q resulting in the loss of at least the *EXT1* and *TRPS1* genes), which also includes learning difficulties and features of trichorhinophalangeal dysplasia [44].

3.3.11 MYH-Associated Polyposis (OMIM 608456)

A colorectal adenoma and carcinoma predisposition syndrome with phenotypes very similar to *FAP* (but usually with a generally later age of onset and slightly less profuse polyposis) has been described recently. This MutYH-associated polyposis (MAP) is an autosomal recessive condition that results from the inheritance of a mutation in each copy of a base excision repair (BER) gene *MutYH* (human MutY homologue, also known as *MYH*) in the absence of inherited mutations in the *APC* gene [45–47]. The mean age at diagnosis of 25 reported unrelated MYH polyposis cases was 46 years (median 48 years, range 13 to 65 years) [46].

3.3.12 Neurofibromatosis Type 1 (OMIM 162200)

Neurofibromatosis type 1 is inherited as an autosomal dominant trait and is caused by a variety of mutations in the *NF1* tumor suppressor gene on chromosome 17q. In around 25–50% of cases, the mutations occur de novo with the parents being unaffected. Many mutations have been described of which around 80% are predicted to disrupt the encoded protein, neurofibromin, loss of which is predicted to cause overactivity of the RAS cell signaling pathway [48]. Affected children are usually recognized by the presence of multiple café-au-lait patches and later skin neurofibromata. The presence of iris hamartomas (Lisch nodules) on slit lamp examination may be helpful for confirmation of the diagnosis. Associated tumors include optic pathway gliomas (present in 15% on CT scan but only one third of these are symptomatic), other brain tumors (1–2%), malignant degeneration of a neurofibroma (1.5%), phaeochromocytomas and rhabdomyosarcomas. In general, around two thirds of patients are only relatively mildly affected. There is no clear genotype–phenotype correlation at present, other than the association of *NF1* gene deletions (rather than point mutations) with dysmorphic features, increased num-bers of neurofibromas and significant developmental delay (in addition to the typical *NF1* manifestations) [49]. In addition, patients with large *NF1* gene deletions may be more predisposed to malignant peripheral nerve sheath tumors (MPNSTs) [50].

3.3.13 Neurofibromatosis Type 2 (OMIM 101000)

Neurofibromatosis type 2, which is generally more serious but approximately 10 times rarer than type 1, is caused by a variety of mutations in the *NF2* tumor suppressor gene on 22q. Bilateral acoustic schwannomas are the most common tumor type but patients may also have spinal schwannoma or meningiomas, falx meningioma, parenchymal astrocytoma or ependymoma, or skin plaques (neurilemmomas). The condition is inherited as an autosomal dominant trait with full penetrance by 60 years of age. Helpful consensus guidelines have been published for the management of patients with neurofibromatosis type 2 and their families [51]. Clinical screening of at-risk individuals can begin from birth and genetic counseling and testing of affected individuals and their at-risk relatives should be offered because presymptomatic diagnosis improves the clinical management of the disease [51].

3.3.14 Perlman's Syndrome (Renal Hamartomas, Nephroblastomatosis and Fetal Gigantism, OMIM 267000)

This rare disorder is inherited as an autosomal recessive trait and is characterized by macrosomia, visceromegaly, hypertrophy of the islets of Langerhans, renal hamartomas with or without nephroblastomatosis, dysmorphic features (enophthalmos, broad depressed nasal bridge and everted upper lip), and cryptorchidism in males. There is a high risk of Wilms' tumor, which is frequently bilateral [52].

3.3.15 Rothmund-Thomson Syndrome (Poikiloderma Atrophicans and Cataract, OMIM 268400)

This condition is inherited as an autosomal recessive trait and, in most cases, appears to be caused by mutations in the gene *RECQL4*, which encodes a DNA helicase that is required for chromosome stability [53, 54]. The syndrome is characterized by skin atrophy, pigmentation and telangiectasia accompanied by juvenile cataract, saddle nose, congenital bone defects, disturbances of hair growth, short stature and hypogonadism. Patients appear to be at increased risk of osteosarcoma [55].

3.3.16 Sotos Syndrome (Cerebral Gigantism, OMIM 117550)

This condition is characterized by excessively rapid growth, acromegalic features and a nonprogressive cerebral disorder with mental handicap. It may be sporadic or inherited as an autosomal dominant trait. About 80–90% of individuals with Sotos syndrome have a demonstrable mutation or deletion of the *NSD1* gene. Around 95% of cases represent new mutations but the risk of transmission to each child of an affected patient is 50%. Tumors occur in fewer than 5% of people with Sotos syndrome but include hepatoblastoma, neuroblastoma, sacrococcygeal teratoma, presacral ganglioma and acute lymphoblastic leukemia [56, 57].

3.3.17 Tuberous Sclerosis (OMIM 191100, 191092)

This condition is inherited as an autosomal dominant trait and is caused by a variety of mutations in one of two genes: *TSC1* and *TSC2*, tumor suppressor genes on the long arm of chromosome 9 and the short arm of chromosome 16, respectively. Affected patients develop a facial fibroangiomatous rash (adenoma sebaceum), white skin patches, skin fibromatous plaques (shagreen patches), enamel pits, whitish retinal phakomata, intracranial calcification, epilepsy and mental handicap. Tumors include renal angiomyolipomata, renal cell carcinoma (occasionally), cardiac rhabdomyomata and malignant gliomas, usually giant cell astrocytomas (in 6%). Clinically, it now appears that mutations in *TSC1* are generally associated with a less severe phenotype than those in *TSC2* [58, 59]. Approximately 60% of cases represent new mutations. In these cases the recurrence risk in a future child (of the normal parents) will be small, but with a residual risk of around 2–3% due to the possibility of gonadal mosaicism in one parent.

3.3.18 WAGR Syndrome (Wilms' Tumor, Aniridia, Genitourinary Anomalies, Mental Retardation Syndrome, OMIM 194072)

This syndrome's name is an acronym of the features of Wilms' tumor, aniridia, genitourinary malformations and mental retardation. It is caused by a microdeletion of chromosome 11p, which encompasses *WT1* (resulting in a high risk of Wilms' tumor) and adjacent genes such as *PAX6* (the loss of which causes aniridia). An affected parent will have a 1 in 2 risk for affected offspring but normal parents with a de novo microdeletion in their child will have a low recurrence risk.

References

1. Aman P, Panagopoulos I, Lassen C, et al. (1996) Expression patterns of the human sarcoma-associated genes *FUS* and *EWS* and the genomic structure of *FUS*. Genomics 37:1–8

2. Janknecht R (2005) EWS-ETS oncoproteins: The linchpins of Ewing tumors. Gene 363:1–14

3. Caron H, van Sluis P, van Hoeve M, et al. (1993) Allelic loss of chromosome 1p36 in neuroblastoma is of preferential maternal origin and correlates with N-*myc* amplification. Nature Genet 4:187–190

4. Simi L, Sestini R, Ferruzzi P, et al. (2005) Phenotype variability of neural crest derived tumours in six Italian families segregating the same founder SDHD mutation Q109X. J Med Genet 42:e52

5. Connor M, Ferguson-Smith M (1997) Essential medical genetics, 5th edn. Blackwell Science, Oxford

6. Harper PS (2004) Practical genetic counselling, 6th edn. Arnold, London

7. Hodgson SV, Maher ER, Eng C, Foulkes W (2006) A practical guide to human cancer genetics. Cambridge University Press, Cambridge

8. Gilchrist DM, Savard ML (1989) Ependymomas in two sisters and a maternal male cousin. Am J Hum Genet 45:A22

9. Yokota T, Tachizawa T, Fukino K, et al. (2003) A family with spinal anaplastic ependymoma: Evidence of loss of chromosome 22q in tumor. J Hum Genet 48:598–602

10. Vieregge P, Gerhard L, Nahser HC (1987) Familial glioma: Occurrence within the "familial cancer syndrome" and systemic malformations. J Neurol 234:220–232

11. Hirschman BA, Pollock BH, Tomlinson GE (2005) The spectrum of APC mutations in children with hepatoblastoma from familial adenomatous polyposis kindreds. J Pediatr 147:263–266

12. Hartley AL, Birch JM, Kelsey AM, et al. (1990) Epidemiological and familial aspects of hepatoblastoma. Med Paediatr Oncol 18:103–109

13. Nagata T, Nakamura M, Shichino H, et al. (2005) Cytogenetic abnormalities in hepatoblastoma: Report of two new cases and review of the literature suggesting imbalance of chromosomal regions on chromosomes 1, 4, and 12. Cancer Genet Cytogenet 156:8–13

14. Mack TM, Cozen W, Shibata DK, et al. (1995) Concordance for Hodgkin's disease in identical twins suggesting genetic susceptibility to the young adult form of the disease. New Engl J Med 332:413–418

15. Goldin LR, McMaster ML, Ter-Minassian M, et al. (2005) A genome screen of families at high risk for Hodgkin lymphoma: Evidence for a susceptibility gene on chromosome 4. J Med Genet 42:595–601

16. Hung KL, Wu CM, Huang JS, How SW (1990) Familial medulloblastoma in siblings: Report of one family and review of the literature. Surg Neurol 33:341–346

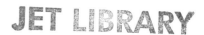

17. Amlashi SF, Riffaud L, Brassier G, Morandi X (2003) Nevoid basal cell carcinoma syndrome: Relation with desmoplastic medulloblastoma in infancy. A population-based study and review of the literature. Cancer 98:618–624

18. De Vos M, Hayward BE, Picton S, et al. (2004) Novel PMS2 pseudogenes can conceal recessive mutations causing a distinctive childhood cancer syndrome. Am J Hum Genet 74:954–964

19. De Vos M, Hayward BE, Charlton R, et al. (2006) PMS2 mutations in childhood cancer. J Natl Cancer Inst 98:358–361

20. Kushner BH, Gilbert F, Helson L (1986) Familial neuroblastoma: Case reports, literature review and etiologic considerations. Cancer 57:1887–1893

21. O'Riordain DS, O'Connell PR, Kirwan WO (1991) Hereditary sacral agenesis with presacral mass and anorectal stenosis: The Currarino triad. Brit J Surg 78:536–538

22. Lynch SA, Bond P, Copp AJ, et al. (1995) A gene for autosomal dominant sacral agenesis maps to the holoprosencephaly region at 7q36. Nature Genet 11:93–95

23. Cretolle C, Zerah M, Jaubert F, et al. (2006) New clinical and therapeutic perspectives in Currarino syndrome (study of 29 cases). J Pediatr Surg 41:126–131; discussion 126–131

24. Simon A, Ohel G, Neri A, Schenker JG (1985) Familial occurrence of mature ovarian teratomas. Obstet Gynecol 66:278–279

25. Gorlin RJ, Cohen MM Jr, Condon LM, Burke BA (1992) Bannayan-Riley-Ruvalcaba syndrome. Am J Med Genet 44:307–314

26. Nagy R, Sweet K, Eng C (2004) Highly penetrant hereditary cancer syndromes. Oncogene 23:6445–6470

27. Pilarski R, Eng C (2004) Will the real Cowden syndrome please stand up (again)? Expanding mutational and clinical spectra of the PTEN hamartoma tumour syndrome. J Med Genet 41:323–326

28. Hatada I, Ohashi H, Fukushima Y, et al. (1996) An imprinted gene p57(KIP2) is mutated in Beckwith-Wiedemann syndrome. Nature 14:171–173

29. Mueller RF (1994) The Denys-Drash syndrome. J Med Genet 31:471–477

30. Little S, Hanks S, King-Underwood L, et al. (2005) A WT1 exon 1 mutation in a child diagnosed with Denys-Drash syndrome. Pediatr Nephrol 20:81–85

31. Wicking C, Shanley S, Smyth I, et al. (1997) Most germline mutations in the nevoid basal cell carcinoma syndrome lead to a premature termination of the PATCHED protein, and no genotype-phenotype correlations are evident. Am J Hum Genet 60:21–26

32. Evans DGR, Ladusans EJ, Rimmer S, et al. (1993) Complications of the naevoid basal cell carcinoma syndrome: Results of a population based study. J Med Genet 30:460–464

33. Frebourg T, Barbier N, Yan Y, et al. (1995) Germ-line p53 mutations in 15 families with Li-Fraumeni syndrome. Am J Hum Genet 56:608–615

34. Moule RN, Jhavar SG, Eeles RA (2006) Genotype phenotype correlation in Li-Fraumeni syndrome kindreds and its implications for management. Fam Cancer 5:129–133

35. Varley JM (2003) Germline TP53 mutations and Li-Fraumeni syndrome. Hum Mutat 21:313–320

36. Barlow JW, Mous M, Wiley JC, et al. (2004) Germ line BAX alterations are infrequent in Li-Fraumeni syndrome. Cancer Epidemiol Biomarkers Prev 13:1403–1406

37. Taconis WK (1988) Osteosarcoma in fibrous dysplasia. Skeletal Radiol 17:163–170

38. Metzler M, Luedecke DK, Saeger W, et al. (2006) Low prevalence of Gs alpha mutations in somatotroph adenomas of children and adolescents. Cancer Genet Cytogenet 166:146–151

39. Christman JE, Ballon SC (1990) Ovarian fibrosarcoma associated with Maffucci's syndrome. Gynecol Oncol 37:290–291

40. Hopyan S, Gokgoz N, Poon R, et al. (2002) A mutant PTH/PTHrP type I receptor in enchondromatosis. Nat Genet 30:306–310

41. Rozeman LB, Sangiorgi L, Briaire-de Bruijn IH, et al. (2004) Enchondromatosis (Ollier disease, Maffucci syndrome) is not caused by the PTHR1 mutation p.R150C. Hum Mutat 24:466–473

42. Blanton SH, Hogue D, Wagner, et al. (1996) Hereditary multiple exostoses: Confirmation of linkage to chromosomes 8 and 11. Am J Med Genet 62:150–159

43. Wicklund CL, Pauli RM, Johnston D, Hecht JT (1995) Natural history study of hereditary multiple exostoses. Am J Med Genet 55:43–46

44. Vaccaro M, Guarneri C, Blandino A (2005) Trichorhinophalangeal syndrome. J Am Acad Dermatol 53:858–860

45. Cheadle JP, Sampson JR (2003) Exposing the MYtH about base excision repair and human inherited disease. Hum Mol Genet 12:R159–165

46. Sampson JR, Dolwani S, Jones S, et al. (2003) Autosomal recessive colorectal adenomatous polyposis due to inherited mutations of MYH. Lancet 362:39–41

47. Sieber OM, Lipton L, Crabtree M, et al. (2003) Multiple colorectal adenomas, classic adenomatous polyposis, and germ-line mutations in MYH. N Engl J Med 348:791–799

48. Arun D, Gutmann DH (2004) Recent advances in neurofibromatosis type 1. Curr Opin Neurol 17:101–105

49. Castle B, Baser ME, Huson SM, et al. (2003) Evaluation of genotype-phenotype correlations in neurofibromatosis type 1. J Med Genet 40:e109

50. De Raedt T, Brems H, Wolkenstein P, et al. (2003) Elevated risk for MPNST in NF1 microdeletion patients. Am J Hum Genet 72:1288–1292

51. Evans DG, Baser ME, O'Reilly B, et al. (2005) Management of the patient and family with neurofibromatosis 2: A consensus conference statement. Br J Neurosurg 19:5–12

52. Greenberg F, Copeland K, Gresik MV (1988) Expanding the spectrum of the Perlman syndrome. Am J Med Genet 29:773–776

53. Petkovic M, Dietschy T, Freire R, et al. (2005) The human Rothmund-Thomson syndrome gene product, RECQL4, localizes to distinct nuclear foci that coincide with proteins involved in the maintenance of genome stability. J Cell Sci 118:4261–4269

54. Larizza L, Magnani I, Roversi G (2006) Rothmund-Thomson syndrome and RECQL4 defect: Splitting and lumping. Cancer Lett 232:107–120

55. Lindor NM, Devries EMG, Michels VV, et al. (1996) Rothmund-Thomson syndrome in siblings: Evidence for acquired in vivo mosaicism. Clin Genet 49:124–129

56. Cole TRP, Hughes HE (1994) Sotos syndrome: A study of the diagnostic criteria and natural history. J Med Genet 31:20–32

57. Tatton-Brown K, Rahman N (2004) Clinical features of NSD1-positive Sotos syndrome. Clin Dysmorphol 13:199–204

58. Lewis JC, Thomas HV, Murphy KC, Sampson JR (2004) Genotype and psychological phenotype in tuberous sclerosis. J Med Genet 41:203–207

59. Sancak O, Nellist M, Goedbloed M, et al. (2005) Mutational analysis of the TSC1 and TSC2 genes in a diagnostic setting: Genotype–phenotype correlations and comparison of diagnostic DNA techniques in Tuberous Sclerosis Complex. Eur J Hum Genet 13:731–741

60. Knudson AG (1993) All in the (cancer) family. Nature Genet 5:103–104

Tumor Markers

4

Robert Carachi, Basith Amjad

Contents

4.1 Introduction

Tumor markers are biological markers, usually proteins associated with a malignancy. They can be detected within a tumor, in circulating tumor cells in peripheral blood, in lymph nodes, bone marrow and in other body fluids including ascites, cerebrospinal fluid, urine, and stool [1]. A tumor marker may be produced by a tumor itself as a by-product of malignant transformation or by the body in response to the tumor. A tumor marker may be used to identify a particular disease, in which case it may be used for diagnosis, staging, or population screening. Markers may also be used to detect the presence of occult metastatic disease, to monitor the response to treatment, or to detect recurrent disease [2]. Recently, they have also been used as targets for therapeutic intervention in clinical trials [3].

Although tumor markers are typically imperfect as screening tests to detect occult (hidden) cancers, once a particular tumor has been found with a marker, the marker may be used to monitor the success or failure of treatment. The tumor marker level may also reflect the extent or stage of the disease, indicate how quickly the cancer is likely to progress and so help determine the prognosis [4].

Examples of tumor markers include alpha-fetoprotein (AFP), carcinoembryonic antigen (CEA), human chorionic gonadotropin (HCG), lactate dehydrogenase (LDH), and neuron-specific enolase (NSE).

In this chapter we shall discuss tumor markers which are practically useful in the management of childhood solid tumors.

4.1.1 Criteria/Sensitivity vs. Specificity of Tumor Markers

Tumor markers are represented by small and large molecules, such as peptides, proteins, glycoproteins, enzymes, hormones, immunoglobulins, mucins, cytokeratins, and low molecular weight metabolites. Table 4.1 summarizes the broad spectrum of the most

Table 4.1 Tumor markers for neuroblastoma and related tumors

Marker	Use	Comments
Catecholamines and metabolites	Diagnosis, follow-up, prognosis	DOPA, dopamine, HVA, VLA are more often high in patients with unfavorable tumors
Neuron-specific enolase	Diagnosis, follow-up, prognosis	Occasionally increased in Wilms' tumor, lymphomas, leukemias, hepatoblastoma, PNET, and dysgerminoma
Lactic dehydrogenase	Follow-up, prognosis	Increased level (>142 ng/ml) is associated with poor prognosis
Ferritin	Prognosis	
Vasoactive intestinal polypeptide	Diagnosis	Increased in patients with severe diarrhea
Disialoganglioside	Diagnosis	
Chromogranin A	Prognosis	
BB isozyme of creatine kinase	Prognosis	Increased level (>190 ng/ml) is associated with poor prognosis
Neuropeptide Y	Prognosis	Increased level (>15 ng/ml) is associated with poor prognosis

commonly used tumor markers, along with their respective clinical potential.

The ideal tumor marker would be produced exclusively by a malignant tissue, or would be elevated in tissue predisposed to progressing towards a malignancy. Such a tumor marker would be elevated in the blood of all patients with this particular cancer. This tumor marker would be highly sensitive to detect early stage disease. It would also be sufficiently specific to safe guard against false-positive results. Unfortunately so far this ideal tumor marker does not exist.

4.2 Tumor Markers for Neuroblastoma and Related Tumors

Neuroblastoma is the most common solid abdominal tumor of childhood comprising approximately 10% of all childhood cancers [5]. Neuroblastomas demonstrate diverse clinical and biological traits and thus a substantial number of tumor markers are now used, both to define disease activity and to monitor the response to therapy. These include catecholamines and their metabolites, lactate dehydrogenase (LDH), ferritin, and neuron-specific enolase (NSE). Of these, the catecholamines are confirmatory indices, while serum NSE is useful in monitoring the disease activity, and both LDH and ferritin are prognostic markers.

A large number of molecular or genetic markers are also known to be associated with neuroblastomas. These include N-myc amplification, gain of chromosome17q, deletion of 1p, DNA-ploidy and index, multidrug resistance associated protein (MRP), CD44 expression and TRKA expression. A systemic review of the use of tumor markers in neuroblastomas was undertaken by Riley, et al. in the UK [5]. A number of conclusions were drawn regarding these potentially important tools and their association with a poor outcome: Amplification of the N-myc gene, expression of the diploid cells (a DNA index of 1) in the tumor, high expression of neurone-specific enolase in the tumor at diagnosis, high serum levels of lactate dehydrogenase and/or ferritin, high multidrug resistance gene-product expression in the tumor, gain of chromosome 1p, low tumor expression of CD44 and/or TRKA, and a low VMA:HVA ratio.

4.2.1 Catecholamines and Metabolites

Neuroblastomas originate from sympathetic neuroblast cells, which are derived from the embryonal neural crest. These neuroblast cells are normally meant to mature and differentiate into sympathetic ganglia and adrenal medulla. Once they turn neoplastic these cells are characterized by defective synthesis of catecholamines and their precursors such as epinephrine (E), norepinephrine (NE), 3,4-dihydroxyphenylalanine (DOPA) and dopamine (DA), and their metabolites like vanillyllmandellic acid (VMA), homovanillic acid (HVA), methoxydopamine (MDA) and methylated catecholamines namely metanephrine (MN), normetanephrine (NMN) and 3-methoxytyramine (3MT). Neuroblastoma cells lack the enzyme phenylethanolamine N-methyltransferase, which converts norepinephrine into epinephrine. The metabolic

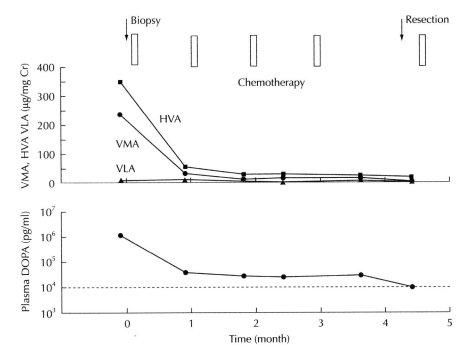

Fig. 4.1 Measurements of urinary levels of VMA, HVA, and VLA, and plasma levels of DOPA are useful not only in making a diagnosis but also in monitoring the course of neuroblastoma.

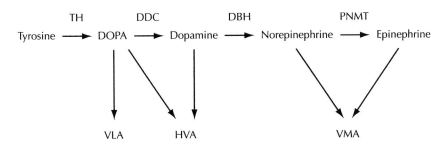

Fig. 4.2 Metabolic pathways of the catecholamines in normal sympathetic nervous tissue and the adrenal gland. TH, Tyrosine hydroxylase; DDC, DOPA decarboxylase; DBH, dopamine-β- hydroxylase; PNMT, phenylethanolamine-N-methyltransferase; DOPA, 3;4 – dihydroxyphenylalanine; VMA, vanillylmandelic acid; HVA, homovanillic acid; VLA, vanillactic acid.

scheme is depicted in Fig. 4.1, thus it can be seen that NE and E are primarily metabolized into VMA while dopamine is metabolized into HVA. Neuroblastoma cells lack the storage vesicles for catecholamines unlike normal neural crest cells, and these catecholamines upon release into the circulation are rapidly degraded into VMA and HVA. Therefore, the analysis of metabolites is considerably more sensitive and they are more useful as tumor markers than the catecholamines themselves [6].

HVA and VMA can be measured in the urine, and are useful in both diagnosis and monitoring disease activity (Fig. 4.2). Urinary catecholamine metabolites are elevated in 90–95% of patients with neuroblastoma

using sensitive assays. Traditionally 24-h urinary values were used but now random assays are also used and these have been found to be equally sensitive. In random estimations, the quantities are expressed as mg/g of creatinine to take into account the urine production rate and make the results more reproducible [7]. Of all the metabolites, VMA and HVA are the ones that are most commonly used and have a sensitivity which exceeds 90% in combination, though their individual sensitivities are below 80% each. Other metabolites with good sensitivity and specificity are NME and DA. Recent studies have suggested reporting a combination of NME with HVA or VMA with a 100% sensitivity and specificity result [8]. DA is not very sensitive and specific in infants but its importance increases with the age of the child. Serum VMA and HVA have been studied in patients with neuroblastoma but the levels are less frequently elevated than the urinary levels.

The catecholamine and their metabolites are not very useful for detecting recurrence during follow-up of patients who have been treated for neuroblastomas previously. In cases with diagnosed recurrence, the levels of these metabolites was found to be raised in only 55% of the patients; this contrasts with more than 90% sensitivity at the time of presentation [9]. Thus, relapse or progression cannot be reliably detected or excluded by monitoring tumor markers alone.

Mass-screening programs carried out in Japan, Germany, and Canada for early detection of neuroblastomas have not been very useful. The tumors detected in this way were found to be biologically favorable with a high tendency for spontaneous regression. Thus, though the program had led to an increase in the number of cases diagnosed, it had not led to a decrease in the mortality attributed to neuroblastomas [10]. The consensus from the results of these programs is that there are two different subsets of neuroblastoma, and the more favorable type presents earlier and is the one that is detected by screening. The poorer prognosis group is not detected by screening; hence, the mortality attributable to neuroblastoma has not decreased [4].

Another issue related to screening is the possibility of unnecessary treatment of biologically favorable tumors destined for regression. In this regard, Yamamoto, et al. have defined criteria for observation of tumors detected on routine screening – small masses on radiography, no invasion of spinal cord or vascular structures, relatively moderate catecholamine excretion, and parental consent [11].

4.2.2 Neuron-Specific Enolase

Neuron-Specific Enolase (NSE) is a specific isoenzyme of the glycolytic enzyme enolase, and is localized within neurons of the central and peripheral nervous tissue. Enolase in mammalian brain is composed of two immunologically distinct subunits, α and γ, and both αγ and γγ dimmers of enolase are specific for the nervous system [12]. NSE is also present in a variety of peripheral and central neuroendocrine cells, which are termed amine precursor uptake, and decarboxylation (APUD) cells. Determination of serum levels of these cells have shown that they are high in patients with neuroblastoma and those with small cell lung cancer [13]. In neuroblastoma, NSE is derived from tumor tissues and the serum level is usually closely correlated with the patient's clinical course. The high level of serum NSE is not always specific for neuroblastoma, and

is occasionally seen in patients with other childhood tumors including Wilm's tumor, lymphomas, leukemias, hepatoblastoma, PNET, and dysgerminoma [14]. It is therefore clear that the serum levels of NSE are not decisive in the differential diagnosis of neuroblastoma and Wilms' tumor. An enzymatic procedure was employed to determine the values of NSE and nonneuronal enolase, permitting the calculation of the ratio of NSE to nonneuronal enolase (NNE). This was reported to enhance the specificity of the NSE determinations for the diagnosis of neuroblastomas. An increase in the ratio characterizes neuroblastomas in advanced stages, whereas low ratios with high NSE are found in other tumors [15].

The upper border of the normal range for serum NSE is approximately 14.6 ng/ml. The serum levels of NSE are higher in widespread and metastatic neuroblastoma than in localized disease. Serum levels higher than 100 ng/ml were thus associated with advanced stage disease and a poor outcome. A useful diagnostic marker, NSE may also be a good indicator of the disease course in children with neuroblastoma [16]. Immunohistochemical investigation showed that the axons of the peripheral nerves were intensely positive for NSE but the Schwann cells were negative. In neuroblastoma the cytoplasm was intensely positive for NSE irrespective of the degree of histologic differentiation. Staining for NSE is of some value in making a differential diagnosis of neural tumors from other morphologically primitive tumors [6].

4.2.3 Lactic Dehydrogenase

Lactic dehydrogenase is a glycolytic enzyme that catalyses the reversible conversion of pyruvate to lactate, and is widely distributed in human tissues. Human LDH is composed of five isoenzymes called LDH1 to LDH5. Each isoenzyme is a tetramer of two subunits, H and M. Total serum LDH activity decreases with age and is higher in children than in adults. The serum level is 434 +/- 164 IU/liter (mean +/- 2SD) in infants, 362 +/- 118 IU/liter in children aged 1–5 years, 312 +/- 108 IU/liter in children aged 6–11 years and 273 +/- 91 in children older than 12 years. A high serum LDH concentration is observed in 70–80% of children with malignant tumors, such as leukemias, lymphomas, Wilms' tumor, hepatoblastoma, and neuroblastoma and is useful in differentiating malignant tumors from benign lesions [17]. An increase in LDH2 and LDH3 is the most frequently encountered malignant pattern and is observed in neuroblastoma [18]. An increase in LDH1 is reported in germ cell tumors including yolk sac tumor, dysgerminoma, and seminoma [17]. In neuroblastoma, serum LDH is increased in patients with advanced disease, and serial measurement of LDH is a useful monitor of tumor activity. There is a correlation between the absolute LDH level and the patient's prognosis, which has been demonstrated in previous studies [19].

4.2.4 Other Markers for Neuroblastoma and Related Tumors

Ferritin is a major iron storage tissue protein composed of a total of 24 subunits of two different sizes, H (molecular weight, 21,000) and L (molecular weight, 19,000). Different combinations of these two subunits yield a variety of isoferritins. In leukemias, lymphomas, liver tumors, breast cancer, and lung cancer, a rise in serum ferritin level is observed, although the precise mechanism by which this happens is not known [20]. In neuroblastoma, increased ferritin in serum was significantly correlated with the presence of active disease and the level returned to normal with remission of the disease. The ferritin level at diagnosis is a prognostic indicator, with high serum ferritin a feature of advanced disease and poor outcome [21].

Children with neuroblastic tumors secrete vasoactive intestinal polypeptide (VIP), often present with severe diarrhea, hypokalemia, dehydration, and malnutrition. In such patients high levels of plasma VIP return to normal and diarrhea ceases following removal of the tumor [22]. Immunohistochemically, VIP is localized exclusively within differentiating and mature ganglion cells of ganglioneuroblastomas, ganglioneuromas, and normal sympathetic ganglia, but not found in undifferentiated neuroblastoma cells.

Scheiben, et al. reported that six of twenty-two (27%) patients with neuroblastic tumors had a high plasma concentration of VIP ranging from 28 to 95 pmol/l (normal limit, 19.0 pmol/l) and that only one, whose plasma level of VIP was 95 pmol/l, had diarrhea [23]. These patients would have their VIP levels monitored for recurrent disease for early detection. Children who present with tumors that secrete VIP have an improved prognosis.

Gangliosides are sialic acid containing glycosphingolipids occurring primarily on the membrane of the cell. A monoclonal antibody (MAB 126) produced against cultured human neuroblastoma cells (LAN-1) was found to react specifically to a disialoganglioside (Gd2) antigen expressed on both cell lines and tissues derived from melanoma and neuroblastoma. Increased levels of Gd2 antigen were demonstrated in sera of patients with neuroblastoma and in primary neuroblastoma tissues. Gd2 maybe inversely related to the degree of differentiation of the tumor because Gd2 was hardly detected in ganglioneuroblastoma and ganglioneuroma. However, the usefulness of ganglioside as a tumor marker has not been fully evaluated [24].

Chromogranin A is an acidic protein costored and coreleased with catecholamines from storage vesicles. Hsiao, et al. measured serum chromogranin A at diagnosis in patients with neuroblastoma. Serum chromogranin A (normal value, ≤52 ng/ml) was a useful marker with a sensitivity of 91% and specificity of 100%, and correlated with the disease stage. The survival rate for patients with low serum chromogranin A levels (less than 190 ng/ml) was 69% but it was only 30% for those with higher levels. This suggests that the serum chromogranin A level at diagnosis is a useful predictor of survival [25].

Creatinine kinase catalyses the transfer of a high-energy phosphate bond from adenosine triphosphate to adenosine diphosphate, and has three isozymes. The BB isozyme of creatinine kinase (CK-BB) is detectable in the serum. Ishigoro, et al. measured the CK-BB level in patients with neuroblastoma and observed that 60% of patients had CK-BB levels higher than 11 ng/ml. There was a correlation between serum CK-BB levels and patient prognosis, and especially those whose serum level was greater than 15 ng/ml had a poor prognosis [26].

Neuropeptide Y (NPY) is a 33 amino acid peptide, found in adrenal medulla and sympathetic nervous system as well as the central nervous system. It has potent biological activities, including smooth muscle relaxation, inhibition of pancreatic secretion, and vasoconstriction. Tumor cells which are immunoreactive for NPY were demonstrated in pheochromocytomas and ganglioneuroblastomas, and NPY concentrations in these tumors were higher than in other endocrine tumors. Rascher, et al. reported that plasma NPY levels had exceeded the normal value, 5.2 pmol/l, in more than 90% of patients with neuroblastoma and the serial determination of the levels had been a sensitive marker of relapse [27]. Kogner, et al. analyzed the plasma concentration of NPY-like immunoreactivity in normal control children and showed that the concentration decreased with age [28]. According to this study, the high plasma NPY was observed in only 42% of neuroblastoma patients. As only neuroblastoma patients with high plasma NPY had a poor outcome, plasma NPY appears to be a sensitive marker in predicting the patient's prognosis, but more data will be needed before plasma NPY is accepted as a tumor marker comparable with catecholamine metabolites or NSE.

4.3 Genetic and Biological Markers for Neuroblastoma

4.3.1 N-myc GENE Amplification

Approximately 30% of neuroblastomas show N-myc gene amplification. According to the initial report by Seegar, et al., all of 11 patients in stage IV with amplified N-myc progressed within 8 months after diagnosis, whereas only 6 of 21 whose tumor had a single had progression at 8 months [29]. This finding suggested a role of N-myc amplification in determining the aggressiveness of neuroblastoma. Initially N-myc amplification was observed only in patients with advanced disease (stages III and IV) and appeared to be indicative of fatality. A recent study, however, showed that 5-year survival for patients with N-myc amplification was 43.9% with a type of intensive induction chemotherapy and that the prognosis of patients with amplified N-myc might be improved by this new intensive treatment. It was also reported that patients with localized neuroblastoma had a favorable prognosis even if they had N-myc amplification [30].

On the other hand, patients without N-myc amplification have a relatively favorable prognosis compared with those with N-myc amplification, but the outlook for stage IV neuroblastomas which lack N-myc amplification is also dismal. It was shown that the cumulative 5-year survival rate for stage IV neuroblastoma without N-myc amplification was only 54.2%, but it was still significantly better than that for stage IV disease with N-myc amplification. The biological mechanisms contributing to the tumor progression in this subset of neuroblastoma are yet to be clarified. In relation to the subject, there are some reports showing that neuroblastomas without N-myc amplification sometimes express N-myc mRNA and N-myc protein. Cohn, et al. demonstrated a prolonged half-life of N-myc protein in a cell line which expressed N-myc mRNA and the protein but lacks N-myc amplification. The half-life of the protein was shorter (30–50 min) in N-myc amplified cell lines such as LA-N-5, Kelly, and IMR-5. The prolonged half-life of N-myc protein may explain the mechanism involved in tumor progression of neuroblastomas without the oncogene amplification [31].

Immunohistochemical detection of N-myc protein expression was reported to be one of the most unfavorable prognostic indicators. It is therefore important to obtain an antibody which specifically reacts to N-myc protein and is suitable for the immunohistochemical detection of the protein. The function of the N-myc gene product is not fully understood. The protein encoded by the oncogene is considered to be involved in DNA binding and protein–protein interaction. Based on its nuclear location and binding to DNA, it is thought that N-myc protein is a transcription factor and is related to the regulation of growth in neuroblastomas [32].

4.3.2 Detection of N-myc Gene Amplification

In some centers such as Japan, patients with stage IV disease are stratified into different therapeutic protocols according to the mode of N-myc amplification, and those with amplified N-myc are treated more intensely than those without amplification. Specimens obtained either by a laparotomy or needle biopsy are examined by Southern blot analysis.

4.3.3 Other Genetic and Biological Markers

Evidence for amplification and/or expression of other oncogenes, including N-ras, H-ras, K-ras, src, fos, and trk, has been sought in neuroblastoma by a number of investigators. For instance, Tanaka, et al. studied H-ras expression and demonstrated that neuroblastomas with higher expression of H-ras gene product (H-ras p21) had a better outcome [33]. Combined analysis of H-ras p21 expression and N-myc gene amplification provides more accurate information pertinent to patients' prognosis.

Recently it was found that most primary neuroblastomas with favorable prognosis expressed high levels of trk-A mRNA, which encodes a receptor for nerve growth factor (NGF-R) [34]. It was also demonstrated that truncated trk-B was preferentially expressed in more differentiated ganglioneuromas and ganglioneuroblastomas, while full-length trk-B was expressed almost exclusively in immature neuroblastomas with N-myc amplification. Detection of trk-A expression is certainly valuable in predicting patients' prognosis [35].

4.4 Screening for Neuroblastoma with Urinary VMA and HVA

In 1985 the Japanese welfare ministry began a national screening program for neuroblastoma with urinary VMA and HVA [36]. When a baby reached 6 months of age, urine was collected by a filter paper and sent to the local laboratory, where urine samples were assayed for the levels of VMA, HVA, and creatinine by HPLC. If VMA and/or HVA levels are higher than the normal range, the child was assessed in a secondary hospital and if a neuroblastoma was detected it was referred to a regional oncological service [37].

4.4.1 Biology of Neuroblastomas Detected on Screening

Numerous studies have looked at the biology of screening-detected neuroblastomas and have revealed that most tumors are biologically favorable. Hachitanda, et al. examined biological factors in a series of 100 neuroblastomas detected by screening. According to the study, 93% had favorable histology and 7% had unfavorable histology showing stroma-poor, undifferentiated histology with a high mitosis-karyorrhexis index. It is generally agreed that 10–20% of neuroblastomas detected by screening have unfavorable biological factors, such as unfavorable histology, DNA diploidy or tetraploidy, and low H-ras p21 expression, but N-myc amplified (>10 copies) tumors are extremely rare. Despite the unfavorable factors tumor progression is hardly seen and the clinical outcome of these patients is unanimously favorable [37].

In contrast, infants with false-negative screening who later present with neuroblastoma, usually children older than 1 year of age, have advanced-stage tumors. Half of them are N-myc amplified tumors and the results of treatment are generally dismal. The pattern of catecholamine metabolism is more often dopaminergic and more HVA than VMA is secreted. Because of these biological studies it appears that the screening is ineffective in detecting unfavorable tumors [10]. It is, however, still unknown whether a low-risk tumor develops into a high-risk tumor if left undetected until it presents clinically.

4.4.2 Treatment of Neuroblastomas Detected on Screening

As the screening-detected tumors are biologically favorable and patients with such tumors survive without recurrence, it is recommended that the treatment should be the minimum even in patients in advanced stages. Aggressive surgery and the administration of high-dose chemotherapy are unnecessary in most cases and should be avoided in asymptomatic patients who have a tumor detected by screening. It has been observed that tumors detected on screening regress spontaneously without treatment [36].

4.4.3 Effects of Neuroblastomas Screening

After implementation of screening programs both in Japan and in Canada, it appears that neuroblastomas detected by screening as well as those detected clinically before the age of 1 year were predominantly of a favorable histology and carried a good prognosis. Tumors missed by screening and detected clinically after 1 year of age were predominantly of unfavorable histology [38].

4.5 Hepatic Tumor Markers

Hepatocellular carcinoma and hepatoblastoma both secrete AFP, a useful tumor marker for diagnosis and follow up of the patient's clinical course [39]. Liver tumors such as hepatoblastoma may also secrete human chorionic gonadotrophin HCG, which could be tracked in the serum [40] (Table 4.2). In fibrolamellar hepatic carcinoma serum, unsaturated vitamin B12 binding capacity can be measured, though the AFP levels are not increased [41]. In mesenchymal hepatic tumors serum, AFP levels are usually within the normal range and only the nonspecific serum tumor marker LDH may be increased.

4.5.1 Alpha-Fetoprotein

AFP, a major plasma protein of the fetus, is synthesized in the yolk sac and the liver of the fetus at an early stage of the development. A trace amount is also synthesized by the fetal gastrointestinal tract. It has a molecular

Table 4.2 Tumor markers for hepatic tumors

Marker	Tumor	Use	Comments
Alpha-fetoprotein	Hepatoblastoma	Diagnosis, follow-up	Increased in >98% of patients
	Hepatocellular carcinoma	Diagnosis, follow-up	Increased in 50%–40% of patients
Beta subunit of HCG	HCG-secreting hepatoblastoma	Diagnosis, follow-up	Approximately 2%–3% of all malignant hepatic tumors
Unsaturated vitamin B12-binding capacity	Fibrolamellar carcinoma	Diagnosis, follow-up	

HCG, human chononic gonadotropin

weight of 70,000 and consists of a single polypeptide chain. Its structural similarities to albumin suggest similar functions as general carriers in plasma and in the maintenance of osmotic pressure. Its production starts at about the 6th week of gestation and trails off at birth. The serum AFP concentration decreases exponentially with a half-life of approximately 5 days from a mean of approximately 50,000 ng/ml to a level of less than 20 ng/ml at 6-8 months of age. Preterm infants have ten times higher levels of AFP than term infants do at birth. The AFP values reach adult levels by 12 months in preterm infants. In adults, 77% of patients with hepatocellular carcinoma have serum AFP levels of >20 ng/ml and the levels exceeded 200 ng/ml in 80% of patients with HbsAG-positive hepatocellular carcinoma, whereas AFP levels were within normal range (<20 ng/ml) in more than 99% of patients with acute and chronic hepatitis B, cirrhosis, and other malignant tumors [42]. Children with hepatic epithelial tumors and yolk sac tumors of germ cell origin have increased serum AFP levels. The AFP concentration is high, beyond the upper border of the normal range for the patients' age in more than 98% of hepatoblastomas and in 50–80% of hepatocellular carcinomas [2]. Although the AFP concentration is relatively higher in hepatoblastomas with embryonal histology than in tumors with fetal histology, there is no prognostic significance. The structure of the carbohydrate portion of AFP produced by the hepatic tumors is different from that of AFP produced by yolk sac tumors. The heterogeneity of the sugar chain structure results in the difference in the AFP subfraction profile demonstrated by means of lectin-affinity immunoelectrophoresis. The reaction of AFP with lens culinaris hemagglutinin (LCH) is related to the fucosylation of the sugar chain; LCH specifically binds the sugar chain with a fucose residue. On the other hand, concanavalin A (Con A) binds the biantennary carbohydrate chain with or without a fucose residue and the modified triantennary or tetra-antennary sugar chain does not bind to Con A. This makes it possible to differentiate AFP derived from hepatic malignancy from AFP derived from yolk sac tumors and a benign hepatic disease, such as hepatitis or cirrhosis [43]. In summary, AFP derived from hepatoblastoma or hepatocellular carcinoma includes a subfraction which binds to LCH, but AFP from a benign hepatic disease does not react with LCH. The presence of a greater amount (>25%) of AFP fraction which is not reactive to Con A differentiates AFP derived from a yolk sac tumor from that of hepatic origin.

Serum AFP levels decline exponentially after complete tumor resection and remain within normal limits (<10 ng/ml) unless recurrence occurs [44]. Failure of high AFP levels to return to normal after surgery with a half-life of approximately 5 days indicates incomplete resection of the tumor or the presence of metastases [39]. AFP may be secreted from the regenerating liver after surgical resection, but this does not interfere with its expected decline. The increase in AFP levels in patients with apparent clinical remission may occur when there is liver dysfunction due to chemotherapy or viral infection. In that case the AFP subfraction profile obtained by lectin-affinity immunoelectrophoresis may give evidence to differentiate an AFP increase due to residual tumor from that which resulted from liver damage. Although caution is necessary, the measurement of AFP is practically useful in monitoring the disease course as well as in making a diagnosis (Fig. 4.3).

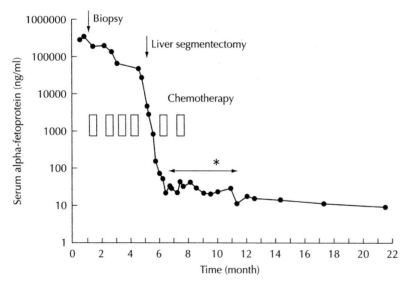

Fig. 4.3 Serum alpha-fetoprotein (AFP) levels in a patient with hepatoblastoma. The AFP levels declined exponentially after tumor resection but remained slightly higher than the normal limits, around 30–50ng/ml (*), for several months. AFP secretion from the regenerating liver or chemotherapy-induced liver dysfunction was a possible reason for the higher levels.

4.5.2 Human Chorionic Gonadotropin

Human chorionic gonadotrophin is a glycoprotein whose molecular weight is approximately 45,000–50,000, and is composed of two subunits, alpha and beta. While the alpha subunit of HCG is structurally similar to the alpha subunit of LH, FSH, and TSH, the beta subunit of HCG (b-hcg) is different from the beta subunit of these pituitary hormones. Because antibodies to beta hcg do not cross-react with LH, beta hcg is usually measured by radioimmunoassay. The half-life of beta hcg is 24 h and its normal range is less than 1.0 ng/ml. Isosexual precocious puberty may develop in male children with hepatoblastoma secreting hcg, which accounts for approximately 2–3% of all malignant hepatic tumors [45]. Virilization with testicular and penile enlargement and growth of pubic hair is seen. It should be emphasized that the serum beta hcg level does not necessarily correspond to the clinical course in some patients [46] (Fig. 4.4).

4.5.3 Other Markers for Hepatic Tumors

In hepatoblastoma it is suggested that interleukine-6 is produced in stromal cells in response to cytokines secreted from tumor cells and that it may be responsible for the thrombocytosis sometimes seen in patients with hepatoblastoma [39]. Hypercholestrolemia is also occasionally seen. Due to poor sensitivity and specificity, however, neither is established as a useful tumor marker in hepatoblastoma. The serum unsaturated vitamin b12-binding capacity is significantly high in fibrolamellar carcinoma (fibrolamellar variant of hepatocellular carcinoma) and rises with disease progression. Fibrolamellar carcinoma occurs in the noncirrhotic livers of older children and young adults [41]. Because the serum AFP level is not increased in the majority of patients, the serial measurement of serum unsaturated vitamin-B12-binding capacity is considerably important in this tumor.

4.6 Tumor Markers for Germ Cell Tumors

Germ cell tumors in children comprise mature and immature teratomas, yolk sac tumors, embryonal carcinoma, germinoma (dysgerminoma), choriocarcinoma, and gonadoblastoma. Embryonal carcinoma is rare in children, but is a major component of the malignant germ cell tumor of the testis and mediastinum in adolescents. Testicular germinoma (seminoma) is usually not seen in children. When a tumor of germ cell origin is among differential diagnosis, serum AFP and beta hcg levels should be included in the measurement of tumor markers.

4.6.1 Alpha-Fetoprotein

Serum AFP levels are increased in patients with yolk sac tumors and correlate well with the clinical course of patients. Immuno-histochemical staining demonstrates tumor cells which are positive for AFP. Although the exact nature of the intracellular and intercellular periodic acid-schiff (PAS)-positive hyaline globules, which are characteristic of yolk sac tumors, is unknown, the globules are frequently positive for AFP. After surgical excision of a yolk sac tumor, serum AFP levels decrease to normal with a half-life of approxi-

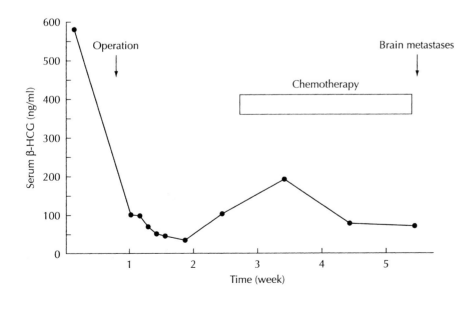

Fig. 4.4 Serum levels of β-subunit of human chorionic gonadotropin (β-HCG) in a patient with choriocarcinoma of the lung; β-HCG levels declined after tumor resection but increased again within a few weeks.

mately 5 days. Sudden elevation of serum AFP levels may indicate the presence of metastatic or recurrent disease [47]. Serum AFP levels may be increased when there are foci of yolk sac tumors in teratomas. Conversely, when teratomas are associated with increased AFP levels, yolk sac tumor elements are somewhere in the tumor. Patients diagnosed with immature teratomas and high AFP at the time of diagnosis have a higher risk of malignant recurrence. Malogolowkin, et al. therefore recommend that immature teratomas with high serum AFP should be treated with similarly to malignant germ cell tumors [48]. Bilik, et al. reported that yolk sac tumors recurred in 8% of patients whose sacrococcygeal teratoma had initially been treated in the neonatal period and that all recurrences were accompanied by an increase in serum AFP [49]. Only in a small number of patients with a huge immature teratoma, a moderate increase in serum AFP occurs due to the gastrointestinal epithelia involved in the tumor.

Serum AFP levels are increased in patients with hepatic tumors as well as germ cell tumors, and the analysis of the AFP subfraction profile is useful in the differential diagnosis as mentioned in the section on hepatic tumors. Aoyagi, et al. measured fucosylation and glycoaminylation indices of AFP in germ cell tumors. The fucosylation index was described as the percentage of AFP whose sugar chain is fucosylated and specifically binds to Lens culinaris agglutinin in total AFP. The glycoaminylation index was defined as the percentage of concanavalin A-nonreactive AFP in total AFP. AFP whose biantennary sugar chain is modified further by glycoaminylation at the mannose core does not bind to Con A. The fucosylation and glucosaminylation indices of AFP in germ cell tumors were 99% +/- 2% and 45%+/- 20%, respectively, and both

indices were significantly higher than those of AFP from hepatic tumors and benign liver disease. These indices may be used to differentiate AFP produced in yolk sac tumors from physiologically increased AFP in early infancy [43].

4.6.2 Human Chorionic Gonadotropin

Choriocarcinoma secrete HCG, and the beta subunit of HCG (βHCG) is measured to monitor the serum levels of HCG (Fig. 4.2). Because the alpha subunit of HCG is identical in amino acid sequence to alpha subunits of pituitary hormones, radioimmunoassay with antibodies to the beta hcg is used to measure serum HCG levels. Microscopically, the coriocarcinoma consists of two components, cytotrophoblasts and syncytiotrophoblasts. The HCG is produced by the latter, which is demonstrated by immunohistochemical staining for beta HCG. When choriocarcinoma occurs in an infant or neonate, the placenta is believed to be the site of the origin of the tumor, and serum beta HCG is always increased [50].

4.6.3 Other Markers for Germ Cell Tumors

The cancer antigen CA 125 is a high-molecular-weight, mucinous glycoprotein which is expressed in celomic epithelium during the embryonic development. In adults the normal values for CA 125 in serum is less than 35 U/ml and the levels are increased in patients with epithelial ovarian cancer. The serum CA 125 is useful in monitoring the clinical course of patients and at the same time it is a potent prognostic factor in ovarian cancer [51] (Fig. 4.5). On the other hand, little is

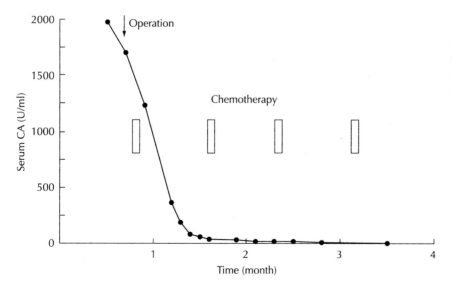

Fig. 4.5 Serum CA-125 levels in a 13-year-old female patient with a ovarian dysgerminoma. The measurement of serum CA-125 levels was useful in monitoring the disease course.

known about the oncologic significance of the marker in children. An increase in serum CA 125 is observed in patients with yolk sac tumor and embryonal carcinoma [52]. The levels decline after the initiation of therapy but re-elevation of the levels was not associated with recurrence [53]. An increase in the marker which is associated with hereditary tyrosinemia in the acute phase of the disease is known. Although the significance of CA 125 in childhood germ cell tumors is not yet fully understood, the measurement of serum levels may sometimes be useful in monitoring the disease process (Fig. 4.3).

Lactate dehydrogenase isoenzyme-1 (LDH-1) increases in the sera of patients with germ cell tumors including yolk sac tumor, dysgerminoma, and choriocarcinoma [54]. Both total serum LDH activity and LDH-1 activity were increased in patients with yolk sac tumor. The relative percentages of LDH-1 isoenzyme ranged from 60% to 88% in these patients and were higher than the normal value of 46%. The increased LDH-1 activity is derived from tumor tissues [2].

4.7 Tumor Markers for Wilms' Tumors

Wilms' tumor is the most common renal tumor in pediatrics. Multidisciplinary treatment of Wilms' tumor has led to a high success rate, with some 90% of patients achieving long-term survival [55]. However, late effects of treatment and management of relapse remain significant clinical problems. If accurate prognostic methods were available, effective therapies could be tailored to optimize care. Few molecular prognostic markers for Wilms' tumor are currently defined, though previous studies have linked allele loss on 1p or 16q, genomic gain of 1q, and overexpression from 1q with an increased risk of relapse [56]. In a prospective study, plasma prorenin and renin concentration were measured in a group of pediatric patients with Wilms' tumor preoperatively. The mean plasma rennin and prorenin concentrations in the patients were raised compared with a control group of patients without nephroblastomas [57]. Four of these patients had recurrence of tumor, and in three, this was associated with an increase in plasma prorenin concentration [58]. Nephroblastoma tissue in this study contained immunoreactive renin and renin messenger RNA, and the renin protein was immunologically and biochemically found to be similar to normal human renin.

4.7.1 Immunohistochemical Study of Wilms' Tumor

An immunohistochemical study of a Wilms' tumor which presented with hypertension showed that renin was localized within neoplastic glomeruloid bodies. The same study also described a patient with congenital mesoblastic nephroma and hypertension that had renin positivity in the juxtaglomerular cells adjacent to the glomeruli, suggesting compression by the tumor. The plasma total renin levels in patients with Wilms' tumor measured by a radioimmunoassay were 547 +/- 298 pg/ml and were significantly higher than the levels in control, 166 +/- 68 pg/ml [59].

4.7.2 Hyaluronic Acid

Hyaluronic acid, a glycosaminoglycan, is usually found connective tissue as ground substance, in synovial fluid, vitreous humor, and the umbilical cord. Its presence in the serum leads to hyperviscosity, and in a reported case of Wilms' was found in a concentration of 8,500 mg/l (normal <10 mg/l) [60]. The serum level is regulated by the influx of the polysaccharide from the tissues via lymph and its receptor-mediated clearance by liver endothelial cells. Markedly high serum levels are noted in inflammatory conditions such as cirrhosis and rheumatoid arthritis, and in patients with septic conditions is a sign of poor prognosis. Certain tumors, notably Wilms' tumor and mesothelioma, produce factors which activate synthesis of hyaluronan and increase its serum level. Lin, et al. measured urinary hyaluronic acid in patients with Wilms' tumor [60]. Urinary hyaluronic acid levels were increased preoperatively in more than 70% of patients and declined after surgery. Increased hyaluronic acid in the late postoperative period indicated tumor relapse and/or recurrence. It is proposed that the increased hyaluronic acid stimulating activity in tumor tissue stimulates hyaluronic acid production in the tissues of patients in an autocrine or endocrine manner.

4.8 Tumor Markers for Other Tumors

4.8.1 Serum Carcinoembryonic Antigen (CEA)

CEA is an oncofetal glycoprotein normally expressed by mucosal cells and overexpressed by adenocarcinomas, particularly colorectal cancer, and contributes to the malignant characteristics of a tumor. It can be measured in serum quantitatively, and its level in plasma can be useful as a marker of disease. Unfortunately, it has not proven to be effective in the pediatric population [61].

4.8.2 Carbohydrate 19-9 (CA 19-9) Antigen

Among various tumor markers, carbohydrate antigen (CA) 19-9 is a tumor-associated, not a tumor-specific, antigen. Although it is usually associated with pancreatic and biliary tract cancers, it has also been reported in cirrhosis, cholangitis, and pancreatitis. Unfortunately, similar to CEA, it also has shown no effectiveness in detecting or keeping track of prognosis in children [61].

4.9 Tumor Markers: The Future

Scientists continue to study tumor markers and their possible role in the early detection and diagnosis of cancer. The NCI is currently conducting the Prostate, Lung, Colorectal, and Ovarian Cancer screening trial, or PLCO trial, to determine if certain screening tests reduce the number of deaths from these cancers. Along with other screening tools, PLCO researchers are studying the use of PSA to screen for prostate cancer and CA 125 to screen for ovarian cancer. Final results from this study are expected in several years.

Cancer researchers are turning to proteomics (the study of protein shape, function, and patterns of expression) in hopes of developing better cancer screening and treatment options. Proteomics technology is being used to search for proteins that may serve as markers of disease in its early stages, or predict the effectiveness of treatment or the chance of the disease returning after treatment has ended.

Scientists are also evaluating patterns of gene expression, for their ability to predict a patient's prognosis or response to therapy. NCI's Early Detection Research Network is developing a number of genomic- and proteomic-based biomarkers, some of which are being validated.

References

1. Ortega JA, Siegel SE (1993) Biological markers in pediatric solid tumours. In: Pizzo PA, Poplack DG (eds) Principles and practice of pediatric oncology. JB Lippincott, Philadelphia, pp 179–194
2. Tsuchida Y (1986) Markers in childhood solid tumours. In: Hays DM (ed) Pediatric surgical oncology. Grune and Stratton, New York, pp 7–62
3. Lindblom A, Liljegren A (2000) Tumour markers in malignancies. BMJ 320:424–427
4. Perkins GL, Slater ED (2003) Serum Tumour markers. Am Fam Physician 68:1075–1082
5. Riley RD, Heney D (2004) A systemic review of molecular and biological tumour markers in neuroblastoma. Clin Cancer Res 10:4–12
6. Singal AK, Agarwala S (2005) Tumour markers in pediatric solid tumours. J Indian Assoc Pediatr Surg 10:183–190
7. Tuchman M, Ramnaraine ML, Woods WG, Krivit W (1987) A three-year experience with random urinary homovanyllic acid and vanyllmandelic acid levels in the diagnosis of neuroblastoma. Pediatrics 79:203–205
8. Monsaingeon M, Perel Y, Simonnet G, Corcuff JB (2003) Comparative value of catecholamines and metabolites for the diagnosis of neuroblastomas. Eur J Pediatr 162:397–402
9. Simon T, Hero B, Hunneman DH, Berthold F (2003) Tumour markers are poor predictors for relapse or progression in neuroblastoma. Eur J Cancer 39:1899–1903
10. Nakagawara A, Zaizen Y, Ikeda K, Suita S, Ohgami H, Nagahara N, et al. (1991) Different genomic and metabolic patterns between mass screening positive and mass screening negative and later presenting neuroblastomas. Cancer 68:2037–2044
11. Yamamoto K, Hanada R, Kikuchi A, Ichikawa M, Aihara T, Oguma E, et al. (1998) Spontaneous regression of localised neuroblastoma detected by neuroblastoma screening. J Clin Oncol 16:1265–1269
12. Brodeur GM, Maris JM, Yamashiro DJ (1997) Biology and genetics of human neuroblastomas. J Pediatr Hematol Oncol 19:93–101
13. Tsuchida Y, Honna T, Iwanaka T, Saeki M, Taguchi N, Kaneko T, et al. (1987) Serial determination of serum neurone specific enolase in patients with neuroblastoma and other pediatric tumours. J Pediatr Surg 22:419–424
14. Viallard JL, Tiget F, Hartmann O, Lemerle J, Demeocq F, Malpuech G, et al. (1988) Serum neuronspecific/nonneuronal enolase ratio in the diagnosis of neuroblastomas. Cancer 62:2546–2553
15. Pritchard J, Cooper EH, Hamilton S, Bailey CC, Ninane J (1987) Serum neuron-specific enolase may be raised in children with Wilm's tumour. Lancet I:110
16. Tsokos M, Linnoila RI, Chandra RS, Triche TJ (1984) Neuron-specific enolase in the diagnosis of neuroblastomas and other small, round-cell tumours in children. Hum Pathol 15:575–584
17. Kinumaki H, Takeuchi H, Ohmi K (1976) Serum lactate dehydrogenase isoenzyme pattern in neuroblastoma. Eur J Pediatr 123:83–87
18. Stenman HU (2005) Testicular cancer: The perfect paradigm for marker combinations. Scand J Clin Lab invest 65:181–188
19. Quinn JJ, Altman AJ (1980) Serum lactic dehydrogenase, an indicator of tumour activity in neuroblastoma. J Pediatr 97:89–91
20. Hann HL, Levy HM, Evans AE (1980) Serum ferritin as a guide to therapy in neuroblastoma. Cancer Res 40:1411–1413
21. Hann HL, Evans AE, Siegel SE, Wong KY, Sather H, Dalton A, et al. (1985) Prognostic importance of serum ferritin in in patients with stages III and IV neuroblastoma: The Childrens Cancer Study Group experience. Cancer Res 45:2843–2848
22. Cooney DR, Voorhess ML, Fisher JE, Brecher M, Karp MP, Jewett TC (1982) Vasoactive intestinal peptide producing neuroblastoma. J Pediatr Surg 17:821–825

23. Scheibel E, Rechnitzer C, Fahrenkrug J, Hertz H (1982) Vasoactive intestinal polypeptide (VIP) in children with neural crest tumours. Acta Paediatr Scand 71:721–725

24. Wu ZL, Schwartz E, Seeger R, Ladisch S (1986) Expression of Gd2 ganglioside by untreated primary human neuroblastomas. Cancer Res 46:440–443

25. Hsiao RJ, Seeger RC, Yu AL, O'Connor DT (1990) Chromogranin A in children with neuroblastoma. J Clin Invest 85:1555–1559

26. Ishiguro Y, Kato K, Akatsuka H, Ito T (1990) The diagnostic and prognostic value of pre-treatment serum creatine kinase BB levels in patients with neuroblastoma. Cancer 65:2014–2019

27. Rascher W, Kremens B, Wagner S, Feth F, Hunneman DH, Lang RE (1993) Serial measurement of neuropeptide Y in plasma for monitoring neuroblastoma in children. J Pediatr 122:914–916

28. Kogner P, Bjork O, Theodorsson E (1994) Plasma neuropeptide Y in healthy children: Influence of age, anaesthesia and the establishment of an age-adjusted reference interval. Acta Paediatr 83:423–427

29. Seegar RC, Brodeur GM, Sather H, Dalton A, Siegel SE, Wong KY, et al. (1985) Association of multiple copies of N-myc oncogene with rapid progression of neuroblastomas. New Engl J Med 313:1111–1116

30. Cohn SL, Look AT, Joshi VV, Holbrook T, Salwan H, Changnovich D, et al. (1995) lack of correlation of N-myc gene amplification with prognosis and localised neuroblastoma: A Pediatric Oncology Group Study. Cancer Res 55:721–726

31. Cohn SL, Salwen H, Quasney NW, Ikegaki N, Cowan JW, Herst CU (1990) Prolonged N-myc protein half life in a neuroblastoma cell line lacking N-myc amplification. Oncogene 5:1821–1827

32. Slamon DJ, Boone TC, Seeger RC, Keith DE, Chazin V, Lee HC (1986) Identification and characterisation of the protein encoded by human neuroblastoma. Science 23:768–772

33. Tanaka T, Seeger RC, Tanabe M, Hiyama E, Shimada H, Ida N (1994) Prognostic prediction in neuroblastoma: Clinical significance of combined analysis for Ha-ras p21 expression and N-myc gene amplification. Cancer Detec Prevent 18:283–289

34. Nakagawara A, Azar CG, Scavarda NJ, Brodeur GM (1994) Expression and function of TRK-B and BDNF in human neuroblastomas. Mol Cell Biol 14:759–767

35. Nakagawara A, Arima-Nakagawara M, Scavarda NJ, Azar CG, Cantor AB, Brodeur GM (1993) Association between high levels of expression of TRK gene and favourable outcome in human neuroblastoma. New Engl J Med 328:847–854

36. Matsumura M, Tsunoda A, Nishi T, Nishihira H, Sasaki Y (1991) Spontaneous regression of neuroblastoma detected by mass screening. Lancet 338:447–448

37. Hachitanda Y, Ishimoto K, Hata J, Simada H (1994) One hundred neuroblastomas detected through a mass screening system in Japan. Cancer 74:3223–3226

38. Takeuchi LA, Hachittanda Y, Woods WG, Tuchman M, Lemieux B, Brisson L, et al. (1995) Screening for neuroblastoma in North America. Cancer 76:2363–2371

39. Herzog CE, Andrassy RJ, Eftekhari F (2000) Childhood Cancers: Hepatoblastomas. The Oncologist 5:445–453

40. Torosian MH (1988) The clinical usefulness and limitations of tumor markers. Surg Gynecol Obstet 166:567–579

41. Paradinas FJ, Melia WM, Willkinson ML, Portmann B, Johnson PJ, Murray-Lyon IM, et al. (1982) High serum Vitamin B 12 binding capacity as a marker of the fibrolamellar variant of hepatocellular carcinoma. Brit Med J 285:840–842

42. Bellet DH, Wands JR, Isselbacher KJ, Bohuon C (1984) Serum alpha-feto protein levels in human disease: Perspective from a highly specific monoclonal radio-immunoassay. Proc Natl Acad Sci 81:3869–3873

43. Tsuchida Y, Terada M, Honna T, Kitano Y, Obana K, Leibundgut K, et al. (1997) The role of sub-fractionation of alpha-feto protein in the management of paediatric surgical patients. J Pediatr Surg 32:514–517

44. Germa JR, Llanos M, Tabernero JM, Mora J (1993) False elevations of alpha-fetoprotein associated with liver dysfunction in germ cell tumors. Cancer 72:2491–2494

45. Murthy ASK, Vawter GF, Lee ABH, Jockin H, Filler RM (1980) Hormonal bioassay of gonadotropin-producing hepatoblastoma. Arch Pathol Lab Med 104:513–517

46. Nakagawara A, Ikeda K, Tsuneyoshi M, Daimaru Y, Enjoji M, Watanabe I, et al. (1985) hepatoblastoma producing both alpha-fetoprotein and human chorionicgonadotropin. Cancer 56:1636–1642

47. Harms D, Janig U (1986) Germ cell tumors of childhood. Virchows Arch 409:223–229

48. Malogolowkin MH, Ortega JA, Krailo M, Gonzalez O, Mahour GH, Landing BH, et al. (1989) Immature teratomas: Identification of patients at risk for malignant recurrance. J Natl Cancer Inst 81:870–874

49. Bilik R, Shandling B, Pope M, Thorner P, Weitzman S, Ein SH (1993) Malignant benign neonatal sacrococcygeal teratoma. J Pediatr Surg 28:1158–1160

50. Belchis DA, Mowry J, Davis JH (1993) Infantile coriocarcinoma. Cancer 72:2028–2032

51. Nagele F, Petru E, Medl M, Kainz C, Graf AH, Sevelda P (1995) Preoperative CA 125:An independent prognostic factor in patients with stage 1 epithelial ovarian cancer. Obstet Gynecol 86:259–264

52. Lahdenne P, Pitkanen S, Rajantie J, Kuusela P, Siimes MA, Lanning M, et al. (1995) Tumour markers CA 125 and CA 19-9 in cord blood and during infancy: Developmental changes and use in pediatric germ cell tumors. Pediatr Res 38:797–801

53. Pitkanen S, Salo MK, Kuusela P, Holmberg C, Simell O, Heikinheimo M (1994) Serum levels of oncofetal markers CA 125, CA 19-9 and alpha-feto protein in children with hereditary tyrosinemia type 1. Pediatr Res 35:205–208

54. Kinumaki H, Takeuchi H, Nakamura K, Ohmi K, Bessho F, Kobayashi N (1985) Serum lactate dehydrogenase isoenzyme-1 in children with yolk sac tumor. Cancer 56:178–181

55. UKCCSG Protocol No WT 2002-02 by United Kingdom Children's Cancer Study Group

56. Brown KW, Malik KTA (2001) The molecular biology of Wilms' tumour. Exp Rev Mol Med 14

57. Carachi R, Lindop GBM, Leckie BJ (1987) Inactive renin: A tumor marker in nephroblastoma. J Pediatr Surg 22:278–280

58. Tsuchida Y, Mochida Y, Kamii Y, Honna T, Saeki M, Hata J, et al. (1990) Determination of plasma total renin levels by RIA with a monoclonal antibody: Value as a marker for nephroblastoma. J Pediatr Surg 25:1092–1094

59. Mochida Y, Tsuchida Y, Hata J, Komura M, Nishiura M (1991) Characterization of a radioimmunoassay to determine plasma total renin. Tumor Biol 12:75–81

60. Wu AHB, Parker OS, Ford L (1984) Hyperviscosity caused by hyaluronic acid in serum in a case of Wilms' tumor. Clin Chem 30:914–916

61. Angel CA, Pratt CB, Rao BN, Schell MJ, Parham DM, Lobe TE, et al. (1992) Carcinoembryonic antigen and carbohydrate 19-9 antigen as markers for colorectal carcinoma in children and adolescents. Cancer 69:1487–1491

Tumor Imaging

5

Melanie Hiorns

5.1 Introduction

Malignant disease in children accounts for approximately 1% of all registered malignancies. While each year approximately 12,500 children and adolescents are diagnosed with cancer in the USA, nearly 80% of children diagnosed with cancer become long-term survivors, and the majority of them are considered cured. Nevertheless, in the USA cancer remains the leading cause of death from disease among children.

Leukemias, tumors of the brain and nervous system, the lymphatic system, kidneys, bones, and muscles are the most common childhood cancers. The solid tumors account for approximately half of all these tumors and it is this group which will be considered in this chapter. Imaging has several important roles in the management of childhood cancer including diagnosis, assessing the local extent and the possible resectability of the tumor, identifying metastases, providing image guidance for biopsy, monitoring treatment, and detecting recurrent disease.

There have been considerable advances in imaging technology over the last few years, and continuing evaluation of these new techniques with an understanding of their use, advantages and limitations is necessary.

5.2 General Principles

Most children dislike hospitals, and busy radiology departments with large pieces of equipment may be especially frightening. It is therefore important for staff to take extra care with the child and family, recognizing their particular needs. Taking time, allowing parents to stay with their child, allowing children to wear their own clothes when possible, toys, videos, and careful explanations will all help to enlist the child's co-operation and result in good quality images. Most pediatric radiology departments have access to specially trained play therapists who can talk a child through a proposed test as a play exercise before the real test takes place. They may also have access to distraction aids such a small portable DVD players in which the child can become absorbed and distracted. Sedative drugs and general anesthesia may be necessary for the infant and young child when longer periods of immobility are necessary. Local anesthetic cream on at least two sites of possible venepuncture will reduce the child's fear and distress at the time of injection of contrast medium or an isotope. Warming the jelly used on the skin surface for ultrasound (US) studies is useful. It is likely that the child will have little understanding of what is taking place, but the parents and family will be anxious and distressed. The referring clinician and radiology staff must carefully explain what is going to happen in order to reduce the parents' and child's fears and anxiety. Allowing the parent to assist with holding the child, as appropriate, can help make the parents feel less alienated and more in control.

Ionizing radiation is an important risk of imaging, even in the child who has cancer. With increasing cure rates and the potential risk of a second malignancy (either iatrogenic or de novo), radiation exposure should be minimized and other diagnostic techniques, such as US and magnetic resonance imaging (MRI) should be used whenever possible, particularly in children who are going to receive multiple radiographic exposures as part of their follow-up over many years.

In most countries children with cancer are treated in specialist centers according to recognized protocols. In Europe and North America, protocols for the diagnostic and follow-up imaging of most tumors exist within organizations such as the International Society of Pediatric Oncology (SIOP), the United Kingdom Children's Cancer Study Group (UKCCSG), and the Children's Oncology Group (COG; formed in 2000 by the amalgamation of four previous groups: the Children's Cancer Group, the Pediatric Oncology Group, the National Wilms' Tumor Study Group, and the Intergroup Rhabdomyosarcoma Study Group), and should be followed in order to provide consistent results which enable treatment, staging, and prognosis to be evaluated. Many clinicians consider it optimal that children are entered into a relevant trial, both for their own benefit and for future patients, and the various organizations listed above have the most up-to-date information regarding specific trials for any particular tumor type.

5.3 Imaging Techniques

5.3.1 Plain Radiography

It is likely that the initial radiographic diagnosis of the child with a tumor will take place at the local hospital with a plain radiograph and US. Computed tomography (CT) may variably be performed at the local hospital but most crosssectional imaging such as CT

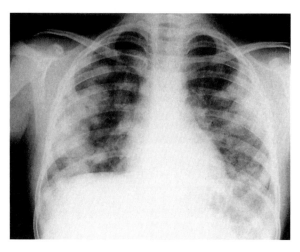

Fig. 5.1 Lung metastases from vaginal rhabdomyosarcoma in a 4-year-old girl presenting with a persistent cough following previous surgical resection of vaginal rhabdomyosarcoma. Chest radiograph demonstrates multiple different-sized pulmonary metastases.

and MRI, and nuclear scintigraphy, should in most instances take place at specialist centers where appropriate expertise and facilities are available.

A plain radiograph may be the first radiological investigation and if interpreted carefully may be helpful in making the diagnosis.

A plain abdominal radiograph in a child with a large abdominal mass may demonstrate calcification, erosion of the pedicles of the spine, and displacement of the paravertebral line, all of which are features of neuroblastoma. The lung bases may be included on the film and demonstrate pulmonary metastases seen in Wilms' tumor, hepatoblastoma, or rhabdomyosarcoma. Plain chest radiographs are essential in the detection of pulmonary metastases in the follow-up of Wilms' tumor, hepatoblastoma, and all sarcomas (Fig. 5.1). Associated features such as pathological fractures or bone infiltration in disseminated neuroblastoma and rarely osteoporosis in hepatoblastoma may be seen. Plain radiographs still have an important role in the diagnosis of primary bone tumors and may provide the diagnosis more easily than other modalities. Characteristic radiographic appearances are described in both benign and malignant bone tumors such as osteochondromas, osteoid osteomas, osteogenic sarcomas, and Ewing's tumor.

5.3.2 Ultrasound

Ultrasound (US) examination lends itself particularly well to the investigation of children with cancer. The technique does not employ ionizing radiation, very rarely requires sedation, and provides excellent images in most children. It is, however, highly operator-dependent, which can be particularly relevant when scanning uncooperative infants. It should be the first investigation in the evaluation of all abdominal masses. US will distinguish between congenital cystic lesions of the kidney, gut or mesentery, and solid tumors. Pelvic tumors are clearly seen with US, particularly intravesical tumors. Extravesical tumors can be distinguished from ovarian cysts, and hematocolpos, and are usually clearly demonstrated although pelvic wall involvement and extension into the sacrum is likely to be underestimated. US has a role in chest pathology, which is limited to determining whether the opaque hemithorax is primarily solid or fluid. Musculoskeletal US is used to determine whether a soft tissue mass is discrete, cystic, or vascular.

5.3.3 Computerized Tomography

Computerized tomography (CT) produces excellent images of the head, neck, thorax, abdomen, and pelvis. It is limited in the peripheral musculoskeletal system where MRI is the imaging of choice for the soft tissues, although CT still gives exquisite bony detail which can be used for 3D reconstructions for surgical planning especially in orthopedics and reconstruction surgery.

Although CT is well established, it utilizes ionizing radiation and therefore modern imaging of most tumors in the pediatric population should preferentially be performed by MRI where this is feasible. Furthermore, MRI has advanced so rapidly in recent years that it is now considered the superior modality (outside the lungs) irrespective of the radiation issues surrounding CT. However, CT is generally more readily available, cheaper, and easier for the patient than MRI and new scanners are now so fast that patients who previously required a general anesthetic for CT may now be able to have the scan performed under sedation or even unsedated. CT provides excellent images of lung parenchyma, mediastinum, head and neck, abdomen, and pelvis. Intravenous injection of contrast medium is essential to delineate mediastinal masses, hepatic tumors, renal masses, and head and neck tumors, and can allow CT angiography providing vessel detail that challenges conventional angiography. Spiral CT rotates the X-ray beam and the diametrically opposing detectors around the patient. Modern scanners have multiple detectors (typically 64 or 128) with the capability of very thin slice thicknesses (as low as 0.625 mm) allowing very rapid scanning of large body areas that can be completed in 5–10 sec which, with extensive image post processing and manipulation, can finally produce reconstructed planar and 3D images.

5.3.4 Magnetic Resonance Imaging

Magnetic resonance imaging (MRI) provides exquisite anatomical detail of many pediatric tumors. It has advantages over CT and US scanning including greater inherent tissue contrast, multiplanar imaging, and noninvasive angiography, and avoids exposure to ionizing radiation. In the past, there have been some practical disadvantages of MRI, which included the reduced availability of MR scanners, the noise and length of time of sequences, as well as the relatively frightening appearances of scanners which resulted in a need for sedation or general anesthesia in many children. However, new super-fast sequences and improving scanner design (i.e., "open-MR") is transforming the feasibility of MRI in the pediatric age group. MRI should be considered the imaging modality of choice for tumors of the musculoskeletal system, central nervous system, including the spine, head and neck tumors, as well as the abdomen, pelvis, and mediastinum. Modern sequences and the use contrast agents can also give information about the vascularity and enhancement characteristics of tumors. This can also be of benefit in the assessment of vascular malformations. Magnetic resonance angiography (MRA) is particularly useful in evaluating tumor proximity or involvement of major vessels. Whole-body MR may also compete with positron emission tomography (PET) imaging to stage abdominal tumors. Specific advantages of MR include determination of resectability of hepatic tumors using combined MR and MRA; staging of neuroblastoma in the bone marrow, lymph nodes, liver and spinal canal; response of bilateral Wilms' tumor and nephroblastomatosis; and detection of pelvic tumors with sagittal sections, and peritoneal tumors with contrast enhancement [46].

Fast spin-echo short inversion time inversion-recovery (STIR) whole-body (MR) imaging is an evolving technique that allows imaging of the entire body in a reasonable time. Its wide availability and lack of radiation exposure makes this method appealing in children. Bone marrow lesions, including marrow infiltration from lymphoma, metastases, and tumor-related edema, are observed with high signal intensity, and are more easily detected on STIR images than with scintigraphy. Focal parenchymal lesions can be distinguished by their slightly different signal intensity, but pathologic lymph nodes cannot at present be differentiated from normal nodes on the basis of signal intensity. The STIR technique is highly sensitive for detection of pathologic lesions, but it is not specific for malignancy; thus, the method cannot be used to differentiate benign conditions from malignant neoplastic lesions with certainty at present [55]. It is, however, already found useful in identifying lesions that otherwise would have been overlooked and these can then be imaged directly with other modalities if necessary. In the near future, MRI is also likely to give reliable information about the cellularity of some types of tumor using ADC (diffusion) maps, further enhancing its advantageous diagnostic utility.

Any patient having an MRI scan must be free of all ferromagnetic materials and should not have a pacemaker as these can be deprogrammed by the radiofrequency field. Some nonferromagnetic materials such as titanium may be present in the patient and while these are not a contraindication, they will still produce significant artifacts on the images. Similarly, all equipment such as anesthetic and resuscitation facilities must be MR compatible.

5.3.5 Nuclear Isotopes

Nuclear scintigraphy is useful in diagnosis, staging, assessment of tumor response, and evaluation of treatment in various pediatric tumors. The technological aspects of radioisotope scanning are particularly important when imaging children.

Careful calculation of dosage of radiopharmaceuticals in proportion to weight is required. Special immobilization of the patient can be achieved by wrapping the patient securely, with sedation and/or general anesthesia. Image magnification and the ability to perform single photon emission computed tomography (SPECT) are essential to performing state-of-the-art pediatric nuclear medicine. Multiple head detector gamma camera systems are available and have the advantages of increased resolution and sensitivity, and decreased time of examination in a child.

Nuclear imaging techniques such as bone scans, meta-iodo-benzyl guanidine (MIBG) scans, and (111) In-diethylenetriaminepentaacetic acid-octreotide scans have greatly increased the sensitivity and specificity of both diagnostic and follow-up protocols for pediatric solid tumors. Molecular targets that are specific for certain pediatric tumors are now being developed. Targets include cell membrane receptors targeted by specific ligands (such as octreotide), subcellular organelles targeted by false transmitters (such as MIBG), and cellular proteins targeted by antibodies [69].

Nonspecific radiopharmaceuticals such as technetium 99m-labeled methylene diphosphonate (Tc99m-MDP) are routinely used in the detection of bone metastases in all children with neuroblastoma, osteogenic sarcoma, Ewing's sarcoma, and bone-metastasizing Wilms' tumor. Although MDP scintigraphy will not necessarily distinguish benign from malignant disease, it is still the appropriate and most sensitive method to survey the skeleton for metastatic disease. However, in the future it may be that this technique is largely surpassed by whole-body MRI sequences specifically

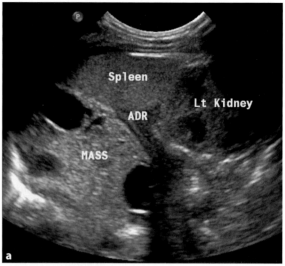

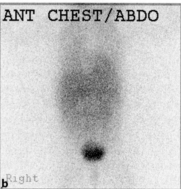

Fig. 5.2 Neuroblastoma in the left suprarenal region. (**a**) US shows the relationship of the left kidney, spleen, and the normal left adrenal to the left-sided suprarenal mass. (**b**) MIBG performed at the same time shows no uptake by the tumor.

designed to detect metastases (STIR sequences) as previously described.

Tumor-specific radiopharmaceuticals including MIBG and gallium-67 (67GA) are used in the management of children with cancer. Of interest is the fact that Tc 99m-MIBG may be taken up by both bone metastases and the primary tumor in instances of neuroblastoma, although not all neuroblastomas are MIBG avid (Fig. 5. 2).

Other isotopes including thallium-201 (201TI), sestamibi, and 2-[fluorine-18]-fluoro-2-deoxy-D-glucose (FDG) PET scanning are being investigated extensively (see below) [16].

5.3.6 Positron Emission Tomography

Positron emission tomography (PET) involves the acquisition of physiologic images based on the detection of radiation from the emission of positrons. Positrons are emitted from a radioactive substance FDG administered to the patient. Different color intensities on a PET image represent different levels of tissue glucose metabolism. Healthy tissue will accumulate some of the tagged glucose, which will show up on the PET images. However, cancers, which use more glucose than normal tissue, will accumulate more of the substance and appear brighter than normal tissue on the PET images (Fig. 5.3). PET scans are useful both in the detection of cancer and in examining the effects of cancer treatment by characterizing biochemical changes in the cancer. PET may be combined with CT to exactly localize areas of abnormal tissue, both for biopsy and to plan surgery.

PET scans are now being used more widely in the pediatric population although usually only in specialized cancer centers.

5.4 Imaging Principals by Body Part

5.4.1 Neck Masses

Tumor-like masses in the neck are unusual in children and are most commonly benign. Most common are congenital cystic lesions including thyroglossal duct cysts, branchial cysts, dermoid cysts, lymphangiomas, and cystic hygromas. Common neoplastic lesions are

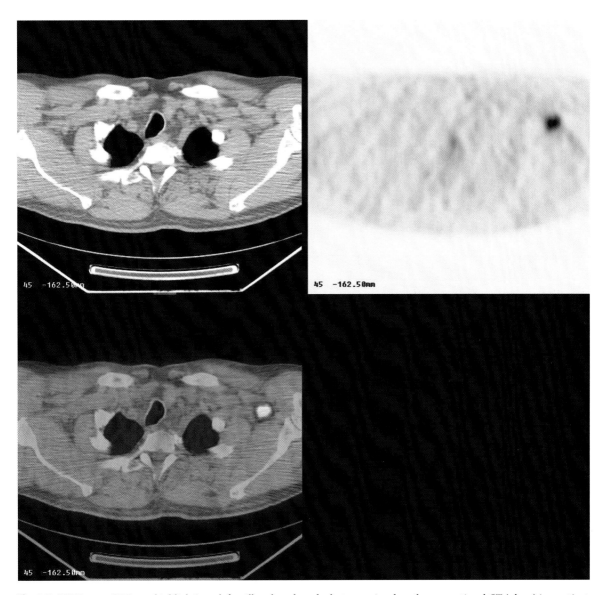

Fig. 5.3 PET image. PET scan highlighting a left axillary lymph node that was missed on the conventional CT (*above*) in a patient with lymphoma (courtesy of Dr Tom Lynch).

hemangiomas and lymphomas. The most common malignant tumors in the head and neck region are lymphomas and rhabdomyosarcomas, but thyroid tumors are also well recognized (Fig. 5.4). Lymph node enlargements, reactive or/and infectious, account for a significant number of cervical masses [51]. Imaging would initially be accomplished by US, which can provide both anatomical and vascular information. If a tumor is identified, MR would be the next imaging modality of choice. As many of these masses contain cystic elements, MR can generally provide better tissue differentiation than CT.

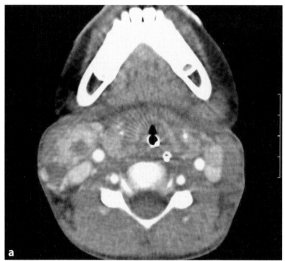
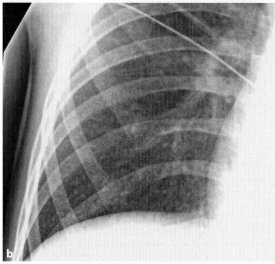

Fig. 5.4 Papillary thyroid cancer. (**a**) CT showing swelling is present on both sides of the neck due to lymph node enlargement. (**b**) Chest x-ray with multiple miliary metastases seen in the lungs typical of papillary thyroid cancer. This tumor carries a relatively good prognosis despite the metastases.

5.4.2 Abdominal Masses

Children may present with abdominal enlargement resulting from a large abdominal or pelvic mass. Nephroblastoma, neuroblastoma, rhabdomyosarcoma, teratoma, and hepatoblastoma frequently present with a large abdominal mass. Acute urinary retention may occur in instances of pelvic tumor. Initial imaging with US is essential and will confirm the presence of a solid echogenic mass and exclude both cystic and congenital renal lesions. The organ of origin of the mass, whether it be renal, suprarenal, hepatic, or pelvic, is often identified, permitting a provisional diagnosis. Further cross-sectional imaging with MRI or CT is then performed. It may be beneficial if this is performed in the center that will be treating the patient as protocols for imaging vary and any individual institution may have a preferred way of imaging the child, or may be entering relevant children into clinical trials that demand a certain imaging protocol. The prime objective is to image the child optimally on the first occasion and avoid repeat imaging once a tertiary referral has been made. Imaging is often performed locally in cases where the diagnosis of malignancy is in doubt, as in some cases of inflammatory disease, e.g., renal abscess, hepatic abscess, xanthogranulomatous pyelonephritis, or if the child is so compromised clinically by the size or effects of the mass that further imaging must be done immediately. Conventionally, an US followed by MRI or CT are performed in all units dealing with these cases.

5.4.3 Image-Guided Biopsy

Either CT or US are suitable for image-guided coreneedle biopsy of the mass, which in most cases (approximately 95%) yields sufficient tissue for both histological diagnostic, and prognostic and cytogenetic markers [44, 78].

5.4.4 Thoracic Masses

Thoracic tumors of childhood arise either in the mediastinum, or from the chest wall and less often from the lung parenchyma.

The mediastinum is the site of the normal thymus which is a relatively large organ in early childhood occupying the anterior and superior mediastinum extending down onto the diaphragm and up into the neck. It is therefore important to recognize the appearance of the normal thymus to avoid confusion with a tumor. On plain chest radiograph the thymus is a bilateral superior mediastinal mass which on the right side may demonstrate a characteristic sail-like shadow with a well-defined inferior and lateral margin. On the left side a wavy lateral margin is produced by adjacent anterior rib compression. Rarely, thymic tissue occurs in the posterior mediastinum either as direct extension from the anterior mediastinum or as ectopic tissue. If there is some doubt as to whether a mediastinal mass in an infant is normal thymus, US is a simple noninvasive technique that will demonstrate the homogeneous, "liver-like" echogenicity of this structure. Tumors of the mediastinum do not demonstrate this homogeneous echogenicity (Fig. 5.5).

The normal thymus imaged by CT is characteristically quadrilateral in shape in the neonate and infant and becomes more classically arrow-head in shape in older children. It is homogeneous in attenuation with a smooth edge and does not compress, distort, or invade underlying structures such as the trachea and major blood vessels. MRI is also useful in distinguishing the normal thymus from an abnormal mediastinal mass [86].

An important cause of an anterior mediastinal mass in neonates is cystic hygroma (Fig. 5.6), which usually arises in the neck and descends into the chest. Clinically, these are soft and echolucent on US. Imaging of the mediastinum with CT demonstrates a mediastinal mass of low, homogeneous attenuation which often encases and appears to displace and compress underlying large blood vessels and may displace the trachea. On MRI it has homogeneous signal intensity, low on T1-weighted sequences and high on T2-weighted sequences. Prior to embarking on a diagnosis of malignancy in an infant it is important that these benign conditions are considered.

Mediastinal masses are classified according to their site of origin into anterior, middle, and posterior mediastinal masses. Lymphomas, teratomas, and cystic hygromas are found in the anterior mediastinum, congenital duplication cysts, and lymphadenopathy in the middle mediastinum and neurogenic tumors, such as ganglioneuroma and neuroblastoma in the posterior mediastinum.

Masses arising from the chest wall include primitive neuroectodermal tumors (PNET), Ewing's tumor and rhabdomyosarcoma

5.5 Imaging of Different Tumor Types

5.5.1 Mediastinal and Chest Wall Tumors

5.5.1.1 Lymphoma

Lymphoma occurs with an incidence of about nine cases per million per annum in children under the age of 15 years, accounting for 6% of all childhood cancers. Hodgkin's lymphoma is slightly more common overall than non-Hodgkin's lymphoma (NHL), but under the age of 10 years and in very young children NHL is much more common. Both Hodgkin's and NHL involve the thorax, and lymphoma is the most common intrathoracic neoplasm in the pediatric age group [92] and as such is an important cause of mediastinal mass. Imaging is important for both diagnosis and management particularly for Hodgkin's lymphoma because therapy and prognosis are very dependent on the location and extent of disease [13, 15]. Diagnostic strategies and treatment approaches for these tumors are largely determined by protocols established by one of the large, multi-institutional cooperative groups and are frequently revised [92].

Clinical presentation may be nonspecific or acute with symptoms and signs of tracheal and superior vena cava obstruction from tumor (Fig. 5.7).

A chest radiograph should be performed on all patients and will demonstrate a mediastinal mass (Fig. 5.8) sometimes with a pleural effusion; a lateral film will confirm the location of the mass in the anterior mediastinum and is useful in the assessment of the airway which is compressed and displaced posteriorly [52, 63]. A US study can be performed to confirm the presence of a pleural effusion and may demonstrate pleural deposits, but is limited and further definitive imaging should be carried out with CT or MRI. A large mediastinal mass, with or without hilar lymphadenopathy and/or involvement of the thymus is usually demonstrated [42]. The airway can be visualized and tracheal compression assessed; this is of particular importance as problems may arise during anesthesia for biopsy, and if symptoms are severe a first cycle of chemotherapy may have to be given to shrink the mass before anesthesia and biopsy. Lung involvement also occurs. It is more common in Hodgkin's lymphoma, and is seen as infiltrates, an area of consolidation or nodules. A pericardial effusion may be present and is evidence of pericardial involvement.

In Hodgkin's lymphoma the presence or absence of disease at other sites must be determined; this is less important in NHL, which is considered to be a disseminated disease. Further imaging with MRI (or CT, if MRI is unavailable) of the abdomen and pelvis is necessary to look for enlarged lymph nodes and involvement of the liver and spleen. Unfortunately, CT is poor at detecting splenic involvement and the presence of splenomegaly on CT does not correlate well with the presence of disease. US scanning may also underestimate splenic involvement and gas in the bowel can interfere with visualization of lymph nodes on US studies. MRI may be the best modality for demonstrating the difference between normal splenic tissue and tumor. At the end of chemotherapy and radiotherapy most patients show no evidence of any residual tumor and surgery is not required.

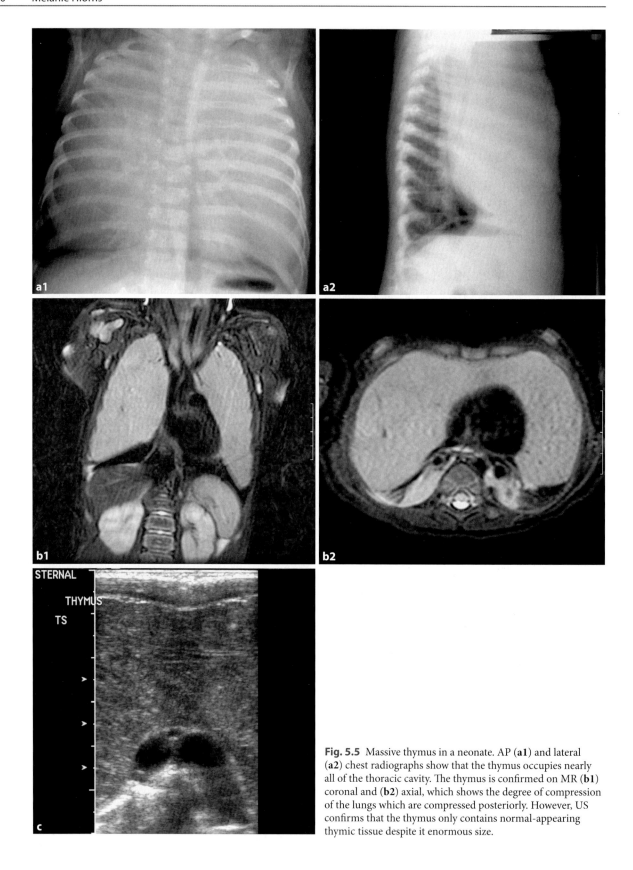

Fig. 5.5 Massive thymus in a neonate. AP (**a1**) and lateral (**a2**) chest radiographs show that the thymus occupies nearly all of the thoracic cavity. The thymus is confirmed on MR (**b1**) coronal and (**b2**) axial, which shows the degree of compression of the lungs which are compressed posteriorly. However, US confirms that the thymus only contains normal-appearing thymic tissue despite it enormous size.

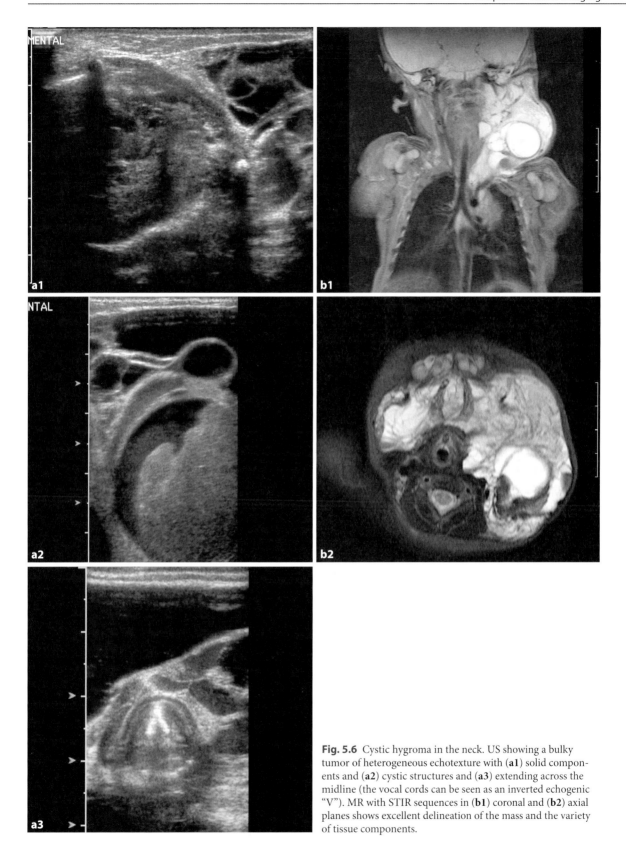

Fig. 5.6 Cystic hygroma in the neck. US showing a bulky tumor of heterogeneous echotexture with (**a1**) solid components and (**a2**) cystic structures and (**a3**) extending across the midline (the vocal cords can be seen as an inverted echogenic "V"). MR with STIR sequences in (**b1**) coronal and (**b2**) axial planes shows excellent delineation of the mass and the variety of tissue components.

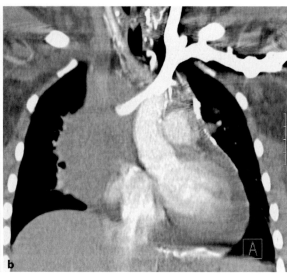

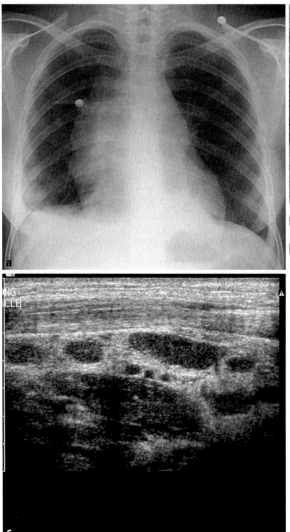

Fig. 5.7 Large B-cell lymphoma of the anterior mediastinum. (**a**) Chest radiograph showing the mass bulging out from the right of the mediastinum and an associated right-sided pleural effusion. (**b**) Coronal CT showing the right-sided mediastinal mass, which is obliterating the superior vena cava just as the left brachiocephalic vein enters; note the collateral drainage in the neck and over the pericardium. (**c**) US showing multiple lymph nodes also present in the neck.

However, in some cases, particularly Hodgkin's lymphoma, a residual mass remains in the mediastinum at the site of the original tumor. This may be due to residual active tumor, or a fibrotic mass, or sometimes cysts in the thymus following treatment [59, 60]. While surgery may be required, it is desirable to avoid this if possible and the yield may be low [87]. Imaging with T2-weighted, and T1-post-contrast sequences on MR has been suggested as a means of differentiating active tumor from fibrotic tissue, with tumor showing high signal intensity and fibrosis low signal intensity. However, results are inconclusive and may confuse areas of inflammation with tumor [91] and MR is likely to be superseded by PET for this particular indication.

The introduction of functional imaging modalities, such as PET scanning, provide the means to correlate tumor activity with anatomic features generated by CT and modify treatment based on tumor response. For centers with access to this modality, PET imaging now plays an important role in staging, evaluating tumor response, planning radiation treatment fields, and monitoring after completion of therapy for pediatric Hodgkin's lymphoma. This trend will likely increase in the future as a result of PET's superior sensitivity in correlating sites of tumor activity compared to other available functional imaging modalities. Ongoing prospective studies of PET in pediatric patients will increase understanding about the optimal use of this modality in children with cancer and define the characteristics of FDG-avid nonmalignant conditions that may be problematic in the interpretation of tumor activity [50]. The fusion of PET with CT provides the most accurate imaging method for disease

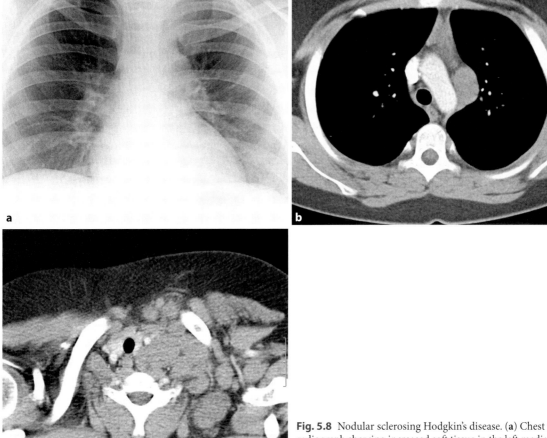

Fig. 5.8 Nodular sclerosing Hodgkin's disease. (**a**) Chest radiograph showing increased soft tissue in the left mediastinum in the region of the aortic knuckle. (**b**) CT confirms tumor lateral to the aortic arch where normally there should be no tissue. (**c**) CT in the neck shows extensive nodal disease, especially on the left side.

characterization and treatment response. Experience with 18F-FDG PET-CT is currently limited in pediatric Hodgkin's disease, but rapidly advancing, and the images must be interpreted with caution as numerous nononcologic processes can mimic recurrent or residual tumor, such as uptake in normal structures, infections, transforming germinal centers, and effects of therapy on normal tissues [54].

5.5.1.2 Teratoma

Mediastinal teratomas occur in the anterior mediastinum and are usually very large at presentation (Fig. 5.9). Imaging with a chest radiograph will demonstrate the mass, which may contain calcification. On further imaging with CT a large irregular and non-

homogeneous mass is seen, often but not necessarily with calcification, and with areas of low attenuation, which may be fat or necrosis and cysts. MRI can also be used to image the mass and will show the different tissue types in great detail and will show the extent of the mass. Initial treatment is by surgical excision and histological examination will determine whether the lesion is benign or malignant. If the tumor is malignant, a CT scan of the chest is required to search for lung nodules.

5.5.1.3 Neuroblastoma

Neurogenic tumors, both benign and malignant, occur in the posterior mediastinum. Neurogenic tumors may be discovered on a chest radiograph as an inci-

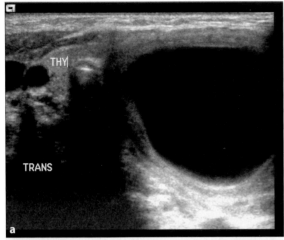

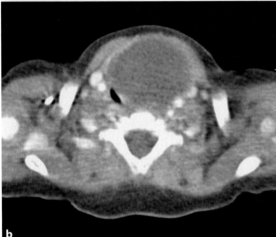

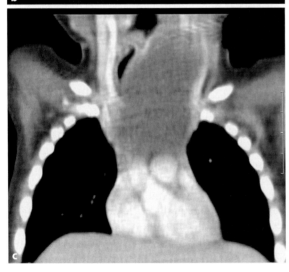

Fig. 5.9 Mature teratoma of the upper anterior mediastinum extending into the neck. (**a**) US of the neck showing a predominantly cystic lesion just lateral to the thyroid. (**b**) CT with contrast in the transverse plan showing displacement of the vessels of the neck and the low attenuation mass. (**c**) Coronal reconstruction of the CT shows the mass to be extending up out of the anterior mediastinum and displacing the vessels.

dental finding or present with signs of cord compression due to extension of tumor into the spinal canal. Imaging of the primary tumor is with CT or MR, although the latter is better at showing the true extent of the mass and its relationship to the ribs, intervertebral foramina, and the spinal canal. More extensive discussion of the imaging of neuroblastoma is covered later in this chapter.

5.5.1.4 Primitive Neuroectodermal Tumor

Primitive neuroectodermal tumors (PNETs) occur most frequently in the central nervous system but also occur in the bones and soft tissues. Histologically, they resemble neuroblastoma and Ewing's tumor. "Askins" tumors are PNETs arising from the chest wall [2].

PNET initial imaging with a chest radiograph will show a large mass often associated with a pleural effusion, rib destruction, and hilar and mediastinal lymphadenopathy. Further imaging with MR or CT is required to demonstrate the true extent of the tumor which may extend into the spinal canal, be closely applied to the heart, major blood vessels, the main bronchi, and be unresectable. Excellent images of these structures and their relationship to the tumor are provided by MR in the coronal plane. Metastatic disease occurs in the lungs and more rarely bones; therefore, a CT scan of the lungs and an isotope bone scan is necessary.

5.5.2 Osteogenic Sarcoma and Ewing's Tumors

Childhood osteogenic sarcoma and Ewing's sarcoma are by far the most common primary bone tumors, together accounting for over 80% of lesions.

Imaging studies are extremely important in identifying the primary site of tumors, providing the differential diagnosis, staging the tumor, and monitoring the response to therapy. As the radiological approach to both tumors is essentially similar, they will be dealt with together.

Most patients will present with symptoms of local pain, a history of trauma, or soft tissue swelling. A plain radiograph of the lesion is extremely important and should be performed in all cases. The characteristic appearances of a malignant tumor are of a poorly defined lesion, bone destruction associated with a periosteal reaction, and a soft tissue mass. Benign bone tumors demonstrate a well-defined margin or narrow zone of transition. Imaging may distinguish between an osteogenic sarcoma and Ewing's sarcoma because although both will have a periosteal reaction and bone destruction, an osteogenic sarcoma is much more likely to have a metaphyseal location with a significant periosteal reaction, and new bone formation and cortical destruction is present in almost all cases. Ewing's sarcoma may occur in both long and flat bones. In the long bones, the location is commonly in the diaphysis and classically the appearance is of a symmetrical lesion with permeative bone destruction, a laminated periosteal reaction, and a soft tissue mass. In the flat bones such as the scapula and the pelvis, the lesion is usually large with extensive bone destruction and a large soft tissue mass. Although crossectional imaging is crucial in demonstrating the extent of tumor and staging, establishing the diagnosis requires biopsy and histopathological examination.

Treatment is with chemotherapy and surgical resection with limb salvage if possible, or radiotherapy in cases of Ewing's sarcoma, usually where resection is not possible. It is therefore very important to accurately delineate the local extent of the tumor and its relationship to the adjacent soft tissues, including normal muscles, blood vessels, and nerves. MR is now the gold standard modality for assessing the true intraosseous and soft tissue extent of a lesion and should be performed early in the work-up of all bone tumors and be the main tool during treatment, at the end of chemotherapy prior to any surgical intervention and in long-term follow-up [10, 32, 45]. While it is true that CT may give a better impression of the bony destruction, it generally underestimates the extent of marrow involvement, and the main purpose of CT in current imaging strategies is for planning orthopedic surgery and/or reconstruction. Compared with CT scanning, MRI is superior in delineating both the soft tissue and bone marrow extent of the tumor [77, 79, 94]. Specific MRI protocols may differ in various tumor centers with preferences for T1-weighted sequences for marrow disease and T2-weighted sequences or T1-weighted sequences with intravenous contrast for soft tissue extent. Fat saturation and STIR sequences also add information. In particular there is some debate as to which is the most accurate way of determining the tumor margin and distinguishing it from adjacent edema. During treatment, MR appearances can be difficult to interpret because tumor necrosis may cause changes in the tumor signal with tissue shrinkage noted early in the treatment, thus giving the erroneous impression of tumor growth [27, 47].

The most common sites of metastatic disease are the lungs and skeleton, and CT scanning of the lungs and radioisotope scintigraphy with Tc99m-MDP is essential in all patients. In osteosarcoma, lung metastases may be calcified. Metastases can occur in other sites, the lymph nodes most commonly, but also the myocardium, pleura, inferior vena cava, kidneys, liver, and brain. If a potential tumor is to be biopsied, this should only be performed after discussion with the surgeon as it is critical that the biopsy be at a site that will subsequently be excised when the definitive surgery is carried out to avoid seeding of tumor and risk subsequent recurrence.

Other rare causes of thoracic masses include inflammatory lesions such as Castleman's syndrome and inflammatory pseudotumors, and other malignant tumors such as pleuropulmonary blastoma, rhabdomyosarcoma, and malignant thymoma. The lungs and the mediastinum are also sites of metastatic spread of tumors arising elsewhere.

Initial imaging of any thoracic lesion includes plain chest radiographs, followed by cross-sectional imaging with CT and/or MR. While CT with intravenous contrast enhancement provides excellent images of the mediastinum and chest wall, MR with the improved inherent soft tissue contrast and multiplanar imaging frequently provides more information about tumor extent and relationship to vital structures.

5.5.3 Musculoskeletal Masses

Primary tumors of the musculoskeletal system in childhood include osteogenic sarcoma, Ewing's tumor, and rhabdomyosarcoma and other soft tissue sarcomas [64]. Primary lymphoma of bone occurs, but only rarely in children. Benign bone tumors such as osteoid osteoma, osteoblastoma, aneurysmal bone cyst, and giant cell tumor are also less common.

Initial clinical presentation includes pain, swelling, and limitation of movement. There is frequently a history of previous trauma. Tumors are usually diagnosed on plain radiographs if they arise from the skeleton and further imaging with MR and nuclear scintographic scans which demonstrate both the local tumor extent and associated skip lesions. Primary soft tissue tumors may or may not show underlying bone erosion and MR scanning is necessary to delineate them. As MRI is highly sensitive to both neoplastic and inflammatory changes in the soft tissues it therefore may not differentiate between malignant and benign or inflammatory lesions, such as infection, post traumatic myositis ossificans, fibromatosis, hemangioma, and lymphangiomatosis. Definite diagnosis usually requires an open biopsy although there are a small number of soft tissue tumors with MR imaging appearances characteristic enough to allow a specific diagnosis, obviating the need for biopsy [84]. If a potential tumor is to be biopsied, this should only be performed after discussion with the surgeon, as it is critical that the biopsy be at a site that will subsequently be excised when the definitive surgery is carried out to avoid seeding of tumor and subsequent recurrence. Central tumors may present with less obvious clinical symptoms such as back pain or painful scoliosis, both

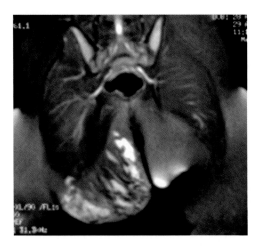

Fig. 5.10 Lymphangioma of the right buttock. MR coronal T2 image showing a heterogeneous lesion of high signal in the right buttock.

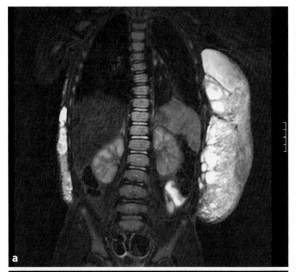

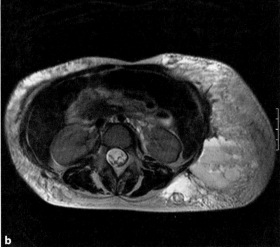

of which are uncommon in children and may be due to a primary tumor of the vertebral body. Pelvic pain is usually related to Ewing's sarcoma.

Other soft tissue masses include all the vascular malformations [arteriovenous malformation, hemangiomas, lymphangiomas (Fig. 5.10), hemangio-lymphangiomas and venous malformations]. Proteus syndrome presents with multiple hamartomatous soft tissue masses of varying size (Fig. 5.11). Lipoblastomatosis and other fatty tumors will also present with a mass lesion. All of these masses are best examined by a combination of US and MR.

5.5.4 Renal Tumors

5.5.4.1 Differential Diagnosis of Pediatric Renal Masses

With the identification of a renal mass Wilms' tumor will inevitably be considered, but a variety of pediatric renal masses may be differentiated from Wilms' tumor on the basis of their combined clinical and imaging features. Wilms' tumor is distinguished by vascular invasion and displacement of structures and is bilateral in approximately 10% of cases. Nephroblastomatosis occurs most often in neonates and is characterized by multiple bilateral subcapsular nodules, often synchronous with a Wilms' tumor. Renal cell carcinoma is unusual in children except in association with von Hippel-Lindau syndrome and typically occurs in the second decade. Mesoblastic nephroma should be a primary consideration in a neonate with a solid renal mass. Multilocular cystic nephroma is suggested by a large mass with multiple cysts and little solid tis-

Fig. 5.11 Proteus syndrome. (**a**) MR (coronal STIR) showing a large, partly pedunculated, soft tissue mass arising from the left lateral chest wall with a smaller component extending to the right side. (**b**) MR (T2-W) demonstrating the full extent of the mass as it wraps around the abdominal wall.

sue. Clear cell sarcoma is distinguished by frequent lung and skeletal metastases, and rhabdoid tumor (Fig. 5.12) is distinguished by its association with brain neoplasms. Angiomyolipoma frequently contains fat and is associated with tuberous sclerosis. Renal medullary carcinoma occurs in patients with sickle cell trait or hemoglobin SC disease and manifests as an infiltrative mass with metastases. Ossifying renal tumor in infancy is differentiated from mesoblastic nephroma by the presence of ossified elements. Metanephric adenoma lacks specific features but is always well defined. Renal lymphoma is characterized by multiple homogeneous masses, often with associated adenopathy [12, 33, 62].

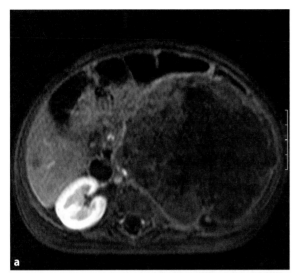

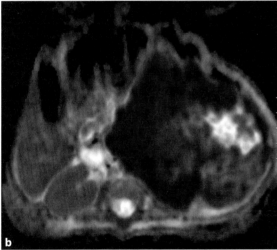

Fig. 5.12 Rhabdoid tumor of the kidney. (**a**) A large left-sided rhabdoid tumor on contrast enhanced T1-W MR, with normal enhancement in the contralateral kidney. Note the associated liver metastasis. (**b**) An ADC map of the same tumor showing that most of the tumor returns low signal, indicating that it is of dense cellularity. Some of the tumor returns a higher signal, indicating that there is more water diffusion between cells and that necrosis may be occurring in these areas.

5.5.4.2 Nephroblastoma (Wilms' Tumor)

Wilms' tumor is the most common malignant renal tumor of children, accounting for 5–6% of childhood cancers in the USA. The survival rate of children with Wilms' tumor has improved dramatically, partly due to large multicenter studies conducted by the National Wilms' Tumor Study Group (NWTSG) and the International Society of Pediatric Oncology [4]. As a result, much of the imaging in Wilms' tumor is now protocol driven and many children participate in large ongoing trials. The initial detection of a renal mass will most commonly be by US, but imaging will usually include MR or CT. Although there is increasing use of MR, CT is still favored by some surgeons for surgical planning.

US characteristically demonstrates a large mass arising from the kidney with or without echolucent lakes [18, 22, 39]. Both CT and MRI demonstrate an intrinsic renal mass with medial distortion of the collecting system which does not enhance, or only minimally, with intravenous contrast medium [30, 73]. Associated pararenal and para-aortic lymphadenopathy may be demonstrated, but may be reactive to, rather than because of, malignant involvement which must be proven by biopsy. Caval thrombosis occurs, and can extend up into the right atrium, and can be demonstrated with US (including transesophageal US), CT, or MRI. IVC thrombus may be difficult to evaluate in the presence of a large right-sided renal mass and should be sought for and excluded with care (Fig. 5.13) [74]. Thrombus confined to the renal vein is difficult to demonstrate reliably but fortunately does not present a major surgical hazard. Direct extension of a right-sided Wilms' tumor into the liver occurs and can be assessed with US, CT, or MRI.

Bilateral Wilms' tumors occur in 5–10% of cases (Fig. 5.14) and present at a younger age than unilateral tumors [8]. The ability of imaging to demonstrate small contralateral lesions is now such that direct manual examination of the contralateral kidney at surgery is unnecessary. CT or MRI are reliable and more accurate than US. Bilateral lesions associated with nephroblastomatosis may not be malignant, and there is some evidence that imaging is useful in determining the need for excision of these lesions, particularly after chemotherapy [38]. Wilms' tumor occurring in a horseshoe kidney is also well recognized [88] (Fig. 5.15), and the presence of a horseshoe kidney confers a slightly increased risk. Imaging will be especially challenging to delineate the extent of the tumor(s) and the vascular supply both to tumor and the kidney overall. In these complicated cases a combination of MR and either CT angiography or conventional angiography will be necessary.

Lung metastases from Wilms' tumor may be detected on plain chest radiograph but CT scanning with its improved resolution is the most sensitive to detect the presence of pulmonary metastases (Fig. 5.16) [15, 23, 93].

The local recurrence rate of Wilms' tumor is low, and following surgery and chemotherapy follow-up with abdominal US and chest radiographs is sufficient. If there is a high risk of recurrence or findings on routine imaging are suspicious, then further investigation with CT and/or MRI is recommended.

Unusual histological variants of Wilms' tumor (considered to be different entities by some investiga-

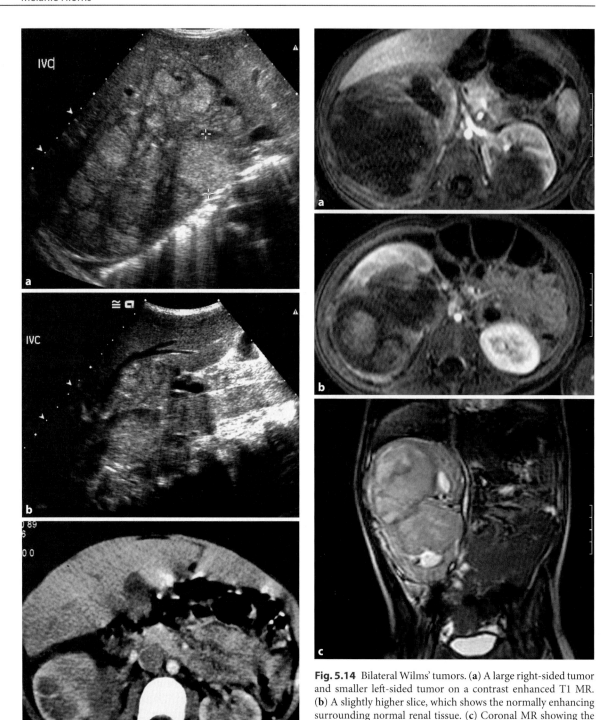

Fig. 5.14 Bilateral Wilms' tumors. (**a**) A large right-sided tumor and smaller left-sided tumor on a contrast enhanced T1 MR. (**b**) A slightly higher slice, which shows the normally enhancing surrounding normal renal tissue. (**c**) Coronal MR showing the coronal extent of the right-sided tumor and deviation of IVC (STIR sequence).

Fig. 5.13 Wilms' tumor with thrombus in the inferior vena cava. (**a**) A large right-sided Wilms' tumor is shown on US in transverse section, with thrombus completely filling the IVC (as shown by the *markers*). (**b**) Longitudinal section on US shows the thrombus to extend up into the base of the right atrium. (**c**) CT shows that thrombus fills the IVC and the right renal vein.

tors) include the sarcomatous type, which frequently metastasizes to the skeleton and therefore requires isotope bone scanning, and the rhabdoid type, which metastasizes to the central nervous system and requires CT or MRI of the brain [85].

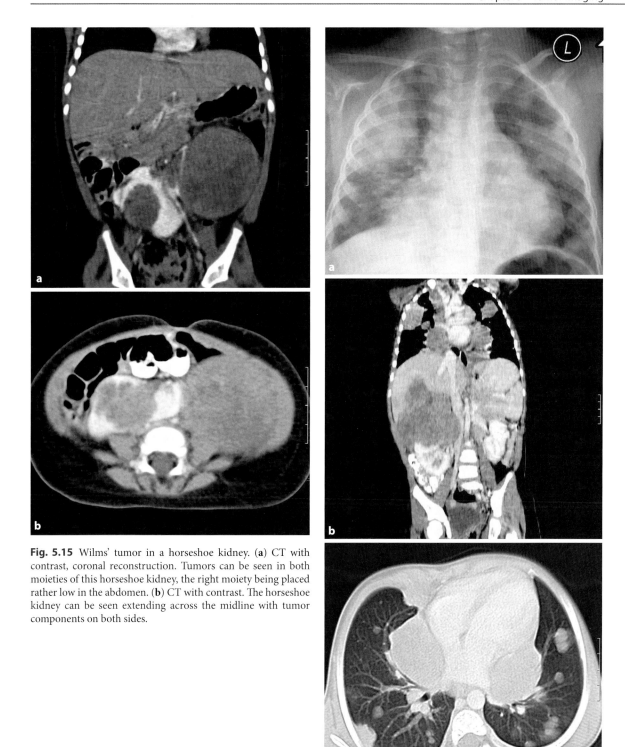

Fig. 5.15 Wilms' tumor in a horseshoe kidney. (**a**) CT with contrast, coronal reconstruction. Tumors can be seen in both moieties of this horseshoe kidney, the right moiety being placed rather low in the abdomen. (**b**) CT with contrast. The horseshoe kidney can be seen extending across the midline with tumor components on both sides.

Fig. 5.16 Lung metastases in Wilms' tumor. (**a**) Chest radiograph showing extensive lung metastases. (**b**) CT demonstrates the extent of the lung metastases and the right-sided Wilms' tumor. (**c**) Lung metastases are best demonstrated on chest CT with dedicated lung windowing.

Patients who are at increased risk of developing a Wilms' tumor require screening. Genitourinary anomalies Denys-Drash syndrome, sporadic aniridia, Beckwith-Wiedemann syndrome, Perlman's syndrome, and hemihypertrophy are anomalies with an increased incidence of Wilms' tumor [31]. Screening is accomplished with regular, 3- or 6-monthly abdominal US examinations.

Genitourinary anomalies are common; however, the incidence of Wilms' tumor in these patients is low. Similarly, true hemihypertrophy is rare and only 3% of these children develop Wilms' tumors. Regular screening in these children may not be cost-effective. However, patients with sporadic aniridia have a 33% risk of developing Wilms' tumor and those with Beckwith-Wiedemann syndrome have a 5–7% risk of developing a tumor, and therefore some centers advocate regular screening with US until the child is 5–10 years of age [3].

There is a divergence in the staging and treatment strategy of Wilms' tumor between North America and Europe. The staging of Wilms' tumor is discussed in Chap. 10. Current practice in North America is that the tumor is first surgically removed and histology of the resection specimen is obtained, followed by chemotherapy. If the tumor is inoperable, it is biopsied at the time of surgery and upstaged to Stage 3.

In Europe it is current practice to biopsy the tumor to establish the tumor type and then to give appropriate chemotherapy before surgery at a later stage. Staging is then at surgery unless imaging shows distant metastases, which indicates that the disease is already Stage IV.

5.5.4.3 Screening for Wilms' Tumor in Children with Beckwith-Wiedemann Syndrome

Wilms' tumor is the most common cancer in children with Beckwith-Wiedemann Syndrome (BWS), occurring in about 5–7% of all children with BWS. Most children develop Wilms tumor prior to their fourth birthday; however, children with BWS can develop Wilms tumor at up to 7 or 8 years of age. By 8 years of age 95% of all Wilms tumor have occurred.

The length of screening interval for US examination is still being established; however, screening by US at intervals of 3 months until the child's seventh birthday

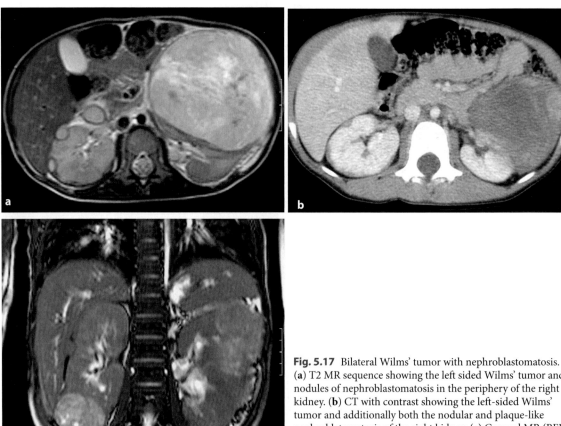

Fig. 5.17 Bilateral Wilms' tumor with nephroblastomatosis. (**a**) T2 MR sequence showing the left sided Wilms' tumor and nodules of nephroblastomatosis in the periphery of the right kidney. (**b**) CT with contrast showing the left-sided Wilms' tumor and additionally both the nodular and plaque-like nephroblatomatosis of the right kidney. (**c**) Coronal MR (BFFE sequence) showing the difference in signal between the Wilms' tumor in the lower pole of the right kidney and the nodule of nephroblastomatosis on the lateral margin of the right kidney. Part of the left-sided tumor can also be seen.

is current practice in many leading centers and is likely to become the established guideline [14, 24, 25, 66].

5.5.4.4 Nephroblastomatosis

Nephroblastomatasis represents persisting nephrogenic rests of fetal renal tissue. Nephrogenic rests are found in approximately 1% of infant kidneys at autopsy and are associated with an increased risk of Wilms' tumor, presumed secondary to neoplastic change. Nephrogenic rests are associated with many syndromes including Beckwith-Wiedemann syndrome, hemihypertrophy, and sporadic aniridia. Children with identifiable syndromes, once diagnosed, should

be screened (usually by US) for the development of Wilms' tumor. Nephrogenic rests are also linked with other lesions such as multilocular cystic nephroma and multicystic dysplasia, usually without malignant complications [61]. Nephroblastomatosis commonly presents as multinodular, peripheral, cortical lesions (Fig. 5.17); the diffuse form of distribution being less common (Fig. 5.18). Foci are usually homogeneous and of low echogenicity, density, or signal intensity. US is the first line examination, but MR is the examination of choice due to its excellent tissue contrast. The lesions can be depicted with contrast-enhanced CT, but T1- and T2-weighted (T1-W, T2-W) MR images are superior. Lesions smaller than 1 cm are rarely identified by US. The most reliable criterion to dif-

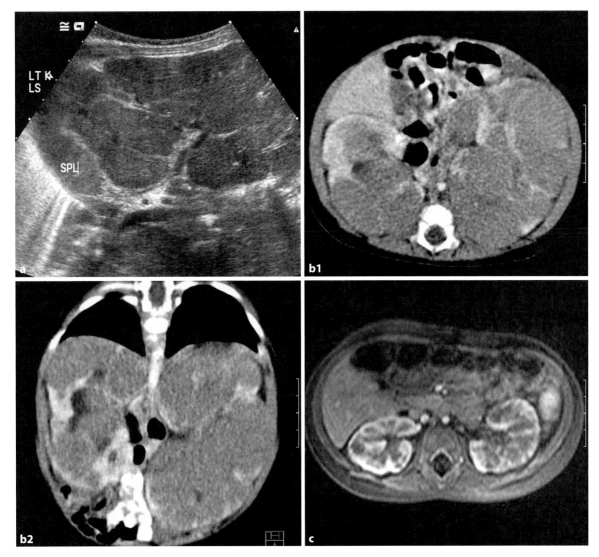

Fig. 5.18 Nephroblastomatosis. (**a**) US showing a diffusely enlarged and infiltrated left kidney, displacing the spleen superiorly. (**b**) Contrast-enhanced CT showing that both kidneys are diffusely affected and occupy much of the abdomen (**b1**) axial and (**b2**) coronal planes. (**c**) MRI with contrast enhancement showing the dramatic reduction in size following treatment.

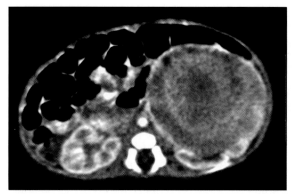

Fig. 5.19 Mesoblastic nephroma. A large left-renal tumor is demonstrated on CT scan of kidneys in this 2-day-old infant. Nephrectomy confirmed mesoblastic nephroma.

ferentiate nephroblastomatosis from Wilms' tumor is their homogeneity. Due to the significant radiation dose of serial CT, MR imaging should be the method of choice wherever it is available. The cost-effectiveness and availability of US makes it ideal for serial follow-up of known lesions.

5.5.4.5 Mesoblastic Nephroma

This renal tumor (Fig. 5.19) is the most common localized renal tumor in the infant under 12 months of age. It is histologically benign, although rare cases with metastases have been described and treatment is with surgical resection alone. Imaging is the same as for Wilms' tumor. Routine postoperative imaging is unnecessary.

5.5.4.6 Others

Other rare causes of renal tumors include renal cell carcinoma, malignant mesenchymal sarcoma, (a malignant form of mesoblastic nephroma), renal lymphoma, angiomyolipoma, and multilocular cystic nephroma. The imaging strategy is essentially the same as for Wilms' tumor. Useful diagnostic features include bilateral involvement with node or other organ involvement in lymphoma; the highly vascular, cystic, and fat components in angiomyolipoma; and the predominantly cystic nature of the multilocular cystic nephroma. Intrarenal neuroblastoma has been described and can be confirmed with urine catecholamine measurements. Infective lesions occasionally present as a renal mass and must be excluded on imaging. Acute infection, with or without abscess formation, may present as a lump on US, which does not enhance following intravenous contrast medium on CT, with a wedge-like, or cystic appearance. Chronic infective lesions such as xanthogranulomatous pyelonephritis are rare in childhood and characteristically give bizarre reniform masses with calculi and perinephric fluid collections. Perinephric inflammatory changes are an important imaging indicator of infection rather than neoplasia.

5.5.5 Neuroblastoma

Neuroblastoma is the most common extracranial pediatric solid tumor and may occur in a number of sites, with most (60%) arising in the abdomen (Fig. 5.20); 20% in the chest (Fig. 5.21), predominantly the posterior mediastinum; and then more rarely in the neck and pelvis (Fig. 5.22). This embryonal neoplasm often encases vascular structures (Fig. 5.23) and, unlike most solid cancers, usually presents with substantial metastatic disease (bone, bone marrow, lymph nodes, liver; spread to lung or brain is rare) and as a result requires a multitude of imaging studies to fully assess the extent of disease at presentation (Fig. 5.24) [57]. Hence, the role of radiological imaging is to assist in making the diagnosis, to demonstrate the extent of the disease, and to demonstrate or exclude the presence of metastases [9, 56].

If the tumor presents in the abdomen, US, CT, and MR scans will all demonstrate a large, irregular, and poorly defined solid mass arising from the suprarenal area or the paravertebral region [5, 11]. However, there is a growing body of literature supporting the use of MRI as the technique of choice for the evaluation of local and regional disease in children with suspected neuroblastoma [67]. The mass frequently crosses the midline and may extend into the spinal canal, and both displace and encase the aorta and inferior vena cava. The ipsilateral kidney is displaced laterally and inferiorly. Rarely, the tumor may extend into the kidney or encase the renal hilum, so that when tumor resection is attempted a nephrectomy may be required. The staging of neuroblastoma is discussed in Chap. 11. Smaller tumors (stage I and II) are often more clearly defined and do not extend beyond the vertebral bodies. Calcification is often present within the mass and may be more obvious after treatment with chemotherapy.

Neuroblastoma arising in the thorax will be seen on the chest radiograph as a posterior mediastinal mass. Displacement and erosion of the posterior ribs and vertebral bodies may be observed with extension into the spinal canal. Both CT and MR are able to demonstrate the tumor, although MR is the imaging method of choice to demonstrate disease in the spinal canal (Fig. 5.25) [26, 82].

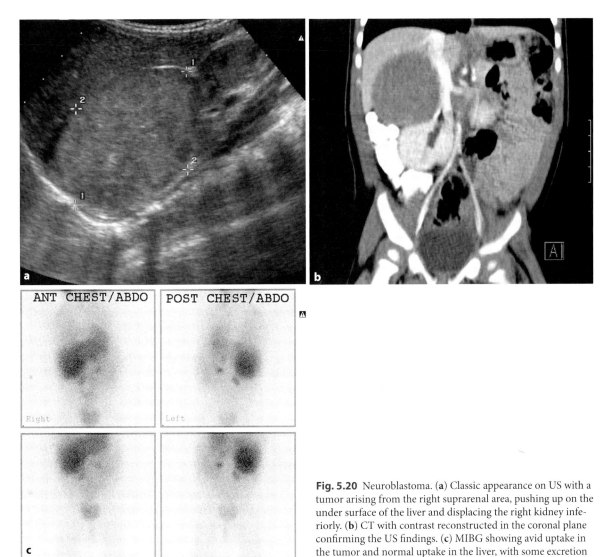

Fig. 5.20 Neuroblastoma. (**a**) Classic appearance on US with a tumor arising from the right suprarenal area, pushing up on the under surface of the liver and displacing the right kidney inferiorly. (**b**) CT with contrast reconstructed in the coronal plane confirming the US findings. (**c**) MIBG showing avid uptake in the tumor and normal uptake in the liver, with some excretion in the collecting systems of both kidneys.

Metastases occur most frequently in the bone and bone marrow. These are detected with 99mTc-MDP isotope bone scanning and (iodine) I[123]-MIBG scanning; MDP bone scanning is a highly sensitive but nonspecific means of detection of bone metastases; MIBG scanning is specific as the isotope is taken up by neurosecretory granules in the neuroblastoma cells. Although this would appear to be the isotope of choice in this tumor, some tumors do not take up MIBG, and the role of the two investigations remains complementary in many institutions [35, 48].

Hence the core imaging in neuroblastoma is an AP chest radiograph, abdominal US, and MRI (or CT if unavailable) of the primary tumor, and isotope scanning using I[123] or preferably I[131] MIBG, supplemented by 99mTcMDP scintigraphy if the MIBG study is ne-

gative. In the high-risk groups follow-up will include repeat MIBG scans which are not required in the standard risk groups.

5.5.6 Adrenocortical Tumors

Clinical manifestations of endocrine abnormalities are common in adrenal cortical tumors and patients who present with Cushing's syndrome, virilization, and others. The distinction between benign and malignant tumors is based primarily on size and the presence of associated lymphadenopathy and metastases. Radiologically, tumors are usually well defined and, if measuring less than 4–6 cm in diameter, are benign, unless there is other evidence such as metas-

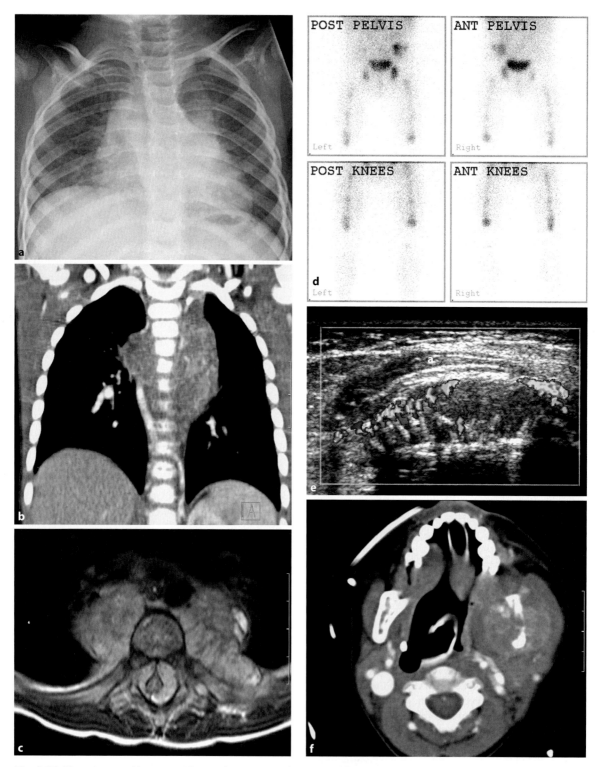

Fig. 5.21 Thoracic neuroblastoma with spinal invasion and mandibular metastasis. (**a**) Chest radiograph showing diffuse widening of the mediastinum and increased soft tissue density in the midline. (**b**) CT with contrast in a coronal reconstruction with tumor seen on both sides of the thoracic spine. (**c**) MR of the spine showing tumor invasion by the primary tumor of the spinal canal bilaterally with the spinal cord compressed in the center. (**d**) MIBG with extensive areas of increased uptake consistent with metastases. (**e**) US of the mandible with an expanding soft tissue mass erupting from the bone, the "sunray" linear echoes represent an intense periosteal reaction. (**f**) CT confirms a destructive lesion in the left mandible with an associated soft tissue mass representing a neuroblastoma deposit.

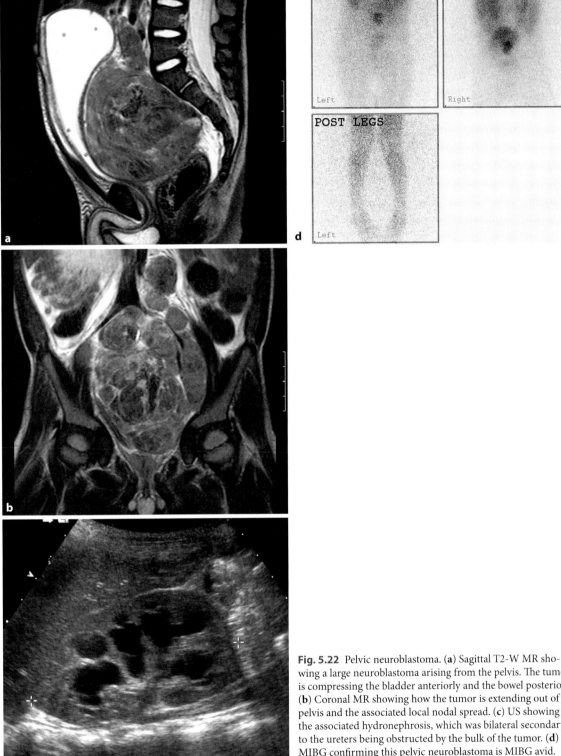

Fig. 5.22 Pelvic neuroblastoma. (**a**) Sagittal T2-W MR showing a large neuroblastoma arising from the pelvis. The tumor
is compressing the bladder anteriorly and the bowel posteriorly.
(**b**) Coronal MR showing how the tumor is extending out of the
pelvis and the associated local nodal spread. (**c**) US showing
the associated hydronephrosis, which was bilateral secondary
to the ureters being obstructed by the bulk of the tumor. (**d**)
MIBG confirming this pelvic neuroblastoma is MIBG avid.
The increased activity superimposed over the tumor represent
isotopes being excreted in the bladder.

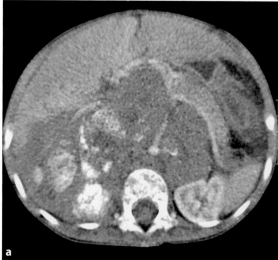

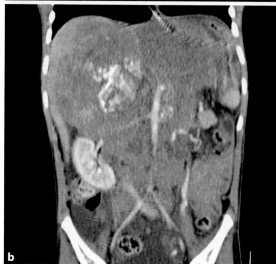

Fig. 5.23 (a) CT in an infant with neuroblastoma. The tumor extends throughout the retroperitoneum and characteristically engulfs vessels and pushes them anteriorly. (b) Coronal reformats showing the tumor has probably arisen from the right suprarenal area and contains typical scattered calcification. The renal arteries are stretched by the mass effect of the tumor.

tases or lymphadenopathy. Characteristically, the tumors are identified by CT scanning, do not enhance following contrast medium injection, and are well defined.

5.5.7 Hemangioma

These usually present in young infants, often in the neonatal period, and may be solitary or diffuse, and are also known as hemangioendothelioma. Clinical

presentation is with an abdominal mass, which may be complicated by cardiac failure, a consumptive coagulopathy (Kasabach-Merritt syndrome) with thrombocytopenia, and hemoperitoneum. The natural history is spontaneous regression, provided the child does not succumb to the complications of the disease. US with Doppler color flow will demonstrate the mass and hypervascularity with dilated hepatic veins and an enlarged hepatic artery [1]. Use of CT demonstrates single or multiple lesions which enhance intensely and peripherally with intravenous contrast medium. This is unlike hepatoblastoma and hepatocellular carcinoma, which do not enhance. However, gadolinium-enhanced MR will also show these lesions with great sensitivity and specificity and is now the imaging modality of choice.

5.5.8 Abdominal B-cell Lymphoma

Lymphoma with involvement of the bowel and mesentery is almost always caused by non-Hodgkin's lymphoma (B-cell origin).

Clinical presentation is varied including diarrhea, weight loss, and intussusception. Plain abdominal radiographs are nonspecific and most commonly show dilated loops of intestine or bowel obstruction. Abdominal CT is probably more accurate than US in achieving a diagnosis, but both studies will show nodular mass lesions, lumen narrowing, focal aneurysmal bowel dilatation, and ascites. On US the mass lesions may be homogeneously hypoechoic. The CT scanning should be carried out after administration of oral contrast medium, and a characteristic appearance of contrast-filled loops of bowel, trapped and encased by large soft tissue masses, is seen. Involvement of the peritoneum and omentum occurs, and CT will show omental cakes lying between the bowel and the anterior abdominal wall, with loss of normal fat planes [83] (Fig. 5.26). If the child presents with nonspecific gastrointestinal symptoms, a barium follow-through may be performed. This will demonstrate bowel dilatation and narrowing with mucosal irregularity, bowel wall thickening, and separation of bowel loops [36] (Fig. 5.27).

Lymphoma may also occur within the liver and spleen and as a nodular infiltrate in the pancreas and both kidneys [80]. Para-aortic lymphadenopathy may also be demonstrated on CT.

5.5.9 Rhabdomyosarcoma

Rhabdomyosarcoma is the most common soft-tissue malignancy in childhood [41], accounting for over 50% of all pediatric soft tissue sarcomas and repre-

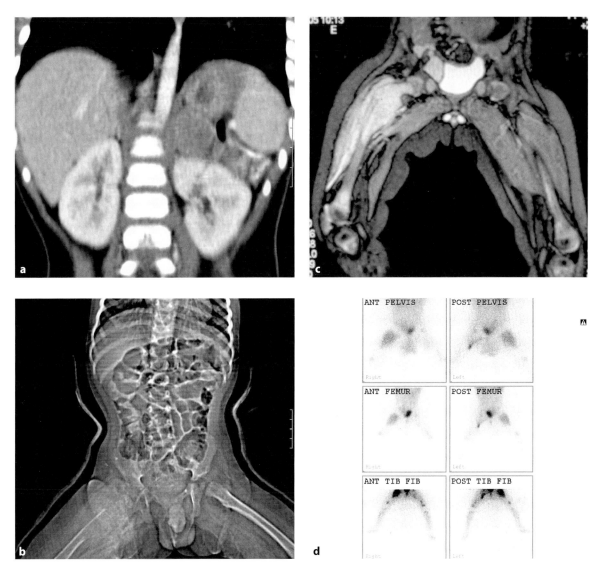

Fig. 5.24 Metastatic neuroblastoma in a child presenting with a femoral fracture. (**a**) CT shows a left suprarenal neuroblastoma displacing the left kidney. (**b**) The topogram for the CT shows the destroyed upper-right femur secondary to metastatic disease and which was associated with a soft tissue mass. (**c**) MR shows the full extent of the upper-right femoral metastatic disease. (**d**) MIBG shows further deposits scattered through both femurs.

senting 4–8% of malignant solid tumors in children, ranking behind CNS tumors, lymphoma, neuroblastoma, and Wilms' tumor. Rhabdomyosarcoma can be found in virtually any organ or tissue in the body including the musculoskeletal system. Diagnostic imaging is important and imaging protocols vary depending on the anatomical location of the primary tumor. The three most common locations in descending order of frequency are the head and neck (Fig. 5.28), the genitourinary system (Fig. 5.29), and the extremities [72]. Rhabdomyosarcoma also occurs in the biliary tree, the chest, and retroperitoneum.

Plain radiographs are of limited value in imaging the primary tumor unless there is destruction and erosion of the adjacent bone which can occur with both extremity and head and neck tumors. Cross-sectional imaging with MR and/or CT is always required. Ideally, first locoregional evaluation should be made with MRI, but CT is acceptable if MRI is not available. MRI is preferable for most locations, other than the chest, including head and neck tumors with possible skull base invasion. MRI is mandatory for genitourinary primaries and paraspinal tumors. CT is occasionally useful for assessing subtle bone destruction, but

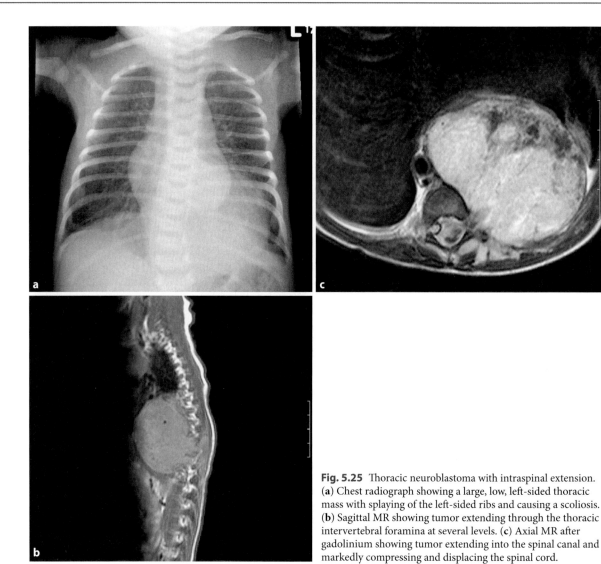

Fig. 5.25 Thoracic neuroblastoma with intraspinal extension. (**a**) Chest radiograph showing a large, low, left-sided thoracic mass with splaying of the left-sided ribs and causing a scoliosis. (**b**) Sagittal MR showing tumor extending through the thoracic intervertebral foramina at several levels. (**c**) Axial MR after gadolinium showing tumor extending into the spinal canal and markedly compressing and displacing the spinal cord.

MRI is sufficient for most head and neck lesions. US is especially useful as an adjunct for genitourinary and biliary tumors.

On CT, rhabdomyosarcoma has a soft tissue attenuation and can be difficult to distinguish from adjacent soft tissues, particularly in the extremities and head and neck, unless intravenous contrast medium is given, and even with contrast CT remains inferior to MRI. Calcification is rare and should suggest an alternative diagnosis. Enhancement is variable and non-homogeneous, and the margins of the tumor are irregular and poorly defined. Use of MRI is significantly better than CT in demonstrating the soft tissue mass, and while lesions are of soft tissue signal intensity on T1-weighted sequences, they are of high signal inten-

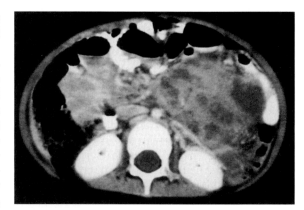

Fig. 5.26 Burkitt's lymphoma. CT scan of mid-abdomen shows soft tissue mesenteric mass is displacing colon anteriorly.

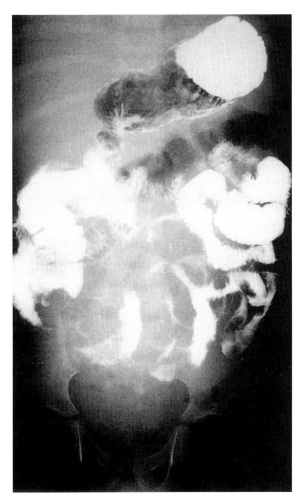

Fig. 5.27 Gastrointestinal lymphoma in a 4-year-old boy with marked weight loss, abdominal pain, and anemia. Barium follow-through examination shows narrowing of distal ileum with bowel wall thickening and separation of bowel loops.

sity on T2-weighted sequences and can therefore be more easily distinguished from adjacent muscle and soft tissue. The tumors can both encase and displace blood vessels and extend into the spinal canal and intracranial fossa either by destruction of the skull base and bone or through the intervertebral and cranial foramina. For showing subtle bone destruction, CT is better than MRI – therefore both CT and MRI are important in these cases [28, 58].

CT of the thorax is mandatory in all patients with rhabdomyosarcoma to assess the presence of lung metastases, and under current protocols most centers also require PA and lateral chest radiographs. Defining pulmonary spread of tumor is critical to staging, although differentiation between metastatic and benign nodules (such as granulomatous disease, hamartomas, intrapulmonary lymph nodes, etc.) can be impossible. One pulmonary/pleural nodule of 1 cm or lesions > 5mm in more than one site should be considered evidence of metastases, provided there is no other clinical explanation for the lesions [37, 71, 81] .A radionuclide bone scan (with plain radiographs and/or MRI of any isolated abnormal site) is mandatory in all patients at diagnosis. Lower limb tumors require evaluation of pelvic lymph nodes by CT/MRI even if femoral nodes are clinically/

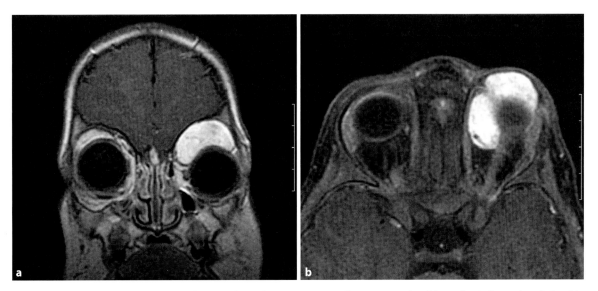

Fig. 5.28 Orbital rhabdomyosarcoma. (**a**) Coronal MR showing a mass in the superior orbit. (**b**) Axial MR shows the relationship to the optic nerve, which is displaced superiorly.

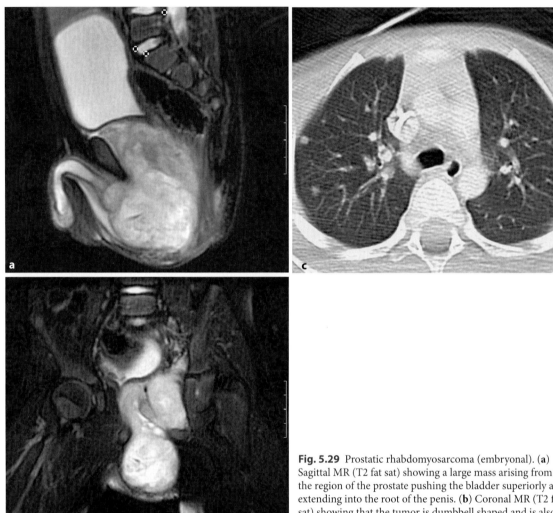

Fig. 5.29 Prostatic rhabdomyosarcoma (embryonal). (**a**) Sagittal MR (T2 fat sat) showing a large mass arising from the region of the prostate pushing the bladder superiorly and extending into the root of the penis. (**b**) Coronal MR (T2 fat sat) showing that the tumor is dumbbell shaped and is also extending inferiorly into the perineum. (**c**) CT with associated lung metastases seen as nodule in the right lung.

radiologically (including US) normal. Upper and lower limb tumors would normally have surgical evaluation of axillary or inguinal nodes, respectively, even if nodes are clinically/radiologically normal.

5.5.10 Liver Tumors

Liver tumors are relatively rare in childhood, representing 1–2% of all tumors. Two thirds of these tumors are malignant [40]. The clinical presentation is usually abdominal enlargement due to an abdominal mass, with associated pain, fever, pallor, anemia, and rarely jaundice or heart failure may occur. Imaging may be critical in distinguishing between benign and malignant tumors [6, 7]. The differential diagnosis of a malignant liver mass in children includes hepatoblastoma, undifferentiated (embryonal) sarcoma, and rarely hepatocellular cancer, and of a benign mass hemangioma, infantile hemangioendothelioma (Fig. 5.30), mesenchymal hamartoma (a benign cystic lesion), focal nodular hyperplasia, adenomas, and germ cell tumors (benign or malignant) [40].

5.5.10.1 Hepatoblastoma

This is the most common primary hepatic malignancy of childhood, although it is quite rare, accounting for only 0.9% of all pediatric cancers [68]. It usually occurs in children younger than 3 years of age. The prognosis is poorest in the neonate. It has been associated

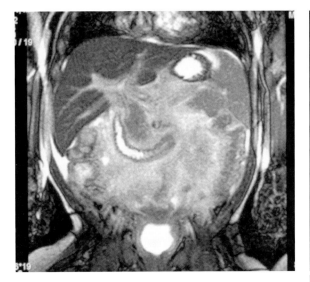

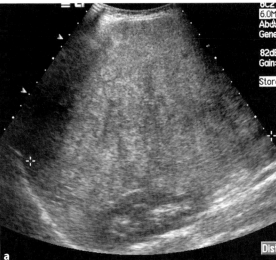

Fig. 5.30 Hemangioendothelioma of the liver. MR in a coronal plane shows the very extensive tumor arising from the liver and extending out to occupy much of the abdomen. A central loop of bowel has been engulfed by the mass.

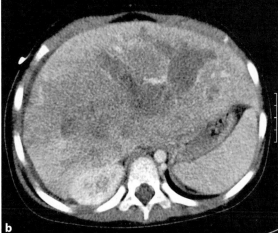

with Beckwith-Wiedemann syndrome, APC mutations (which occur in familial adenomatosis polypi), and low birth weight [43].

Hepatoblastoma is most frequently located in the right lobe of the liver (approximately 50%), but may be in the left lobe or be centrally located, and may be unifocal or multifocal. US imaging is the initial investigation of choice and will demonstrate a solid mass of variable echogenicity sometimes with thrombosis of the portal or hepatic vein branches [21]. Thrombus in the inferior vena cava is also recognized. Calcification is often present. Both CT and MRI will demonstrate the anatomy and the extent of the tumor in more detail (Fig. 5.31). In order to plan for surgical excision it is necessary to delineate the hepatic veins and the segmental anatomy; while this can be shown on CT,

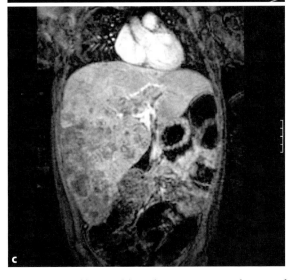

Fig. 5.31 Hepatoblastoma. (**a**) US shows extensive involvement of the liver, which is enlarged. (**b**) CT shows a diffuse infiltrative pattern. (**c**) Coronal MR (T1-weighted post contrast) showing the extent of liver enlargement. Much of the left lobe is unaffected.

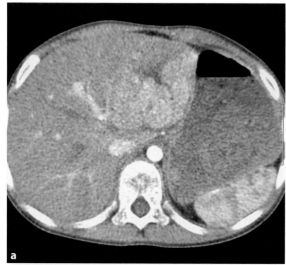

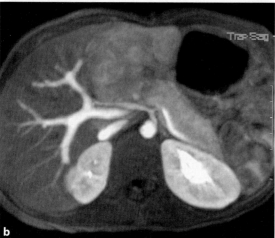

Fig. 5.32 Hepatoblastoma. (**a**) CT of hepatoblastoma showing the tumor but not clarifying its relationship to the hepatic vessels, which is essential for staging. (**b**) MR in the same patient with a maximum intensity projection (MIP). This reconstruction technique allows the "sandwiching" together of several slices to give a better overall impression of the anatomy. The relationship of the tumor to the hepatic artery and portal vessels can now be clearly delineated.

MRI is considered to be more accurate (Fig. 5.32) [29]. The exact delineation of the extent of the tumor and the number and location of liver segments involved is crucial for surgical planning and management (Fig. 5.33) [19, 20] and especially in children who are treated according to the protocols of the International Childhood Liver Tumor Strategy Group (SIOPEL) [75]. Extrahepatic disease may also be demonstrated on CT or MRI.

CT of the chest is also necessary to exclude the presence of pulmonary metastases. Following treatment with preoperative chemotherapy imaging is essential

prior to surgical resection in order to assess tumor resectability. In addition to the imaging already described, most units have replaced conventional angiography with MRA. Angiography is occasionally helpful for planning complicated surgery, or for hepatic artery chemoembolization.

Follow-up of hepatoblastoma is by MRI, but interpretation can be difficult. It is possible that FDG-PET (and/or PET CT) may have an important role to play in the assessment of recurrence in the near future [70]. Scintigraphy with 99mTc-labeled monoclonal anti-AFP has been proposed as a method of staging children with hepatoblastoma, but the clinical usefulness of this technique is not yet known [53].

5.5.10.2 Hepatocellular Carcinoma

Hepatocellular carcinoma is less common than hepatoblastoma and usually occurs in the second decade and in children with chronic liver disease, such as cirrhosis secondary to diseases like biliary atresia, Byler's disease, and tyrosinemia. It is more often multifocal and invasive when compared with hepatoblastoma with evidence of tumor thrombi in main hepatic veins and portal veins. Imaging and preoperative work-up is the same as quoted for hepatoblastoma with more emphasis on the portal and venous systems, which often require careful US examination and Doppler scanning.

Metastatic spread is to the lungs primarily but other sites are involved depending on the primary site. Scanning of the lung by CT is essential; bone marrow metastases are usually detected by bone marrow aspirates or trephines, and liver or lymph node spread is imaged with CT or MR.

Response to therapy is assessed with repeat cross-sectional imaging and reduction in tumor size; timing is controversial with some debate about the most optimal time, as some rhabdomyosarcomas are relatively slow to shrink initially but demonstrate a good response eventually. At the end of chemotherapy, small residual masses at the primary site may remain surgically inaccessible, e.g., in the orbit or bladder. Imaging and histology may find it difficult to establish definite evidence of residual viable tumor and in some instances conservative surgery with vigilant postoperative follow-up is useful. This requires full imaging of the primary site with MR and/or CT.

Rhabdomyosarcoma of the liver is rare and arises in the major biliary ducts. The tumor has a botyroid appearance and causes biliary duct dilatation, resulting in a characteristic clinical presentation of jaundice and an abdominal mass. If the tumor arises in the distal biliary ducts, it is indistinguishable from other primary tumors of the liver. Imaging is with a combination of

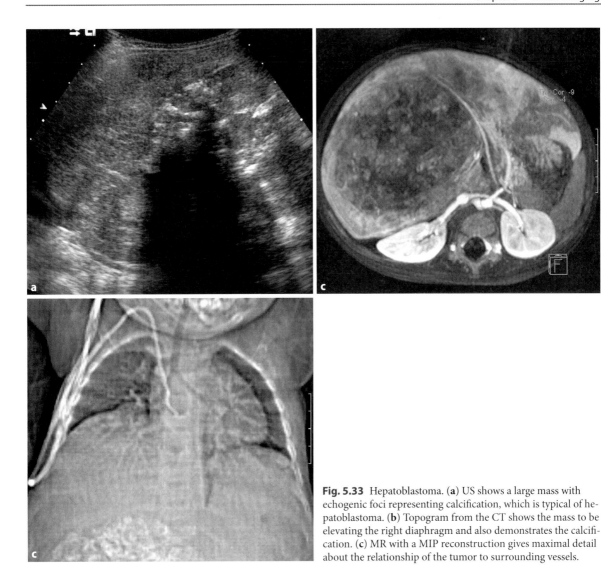

Fig. 5.33 Hepatoblastoma. (**a**) US shows a large mass with echogenic foci representing calcification, which is typical of hepatoblastoma. (**b**) Topogram from the CT shows the mass to be elevating the right diaphragm and also demonstrates the calcification. (**c**) MR with a MIP reconstruction gives maximal detail about the relationship of the tumor to surrounding vessels.

US, CT, and MR. The prognosis is very poor and surgical excision rarely possible. Surgical relief of the biliary obstruction may be necessary and percutaneous or peroperative cholangiography will demonstrate the intraluminal and botyroid tumor.

5.5.11 Pelvic Tumors

5.5.11.1 Rhabdomyosarcoma

Genitourinary tumors occur at the base of the bladder and prostatic region, the vagina, the testes, penis, and perineum. US is a very useful modality in bladder tumors and should be performed while the patient has a full bladder. Tumors may arise within the bladder, at the base or at the dome and characteristically have a lobulated, polypoid appearance and are described as botyroid tumors. This appearance is also true of vaginal lesions. Tumors arising from the prostatic region displace the bladder anteriorly and superiorly and have a more defined uniform structure. Compression of the ureters and bilateral hydronephrosis may occur [65]. Both CT and MRI can be used to further delineate the extent of the tumor, including spread beyond the bladder into the perivesical fat, lymph nodes, soft tissues, and rectum [34, 89]. MRI is by far a superior modality as multiplanar imaging is an advantage when assessing pelvic lesions and in particular is helpful in demonstrating the relationship of the tumor to other organs and the sacral foramina and spinal canal. MRI of genitourinary tumors is mandatory (Fig. 5.34). Paratesticular tumors must have evaluation of regional (para aortic) lymph nodes by CT/MRI and US. CT of

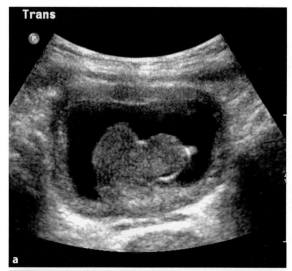

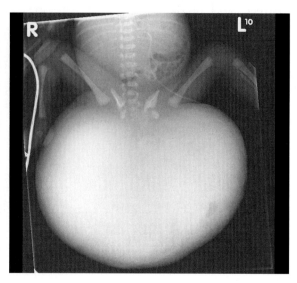

Fig. 5.35 Sacrococcygeal teratoma. Pelvis x-ray in a neonate showing a huge exophytic sacrococcygeal teratoma splaying the pubic symphysis and the legs.

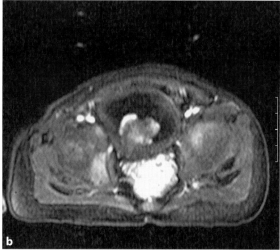

Fig. 5.34 Bladder rhabdomyosarcoma. (**a**) US showing the tumor arising from the bladder base and having a significant exophytic component. (**b**) MR showing variable enhancement of the bladder mass after gadolinium.

ses or intraspinal extension, MRI in the sagittal plane provides useful anatomical information and is recommended. Teratomas may also occur in the abdomen (Fig. 5.37).

Testicular teratomas also occur in the young infant, whereas ovarian and some testicular tumors occur at puberty. Pelvic US with a full bladder will demonstrate an ovarian mass and CT will often confirm the diagnosis in a mass with cysts, calcification, and fat.

Metastatic disease is rare as many pelvic teratomas are benign. However, metastases can occur in both local lymph nodes and the lungs. Therefore, an abdominal CT or MRI is recommended in patients with testicular teratomas to look for spread to regional lymph nodes, although there is some doubt in the accuracy and significance of the results [49].

the thorax is also a prerequisite in genitourinary rhabdomyosarcomas (see above).

5.5.11.2 Teratoma

Sacrococcygeal tumors occur in the neonate and are readily identified at birth as tumors that are exophytic, usually with a significant external component (Fig. 5.35). Most are benign and imaging is required to enable surgical planning. While the lesion will be apparent on US, CT will more clearly demonstrate cysts, fat, and calcification as well as the rare cases with erosion of the sacrum (Fig. 5.36). For suspected metasta-

5.5.12 Second Malignant Neoplasms

Therapeutic advances in the treatment of pediatric cancers have improved the prognosis but have also increased the risk of developing rare second malignant neoplasms (SMNs). Primary neoplasms that are often associated with SMNs include lymphoma, retinoblastoma, medulloblastoma, neuroblastoma, and leukemia. The most common SMNs are CNS tumors, sarcomas, thyroid and parotid gland tumors, and leukemia, especially acute myeloid leukemia. Genetic predisposition, chemotherapy, and particularly radiotherapy are all implicated as pathogenic factors in SMN. It is therefore especially important in the life-long follow

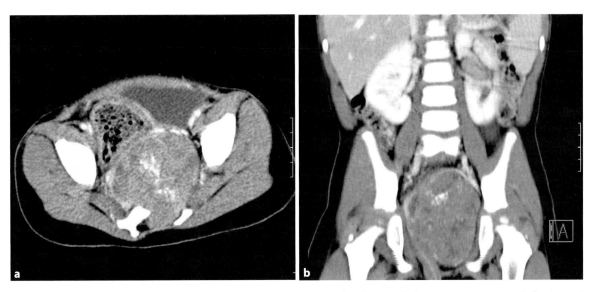

Fig. 5.36 Sacrococcygeal teratoma in a neonate. (**a**) CT through the low pelvis showing the large mass containing calcification and disrupting the sacrum. Note both the rectum and the bladder are pushed anteriorly, identifying this as a presacral mass. (**b**) Coronal reconstruction in the same patient demonstrating the diastasis of the pubic symphysis.

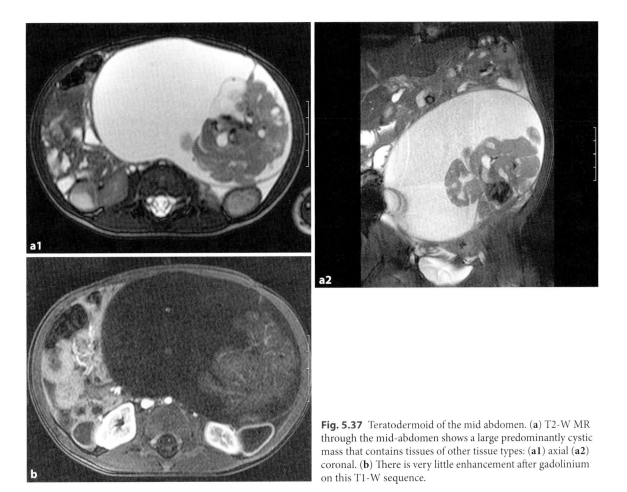

Fig. 5.37 Teratodermoid of the mid abdomen. (**a**) T2-W MR through the mid-abdomen shows a large predominantly cystic mass that contains tissues of other tissue types: (**a1**) axial (**a2**) coronal. (**b**) There is very little enhancement after gadolinium on this T1-W sequence.

up of these patients that any imaging should avoid ionizing radiation where at all possible. MRI is the optimal investigation as it can cover small or large body areas and provides excellent anatomic detail, particularly in the head and neck [90]. In the abdomen, follow-up can be by a combination of US and MRI.

References

1. Abramson SJ, Lack EE, Teele RL (1982) Benign vascular tumors of the liver in infants: Sonographic appearance. AJR Am J Roentgenol 138:629–632

2. Askin FB, Rosai J, Sibley RK, Dehner LP, Mcalister WH (1979) Malignant small cell tumor of the thoracopulmonary region in childhood: A distinctive clinicopathologic entity of uncertain histogenesis. Cancer 43:2438–2451

3. Azouz EM, Larson EJ, Patel J, Gyepes MT (1990) Beckwith-Wiedemann syndrome: Development of nephroblastoma during the surveillance period. Pediatr Radiol 20:550–552

4. Blakely ML, Ritchey ML (2001) Controversies in the management of Wilms' tumor. Semin Pediatr Surg 10:127–131

5. Boechat MI, Ortega J, Hoffman AD, Cleveland RH, Kangarloo H, Gilsanz V (1985) Computed tomography in stage III neuroblastoma. AJR Am J Roentgenol 145:1283–1287

6. Boechat MI, Kangarloo H, Gilsanz V (1988) Hepatic masses in children. Semin Roentgenol 23:185–193

7. Boechat MI, Kangarloo H, Ortega J, Hall T, Feig S, Stanley P, Gilsanz V (1988) Primary liver tumors in children: Comparison of CT and MR imaging. Radiology 169:727–732

8. Bond JV (1975) Bilateral Wilms' tumour. Age at diagnosis, associated congenital anormalies, and possible pattern of inheritance. Lancet 2:482–484

9. Bousvaros A, Kirks DR, Grossman H (1986) Imaging of neuroblastoma: An overview. Pediatr Radiol 16:89–106

10. Boyko OB, Cory DA, Cohen MD, Provisor A, Mirkin D, Derosa GP (1987) MR imaging of osteogenic and Ewing's sarcoma. AJR Am J Roentgenol 148:317–322

11. Brodeur GM, Pritchard J, Berthold F, Carlsen NL, Castel V, Castelberry RP, De Bernardi B, Evans AE, Favrot M, Hedborg F, et al. (1993) Revisions of the international criteria for neuroblastoma diagnosis, staging, and response to treatment. J Clin Oncol 11:1466–1477

12. Broecker B (2000) Non-Wilms' renal tumors in children. Urol Clin North Am 27:463–469, ix

13. Castellino RA (1986) Hodgkin disease: Practical concepts for the diagnostic radiologist. Radiology 159:305–310

14. Choyke PL, Siegel MJ, Craft AW, Green DM, Debaun MR (1999) Screening for Wilms tumor in children with Beckwith-Wiedemann syndrome or idiopathic hemihypertrophy. Med Pediatr Oncol 32:196–200

15. Cohen MD, Siddiqui A, Weetman R, Provisor A, Coates T (1986) Hodgkin disease and non-Hodgkin lymphomas in children: Utilization of radiological modalities. Radiology 158:499–505

16. Connolly LP, Drubach LA, Ted Treves S (2002) Applications of nuclear medicine in pediatric oncology. Clin Nucl Med 27:117–125

17. Couinaud C (1994) The paracaval segments of the liver. J Hepatobiliary Pancreat Surgery: 2:145–151

18. Cremin BJ (1987) Wilms' tumour: Ultrasound and changing concepts. Clin Radiol 38:465–474

19. Czauderna P, Otte JB, Aronson DC, Gauthier F, Mackinlay G, Roebuck D, Plaschkes J, Perilongo G (2005) Guidelines for surgical treatment of hepatoblastoma in the modern era – Recommendations from the childhood liver Tumour Strategy Group of the International Society Of Paediatric Oncology (SIOPEL). Eur J Cancer 41:1031–1036

20. Czauderna P, Otte JB, Roebuck DJ, Von Schweinitz D, Plaschkes J (2006) Surgical treatment of hepatoblastoma in children. Pediatr Radiol 36:187–191

21. Dachman AH, Pakter RL, Ros PR, Fishman EK, Goodman ZD, Lichtenstein JE (1987) Hepatoblastoma: Radiologic-pathologic correlation in 50 cases. Radiology 164:15–19

22. D'angio GJ, Beckwith JB, Breslow N (1989) Wilms' tumor (nephroblastoma, renal embryoma). In: Pizzo PA Poplack DG (eds) Principles and practice of pediatric oncology. Lippincott, Philadelphia, pp 553–606

23. D'angio GJ, Breslow N, Beckwith JB, Evans A, Baum H, Delorimier A, Fernbach D, Hrabovsky E, Jones B, Kelalis P, et al. (1989) Treatment of Wilms' tumor. Results of the third national Wilms' tumor study. Cancer 64:349–360

24. Debaun MR, Brown M, Kessler L (1996) Screening for Wilms' tumor in children with high-risk congenital syndromes: Considerations for an intervention trial. Med Pediatr Oncol 27:415–421

25. Debaun MR, Tucker MA (1998) Risk of cancer during the first four years of life in children from the Beckwith-Wiedemann syndrome registry. J Pediatr 132:398–400

26. Dietrich RB, Kangarloo H, Lenarsky C, Feig SA (1987) Neuroblastoma: The role of MR imaging. AJR Am J Roentgenol 148:937–942

27. Erlemann R, Sciuk J, Bosse A, Ritter J, Kusnierz-Glaz CR, Peters PE, Wuisman P (1990) Response of osteosarcoma and Ewing sarcoma to preoperative chemotherapy: Assessment with dynamic and static MR imaging and skeletal scintigraphy. Radiology 175:791–796

28. Feldman BA (1982) Rhabdomyosarcoma of the head and neck. Laryngoscope 92:424–440

29. Finn JP, Hall-Craggs MA, Dicks-Mireaux C, Spitz L, Howard ER, Pritchard J, Vergani GM (1990) Primary malignant liver tumors in childhood: Assessment of resectability with high-field MR and comparison with CT. Pediatr Radiol 21:34–38

30. Fishman EK, Hartman DS, Goldman SM, Siegelman SS (1983) The CT appearance of Wilms tumor. J Comput Assist Tomogr 7:659–665

31. Friedman AL (1986) Wilms' tumor detection in patients with sporadic aniridia. Successful use of ultrasound. Am J Dis Child 140:173–174

32. Frouge C, Vanel D, Coffre C, Couanet D, Contesso G, Sarrazin D (1988) The role of magnetic resonance imaging in the evaluation of Ewing sarcoma. A report of 27 cases. Skeletal Radiol 17:387–392

33. Geller E, Smergel EM, Lowry PA (1997) Renal neoplasms of childhood. Radiol Clin North Am 35:1391–1413

34. Geoffray A, Couanet D, Montagne JP, Leclere J, Flamant F (1987) Ultrasonography and computed tomography for diagnosis and follow-up of pelvic rhabdomyosarcomas in children. Pediatr Radiol 17:132–136

35. Gordon I, Peters AM, Gutman A, Morony S, Dicks-Mireaux C, Pritchard J (1990) Skeletal assessment in neuroblastoma – The pitfalls of iodine-123-MIBG scans. J Nucl Med 31:129–134

36. Gourtsoyiannis NC, Nolan DJ (1988) Lymphoma of the small intestine: Radiological appearances. Clin Radiol 39:639–645

37. Grampp S, Bankier AA, Zoubek A, Wiesbauer P, Schroth B, Henk CB, Grois N, Mostbeck GH (2000) Spiral CT of the lung in children with malignant extra-thoracic tumors: Distribution of benign vs malignant pulmonary nodules. Eur Radiol 10:1318–1322

38. Gylys-Morin V, Hoffer FA, Kozakewich H, Shamberger RC (1993) Wilms tumor and nephroblastomatosis: Imaging characteristics at gadolinium-enhanced MR imaging. Radiology 188:517–521

39. Hartman DS, Sanders RC (1982) Wilms' tumor versus neuroblastoma: Usefulness of ultrasound in differentiation. J Ultrasound Med 1:117–122

40. Helmberger TK, Ros PR, Mergo PJ, Tomczak R, Reiser MF (1999) Pediatric liver neoplasms: A radiologic-pathologic correlation. Eur Radiol 9:1339–1347

41. Hensle TW, Chang DT (2000) Reconstructive surgery for children with pelvic rhabdomyosarcoma. Urol Clin North Am 27:489–502, ix

42. Heron CW, Husband JE, Williams MP (1988) Hodgkin disease: CT of the thymus. Radiology 167:647–651

43. Herzog CE, Andrassy RJ, Eftekhari F (2000) Childhood cancers: Hepatoblastoma. Oncologist 5:445–453

44. Hoffer FA, Chung T, Diller L, Kozakewich H, Fletcher JA, Shamberger RC (1996) Percutaneous biopsy for prognostic testing of neuroblastoma. Radiology 200:213–216

45. Hoffer FA (2002) Primary skeletal neoplasms: Osteosarcoma and Ewing sarcoma. Top Magn Reson Imaging 13:231–239

46. Hoffer FA (2005) Magnetic resonance imaging of abdominal masses in the pediatric patient. Semin Ultrasound CT MR 26:212–223

47. Holscher HC, Bloem JL, Nooy MA, Taminiau AH, Eulderink F, Hermans J (1990) The value of MR imaging in monitoring the effect of chemotherapy on bone sarcomas. AJR Am J Roentgenol 154:763–769

48. Howman-Giles RB, Gilday DL, Ash JM (1979) Radionuclide skeletal survey in neuroblastoma. Radiology 131:497–502

49. Huddart SN, Mann JR, Gornall P, Pearson D, Barrett A, Raafat F, Barnes JM, Wallendsus KR (1990) The UK children's cancer study group: Testicular malignant germ cell tumours 1979–1988. J Pediatr Surg 25:406–410

50. Hudson MM, Krasin MJ, Kaste SC (2004) PET imaging in pediatric Hodgkin's lymphoma. Pediatr Radiol 34:190–198

51. Imhof H, Czerny C, Hormann M, Krestan C (2004) Tumors and tumor-like lesions of the neck: From childhood to adult. Eur Radiol 14 (Suppl) 4:1155–1165

52. Jeffery GM, Mead GM, Whitehouse JM (1991) Life-threatening airway obstruction at the presentation of Hodgkin's disease. Cancer 67:506–510

53. Kairemo KJ, Lindahl H, Merenmies J, Fohr A, Nikkinen P, Karonen SL, Makipernaa A, Hockerstedt K, Goldenberg DM, Heikinheimo M (2002) Anti-alpha-fetoprotein imaging is useful for staging hepatoblastoma. Transplantation 73:1151–1154

54. Kaste SC, Howard SC, Mccarville EB, Krasin MJ, Kogos PG, Hudson MM (2005) 18f-FDG-avid sites mimicking active disease in pediatric Hodgkin's. Pediatr Radiol 35:141–154

55. Kellenberger CJ, Epelman M, Miller SF, Babyn PS (2004) Fast stir whole-body MR imaging in children. Radiographics 24:1317–1330

56. Kiely EM (1994) The surgical challenge of neuroblastoma. J Pediatr Surg 29:128–133

57. Kushner BH (2004) Neuroblastoma: A disease requiring a multitude of imaging studies. J Nucl Med 45:1172–1188

58. Latack JT, Hutchinson RJ, Heyn RM (1987) Imaging of rhabdomyosarcomas of the head and neck. AJR Am J Neuroradiol 8:353–359

59. Lewis E, Bernardino ME, Salvador PG, Cabanillas FF, Barnes PA, Thomas JL (1982) Post-therapy CT-detected mass in lymphoma patients: Is it viable tissue? J Comput Assist Tomogr 6:792–795

60. Lindfors KK, Meyer JE, Dedrick CG, Hassell LA, Harris NL (1985) Thymic cysts in mediastinal Hodgkin disease. Radiology 156:37–41

61. Lonergan GJ, Martinez-Leon MI, Agrons GA, Montemarano H, Suarez ES (1998) Nephrogenic rests, nephroblastomatosis, and associated lesions of the kidney. Radiographics 18:947–968

62. Lowe LH, Isuani BH, Heller RM, Stein SM, Johnson JE, Navarro OM, Hernanz-Schulman M (2000) Pediatric renal masses: Wilms tumor and beyond. Radiographics 20:1585–1603

63. Mandell GA, Lantieri R, Goodman LR (1982) Tracheobronchial compression in Hodgkin lymphoma in children. AJR Am J Roentgenol 139:1167–1170

64. Mankin HJ, Hornicek FJ (2005) Diagnosis, classification, and management of soft tissue sarcomas. Cancer Control 12:5–21

65. Mcleod AJ, Lewis E (1984) Sonographic evaluation of pediatric rhabdomyosarcomas. J Ultrasound Med 3:69–73

66. McNeil DE, Brown M, Ching A, Debaun MR (2001) Screening for Wilms tumor and hepatoblastoma in children with Beckwith-Wiedemann syndromes: A cost-effective model. Med Pediatr Oncol 37:349–356

67. Meyer JS, Harty MP, Khademian Z (2002) Imaging of neuroblastoma and Wilms' tumor. Magn Reson Imaging Clin N Am 10:275–302

68. Miller RW, Young JLJ, Novakovic B (1995) Childhood cancer. Cancer 75:398–405

69. Pashankar FD, O'dorisio MS, Menda Y (2005) MIBG and somatostatin receptor analogs in children: Current concepts on diagnostic and therapeutic use. J Nucl Med 46 (Suppl) 1:55s–61s

70. Philip I, Shun A, Mccowage G, Howman-Giles R (2005) Positron emission tomography in recurrent hepatoblastoma. Pediatr Surg Int 21:341–345

71. Picci P, Vanel D, Briccoli A, Talle K, Haakenaasen U, Mala-guti C, Monti C, Ferrari C, Bacci G, Saeter G, Alvegard TA (2001) Computed tomography of pulmonary metastases from osteosarcoma: The less poor technique. A study of 51 patients with histological correlation. Ann Oncol 12:1601–1604

72. Raney RB, Hays DM, Teftt M (1989) Rhabdomyosarcome and the undifferentiated sarcomas. In: Pizzo PA, Poplack DG (eds) Principles and practice of pediatric oncology. Lippincott, Philadelphia, pp 636–658

73. Reiman TA, Siegel MJ, Shackelford GD (1986) Wilms tumor in children: Abdominal CT and US evaluation. Radiology 160:501–505

74. Ritchey ML, Kelalis PP, Breslow N, Offord KP, Shochat SJ, D'angio GJ (1988) Intracaval and atrial involvement with nephroblastoma: Review of national Wilms tumor study-3. J Urol 140:1113–1118

75. Roebuck DJ, Olsen O, Pariente D (2006) Radiological staging in children with hepatoblastoma. Pediatr Radiol 36:176–182

76. Rosen EM, Cassady JR, Frantz CN, Kretschmar CS, Levey R, Sallen SE (1985) Stage IV-V: A favourable subset of children with metastatic neuroblastoma. Med Pediatr Oncol 13:194–198

77. Schreiman JS, Crass JR, Wick MR, Maile CW, Thompson RC Jr (1986) Osteosarcoma: Role of CT in limb-sparing treatment. Radiology 161:485–488

78. Sebire NJ, Roebuck DJ (2006) Pathological diagnosis of paediatric tumours from image-guided needle core biopsies: A systematic review. Pediatr Radiol 36:426–431

79. Seeger LL, Eckardt JJ, Bassett LW (1989) Cross-sectional imaging in the evaluation of osteogenic sarcoma: MRI and CT. Semin Roentgenol 24:174–184

80. Sekiya T, Meller ST, Cosgrove DO, McCready VR (1982) Ultrasonography of Hodgkin's disease in the liver and spleen. Clin Radiol 33:635–639

81. Seo JB, Im JG, Goo JM, Chung MJ, Kim MY (2001) Atypical pulmonary metastases: Spectrum of radiologic findings. Radiographics 21:403–417

82. Siegel MJ, Jamroz GA, Glazer HS, Abramson CL (1986) MR imaging of intraspinal extension of neuroblastoma. J Comput Assist Tomogr 10:593–595

83. Siegel MJ, Evans SJ, Balfe DM (1988) Small bowel disease in children: Diagnosis with CT. Radiology 169:127–130

84. Siegel MJ (2001) Magnetic resonance imaging of musculoskeletal soft tissue masses. Radiol Clin North Am 39:701–720

85. Sisler CL, Siegel MJ (1989) Malignant rhabdoid tumor of the kidney: Radiologic features. Radiology 172:211–212

86. St. Amour TE, Siegel MJ, Glazer HS, Nadel SN (1987) CT appearances of the normal and abnormal thymus in childhood. J Comput Assist Tomogr 11:645–650

87. Stolar CJ, Garvin JH Jr, Rustad DG, Amodio JB, Lipton JM (1987) Residual or recurrent chest mass in pediatric Hodgkin's disease. A surgical problem? Am J Pediatr Hematol Oncol 9:289–294

88. Talpallikar MC, Sawant V, Hirugade S, Borwankar SS, Sanghani H (2001) Wilms' tumor arising in a horseshoe kidney. Pediatr Surg Int 17:465–466

89. Tannous WN, Azouz EM, Homsy YL, Kiruluta HG, Grattan-Smith D (1989) CT and ultrasound imaging of pelvic rhabdomyosarcoma in children. A review of 56 patients. Pediatr Radiol 19:530–534

90. Vazquez E, Castellote A, Piqueras J, Ortuno P, Sanchez-Toledo J, Nogues P, Lucaya J (2003) Second malignancies in pediatric patients: Imaging findings and differential diagnosis. Radiographics 23:1155–1172

91. Webb WR (1989) MR imaging of treated mediastinal Hodgkin disease. Radiology 170:315–316

92. White KS (2001) Thoracic imaging of pediatric lymphomas. J Thorac Imaging 16:224–237

93. Wilimas JA, Douglass EC, Magill HL, Fitch S, Hustu HO (1988) Significance of pulmonary computed tomography at diagnosis in Wilms' tumor. J Clin Oncol 6:1144–1146

94. Williams MP, Husband JE, Mcelwain TJ (1989) Role of computed tomography scanning in the management of Ewing's sarcoma. Med Pediatr Oncol 17:414–417

Tumor Pathology – General Principles

6

Allan G. Howatson

Contents

6.1 Introduction

The multidisciplinary approach to the management of pediatric neoplasia has resulted in dramatic improvements in outcome for children with cancer. The success of this approach demands close co-operation between specialists from several disciplines and this is best facilitated by good communication and the development of a clear mutual understanding of the nature of the work of these disciplines.

The purpose of this chapter is to establish the role of the pathologist in this multidisciplinary process, to explain the procedures involved, and to indicate the ways in which the surgeon can facilitate this effort. More detailed consideration of the pathology of individual neoplasms can be found in the relevant chapters of this book.

The role of the pathologist goes beyond providing histological diagnosis and includes provision of prognostic information and facilitation of ancillary studies and research.

It is important for surgeons and oncologists to appreciate that the pathological diagnosis is a clinical opinion, not a "result," and like all opinions its formulation is the product of integration of clinical information, imaging studies and other laboratory investigations, as well as gross and microscopic study. It should be obvious that this may take time and that denial of access to such information can only delay the process at best or lead to a diagnosis which results in inappropriate therapy at worst.

6.2 The Diagnostic Specimen

It should be axiomatic that all tumor tissue or suspected tumor tissue, with the sole exception of cytology specimens, should be submitted to the pathology laboratory promptly, unfixed, and in a dry, sterile container.

There are potentially five types of specimens which might be submitted to the pathologist:

1. Cytology specimen;
2. Needle biopsy;
3. Incisional biopsy;
4. Excisional biopsy;
6. Resected specimen.

The latter may be either pre- or post treatment and may or may not be an attempt at complete surgical extirpation of the tumor – in which case assessment of margins is important.

6.3 The Request Form

In each instance it is essential that a request form, paper or electronic, is correctly completed and submitted with a properly labeled and identified specimen. The importance of a correctly completed request cannot be overemphasized. Full patient identification details are necessary if errors of attribution of specimens are to be avoided.

The accurate spelling of a name and also of unique patient identifiers such as date of birth and hospital number are essential. The significance of the site of biopsy is self-evident. Frequently the clinical history is omitted or inadequate. This omission should be unacceptable in modern practice. The pathologist, as a medical consultant, requires clinical information to assist in the integration of evidence derived from gross and histological examination of a specimen if an accurate and clinically meaningful opinion and diagnosis are to be proffered. It is also very useful for the surgeon to indicate specific features of the case which he particularly needs resolved. As always, communication with the pathologist in advance of taking the specimen is good practice and in the best centers is routine.

6.4 Cytology

In general, cytological techniques have not been much employed in the diagnosis of pediatric neoplasia. This probably reflects the relative rarity of pediatric tumors and may be a hangover from the concept of the "small blue cell tumor of childhood" in which various neoplasms of differing biological potential can appear somewhat similar histologically. In addition, most pediatric lesions were not directly amenable to the surface scraping and fluid aspiration methodologies of classical cytology (Fig. 6.1). However, with the advent of fine needle aspiration this situation is changing rapidly and the move towards smaller diagnostic samples will lead to a greater use of cytology for primary diagnosis and review of progress in the future [1].

The most useful cytological investigation with regard to pediatric neoplasia is fine needle aspiration cytology in which both superficial and deeply sited lesions become accessible either by palpation and direct puncture or radiologically [ultrasound or computed tomography (CT)] guided techniques. Most areas of the body are now accessible, by means of imaging, to the technique of fine needle aspiration [2–5].

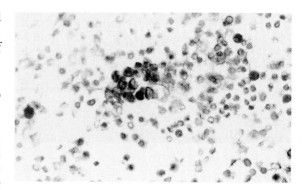

Fig. 6.1 Smear of rhabdomyosarcoma cells stained for desmin, found in ascitic fluid.

The question as to who should perform the aspiration is dependant on local circumstances. In the case of palpation and direct puncture, what is more important is that the operator is experienced in the technique of sampling and this can either be a surgeon or a pathologist. Several passages through the lesion with aspiration are required to ensure an adequate sample, and the use of a needle of appropriate gauge (23 or 25) and an aspiration gun to allow single-handed manipulation of needle and syringe are obviously important (Figs. 6.2a, b). In the case of deeply seated lesions which require imaging guidance, these can be performed by radiologists or other clinicians with expertise in interventional techniques (Fig. 6.3).

A significant feature of a fine needle aspiration is the potential for obtaining "microbiopsies" with preserved histological microanatomy which pathologists frequently find useful in the diagnosis of many pediatric tumors. It is also possible to make cell pellets from an aspiration specimen if pathologists are less experienced in dealing with cytological preparations [6]. These pellets can be then processed and sectioned as histological blocks in the more usual way.

Central to the success of fine needle aspiration is the adequacy of the aspirate and the subsequent production of good smears and cytocentrifuge preparations and it is therefore necessary that the surgeon notifies the laboratory well in advance in order that a cytotechnician can be on hand to facilitate the preparation of air-dried and alcohol-fixed smears. A poorly prepared slide can negate the entire procedure and it is frequently difficult to get an adequate smear, particularly if one is not experienced in the preparation of these slides.

Great care is needed if a potentially confusing artifact is to be avoided in the case of alcohol-fixed preparations. Any degree of air drying in a poorly fixed smear preparation causes artifactual nuclear enlargement and irregularity of chromatin distribution – fea-

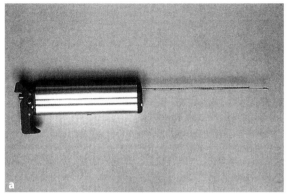

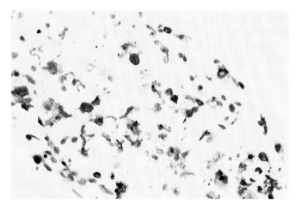

Fig. 6.3 Fine needle aspiration of an embryonal rhabdomyosarcoma stained for desmin.

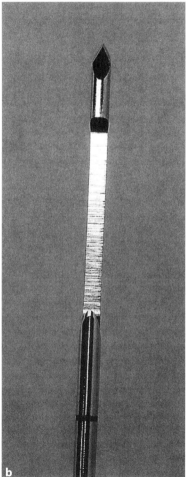

Fig. 6.2 a Biopsy using an automatic cutting device with a 2.2-cm long needle throw (Pro-Mag 2.2 Manan Medical Products, Inc. Northbrook, USA) and a 14-gauge cutting needle (Manan Medical Products Inc). The biopsy is taken during suspended inspiration. **b** Close up of needle tip.

tures seen in malignant cells. It is preferred to have both alcohol-fixed slides stained by the Papanicolaou method and air-dried slides stained by the May-Grunwald-Giemsa or Diff-Quick methods. These can be either on smears or cytocentrifugation preparations. Cytocentrifugation has the advantage, in fluids and hypocellular samples, of concentrating the cellular component to be studied.

In addition to the standard cellular morphology that can be expected in aspirates of pediatric tumors, it is also possible to apply ancillary techniques to these specimens [7].

Therefore, prior to the aspiration procedure, consideration should be given to the possibility that the diagnosis of a case may benefit from investigations other than morphology. Of particular value are cytogenetics and molecular genetics, immunocytochemistry, and electron microscopy. Portions of the aspirate can be allocated to these purposes in order of priority as determined by the clinical presentation of the individual case and presumptive clinical diagnosis.

It should be understood that the cytological diagnosis of pediatric neoplasms is a difficult area and expertise is developed over a period of time. It is not possible for a pathologist without experience of this technique to receive a specimen and be expected to make an erudite diagnosis at once. The learning curve is long, and with the paucity of material resulting from small numbers of cases it can be an area fraught with difficulty. It is often sound practice for the pathologist to aspirate resected specimens in the laboratory in order to practice looking at more material than otherwise would be submitted for primary diagnosis.

The complications of fine needle aspiration are minimal. Local bleeding is usually of minor significance even with substantial vascular lesions and needle aspiration of lesions in the lung very seldom lead to pneumothorax.

Cytology has another significant use in cases of pediatric neoplasia and that is to identify infections related to immunocompromise resulting from therapy. Cytological preparations of skin scrapings can identify viral infections such as herpes simplex and infections of the respiratory tract, e.g., Pneumocystis carnii, fungal infections, and viral infections such as cytomegalovirus (CMV), are also amenable to diagnosis in bronchial lavage specimens by cytological techniques.

It is clear that cytological diagnosis will become an increasingly important part of the pediatric pathologist's workload because it is a relatively noninvasive technique and reduces the use and risk of anesthesia.

Cases which will benefit most from cytological diagnosis involve "neck lumps" and in particular the assessment of cases of lymph node enlargement. Nodal pathologies with persisting node enlargement are a frequent cause of referral to pediatric surgeons. These can be either reactive or neoplastic (usually Hodgkin's or non-Hodgkin's lymphoma) and with adequate sampling are amenable to cytological diagnosis thus avoiding open biopsy with resulting scar and risks related to anesthesia. If cytological techniques are to be applied in such cases, a clear protocol for the prebiopsy assessment of the child, the obtaining of an adequate sample by a competent experienced operator, the performance of ancillary studies (particularly microbiology) and a plan for follow-up and open biopsy in cases of persistence of the mass must be in place and followed in all instances if false negative diagnoses are not to be detrimental to the patient. Kardos et al. [8] laid out such a protocol which fulfils these requirements and provides a model of sound practice – it is highly recommended.

It must be emphasized that cytology alone cannot provide all the answers required of a tissue diagnosis and the need for larger biopsy samples will remain with us for the foreseeable future especially when fresh tissue is required for special biological and cytogenetic investigations that may influence therapy.

6.5 The Diagnostic Needle Biopsy

The core of tissue derived from a needle biopsy either by use of a Tru-cut needle [9] or the more recently available biopsy gun can provide adequate tissue to allow accurate diagnosis of the majority of pediatric neoplasms [10]. More than one core, and preferably at least three, should be taken to allow for tumor heterogeneity and to permit ancillary investigations. With the modern instruments, trauma of the tissue core is usually minimal and although the sample is small, typically 10 x 1 x 1 mm, it is usually possible to obtain material for ancillary studies and for immunohistochemistry. The paucity of material does, however, frequently make it difficult for the pathologist to provide other information, for instance in relation to the presence or absence of anaplasia in nephroblastoma, tumor grading in soft tissue sarcoma or the mitosis/

karyorrhexis index (MKI) and other prognostic features in neuroblastoma.

In general, directed biopsies using ultrasound and CT guidance give better samples than a blind biopsy performed either percutaneously or under direct vision at surgery. Drying artifact during transit of fresh samples to the laboratory is a potential problem and rapid transfer in a closed container is essential.

6.6 Incisional Biopsy

Incisional biopsies under direct vision provide very adequate tissue samples which permit all necessary ancillary studies to be performed in the majority of cases. The surgeon will of course have placed his incision to avoid any potential compromise of subsequent resection and to minimize contamination of surrounding structures and tissue compartments. The surgeon should avoid crushing the tissue with forceps during removal. In the archetypical small blue cell tumors of childhood the cells are fragile and injudicious application of force renders the tumor cells into an amorphous smear of nuclear material impervious to diagnosis (Figs. 6.4a, b). The surgeon should also

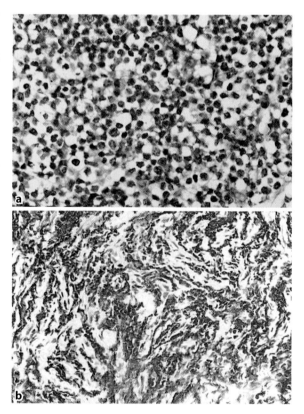

Fig. 6.4 a Intact biopsy of Ewing's sarcoma. **b** Surgical crush artifact of a biopsy of a Ewing's sarcoma.

avoid placing the tissue on any surface which might dry out the tissue during transit to the laboratory. The skin incision must be placed such that further surgery will include this area, as the biopsy will inevitably have seeded cells into the wound.

6.7 Excisional Biopsy

Excisional biopsy entails the apparent complete removal of a small lesion, perhaps up to 5 cm in its greatest dimension. Very frequently this involves the "shelling-out" of a lesion such as lymph node or soft tissue tumors of the limbs. It is usual in the latter situation for tumor to be left behind as the plane of dissection is frequently through the tumor pseudocapsule and not through noninvolved healthy tissue [11]. Once again, this technique provides very adequate material for ancillary studies such as cytogenetics, molecular genetics, and other research activities. The surgeon should consider marking the margins of specific interest if he or she believes that the excisional biopsy represents a clearance of the tumor, and the tumor should not be incised prior to transfer to the pathology department as excision margins will be compromised or contaminated by tumor, giving rise to a risk of a false diagnosis of incomplete excision resulting in inappropriate further surgery or adjuvant therapy.

6.8 Surgical Resection

Definitive surgical resection can either be performed as a primary surgical procedure or following preoperative chemotherapy or radiotherapy. The advent of preoperative therapy allows tumor shrinkage and reduction in vascularity. Many tumors which were deemed not amenable to resection prior to therapy may become resectable after chemotherapy (Fig. 6.5) [12, 13].

The margins of the resected specimens should be marked in all cases. It is important that the surgeon should not incise these specimens prior to receipt in the pathology department since this may lead to capsular retraction and render the margins contaminated, making it impossible for the pathologist to be sure that the tumor is completely excised with a margin of clear noninvolved tissue. Any lymph nodes or other tissues removed at the time of primary or post therapy resection should be specifically labeled with their site clearly indicated in the request form and on the specimen containers. It is insufficient to say "lymph node" and not to specify the site from which it is taken because the site of lymph node involvement may determine the stage of the disease and fields for any subsequent radiotherapy.

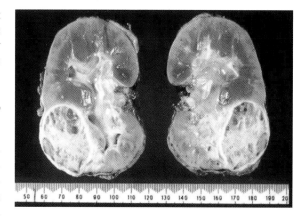

Fig. 6.5 Nephroblastoma after chemotherapy.

6.9 Specimen Handling in the Pathology Department

The assessment of a specimen submitted for diagnosis involves both gross and microscopic examinations. Even the smallest of biopsy specimens can yield useful information on gross examination [14]. The presence of necrosis, hemorrhage, or a variegated appearance may indicate a heterogeneous histological structure. In the case of larger specimens, the gross examination takes on more importance, particularly with regard to the surgical margins of excision and the vascular and neural margins if appropriate.

All tumor specimens, biopsies and resections, should be submitted to the laboratory fresh, i.e., not in fixative. There should be no delay in the receipt of this material in the laboratory and prior notification is essential if appropriate preparations for taking ancillary study samples are to be made in the laboratory. The range of investigations and sampling will obviously be dependent on the size of the sample submitted for diagnosis. In the case of a cytology fine needle aspirate, it is often possible to have some cells submitted for cytogenetic analysis and some for electron microscopy, but often the entire specimen is used for primary cytologic diagnosis. Needle biopsies represent a larger sample, but the volume of material is still extremely small and it may be that only a small piece for cytogenetics can be spared, with the remainder being submitted for histological examination. Incisional biopsies, excisional biopsies, and resected specimens should all provide sufficient material for histological diagnosis, cytogenetics, electron microscopy, and storage of tissue for subsequent molecular studies if required. In addition, it is also often appropriate to submit material for microbiological investigation, particularly in instances of lymphadenopathy.

The use of intraoperative frozen section for histological diagnosis in pediatric neoplasia should be confined to very specific indications. The desire of the surgeon to be able to tell the parents of the nature of the diagnosis and likely prognosis at the end of the operation is not a sufficient reason for a frozen section to be performed. The only uses for a frozen section during operation are to confirm the presence of tumor, to ascertain that adequate diagnostic material of the native lesion is present in the sample excised, and to assess the need to take wider margins if required. It is often difficult, as a result of artifact related to the frozen section process, to come to a specific histological diagnosis in some of the small, round cell type and spindle cell type pediatric neoplasms. It is wholly inappropriate to use the frozen section diagnosis as a definitive statement for discussions with parents. Such discussions should await the formulation of a definitive paraffin histology-based diagnostic opinion and report.

In the case of excisional biopsy and resection specimens in which complete surgical extirpation of the tumor is intended, evaluation of the surgical margins is important with regard to decisions for further local and systemic therapy. One technique which is widely used to determine true surgical margins is to paint the specimen with indian ink ("inking") or other suitable dyes prior to the incision of a specimen. The dye must be dried onto the surface of the specimen before the specimen is placed in fixative, but if the margin is in question it is a valuable technique. It is axiomatic that the surgeon should not compromise the margins of excision by incising the specimen prior to submission to the pathologist.

Gross examination is vitally important in order that one can be sure that the blocks being sampled from the specimen relate to true surgical margins and not to areas of artifact. It is therefore important that the specimen should be thoroughly examined macroscopically, weighed where appropriate, measured, and photographed, preferably prior to fixation. Where fresh tumor samples must be taken for ancillary studies prior to fixation it is best to incise the specimen through an area in which there is no doubt that excision is complete, i.e., one with a thick intact capsule or covering layer of normal tissue.

6.10 Ancillary Studies

Ancillary studies are essential, not optional, in all cases of pediatric neoplasia in which material is submitted for diagnosis. The majority of new SIOP trial protocols include mandatory sampling for biological studies. It is routine practice in our laboratory to take samples in culture medium for cytogenetics as the minimum

additional investigation in every case. With more substantial specimens, i.e., open biopsies or resections, a more detailed protocol is applied (Table 6.1). In taking these samples, every effort should be made to use "sterile technique" and sterile disposable instruments, etc. This is particularly important for those samples to be cultured for cytogenetic studies. In the USA, the Children's Cancer Group (CCG) provide kits for specimen procurement in cases of pediatric neoplasia thus facilitating diagnostic studies and ongoing biological research into these complex and fascinating conditions.

Both normal and tumor tissue should be sampled and stored whenever possible.

The samples should be taken as promptly as possible after removal of the specimen from the patient, but this must be done by the person reporting the specimen, i.e., the pathologist. Therefore, a short delay in transit to the laboratory is acceptable. Our procedure is to leave the photography until after samples have been taken. With a large specimen it is possible to section it and, if homogeneous, take the samples from one half leaving the other for photography. It is always possible to take the samples without compromising assessment of margins. If studies of mRNA are contemplated, then the tissue sample should be stored in sterile conditions on water ice prior to uplift. The delay in taking the sample should be as short as practicable as mRNA is susceptible to relatively rapid deterioration.

In the case of heterogeneous lesions, the sampling should incorporate multiple areas. Foci of obvious necrosis can be avoided but hemorrhagic areas are often the most viable, and firm fleshy areas may be more fibrous and contain fewer tumor cells. The concept of heterogeneity does not apply to macroscopic appearances only. Within a large tumor mass there is the possibility of clonal heterogeneity and this may be significant if assessment of prognostic features is to have a bearing on the intensity of therapy. Examples would be the identification of n-myc amplification in composite nodular ganglioneuroblastoma or 1p deletion in neuroblastoma [15] – bad prognostic features which can be variably present in different parts/cellular nodules of a tumor, and if only one area is examined a false negative result may be obtained. It is therefore good practice to take tissue from several areas of all substantial tumor specimens in order to minimize this potential problem.

The number of blocks that should be taken for histological examination from a large specimen varies according to the individual case. A useful rule of thumb is to take a minimum of one block for each centimeter of the largest dimension of the lesion, but this should not be regarded as an absolute and in most instances many more blocks are indicated. Points of interest and resection edges of nerves, vessels, and soft tissue mar-

Table 6.1 Pediatric neoplasia: ancillary studies (excluding "routine" paraffin section immunohistochemistry)

Investigation	Samples required
Cytogenetics	Tumor and normal tissue in cytogenetics medium
Molecular genetics	Tumor and normal tissue snap frozen in liquid nitrogen and stored in liquid nitrogen (gaseous phase) or at –80oC. Sample held on water ice for mRNA studies to be dealt with without delay
Immunohistochemistry/Fluorescent in situ hybridization (FISH)	Snap frozen in OCT medium, store at –80oC
Touch imprints (>10) for FISH	Air dry
Electron microscopy	Paper-thin section or 1 mm cubes in 4% gluteraldehyde
Tissue storage (long term)	Tumor and normal tissue for research, flow cytometry, etc., s stored in liquid nitrogen (gaseous phase) or at –80oC

gins of questionable clearance which have been indicated by the surgeon by means of marker sutures or in the request form should receive particular attention and will require a larger number of blocks to be taken. Tissue blocks should be taken from normal tissue as well as the lesion. Sectioning of a block of appropriate size is much easier after fixation. The site of origin of individual blocks should be recorded on an appropriate diagram or photograph of the specimen at the time of sampling. This allows the pathologist to return to a specific area of the specimen if initial histological examination identifies additional features requiring further detailed assessment, e.g., focal or diffuse anaplasia in nephroblastoma [16]. It is good practice to take "mirror image" blocks from the tumor with one block frozen down in liquid nitrogen for research purposes while the other is processed for histology. This allows molecular studies, preparations of microarrays, and morphological studies to be conducted on the same potentially clonal areas of an individual tumor.

6.11 Fixation and Processing

A number of standard fixatives are available to the pathologist, but the most flexible given the need for speed of fixation, lack of toxicity, etc., is 10% buffered formalin solution. It is possible to perform electron microscopy on tissues which have been in 10% formalin fixative even although ultrastructure is degraded. This fixative is also ideal for most immunohistochemical studies.

In North America, the fixative B5 (sublimate sodium acetate formalin) is widely used for lymph node and renal biopsies.

Other commonly used fixatives include Bouin's, Zenker's, and Carnoy's. All have advantages for specific

indications but for general use these are outweighed by problems of cost, preparation, and disposal.

Heat fixation by microwave using a standard domestic microwave oven is effective for specimens of substantial size, but we have found a significant frequency of unacceptable cellular artifact and do not use this method as routine.

The volume of fixative is critical. A ratio of 10:1 fixative to specimen is an acceptable minimum. It is important that the specimen should be entirely immersed in the fixative solution. The purpose of these fixatives is to complex the proteins in the tissue, stabilizing tissue and thus stopping the autolytic processes which would degrade tissue structure and ultrastructure.

The penetration of fixative into tissue blocks is one of the most significant rate-limiting factors in determining how long it takes to have material available for the pathologist to study under the microscope. In general terms formalin will penetrate at a rate of 1 mm/h and will go on for a considerable period slowly penetrating into the middle of large tissue specimens. Other fixatives penetrate much more slowly or only penetrate the surface of the tissue sample to any great degree.

The penetration of formalin is temperature-dependant and while it is entirely satisfactory at as low as 4°C it is probably accelerated at higher temperatures and this is one means by which the fixation time can be reduced if there is an urgent requirement for a tissue diagnosis. Standard vacuum embedding processing machines also accelerate both fixation and processing and save time. One can process needle core biopsy samples over a period of only 4 hand have a paraffin section cut and stained for viewing within 5 h of the biopsy having been taken. However, this means that we must accept some degradation in morphology and perhaps also compromise immunohistochemical studies as

Table 6.2 Typical tissue processing cycles (vacuum embedding)

Overnight (standard blocks)			Rapid (small biopsies)		
Phase	Duration (min)	Temperature 8C	Phase	Duration (min)	Temperature 8C
1	120	45	1 Formalin	Passed	
2	30	No heating	2 Water	Passed	
3	60	No heating	3 70% Spirit	Passed	
4	60	No heating	4 Methylated spirit	25	45
5	60	No heating	5 Methylated spirit	25	45
6	60	No heating	6 Methylated spirit	25	45
7	60	45	7 Methylated spirit	30	45
8	90	45	8 Absolute alcohol	30	45
9	90	No heating	9 Xylene	30	45
10 Xylene	90	No heating	10 Xylene	30	45
11 Wax	45	60	11 Wax	15	60
12 Wax	45	60	12 Wax	15	45
13 Wax	45	60	13 Wax	15	45
14 Wax	45	60	14 Wax	30	45

the fixation is not as good as it would be with a longer fixation, and processing period and protein linkages which expose or mask antigens are not optimal. More usually, tissue samples are fixed for approximately 24 h before being processed on a cycle which takes between 16 and 18 h to remove tissue water and fat and to replace these with paraffin, providing a paraffin block for sectioning. Dehydration is achieved by use of alcohols and fat is removed by alcohols and xylene (Table 6.2). For bone lesions, decalcification may be necessary and will delay block sampling and subsequent histological examination by several days.

The new generation of tissue processors utilize microwaves to accelerate fixation and this together with use of alternative solvents allows needle biopsies to be processed within 1 h, or a block of a tumor resection (5 mm thickness) to be processed in 3 h. Decalcification of a bone tumor sample can be completed in 12 h.

6.12 The Preparation of Histological Material

The histological examination of surgical material is an essential part of the diagnostic process. This requires the cutting of sections from the paraffin block, usually at a thickness of 4–5 microns and these sections are then stained with a variety of dyes which can demonstrate the various component parts of the tissue sample in question. The standard histological stain for daily use is the hemotoxylin and eosin (H & E) stain, which provides a very good demarcation between nuclei, stained blue with hematoxylin, and the cytoplasm, stained varying degrees of pink with eosin.

The diagnostic utility of other special stains has been to a considerable extent superseded by the development of immunohistochemistry. However, a limited number of these stains remain useful in specific tumors (Fig. 6.6, Table 6.3).

Formalin-fixed paraffin-embedded tissue sections are also utilized for immunohistochemical studies. Cytology touch preparations and frozen sections are better for in situ hybridization studies and are also essential for immunofluorescence studies when appropriate.

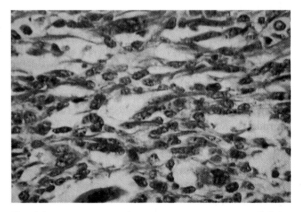

Fig. 6.6 PTAH staining showing cross-striations in a rhabdomyosarcoma.

Table 6.3 Special stains in pediatric neoplasia

Stain	Demonstrates
Periodic acid-Schiff (PAS) ± diastase	Glycogen in Ewing's sarcoma
Reticulin	Reticulin fibers (types III and IV collagen) in soft tissue tumors
Phosphotungstic acid-hematoxylin (PTAH)	Cross-striation in rhabdomyoblasts (little used)
Masson-Fontana	Melanin pigment in clear cell sarcoma and melanoma
Grimelius	Argyrophilic reaction in paraganglionoma
Perls Prussian Blue	Ferric iron pigment
von Kossa	Calcium
Alkaline phosphatase	Positive in osteoblasts in osteosarcoma

6.13 The Diagnostic Process

The development of a final diagnostic opinion is the result of consideration and integration of several sources of information, i.e., clinical presentation, anatomic localization (clinical and imaging), laboratory investigations (e.g., biochemistry) and operative appearances. With this information on hand, the macroscopic examination and sampling of a specimen leads to the final step of histological examination.

While it is true that a diagnosis can be inferred from any or all of the steps outlined above, there is no doubt that only histology can provide a definitive diagnostic opinion and this examination will also deliver prognostic information relevant to the individual case.

In making a histological diagnosis the pathologist assesses the presence of features of malignancy and seeks evidence of differentiation, i.e., the development of features indicative of the cell lineage of origin which can be recognized by H & E staining, special stains, and immunohistochemical studies.

The histological diagnosis of malignancy is based on assessment of a lesion with regard to the age of the patient, the site or organ of origin, the nature of the lesion in relation to surrounding structures, the presence of necrosis, degree of organization/differentiation, and cellular morphology. For example, a highly cellular mass in the middle of the kidney is likely to be a neoplasm. Necrosis of a spindle cell proliferative lesion of soft tissue is a strong indicator that one is dealing with a sarcoma. In all instances infiltrative invasive lesional margins as opposed to encapsulated/pseudo-encapsulated expansile margins suggests malignancy. These features and the presence or absence of differentiation do not absolutely predict behavior and the cellular morphology is important. Nuclear enlargement with increased hematoxylin staining density (hyperchromatism) and variation in nuclear and cellular size and shape (pleomorphism) are typical features of neoplasms. An increased mitotic rate with atypical and abnormal mitotic figures is frequently but not invariably seen. Thus it is the assessment of the lesion both in isolation and in the context of its surroundings that leads to a diagnosis. Frequently, however, the tumor may present as a lesion of small blue cells or an apparently undifferentiated sarcoma. In these instances the search for evidence of differentiation indicating the cell lineage of the tumor requires studies of molecular or ultrastructural differentiation by immunohistochemistry and electron microscopy.

Patterns of regression in childhood tumors can be spontaneous or treatment-induced and may present as either maturation or true regressive changes, e.g., necrosis, fibrosis, cystic degeneration, myxoid degeneration, or calcification [17–19].

Spontaneous regressive features, i.e., not related to therapy, can indicate some prognostic potential. Necrosis is generally regarded as a feature of aggressive, fast-growing malignant tumors but may also indicate the potential for a good response to chemotherapy because of the high cell turnover rate, although this is not true for rhabdoid tumors. The presence of a significant lymphoid cell infiltrate is sometimes an indication of a better prognosis lesion, e.g., inflammatory fibrosarcoma, or a pseudotumor. Myxoid change tends to be a feature of benign or slow-growing tumors of low malignant potential. Myxoid change in botyroid rhabdomyosarcoma is associated with better prognosis lesions.

Maturation of untreated tumors is characterized by increasing differentiation towards mature tissue phenotype. The classical example is neuroblastoma where spontaneous maturation to ganglioneuroblastoma or ganglioneuroma is well recognized. In the case of ovarian teratomas the presence of gliomatosis peritonei is a marker of a good prognosis.

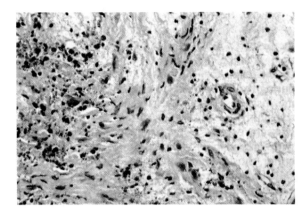

Fig. 6.7 Histology of an embryonal rhabdomyosarcoma showing postchemotherapy changes. Foamy macrophages, hemosiderin-laden macrophages, and fibrosis.

Similar patterns of regression and maturation are seen as an effect of therapy and can pose problems for the pathologist if they are so marked as to preclude most of the prognostic assessment of a tumor (Fig. 6.7). Chemotherapy frequently downstages a tumor – an effect most often seen in nephroblastoma. Postchemotherapy cystic change in nephroblastoma is common and care must be taken not to mistake this feature and make a diagnosis of cystic partially differentiated nephroblastoma. In osteosarcoma the postchemotherapy assessment of tumor response is a very accurate predictor of prognosis. If 10% or more of the tumor cells remain viable after a course of intensive therapy then the prognosis is poor.

It should be remembered that tumors are composed of clones of cells which as a result of mutation during tumorigenesis may have different patterns and degrees of response to therapy. This may result in a very heterogeneous response with fibrosis of tumor adjacent to viable lesional tissue. Occasionally the therapy seems to select out a particularly "resistant" aggressive clone and the pattern of dedifferentiation is seen. The prognostic implications of maturation under the influence of therapy are not yet clear and similarly metaplasia is not thought to have prognostic significance.

6.14 Immunohistochemistry

The introduction of immunohistochemistry to the armamentarium of diagnostic histopathology has revolutionized the subject and has significantly contributed to the management of pediatric neoplasia. In recent years there has been a massive expansion in the use of antibodies in tissue diagnosis. The principal influence has been in adding a degree of objectivity into the essentially subjective area of histological diagnosis by

confirming lineage differentiation in embryonal and undifferentiated neoplasms (Fig. 6.8a–g).

Immunohistochemistry is based on the premise that a particular component of a tissue, acting as an antigen, can be identified by a specific antibody carrying a label which can be rendered visible. A number of techniques are routinely used, but the underlying philosophy is the same for all. The variation in technique relates to attempts to maximize the intensity of the label signal indicating the presence of a specific antigen of interest.

Two types of antibodies are used. The first are polyclonal and tend to be less specific and sensitive while the second, which are now more commonly used, are monoclonal antibodies which allow for the use of very sensitive and highly specific detection techniques. The most commonly used methods of demonstrating the presence of antibody binding to tissue antigen are the peroxidase-antiperoxidase immune complex method and the avidin-biotin immunoenzymatic method. More detailed consideration of the principles and techniques can be found in a variety of specialist texts [20, 21].

The antibodies are named either by reference to the antigen (protein product/structure) to which they bind or in the case of leukocytes and related antigens, by the cluster differentiation antigen designation (CD) which have been determined at a series of international workshops.

Sensitivity and specificity are of vital importance. A number of techniques have been employed to increase sensitivity and, in general, these attempt to unmask antigens which are hidden during tissue processing presumably by the complexing of proteins during fixation. This can be achieved by digestion of the tissue sections by proteolytic enzymes, e.g., trypsin, by a combination of heat and pressure in a pressure cooker, or by treatment with microwaves with and without the use of additional chemical buffer, most commonly citrate. This process of so-called antigen retrieval using microwaving of sections in citrate or other buffers is now widely used and is extremely successful in allowing low antigen concentrations to be exposed for antibody binding thus increasing the frequency and intensity of positive reactions. Care must be exercised in the use of antigen retrieval as it is possible to produce very convincing and wholly inappropriate false-positive reactions with several antibodies. Meticulous attention to the practical and technical aspects is essential and each laboratory has to establish its own specific methodological conditions, within general principles, for each antibody whichever technique is employed.

Antibodies are used in panels, i.e., several different antisera are individually applied to separate, usually consecutive, sections of a block or blocks of tumor in

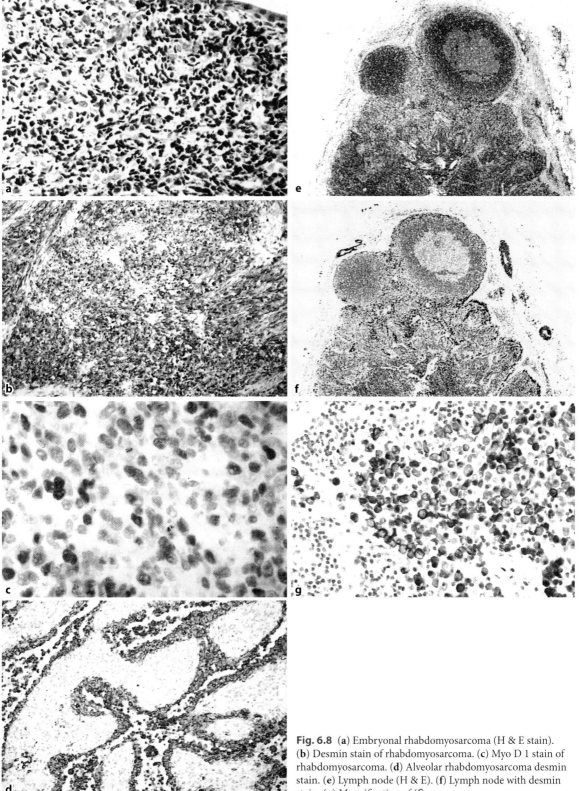

Fig. 6.8 (**a**) Embryonal rhabdomyosarcoma (H & E stain). (**b**) Desmin stain of rhabdomyosarcoma. (**c**) Myo D 1 stain of rhabdomyosarcoma. (**d**) Alveolar rhabdomyosarcoma desmin stain. (**e**) Lymph node (H & E). (**f**) Lymph node with desmin stain. (**g**) Magnification of (**f**).

Table 6.4 Examples of antibodies useful in pediatric tumor diagnosis

Antibody	Antisera/cell lineage marked	Tumor
CD45 Leukocyte common antigen	Leukocytes	Lymphomas
CD20 (L26)	B lymphocytes	Lymphomas
CD45RO(UCHL-1)	T lymphocytes	Lymphomas
CD30 (Ber H-2)	Activated lymphocytes/macrophages/ Reed-Sternberg cells	Hodgkin's disease/Anaplastic large cell lymphoma
CD15 (LeuM1)	Reed-Sternberg cells	Hodgkin's disease
CD68 (KP1)	Macrophages	Histiocytic neoplasms
Kappa/Lambda	Ig light chains	Lymphoid clonal proliferation
Neuron-specific enolase (NSE)	Neuroectoderm	Neuroblastoma
S100	Glial/Schwann cells/others	Neurofibroma, etc., Langerhan's cells
β2-microglobulin	β2-microglobulin	PNET
Synaptophysin	Neuroectoderm/neuroendocrine	Ewing's/PNET
MIC-2 (CD99)	MIC-2 gene product (glycoprotein P30/32)	Ewing's/PNET
Vimentin	Intermediate filaments/mesenchyme	Ewing's/soft tissue sarcoma
Actin (common, smooth muscle, sarcomeric)	Muscle filaments	Rhabdomyosarcoma
Desmin	Muscle (smooth/striated)	Rhabdomyosarcoma
Myoglobin	Striated muscle	Rhabdomyosarcoma
Myo D-1	Skeletal muscle	Rhabdomyosarcoma
Cytokeratins (AE1-AE3, CAM 5.2,etc.)	Epithelial	Synovial sarcoma
CD1a	Langerhan's cells	Langerhan's cell histiocytosis

order to demonstrate evidence of lineage differentiation.

It is vital to avoid false-positive and false-negative staining and to that end standard positive controls and negative controls are always included in staining batches. Pediatric neoplasms commonly exhibit pluripotent differentiation [22] and this potential pitfall is partly negated by the use of multiple antibodies. Example panels of some antibodies commonly used in the diagnosis of pediatric tumors are provided in Table 6.4. The use of more than one antibody specific for a particular cell lineage is recommended when diagnostic confirmation is sought.

A common problem in immunohistochemistry is the need to recognize and avoid blind overreliance on the presence of a "positive" reaction. There is much crossreaction and variable expression of antigens in pediatric tumors. For example, in primitive rhabdomyosarcomas it is not uncommon to see positive staining for neuron-specific enolase, which is generally regarded as a marker useful in the diagnosis of neuroblastoma. Similarly, the MIC2 (CD99) Ewing's/primitive neuroectodermal tumor (PNET) marker can be expressed in other pediatric tumors, in particular lymphoma and rhabdomyosarcoma. It is therefore not sufficient merely to expose the section to the antibody, blindly identify a positive labeling signal, and attribute a diagnosis. The positive staining must be in the correct tissue fraction and must correlate with the morphology of the lesion and the clinical presentation of the case. Evaluation of these studies requires an experienced medical practitioner to correlate the data. Blind adherence to immunohistochemical staining may lead to erroneous diagnosis.

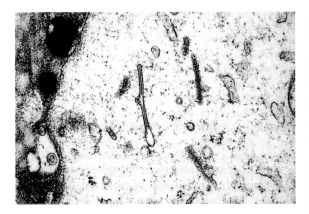

Fig. 6.9 Electron micrographs showing diagnostic Birbeck granules in Langerhan's cells.

6.15 Electron Microscopy

The advent of immunohistochemical techniques has been associated with a dramatic reduction in the utilization of electron microscopy in the diagnosis of pediatric neoplasia. There are instances, however, where ultrastructure can indicate lineage specificity of otherwise undifferentiated tumors and clarify its true nature (i.e., neuroendocrine "granules" in neuroblastoma, cytoplasmic glycogen in Ewing's sarcoma, cytoplasmic filaments with Z bands in rhabdomyosarcoma). Electron microscopy is particularly important in the diagnosis of Langerhan's cell histiocytosis where the identification of Birbeck granules is diagnostic (Fig. 6.9).

Tissue submitted for electron microscopy studies must be placed in special fixatives, e.g., gluteraldehyde 4%. The processing of tissue for electron microscopy requires only very small tissue samples because gluteraldehyde penetrates so poorly. It is labor-intensive and expensive. In tumor diagnosis, we reserve electron microscopy for very specific indications and do not perform these studies as routine in all pediatric neoplasms, although we take appropriate samples in gluteraldehyde fixative from all tumors if sufficient tissues are submitted and additional studies are required.

6.16 Cytogenetics

Several pediatric tumors are characterized by specific chromosomal translocations which, in those cases which are diagnostically difficult on light microscopy, can help clarify the diagnosis. Examples include t(2:13) (q35: q14) in alveolar rhabdomyosarcoma [23], t(11:22) (q24:q12) in Ewing's sarcoma, and peripheral PNETs [24], t(x:18) (p11.2:q11.2) in synovial sarcoma [25]. Many other tumors also express consistent chromosomal abnormalities and more examples are being identified almost with every passing week.

Previously these were identified by classical G-banding studies of metaphase spreads of cultured tumor cells, but more recently the use of specific probes and the fluorescent in situ hybridization (FISH) technique has been employed in the rapid identification of chromosomal abnormality such as translocations. FISH can be done on cytological samples and frozen sections thus avoiding the need for expensive and time-consuming tumor cell culture. Interphase FISH studies can also be performed on formalin fixed paraffin embedded sections, including sections from archived tumor cases. The procedure is more technically demanding than that with nonformalin fixed material and requires careful attention to protein digestion and chemical pretreatments to increase cellular permeability and facilitate entry and binding of the DNA probes.

A more detailed review of these cytogenetic lesions and the methodologies employed in their investigation is provided in subsequent chapters of this book.

6.17 Molecular Genetics

As diagnostic samples become ever smaller, the provision of adequate tissue for classical cytogenetic analysis becomes problematic. This challenge has been met by the now routine application of polymerase chain reaction (PCR) techniques to amplify tumor DNA or RNA (reverse-transcriptase polymerase chain reaction, RT-PCR) in small tumor samples, thus allowing identification of tumor specific translocations and their fusion transcripts [26–28]. Once again, both standard PCR (DNA) or RT-PCR (RNA) is easier on unfixed samples, fresh or snap frozen in liquid nitrogen, but results can also be achieved on archived tumor paraffin blocks.

6.18 The Prognostic Process

Increasingly, in cases of pediatric neoplasia, it is necessary for the pathologist to provide prognostic information as well as a histological diagnosis. This is done by further detailed evaluation of the histology and, in the case of some tumors, by molecular and cytogenetic studies of tumor tissue samples.

6.19 Standard Histological Criteria

In many types of tumor the histological subtype alone carries prognostic implications. For example, alveolar rhabdomyosarcoma is known to carry more serious prognosis stage for stage than embryonal rhabdomyo-

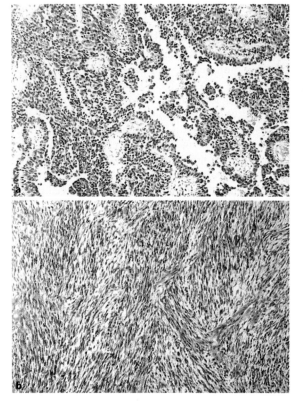

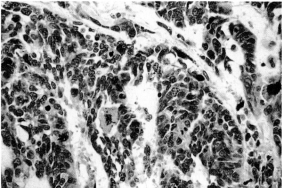

Fig. 6.11 Unfavorable nephroblastoma.

Fig. 6.10 (**a**) Alveolar rhabdomyosarcoma; (**b**) spindle cell variant.

nodal metastases, and "M" to the presence or absence of distant metastases. A 2, i.e., similarity or otherwise to normal tissue of the same lineage, are assessed. The grading system of Coindre et al. [32] as used by review pathologists in United Kingdom Children Cancer Study Group trials is shown in Table 6.5 for illustration. The reader is directed to references to the grading systems of Markhede, Myhre Jensen, Costa, and Trojani at the end of this chapter for further information [33–36].

6.20 Cytogenetics and Molecular Genetics

Vital prognostic information which has a significant bearing on intensity and duration of therapy in certain pediatric neoplasms is obtained from genetic analyses. For example, in rhabdomyosarcoma the confirmation of the alveolar subtype by demonstration of t(2:13) in a lesion previously considered embryonal on light microscopy will result in a more intensive therapeutic regimen. In neuroblastoma the identification of 1p deletion15 and N-myc amplification [37] are proven indicators of more aggressive tumors with a worse prognosis which require intensive therapy compared with neuroblastomas without these features. High trk-A proto-oncogene expression is associated with a better prognosis and is inversely related to N-myc amplification [38].

An important advance in prognostication has resulted from the capacity of molecular genetic techniques, particularly RT-PCR, to identify previously undetectable tumor cells in peripheral blood or bone marrow samples [39].

Tumors will spread via the blood stream as they metastasize. There is now clear evidence that the presence of this otherwise occult tumor spread is associated with increased incidence of established me-

sarcoma. Spindle cell rhabdomyosarcoma has a better prognosis than any other variant (Figs. 6.10, 6.11).

It is important to search for prognostic features in individual tumor types, e.g., anaplasia/unfavorable histology in nephroblastoma, the MKI and extent of cellular and stromal differentiation in neuroblastoma [29–30], because features such as these can influence therapy in individual tumors of a given stage. These and other examples will be discussed in more detail in the chapters relating to individual tumor types.

The more general principles regarding prognostication relate to assessment of tumor stage and, particularly in soft tissue sarcomas, the histological grade. Staging is based on the gross anatomical distribution of disease modified by histological assessment of local excision margins and confirmation/identification of nodal and distal metastases. Specific staging systems apply to several of the organ-specific pediatric tumors, e.g., nephroblastoma, and the National Wilms' Tumor Study (NWTS) definitions of stage are described elsewhere in this book.

An alternative staging system applicable to tumors of all sites is the TNM system: "T" related to the size of the primary tumor, "N" to the presence or absence of

Table 6.5 Histological grading in soft tissue sarcoma [32]

Feature		Score
Mitoses	0–9 (per 10 high power fields	1
	10–19 (per 10 high power fields)	2
	>20 (per 10 high power fields)	3
Necrosis	None	1
	<50% of the tumor	2
	>50% of the tumor	3
Differentiation	Very highly differentiated	2
	Moderately differentiated but cell type easily recognizable	3
	Poorly differentiated or cell type uncertain	

Grade is determined by aggregate score for all these features, i.e., Grade I, Score 3–4; Grade II, Score 5–6; Grade III, Score 7–9

Table 6.6 Some pediatric tumors with specific, diagnostic chromosomal translocations

Tumor	Translocation	Gene fusion transcript
Ewing's sarcoma group	t(11;22)(q24:q12)	EWS-FLI1
	t(21;22)(q22;q12)	EWS-ERG
	t(7;22)(p22;q12)	EWS-ETV1
	t(17;22)q12;q12	EWS-E1AF
	t(2;22)q33;q12	EWS-FEV
Desmoplastic small round cell tumor	t(11;22)q13;q12	EWS-WT1
Alveolar rhabdomyosarcoma	t(2;13)(q35;q14)	PAX3-FKHR
	t(2;13)(q335;q14)	PAX7-FKHR
Synovial sarcoma	t(x;18)(p11.2;q11.2)	SYT-SSX1
		SYT-SSX2
		SYT-SSX4
Congenital fibrosarcoma	t(12;15)(p13;q25)	ETV6-NTRK3

tastases, reduced disease-free interval, and reduced survival [40]. In those tumors characterized by specific chromosomal translocations and resultant gene fusion transcripts (Table 6.6) the use of RT-PCR can detect this tumor spread in blood and marrow thus providing objective evidence for upstaging or intensification of chemotherapy. Some SIOP tumor protocols now include this investigation as part of patient surveillance.

A more detailed review of this area is given in subsequent chapters of this book.

6.21 Additional Techniques

There are a number of techniques, which are non-standard, but which can provide further valuable diagnostic and prognostic information in pediatric neoplasms.

6.22 Flow Cytometry

Flow cytometry is a technique which allows cell suspensions to be analyzed for the presence or absence of a number of features including cell size, DNA content (ploidy), and the presence or absence of cell surface or cytoplasmic antigens [41].

The general principle is that the sample is a suspension of cells stained with dyes or labeled by antibodies to specific cellular antigens which are passed through a beam of laser light. The cells and their constituent parts reflect back the light which is picked up by detectors which count the number of "events" and analyze the different constituent populations of the cell suspension. The data obtained is presented in a digitized form, usually as a scatter curve or as a histogram.

In the case of neoplasia, the features which are most usefully measured using flow cytometry are ploidy and cell surface marker phenotype. Neoplasms can be either diploid, that is with a normal DNA content or aneuploid, i.e., those which have other than a normal content. Aneuploidy usually correlates with tumor aggressiveness and a worse prognosis; however, in neuroblastoma hyperdiploid tumors have a better prognosis [42].

The other major use for flow cytometry is in the study of lymphoid tissue enlargement where one cannot be sure if the process is a bizarre reaction or a lymphoma. If the cells are exposed to antisera which bind to cell surface markers it is possible to define the presence of small clones of atypical cells, frequently aneuploid or abnormally large, within a more heterogeneous cell population within the lymph node and also determine the specific lineage, e.g., T or B lymphocyte in non-Hodgkin's lymphoma or CD30 positive Reed-Sternberg cells in Hodgkin's disease. We have used this technique with some success in patients with lymphadenopathy who present with bizarre lymphoproliferative pathology in various inherited immune deficiency disorders.

Flow cytometry with analysis of DNA content/ploidy can also be performed in paraffin-embedded tissues in which the nuclei are released from the paraffin and rendered in suspension. The DNA is then stained, the nuclei can be counted and the nucleic acid content and therefore ploidy determined.

6.23 Indices of Cell Proliferation in Tumors

Attempts have been made to correlate growth fraction and other indicators of cell proliferation in tumor samples with prognosis. The S phase fraction, i.e., that committed to mitosis, may correlate with prognosis. Modern techniques of assessment of cell proliferation are based on immunohistochemical principles using antibodies to proteins involved in the mitotic phase of the cell cycle, or in the phase of cell cycle prior to mitoses, or on the identification of features which correlate with proliferation.

It is known that Ki-67 is a nuclear protein expressed in cells in the proliferate phases of the cell, G1, G2, M, and S. It is now widely used for the immunohistochemical assessment of growth faction in paraffin sections and appears to correlate with increased tumor aggressiveness [43]. Ki-67 is the standard proliferation marker used in my department. PCNA is another of these proteins but it is less specific, being present in a proportion of cells in the resting phase of the cell.

AgNOR proteins were previously fashionable as potential indicators of tumor aggressiveness and proliferation [44]. NORS are nucleolar organizing regions which contain ribosomal genes and related proteins and represent sites of increased DNA transcription.

They are normally identified by their capacity to bind silver, which allows them to be counted in cells, and the mean AgNOR count in a cell population can be used as a prognostic indicator with a higher AgNOR count correlating with a more aggressive lesion and a worse prognosis.

In the case of pediatric tumors, AgNORs have little place as there are other more robust and reliable prognostic indicators as previously described.

6.24 p53

The p53 tumor suppressor gene product is involved in many cellular pathways including cell cycle control, DNA repair, and programmed cell death (apoptosis) [45, 46]. In human cancers p53 is the most frequently detected mutated gene, and loss of gene product function by mutation or allelic loss is regarded as a central part of the process of tumorigenesis. The Li-Fraumeni familial cancer syndrome is the result of autosomal dominant transmission of germ line abnormalities of the p53 gene [47, 48] and this syndrome is now recognized as having implications for pediatric neoplasia, particularly rhabdomyosarcoma and adrenocortical carcinoma, as well as several different carcinomas and sarcomas in adults.

Given the key role of p53 there has been, over recent years, considerable interest in the potential of this gene as a prognostic factor in tumors. Most activity has been in the use of immunohistochemistry employing antisera to p53 protein and assessing the proportion of positive cells and the intensity of staining. Abnormal p53 protein accumulates in cells bearing p53 gene mutations. The results are mixed and mostly relate to adult malignant neoplasms. It appears likely that increased p53 immunostaining does correlate with more aggressive, poor prognosis tumor in many tumor types, but there is no convincing evidence that this is an independent predictive prognostic variable, and assessment of p53 status remains, for the present, confined to the research end of the spectrum of tumor pathology.

6.25 Future Perspectives

The key challenges for pathology in the near future will lie in the need to support more complex and detailed ancillary investigations of pediatric tumors principally for prognostic purposes, which will increasingly select and direct the therapeutic options in any given case. This challenge will be faced in light of increasingly small diagnostic samples and presurgical therapy. Cytological diagnosis, particularly the use of fine needle aspiration, will increasingly become the primary diagnostic methodology providing samples for histological diagnosis and genetic studies. Surgeons will have to appreciate the pressures placed on the pathologist in these circumstances and develop with their colleagues appropriate protocols to ensure that the essential diagnostic and prognostic processes are not compromised to the detriment of the clinical care of our patients.

Surgeons and pathologists have a responsibility to ensure the supply and retention of tumor and normal tissue samples for research purposes if progress in diagnosis, prognostication, and treatment is to be maintained. The application of RT-PCR and the generation of tissue microarrays is a revolution in cancer research with massive potential for early therapeutic gain. The role of diagnostic histopathology in the management of pediatric neoplasia is greater today than ever. The constant desire to improve survival with highly toxic therapies has led to a demand for a more detailed assessment of individual neoplasms in terms of specific histological types and their variants, stage, and histological grade. The remarkable and rapidly accruing insights into the molecular biology and cytogenetics of tumors and tumorigenesis has not reduced the role of pathology. Rather it has imposed a need for pathologists to do more with tumor samples submitted for examination.

The result of the advances in knowledge of pediatric cancer is the need for all specialists to work together in an organized and coherent team approach. Pathologists, as part of this team, have a vital contribution to make which is at the fulcrum of clinical management.

References

1. Buchino JJ (1991) Cytopathology in pediatrics. Karger, Basel

2. Schaller RT, Schaller JF, Buschmann C, Kiviat N (1983) The usefulness of percutaneous fine-needle biopsy in infants and children. J Pediatr Surg 18:398–405

3. Wakely PE, Kardos TF, Frable WJ (1988) Application of fine needle aspiration biopsy to pediatrics. Hum Pathol 19:1383–1386

4. Cohen MB, Bottles, K, Ablin AR, Miller TR (1989) The use of fine needle aspiration biopsy in children. West J Med 150:665–667

6. McGahey BE, Nelson WA, Hall MT (1989) Fine needle aspiration biopsy of small round blue cell tumors of childhood: A three and a half year study. Lab Med 60:5P

6. Leung SW, Bedard YC (1993) Simple miniblock technique for cytology. Mod Pathol 6:630–632

7. Silverman JF, Joshi VV (1994) FNA biopsy of small round cell tumours of childhood: Cytomorphologic features and the role of ancillary studies. Diagn Cytopathol 10:245–255

8. Kardos TF, Maygarden SJ, Blumberg AK, Wakely PE, Frable WJ (1989) Fine needle aspiration biopsy in the management of children and young adults with peripheral lymphadenopathy. Cancer 63:703–707

9. Ball AB, Fisher C, Pittam M, Watkins RM, Westburg G (1990) Diagnosis of soft tissue tumours by Tru-cut biopsy. Brit J Surg 77:756–758

10. Barth RJ, Merino MR, Solomon D, Yang JC, Baker AR (1992) A prospective study of the value of core needle biopsy and fine needle aspiration in the diagnosis of soft tissue masses. Surgery 112:56–43

11. Giuliano AE, Eilber FR (1985) The rationale for planned reoperation after unplanned total excision of soft tissue sarcomas. J Clin Oncol 3:1344–1350

12. Bannayan GA, Huvos AG, D'Angio GJ (1971) Effect of irradiation on the maturation of Wilms' tumor. Cancer 27:812–818

13. Zuppan CW, Beckwith JB, Weeks DA, Luckey DW, Pringle KC (1991) The effect of preoperative therapy on the histologic features of Wilms' tumor: An analysis of cases from the third National Wilms' Tumor Study. Cancer 68:384–394

14. Smith JC (1974) In praise of the gross examination. Hum Pathol 5:505–506

15. Hayashi Y, Kanda N, Inaba T, Hanada R, Nagahara N, et al. (1989) Cytogenic findings and prognosis in neuroblastoma with emphasis on marker chromosome 1. Cancer 63:126–132

16. Beckwith JB (1998) National Wilms' Tumour Study: An update for pathologists. Pediatr Develop Pathol 1:79–84

17. Bolande RP (1985) Spontaneous regression and cytodifferentiation of cancer in early life: The oncogenic grace period. Surv Synth Pathol Res 44:296–311

18. Evans AE, Gerson J, Schnaufer L (1976) Spontaneous regression of neuroblastoma. NCI Monogr 44:49–54

19. Griffin ME, Bolande RP (1969) Familial neuroblastoma with regression and maturation to ganglioneuroblastoma. Paediatrics 43:377–382

20. Beesley JE (1993) Immunocytochemistry – A practical approach. Oxford University Press, Oxford

21. Polak JM, van Noorden S (1986) Immunocytochemistry. Modern methods and applications, 2nd edn. J Wright, Bristol

22. Parham DM, Weeks DA, Beckwith JB (1994) The clinicopathological spectrum of putative extrarenal rhabdoid tumours: An analysis of 42 case studies with immunohistochemistry and/or electron microscopy. Am J Surg Pathol 18:1010–1029

23. Douglass EC, Valentine M, Etcubanas E, Parham D, Weber BL, et al. (1987) A specific chromosomal abnormality in rhabdomyosarcoma. Cytogenet Cell Genet 45:148–155

24. Douglass EC, Valentine M, Green AA, Hayes FA, Thompson EI (1986) t(11: 22) and other chromosomal rearrangements in Ewing's sarcoma. J Natl Cancer Inst 77:1211–1215

25. Peter M, Gilbert E, Delattre O (2001) A multiplex real-time pcr assay for the detection of gene fusions observed in solid tumours. Lab Invest 81:905–912

26. Gilbert J, Haber M, Bordon SB, Marshall GM, Norris MD (1999) Use of tumour-specific gene expression for the differential diagnosis of neuroblastoma from other pediatric small round-cell malignancies. Am J Pathol 155:17–21

27. Anderson J, Gordon T, McManus A, Mapp T, Gould S, et al. (2001) Detection of the PAX3-FKHR fusion gene in paediatric rhabdomyosarcoma: A reproducible predictor of outcome? Br J Cancer 85:831–835

28. Limon J, Mrozek K, Mandahl N (1991) Cytogenetics of synovial sarcoma; presentation of ten new cases and review of the literature. Genes Chrom Cancer 3:338–345

29. Shimada H, Chatten J, Newton WA, Sachs N, Hamoudi AB, et al. (1984) Histopathologic prognostic factors in neuroblastic tumors: Definition of subtypes of ganglioneuroblastoma and an age-linked classification of neuroblastomas. J Natl Cancer Inst 73:405–416

30. Joshi VV, Cantor AB, Altshuler G, Larkin EW, Neill JSA, et al. (1992) Age-linked prognostic categorization based on a new histologic grading system of neuroblastomas. A clinicopathologic study of 211 cases from the Pediatric Oncology Group. Cancer 69:2197–2211

31. Beahrs OH, Henson DE, Hutter RVP (1992) Manual for staging of cancer, 3rd edn. Lippincott, Phildelphia

32. Coindre JM, Trojani M, Contesso G, David M, Rouesse J, et al. (1986) Reproducibility of a histopathological grading system for adult soft tissue sarcoma. Cancer 58:306–309

33. Markhede G, Angervall L, Stener B (1982) A multivariate analysis of the prognosis after surgical treatment of malignant soft tissue tumors. Cancer 49:1721–1733

34. Myhre Jensen O, Hogh J, Ostgaard SE, Nordentoft AM, Sneppen O (1991) Histopathological grading of soft tissue tumors: Prognostic significance in a prospective study of 278 consecutive cases. J Pathol 163:19–24

35. Costa J, Wesley RA, Glatstein E, Rosenberg SA (1984) The grading of soft tissue sarcomas: Results of a clinico-histopathologic correlation in a series of 163 cases. Cancer 53:530–541

36. Trojani M, Contesso G, Coindre JM, Rouesse J, Bui NB, et al. (1984) Soft tissue sarcomas of adults: Study of pathological and prognostic variables and definition of a histological grading system. Int J Cancer 33:37–42

37. Schwab M (1993) Amplification of N-myc as a prognostic marker for patients with neuroblastoma. Semin Cancer Biol 4:13–18

38. Nakagawara A, Arima M, Azar CG, Scavarda N, Brodeur GM (1992) Inverse relationship between trk expression and N-myc amplification in human neuroblastomas. Cancer Res 52:1364–1368

39. Burchill SA, Lewis IJ, Abrams K, Riley R, Imeson J, et al. (2001) Circulating neuroblastoma cells detected by reverse transcriptase polymerase chain reaction for tyrosine hydroxylase mRNA are an independent poor prognostic indicator in stage 4 neuroblastoma in children over 1 year. J Clin Oncol 19:1795–1801

40. Burchill SA, Selby PJ (2000) Molecular detection of low level disease in patients with cancer. J Pathol 190:6–14

41. Shapiro HM (1995) Practical flow cytometry, 3rd edn. Wiley-Liss, New York

42. Look AT, Hayes FA, Nitschke R, McWilliams NB, Green AA (1984) Cellular DNA content as a predictor of response to chemotherapy in infants with unresectable neuroblastoma. New Engl J Med 311:231–235

43. Jay V, Parkinson D, Becker L, Chan F-W (1994) Cell kinetic analysis in pediatric brain and spinal tumors: A study of 117 cases with Ki-67 quantitation and flow cytometry. Pediatr Pathol 14:253–276

44. Crocker J (1995) The trials and tribulations of interphase AgNORs. J Pathol 175:367–368

45. Dowell SP, Hall PA (1995) The p53 tumour suppressor gene and tumour prognosis: Is there a relationship? J Pathol 177:221–224

46. Wynford-Thomas D (1996) p53: Guardian of cellular senescence. J Pathol 180:118–121

47. Kleihues P, Schiauble B, zur Hausen A, Estieve J, Ohgaki H (1997) Tumours associated with p53 germline mutations: A synopsis of 91 families. Am J Pathol 150:1–13

48. Birch JM, Hartley AL, Tricker KJ, Prosser J, Condie A, et al. (1994) Prevalence and diversity of constitutional mutations in the p53 gene among 21 Li-Fraumeni families. Cancer Res 53:1298–1304

Chemotherapy and Novel Cancer Targeted Therapies

7

Milind Ronghe, Dermot Murphy

Contents

7.1 Introduction

Children's cancers are rare and account for 1% of all malignancies. Within Europe this represents some 12,000 new cases each year, with approximately 1,600 per year in the UK. In the UK, 1 in every 600 children under 15 years of age develop cancer. Although rare, childhood cancer is the second commonest cause of death in children between 1–14 years of age. These cancers are quite different from cancers affecting adults. Most adult tumors are carcinomas and are usually classified by their site of origin, whereas pediatric tumors occur in different parts of the body, look different under the microscope, and are classified by histological subtypes. Tumor types that are common to both adults and children, such as lymphomas and leukemia, differ in their biology, behavior, and prognosis and hence demand different treatment. They also respond differently to treatment. Some embryonal tumors presenting in infancy undergo spontaneous remission or maturation (e.g., Stage IVS neuroblastoma).

Survival rates for childhood cancer have improved dramatically over the last 20 years, such that approximately 70% of children can expect to become long-term survivors [1, 2]. This is reflected by the fact that today, 1 in 750 of the young adult population is now a survivor of childhood cancer. Treatments used to achieve this success are surgery, chemotherapy, and/or radiotherapy. Factors contributing to these improved survival rates are: the development of dedicated pediatric oncology centers, advances in surgical techniques, novel chemotherapy agents and regimens, targeted radiotherapy, and improvements in supportive care (early treatment of febrile neutropenia, better intensive care, improved transfusion services).

Surgery was the mainstay of treatment of solid tumors in children before the advent of effective chemotherapy. Cure could be obtained by surgery alone in the proportion of children with localized disease, and good palliation obtained in many others, and the surgeon was often the key clinician in the management of pediatric solid tumors. However, very few tumors present as a purely localized surgical problem. The surgeon becomes part of a larger team, needing to integrate surgical procedures with chemotherapy and/or radiotherapy. Although improvements in radiotherapy and surgery have reduced the late sequelae of curative therapy, chemotherapy now remains the mainstay of treatment for most childhood cancers. This chapter aims to discuss the factors which affect the way the pediatric surgeon interacts with a multidisciplinary team of experts, including the pediatric oncologist, radiologist, pathologist, and radiotherapist. The best outcome will be achieved by collaboration of interested specialists clearly understanding the efficacies and limitations of various forms of treatment.

Although complete tumor resection is of paramount importance for cure, most pediatric cancers are advanced at presentation (e.g., 55–60% sarcomas are high risk at diagnosis, 25% of bone tumors are metastatic at diagnosis, 90% of neuroblastomas occurring after infancy are Stage IV) and require systemic treatment. The prognosis for malignant solid tumors has improved since the introduction of effective chemotherapy capable of reducing the tumor volume and making previously unresectable tumors resectable. The operation also becomes safer and easier after preoperative chemotherapy. Furthermore, there is no delay in treating metastatic disease, which is detectable at diagnosis in a significant proportion of patients.

Some diseases, such as osteosarcoma, cannot be cured except with surgery to remove the local tumor, whereas in others such as lymphoma, biopsy followed by chemotherapy is all that is needed. In others, such as Ewing's sarcoma and rhabdomyosarcoma, the best treatment results may be obtained with systemic chemotherapy and a combination of surgery and/or radiotherapy for local control. In Europe, since the early 1990s, the concept of preoperative chemotherapy and delayed surgery for solid tumors of childhood became standard clinical practice due to successful Wilms' tumor trials of the SIOP (International Society of Pediatric Oncology) Group [3–5].

Children presenting with malignant diseases other than leukemia often present with palpable masses and are usually seen first by a surgeon. Except in emergencies, a thorough consideration of the possible differential diagnosis should be made before any surgical procedures are undertaken. This should ideally be done in discussion with the pediatric oncology team. Any necessary presurgical staging or investigations can then be planned, depending on the nature of the suspected lesion and the facilities available. Biopsy should ideally be performed in the regional specialist centers, where the necessary support services are available (e.g., molecular biology services) and once radiological examination of the lesion is complete. If appropriate, a number of interventions (such as bone marrow aspiration/trephine for staging) can be carried out while the child is anesthetized for biopsy/surgery.

In nearly all cases of malignancy, diagnosis must be confirmed by biopsy of the primary tumor. Traditionally, tumor material would be obtained by incisional or excisional biopsy at open operation, but advances in imaging techniques have led to much greater use of trucut biopsies obtained with ultrasound or computerized tomography (CT) guidance. In a tumor with obvious heterogeneity on initial imaging, open biopsy may still be preferable, to ensure that a representative sample is obtained. Biopsy sites must be within potential radiation fields, as malignant cells may seed along the biopsy track. In rare instances, a combination of radiological and biochemical or molecular biological findings may enable a definitive diagnosis to be made without biopsy, e.g., a tumor in the characteristic site, such as the anterior mediastinum or pineal region, with high alphafetoprotein (AFP) levels in the blood can be confidently diagnosed as a germ cell tumor, and a heterogeneous abdominal mass with calcification, raised urinary catecholamines, and infiltration of the bone marrow is a neuroblastoma. However, failure to obtain tissue makes it impossible to acquire important information regarding the biological and genetic characteristics of the tumor that often determine the risk factors affecting therapeutic decisions. Although the overall cure rate for childhood tumors is now around 70%, it is only by increased understanding at the biological level that further progress will be made, particularly in an appropriate risk stratification of current intensive treatments and in the development of novel therapies. With increased survival rates for childhood cancer, philosophy of treatment has changed over the years from "Cure at any cost" to "Cure at least possible cost."

7.2 Staging

Once the diagnosis has been confirmed, the extent of the tumor (size, position, relationship to surrounding structures, appearance of lymph nodes) must be established. Unfortunately, there is no single uniform staging approach for childhood malignancies and the surgeon will need to be aware of the requirements for staging of each tumor type according to the current protocols (see Table 7.1).

1. The staging of disease directs the treatment given and should help to avoid excessive therapy: in easily curable conditions excessive therapy is known to put the child at increased risk of adverse late effects of treatment.
2. The stage of the disease also tends to reflect the prognosis and, consequently, aids counseling of the family.
3. Staging systems generally progress from localized disease (Stage I) to widespread disease (Stage IV) and are based on the results obtained from clinical examination, radiology, and pathology.

More extensive tissue sampling and biopsy is usually only needed at the time of definitive operation. This information will determine what type of further treatment is required postoperatively. For example, in the current SIOP Wilms' tumor trial, pathologists make precise evaluation of the stage of the disease post nephrectomy. Children are then risk stratified and treated according to different therapy, depending on tumor histological subtype and stage of disease.

Table 7.1 Staging procedures for pediatric tumors

Germ cell	Wilms'	Neuro-blastoma	Lymphoma	Rhabdomyo-sarcoma	Hepato-blastoma	Osteo-sarcoma	Ewing's
AFP level	USS Abdo CT/MRI Abdo	Urinary Catecholamines	Bone marrow aspirate and trephine	CT/MRI scan local tumor	CT/MRI liver and abdo	MRI (or primary) before biopsy	CT or MRI (of primary) before biopsy
HCG	Chest x-ray; CT chest	Bone marrow aspirate/ trephine	CSF exam	CT chest; MRI abdo/ pelvis	MR angiography; CT chest	CT chest	CT chest
MRI/CT; Abdo/chest		Bone/ MIBG scan; CT chest/MRI abdo; Estimation of N-myc copy; +1p deletion (from fresh tumor)	CT chest; MRI of abdo/ pelvis; bone scan	CT/MRI brain scan (for head/ neck disease); Bone scan; Bone marrow; aspirate/ trephine	Bone marrow; aspirate/ trephine	Bone scan	Bone scan; bone marrow; aspirate/ trephine; fresh tumor for chromosome analysis

In some cases a presumptive diagnosis may be confirmed by tests other than biopsy of the primary tumor. Fresh material is often required from the biopsy to determine which protocol is used for treatment. AFP, Alpha Feto Protein; HCG, Human Chorionic Gonadotrophin; CSF, Cerebrospinal fluid

Staging for pediatric CNS tumors involves preoperative MRI of brain and spine, postoperative scan (usually within 48–72 h after resection) to assess the degree of residual disease, plus CSF sampling for malignant cells.

Increasingly, the chemotherapy response of the primary tumor in the postsurgical specimen is used in deciding postoperative treatment for a number of malignant solid tumors (e.g., in osteosarcoma and Ewing's sarcoma <90% necrosis of the tumor is considered a poor response and these patients are now randomized to receive more intensive treatment to improve the chances of long-term survival).

Intraoperative photography or clear diagrams can be very helpful to the radiotherapist and, even in the era of three-dimensional imaging, a description of the tumor in relation to fixed anatomical points is also useful. The use of titanium clips is valuable to delineate tumor margins and does not affect subsequent imaging.

Although chemotherapy is needed for nearly all tumors in childhood and is often given before definitive surgery, primary surgical excision is still indicated for a number of malignancies. These include Stage I testicular tumors, where no further treatment is needed if an associated raised AFP titre falls to normal with an expected half-life of 2.7 days postoperatively, Stage I or II neuroblastoma (abdominal or thoracic), some adult-type soft tissue sarcomas, most brain tumors such as astrocytomas and medulloblastomas.

Debulking of tumors are rarely indicated as primary surgical procedures, except for some brain tumors. In particular, they confirm no advantage in the treatment of lymphoma, which may present with widespread intra-abdominal disease, although surgery may be necessary if chemotherapy results in a complication such as perforation or bleeding, or if the patient presents with intestinal obstruction. It is important that the surgeon is then as conservative as possible in his approach, since the chance of complete remission of disease following chemotherapy is high and surgery performed at any stage in the disease does not lead to improved cure rates.

Emergency operations are unavoidable for intussusceptions, torsion of the tumor, perforation, and some rapid enlargement due to intratumoral bleeding, cystic degeneration, or necrosis.

Insertion of central venous catheter is probably the single most frequent operation that pediatric surgeons perform while caring for a child with malignancy. Centrally placed, long-term venous catheters are used for the administration of chemotherapy and antibiotics and for blood sampling. Central venous catheters make the care of the child easier, both for the child and for the medical team. Currently there are two main types of catheters used in clinical practice – tunneled, external catheters (Hickman line, Broviac line, Groshong catheters) and totally implanted access devices such as a portocath. External, tunnel catheters are generally easier to access, are less expensive than portocaths, offer less risk of extravasation into sub-

Table 7.2 Percentages of children with cancer or nonmalignant CNS tumor initially referred to UKCCSG, classified by age at diagnosis, Great Britain 1978–2000

Age at Diagnosis	1978–1982	1983–1987	1988–1992	1993–1997	1998–2002
0–9	62	74	81	90	92
10–12	55	63	67	81	86
13–14	36	46	51	71	76
Total	57	69	76	86	89

cutaneous tissue, allow more rapid infusions, and can be removed easily at the end of treatment. However, the portocath offers an improved cosmetic result, less restriction in normal activities, less maintenance care, and they are well protected, thus decreasing the chance of damage, and are associated with a lower risk of infection. Numerous methods of catheter care, e.g., flushing, are practiced in various pediatric oncology centers and none have proved superior when the literature is taken as a whole.

In addition to the insertion of central venous lines, diagnostic biopsies, and resection of individual tumors, the surgeon has a role in facilitating treatment given by other members of the oncology team, i.e., insertion of a mesh to displace the bowel out of the future field of radiation or insertion of pain control devices and surgical exposure for brachytherapy.

Furthermore, a surgeon also has a role in providing enteral access in patients receiving intensive chemotherapy. Children with cancer often have associated cachexia, with significant weight loss and malnutrition. The intensity and type of primary therapy (chemotherapy, surgery, and/or radiotherapy) is associated with decline in the nutritional status. Furthermore, patients receiving intensive chemotherapy have prolonged illnesses – mucositis, diarrhea, suboptimal dietary intake, and decreased appetite – all are side effects of chemotherapy that contribute to further weight loss. Numerous studies have demonstrated that a nutritionally-repleted patient tolerates therapy better and with fewer complications [6–8]. In addition to providing nutritional requirements, gastrostomy tubes can perform other functions. Clinical experience has demonstrated that gastrostomy tubes are an effective way to deliver medications and to provide hydration to children experiencing excessive emesis. The quality of life of both the child and family also appears to improve, as eating is a frequent source of conflict between the child and parents. Providing nutrition through a gastrostomy tube alleviates the frustration associated with forced feeding of the child via the mouth. Maintenance of normal patient nutrition throughout cancer treatment allows normal growth and improves quality of life.

In many cases of solid tumors, surgical excision of primary tumor is the preferred local treatment since radiotherapy has a much greater risk of long-term sequelae. The general principles of choice of local treatment are that surgical excision is the treatment of choice where: (1) complete excision is possible and results in improved survival and cure; (2) it will give functional and cosmetic results better than those obtained by other treatment.

Surgeons may also be consulted to deal with complications related to other forms of treatment: extravasation of chemotherapy agents causing tissue necrosis, typhilitis (neutropenic enterocolitis), intestinal perforation, strictures or avascular necrosis, or other damage due to late effects of radiotherapy.

Surgical decisions, as well as those concerning chemotherapy, radiotherapy, and overall treatment strategies are best made after joint discussion, which is facilitated by a formal system of consultations such as regular multidisciplinary oncology team meetings (Tumor Board), as well as maintaining communication between the key team members during the treatment.

In the UK, more than 80% of children with malignant disease are registered with the United Kingdom Children's Cancer Study Group (UKCCSG) (Table 7.2) [9] and are treated according to agreed tumor protocols. Although there are approximately 1,600 cases of childhood cancer diagnosed in the UK annually, when broken down into individual tumor types, the numbers, even for the commonest childhood tumors, are often too small to ensure that clinical trials can be completed satisfactorily at a national level. It is for this reason that the majority of the Phase III clinical trials in childhood cancer are now increasingly conducted at an international or collaborative basis (see Table 7.3). The power of such collaboration is the ability to conduct large trials with rapid accrual, which would allow the investigation of new agents to be undertaken quickly and effectively and thus be able to answer more rapidly some still unanswered questions regarding the treatment of children with malignant tumors. Active participation of all the interested clinicians treating childhood cancer in a group such as the

Table 7.3 Commonly used protocols for solid tumors

Tumor	Current protocol	Drugs	Acronyms
Neuroblastoma (stage IV)	HR-NBL-1/ESIOP (Induction)	Vincristine Cyclophosphamide Etoposide Cisplatin Carboplatin	RAPID COJEC
	(Myeloablative Treatment)	Busulphan Melphalan or Carboplatin Etoposide Melphalan	Bu-Mel CEM
Unresectable/Refractory	TVD protocol	Topotecan Vincristine Doxorubicin	TVD
Wilms'	SIOP WT 2002	Vincristine/ Actinomycin Doxorubicin	AV AVD
	(High risk)	Etoposide Carboplatin Cyclophosphamide	
Sarcoma	EpSSG RMS-2005 for Rhabdomyosarcoma	Ifosfamide Vincristine Actinomycin Doxorubicin	IVADO
	EpSSG – Non-Rhabdomyosarcoma	Ifosfamide Doxorubicin	
Ewing's	EURO-EWING'S (Induction)	Vincristine Ifosfamide Doxorubicin Etoposide	VIDE
	(Consolidation)	Cyclophosphamide	VAC; VAI
Hepatoblastoma	SIOPEL-3	Cisplatin	PLADO
Germ cell GC3	(Standard risk) SIOPEL-4 (High risk) SIOPEL-3 GC-3	Doxorubicin Cisplatin Doxorubicin Cisplatin Etoposide	JEB
Osteosarcoma	EURAMOS	Carboplatin Bleomycin Methotrexate	MAP
Hodgkin's	Hodgkin 2000	Adriamycin CisPlatinum Ifosfamide Etoposide Vincristine	MAPIE

Table 7.3 *(Continued)* Commonly used protocols for solid tumors

Tumor	Current protocol	Drugs	Acronyms
Non Hodgkin's lymphoma		Prednisolone	OEPA
		Etoposide	
		Adriamycin	
	EURO-LB 02	Cyclophosphamide	
		Procarbazine	COPP
		Prednisolone	COP
Medulloblastoma		Vincristine	COP
		Daunorubicin	COPADM
		Asparaginase	CYM
		Cyclophosphamide	
		Methotrexate	
	SIOP PNET4 (avg risk)	Vincristine	Packer
High grade anaplastic Astro-cytoma		Cisplatin	
		CCNU (Lomustine)	
	Cis Tem	Cisplatin	CISTEM
Low grade glioma		Temozolomide	
	LGG-2	Vincristine	VCE
		Carboplatin	
		Etoposide	

UKCCSG or SIOP is therefore essential to keep up to date with the various protocols/clinical trials, which in turn will continue to improve the outcome of childhood cancer.

7.3 Chemotherapy

The effective use of cancer chemotherapy requires a thorough understanding of principles of neoblastic cell growth kinetics, basic pharmacologic mechanisms of drug action, and pharmaco-kinetic and pharmaco-dynamic variability. Development of selective, highly effective therapy for cancer has been hindered by lack of understanding of the molecular mechanisms, malignant transformation, and de novo or acquired drug resistance. In spite of scientific advances in the field of molecular oncology, information remains incomplete, therefore therapy continues to be largely empiric.

7.3.1 The Cell Cycle and Tumor Growth Kinetics

The growth pattern of individual neoplastic cells may greatly affect the overall biological behavior of human tumors and their responses to specific types of cancer therapy. Tumor cells can be subdivided into three general populations: (1) cells that are not dividing and are terminally differentiated; (2) cells that continue to proliferate; and (3) nondividing cells that are currently quiescent but may be recruited into the cell cycle. The kinetic behavior of dividing cells is best described by the concept of the cell cycle.

The cell cycle is composed of four distinct phases during which the cell prepares for and undergoes mitosis. The G1 phase consists of cells that have recently completed division and are committed to continued proliferation. After a variable period of time, these cells begin to synthesize DNA, marking the beginning of the S phase. After DNA synthesis is complete, the end of the S phase is followed by the premitotic rest interval called the G2 phase. Finally, chromosome condensation occurs and the cells divide during the mitotic M phase. Resting diploid cells that are not actively dividing are described as being in the G0 phase. The transition between cell cycle phases is strictly regulated by specific signaling proteins; however, these cell cycle checkpoints may become aberrant in some tumor types.

The most common anticancer drugs are cytotoxic agents which are cell poisons that act indiscriminately on most cells, either causing direct damage to DNA or inhibiting cell replication. The mechanism of action of most current anticancer drugs are nonselective and target vital micromolecules (e.g., nucleic acid) or metabolic pathways that are critical to malignant and normal cells. The molecular basis of cytotoxic-induced cell death is the subject of considerable interest, and it is becoming clear that one of the important common pathways is that of programmed cell death or apoptosis [10].

Cancer chemotherapy relies on exploiting the therapeutic index – the ratio of cell killing in the malignant cell population compared with killing of normal cells. Mechanisms for recovery from damage are generally more efficient in normal cells than in their malignant counterparts and, if time is allowed between courses of treatment for this recovery to occur, malignant cells can be differentially killed by repeated courses of chemotherapy.

In the clinical development of anticancer drugs, the initial dose finding trials (Phase I), and subsequent studies to define the spectrum of activity of a new agent (Phase II), employ an empirical methodology. Phase I trials can be seen as toxicity-screening studies where a new drug is administered for the first time to humans in order to determine the maximum tolerated dose. There are usually two aims of the Phase I trial – to establish the optimal dose to be used in the Phase II trial for drug efficacy, and to determine the type and degree of toxicity (adverse effects) associated with the drug. In Phase II trials, the response is evaluated in patients with different forms of cancer to determine which tumors the drug may have activity against. The end points of such trials are the response rate and toxicity. After a drug is found to have some activity in Phase II trials, the next step is to determine its relative efficacy in a larger Phase III trial, where the drug is compared – either alone or in combination – with other drugs, i.e., to a control group, usually the best available treatment, or a historical control. Most UKCCSG trials are Phase III, comparing patients on a new treatment versus standard treatment, to try and establish whether new treatment is better than standard treatment. The dose and schedule of the anticancer drugs are empirically based. All patients receive the same fixed dose of drugs, adjusted for body weight or surface area, with subsequent dose or schedule modifications based only on ensuing toxicities, rather than on achieving a therapeutic plasma drug concentration. Commonly used cytotoxic agents and their metabolism use and side effects are listed in Table 7.4. Despite various limitations, several principles of cancer chemotherapy have evolved from clinical experience, including the use of multidrug combination chemotherapy regimens, the administration of chemotherapy before the development of clinically evident metastatic disease (adjuvant chemotherapy), and administration of drugs in maximally tolerated doses (dose intensity).

7.3.2 Combination Chemotherapy

Multiagent therapy has three important theoretical advantages over single-agent therapy. Firstly, it maximizes the cell kill, while minimizing host toxicities by using agents with nonoverlapping dose-limiting toxicities. Secondly, it may increase the range of drug activity against tumor cells with endogenous resistance to specific types of therapy. Finally, it may also prevent or slow the development of newly resistant tumor cells. Specific principles for selecting agents for use in combination chemotherapy regimens are listed in Table 7.5 [11].

7.3.3 Adjuvant Chemotherapy

The aim of adjuvant chemotherapy is to prevent metastatic recurrence by eliminating micrometastatic tumor deposits in the lungs, bone, bone marrow, or other sites at the time of diagnosis. Adjuvant chemotherapy has been demonstrated to be efficacious for most of the common pediatric cancers, including Wilms' tumor, Ewing's sarcoma, osteosarcoma, and rhabdomyosarcoma. Adjuvant chemotherapy should be given as soon as possible after definitive local therapy. A delay to allow for recovery from surgery or radiation therapy may compromise the chance of curing the patient.

Increasingly, chemotherapy is now used in a neoadjuvant setting (before the definitive treatment) in pediatric solid tumors as chemotherapy shrinks the tumor and the operation becomes safer and easier. Neoadjuvant chemotherapy also provides earlier set treatment for micrometastases.

7.3.4 Dose Intensity

Most anticancer drugs have a steep dose response curve, and a small increment in the dose can significantly enhance the therapeutic effect of the drug. The maximum tolerated dose of the drug combination should be given as frequently as possible to achieve optimal cell kill at a time when the size of the drug-resistant population is limited. Methods for maximizing dose intensity include: greater physician and patient willingness to tolerate drug toxicities, more aggressive supportive care, selective rescue of the patient from toxicity such as with peripheral stem cell transplantation or the administration of colony-stimulating factors such as G-CSF, use of regional chemotherapy (intra-arterial, intrathecal delivery) to achieve high drug concentrations at local tumor sites, and the development of new treatment schedules such as long-term continuous infusions that may allow more drugs to be administered over a given period.

Whatever the final pathway of cell death, there remains a correlation between sensitivity to anticancer drugs and the stage of the cell cycle at the time of drug exposure. During the S-phase most agents are

Table 7.4 Classification of the commonly used cytotoxic agents

Agent Type	Substance name	Major clinical use	Metabolism	Excretion	Toxicities
1. Antimetabolites	Methotrexate	Leukemia, lymphoma, CNS, osteosarcoma	Hepatic	Renal, 50–90% excreted unchanged; biliary	BM, M, kidney, lung liver, CNS
	5-Fluorouracil	Colorectal, liver	Hepatic	Renal	BM, M, diarrhea
	6-Mercaptopurine (6-MP)	Leukemia, lymphoma	Hepatic; allopurinol inhibits metabolism	Renal	BM, liver
	6-Thiogranine (6-TG)	Leukemia, lymphoma	Hepatic	Renal	BM
	Cytarabine	Leukemia, lymphoma, CNS	Hepatic	Renal	BM, M, cholestasis, N+V, diarrhea, CNS, lung, conjunctivitis
2. Alkylating agents	Nitrogen mustard	Hodgkin's disease	Hepatic	Biliary	BM, N+V, alopecia, sterility
	Cyclophosphamide	Leukemia, lymphoma, neuroblastoma, rhabdomyosarcoma, Ewing's sarcoma, germ cell tumors	Hepatic	Renal	BM, cystitis, alopecia, lung, heart, sterility
	Ifosfamide	Neuroblastoma, sarcomas, leukemia, Hodgkin's disease	Hepatic	Renal	BM, alopecia, cystitis encephalopathy, kidney, sterility, heart
	Melphalan		Hepatic	Renal	BM, M, alopecia, heart, sterility
	Busulphan	Leukemia	Hepatic	Renal	VOD; lung fibrosis; sterility; Addisonian-like state
	BCNU (Carmustine)	Brain tumors, lymphomas	Hepatic	Renal	Late bone marrow toxicity (up to 6/52), sterility, lung, heart
	CCNU (Lomustine)				
	Cisplatin	Germ cell tumors, neuroblastoma, sarcomas, CNS, liver	–	Renal	N+V, renal, hearing loss
	Carboplatin				
4. Vinca a lkaloids	Vincristine Vinblastine	Leukemia, lymphoma, Wilms' tumor, neuroblastoma, rhabdomyosarcoma, Ewing's sarcoma Lymphoma	Hepatic Hepatic	Biliary Biliary	Neurotoxicity, jaw pain, constipation, inappropriate ADH secretion Jaw pain, mucositis
	Vindesine	Sarcomas	Hepatic	Biliary	BM

effective, in contrast to the G0-resting phase, during which most tumor cells will be chemo-resistant. Anticancer drugs can be classified on the basis of the cell cycle phase during which they are more effective. For example, Nitrogen mustard, alkylating agents, and gamma radiation are noncycle-specific, being effective at most phases of the cell cycle and in some cases including the G0 population. Phase-specific

Table 7.4 (*Continued*) Classification of the commonly used cytotoxic agents

Agent Type	Substance name	Major clinical use	Metabolism	Excretion	Toxicities
5. Epipodo-phylotoxins	Etoposide (VP-16)	Leukemia, lymphoma, neuroblastoma, germ cell tumors	–	Renal	BM, N+V, neurotoxicity, leukemia, alopecia
	Teniposide (VM026)				
	Doxorubicin	Leukemia, lymphoma, neuroblastoma, rhabdomyosarcoma, Ewing's sarcoma, Wilms' tumor	Hepatic	Biliary, renal	BM, N+V, heart, mucositis, alopecia, radiation recall
	Daunorubicin	Leukemia	Hepatic	Biliary, renal	BM, N+V, heart, alopecia, radiation recall
	Epirubicin	Lymphoma, sarcoma	Hepatic	Biliary, renal	BM, alopecia, heart
	Mitozantrone	Lymphoma, leukemia	Hepatic		BM, cholestasis
	Actinomycin D	Wilms' tumor, Ewing's sarcoma, rhabdomyo-sarcoma	–	Renal	BM, N+V, skin (with radiation), liver, alopecia
7. Miscel-laneous	Bleomycin	Germ cell tumors, lymphoma	Hepatic	Renal	Lung fibrosis, fever, pigmentation, Raynaud's Phenomenon
	Dacarbazine	Sarcoma, Hodgkin's disease	Hepatic	Renal	"Flu" symptoms, liver
	Procarbazine	Hodgkin's disease	Hepatic	Renal	Liver, "flu" symptoms
	L-Asparaginase	Leukemia	–	Reticulo-endothelial system	Hypersensitivity, liver, CNS
	Prednisolone	Leukemia, lymphoma	Hepatic	Renal	Hypertension, blood sugar diabetes, cataracts, Cushing's, osteoporosis, immunosuppression

Table 7.5 Principles for selecting agents for use in combination chemotherapy regimens

Drugs known to be active as single agents should be selected for use in combinations; preferentially drugs that induce complete remission should be included.

Drugs with different mechanisms of action and with additive or synergistic cytotoxic effects on the tumor should be combined.

Drugs with different dose-limiting toxicities should be combined so that full or nearly full therapeutic doses can be utilized.

Drugs should be used at their optimal dose and schedule.

Drugs should be given at consistent intervals, and the treatment-free time period should be as short as possible to allow for recovery for the most sensitive normal tissues.

Drugs with different patterns of resistance should be used to minimise cross-resistance.

agents include Vinblastine and Vincristine, which are active during the mitotic phase; Etoposide and Tenoposide effective during the G2 premitotic phase; and Methotrexate, 6-Mercaptopurine and Cytosine Arabinoside effective during the S-phase. Agents that are cycle- but not phase-specific include 5-Fluorouracil, Actinomycin D, and Doxorubicin (Table 7.6) (Fig. 7.1).

Table 7.6 Cell-cycle-phase-specific drugs

S phase-dependent	M phase-dependent
Antimetabolites	Vinca alkaloids[a]
Cytarabine	Vinblastine
Doxorubicin	Vincristine
Fludarabine	Vinorelbine
Gemcitabine	Podophyllotoxins
Hydroxyurea	Etoposide
Mercaptopurine	Teniposide
Methotrexate	
Prednisolone	Taxanes
Procarbazine	Docetaxel
Thioguanine	Paclitaxel
	G_2 phase-dependent
	Bleomycin
	Irinotecan
	Mitoxantrone
	Topotecan
	G_1 phase-dependent
	Asparaginase
	Corticosteroids

[a] Have greatest effects in S phase and possibly late G_2 phase; cell blockade or death; however, occurs in early mitosos.
BM, bone marrow; M, mucositis; N+V, nausea and vomiting

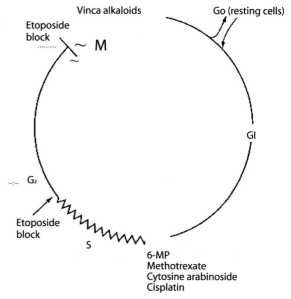

Fig. 7.1 Cell cycle and phase-specific drugs

All cytotoxic drugs produce DNA damage but by different mechanisms. Alkylating agents induce arrest of DNA transcription regulation. Antimetabolites produce DNA injury by inhibiting thymidine synthetase, or blocking purine synthesis or DNA repair. Anthracyclines produce intercalation (crosslinking) between strands of DNA, may generate free radicals, or interact with DNA-modifying enzymes. The final common pathway of cytotoxic induced cell death is apoptosis but, by exploiting these different mechanisms of damage, greater tumor cell kill can be achieved. One of the main reasons why chemotherapy may fail to kill all tumor cells is that clones of "resistant" cells may develop. Tumor resistance is related to a genetic event in the cell – a mutation, gene amplification, deletion, or chromosome translocation which may affect drug transport, intracellular drug activation, or efflux from the cell.

Three genes have so far been implicated in multiple drug resistance (MDR) – IP glycoprotein, which acts as a transmembrane pump to reduce the intracellular drug concentration; multiple drug resistance-associated protein gene (MRP), which is related to non=p-glycoprotein-mediated resistance; and DNA topoisomerase II mutations, which affect DNA conformation [12, 13].

Irrespective of the precise mechanism of drug resistance, it has been suggested by the Goldie-Cold-man hypothesis [14] that there is a high likelihood of drug-resistant mutants at the time of initial diagnosis, and that two important considerations must therefore be taken into account in protocol design. Firstly, the earliest use of noncross resistant drugs (combination chemotherapy), and secondly the maximum tolerated dose of the drug combinations should be given as frequently as possible to achieve optimum cell kill, at a time when the size of the drug-resistant population and number of mechanisms are limited.

High-dose chemotherapy offers a strategy for overcoming multiple drug resistance and is feasible as long as bone marrow suppression, which can be overcome by bone marrow or peripheral stem cell rescue, is the only dose-limiting toxicity.

In adults, local perfusion of cytotoxic agents has been attempted in a number of situations. Isolated limb perfusion has achieved some success as a treatment for melanoma, but this tumor is extremely uncommon in children. Hepatic artery infusion has been used to treat liver metastases, particularly from colonic cancers in adults. Again, the usefulness of this approach is limited in children where systemic therapy is needed for most tumors because of the pattern of tumor spread. It may have some place in the treatment of hepatoblastoma. Randomized trials comparing regional perfusion with systemic therapy have not shown a specific advantage for localized therapy.

For solid tumors, chemotherapy has two main goals – to eliminate overt metastases or microscopic spread, and to destroy or reduce the primary tumor mass so that, with or without further local treatment, complete response (CR) can be obtained. Without complete response, cure will never be possible. For the purposes of comparison in trials, different categories of response criteria are used to assess the effectiveness of systemic treatment. In general these are as follows:

7.4 Response Criteria for Solid Tumors

– Complete Response (CR): Complete disappearance of all visible disease.
– Very Good Partial Response (VGPR): Tumor volume reduction ≥90% but <100%.
– Partial Response (PR ≥2/3): Tumor volume reduction ≥66% but <89%.
– Minor Partial Response (PR<2/3): Tumor volume reduction >33% but <66%.
– Stable Disease (SD): No criteria for PR or PD (<33% tumor volume reduction).
– Progressive Disease (PD): Any increase of more than 40% in volume (or > 25% in area) of any measurable lesion, or appearance of new lesions.

7.5 Response Criteria for CNS Tumors

– Complete Response (CR): Disappearance of all enhancing tumor.
– Partial Response (PR): ≥50% reduction in size of enhancing tumor.
– Progressive Disease (PD): ≥25% increase in size of enhancing tumor.
– Stable Disease (SD): All other situations.

7.6 Management of Side Effects of Chemotherapy

7.6.1 Acute Complications

Early complications include metabolic disorders (tumor lysis syndrome), bone marrow suppression, immunosuppression, nausea and vomiting.

7.6.1.1 Tumor Lysis Syndrome

Patients with large tumor burden may have substantial breakdown of tumor cells following the start of treatment and renal function may be impaired from uric acid nephropathy. This problem is seen most often in hematological malignancies, but can occur in solid tumors (Burkitt's lymphoma, germ cell tumors, metastatic neuroblastoma). Before initiating treatment for these malignancies, renal function should be measured, adequate hydration should be ensured,

and Allopurinol (xanthine-oxidase inhibitor) should be given. In patients with very high risk of tumor lysis [bulky disease, high white cell count in acute leukemia, high lactate dehydrogenase (LDH) and uric acid, those presenting with oliguria], Rasburicase (urate oxidase inhibitor) should be used to avoid tumor lysis syndrome. In the tumor lysis syndrome the phosphates and potassium are released into the circulation from cells that are lysed by chemotherapy, leading to hyperkalemia, hyperphosphatemia, hypocalcemia. It is prudent to inform the renal team as the treatment is initiated in these high-risk cases. It is also important to remember that there other causes of renal failure (obstruction of urinary tract, sepsis, fluid shifts) apart from tumor lysis in these patients.

7.6.1.2 Bone Marrow Suppression

Tumors that invade the bone marrow can cause pancytopenia. The majority of chemotherapy drugs produce myelosuppression. Anemia can be corrected by transfusions of packed red cells and thrombocytopenia by platelet transfusions. Neutropenia (ANC <0.5 × 109/l) poses a significant risk of life-threatening infection. Febrile neutropenia patients should be hospitalized and treated as an emergency with empirical broad spectrum intravenous antibiotics pending the results of appropriate cultures. Treatment should be continued until the fever resolves or neutrophil count rises. If there is no response to antibiotics, antifungal or antiviral drugs may be required. Fever may be related to sepsis from indwelling central venous line requiring its removal. Bone marrow recovery may be facilitated by the use of G-CSF (granulocyte colony stimulating factor).

7.6.1.3 Infection

Opportunistic infections with pneumocystis carinii can produce fatal interstitial pneumonitis and prophylaxis with Trimethoprim/Sulfa-methoxazole is recommended where severe immunosuppression is anticipated from chemotherapy.

Children receiving chemotherapy and exposed to chicken pox contact require zoster immunoglobulin and if clinical disease develops, they require hospitalization and treatment with intravenous high dose Aciclovir.

7.6.1.4 Nausea and Vomiting

This is often the most troubling side-effect from the patient's point of view and should be treated effectively from the first course of chemotherapy. Protocols containing Cisplatin, Actinomycin-D, and Cyclophosphamide or Ifosfamide are associated with the highest incidence of vomiting, but sickness is also a problem with Procarbazine, Adriamycin (Doxorubicin), Daunorubicin, and Carboplatin. The new 5-hydroxytryptamine (5-HT3) antagonists such as Ondansetron and Granisetron act centrally in the chemo-receptor trigger zone in the brain and are effective in preventing vomiting with most agents. These drugs are given intravenously at the time of chemotherapy and orally for 5 days until the gastrointestinal side-effects resolve. Dexamethasone is often added, also for 5 days, and is effective, though its mechanism of action is uncertain. Additional sedation, and relative amnesia, can be obtained by including Benzodiazepine such as Lorazepam in the anti-emetic regimen. If emesis is less severe, Domperidone, Prochlorperazine, Chlorpromazine, or Metoclopramide have been used but are less effective and may have troublesome side-effects.

7.6.1.5 Malnutrition/Mucositis

This is a particular risk in patients receiving intensive chemotherapy, or radiotherapy to the abdomen or head and neck. As these treatments cause mucositis, careful oral hygiene is important during this phase. If oral or enteral intake is inadequate then patients may require intravenous fluid and electrolyte supplementation or total parenteral nutrition. Intravenous opiate analgesia may also be required at this time.

7.6.2 Late Effects

Successful treatment of childhood cancer with multiagent chemotherapy in combination with surgery or radiotherapy causes significant morbidity in later life [15]. Successful surgical resection may require the loss of important functional structures. Radiotherapy can produce irreversible organ damage with symptoms and functional limitations depending on the organ involved and the severity of damage. Endocrine consultation regarding growth, sex maturation, and thyroid function is necessary for any child who has received cranial or total body irradiation, or who has chemotherapy-induced ovarian or testicular damage.

Chemotherapy also carries the risk of severe organ damage. Of particular concerns are leukoencephalopathy after high-dose Methotrexate therapy, myocardial damage from anthracyclines, pulmonary fibrosis after Bleomycin, sterility in patients treated with alkylating agents, hearing loss after Cisplatin chemotherapy, and renal tubular damage from Ifosfamide. Patients must be closely monitored by obtaining baseline and sequential measurements during their treatment, wherever possible.

Psychosocial evaluation and educational support is often needed especially following treatment of brain tumors in children. Periods of physiological stress, for example pregnancy, may lead to overt expression of subclinical damage [e.g., heart failure after Adriamycin (doxorubicin) or fetal loss after uterine muscle irradiation]. Long-term follow-up of all children treated for cancer is essential if we are to improve the cure rates and minimize harmful effects of treatment including the increased risk of second malignancy.

7.7 Novel Cancer Targeted Therapies

The overall cure rate for children's cancers now approaches 75%. Although this means one-quarter of children with tumors still die, this still represents one of the most remarkable improvements in outcome in modern medical history. Thirty years ago cure rates were <20% and it is only 50 years ago that the outcome for children with cancer was so appalling that there were strong debates about the ethics of giving children chemotherapy at all.

As alluded to earlier in this chapter, part of this turnaround can be attributed to improvements in surgery, radiotherapy, and supportive care. As a consequence, it is now rare for children to die during their anticancer therapy. Much of the turnaround, however, has been as a direct consequence of a better use of standard chemotherapeutic drugs. It is unlikely that further improvements in cure rates will be achieved by modification of existing modalities of treatment. Novel compounds as well as novel approaches to treatment will be required to help children who are currently incurable.

The explosion of molecular biological knowledge and techniques coupled with a better understanding of host/tumor interactions has spurred on a whole new area of drug development. However, host/tumor interactions have long been recognized. Coley, in the 1800s, demonstrated tumor regression following infection in some of his patients [16]. Donor Lymphocyte Infusions (DLI) post transplantation is now standard hematological practice (see below).

The drive for all new therapies is to devise compounds that maximally target the tumor, avoiding systemic side effects. An in-depth analysis of the pharmacology, pharmaco-dynamics, and pharmaco-genetics of novel compounds is beyond the scope of this book but readers wanting further information can read the excellent recent reviews by Arceci [17] or Krause [18].

7.7.1 Monoclonal Antibody Therapy

The 30 years since Kohler and Millstone's landmark publication [19] describing, for the first time, a generation of humanized monoclonal antibodies from mice has been frustrating. This tantalizing paper opened the promise of "magic bullet" therapy. Unfortunately, this initial enthusiasm gave way to the harsh reality of drug development. For a biological agent to be effective many hurdles have to be overcome. Tumor antigens need to be expressed on cell surfaces, there needs to be a high binding affinity, and the antigens themselves should be specific-specific. Significant problems with allergy and toxicity also have to be overcome. However, much has been learned during this time and that knowledge in itself has spurred further drug development.

It is also important to understand whether the target for monoclonal antibody therapy is present on the tumor mass alone or on the tumor stem cells (e.g., CD33 is present on committed AML blasts but absent from the leukemic stem cell). If the target is only expressed on mature tumor cells the monoclonal therapy should be seen as cytoreductive therapy. However, if the stem cell expresses the antigen, monoclonal antibody therapy can be used in the setting of minimal residual disease where a successful result is more likely.

The era of monoclonal therapy has firmly arrived: Rituximab, a monoclonal antibody targeting cells expressing CD20 antigens, is licensed for use against follicular lymphoma and diffuse large B-cell non-Hodgkin's lymphoma (NHL) [20]. Cetuximab is active against tumors expressing epidermal growth factor (EGFR). It has been used in adult practice against metastatic colorectal cancer and advanced squamous cell cancer in the head and neck [21]. It is undergoing Phase I and Phase II trials in the USA against soft tissue sarcomas in children. The chimeric antibody, ch14.18 anti GD2, is undergoing evaluation in the latest Pan-European High Risk Neuroblastoma study.

7.7.2 Other Immunomodulators

Other biological agents act by immunostimulation or by driving differentiation: Muramyl tripeptide phosphatidylethanolamine (MTP-PE) induces phagocytosis and costimulation of cytokines. Some useful effect has been seen in osteosarcoma [22] and it is likely to form part of the next international Phase III trial in that disease.

All-Transretinoic acid (ATRA) drives differentiation of the promyelocytes in the APML variant of Acute Myeloid Leukemia. Cis-retinoic acid drives differentiation of primitive neuroblasts to mature ganglioneuronal cells. Both of these retinoids are now incorporated into the standard treatment of these diseases in children.

7.7.3 Small Molecule Therapy

Tyrosine kinase inhibitors act on genes that are responsible for many aspects of cell survival. These genes are important in cellular proliferation, differentiation, motility, and apoptosis. There are two main classes of tyrosine kinases: transmembrane proteins and those found within the cell (see Fig. 7.2). Both have enzymatic properties under strict regulation so that cells that are not rapidly dividing have very low levels of tyrosyl phosphorolated protein [17]. The first successful clinical use of a tyrosine kinase inhibitor was imatinib in chronic myeloid leukemia (CML) [23]. This dramatic response accelerated research into tyrosine kinase inhibitors for solid tumors. The most successful use so far has been in adults with gastrointestinal stromal tumors (GISTs) where Imatinib has been used to target mutations in c-KIT. Preclinical data show expression of c-KIT and platelet-derived growth factors (PDGF) in other solid tumors. Many of these affect children and include glioblastoma, sarcomas, and chondromas.

Other targets that may be inhibited by small molecules include endothelial and vascular endothelial growth factors (EGF/VEGF) and once again evidence of expression has been found in cell lines in many pediatric tumors. Drugs targeting these pathways are currently undergoing Phase I and II trials in the pediatric setting.

7.7.4 Cancer Vaccination and T-cell Therapy

Vaccination works by stimulating host T-cells to fight off disease. Anticancer vaccines have been worked on for many years and recent increased understanding of cellular biology has meant there have been crucial developments in producing useful anticancer vaccines. Vaccination strategy is not only dependent on optimizing antigen presentation but also the interaction of that presenting cell with disease-modulating T-cells. The most exciting results have been seen using patient-specific vaccines derived from autologous tumor cell lines. Melanoma, which increasingly affects teenagers and young adults, has shown the most susceptibility to a vaccination approach. A recent report of patient-specific dendritic cell vaccines in a cohort of heavily pretreated patients with metastatic disease, will hopefully prove to be a large step forward in the long search for a successful anticancer vaccine [24].

The pattern of infusion of donor lymphocytes following bone marrow transplant in patients with re-

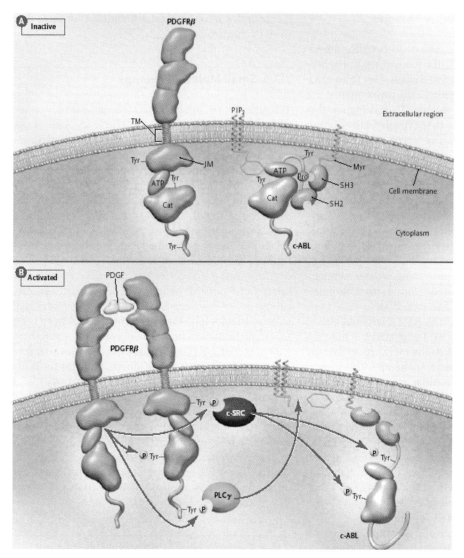

Fig. 7.2 Mechanisms of activation of normal TKs. A typical receptor TK [platelet-derived growth factor receptor β (PDGFR β)] and nonreceptor TK (c-ABL) are depicted, with the ATP-binding (ATP) and catalyic (Cat) lobes of the kinase domains and the transmembrane (TM) region of PDGFRβ indicated. **Panel A** shows both kinases in their inactive states. Inactive PDGFRβ is monomeric and unphosphorylated, and the catalytic domain is inhibited by protrusion of a regulatory tyrosine (Tyr) in the activation loop into the substrate cleft and by an intramolecular interaction with the juxtamembrane (JM) domain. Inactive c-ABL is associated with the membrane through a covalent N-terminal myristate group (Myr) and is inhibited through intramolecular interaction of the Src homology-3 (SH3) domain with an adjacent proline (Pro) residue and by direct interaction of the catalytic domain with an inhibitory membrane lipid, phosphatidylinositol-4,5-bisphosphate (PIP_2). In **Panel**

B, PDGFRβ is activated upon binding of the ligand (dimeric platelet-derived growth factor (PDGF), which induces oligomerization of the receptor and intermolecular phosphorylation (P, in *yellow*) of the activation on-loop tyrosine. This leads to a conformational change in the catalytic domain and increased enzymatic activity, while phosphorylation of other tyrosines within the intracellular domain of the receptor creates binding sites for SH2 domain-containing signaling proteins, including c-SRC (*red oval*) and phospholipase Cγ (PLCγ) (*green oval*). c-ABL is activated through the phosphorylation of two regulatory tyrosines, one in the activation loop and the other near the SH3 binding site, which can be phosphorylated by another TK, such as c-SRC. In addition, activated PLCγ can hydrolyze and destroy the lipid inhibitor PIP_2. Further detail is provided in the review by Van Etten [18].

lapsed leukemia has become standard practice in pediatric patients. These T-cells are not specific-specific and are associated with the development of significant graft-versus-host-disease (GVHD). Indeed, it is believed that the mechanism for GVHD is closely related to the mechanism for the graft-versus-leukemia-effect (GVL) and clinicians view mild GVHD post DLI as a marker of effect. However, specific-specific T-cell populations have the advantage of destroying the disease with less systemic side effects. Manipulated cytotoxic T-cells have been successful in eradicating viral-induced cancers: EBV-driven lymphoproliferative disease, Hodgkin's disease, and nasopharyngeal carcinomas have all responded to EBV-specific cytotoxic T-cell therapy [25].

Despite the excitement generated by novel therapies, there are of course challenges to their use. Although their toxicity should be less than a conventional chemotherapeutic agent, this does not mean they are without significant side effects. Allergic reactions and cytokine release syndromes are common following monoclonal therapy. Cytokine storms have resulted in life-threatening events [26].

Immune disregulation, cardiotoxicity, and skin problems have all been noted as side effects of targeted small molecules. Resistance to therapy is increasingly recognized.

7.8 Future Challenges

We are unlikely to see the large step change in cure rates that has characterized the last 30 years of anticancer therapy in children. As important as an increased understanding of molecular biology will be a regulatory and fiscal environment that encourages new drug development in rare tumors. There will also need to be improvements in trial design and analysis to be able to identify real but small improvements in outcome. Long-term follow up will be crucial in identifying any as yet unrecognized late effects.

So what does the future hold? It is likely that gross disease will continue to be debulked by traditional treatment modalities. This may be followed by establishing a patient-specific, molecular tumor profile with microarray technology, allowing a targeted attack of disease residuum with small molecules, immunomodulation, or vaccination.

References

1. Wallace WHB (1997) Growth and endocrine function following the treatment of childhood malignantand disease. In: Pinkerton CR, et al. (eds) Paediatric oncology: Clinical practice and controversies, 2nd edn. Chapman and Hall Medical, London, pp 706–731
2. Bleyer WA (1990) The impact of childhood cancer on the United States and the world. Cancer 40:355–367
3. Lemerle J, Voûte PA, Tournade MF, et al. (1983) Effectiveness of preoperative chemotherapy in Wilms' tumour: Results of an international society of paediatric oncology (SIOP) clinical trial. J Clin Onc 1(10):604–609
4. Voûte PA, Tournade MF, Delemarre JFM, et al. (1987) Preoperative chemotherapy as first treatment in children with Wilms' tumour. Results of SIOP nephroblastoma trials and studies. SIOP proceedings. (Abstr) 123, Jerusalem
5. Tournade MF, Com-Nougue C, Voute PA, Lemerle J, De Kraker J, et al. (1993) Results of the Sixth International Society of Pediatric Oncology Wilms' Tumour Trial and Study: A risk-adapted therapy approach in Wilms' tumour. J Clin Oncol 11:1014–1023
6. Rickard KA, Loghman ES, Grosfeld JL, et al. (1985) Short and long-term effectiveness of enteral and parenteral nutrition in reversing or preventing protein energy malnutrition in advanced neuroblastoma; a prospective randomised study. Cancer 56:2881
7. Rickard KA, Coates TD, Grosfeld JL, et al. (1986) The value of nutritional support in children with cancer. Cancer 48:1904
8. Capra S, Ferguson M, Ried K (2001) Cancer: Impact of nutrition intervention outcome – Nutrition issues for patients. Nutrition 9:769–772
9. UKCCSG (2006) Annual Scientific Report. United Kingdom Children's Cancer Study Group
10. Wyllie AH (1993) Apoptosis. Br J Cancer 67:205–208
11. Takimoto C, Page R (1991) Principles of chemotherapy. In: Pazdur R, Coia LR, Hoskins WJ, Wagman LD (eds) Cancer management: A multidisciplinary approach 5th edn. PRR, Melville, NY, pp 21–38
12. Lum BL, Fisher GA, Brophy NA, Yahanda AM, Alder KM, et al. (1993) Clinical trials of modulation of multidrug resistance. Pharmacokinetic and pharmacodynamic considerations. Cancer 72(Suppl):3502–3514
13. Pinkerton CR, Hardy JR (1997) Cancer chemotherapy and mechanisms of resistance. In: Pinkerton CR, Plowman, et al. Paediatric oncology: Clinical practice and Controversies, 2nd edn. Chapman and Hall Medical, London, pp 159–188
14. Goldie JH, Coldman AJ (1979) A mathematic model for relating the drug sensitivity of tumours to their spontaneous mutation rate. Cancer Treat Rep 63:1727
15. Wallace WHB, Blacklay A, Eiser C, et al. (2001) Developing strategies for long term follow up of survivors of childhood cancer. Br Med J 323:271–274
16. Coley W (1893) The treatment of malignant tumours by repeated inoculation of Erysipelas: With a report of 10 original cases. AM J Med Sci 105:487–511
17. Arceci RJ, Cripe TP (2002) Emerging cancer-targated therapies. Pediatr Clin N Am 49:1339–1368
18. Krause D, Van Etten RA (2005) Tyrosine Kinases as targets for cancer therapy. NEJM 353:172–187
19. Kohler G, Milstein C (1975) Continuous cultures of fused cells secreting antibody of pre-defined specificity. Nature 256:495–497
20. Lynch DA, Yang XT (2002) Therapeutic potential of ABX-EGA: A fully human anti-epidermal growth factor receptor monoclonal antibody for cancer treatment. Semin Oncl 29:47–50
21. Waksal HW (1999) Role of anti-epidermal growth factor receptor in treating cancer. Cancer Metastases Rev 18(4):427–436

22. Worth LL, Jeha SS, Kleinermann ES (2001) Biologic response modifiers in pediatric cancer. Hematol Oncol Clin N Am 15:723–740

23. Buchdunger E, Zimmermann J, et al. (1996) Inhibition of the Abl protein-tyrosine kinase in vitro and in vivo by a 2-Phenylaminopyrimidine derivative. Cancer Ref 56(1):100–104

24. Dillman R, Dselvan F, Schiltz D (2006) Patient-specific dendritic cell vaccines for metastatic melanoma. N Eng J Med 355:1179–1181

25. Foster A, Rooney C (2006) Improving T cell therapy for cancer. Exper Opin Biol Ther 6(3):215–229

26. Suntharalingan G, Perry MR, Ward S, et al. (2006) Cytokineand storm in a Phase I trial of the anti-CD28 monoclonal antibody PDN1412. N Eng J Med 335:1018–1028

Radiotherapy

8

Fiona Cowie

Contents

8.1 Introduction

With improvements in staging, surgery, and systemic therapies, the role of radiation treatment in children has changed dramatically over the past few decades. Improved cure rates as demonstrated in sequential clinical trials have shifted the focus from cure alone to cure with best long-term function and quality of life. This has particular implications for radiotherapy where the long-term consequences are well recognized. Over the same period pediatric radiotherapy has become more refined as a result of improvements in techniques for both planning and delivery of treatment. Whenever radiation therapy is being considered for a child the indications should be very carefully thought through and the role of radiotherapy in that child's management continually appraised.

Radiation can now be (almost) completely omitted from the treatment of some disease types, for example non-Hodgkin's lymphoma where it's only role is in palliation, relapsed or CNS disease.

8.2 What is Radiotherapy

Radiotherapy (RT) is the treatment of disease (almost exclusively malignant tumors) with electromagnetic and particle radiation. This may be delivered as beams from outside the body (like an x-ray) often called XRT, or by using radioactive material, which is inserted (e.g., radioactive source), ingested (Iodine) or injected (mIBG). Most radiation treatment is external beam radiation and is delivered using a machine called a linear accelerator, which delivers photon radiation; some machines can also produce electrons. Rarely now cobalt sources are used, although historically they were very important. Some departments may have a proton beam treatment unit.

The energy from radiation is ionizing. This means that it disrupts the atomic structure of material it passes through, in this case human tissue. Ionization produces chemical and biological changes in tissues. These changes may be to any molecular cell component; however, the most important is damage to DNA, especially bonds between molecules.

This DNA damage may not be expressed biologically for years. Some cells will die quickly (apoptosis); however, others will do so at a later date when a damaged region of DNA is "used." Some cells function too poorly to divide but may die earlier than expected.

Normal tissue is affected in the same way as malignant tissue, but normal cells initially have more intact DNA and their DNA repair is better (especially in tissues with rapid turnover, for example, mucosa).

8.3 Radiobiology

Radiobiology is the study of the effects of radiation on tissues and how particular cells or tissue types are affected by the type of radiation, total dose given, dose per fraction, interval between fractions, and overall duration of treatment [4]. This has allowed the development of radiotherapy schedules; initially these were empirical but have now evolved with a strong scientific basis. Much of this data is from cell line work and may be expressed as SF2; this is the surviving fraction (of cells) after 2 Gy. Using this type of experimental data a comparison can be made between tumor types or treatment conditions.

8.3.1 Type of Radiation

The energy of a radiotherapy beam and what it is made up of (photons, electrons, or protons) will affect the way in which this energy is deposited in tissue and thus affect the tissue response to it. For example, low energy photons (orthovoltage or kilovoltage) are preferentially absorbed in bone and do not exhibit the skin-sparing phenomenon seen with megavoltage photon irradiation. For this reason orthovoltage radiotherapy can be particularly useful for treating skin or bone lesions. In children, however, it may cause greater disruption of bone growth in the longer term than higher energy treatment.

8.3.2 Total Dose

The total dose needed for different tumor types varies; some are more sensitive (e.g., lymphoma, leukemia), others are relatively resistant (e.g., osteosarcoma), many, however, are between these extremes. For example, we know that the dose needed to treat Ewing's sarcoma is greater than that needed for Wilms' tumor. This knowledge guides the recommended total dose delivered. The dose required doesn't vary with the age of the child – though the biology of a particular tumor

may vary between a very young child compared with an older child (e.g., neuroblastoma). Radiation dose is commonly expressed as Gray (Gy) or centigray (cGy), where 100 cGy = 1 Gy.

8.3.3 Dose Per Fraction

If the total dose were delivered in a single treatment the antitumor effect would be excellent; however, the effect on normal supporting tissues would unfortunately be devastating. For the majority of situations where a large area or volume of the patient has to be treated this is unacceptable. There are two main exceptions to this, palliative treatment (where the total dose is lower), and small brain lesions. The latter can be treated with stereotaxic radiosurgery (single treatment to a small area with a high dose) though this is not employed as often in children as in adults.

The total dose is therefore divided into a number of small doses or fractions, which are delivered on a daily (or more rarely twice a day) basis. This allows the normal tissues (and the tumor cells) a chance to repair some of the DNA damage. The reason radiotherapy works to kill tumor cells is that they do not repair DNA damage as efficiently as normal cells.

As the dose per fraction gets smaller, there is greater relative sparing of normal tissues, but a higher risk that tumor cells are also spared permanent damage.

This illustrates the reason why gaps or breaks in treatment are detrimental to clinical outcome; a break in treatment will allow time for more DNA repair. Clinical data bears this out, e.g., medulloblastoma, survival is linked to overall time of radiation treatment.

8.3.4 Interval Between Fractions

Traditionally a dose of radiotherapy is given daily with a 24 h interval between treatments. Shortening the interval between fractions, for example to 6–8 h, should result in a greater biological effect on both normal and tumor cells. If the interval is long enough for the normal tissue to recover, but not long enough for tumor tissue recovery, there will be a greater amount of damage to tumor cells. This type of radiotherapy delivery is called hyperfractionation. It poses logistic problems, as the working day is typically 8 h long. Treatment therefore has to be given first thing in the morning and last thing at night. It is difficult to deliver this type of treatment to an anesthetized child. As there are theoretical advantages in this approach it has been used in both Ewing's sarcoma and medulloblastoma, but does not yet represent a standard treatment approach.

8.3.5 Overall Time

Most radiotherapy departments' work only 5 days a week and some are unable to treat on bank holidays. These gaps in treatment are inevitable; however, it is important to make every attempt to avoid any other gaps in treatment, for example due to transport problems, the patient being too ill to receive treatment, or machine breakdown. When such gaps do occur an adjustment to the remaining treatment may need to be made, although this is not always possible. The result may be a poorer chance of disease control or a greater chance of long-term toxicity.

8.3.6 Typical Pediatric Treatment Schedules

Most children will be treated with fraction sizes of 1.8 Gy (range 1.5–2 Gy) per day, 5 days per week for 2–6 weeks, depending upon the indications for radiotherapy and the disease type.

8.4 Challenges of Pediatric Radiotherapy

When radiation treatment is delivered to a child there are a number of aspects that differ from an adult's treatment. These need to be taken into account by the radiotherapy team and department and may necessitate a change in practice compared with "normal" departmental policy [5].

Ensuring the cooperation and compliance of the child is vital if accurate high quality treatment is to be given. This is generally much easier in adult patients who can understand what they are being asked to do and follow instructions, even if they are uncomfortable or scared.

Most pediatric treatment regimens are complex and require different treatments to be dovetailed together. This may cause difficulties in booking radiotherapy as occasionally little warning can be given or dates need to be changed at short notice.

Children are particularly prone to long-term consequences of radiotherapy; growing tissues will ultimately display changes that will never be observed in a fully grown person. Many parts are immature and have to both develop and grow; both of these processes are liable to be affected by irradiation. A particular point of concern is the developing CNS, which is very sensitive to the detrimental effect of radiotherapy. Children under 3 years of age are at particular risk of neurocognitive changes; however, older children may also be affected.

These detrimental effects may be minimized by following the principles of radiotherapy to children, which encourage:

1. Using the lowest effective total dose
2. Using the smallest possible treatment volume
3. Using a low dose rate or dose per fraction
4. Treating over an appropriate overall time

8.4.1 Lowest Effective Total Dose

Dose response curves in radiotherapy are a sigmoid shape (see Fig. 8.1). A small decrease in dose may result in a big reduction in the antitumor effect. The risk of side effects can also be expressed with a curve of this shape. Although the total dose used has to be effective at dealing with the tumor, if it can be reduced a little this may significantly decrease the long-term toxicity.

The small bowel, for example, presents a problem; toxicity is expressed rapidly and bowel is often unavoidably treated. Here, however, a small reduction in dose can result in a significant reduction in toxicity.

8.4.2 Smallest Possible Treatment Volume

Careful use of shielding and consideration of field arrangement will help to avoid structures at greatest risk of side effects. In this way the lens of the eye may be spared, or the jaw and developing teeth. The dose received by any area or organ at risk can be estimated during planning and in some cases measured during treatment.

Due to the known effects of radiotherapy on growing and developing tissues, symmetrical irradiation of the neck and spine is generally encouraged. For example, stage 1A Hodgkin's of the neck can be treated

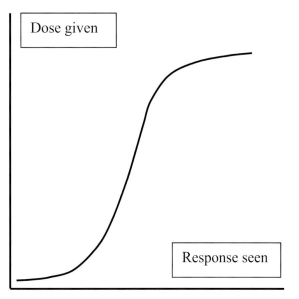

Fig. 8.1 Graph showing sigmoid curve

with radiotherapy alone, but conventionally the whole neck is irradiated even if the disease is unilateral.

In order to avoid an "organ at risk" (OAR), the beam arrangement or shape of the field may be manipulated, providing the target area is still treated appropriately. There may need to be a clinical decision about which toxicity is "preferable," or whether the target can be compromised. An example of this would be avoiding the femoral epiphyses at the expense of a higher rectal dose in a pelvic treatment.

8.4.3 Low Dose Rate or Dose Per Fraction

As previously discussed, small fraction sizes allow greater normal tissue repair, although if the dose per fraction is too low the desired effect on tumor cells will be reduced. Taken to its extreme, continuous irradiation at a low dose rate allows both recovery of normal tissues and tumor cell death. This is employed in low dose rate brachytherapy.

8.4.4 An Appropriate Overall Time

If treatment is extended over a prolonged time period (e.g., due to patient illness or machine breakdown) the antitumor effect is reduced.

Some protocols are looking at shortening the overall time a treatment is delivered over (e.g., hyperfractionated accelerated radiotherapy in medulloblastoma) to increase the antitumor effect.

8.5 Procedures

8.5.1 Decision to Irradiate

This is often made after discussion at a Multi Disciplinary Team (MDT) meeting where response on radiological, pathological, or clinical grounds is examined. Many therapeutic protocols specify that radiotherapy needs to be considered at a particular point in the child's overall management. In other cases radiotherapy may be one of the options when management strategy is being formulated [5].

No one takes this decision lightly. There are times when radiotherapy is technically easy but may not be in the child's best interests. On other occasions, radiotherapy may be the most appropriate choice but technically very challenging.

8.5.2 Booking

All departments will have a system for arranging or booking radiotherapy planning and treatment. This will not only require patients demographic details (name, date of birth, address, etc.) but also the tumor type, site to be treated, need for anesthetic, and much more. A booking request can generally only be completed after a clinical oncologist (radiotherapist) has seen the patient. Departmental policy regarding prioritization varies. There is usually a classification into routine, urgent, and emergency treatments, based upon clinical need and tumor biology. Booking radiotherapy generally authorizes exposure to ionizing radiation (in the form of scans and x-rays), though formal written consent will be required for treatment.

8.5.3 Information Giving and Preparation

Before the child and parents or caregivers visit the department to begin the planning process they need to understand what will happen and what is expected of the child. Many departments will have information sheets or leaflets; some will have videos or websites. An initial visit to the department can be invaluable for children of all ages. This allows them to look around, see into the different areas and rooms they will need to enter, perhaps handle an immobilization device or to move the couch and obviously to ask questions.

Most departments will have an identified person who can act as a link for the family. This may be a radiographer, nurse, play specialist, or doctor.

It is increasingly recognized that pretreatment preparation is vital and may enable children who would otherwise need a general anesthetic (GA) to receive radiotherapy to manage without. Time spent at this stage can result in huge benefits later.

8.5.4 Anesthetic

There will always be some children who are not able to receive radiotherapy without sedation or GA. As children receiving treatment will be alone in the treatment room they need to be remotely supervised, completely still, and may need to wear a restraining/immobilization mask or device. General anesthetic with appropriate telemetry and support/recovery is usually preferred over sedation. For this to be a viable option all rooms used (mould room, simulator, treatment room with back-up room) must be fitted out appropriately. For instance, adequate lighting, anesthetic machine availability, available oxygen and suction, an induction and recovery area. Marks on the shell are used to accurately set up the treatment fields. Telemetry is in place and remotely viewed on a linked screen outside the room.

Venous access is desirable for anesthetic delivery and central venous access in the form of a tunneled line can be justified for daily anesthetics over a week or more. The alternative of using peripheral access will be preferred in some departments.

Pediatric anesthetists obviously play a central role in this part of the service. They must be adequately supported during the procedure and able to ensure the child recovers safely and appropriately each day. As many radiotherapy facilities are remote from a pediatric hospital there are obviously logistic difficulties that must be overcome.

8.5.5 Immobilization

Radiation treatment is planned with very little margin allowed for movement of the patient. It is known that if the patient stays "still" a margin of up to 10 mm needs to be added to the target volume depending upon the site treated. This can be challenging in adults but is more so in children, their smaller overall size means adding this extra margin will irradiate a proportionally larger amount of them.

In all patients, however, accurate and reproducible set up in a comfortable and stable position offers the best chance to get things right. A variety of aids are used here: knee bolsters, vacuum bags, body casts, foam wedges, and beam directing shells all have a place. Vacuum bags are plastic bags full of polystyrene beads that mould to the shape of the patient when the air is sucked out. They retain their shape over the course of treatment (a plug is put in) and can then be reused.

Plastic (or other rigid material) can be used to make a body cast in a similar way. These support part of body in the desired position and can be marked to aid set up.

Plastic beam directing shells (BDS) or masks are used for all head and neck treatments (Fig. 8.2). Here accuracy is more vital and small movements detrimental. Marks drawn on the shell mean that no marks need to be drawn on the patient.

8.5.6 Planning

All planning and treatment is done with the child in the chosen position and immobilization device. All couch tops are identical in terms of geometry with respect to simulator and treatment beams. Simple planning can be done in a simulator using radiography to define the field to be treated, or by looking at the patient [1].

More complex plans require a CT scan first. Marks are drawn on the patient or radio-opaque markers stuck onto the skin. These will be used to make shifts in position (side to side or up and down) once the plan has been created. These all have to stay on until the patient comes for the next visit (often a week later).

CT scans are used to delineate the treatment volume on a computer-based system. The physics-planning department then creates a plan. This can be viewed on a computer system to look at dose distribution, hot spots, normal tissue doses, etc. before the patient attends for a treatment verification visit.

Verification is carried out before the patient starts treatment; often this is done using beams eye x-ray pictures, which can be checked against the physics plan. An example of this is seen in Fig. 8.3; this shows the field that will be treated for para-aortic nodal irradiation in Wilms' tumor; note the whole vertebral bodies are included to ensure uniform growth. Any

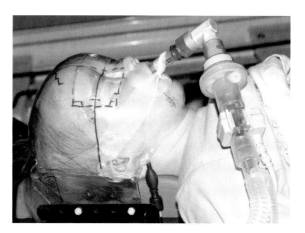

Fig. 8.2 An anesthetized child wearing a plastic beam directing shell with marks to guide field set up

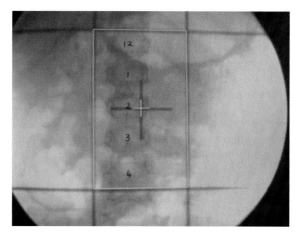

Fig. 8.3 Simulator film for nodal irradiation

changes to be made can be done at this stage. Permanent marks are needed to guide treatment set up on a daily basis. Tattoos are commonly used; these are pinprick marks made at one or more sites. While there is no difficulty performing a tattoo on an anesthetized or older compliant child, younger children may present a problem. Unfortunately, it is not possible to use topical local anesthetic as the precise position of the marks is critical and the location is not certain until the simulation visit is nearly completed. Play specialist input may be helpful for fearful children and many need some preparation.

8.5.7 Consent

Written informed consent prior to any radiation exposure is vital. It is required for all treatments, palliative and radical. The child will have been involved in discussions regarding treatment aims, side effects, and alternatives in an age-appropriate fashion. For those girls who could potentially become pregnant (over the age of 12 years in the UK) a signed declaration that they are not pregnant is required. No pregnancy test is undertaken unless there is uncertainty, in which case a spot urine test is performed.

8.5.8 Treatment

While the planning sessions may take 20–40 min, a treatment session is generally quicker. The total length of time a child is in the treatment room may be 10–30 min, depending upon their cooperation, how quickly the correct treatment position can be obtained, and the number of fields to be treated.

While the treatment beam is on, no one else is allowed in the treatment room. Unlike the simulator or CT simulator, the linear accelerator beam energy means that there is no window into the room. Patient observation is by closed circuit television (CCTV). There may be no physical door, just a long, curved corridor, so a shouted conversation is possible, or an intercom may be used.

Music or a story can be played on a CD player or the radio can be on. In some cases prior preparation is invaluable, for instance, asking the parents to practice with the child lying on a table at home, while listening to their chosen music with the parents waiting outside the door. The child can judge how far into the music or story they need to lie for.

It does not hurt to receive radiotherapy. Most patients are not aware of anything during exposure. Side effects may occur hours or days later.

8.6 Palliative Treatment

Palliative radiotherapy needs to be quick, simple, and effective. There is much less need to be concerned about the long-term side effects, providing short-term toxicity can be minimized and remain acceptable. Palliative treatments may be given in a single dose or a daily dose over a shorter period of time (a week for example). It is generally possible to get palliative treatment started within a few days of making the decision to irradiate.

In some cases where cure is unlikely aggressive palliative radiotherapy is called for, in the same way that intensive chemotherapy regimens may be used in this situation. For instance, irradiating as many of the disease sites as possible after completion of chemotherapy is suggested for metastatic Ewing's sarcoma, even though this may call for several areas to be treated. Decisions about how this type of recommendation is interpreted need to be made carefully.

8.7 Surgical Procedures to Reduce Toxicity of Radiotherapy

In some cases it is possible to insert a sling or mesh to lift small bowel away from the area to be irradiated; tissue expanders can be used in a similar way to push small bowel or other organs away from the irradiated area. Figure 8.4 shows a patient with a tissue expander in his pelvis. The red line shows the target volume and the treatment beams are indicated. The tissue expander helped to keep small bowel out of the treated area. Tissue expanders can be removed after treatment has been completed; a mesh may be absorbable. This approach is only valuable if it is possible to move structures such as the bowel away from the area to be treated. Early and comprehensive discussions between the surgeon, radiotherapist, and radiologist are needed if this is being considered.

Gonads can occasionally be moved to a safer area. If this is being considered it is important to discuss the proposed new location with the radiation therapist prior to surgery. It may be helpful to mark their new position with a clip for localization purposes on the planning images. In this way a dose estimate can be calculated prior to irradiation.

If any clips are placed at the time of surgery these will be seen at radiotherapy planning. If the operation record states where these are in relation to the tumor bed or at-risk area it can allow the radiation target to be placed with greater certainly. If, however, the clips were placed for hemostasis this should be annotated, as they would not need to be included in the target. Titanium clips are preferred.

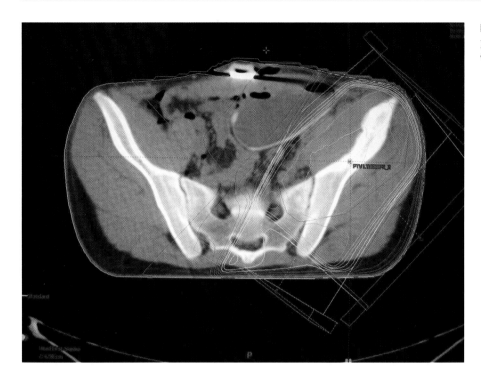

Fig. 8.4 Child with pelvic tissue expander to displace some bowel

Patients with a cystic component to a brain tumor will benefit from aspiration of the cyst to reduce its volume, even if debulking of the tumor is not feasible. The benefit may be seen in terms of clinical improvement; however, from a radiation treatment point of view a large cyst will require larger radiation treatment fields than a small cyst. Care must be taken in this situation to monitor the cyst for reaccumulation as this might push the edge of the cyst or tumor outside the volume being treated.

Surgeons have a common role in placing tunneled central lines or ports and occasionally enterostomy tubes. When required these allow the treatment to be given with a minimum of delay or upset to the child.

8.8 Timing of Radiotherapy with Respect to Surgery

Many pediatric oncology treatment protocols specify the sequencing of different treatment modalities, in particular if surgery should precede radiotherapy. There are some situations where preoperative radiotherapy can be considered and may have advantages. This predominantly occurs in the management of those soft tissue sarcomas where both radiotherapy and surgery are required. In adult sarcoma practice there does not appear to be any difference in survival or limb function for patients treated with preoperative compared with postoperative radiation for limb tumors. There is, however, a greater risk of serious post-operative wound complications in the group treated with preoperative radiotherapy. This result may not be directly applicable to pediatric practice as postoperative wound complications are much less common than in adults.

8.9 Adverse Effects and Management

Side effects are well recognized and depend a great deal on the area being treated. They are usually divided into acute effects (those seen during the period of irradiation or shortly after) and late effects (these may take months or years to become apparent) [5].

8.9.1 Acute Effects

These are not significantly worse in children than in adults – though they may cause greater distress and require careful management.

Most of these only affect the regions through which the irradiation passes. General side effects, however, occur, such as lethargy or tiredness regardless of the region treated. These are seldom severe in children and many experience no change in their activity levels. Nausea and vomiting may occur if the bowel, stomach, or liver are treated and can also be a problem with some CNS treatments. A standard antiemetic approach with an HT3 antagonist such as ondansetron or granisetron without steroids is usually sufficient. In some cases anorexia due to treatment may necessitate enteral feeding (e.g. craniospinal irradiation).

Skin and mucosal reactions develop during the course of treatment and generally settle rapidly without sequelae, the exception being some severe reactions, which may heal with scarring. It is rare for skin reactions to become severe in children; the doses used are lower than for many adult treatments and recovery more rapid. There are of course exceptions to this, which are usually predictable and dose related. The mucosa affected includes the lining of GI tract, GU tract, and respiratory system. Mucositis may be severe, particularly in those children who are receiving concomitant chemotherapy; occasionally parenteral opiate analgesia and feeding are needed.

Hair loss when a hair bearing area is irradiated develops after 10–14 days. Many children will already have alopecia due to chemotherapy. In rare cases radiotherapy causes permanent hair loss or thinning; this depends upon the total dose, comorbid factors, concomitant chemo, and dose received by hair follicles. Some treatments predictably cause a recognizable pattern of permanent thinning (e.g. posterior fossa boost for medulloblastoma treatment).

Those patients who have received prior or concomitant chemotherapy with drugs that may exacerbate the side effects of radiotherapy should be monitored with extra vigilance. They may develop radiation reactions of greater severity than expected.

Very few patients have a genetic radiation hypersensitivity syndrome (e.g., Ataxia Telangiectasia). Radiation should be avoided in these patients as acute side effects can be devastating or life threatening.

8.9.2 Late Effects

These occur after a time lag of several years or decades. DNA damage during radiotherapy may not be manifested until many years later. Many long-term side effects are a result of damage to endothelial cells lining small blood vessels. This leads to proliferation of small vessels, fibrosis, necrosis, or end organ failure.

The range of problems a child might be at risk of can be predicted from the treatment plan. However, while some of the problems are inevitable, their extent or severity may vary (for example, organ function, growth, or neurocognitive impairment). Other problems are not inevitable, but potentially very serious if they occur (for example, second malignancy).

Impairment to organ function after irradiation depends upon the type of organ involved. In some cases a small part of the organ (e.g., liver or kidney) can be irradiated to a high dose providing enough is left untreated. This is particularly important in those patients with only one kidney after a nephrectomy for Wilms'

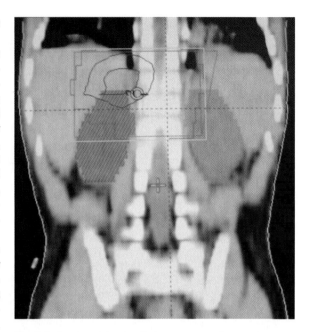

Fig. 8.5 Renal position in relation to target volume

tumor or neuroblastoma. In other cases (such as spinal cord) no part of the structure can receive a high dose without significant risk of serious sequelae. Figure 8.5 shows a CT planning scan of a child with neuroblastoma; both kidneys are functioning and preserved after surgery. Unfortunately, the tumor bed and resected nodal area need to be irradiated. The red outline shows the tumor bed; the nodal area is not seen on this view as it is situated more anteriorly. The yellow rectangle shows the treatment field that has been further shaped by a multileaf collimator (MLC) indicated by the orange line. In this case treating part of both kidneys is unavoidable, but manageable as the total dose needed is low and enough of each kidney is left unirradiated.

Doses of 25–30 Gy result in failure of soft tissue development (rather than true atrophy). Thirty Gy will inhibit future bone growth, although within a bone there will be cells already committed to "growing" which may produce a further 1–1.5 cm of postirradiation bone lengthening. Less than 30 Gy to bone will also affect growth, but not so severely and as little as 10 Gy can still impair bone and soft tissue growth; this may result in visible cosmetic asymmetry, absence of breast development, scoliosis, or functional problems (e.g. length discrepancy).

As the developing CNS is very sensitive to irradiation, particularly in younger children, developmental delay and neuropsychological impairment are a significant concern. Irradiation is avoided wherever possible. When it is required to effect a cure, careful

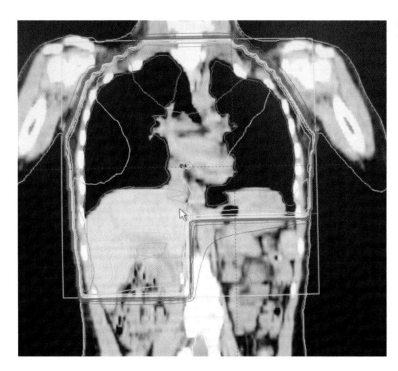

Fig. 8.6 Whole lung and flank fields for Wilms' tumor

monitoring and appropriate counseling and advice are imperative.

Second tumors are a devastating consequence of therapy. When they occur, there is generally a lag time of several years and they occur in the region exposed to irradiation [7]. These patients may be susceptible to developing more than one malignancy for a number of additional reasons: genetic factors, use of alkylating and other agents in chemotherapy, and if cured the prospect of a long life ahead.

Figure 8.6 illustrates the fields required for whole lung and renal bed irradiation in a patient with Wilms' tumor and pulmonary metastases. It can be seen from these treatment fields that the large treated area leads to the possibility of serious late effects – especially if the child is very young at the time of treatment. In a girl, both breast buds will be included in these fields; this may result in breast hypoplasia or poor development during puberty and in some cases requires breast augmentation in later life.

8.10 New Advances/Other Modalities

8.10.1 Brachytherapy

This term encompasses treatment that is given by a source emitting radiation; this is inserted into the body or less frequently placed on the outside [2 ,6]. These sources are made into a solid object such as wire (iridium), seed (gold), or a flat plaque (ruthenium).

There are a number of different ways this type of treatment can be administered; insertion or application under anesthesia is generally required. Whenever an active source is used, full radiation protection procedures are employed.

The advantage of this approach is that a high dose can be delivered to a small, defined volume. This is particularly advantageous in children, as surrounding organs at risk will receive a lower dose than with conventional external beam radiotherapy. However, there are a number of problems and brachytherapy is not suitable in many situations requiring radiotherapy. The major difficulties are compliance (treatment may require several days in a protected room, with limited close family contact and uncomfortable tubes or sutures), clinical experience, low level of supporting published evidence and concern about long-term effects (these will still occur). Close collaboration between all involved specialties is obviously required, as is specialist accommodation and experience in dealing with this type of treatment. As a result there are only a few very specialized centers where this treatment is offered.

8.10.2 Stereotactic Radiosurgery

This refers to the very accurate delivery of a single high dose of radiotherapy using multiple thin beams [2]. At present it is only possible to do this if the area to be treated is in an intracranial site (immobilization is better and localization more accurate), small enough (a few centimeters), and not too close to a critical structure (brainstem or optic nerves, for example). This type of treatment causes radionecrosis and there are biological uncertainties about the effect of such a treatment on adjacent normal structures. There are a limited number of suitable situations in pediatric practice, but some small brain lesions may be suitable.

8.10.3 Proton Beam Irradiation

Protons are another type of energy (charged particles) that can be artificially produced (by a cyclotron) and used therapeutically [2]. They are available in a few centers and have very different physical characteristics to photons. Their principle advantage is that the energy deposition within tissue falls off abruptly at a defined depth within tissue. This may greatly reduce the volume of tissue exposed to the damage caused by radiation and hence the acute and long-term side effects. Not all situations requiring radiotherapy would be suitable for proton beam irradiation, and in many cases it would offer limited advantages over conventional therapy. However, there are an increasing number of situations where its advantages are being recognized as a way of reducing exposure of normal tissue and increasing dose to a focused target area. Unfortunately, there are few facilities in the world that are capable of delivering this treatment and some are only able to treat patients with a fixed treatment beam. The usefulness of proton beam irradiation in pediatric oncology still needs to be determined.

8.10.4 Intensity Modulated Radiotherapy (IMRT)

This term refers to a way of delivering conventional fractionated radiotherapy that may have significant advantages over treatments using fixed beam shaping [2]. It aims to create a uniform dose distribution in the target area by delivering a nonuniform dose to the treatment fields. It requires the shape of the treatment field to constantly change during a treatment and typically the number of treatment fields is increased from the usual 2–4. The advantage in shaping the high dose treatment region around the target while sparing adjacent normal structures may allow the dose to tumor to be increased; this is particularly important in those situations where the tumor is relatively resistant. Equally important is the ability to spare a critical structure that is sensitive to radiation (for example, the spinal cord). There is, however, concern about the integral dose of radiation received by the whole body from this type of approach which may ultimately be expressed as a higher number of patients developing second tumors in the decades to come [3].

Whilst IMRT is increasingly available it is still not routine practice everywhere, and in some situations will not offer advantages over conventional treatment. Its place in pediatric radiotherapy is increasing but continues to be evaluated.

8.10.5 Therapeutic Radioisotopes

This refers to the administration of a radiolabeled target molecule that is specific to certain cells. These cells will be irradiated and therefore damaged. These compounds may be injected or ingested, and may be given alone or in combination with conventional chemotherapy.

The commonest of these is mIBG therapy for neuroblastoma. This is a useful palliative treatment and currently under investigation as part of a curative approach for advanced disease. It requires appropriate care and isolation of the child after treatment to comply with radiation protection legislation. Typically a child needs to be isolated with limited close contact for 5 days. Thyroid blockade with iodine is needed. It is, however, a tolerable and often very effective treatment.

References

1. Dobbs J, Barrtt A, Ash D (1999) Practical radiotherapy planning. Arnold, London
2. Habrand J-L, Abdulkarim B, Roberti H (2004) Radiotherapeutic innovations in pediatric solid tumours. Ped Blood Cancer 43:622–628
3. Hall EJ (2006) Iatrogenic cancer: The impact of intensity modulated radiotherapy. Clin Onc 18:277–282
4. Hall E, Giaccia A (2006) Radiobiology for the radiologist, 6th edn. Lippincott, Philadelphia
5. Halperin E, Constine L, Tarbell N, et al. (2005) Pediatric radiation oncology, 4th edn. Lippincott, Philadelphia
6. Martinez-Monge R, Camberio M, San-Julian M, et al. (2006) Use of brachytherapy in children with cancer: the search for an uncomplicated cure. Lancet Oncol 7:157–166
7. Meadows AT (2001) Paediatric update: Second tumours. Eur J Can 37:2074–2081

Part B

Perinatal Tumors

9

Richard G. Azizkhan

Contents

9.1 Introduction

Most solid tumors observed in early infancy are benign. Malignant tumors diagnosed during the neonatal period are rare. They account for only 2% of all childhood cancers and have a reported incidence of 1:27,000 live births in the USA [1]. Management of affected infants is extremely challenging. Because factors such as drug absorption, metabolism, distribution, and elimination are affected by age and physiologic maturity, complications associated with the immature physiology of the neonate are common. Age-dependent maturation of the renal, hepatic, hematopoietic, and neurodevelopmental systems make the neonate particularly vulnerable to the deleterious effects of aggressive multimodal therapy involving extirpative surgery, chemotherapy, and radiotherapy [2, 3]. Over the past three decades, the long-term effects of administering anticancer therapies to neonates have become increasingly evident [2–9]. An additional complicating factor is that many neonatal malignancies differ significantly from similar tumors in older children with respect to their biological behavior [10–12]. Certain benign tumors (e.g., sacrococcygeal teratoma) may have malignant potential and undergo malignant change if untreated. Other tumors that are histologically malignant (e.g., fibrosarcoma) may exhibit benign behavior. Some benign tumors may be life threatening because of their size, anatomic location, and impact on infant physiology. Additionally, congenital neuroblastoma may have an unpredictable course, with many tumors involuting spontaneously and others progressing to a fatal outcome.

Due to the rarity of malignant neoplasms in neonates, existing treatment protocols are based on studies that predominantly comprise older children. These protocols may not consider the unique aspects of treating perinatal tumors. In an effort to shed light on this topic, I will address the distinguishing clinical features, management, and prognosis of the most common perinatal neoplasms, including teratomas, neuroblastoma, sarcomas, renal and hepatic tumors, and retinoblastoma.

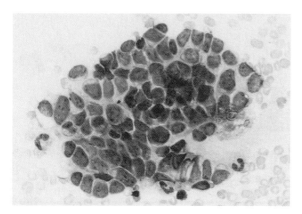

Fig. 9.1 Neuroblastoma cells in bone marrow.

9.2 Overview

9.2.1 Clinical Presentation

Nearly 50% of tumors occurring in neonates are observed at birth; another 20–29% become evident within the first week of life [13, 14]. Although there is variation in the reported frequency of specific tumor diagnoses across neonatal series [14–19], teratomas and neuroblastoma account for approximately two thirds of reported neoplasms. The most common finding on physical examination is a palpable mass. Nonspecific symptoms such as irritability, lethargy, failure to thrive, and feeding difficulties may indicate the presence of an occult neoplasm. Petechial hemorrhages and other hematologic abnormalities may indicate extensive bone marrow replacement by tumor cells such as neuroblastoma or leukemia (Fig. 9.1).

The association between congenital abnormalities and tumors is well documented, with concurrence reported in as many as 15% of neonatal tumors [17, 20, 21]. Many such associations are related to chromosomal defects, particularly trisomies 13, 18, and 21. An increased incidence of leukemia and retroperitoneal teratoma has been reported in neonates with Down syndrome [21], and teratomas are associated with regional and distal congenital anomalies including cloaca, limb hypoplasia, and spina bifida [22].

9.2.2 Oncogenesis and Genetic Risk Factors

Many neonatal malignancies are inherited or occur spontaneously as the result of a de novo mutational event. The etiology of these tumors is likely multifactorial, including both genetic and environmental factors. Both genetically determined syndromes and constitutional chromosomal defects may result in an increased risk of malignancy. This includes single-gene malignancy-related syndromes and the familial associations of tumors [22]. Particular constitutional chromosome anomalies specifically favor neoplasms occurring in the fetal and neonatal period. These anomalies have been identified in retinoblastoma (13q) and nephroblastoma (11p) [23]. In patients with Denys-Drash syndrome, there is an association with genetic mutations located at 11p13 and WT1. These patients commonly have Wilms' tumor. The specific site of the point mutation identified in most cases is located on the WT1 gene exon 9 [24]. Other examples of constitutional chromosomal anomalies associated with neoplasms include an increased risk of leukemia in patients with Down syndrome [25, 26] and a high frequency of poor-prognosis neonatal leukemia involving the 11q23 locus of the MLL gene. This specific genetic defect is rare in older children [27]. Genes that confer a higher risk of neoplasia by enhancing susceptibility to oncogenic factors are likely to exist and may play a role in certain inherited syndromes. For example, there is an increased risk of hepatoblastoma and rhabdomyosarcoma in patients with Li-Fraumeni syndrome (p53 mutation) [22].

9.2.3 Diagnostic Investigations

The selection of imaging studies is dependent upon suspected pathology, affected anatomic site, and differential diagnosis. Dramatic improvements in prenatal ultrasonography (US) and magnetic resonance imaging (MRI) have had a significant impact on prenatal diagnosis, management, and fetal outcome [28–30]. Prenatal US has been particularly useful in identifying large sacrococcygeal or cervical teratomas that may complicate vaginal delivery or be responsible for intrauterine fetal demise or postnatal complications. US can also detect adrenal or thoracic masses in the fetus, providing useful information regarding both the nature of the mass and, in most cases, its origin. Fetal MRI can better characterize and delineate specific anatomic details and the extent of tumor involvement. These complementary techniques help to facilitate the development of a comprehensive plan of action that determines the mode, timing, and location of delivery as well as the initial postnatal management strategy. Fetal surgery and the ex utero intrapartum treatment (EXIT) procedure have proven useful in treating non-immune hydrops and congestive heart failure caused by neoplasms. The EXIT procedure has also been successfully used to salvage infants with high-grade airway obstruction caused by tumors [31].

Contrast-enhanced computed tomography (CT) provides excellent postnatal images of most neoplasms, though it has limitations in evaluating intraspinal involvement. MRI, however, is particularly useful for evaluating tumors that involve the central nervous system or spinal canal. It is also extremely useful in the preoperative delineation of the vascular anatomy of the tumor and adjacent organs. Although limited information is available concerning the use of positron emission tomography (PET) in neonates, evidence suggests that it is helpful in determining cerebral glucose metabolism and, more importantly, holds promise in the management of selected pediatric patients with malignancy [32].

Cytogenetics is playing an increasingly important role in the diagnosis, risk stratification, and monitoring of patients with neonatal tumors. Most cancer cells are thought to have a high incidence of chromosomal changes and genetic mutations that frequently are identifiable and, in some cases, are prognostically important. For example, N-myc amplification is a specific molecular marker that characterizes a subset of aggressive neuroblastomas that usually has a poor prognosis [33].

9.2.4 Therapeutic Interventions

9.2.4.1 Surgical Management

Surgical extirpation remains the definitive treatment modality in most neonates with solid tumors. The timing of the surgical procedure and the surgical strategies employed must take into account the physiologic and metabolic needs of the neonate. Avoidance of hypoglycemia and hypothermia, especially if significant fluid or blood replacement is required or prolonged exposure occurs are important considerations.

The impact of surgery on the subsequent growth and development of the neonate can be profound, especially when major tumor extirpations are extensive or resection of unaffected tissues integral for normal structure and function has occurred. In some patients, appropriate surgical management may result in impairment of gastrointestinal or bladder function, ambulation, or future sexual function, thereby creating life-long physical and emotional burdens for patients. Interrupting or traversing normal growth centers in order to resect tumors can have a profound effect on structural symmetry and function. For example, intrathecal tumor removal extending over several vertebral segments often results in some degree of postlaminectomy scoliosis later in childhood. Preserving function and structure without compromising survival is thus the paramount principle guiding contemporary surgical and multimodal treatment strategies. For many patients in whom a tumor is initially unresectable (e.g., those with stage 3 neuroblastoma) or involves important structures that should be preserved, the administration of several courses of preoperative chemotherapy has been extremely beneficial. This approach has allowed delayed complete primary resection with preservation of vital structures, thus improving surgical outcomes and quality of life.

9.2.5 Radiotherapy

Because many malignant tumors in childhood are radiosensitive, radiotherapy plays an important role in the management of advanced-stage tumors. In light of the scarcity of neonatal data, however, treatment parameters such as dosing schedules have been extrapolated largely from data in older children. Because the neonate experiences rapid growth of organs and structures, radiotherapy has a profound impact on subsequent development. The sensitivity and detrimental effects of radiation therapy on the central nervous system, skeletal growth, and visceral organs appear to be inversely related to the child's age and directly related to the radiation dose [6].

In a seminal study of children younger than age 2 years, Meadows, et al. [6] found that growth disturbances and musculoskeletal abnormalities were the most common late effects of radiation therapy. Approximately 85% of patients had some degree of bone or soft tissue abnormality; this problem was most severe in children who had received thoracic or spinal irradiation. Other authors have documented a wide spectrum of significant late radiation effects, including scoliosis and severe bony deformities (70%) and delayed physical development [14, 34]. Children receiving radiation to the cerebrospinal axis for leukemia or brain tumors reportedly experience major delays in cognitive development, and infants treated with cranial irradiation have a high incidence of learning disabilities and mental retardation [35, 36]. The severity of these disabilities is strongly correlated with radiation dose. As in older children, other significant late effects of radiation therapy in neonates include breast agenesis, aortic arch dysgenesis, second malignancies (particularly leukemias and breast and thyroid cancer), and chronic renal and hepatic insufficiency [36–40].

9.2.6 Chemotherapy

The lack of substantial pharmacologic data on newborns significantly complicates the administration of chemotherapeutic agents. Knowledge of drug interactions, metabolism and clearance, and toxicity are all areas of notable deficiency. They remain the focus of intense ongoing discussion and contemporary investigation. In an overview of a recent (2003) workshop concerning cancer pharmacology in infants and young children, a significantly greater incidence of neurotoxicity for vincristine, hepatic toxicity for actinomycin D, and ototoxicity for cisplatin [41] was observed in infants and young children For virtually all of these older agents and the newer camptothecin agents, the limited available data indicate that weight-based dosing in young children normalizes the drug clearance profiles and may improve the toxicity profiles, bringing them in line with that of older children [41].

During the course of the second National Wilms' Tumor Study, the prescribed doses of actinomycin D, vincristine, and doxorubicin were reduced by 50% due to observed excessive myelodepression in infants younger than 1 year of age. Interestingly, reduction of dose did not compromise therapeutic effectiveness [42]. A similar dose reduction approach was followed in the Intergroup Rhabdomyosarcoma Study protocols [43]. Excessive drug-related toxicity has not been observed in infants with leukemia. Moreover, reduced dosage protocols have had a detrimental effect on clinical response and outcome [44].

9.3 Teratomas

Teratomas are embryonal neoplasms that contain tissues from at least two of the three germ layers (ectoderm, endoderm, and mesoderm). These neoplasms arise in both gonadal and extragonadal sites, with location thought to correspond to the embryonic resting sites of primordial totipotential germ cells. Tumor location correlates with the age of the patient. Teratomas occurring in infancy and early childhood are generally extragonadal, whereas those presenting in older children more commonly occur in the ovary or testis [45]. More than 50% of teratomas are evident at birth and are most commonly seen in the sacrococcygeal area. Although more than one third of teratomas of the testis are recognized in the first year of life, these lesions are rarely diagnosed in the neonatal period. The sacrococcyx is also the most common extragonadal location irrespective of age (45–65%) [46]. Cervicofacial and central nervous system tumors and tumors of the retroperitoneum are seen less frequently. Teratomas presenting in the mediastinum, heart, and liver are rarely seen. Excluding testicular teratomas, 75–80% of teratomas occur in females. Approximately 20% of tumors contain malignant components, the most common being endodermal sinus tumor [46].

A wide range of congenital anomalies is seen in association with teratomas, and the type of anomaly frequently depends on the tumor site and size. Single or combined malformations of the genitourinary tract, rectum, anus, vertebrae, and caudal spinal cord are sometimes found in patients with extensive sacrococcygeal teratomas [16, 47–49]. Disfiguring cleft palate

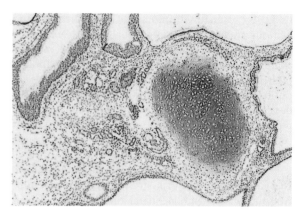

Fig. 9.2 Microphotograph of a benign teratoma showing differentiated cartilage, respiratory epithelium, mucinous epithelium, and salivary gland acini.

defects are found in newborns with massive cranial and nasopharyngeal teratomas [50].

Teratomas can present as solid, cystic, or mixed solid and cystic lesions. Most teratomas that are present at birth consist of ectodermal and mesodermal components. Epidermal and dermal structures such as hair, sebaceous glands, sweat glands, and teeth are frequently present. Virtually all teratomas have mesodermal components, including fat, cartilage, bone, and muscle. Endodermal components commonly include intestinal epithelium and cystic structures lined by squamous, cuboidal, or flattened epithelium [51]. Pancreatic, adrenal, and thyroid tissue, as well as mature and immature neuroepithelial and glial tissue is also frequently seen (Fig. 9.2).

Tumors are histologically classified as either mature or immature, with most pediatric teratomas classified as mature. These tumors exhibit an absence of coexisting malignant cells and little or no tendency to malignant degeneration. They nevertheless may be fatal if the airway is compromised or if vital structures such as the brain or heart are involved. Moreover, depending on location and size, even benign tumors may be inoperable and incompatible with extrauterine life.

Although useful tumor grading systems have been developed [52, 53], these systems are of limited use in regard to the fetus or newborn in that embryonic or immature elements may be appropriate for the stage of development [54, 55]. Regardless of tumor grade in these patients, immature teratomas are associated with a favorable prognosis, and only in rare cases does immature neuroglial tissue metastasize to adjacent lymph nodes, lungs, and other distant organs from an immature primary site [56, 57]. (For additional information on germ cell tumor staging and grading systems, refer to Chap. 13.)

The most important predictor of recurrence in pediatric immature teratomas appears to be the presence of microscopic foci of yolk sac tumor [58]. Because of their small size, these tumors may be missed by the pathologic sampling process. Such oversights may account for metachronous metastases after resection of the immature teratoma metastasis.

In general, the prognosis of neonates depends upon the resectability of the tumor and the presence of metastases or metastatic potential.

9.3.1 Sacrococcygeal Teratoma (SCT)

9.3.1.1 Clinical Presentation and Diagnosis

SCT is the predominant teratoma as well as the most common neoplasm of the fetus and newborn. The tumor has an estimated incidence of 1:20 000 to 1:40 000 live births and a female predominance ranging from 2:1 to 4:1 [47, 59–61]. Ten percent to 20% of patients with SCT have coexisting congenital anomalies such as tracheoesophageal fistula, imperforate anus, anorectal stenosis, spina bifida, genitourinary malformations, meningomyelocele, and anencephaly [16, 57, 62–64]. Also, many patients have significant structural abnormalities of juxtaposed organs resulting from displacement by a large teratoma.

A classification system developed by Altman, et al. [65] divides SCTs into four distinct anatomic types that differ in the degree of intra- and extrapelvic extension (Fig. 9.3). Type I (46.7%) is predominantly external, with minimal presacral extension. Type II (34.7%) arises externally and has a significant intrapelvic component. Type III (8.8%) is primarily pelvic and abdominal but is apparent externally. Type IV (9.8%) is presacral and has no external manifestation. The incidence of malignant components not only correlated with anatomic type (8% in type I vs. 38% in type IV) but also with age at diagnosis and gender; however, the size of the tumor was unrelated. The rate of malignancy of tumors in older infants (>6 months) and children is significantly higher than that of the visible exophytic tumors seen in neonates. Malignant change appears to be more frequent in males, particularly those with solid versus complex or cystic tumors [66–67]. The most common malignant elements identified within sacrococcygeal lesions are yolk sac tumor and embryonal carcinoma (Fig. 9.4) [68].

In countries where antenatal US screening is carried out, most large SCTs are diagnosed before birth. Uterine size larger than expected for a gestational date (polyhydramnios or tumor enlargement) is the most common obstetrical indication for initiating maternal-fetal US examination. Sonography may reveal an external mass arising from the sacral area of the fetus (Fig. 9.5). This mass is composed of solid and cystic areas, with foci of calcification sometimes apparent.

Most prenatally diagnosed SCTs are extremely vascular and can be seen on color-flow Doppler studies.

Lumbosacral myelomeningocele is the most likely condition to be confused with SCT. Lumbosacral myelomeningocele and cystic SCT may show similar findings on US. Since both are associated with elevated maternal levels of alpha fetoprotein (AFP), these levels are not helpful in distinguishing between the two entities. Other critical information gained from US includes the possible presence of abdominal or pelvic extension, evidence for bowel or urinary tract obstruction, assessment of the integrity of the fetal spine, and documentation of fetal lower extremity function [69]. Imaging of the fetal brain is helpful in establishing the diagnosis in that most fetuses with lumbosacral myelomeningocele have cranial findings such as Arnold-Chiari malformation [70]. When there is doubt, performing a fetal MRI can be extremely valuable in clarifying fetal anatomy and in making a definitive diagnosis (Fig. 9.6). Other soft tissue tumors that may mimic SCT include neuroblastoma, hemangioma, leiomyoma, and lipoma [70].

Tumors can grow at an unpredictable rate to tremendous dimensions and may extend retroperitoneally displacing pelvic or abdominal structures (Fig. 9.7). Large tumors can cause placentomegaly, nonimmune fetal hydrops, and the mirror syndrome [59, 71]. These conditions are thought to result from a hyperdynamic state induced by low-resistance vessels in the teratoma. Without fetal intervention, high-output cardiac failure and hydrops resulting in fetal demise is almost certain. Thus, in a select subset of fetuses that meet specific criteria, restoring more normal fetal physiology may be achieved by surgical debulking of the SCT in utero [72].

Neonatal death may occur due to obstetric complications from tumor rupture, preterm labor, or dystocia [73–75]. Impending preterm labor from polyhydramnios or uterine distension from tumor mass may therefore require treatment by amnioreduction or cyst aspiration. Dystocia and tumor rupture can be avoided by planned cesarean section delivery for infants with tumors larger than 5 cm [45].

Antenatal diagnosis carries a significantly less favorable outcome than diagnosis at birth, and prognostic factors outlined in the current SCT classification system are not applicable to fetal cases. While the mortality rate for SCT diagnosed in neonates is 5% at most, that for fetal SCT is close to 50% [71, 73, 74]. Results of most clinical series indicate that hydrops and/or polyhydramnios and placentomegaly portend a fatal outcome. The indication for maternal-fetal US has also been shown to be a predictive factor [73]. If SCT is an incidental finding on routine prenatal US, the prognosis is favorable at any gestational age. Many of these lesions are predominantly cystic and relatively avascular

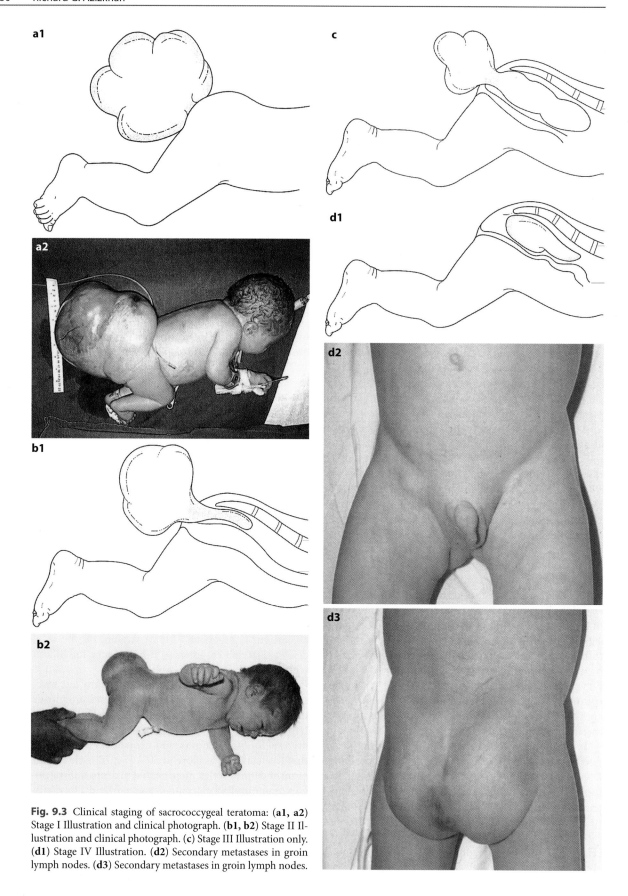

Fig. 9.3 Clinical staging of sacrococcygeal teratoma: (**a1, a2**) Stage I Illustration and clinical photograph. (**b1, b2**) Stage II Illustration and clinical photograph. (**c**) Stage III Illustration only. (**d1**) Stage IV Illustration. (**d2**) Secondary metastases in groin lymph nodes. (**d3**) Secondary metastases in groin lymph nodes.

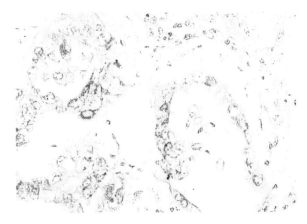

Fig. 9.4 Histology of an endodermal sinus tumor with alpha-fetoprotein stain.

and can be managed postnatally with surgical resection. If US is initiated due to maternal indications, the outcome is much less favorable. Additionally, prematurity from polyhydramnios or cesarean section performed before 30–32 weeks' gestation results in increased mortality [45]. In light of these factors, antenatal diagnosis requires referral to a high-risk obstetric center, with immediately available neonatal intensive care and qualified pediatric surgical and anesthesia expertise.

Postnatal diagnosis is determined by clinical findings on physical examination, serum levels of AFP and ß-human chorionic gonadotropin (ß-HCG), and a number of radiographic imaging studies. Ninety percent of SCTs are noted at delivery, with a protruding caudal mass extending from the coccygeal region.

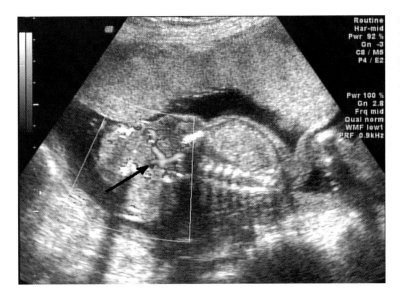

Fig. 9.5 Antenatal maternal-fetal Doppler ultrasound of a 21-week gestation fetus with a sacrococcygeal tumor showing solid and cystic components. *Black arrow* marks vessel with high blood flow within the tumor on the Doppler image. Courtesy of Dr. Timothy Crombleholme, M.D.

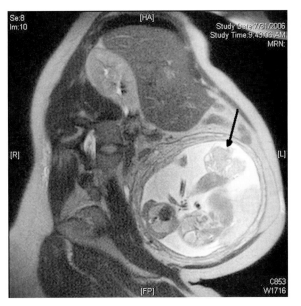

Fig. 9.6 MRI of twin gestation at 21 weeks with one twin having a large sacrococcygeal teratoma (*black arrow*) associated with hydrops and high output failure. Courtesy of Dr. Timothy Crombleholme, M.D.

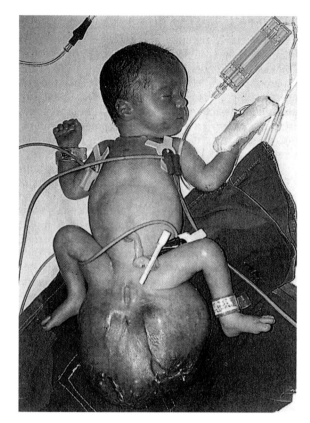

Fig. 9.7 Neonate with a large sacrococcygeal teratoma.

These tumors are easily recognized and a diagnosis can generally be made by physical examination alone. Intrapelvic components can be diagnosed by a rectal digital examination. SCTs seen at birth are predominantly benign, and many are functionally asymptomatic.

Intrapelvic variants may have a delayed postnatal presentation [59, 65, 71]. They are typically noted in infants and children from ages 4–6 months to 4 years. In contrast to the SCTs seen in neonates, these tumors are located in the pelvis and have no external component. More than one third are associated with malignancy. Clinical presentation may include constipation, anal stenosis or symptoms related to the tumor compressing the bladder or rectum and a palpable mass. Presacral tumors are associated with sacral defects and anorectal malformations (Currarino triad) [46].

Radiographs of the pelvis identify any sacral defects or tumor calcifications. CT with intravenous and rectal contrast material defines the intrapelvic extent of the tumor, identifies any nodal or distant metastases, and demonstrates possible urinary tract displacement or obstruction. CT imaging also identifies liver metastasis and periaortic lymph node enlargement. MR imaging is useful when spinal involvement is suspected or if the diagnosis is in doubt. A chest radiograph

is useful in revealing obvious pulmonary metastases. Because chest CT is more reliable in identifying smaller metastatic lesions, it should be performed when there is a high index of suspicion.

9.3.1.2 Operative Treatment

9.3.1.3 Open Fetal Surgery

In a fetus with a large SCT, signs of cardiovascular compromise and early hydrops are indications for open fetal surgery. Since the first reported fetal resection of SCT in 1997 [76], this approach has had several long-term survivors. Because in utero SCT resection commonly precipitates preterm labor, meticulous monitoring and tocolytic therapy during the immediate postoperative period is essential. Hospitalized patients undergo daily US and fetal echocardiography as indicated. Although signs of hydrops generally begin to resolve within several days of tumor resection, complete resolution may take weeks [29]. Since the intrauterine procedure is not designed to completely remove the teratoma, patients often require a second operation postnatally to remove the coccyx and any residual tumor mass. At surgery, the exophytic tumor is dissected free of the anus and rectum. The tumor is then removed by dividing it near the coccyx with a thick tissue-stapling device [29].

A rapidly enlarging macrocystic SCT results in polyhydramnios and placentomegaly, with associated mirror syndrome. Because this syndrome resembles severe pre-eclampsia and is life threatening to the mother, immediate delivery of the fetus or infant is essential.

9.3.1.4 Postnatal Intervention

The treatment of choice for infants with SCT is complete surgical resection, with the exception of emergencies related to tumor rupture or hemorrhage that adversely affect the neonate's hemodynamic status. The operative procedure can be performed on an elective basis early in the newborn period. The anatomic location of the tumor determines the operative approach. Tumors with extensive intrapelvic extension or a dominant abdominal component (type III or IV) are initially approached through the abdomen. A posterior sacral approach is sufficient for most type I tumors and type II tumors.

Operative goals include: (a) complete and prompt tumor excision. A significant delay may result in serious complications, including pressure necrosis, tumor hemorrhage, and malignant degeneration; (b) resection of the coccyx to prevent tumor recurrence; (c) reconstruction of the muscles of anorectal continence; and (d) restoration of a normal perineal and gluteal appearance [77, 78].

Initial control of the middle sacral and hypogastric arteries may be required in order to safely remove tumors in these fragile infants. The procedure is performed in a temperature-controlled environment, and infants are protected from heat loss with appropriate measures. The urinary bladder is catheterized and the operation is generally performed with the patient in a prone jackknife position, cushioned in a sterile foam ring. After skin preparation and sterile draping, a frown-shaped or inverted chevron incision is made superiorly to the tumor (Fig. 9.8a). This incision provides excellent exposure and keeps later wound closure some distance from the anal orifice. To delineate the rectum, the surgeon's finger and/or a Hegar dilator also may be inserted 3 cm into the anal canal. After raising skin flaps off the tumor, the attenuated retrorectal muscles are carefully identified and preserved. The mass is mobilized close to its capsule, and hemostasis is achieved with electrocautery or ligatures. To retard heat loss, warm gauze pads are placed over the exposed dissection and the tumor mass. The main blood supply to the tumor usually arises from a primitive middle sacral artery or from branches of the hypogastric artery. After division of the coccyx from the sacrum, the vessels can be observed exiting the presacral space ventral to the coccyx. For patients with extremely large or vascular lesions in which excessive fluid shifts or hemorrhage may result in operative mortality, surgeons occasionally use extracorporeal membrane oxygenation (ECMO) in conjunction with hypothermia and hypoperfusion to facilitate better control of bleeding during resection [79].

As failure to remove the coccyx is associated with a recurrence rate as high as 37% [80], the coccyx is excised in continuity with the tumor (Fig. 9.8b). The tumor is dissected free from the rectal wall and the anorectal muscles are reconstructed. The levator muscles are attached superiorly, providing support to the rectum and positioning the anus in the normal location. A closed-suction drain may be placed below the subcutaneous flaps. The wound is then closed in layers with interrupted absorbable sutures. A urinary catheter is left in position for several days. To maintain cleanliness of the wound, the patient is kept prone for several days after surgery.

Premature newborns with large teratomas are challenging to manage. Due to lung immaturity, increased tumor vascularity, and poor tolerance of blood loss, surgical risks are high [81]. In these patients, devascularization and staged resection may be considered to avoid excessive blood loss. The fetus with a large SCT presents an even greater management challenge. As

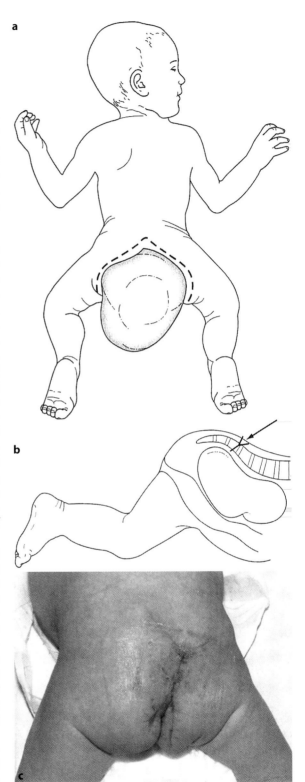

Fig. 9.8 Operative details. (**a**) Position of the patient for surgery. The chevron incision is used. (**b**) Cross-section of tumor and excision of coccygeal segment to ensure complete incision. (**c**) Postoperative cosmetic result.

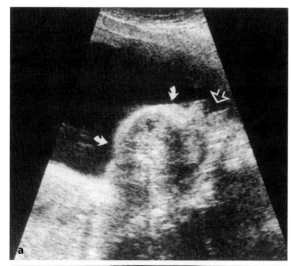

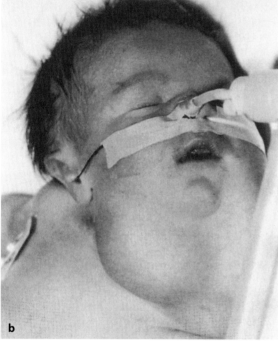

Fig. 9.9 (a)Antenatal ultrasound of a cervical teratoma (b) Infant with a cervical teratoma causing respiratory distress.

mentioned earlier, fetal hydrops and placentomegaly are associated with fetal demise.

The most serious complication of excision is intraoperative hemorrhage, and the major cause of mortality is hemorrhagic shock. One successful preoperative strategy for stabilizing patients with vascular tumors in which there is significant bleeding is to tightly wrap the teratoma with an elastic bandage. As a salvage approach for acute life-threatening hemorrhage, performing an emergent laparotomy and temporarily cross-clamping the distal abdominal aorta has been reported [82].

As with any surgical procedure, wound complications can occur. Resection of teratomas with significant intrapelvic and intraperitoneal extension may be associated with temporary or persistent urinary retention in the postoperative period, but these symptoms generally resolve. Although patients with small tumors usually have normal anorectal continence, 30–40% of premature infants with large SCTs and in whom the levator and gluteal muscles are severely attenuated, have fecal incontinence. Long-term bowel management strategies allow most patients to achieve socially manageable bowel function.

9.3.1.5 Adjuvant Chemotherapy

Detection of malignant elements necessitates adjuvant multiagent chemotherapy. The most active antineoplastic drugs include cisplatin, etoposide, and bleomycin. Reports indicate impressive survival after administration of intensive chemotherapy both in children with locally advanced disease and in those with metastatic disease [83–85]. Even with malignant transformation of SCT, reported survival is 88% with local disease and 75% with distant metastases [86]. Moreover, it appears that stage, extent of metastasis, and extension into bone have no prognostic significance when children are treated with platinum-based regimens [87].

For patients in whom the primary malignant tumor is unresectable, a course of multiagent chemotherapy is administered to facilitate subsequent resection. If a good tumor response is indicated by a diminishing serum AFP level, CT imaging, and a chest radiograph, resection is undertaken after several cycles of chemotherapy.

In patients with localized malignant recurrence, complete resection remains the cornerstone of salvage treatment. This is carried out in conjunction with adjuvant chemotherapy.

Chemotherapy also has been effective in the treatment of metastatic foci in the lungs and liver. However, to ensure removal of any malignant elements, residual lesions must be excised. Although radiation therapy is uncommon and used selectively, it may have a role in controlling unresectable disease.

9.3.1.6 Long-Term Outcomes

Research over the past several decades indicates that age at diagnosis is the dominant prognostic factor for SCT. Fetuses diagnosed with SCT after 30 weeks' gestation tend to have better outcomes than those diagnosed earlier [74, 88]. When the diagnosis is made prior to 2 months of age or excision is performed prior to 4 months of age, the malignancy rate is 5–10% [89,

90]. Additionally, cystic tumors, which are generally mature, carry a better prognosis. Complications related to hemorrhage, vascular steal, and malignancy are seen more frequently in patients with solid tumors.

The long-term survival of newborns who have undergone complete resection is generally excellent regardless of tumor histology [91]. Nevertheless, because all SCTs have a risk of local and/or distant recurrence, close follow-up at 3-month intervals for a 3- to 4-year period is essential. An 11% tumor recurrence with mature teratoma and a 4% recurrence with immature teratoma have been reported [63]. Although 43–50% of these occurrences are malignant, the chemosensitivity of yolk sac (endodermal sinus) tumor results in a high survival rate. Serum AFP levels are monitored and physical examinations are performed. Special attention is given to rectal examination in that it may detect a presacral recurrence. When serum AFP levels do not fall appropriately, abdominal US is performed. When there is an index of suspicion, an abdominopelvic CT or MR imaging and a lung CT are performed. Recurrent tumor may be benign, but should be re-excised to minimize the long-term risk of malignant transformation.

9.3.2 Head and Neck Teratomas

Head and neck teratomas account for 5% of all neonatal teratomas. These neoplasms have no sex or race predilection. They can occur in the brain, orbit, oropharynx, and neck.

9.3.2.1 Intracranial Teratomas

Intracranial teratomas account for approximately 50% of all brain tumors in early infancy [59]. These tumors occur most commonly in the pineal region but also are found in the hypothalamus, ventricles, and suprasellar and cerebellar regions. Unlike intracranial teratomas in older children, most intracranial teratomas in neonates are benign. The most common presenting symptoms and findings are related to the presence of obstructive hydrocephalus. On imaging studies, these lesions may be suspected by visualizing midline or paraxial intracranial calcifications.

Although resection is the treatment of choice, many neonatal intracranial teratomas are not resectable. Palliative shunting to alleviate intracranial pressure and hydrocephalus has little long-term benefit. Moreover, in some infants, shunting has been associated with extracranial spread of tumor. The role and effectiveness of chemotherapy remain undefined for this subgroup of patients.

Long-term survival is predicated on complete tumor removal. Outcomes are significantly worse for patients with extensive intracranial involvement that is not amenable to complete resection. Survival for these patients is reportedly between 15% and 20% [92].

9.3.2.2 Cervicofacial Teratomas

Cervical teratomas are extremely rare neoplasms. They occur with an estimated incidence of 1:40 000 to 1:80 000 live births and account for 2% of all neonatal tumors [93, 94]. Although most cervical teratomas are histologically benign, they frequently cause significant airway and esophageal obstruction in the perinatal period and are thus potentially fatal. Primary tumor sites include the tongue, nasopharynx, palate, sinus, mandible, tonsil, anterior neck, and thyroid gland. Males and females are equally affected.

Prenatal US is a reliable and essential diagnostic tool for detecting these lesions in utero, allowing for careful arrangement of the time, mode, and place of delivery (Fig. 9.9). When large cervical teratomas are prenatally detected, findings generally reveal multiloculated irregular masses with both solid and cystic components [95]. To delineate anatomy more clearly, fetal MR imaging is the diagnostic imaging study of choice. Of cases detected prenatally, lymphatic malformation (cystic hygroma) is the most likely entity to be mistaken for cervical teratoma. Similarities in size, sonographic findings, clinical characteristics, location, and gestational age at presentation can make this distinction difficult [96]. Other lesions to be considered in the differential diagnosis include large branchial cleft cyst and congenital thyroid goiter. Because fewer than 30% of cervical teratomas are associated with elevated serum AFP levels, this assay is not particularly helpful in the differential diagnosis of fetal cervical masses [70]. Approximately one third of prenatally diagnosed cases are complicated by maternal polyhydramnios, due to esophageal obstruction and/or interference with fetal swallowing. There is a high incidence of preterm labor and delivery that may be related to increased uterine size resulting from polyhydramnios and/or tumor.

Cervical teratomas are generally large and bulky, often measuring 5–12 cm in diameter (Fig. 9.9b). Tumor masses greater than the size of the fetal head have been reported [96–98], as has involvement of the oral floor, protrusion into the oral cavity (epignathus), and extension into the superior mediastinum [97]. Massive lesions may cause dystocia, requiring a cesarean section to deliver the baby. Various anomalies occurring in association with cervical teratomas have been reported. These include craniofacial and central nervous system anomalies, hypoplastic left ventricle, trisomy

13, and a case each of chondrodystrophia fetalis and imperforate anus [93]. Mandibular hypoplasia also has been seen as a direct result of mass effect on the developing mandible [70].

Up to 50% of cervicofacial teratomas have calcifications present and these are often seen more easily on postnatal plain radiographs [95]. When calcifications are present in a partially cystic and solid neck mass, they are virtually diagnostic of cervical teratoma [95]. A postnatal CT scan is particularly useful in delineating the anatomic extent and precise involvement of the neoplasm.

As shown in a number of series [93, 97–101], airway obstruction at birth is life threatening and associated with a high mortality rate. In patients with massive fetal neck masses, this is generally associated with a delay in obtaining an airway and ineffective ventilation. Delay in acquiring an adequate airway can result in hypoxia and acidosis and if longer than 5 min, can result in anoxic injury. In light of these concerns, most cervicofacial teratomas are definitively treated immediately after delivery, which preferably should take place at a tertiary care center with an expert perinatal team that includes a pediatric surgeon. Optimally, if a cesarean section is performed, maternal-fetal placental circulation should be maintained while an airway is secured. This is accomplished by employing an EXIT procedure; this allows time to perform procedures such as direct laryngoscopy, bronchoscopy, tracheostomy, surfactant administration, and cyst decompression, which may be required to secure the airway [70]. Because precipitous airway obstruction may occur due to hemorrhage into the tumor, orotracheal intubation is indicated in all patients, regardless of the presence or absence of symptoms.

In some reported series [101–103], infants have either had acute airway obstruction or lost a previously secure orotracheal airway within a few hours or days after delivery. Because early resection after stabilization is the most effective method of achieving total airway control, it is the treatment of choice. Delaying surgery can have other serious ramifications, including retention of secretions, atelectasis, and/or pneumonia due to interference with swallowing [49, 96]. Resection also removes the risk of malignant degeneration, which occurs at much higher frequencies (>90%) in cases of cervical teratomas that are not diagnosed or treated until late adolescence or adulthood [104].

To minimize operative morbidity, dissection of the teratoma should begin in areas distant to important regional nerves. Cervical teratomas often have a pseudocapsule, which facilitates gentle elevation of the tumor out of the neck. If the tumor arises from the thyroid gland, the involved thyroid lobe is excised in continuity with the teratoma. As glial metastases may be present, any enlarged lymph nodes should be excised with the tumor. After excision, a drain is left in place for 24–48 h. Because these tumors are often large, envelopment of vital anatomic structures in the neck is common. In some cases, complete tumor excision with acceptable functional and cosmetic results can be achieved only by staged procedures.

In contrast to the high incidence of malignancy (>60%) in adults, malignant cervicofacial teratomas with metastases are comparatively uncommon in neonates, with a reported incidence of 20% [93]. Despite the existence of poorly differentiated or undifferentiated tissue in the primary tumor, many infants remain free from recurrence following complete resection of a cervical teratoma. Such cases suggest that malignant biologic behavior is uncommon in this population [95, 96]. Reported findings show a number of consistent histologic patterns [93]. Neuroectodermal elements and immature neural tissue are the most commonly observed tissues in metastatic foci. In approximately one third of cases, the metastases are more differentiated but confined to regional lymph nodes. Patients with isolated regional lymph node metastases who are treated with excision of the primary tumor generally survive free of disease [46]. This supports the concept that the presence of metastases containing only differentiated tumor usually correlates with a good prognosis.

There are currently no chemotherapy guidelines for neonates with malignant cervical teratomas. Based on results in their series, however, Azizkhan, et al. [93] have recommended that this modality be reserved for infants with disseminated disease (undifferentiated lesions) and those who have invasive tumors and residual disease after resection.

Although cervical teratoma is generally a benign tumor, the possibility of malignant transformation mandates close surveillance for tumor recurrence. Serum AFP levels should be monitored at 3-month intervals in infancy and annually thereafter, with a rising level alerting the clinician to possible tumor recurrence. As previously discussed, serum AFP levels must be interpreted with caution and viewed within the framework of their natural half-life. Imaging studies twice a year for the first 3 years of life are also recommended. Since the thyroid and parathyroid glands may be removed or affected by tumor excision, the risk of temporary or permanent hypothyroidism must be considered. If encountered, these complications must be monitored and managed appropriately.

9.3.2.3 Retroperitoneal Teratomas

The retroperitoneum is the third most common extragonadal site for occurrence of teratoma, accounting for 2–5% of all pediatric cases [105, 106]. Most lesions are observed in early infancy and 50% are identified in the first year of life [59, 92]. Females are more commonly affected (2:1) than males. Infants generally present with a palpable abdominal mass. CT or MR imaging of the abdomen helps differentiate this neoplasm from the more commonly occurring neuroblastoma or Wilms' tumor. Laparotomy or a minimally invasive laparoscopic approach is used to achieve complete tumor resection; however, larger lesions are more likely to require an open procedure. Although an overall malignancy rate of 7% has been documented in children with teratomas, approximately 24% of retroperitoneal teratomas diagnosed during the first postnatal month have been found to be malignant, based on histology or clinical course [107]. Additionally, 30–40% of tumors have histologically immature elements. Malignant recurrence has been reported in patients with benign retroperitoneal teratomas containing immature components. As such, malignant lesions and lesions containing high-grade immature elements should be treated with adjuvant cisplatin-based chemotherapy following resection [106].

9.4 Neuroblastoma

Neuroblastoma arises from neural crest cells and can present anywhere along the sympathetic chain, including the adrenal medulla and sympathetic ganglia. It is the second most common tumor diagnosed in the neonatal period, with a reported incidence of 5–8 per million live births [108, 109]. It is also the most common neonatal malignancy, accounting for nearly one third of all malignancies diagnosed in newborns [108, 109]. Autopsy series of infants who have died from unrelated causes indicate an occurrence rate (in situ neuroblastomas) far exceeding the reported incidence of neuroblastoma [110, 111]. Most of these tumors are occult and known to regress spontaneously.

Up to 80% of neuroblastomas have recognizable and abnormal chromosomal patterns. In most cases, the defect is found on chromosomes 1 and 17 [18]; however, other abnormalities have been identified at 4p, 6q, 9q, 10q, 11q, 12q, 13q, 14q, 16q, 22p, and 22q [112]. The most important of these abnormalities are N-myc amplifications, deletions of chromosome 1p, and aneuploidy [18, 113–115]. Amplification of the N-myc oncogene is associated with a more aggressive tumor type that often presents with advanced stage disease. As such, it is considered a critical prognostic factor [18, 33, 113–115].

9.4.1 Clinical Presentation

The most common presentation of neonatal neuroblastoma is an abdominal mass arising from the adrenal gland. Primary lesions also can occur in the neck, mediastinum, retroperitoneum, and pelvis. Symptoms vary, depending on the anatomic location of the tumor, its physiology, and its mass effect. Nearly half of tumors have metastases at diagnosis, most commonly to the liver [116]. Hepatomegaly or massive abdominal distention associated with respiratory compromise may be the initial findings in patients with disseminated disease. These patients also may have skin nodules and bone marrow involvement (stage 4S).

Most neuroblastomas diagnosed during the neonatal period present as solid lesions, although cystic lesions have been described; such lesions may arise from an adrenal cyst or develop as a result of hemorrhage or degeneration within a solid neuroblastoma [117].

9.4.2 Diagnostic Evaluation

9.4.3 Antenatal

The routine use of antenatal US has increasingly identified the presence of adrenal tumors and other intra-abdominal masses [118–121]. Fetal MRI may be required to help distinguish neuroblastomas from other mass lesions [122]. Unlike neuroblastomas diagnosed during the neonatal period, prenatally diagnosed lesions often have a cystic component [119]. More than 90% of these cystic tumors arise in the adrenal grand, suggesting a link between perinatal tumors and the nodular collections of neuroblasts that are part of normal adrenal development [123]. Moreover, there is evidence that cystic tumors are caused by a disturbance in the natural course of neuroblastic nodule regression [123]. Most antenatally diagnosed cystic tumors are stage 1, 2, or 4S and usually have favorable biological characteristics. Evidence indicates that these lesions have a tendency to regress spontaneously [124].

Although increased urinary excretion of catecholamine metabolites is found in most children with neuroblastoma, a significant percentage of infants in whom there is a fetal diagnosis of intra-abdominal neuroblastoma have negative markers, reflecting the presence of a nonfunctioning tumor [117, 125, 126.]. Catecholamine-secreting fetal tumors are sometimes recognized, however, by the onset of maternal hypertension or pre-eclampsia appearing in the last trimester of pregnancy [127]. These offspring usually have either stage 4 or 4S disease or multiple metastases to the placenta [118].

9.4.4 Postnatal

Imaging studies are required during the postnatal period to differentiate neuroblastomas from adrenal hemorrhage, renal masses, and intra-abdominal extralobar sequestration. Diagnosis is confirmed by biopsy of the primary or metastatic tumor foci. As most neuroblastomas secrete varying quantities of catecholamine metabolites such as vanillylmandelic acid (VMA) and homovanillic acid (HVA), these values should be checked by random urine studies [128, 129]. Open biopsy should be avoided in neonates with massive liver involvement and in those that are high surgical risks due to impaired ventilation or concern about wound closure. In such patients, elevated urinary catecholamine levels and a positive bone marrow aspirate are sufficient to confirm the diagnosis. Tissue samples also should be analyzed for histology, amplification of the N-myc oncogene, chromosome IP, other tumor markers (e.g. TrK-A) and for ploidy, which significantly affect prognosis [113–115].

Staging requires CT or MRI scans of the primary lesion and suspected metastatic sites. A technetium or MIGB bone scan should be obtained to identify possible cortical bone metastases.

9.4.5 Stage 4S Disease

Infants younger than 1 year of age often present with a pattern of metastatic disease (stage 4S) that is unique to this age group. Stage 4S infants may have a small or undetectable primary neuroblastoma with metastases to the liver, skin, and bone marrow [130, 131]. The adrenal is the most common primary site. Skin lesions typically present as multiple bluish subcutaneous nodules. Stage 4S tumors exhibit particularly interesting biologic behavior. Most (75%) of these tumors regress spontaneously during infancy [132, 133]. Frequently, however, newborns with massive hepatic involvement are subject to a wide spectrum of significant respiratory and cardiovascular problems that may be fatal.

9.4.6 Treatment and Prognosis

Treatment strategies are based on stage and biologic features. As most oncologic studies do not segregate neonates from the broader grouping of infants younger than age 1 year, information pertaining to both treatment and prognosis in this specific age group is scant. Overall survival rates of infants younger than age 1 year, however, are known to be significantly greater than those of older children.

9.4.6.1 Stages 1 and 2

Neonates with stage 1 or 2 disease are considered to be at low risk regardless of biologic tumor features. Surgery alone is generally sufficient to control disease, and survival is nearly 100% [116]. In patients with stage 2 disease without N-myc amplification, residual microscopic disease usually regresses without additional intervention.

9.4.6.2 Cystic Neuroblastoma

Most prenatally diagnosed cystic neuroblastomas are localized and exhibit favorable biologic features. These tumors are usually associated with an almost universally favorable outcome [119, 121, 124]. As with low-stage solid tumors, cystic tumors are typically managed with resection.

Because of uniformly positive outcomes, as well as evidence that some cystic lesions regress spontaneously [124], the Children's Oncology Group (COG) has initiated a prospective study to investigate the effectiveness of observation alone as a management strategy. In the current protocol, serial sonograms are used to monitor the mass during the first few months of life to determine if tumor regression is ongoing. Surgical resection is reserved only for cystic tumors that fail to regress or increase in size [123]. To date, results of this study have not been reported.

9.4.6.3 Stages 3 and 4

The incidence of stage 3 and 4 tumors in neonates and infants younger than 1 year is lower than that in older children [131]. Infants with stage 3 disease generally undergo several cycles of combination chemotherapy followed by delayed primary resection. Those without N-myc amplification have an excellent prognosis and enjoy a 90% event-free survival [134]. Infants with stage 4 disease without N-myc amplification do not fare as well. Although studies show variable survival rates, these rates exceed 50% [135–137].

Infants with stage 3 or 4 disease and N-myc amplification are considered to be a particularly high-risk group, requiring more intensive high-dose chemotherapy and radiation therapy and possible bone marrow rescue. Despite this approach, those with more than 10 copies of the N-myc oncogene have rapidly progressive disease and frequently die [137].

9.4.6.4 Stage 4S

The survival rate of infants with stage 4S disease is greater than 80%, often without specific treatment [138, 139]. Most patients have favorable genetic and biologic factors, including high proto-oncogene Trk-A expression, absence of N-myc amplification, favorable histology, and no evidence of allelic loss of chromosome 1p [138.].

Despite the high rate of spontaneous tumor regression, progressive hepatomegaly may lead to respiratory embarrassment or inferior vena caval compression. In these patients, low-dose radiation to the liver (1–1.5 Gy per day over several days, with a total dose of 6–12 Gy) and low-dose chemotherapy (cyclophosphamide, 5 mg/kg per day) are used to accelerate tumor regression. As a measure of last resort, some surgeons have released the intra-abdominal compartment syndrome by creating a ventral hernia, using a large silastic patch to cover the surgical defect. This approach is generally not effective and therefore is no longer advocated.

A small subset of stage 4S patients with adverse genetic and biologic prognostic factors (e.g., more than 10 copies of N-myc and chromosome 1p deletion) require more aggressive therapy, including resection of the primary tumor, if identified. In cases with massive hepatic involvement, resection of the primary tumor confers no benefit in terms of survival. Most deaths in stage 4S occur in infants younger than 2 months of age with severe symptoms due to hepatomegaly. As compared to older infants, this younger group exhibits less tolerance to therapy [131, 139].

9.5 Soft Tissue Sarcomas

More than 75% of soft tissue masses in children younger than age 1 year are benign lesions of vascular or fibromuscular origin. Soft tissue sarcomas diagnosed during the neonatal period are extremely rare, accounting for approximately 10% of all neonatal malignant tumors and only 2% of all childhood sarcomas [3, 14, 140]. (Fig. 9.10) These tumors falls into three diagnostic groups, including congenital fibrosarcoma, rhabdomyosarcoma, and an exceedingly rare and diverse group of tumors sometimes collectively referred to non-rhabdomyosarcoma soft tissue sarcomas. Soft tissue sarcomas usually present as a mass on physical examination. Imaging studies are used to assess evidence of local or distant spread. In some patients, diagnostic bone marrow aspiration also may be used to rule out bone marrow involvement.

Soft tissue sarcomas differ in their natural history and their response to chemotherapy and radiotherapy. In view of the known long-term effects of radiothe-

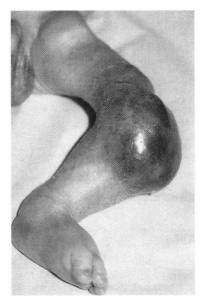

Fig. 9.10 Clinical photograph of a neonate with a sarcoma of the knee with metastatic spread to groin lymph nodes.

rapy, this should be used only as a treatment of last resort. Surgery plays a major role both in establishing the diagnosis and in tumor management, especially in neonates. Optimally, localized soft-tissues masses are treated by wide excision with a clear margin, if this can be achieved without compromising function, growth, or appearance [141].

9.5.1 Congenital Fibrosarcoma

Congenital fibrosarcoma is a well-recognized tumor with a low metastatic rate and a five-year disease-free survival greater than 90% [142–144]. It is characterized by the t (12;15) chromosomal translocation involving the ETV6 and NTRK3 genes, which is not found in fibrosarcomas that occur later in childhood [145, 146]. Congenital fibrosarcoma most commonly occurs in the extremities, but may arise in the back, retroperitoneum, sacrococcyx, and head and neck. The incidence of this tumor is higher in the first 6 months of life, and approximately one third of tumors diagnosed before age 5 are diagnosed shortly after birth [142, 147]. Spontaneous resolution of congenital fibrosarcomas has been documented [141].

Primary excision is the first line of treatment. Large bulky neoplasms that are not amenable to limb-sparing surgical procedures can be managed with perioperative chemotherapy (vincristine, actinomycin D, and cyclophosphamide) [141, 144]. This approach allows for delayed and less extensive resection that might otherwise result in significant mutilation or morbidity.

In some cases, chemotherapy may even lead to complete remission, thus eliminating the need for excision [141]. Although metastases are uncommon, local tumor control may be exceedingly difficult, with tumor recurrence reported as high as 40% [140, 142, 143, 147, 148]. In general, prognosis is not adversely affected by local tumor recurrence or metastatic spread, although exceptions have been reported [149].

9.5.2 Rhabdomyosarcoma

Because less than 5% of all rhabdomyosarcomas present in patients younger than age 1 year, data pertaining to neonatal rhabdomyosarcoma is extremely limited. In an Intergroup Rhabdomyosarcoma Study (IRS) reported in 1994, there were only 14 neonates in a study group of 3,217 patients, an incidence of 0.4% [43].

Two histologic subtypes of rhabdomyosarcoma have been described: embryonal and alveolar. These subtypes have differing clinical behaviors and are associated with distinct chromosomal translocations. The predominant histologic subtype in rhabdomyosarcomas presenting in neonates is embryonal. These lesions are associated with allelic loss of the 11p15 region [150].

Approximately half of neonatal rhabdomyosarcomas arise in the bladder, vagina, testicular, and sacrococcygeal regions [151]. In a multi-institutional Children's Cancer Group (CCG) study reported in 1995, a common characteristic of neonatal rhabdomyosarcoma was its aggressive biologic behavior as half of the patients had widespread disease at the time of diagnosis [140]. Metastatic disease can appear in the lungs, lymph nodes, liver, bone marrow, bone, and brain [152, 153].

Treatment of rhabdomyosarcoma comprises multimodal therapy with surgery and combination chemotherapy. The most effective chemotherapy regimen is considered to be vincristine, actinomycin D, and cyclophosphamide [154, 155]. Complete resection of nonmetastatic primaries is recommended if it can be accomplished with acceptable morbidity. Radiotherapy is reserved for infants with gross or microscopic residual disease. Prognosis depends on stage at presentation, histologic characteristics of the lesion, and the location of the primary tumor. Infants with embryonal histology and complete surgical resection do well, with cure rates higher than 90% [154]. Those with primary tumors in the head and neck (except parameningeal) and genitourinary region enjoy this same favorable prognosis [154]. Infants with metastatic disease at diagnosis do not fare well, with long-term survival rates of 25% [155].

9.5.3 Non-Rhabdomyosarcoma Soft Tissue Sarcomas

Other neonatal soft tissue sarcomas are exceedingly rare, with published experiences consisting only of small series or case reports. The previously cited CCG study reported nine neonates with non-rhabdomyosarcoma soft tissue sarcomas [140]. In seven of these nine patients, tumors were diagnosed at birth. Four patients had evidence of extensive regional spread or metastatic disease at the time of diagnosis. The pathology included malignant mesenchymal sarcoma (n=4), primitive sarcoma (n=1), angiosarcoma (n=1), chondrosarcoma (n=1), rhabdoid sarcoma (n=1), and the remaining tumor was unclassified. Primary tumor sites were head and neck, extremities, and trunk. Tumor management was based on location, biology, and resectability. Five of the nine newborns in this study survived (mean follow-up, 9 years). These patients had localized disease at the time of surgery. Four infants had complete surgical resections, and one had microscopic disease at the surgical site; this patient was treated with chemotherapy. All patients with unresectable regional or metastatic disease died despite adjuvant chemotherapy.

9.6 Renal Tumors

Solid renal neoplasms are extremely rare in neonates, accounting for only 8% of neonatal tumors [15, 16]. The most common tumor of the kidney in the neonate is congenital mesoblastic nephroma (CMN), which accounts for approximately 75% of the renal neoplasms in this age group [156]. This is followed by Wilms' tumor, which has an incidence in neonates lower than 0.2% [156, 157].

9.6.1 Congenital Mesoblastic Nephroma

CMN is a benign mesenchymal renal tumor that is histologically characterized by the proliferation of spindle-shaped cells arranged in fascicles that separate normal renal parenchymal tissue. This tumor occurs more commonly in males (2:1). Most neonates with CMN present with a palpable, nontender abdominal mass but hematuria, hypertension, and vomiting can occur (Fig. 9.11a, b). Although prenatal US has enabled detection of some renal neoplasms in utero, there are no specific prenatal sonographic characteristics that reliably distinguish between CMN and Wilms' tumor [158]. Based on incidence alone, however, a renal tumor presenting during the newborn period is more likely to be a CMN. Postnatal imaging modalities such as MRI can be useful in making a more precise diag-

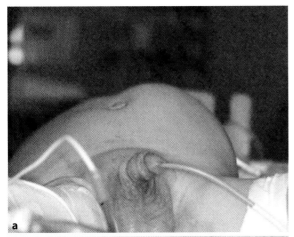

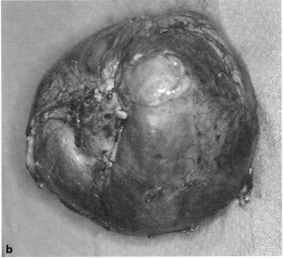

Fig. 9.11 (**a**) A 3-week-old infant with a congenital mesoblastic nephroma (**b**) Operative specimen

nosis but also are limited in distinguishing between the two tumors. Histologic assessment thus remains essential for establishing a definitive diagnosis [159].

Most cases of CMN are confined to the renal capsule, and as such, nephrectomy is curative. In some patients, however, the growth pattern is one of local invasion and extension through the renal capsule. During the course of resection, these tumors may be particularly friable and prone to intraoperative bleeding and rupture [15, 160]. Despite these possible complications, a survival rate exceeding 90% has been reported [15]. Metastases, which rarely occur, are managed with chemotherapy [161].

9.6.2 Wilms' Tumor

Wilms' tumor is thought to arise from nephrogenic rests that persist beyond 36 weeks of gestation [162].

Unlike CMN, this tumor affects both sexes equally [163, 164]. Both WAGR syndrome (Wilms, aniridia, genitourinary tract abnormalities, mental retardation) and Beckwith-Wiedemann syndrome (gigantism, omphalocele, macroglossia, hemihypertrophy) are associated with an increased risk of developing Wilms' tumor. These syndromes are associated with a loss of function of the WT1 gene at chromosome band 11p13 (WAGR) [165] or WT2 at chromosome band 11p15 (BWS) [166]. Among patients with Wilms' tumor who have no identifiable syndrome, approximately 40% have abnormalities in expression of WT1 and WT2 [167].

As with CMN, Wilms' tumor in neonates usually presents as a nontender abdominal mass. Most tumors are low stage and have favorable histology, however, metastatic disease can occur [157, 168]. The most common site of metastasis is the lungs. Primary excision of the tumor and chemotherapy are currently the mainstay of treatment, resulting in cure rates of greater than 90% [157, 168]. In light of this favorable prognosis, a recent COG protocol for infants with small (<550 g) stage I tumors compared treatment with surgery alone to treatment with surgery and a brief course of adjuvant chemotherapy [169]. Recurrence rates in the cohort who received surgery alone approached 15%, thus resulting in early closure of this arm of the study. Fortunately, most of these patients were treated successfully with salvage chemotherapy. Higher stage disease mandates more intensive chemotherapy, and in some patients, radiation therapy.

9.7 Liver Tumors

Primary liver tumors are extremely rare and account for only 2% of neonatal neoplasms [170]. They include a wide spectrum of benign and malignant neoplasms that occur with a distribution that is different from that in older children [171]. Most benign neonatal liver tumors are of vascular origin. The nosology of these tumors remains inconsistent and confusing. Many liver lesions that were formerly referred to as infantile hemangioendotheliomas are now considered to be hepatic hemangiomas. These lesions are generally asymptomatic and are incidental findings on prenatal or postnatal US. When symptomatic, however, hepatic hemangiomas are associated with serious and/or life-threatening complications. The second most common benign liver tumor of neonates and infants is mesenchymal hamartoma. The most common neonatal malignant liver tumor is hepatoblastoma; however, less than 10% of these tumors occur during the neonatal period [171].

9.7.1 Infantile Hepatic Hemangiomas

Unlike cutaneous hemangiomas of infancy, hepatic hemangiomas are rarely seen. These lesions follow a natural history similar to that of cutaneous lesions, and as with cutaneous lesions, they occur more commonly in females. Most hepatic hemangiomas are asymptomatic and incidentally discovered during imaging of the abdomen. Diffuse involvement of the liver is more often associated with severe complications during the proliferative phase, such as high output cardiac failure, hepatic dysfunction, abdominal compartment syndrome, and hypothyroidism. Significant symptoms or complications generally become evident during the first 3–4 months of life. Cutaneous hemangiomas are frequently the first indication of potential visceral involvement; however, hepatic and other visceral hemangiomas also can occur without cutaneous involvement [172].

Hepatic hemangiomas present variably, from tiny asymptomatic tumors that are detected incidentally to large (>5 cm in diameter) single, or multiple tumors that may or may not be associated with high output cardiac states. Infants are frequently seen with a triad of hepatomegaly, anemia, and high-output cardiac failure [173]. A systolic bruit may occasionally be heard over the enlarged liver. In rare cases, progressive and massive liver enlargement may cause abdominal compartment syndrome, resulting in life-threatening visceral ischemia and ventilatory failure [174].

US of the liver in infants with multiple or solitary lesions is useful both for initial screening and for following up of lesions that are well characterized. US demonstates either a single lesion or multiple lesions with draining veins and often a dilated proximal abdominal aorta. There may also be signs of significant intrahepatic shunting. US may also detect large hepatic lesions antenatally [175].

MRI is the imaging technique of choice for completely defining the extent and location of hepatic hemangiomas and their relationship to vascular structures. Although imaging features vary, most lesions appear as focal or multifocal T2-hyperintense spheres with centripetal contrast enhancement and dilated feeding and draining vessels (Fig. 9.12a). Three atypical patterns have also been found which include focal mass lesions with a large central varix with or without direct shunts, focal mass lesions with central necrosis or thrombosis, and massive hemangiomatous involvement of the liver with abdominal vascular compression [176]. The latter pattern of massive replacement of liver is associated with abdominal compartment syndrome, hypothyroidism, and a high mortality rate. Hypothyroidism is attributed to high levels of type 3 iodothyronine deiodinase activity produced by hemangiomas; this activity inactivates circulating thyroid hormone [177]. Patients

with diffuse liver hemangiomatosis should undergo screening for hypothyroidism. Because an abnormal thyroid-stimulating hormone level may not develop until a hemangioma proliferates, repeat testing is indicated when lesions undergo considerable growth. For patients with diffuse hemangiomatosis, high-output cardiac failure, and compartment syndrome the mortality rate exceeds 50%.

Angiography also is performed to define lesions prior to instituting embolic therapy. Angiographic features of hepatic hemangiomas are variable, ranging from discrete hypervascular tumors to diffuse tumors with macroscopic arteriovenous, arterioportal, and portosystemic shunting [173, 178]. Because hepatic hemangioma and arteriovenous malformations are rheologically fast flow, they may be mistaken for one another; however, arteriovenous malformations are extremely rare. Large solitary lesions diagnosed antenatally or soon after birth are likely to be congenital hemangiomas that are characterized by central necrosis of the lesion, capillary proliferation in the periphery of the lesion, and indistinct lesion margins due to abnormally large vessels extending into the adjacent liver tissue (Fig. 9.12b).

When imaging features are atypical and the diagnosis is unclear, incisional or excisional biopsies are extremely helpful in determining the pathology of a lesion and the most appropriate course of treatment. Differential diagnosis includes neuroblastoma, hepatoblastoma, and mesenchymal hamartomas, as well as a number of other neoplasms.

Most infantile hepatic hemangiomas, including those detected incidentally on imaging studies, remain asymptomatic throughout their natural clinical course. Patients with focal lesions without high flow seen on Doppler US generally do not require treatment [176]. Those patients with small, asymptomatic lesions should be followed with sequential physical examinations and US studies. Treatment should be reserved for infants with enlarged lesions that cause significant symptoms or complications.

Either systemic oral or intravenous corticosteroid therapy is the initial treatment of choice, depending on the severity of symptoms. For unstable patients, intravenous corticosteroids are preferred. In the protocol currently followed at Cincinnati Children's Hospital Medical Center, high doses of methylprednisolone are administered at a daily dose of 30 mg/kg for 3 days. This is followed by a daily dose of 20 mg/kg for 4 days and then a daily dose of 10, 5, 2, and 1 mg/kg for 1 week, with each dose given once daily before 8:00 am. Patients who are relatively stable are treated with oral corticosteroid therapy. Oral prednisone or prednisolone is administered at an initial dose of at least 3 mg/kg/day for 1 month. If the lesion responds to treatment, the patient is continued on this dose for

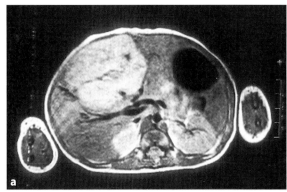

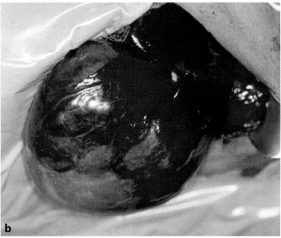

Fig. 9.12 (**a**) MRI of the liver demonstrating a large intrahepatic hemangioma (**b**) Operative photograph showing large hemangioma of the liver in a 1-month-old infant

another 4 weeks. The daily dose is then gradually lowered to 1 mg/kg/day, and is generally maintained for up to 4 months, and occasionally 6 months. If no response is seen with this dosing regimen, an attempt is made to titrate the dose to an upper limit of 5 mg/kg/day in order to effect a response. If this fails, the dose is rapidly tapered, the infant is taken off the medication, and other treatment approaches are instituted. Because rebound growth can occur if the steroids are discontinued before the end of the proliferative phase, patients should be monitored while being weaned from medication.

For lesions that are unresponsive to steroids, vincristine is the current drug of choice. Because it is a vesicant, it is best delivered through central venous access. An initial weekly dose of 0.05–1 mg/m2 is administered by intravenous injection. This dose is then tapered, increasing the interval between injections depending on the clinical response. Treatment is administered for 4–6 months.

The angiogenesis inhibitor interferon-α is also occasionally used for lesions that are refractory to corticosteroid therapy. It is typically administered as a daily subcutaneous injection at a dosage range of 1–3 million units/m2. Because of its known neurotoxicity, particularly its association with spastic diplegia [179, 180], the use of interferon-α in children younger than age 1 year should be avoided.

In patients with persistent high-output cardiac failure, angiography and embolization may be performed, with the latter being useful only if there are direct macrovascular shunts through the lesion. Because angiography and embolization are associated with risk of injury to the femoral access vessel or inadvertently embolized visceral vessels, it should be performed only by an interventional radiologist with skill and experience with these techniques in infants.

Other treatment options reserved for refractory lesions include surgical resection of large solitary lesions, hepatic artery ligation, and liver transplantation. Prior to contemporary pharmacologic therapy, resection of solitary lesions and embolization were frequently the only viable treatment options. Because they are associated with extremely high mortality, however, they are now infrequently performed. A review of the literature reported in 2003 described 35 cases treated by hepatic artery ligation with a survival rate of 80% [181]. Liver transplantation is rarely performed, and is reserved for patients in whom there is diffuse hepatic involvement and an imminent risk of death [182].

9.7.2 Mesenchymal Hamartomas

Mesenchymal hamartomas typically present as a large, palpable, nontender cystic liver mass, more common in the right lobe. Lesions are generally diagnosed during the first 2 years of life but have been reported in the newborn [171]. The mass is usually encapsulated, although occasionally it can infiltrate into the hepatic parenchyma and can cause respiratory distress or heart failure resulting from arteriovenous shunting. Although spontaneous tumor regression can occur, cases of massive local recurrence and later transformation to undifferentiated sarcoma have been reported [183–185]. Thus, when feasible, complete surgical resection is the treatment of choice.

9.7.3 Hepatoblastoma

Hepatoblastoma is an embryonal neoplasm composed of malignant epithelial tissue with variable differentiation, most often with embryonal or fetal components [171]. There is an increased incidence of this tumor among patients with Beckwith-Weidemann syndrome, Li-Fraumeni syndrome, or hemihypertrophy [186–188], and familial adenomatous polyposis [189].

There also is an increased incidence of hepatoblastoma among surviving premature infants [190, 191], with risk increasing with lower birth weight [192].

Hepatoblastomas can be detected prenatally by abdominal US and can cause polyhydramnios and stillbirth [193]. Tumor rupture and massive hemorrhage have been described following delivery [194, 195]. Postnatally, hepatoblastoma presents with abdominal enlargement and hepatomegaly. The lungs are the primary site of metastasis, though bone and brain involvement can occur. AFP levels are elevated in most patients and are especially useful in monitoring disease status following treatment.

Complete surgical resection and subsequent chemotherapy with cytotoxic agents (e.g., cisplatin and doxorubicin) is the treatment of choice [196, 197]. For neonates with lesions that initially are not resectable, preoperative chemotherapy can be beneficial. For patients with unresectable tumors confined to the liver, hepatic transplantation is an alternative [182]. Prognosis is largely dependent on resectability. Approximately two thirds of patients with tumors that are initially unresectable can be cured with chemotherapy followed by surgical resection and additional postoperative chemotherapy [198, 199].

9.8 Retinoblastoma

Retinoblastoma is a rare tumor that presents occasionally at birth. Forty percent of cases have been shown to result from inheritance of a germline mutation in the RB1 gene [200, 201]. The tumor is detected by absence of the normal red reflex when the infant's eyes are examined with an ophthalmoscope. All newborns should be screened for this reflex and any infant with a family history of retinoblastoma should undergo a comprehensive ophthalmologic examination. These patients are at risk for bilateral involvement.

When detected early, retinoblastoma usually is curable [202–204]. When disease is intraocular, laser therapy or cryotherapy are used either with or without adjuvant chemotherapy, depending on the size of the lesion. In selective cases, radiotherapy is also used to salvage vision. Extensive intraocular disease can be managed with enucleation [205]. Metastatic disease requires aggressive chemotherapy [206, 207].

References

1. Bader JL, Miller RW (1979) US cancer incidence and mortality in the first year of life. Am J Dis Child 133:157–159
2. Littman P, D'Angio GJ (1981) Radiation therapy in the neonate. Am J Pediatr Hematol Oncol 3:279–285
3. Reaman GH, Bleyer A (2002) Infants and adolescents with cancer: Special considerations. In: Pizzo PA, Poplack DG (eds) Principles and practice of pediatric oncology, 4th edn. Lippincott, Philadelphia
4. Bhatia S, Landier W, Robison LL (2002) Late effects of childhood cancer therapy. In: DeVita VT, Hellman S, Rosenberg SA (eds) Progress in oncology. Jones and Bartlett Publishers, Sudbury, MA, pp 171–213
5. Pintér AB, Hock A, Kajtár P, Dober I (2003) Long-term follow-up of cancer in neonate and infants: A national survey of 142 patients. Pediatr Surg Int 19:233–239
6. Meadows AT, Gallagher JA, Bunin GR (1992) Late effects of early childhood cancer therapy. Br J Cancer (Suppl) 18: S92–S95
7. Paulino AC, Wen BC, Brown CK, et al. (2000) Late effects in children treated with radiation therapy for Wilms' tumor. Int J Radiat Oncol Biol Phys 46:1239–1246
8. Dreyer ZE, Blatt J, Bleyer A (2002) Late effects of childhood cancer and its treatment. In: Pizzo PA, Poplack DG (eds) Principles and practice of pediatric oncology, 4th edn. Lippincott, Philadelphia
9. Robison LL (2005) The Childhood Cancer Survivor Study: A resource for research of long-term outcomes among adult survivors of childhood cancer. Minn Med 88:45–49
10. Crom DB, Wilimas JA, Green AA, Pratt CB, Jenkins JJ 3rd, Behm FG (1989) Malignancy in the neonate. Med Pediatr Oncol 17:101–104
11. Campbell AN, Chan HS, O'Brien A, Smith CR, Becker LE (1988) Malignant tumors in the neonate. Arch Dis Child 62:19–23
12. Davis CF, Carachi R, Young DG (1988) Neonatal tumors: Glasgow 1955–1986. Arch Dis Child 63:1075–1078
13. Xue H, Horwitz JR, Smith MB, et al. (1995) Malignant solid tumors in neonates: A 40-year review. J Pediatr Surg 30:543–545
14. Moore SW, Kaschula ROC, Albertyn R, Rode H, Millar AJW, Karabus C (1995) The outcome of solid tumours occurring in the neonatal period. Pediatr Surg Int 10:366–370
15. Dillon PW, Azizkhan RG (1997) Neonatal tumors. In: Andrassy RJ (ed) Pediatric surgery oncology. WB Saunders, Philadelphia
16. Parkes SE, Muir KR, Southern L, Cameron AH, Darbyshire PJ, Stevens MC (1994) Neonatal tumors: A thirty-year population-based study. Med Pediatr Oncol 22:309–317
17. Halperin EC (2000) Neonatal neoplasms. Int J Radiat Oncol Biol Phys 47:171–178
18. Moore SW, Plaschkes J (2003) Epidemiology and genetic associations of neonatal tumors. In: Puri P (ed) Newborn surgery, 2nd edn. Oxford University Press, New York
19. Buyukpamukcu M, Varan A, Tanyel C, et al. (2003) Solid tumors in the neonatal period. Clin Pediatr 42:29–34
20. Moore SW (1996) Genetic and clinical associations of neonatal tumours. In: Puri P (ed) Neonatal tumours. Springer, New York, pp 11–22
21. Altmann AE, Halliday JL, Giles GG (1998) Associations between congenital malformations and childhood cancer: A register-based case-control study. Br J Cancer 78:1244–1249

22. Moore SW, Satgé D, Sasco AJ, Zimmermann A, Plaschkes J (2003) The epidemiology of neonatal tumours: Report of an international working group. Pediatr Sug Int 19:509–519

23. Satgé D, Van Den Berghe H (1996) Aspects of the neoplasms observed in patients with constitutional autosomal trisomy. Cancer Genet Cytogenet 87:63–70

24. Coppes MJ, Campbell CE, Williams BR (1993) The role of WT1 in Wilms tumorigenesis. FASEB J 7:886–895

25. Holland WW, Doll R, Carter CO (1962) The mortality from leukaemia and other cancers among patients with Down's syndrome (Mongols) and among their parents. Br J Cancer 16:177–186

26. Weinberg AG, Schiller G, Windmiller J (1982) Neonatal leukemoid reaction. An isolated manifestation of mosaic Trisomy 21. Am J Dis Child 136:310–311

27. Bresters D, Reus AC, Veerman AJ, van Wering AR, van der Does-van den Berg A, Kaspers GJ (2002) Congenital leukaemia: The Dutch experience and review of the literature. Br J Haematol 117:513–524

28. Rahbar R, Vogel A, Myers LB, et al. (2005) Fetal surgery in otolaryngology: A new era in the diagnosis and management of fetal airway obstruction because of advances in prenatal imaging. Arch Otolaryngol Head Neck Surg 131:393–398

29. Coleman BG, Adzick NS, Crombleholme TM, et al. (2002) Fetal therapy: State of the art. J Ultrasound Med 21:1257–1288

30. Sauvat F, Sarnacki S, Brisse H, et al. (2002) Outcome of suprarenal localized masses diagnosed during the perinatal period: A retrospective multicenter study. Cancer 94:2474–2480

31. Mychaliska GB, Bealer JF, Graf JL, Rosen MA, Adzick NS, Harrison MR (1997) Operating on placental support: The ex utero intrapartum treatment procedure. J Pediatr Surg 32:227–230

32. Wegner EA, Barrington SF, Kingston JE, et al. (2005) The impact of PET scanning on management of paediatric oncology patients. Eur J Nucl Med Mol Imaging 32:23–30

33. Brodeur GM, Maris JM (2002) Neuroblastoma. In: Pizzo PA, Poplack DG (eds) Principles and practice of pediatric oncology, 4th edn. Lippincott, Philadelphia

34. Silber JH, Littman PS, Meadows AT (1990) Stature loss following skeletal irradiation for childhood cancer. J Clin Oncol 8:304–312

35. Meadows AT, Gordon J, Massari DJ, Littman P, Fergusson J, Moss K (1981) Declines in IQ scores and cognitive dysfunctions in children with acute lymphocytic leukaemia treated with cranial irradiation. Lancet 2:1015–1018

36. Farwell JR, Dohrmann GJ, Flannery JT (1978) Intracranial neoplasms in infants. Arch Neurol 35:533–537

37. Littman PS, D'Angio GJ (1979) Growth considerations in the radiation therapy of children with cancer. Annu Rev Med 30:405–415

38. Guibout C, Adjadj E, Rubino C, et al. (2005) Malignant breast tumors after radiotherapy for a first cancer during childhood. J Clin Oncol 23:197–204

39. Maier JG (1972) Effects of radiation on kidney, bladder and prostate. In: Vaeth JM (ed) Frontiers of radiation therapy and oncology, vol 6. Karger, Basel and University Park Press, Baltimore, pp 196–207

40. Kraut JW, Bagshaw MA, Glatstein EJ (1972) Hepatic effects of irradiation. In: Vaeth JM (ed) Frontiers of radiation therapy and oncology, vol 6. Karger, Basel and University Park Press, Baltimore, pp 182–195

41. Cancer Pharmacology in Infants and Young Children (2003) Online summary of meeting sponsored by the Children's Oncology Group (COG) and National Cancer Institute-Cancer Therapy Evaluation Program (CTEP). Arlington, VA

42. Morgan E, Baum E, Breslow N, Takashima J, D'Angio G (1988) Chemotherapy-related toxicity in infants treated according to the Second National Wilms' Tumor Study. J Clin Oncol 6:51–55

43. Lobe TE, Wiener ES, Hays DM et al. (1994) Neonatal rhabdomyosarcoma: The IRS experience. J Pediatr Surg 29:1167–1170

44. Reaman G, Zeltzer P, Bleyer WA, et al. (1985) Acute lymphoblastic leukemia in infants less than one year of age: A cumulative experience of the Children's Cancer Study Group. J Clin Oncol 3:1513–1521

45. Shamberger RC (2004) Teratomas and germ cell tumors. In: O'Neill JA, Grosfeld JL, Fonkalsrud EW, et al. (eds) Principles of pediatric surgery, 2nd edn. Mosby, St. Louis

46. Azizkhan RG (2006) Teratomas and other germ cell tumors. In: Grosfeld JL, O'Neill JA, Coran AG, Fonkalsrud EW (eds) Pediatric surgery, 6th edn. Mosby, Philadelphia

47. Bale PM (1984) Sacrococcygeal developmental abnormalities and tumors in children. Perspect Pediatr Pathol 8:9–56

48. Lemire RJ, Beckwith JB (1982) Pathogenesis of congenital tumors and malformations of the sacrococcygeal region. Teratology 25:201–213

49. Noseworthy J, Lack EE, Kozakewich HP, Vawter GF, Welch KJ (1981) Sacrococcygeal germ cell tumors in childhood: An updated experience with 118 patients. J Pediatr Surg 16:358–364

50. Gonzalez-Crussi F (1982) Extragonadal teratomas. In: Atlas of tumor pathology, 2nd series. Armed Forces Institute of Pathology, Washington, DC, fascicle 18

51. Cushing B, Perlman EJ, Marina NM, Castleberry RP (2002) Germ cell tumors. In: Pizzo PA, Poplack DG (eds) Principles and practice of pediatric oncology, 4th edn. Lippincott, Philadelphia

52. Norris HJ, Zirkin HJ, Benson WL (1976) Immature (malignant) teratoma of the ovary: A clinical and pathologic study of 58 cases. Cancer 37:2359–2372

53. Robboy SJ, Scully RE (1970) Ovarian teratoma with glial implants on the peritoneum. An analysis of 12 cases. Hum Pathol 1:643–653

54. Isaacs H Jr. Germ cell tumors (1997) In: Tumors of the fetus and newborn (major problems in pathology series), vol 35. WB Saunders, Philadelphia

55. Valdiserri RO, Yunis EJ (1981) Sacrococcygeal teratomas: A review of 68 cases. Cancer 48:217–221

56. Baumann FR, Nerlich A (1993) Metastasizing cervical teratoma of the fetus. Pediatr Pathol 13:21–27

57. Dehner LP, Mills A, Talerman A, Billman GF, Krous HF, Platz CE (1990) Germ cell neoplasms of head and neck soft tissues: A pathologic spectrum of teratomatous and endodermal sinus tumors. Hum Pathol 21:309–318

58. Heifetz SA, Cushing B, Giller R, et al. (1998) Immature teratomas in children: Pathologic considerations: A report from the combined Pediatric Oncology Group/Children's Cancer Group. Am J Surg Pathol 22:1115–1124

59. Rowe MI, O'Neill JA, Grosfeld JL, Fonkalsrud EW, Coran AG (1995) Teratomas and germ cell tumors. In: Rowe MI, O'Neill JA, Grosfeld JL, Fonkalsrud EW, Coran AG (eds) Essentials of pediatric surgery. Mosby-Year Book, St Louis

60. Magee JF, McFadden DE, Pantzar JT (1992) Congenital tumors. In: Dimmick JE, Kalousek DK (eds) Developmental pathology of the embryo and fetus. Lippincott, Philadelphia. p 235

61. Schropp KP, Lobe TE, Rao B, et al. (1992) Sacrococcygeal teratoma: The experience of four decades. J Pediatr Surg 27:1075–1079

62. Goto M, Makino Y, Tamura R, Ikeda S, Kawarabayashi T (2000) Sacrococcygeal teratoma with hydrops fetalis and bilateral hydronephrosis. J Perinat Med 28:414–418

63. Rescorla FJ, Sawin RS, Coran AG, Dillon PW, Azizkhan RG (1998) Long-term outcome for infants and children with sacrococcygeal teratoma: A report from the Children's Cancer Group. J Pediatr Surg 33:171–176

64. Werb P, Scurry J, Ostor A, Fortune D, Attwood H (1992) Survey of congenital tumors in perinatal necropsies. Pathology 24:247–253

65. Altman RP, Randolph JG, Lilly JR (1974) Sacrococcygeal teratoma: American Academy of Pediatrics Surgical Section Survey–1973. J Pediatr Surg 9:389–398

66. Carney JA, Thompson DP, Johnson CL, Lynn HB (1972) Teratomas in children: Clinical and pathologic aspects. J Pediatr Surg 7:271–282

67. Fraumeni JF Jr, Li FP, Dalager N (1973) Teratomas in children: Epidemiologic features. J Natl Cancer Inst 51:1425–1430

68. Hawkins E, Perlman EJ (1996) Germ cell tumors. In: Parham DM (ed) Pediatric neoplasia: Morphology and biology. Lippincott-Raven, Philadelphia

69. Shaaban AF, Kim HB, Flake AW (2003) Fetal surgery, diagnosis, and intervention. In: Ziegler MM, Azizkhan RG, Weber TR (eds) Operative pediatric surgery. McGraw-Hill, New York, NY

70. Bianchi DW, Crombleholme TM, D'Alton ME (2000) Fetology: diagnosis and management of the fetal patient. McGraw-Hill, New York

71. Flake AW (1993) Fetal sacrococcygeal teratoma. Semin Pediatr Surg 2: 113–120

72. Hedrick HL, Flake AW, Crombleholme TM, et al. (2004) Sacrococcygeal teratoma: Prenatal assessment, fetal intervention, and outcome. J Pediatr Surg 39:430–438

73. Bond SJ, Harrison MR, Schmidt KG, et al. (1990) Death due to high-output cardiac failure in fetal sacrococcygeal teratoma. J Pediatr Surg 25:1287–1291

74. Flake AW, Harrison MR, Adzick NS, Laberge JM, Warsof SL (1986) Fetal sacrococcygeal teratoma. J Pediatr Surg 21:563–566

75. Musci MN Jr, Clark MJ, Ayres RE, Finkel MA (1983) Management of dystocia caused by a large sacrococcygeal teratoma. Obstet Gynecol 62:10s–12s

76. Adzick NS, Crombleholme TM, Morgan MA, Quinn TM (1997) A rapidly growing fetal teratoma. Lancet 349:538

77. Azizkhan RG (1999) Neonatal tumors. In: Carachi R, Azmy A, Grosfeld JL (eds) The surgery of childhood tumors. Oxford University Press, New York

78. Fishman SJ, Jennings RW, Johnson SM, Kim HB (2004) Contouring buttock reconstruction after sacrococcygeal teratoma resection. J Pediatr Surg 39:439–441

79. Lund DP, Soriano SG, Fauza D, et al. (1995) Resection of a massive sacrococcygeal teratoma using hypothermic hypoperfusion: A novel use of extracorporeal membrane oxygenation. J Pediatr Surg 30:1557–1559

80. Gross RW, Clatworthy HW Jr, Meeker IA Jr (1951) Sacrococcygeal teratomas in infants and children: A report of 40 cases. Surg Gynecol Obstet 92:341–354

81. Robertson FM, Crombleholme TM, Frantz ID 3rd, Shephard BA, Bianchi DW, D'Alton ME (1995) Devascularization and staged resection of giant sacrococcygeal teratoma in the premature infant. J Pediatr Surg 30:309–311

82. Teitelbaum D, Teich S, Cassidy S, Karp M, Cooney D, Besner G (1994) Highly vascularized sacrococcygeal teratoma: Description of this atypical variant and its operative management. J Pediatr Surg 29:98–101

83. Göbel U, Schneider DT, Calaminus G, et al. (2001) Multimodal treatment of malignant sacrococcygeal germ cell tumors: A prospective analysis of 66 patients of the German cooperative protocols MAKEI 83/86 and 89. J Clin Oncol 19:1943–1950

84. Göbel U, Calaminus G, Schneider DT, Schmidt P, Haas RJ (2002) Management of germ cell tumors in children: Approaches to cure. Onkologie 25:14–22

85. Rescorla F, Billmire D, Stolar C, et al. (2001) The effect of cisplatin dose and surgical resection in children with malignant germ cell tumors at the sacrococcygeal region: A pediatric intergroup trial (POG 9049/CCG 8882). J Pediatr Surg 36:12–17

86. Misra D, Pritchard J, Drake DP, Kiely EM, Spitz L (1997) Markedly improved survival in malignant sacro-coccygeal teratomas – 16 years' experience. Eur J Pediatr Surg 7:152–155

87. Calaminus G, Schneider DT, Bokkerink JP, et al. (2003) Prognostic value of tumor size, metastases, extension into bone, and increased tumor marker in children with malignant sacrococcygeal germ cell tumors: A prospective evaluation of 71 patients treated in the German cooperative protocols Maligne Keimzelltumoren (MAKEI) 83/86 and MAKEI 89. J Clin Oncol 21:781–786

88. Kuhlmann RS, Warsof SL, Levy DL, Flake AJ, Harrison MR (1987) Fetal sacrococcygeal teratoma. Fetal Ther 2:95–100

89. Donnellan WA, Swenson O (1968) Benign and malignant sacrococcygeal teratomas. Surgery 64:834–846

90. Waldhausen JA, Kolman JW, Vellios F, Battersby JS (1963) Sacrococcygeal teratoma. Surgery 54:933–949

91. Marina NM, Cushing B, Giller R, et al. (1999) Complete surgical excision is effective treatment for children with immature teratomas with or without malignant elements: A Pediatric Oncology Group/Children's Cancer Group Intergroup Study. J Clin Oncol 17:2137–2143

92. Azizkhan RG, Caty MG (1996) Teratomas in childhood. Curr Opin Pediatr 8:287–292

93. Azizkhan RG, Haase GM, Applebaum H, et al. (1995) Diagnosis, management, and outcome of cervicofacial teratomas in neonates: A Children's Cancer Group Study. J Pediatr Surg 30:312–316

94. Lack EE (1985) Extragonadal germ cell tumors of the head and neck region: Review of 16 cases. Hum Pathol 16:56–64

95. Gundry SR, Wesley JR, Klein MD, Barr M, Coran AG (1983) Cervical teratomas in the newborn. J Pediatr Surg 18:382–386

96. Batsakis JG, Littler ER, Oberman HA (1964) Teratomas of the neck. A clinicopathologic appraisal. Arch Otolaryngol 79:619–624

97. Jordan RB, Gauderer MW (1988) Cervical teratomas: An analysis, literature review and proposed classification. J Pediatr Surg 23:583–591

98. Liechty KW, Hedrick HL, Hubbard AM, et al. (2006) Severe pulmonary hypoplasia associated with giant cervical teratomas. J Pediatr Surg 41:230–233

99. Elmasalme F, Giacomantonio M, Clarke KD, Othman E, Matbouli S (2000) Congenital cervical teratoma in neonates. Case report and review. Eur J Pediatr Surg 10:252–257

100. Sbragia L, Paek BW, Feldstein VA, et al. (2001) Outcome of prenatally diagnosed solid fetal tumors. J Pediatr Surg 36:1244–1247

101. De Backer A, Madern GC, van de Ven CP, Tibboel D, Hazebroek FW (2004) Strategy for management of newborns with cervical teratoma. J Perinat Med 32:500–508

102. Langer JC, Tabb T, Thompson P, Paes BA, Caco CC (1992) Management of prenatally diagnosed tracheal obstruction: Access to the airway in utero prior to delivery. Fetal Diagn Ther 7:12–16

103. Touran T, Applebaum H, Frost DB, Richardson R, Taber P, Rowland J (1989) Congenital metastatic cervical teratoma: Diagnostic and management considerations. J Pediatr Surg 24:21–23

104. Buckley NJ, Burch WM, Leight GS (1986) Malignant teratoma in the thyroid gland of an adult: A case report and a review of the literature. Surgery 100:932–937

105. Mahour GH, Landing BH, Woolley MM (1978) Teratomas in children: Clinico-pathologic studies in 133 patients. Z Kinderchir 23:365–380

106. Gatcombe HG, Assikis V, Kooby D, Johnstone PA (2004) Primary retroperitoneal teratomas: A review of the literature. J Surg Oncol 86:107–113

107. Auge B, Satge D, Sauvage P, Lutz P, Chenard MP, Levy JM (1993) Retroperitoneal teratomas in the perinatal period. Review of the literature concerning a neonatal, immature, aggressive teratoma. Ann Pediatr (Paris) 40:613–621

108. Isaacs H Jr (1985) Perinatal (congenital and neonatal) neoplasms: A report of 110 cases. Pediatr Pathol 3:165–216

109. Dehner LP (1981) Neoplasms of the fetus and neonate. In: Naeye RL, Kissane JM, Kaufman N (eds) Perinatal diseases. International Academy of Pathology Monograph Number 22. Williams and Wilkens, Baltimore, pp 286–345

110. Beckwith JB, Perrin EV (1963) In situ neuroblastomas: A contribution to the natural history of neural crest tumors. Am J Pathol 43:1089–1104

111. Guin GH, Gilbert EF, Jones B (1969) Incidental neuroblastoma in infants. Am J Clin Pathol 51:126–136

112. Woods WG, Lemieux B, Tuchman M (1992) Neuroblastoma represents distinct clinical-biologic entities: A review and perspective from the Quebec Neuroblastoma Screening Project. Pediatrics 89:114–118

113. Look AT, Hayes FA, Shuster JJ, et al. (1991) Clinical relevance of tumor cell ploidy and N-myc gene amplification in childhood neuroblastoma: A Pediatric Oncology Group study. J Clin Oncol 9:581–591

114. Brodeur GM, Maris JM, Yamashiro DJ, Hogarty MD, White PS (1997) Biology and genetics of human neuroblastomas. J Pediatr Hematol Oncol 19:93–101

115. Seeger RC, Brodeur GM, Sather H, et al. (1985) Association of multiple copies of the N-myc oncogene with rapid progression of neuroblastomas. N Engl J Med 313:1111–1116

116. Azizkhan RG, Haase GM, Coran AG, et al. (1995) Diagnosis, management and outcome of neuroblastoma in neonates: A Children's Cancer Group study. 36th World Congress of Surgery Abstract Book; 134

117. Richards ML, Gundersen AE, Williams MS (1995) Cystic neuroblastoma of infancy. J Pediatr Surg 30:1354–1357

118. Jennings RW, LaQuaglia MP, Leong K, Hendren WH, Adzick NS (1993) Fetal neuroblastoma: Prenatal diagnosis and natural history. J Pediatr Surg 28:1168–1174

119. Ho PT, Estroff JA, Kozakewich H, et al. (1993) Prenatal detection of neuroblastoma: A ten-year experience from the Dana-Farber Cancer Institute and Children's Hospital. Pediatrics 92:358–364

120. Saylors RL 3rd, Cohn SL, Morgan ER, Brodeur GM (1994) Prenatal detection of neuroblastoma by fetal ultrasonography. Am J Pediatr Hematol Oncol 16:356–360

121. Acharya S, Jayabose S, Kogan SJ, et al. (1997) Prenatally diagnosed neuroblastoma. Cancer 80:304–310

122. Aslan H, Ozseker B, Gul A (2004) Prenatal sonographic and magnetic resonance imaging diagnosis of cystic neuroblastoma. Ultrasound Obstet Gynecol 24:693–694

123. Nuchtern JG (2006) Perinatal neuroblastoma. Semin Pediatr Surg 15:10–16

124. Holgersen LO, Subramanian S, Kirpekar M, Mootabar H, Marcus JR (1996) Spontaneous resolution of antenatally diagnosed adrenal masses. J Pediatr Surg 31:153–155

125. Hosoda Y, Miyano T, Kimura K, et al. (1992) Characteristics and management of patients with fetal neuroblastoma. J Pediatr Surg 27:623–625

126. Laug WE, Siegel SE, Shaw KN, Landing B, Baptista J, Gutenstein M (1978) Initial urinary catecholamine metabolite concentrations and prognosis in neuroblastoma. Pediatrics 62:77–83

127. Newton ER, Louis F, Dalton ME, Feingold M (1985) Fetal neuroblastoma and catecholamine-induced maternal hypertension. Obstet Gynecol 65:49S–52S

128. Tuchman M, Morris CL, Ramnaraine ML, Bowers LD, Krivit W (1985) Value of random urinary homovanillic acid and vanillylmandelic acid levels in the diagnosis and management of patients with neuroblastoma: Comparison with 24-hour urine collections. Pediatrics 75:324–328

129. Tuchman M, Ramnaraine ML, Woods WG, Krivit W (1987) Three years of experience with random urinary homovanillic and vanillylmandelic acid levels in the diagnosis of neuroblastoma. Pediatrics 79:203–205

130. D'Angio GJ, Evans AE, Koop CE (1971) Special pattern of widespread neuroblastoma with a favourable prognosis. Lancet 1:1046–1049

131. Grosfeld JL, Rescorla FJ, West KW, Goldman J (1993) Neuroblastoma in the first year of life: Clinical and biologic factors influencing outcome. Semin Pediatr Surg 2:37–46

132. van Noesel MM, Hahlen K, Hakvoort-Cammel FG, Egeler RM (1997) Neuroblastoma 4S: A heterogeneous disease with variable risk factors and treatment strategies. Cancer 80:834–843

133. Evans AE, Chatten J, D'Angio GJ, Gerson JM, Robinson J, Schnaufer L (1980) A review of 17 IV-S neuroblastoma patients at the Children's Hospital of Philadelphia. Cancer 45:833–839

134. Matthay KK, Perez C, Seeger RC, et al. (1998) Successful treatment of stage III neuroblastoma based on prospective biologic staging: A Children's Cancer Group study. J Clin Oncol 16:1256–1264

135. Strother D, Shuster JJ, McWilliams N, et al. (1995) Results of pediatric oncology group protocol 8104 for infants with stages D and DS neuroblastoma. J Pediatr Hematol Oncol 17:254–259

136. Paul SR, Tarbell NJ, Korf B, et al. (1991) Stage IV neuroblastoma in infants: Long-term survival. Cancer 67:1493–1497

137. Schmidt ML, Lukens JN, Seeger RC, et al. (2000) Biologic factors determine prognosis in infants with stage IV neuroblastoma: A prospective Children's Cancer Group study. J Clin Oncol 18:1260–1268

138. Grosfeld JL (2006) Neuroblastoma. In: Grosfeld JL, O'Neill JA Jr, Coran AG, Fonkalsrud EW (eds) Pediatric surgery, vol 1, 6th edn. Mosby, Philadelphia

139. Nickerson HJ, Matthay KK, Seeger RC, et al. (2000) Favorable biology and outcome of stage IV-S neuroblastoma with supportive care or minimal therapy: A Children's Cancer Group study. J Clin Oncol 18:477–486

140. Dillon PW, Whalen TV, Azizkhan RG, et al. (1995) Neonatal soft tissue sarcomas: The influence of pathology on treatment and survival. J Pediatr Surg 30:1038–1041

141. Lloyd DA (2003) Soft-tissue sarcoma. In: Puri P (ed) Newborn surgery, 2nd edn. Oxford University Press, New York

142. Soule EH, Pritchard DJ (1977) Fibrosarcoma in infants and children: A review of 110 cases. Cancer 40:1711–1721

143. Blocker S, Koenig J, Ternberg J (1987) Congenital fibrosarcoma. J Pediatr Surg 22:665–670

144. Ninane J, Gosseye S, Panteon E, Claus D, Rombouts JJ, Cornu G (1986) Congenital fibrosarcoma: Preoperative chemotherapy and conservative surgery. Cancer 58:1400–1406

145. Knezevich SR, McFadden DE, Tao W, Lim JF, Sorensen PH (1998) A novel ETV6-NTRK3 gene fusion in congenital fibrosarcoma. Nat Genet 18:184–187

146. Rubin BP, Chen CJ, Morgan TW, et al. (1998) Congenital mesoblastic nephroma t (12;15) is associated with ETV6-NTRK3 gene fusion: Cytogenetic and molecular relationship to congenital (infantile) fibrosarcoma. Am J Pathol 153:1451–1458

147. Chung EB, Enzinger FM (1976) Infantile fibrosarcoma. Cancer 38:729–739

148. Coffin CM, Dehner LP (1990) Soft tissue tumors in first year of life: A report of 190 cases. Pediatr Pathol 10:509–526

149. Salloum E, Flamant F, Caillaud JM, et al. (1990) Diagnostic and therapeutic problems of soft tissue tumors other than rhabdomyosarcoma in infants under 1 year of age: A clinicopathological study of 34 cases treated at the Institut Gustave-Roussy. Med Pediatr Oncol 18:37–43

150. Barr FG (1997) Molecular genetics and pathogenesis of rhabdomyosarcoma. J Pediatr Hematol Oncol 19:483–491

151. Raney RB Jr, Hays DM, Tefft M, Triche TJ (1989) Rhabdomyosarcoma and the undifferentiated sarcomas. In: Pizzo PA, Poplack DG (eds) Principles and practice of pediatric oncology. Lippincott, Philadelphia, pp 635–658

152. King DR, Clatworthy HW Jr (1981) The pediatric patient with sarcoma. Semin Oncol 8:215–221

153. Grosfeld JL, Weber TR, Weetman RM, Baehner RL, et al. (1983) Rhabdomyosarcoma in childhood: Analysis of survival in 98 cases. J Pediatr Surg 18:141–146

154. Crist WM, Anderson JR, Meza JL, et al. (2001) Intergroup rhabdomyosarcoma study-IV: Results for patients with nonmetastatic disease. J Clin Oncol 19:3091–3102

155. Crist W, Gehan EA, Ragab AH, et al. (1995) The Third Intergroup Rhabdomyosarcoma Study. J Clin Oncol 13:610–630

156. Hrabovsky EE, Othersen HB Jr, deLorimier A, Kelalis P, Beckwith JB, Takashima J (1986) Wilms' tumor in the neonate: A report from the National Wilms' Tumor Study. J Pediatr Surg 21:385–387

157. Ritchey ML, Azizkhan RG, Beckwith JB, Hrabovsky EE, Haase GM (1995) Neonatal Wilms tumor. J Pediatr Surg 30:856–859

158. Giulian BB (1984) Prenatal ultrasonographic diagnosis of fetal renal tumors. Radiology 152:69–70

159. Riccabona M (2003) Imaging of renal tumours in infancy and childhood. Eur Radiol 13:L116–L129

160. Leclair MD, El-Ghoneimi A, Audry G, et al. (2005) The outcome of prenatally diagnosed renal tumors. J Urol 173:186–189

161. Gonzalez-Crussi F, Sotelo-Avila C, Kidd JM (1980) Malignant mesenchymal nephroma of infancy: Report of a case with pulmonary metastases. Am J Surg Pathol 4:185–190

162. Machin GA (1980) Persistent renal blastoma (nephroblastomatosis) as a frequent precursor of Wilms' tumor: A pathological and clinical review. Part 2. Significance of nephroblastomatosis in the genesis of Wilms' tumor. Am J Pediatr Hematol Oncol 2:253–261

163. Bolande RP, Brough AJ, Izant RJ Jr (1967) Congenital mesoblastic nephroma of infancy: A report of eight cases and the relationship to Wilms' tumor. Pediatrics 40:272–278

164. Beckwith JB (1970) Mesenchymal renal neoplasms of infancy. J Pediatr Surg 5:405–406

165. Riccardi VM, Sujansky E, Smith AC, Francke U (1978) Chromosomal imbalance in the Aniridia-Wilms' tumor association: 11p interstitial deletion. Pediatrics 61:604–610

166. Weksberg R, Squire JA (1996) Molecular biology of Beckwith-Wiedemann syndrome. Med Pediatr Oncol 27:462–469

167. Grundy P, Telzerow P, Moksness J, Breslow NE (1996) Clinicopathologic correlates of loss of heterozygosity in Wilms' tumor: A preliminary analysis. Med Pediatr Oncol 27:429–433

168. Green DM, Breslow NE, Beckwith JB, Takashima J, Kelalis P, D'Angio GJ (1993) Treatment outcomes in patients less than two years of age with small, stage I, favorable-histology Wilms' tumors. A report from the National Wilms' Tumor Study. J Clin Oncol 11:91–95

169. Green DM, Breslow NE, Beckwith JB, et al. (2001) Treatment with nephrectomy only for small, stage I/favorable histology Wilms' tumor: A report from the National Wilms' Tumor Study Group. J Clin Oncol 19:3719–3724

170. Campbell AN, Chan HS, O'Brien A, Smith CR, Becker LE (1987) Malignant tumors in the neonate. Arch Dis Child 62:19–23

171. von Schweinitz D (2003) Neonatal liver tumours. Semin Neonatol 8:403–410

172. Douri T (2005) Multiple cutaneous hemangiomas accompanied by hepatic hemangiomas. Dermatol Online J 11:21

173. Boon LM, Burrows PE, Paltiel HJ, et al. (1996) Hepatic vascular anomalies in infancy: A twenty-seven-year experience. J Pediatr 129:346–354

174. Mulliken JB, Fishman SJ, Burrows PE (2000) Vascular anomalies. Curr Probl Surg 37:517–584

175. Marler JJ, Fishman SJ, Upton J, et al. (2002) Prenatal diagnosis of vascular anomalies. J Pediatr Surg 37:318–326

176. Kassarjian A, Zurakowski D, Dubois J, Paltiel HJ, Fishman SJ, Burrows PE (2004) Infantile hepatic hemangiomas: Clinical and imaging findings and their correlation with therapy. Am J Roentgenol 182:785–795

177. Huang SA, Tu HM, Harney JW, et al. (2000) Severe hypothyroidism caused by type 3 iodothyronine deiodinase in infantile hemangiomas. N Engl J Med 343:185–189

178. Kassarjian A, Dubois J, Burrows PE (2002) Angiographic classification of hepatic hemangiomas in infants. Radiology 222:693–698

179. Barlow CF, Priebe CJ, Mulliken JB, et al. (1998) Spastic diplegia as a complication of interferon Alfa-2a treatment of hemangiomas of infancy. J Pediatr 132:527–530

180. Michaud AP, Bauman NM, Burke DK, Manaligod JM, Smith RJ (2004) Spastic diplegia and other motor disturbances in infants receiving interferon-alpha. Laryngoscope 114:1231–1236

181. Yoon SS, Charny CK, Fong Y, et al. (2003) Diagnosis, management, and outcomes of 115 patients with hepatic hemangioma. J Am Coll Surg 197:392–402

182. Tiao GM, Alonso M, Bezerra J, et al. (2005) Liver transplantation in children younger than 1 year – The Cincinnati experience. J Pediatr Surg 40:268–273

183. Barnhart DC, Hirschl RB, Garver KA, Geiger JD, Harmon CM, Coran AG (1997) Conservative management of mesenchymal hamartoma of the liver. J Pediatr Surg 32:1495–1498

184. Stringer MD, Alizai NK (2005) Mesenchymal hamartoma of the liver: A systematic review. J. Pediatr Surg 40:1681–1690

185. Ramanujam TM, Ramesh JC, Goh DW, et al. (1999) Malignant transformation of mesenchymal hamartoma of the liver: Case report and review of the literature. J Pediatr Surg 34:1684–1686

186. Berry CL, Keeling J, Hilton C (1970) Coincidence of congenital malformation and embryonic tumours of childhood. Arch Dis Child 45:229–231

187. Fraumeni JF Jr, Miller RW (1967) Adrenocortical neoplasms with hemihypertrophy, brain tumors, and other disorders. J Pediatr 70:129–138

188. Sotelo-Avila C, Gooch WM 3rd (1976) Neoplasms associated with the Beckwith-Wiedemann syndrome. Perspect Pediatr Pathol 3:255–272

189. Bodmer WF, Bailey CJ, Bodmer J, et al. (1987) Localization of the gene for familial adenomatous polyposis on chromosome 5. Nature 328:614–616

190. Ikeda H, Hachitanda Y, Tanimura M, Maruyama K, Koizumi T, Tsuchida Y (1998) Development of unfavorable hepatoblastoma in children of very low birth weight: Results of a surgical and pathologic review. Cancer 82:1789–1796

191. Ikeda H, Matsuyama S, Tanimura M (1997) Association between hepatoblastoma and very low birth weight: A trend or a chance? J Pediatr 130:557–560

192. Tanimura M, Matsui I, Abe J, et al. (1998) Increased risk of hepatoblastoma among immature children with a lower birth weight. Cancer Res 58:3032–3035

193. Ammann RA, Plaschkes J, Leibundgut K (1999) Congenital hepatoblastoma: A distinct entity? Med Pediatr Oncol 32:466–468

194. Cremin BJ, Nuss D (1974) Calcified hepatoblastoma in a newborn. J Pediatr Surg 9:913–915

195. Sinta L, Freud N, Dulitzki F (1992) Hemoperitoneum as the presenting sign of hepatoblastoma in a newborn. Pediatr Surg Int 7:131–133

196. Ortega JA, Douglass EC, Feusner JH, et al. (2000) Randomized comparison of cisplatin/vincristine/fluorouracil and cisplatin/continuous infusion doxorubicin for treatment of pediatric hepatoblastoma: A report from the Children's Cancer Group and the Pediatric Oncology Group. J Clin Oncol 18:2665–2675

197. Pritchard J, Brown J, Shafford E, et al. (2000) Cisplatin, doxorubicin and delayed surgery for childhood hepatoblastoma: A successful approach – Results of the first prospective study of the International Society of Pediatric Oncology. J Clin Oncol 18:3819–3828

198. Fuchs J, Rydzynski J, Hecker H, et al. (2002) The influence of preoperative chemotherapy and surgical technique in the treatment of hepatoblastoma: A report from the German Cooperative Liver Tumour Studies HB 89 and HB 94. Eur J Pediatr Surg 12:255–261

199. Fuchs J, Rydzynski J, von Schweinitz D, et al. (2002) Pretreatment prognostic factors and treatment results in children with hepatoblastoma: A report form the German Cooperative Pediatric Liver Tumor Study HB 94. Cancer 95:172–182

200. Knudson AG Jr (1971) Mutation and cancer: Statistical study of retinoblastoma. Proc Natl Acad Sci USA 68:820–823

201. Bonaiti-Pellie C, Briard-Guillemot ML (1981) Segregation analysis in hereditary retinoblastoma. Hum Genet 57:411–419

202. Shields CL, Shields JA, Needle M, et al. (1997) Combined chemoreduction and adjuvant treatment for intraocular retinoblastoma. Ophthalmology 104:2101–2111

203. Shields JA, Shields CL (1994) Current management of retinoblastoma. Mayo Clin Proc 69:50–56

204. Dudgeon J (1995) Retinoblastoma: Trends in conservative management. Br J Ophthalmol 79:104

205. Lamkin TD, Gamis AS (2005) Neonatal oncology. In: deAlarcon PA, Werner E (eds) Neonatal hematology. Cambridge University Press, New York

206. Doz F, Neuenschwander S, Plantaz D, et al. (1995) Etoposide and carboplatin in extraocular retinoblastoma: A study by the Société Française d'Oncologie Pédiatrique. J Clin Oncol 13:902–909

207. Pratt CB, Fontanesi J, Chenaille P, et al. (1994) Chemotherapy for extraocular retinoblastoma. Pediatr Hematol Oncol 11:301–309

Renal Tumors

10

Robert C. Shamberger

Contents

10.1 Introduction

A broad spectrum of tumors arise in the kidney in infants and children ranging from benign to some of the most malignant tumors seen in children. Wilms' tumor is the most common renal tumor in childhood and is the second most common abdominal tumor presenting in infants and children after neuroblastoma. Today the vast majority of children with Wilms' tumor can be cured by multidisciplinary therapy. Their treatment is in fact the paradigm for management of most childhood tumors and is based upon evidence obtained from three cooperative group organizations, the National Wilms' Tumor Study Group (NWTSG), the United Kingdom Children's Cancer Study Group (UKCCSG), and the Sociètè Internationale d'Oncologie Pèdiatrique (SIOP). These organizations have performed multiple randomized therapeutic trials which have established the basis for current therapy. Current pathologic classification and staging was established by central pathologic review of the specimens of patients enrolled in these studies. It could never have been established without multi-institutional participation due to the relative rarity of pediatric renal tumors. In this chapter the early history of treatment of pediatric renal tumors will be presented followed by a discussion of their etiologic factors, pathologic subtypes, and premalignant syndromes. Current treatment algorithms for Wilms' tumors and other tumors of the kidney will be reviewed.

10.2 History

The first descriptions of Wilms tumor have been variably attributed to either Rance in 1814 or Wilms' in 1899 [125, 177]. Ironically, however, the first known specimen of this tumor was collected by the British surgeon John Hunter between 1763 and 1793 when he was assembling specimens for his museum [11]. This case of a bilateral tumor in a young infant remains in the Hunterian Museum of the Royal College of Surgeons in London to this day (Fig. 10.1). Wilms' name became indelibly linked to the mixed renal embryonal tumor following publication of his comprehensive monograph on mixed tissue tumors of the kidney in 1899 where he described seven children suffering from nephroblastomas. Early surgery for this tumor was fraught with challenges. The first successful resection is attributed to Thomas Richard Jessop at the General Infirmary in Leeds in 1877 [176]. Czerny reported an early series of 150 patients resected before 1891 [176]. The operative mortality of this series was about 75% and only five children survived for greater than 5 years.

William E. Ladd and Robert E. Gross [71, 95] established the principles of surgical therapy for Wilms'

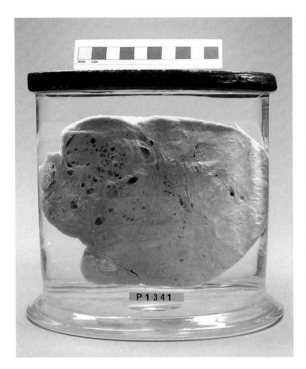

Fig. 10.1 First documented specimen of a nephroblastoma collected by John Hunter for inclusion in the "Hunterian Museum" of the Royal College of Surgeons of England. This specimen is one of two from a child with bilateral renal tumors. (Photo courtesy of the Hunterian Museum at the Royal College of Surgeons.)

tumor including transperitoneal exposure and preliminary ligation of the renal pedicle. They stressed the need to remove the perirenal fat to include lymphatic extensions of the tumor and to avoid rupture of the renal capsule, principles we continue to follow to this day. Adoption of their techniques significantly lowered the operative mortality of nephrectomy in children. Gross and Neuhauser later proposed the routine addition of abdominal radiation to the therapy of Wilms' tumors and reported an estimated 47% frequency of cure [71]. Under Gross's tutelege, pediatric surgeons in North America generally performed primary resection of Wilms' tumors, while in Europe the Paris school lead by Schweisguth and Bamberger reported early success with preoperative irradiation, establishing a precident for preoperative therapy [148].

From 1931 to 1939, survival following surgical resection alone involving ligation of the renal pedicle before removal was 32% at Children's Hospital in Boston [47]. After 1940, most of the patients received postoperative radiation to the renal fossa, achieving lower local recurrence rates, but radiation did not significantly impact the frequency of pulmonary metastases or improve the long-term survival. Actinomycin D was the first active agent identified for the treatment of Wilms' tumor. An 89% 2-year disease-free survival

was achieved from 1957 to 1964 in 53 patients without demonstrable metastasis treated with combined therapy of surgery, local radiation, and actinomycin-D [47]. This would be a very acceptable survival even today. Eighteen of 31 children with metastasis (58%) were alive and free of disease greater than 2 years later. Subsequently, vincristine sulfate was identified as an active agent in Wilms' tumor and was added to its standard therapy [161]. In the ensuing decades other agents were added to the management of the unfavorable histology subtypes and recurrent tumors.

Wilms' tumor was the first malignancy in which the importance of adjuvant treatment of the tumor was recognized, and Sidney Farber espoused its use decades before it would be applied to other pediatric and adult solid tumors [47]. Adjuvant therapy "was based upon the supposition that in the children with Wilms' tumor who died, the tumor must have metastasized already at the time of discovery of the primary tumor" although no evidence of spread was available.

10.3 Wilms' Tumor Incidence and Etiology

Wilms' tumor is the most frequent tumor of the kidney in infants and children. Its incidence is 7.6 cases for every million children less than 15 years of age or 1 case per 10,000 infants [16]. Its frequency varies by race; it's rarer in East Asian populations than in Caucasians, but more frequent in Africa and in African American children [159]. The frequency of Wilms' tumor far outstrips the occurrence of renal cell carcinoma in children until the age range of 15 to 19, when renal cell carcinoma becomes more frequent [16] (Fig. 10.2).

Wilms' tumor is associated with several congenital syndromes in just under 10% of cases, including sporadic aniridia, isolated hemihypertrophy, the Denys-Drash syndrome (nephropathy, renal failure, male pseudohermaphroditism, and Wilms' tumor), genital anomalies, Beckwith-Wiedemann syndrome [visceromegaly, macroglossia, omphalocele, and hyperinsulinemic hypoglycemia in infancy (Fig. 10.3)], and the WAGR complex (Wilms' tumor with aniridia, genitourinary malformations, and mental retardation) which suggested a genetic predisposition to this tumor [86]. Wilms' tumor is also reported in individuals with Simpson-Golabi-Behmel syndrome, another overgrowth syndrome similar to Beckwith-Wiedemann in many respects [84]. These congenital disorders have now been linked to abnormalities at specific genetic loci implicated in Wilms' tumorigenesis.

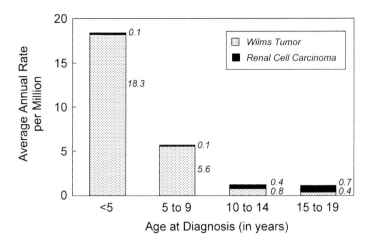

Fig. 10.2 Age-specific occurrence of Wilms' tumor and renal cell carcinoma is depicted in this chart derived from SEER data for 1975–1995. The marked dominance of Wilms' tumor in children up to 9 years of age is well demonstrated. Only in children over 15 years of age does renal cell carcinoma become more prevalent than Wilms' tumor.

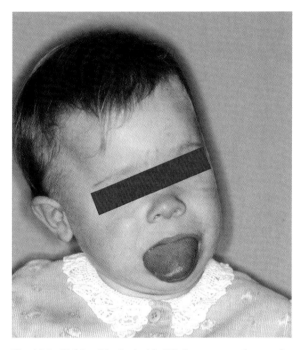

Fig. 10.3 Child with Beckwith-Wiedemann syndrome demonstrating the macroglossia characteristic of this syndrome as well as the mild midface deficiency which produces a sleepy appearance in children with this syndrome.

10.3.1 Genetic Origins

The identification of a large chromosomal deletion of band p13 of the eleventh chromosome in children with the WAGR syndrome led to a search at this site for a gene producing the Wilms' tumor [51, 129]. This deletion includes the aniridia gene *(PAX6)* and a putative Wilms' tumor suppressor gene *(WT1)*. It should be recognized that children can lack the *PAX6* gene but not the *WT1* gene and are then not at increased risk

for the development of Wilms' tumors. In fact, from the Danish aniridia registry 44 of 144 cases of aniridia were sporadic. Of the sporadic cases 5 included a deletion of the *WT1* gene and of those only 2 developed a Wilms' tumor [70]. None of the familial cases lacked the *WT1* site. The risk of Wilms' tumor occurring in all patients with aniridia is low, but it is estimated that in the children with sporadic aniridia the risk of developing a Wilms' tumor was 67 times higher than a normal population, but it is entirely attributable to the small proportion who lack the *WT1* gene. It is estimated that between 45% and 57% of children with the WAGR syndrome will develop a Wilms' tumor [50, 113].

The protein product of the *WT1* gene is a developmentally regulated transcriptional factor of the zinc finger family which regulates the expression of other genes including growth-inducing genes such as those encoding early growth response, insulin-like growth factor II, and platelet-derived growth factor A chain [127, 126]. Suppression of these growth associated genes may explain the tumor suppressor role of *WT1*. Recently, the *WT1* gene product has been found to physically bind to the p53 protein [104]. Children with the WAGR syndrome have constitutional deletions of band 11p13 while virtually all patients with Denys-Drash syndrome carry point mutations of *WT1* in the germline [129]. These result in a dominant negative oncogene and more severe somatic abnormalities than in the WAGR syndrome attributed to the inhibition by the mutated protein on the action of the normal wild-type protein produced by the normal chromosome [102]. The second *WT1* allele is lost in the Wilms' tumor cells in patients with WAGR and similarly the tumor in children with Denys-Drash syndrome have loss of the remaining wild-type allele [98]. The most common phenotypic abnormality in the WAGR syndrome besides aniridia is cryporchidism, found in 60% of male patients, while abnormalities of the internal reproductive organs including streak ovaries and bicornuate uterus are seen in 17% of females followed by ambiguous genitalia in boys and girls [50]. Mental retardation was seen in 70% of children and renal failure in 29%, which was produced by both nephrectomy and glomerulonephritis predominantly focal segmental glomerulosclerosis (FSGS). Studies have demonstrated that children with WAGR syndrome more frequently have bilateral tumors (17% vs. 6%) and are younger at diagnosis (22 vs. 39 months) than children without WAGR [26].

The Beckwith-Wiedemann syndrome has been associated with a 5–10% incidence of Wilms' tumor and other embryonal tumors. Abnormalities at the 11p15 locus, particularly loss of heterozygosity, have been associated with Beckwith-Wiedemann patients [91, 122, 128]. The locus for a putative second Wilms' tumor gene (*WT2*) has not been defined nor is it known whether the Beckwith-Wiedemann locus and *WT2* are the same or contiguous loci [157]. At the *WT2* site, there are several imprinted genes which are expressed preferentially from one of the parental alleles [157]. In some cases, a constitutional duplication of the paternal 11p15 chromosomal fragment has been identified (trisomy at 11p15) [172]. In other cases, both copies are from the father with none from the mother (uniparental isodisomy) [72, 78]. These findings led to speculation that the Beckwith-Wiedemann gene is expressed only by the paternal allele and these genetic abnormalities which lead to the presence of two paternal alleles would double the expression of this gene and may result in the overgrowth.

Two *WT2* candidate genes are the insulin-like growth factor 2 gene and the *H19* gene. The insulin-like growth factor 2 (*IGF2*) gene is present at the 11p15 locus. It is an embryonal growth-inducing gene with expression restricted to the paternal allele [43]. However, there is no direct evidence to link the *IGF2* gene to the causation of the Beckwith-Wiedemann syndrome [36]. Loss of expression of *H19*, a tumor-suppressor gene of uncertain function, has also been reported in Wilms' tumors [158]. The *H19* gene is expressed preferentially from the maternal allele. With loss of heterozygosity, the cell may loose the maternal (active) copy and hence its tumor suppressor function.

Children whose manifestations of the Beckwith-Wiedemann syndrome include hemihypertrophy appear to have a greater risk for the occurrence of malignancy than those who do not. In a series reported by Wiedemann, cancer was reported in 7.5% of all children with the syndrome, but in more than 40% of children with both the syndrome and hemihypertrophy [174].

The Simpson-Golabi-Behmel syndrome is an overgrowth syndrome phenotypically similar to Beckwith-Wiedemann syndrome with macroglossia, coarse facial features, and visceromegally The less frequent manifestations of diaphragmatic and heart defects and polydactyly are unique to Simpson-Golabi-Behmel syndrome. It is a sex-linked syndrome localized to Xq25-27, and the protein product Glypican 3 may interact with the *IGF-II* receptor [83, 177]. Expression of this protein is seen primarily in mesodermal fetal tissues including lung, liver, and kidney [54].

Familial cases of Wilms' tumor account for only 1–2% of cases and have not been associated with the above syndromes. Analysis of two kindreds revealed a link with chromosome band 17q12-21, and the putative tumor gene at this locus has been named *FWT1* [124]. In addition, loss of heterozygosity was seen at 19q in tumors from individuals from two families whose predisposition is not due to the previously defined 17q locus, suggesting that alterations at two distinct loci are critical rate-limiting steps in the etiology of these familial Wilms' tumors involving both germline predisposing mutations and somatic alteration at a second locus. Subsequent studies demonstrated in five kindreds an inherited Wilms' tumor predisposition gene at 19q13.3-q13.4 called *FWT2* [107].

WT1 and *WT2* do not appear to have any prognostic significance for children with Wilms' tumor in marked contrast with the *nMYC* gene in neuroblastoma. These genes are also noted in a small percentage of children with Wilms' tumor who have the associated syndromes. Recent studies have suggested that loss of heterozygosity on chromosome 16q in Wilms' tumors (observed in 15–20% of cases) was associated with a 3.3 times greater incidence of relapse and a 12 times greater incidence of mortality as compared to children without these chromosomal changes [73]. This region of loss has now been localized to an area of 6.7 megabases which contain three recognized tumor suppressor genes, and one of them, *E-cadherin*, has been shown to have reduced expression in Wilms' tumors with LOH at 16q [144]. A similar trend was seen for children with loss of heterozygosity for 1p, which occurs in approximately 10% of Wilms' tumors, but these trends were not statistically significant. Identification of increased expression of the *p53* has also been associated with advanced stage at presentation and increased disease relapse [156]. One of the primary goals of the fifth NWTS study was to assess whether identified chromosomal abnormalities were of prognostic significance in Wilms' tumor and might provide guidance for future therapeutic recommendations.

Routine radiographic screening of children with syndromes associated with Wilms' tumor has been recommended. Surveillance ultrasonograms are generally obtained every 3 months until the children are 5 years of age. No prospective studies, however, have been performed to evaluate the cost effectiveness or efficacy of following this recommendation [32, 58]. Retrospective reviews of routine ultrasonographic screening report conflicting results on its purported benefits as assessed by the stage distribution at presentation or the outcome of the children with prospective screening [31, 39].

10.3.2 Pathologic Precursors: Nephrogenic Rests, Nephroblastomatosis, and Multicystic Dysplastic Kidneys

The presence of nephrogenic rests (NR: persistent metanephric tissue in the kidney after the 36th week of gestation) has been associated with the occurrence of Wilms' tumor. The rests may occur in a perilobular (PLNR) or intralobular (ILNR) location and may be single or multiple. In children with aniridia or the Denys-Drash syndrome, the lesions are primarily ILNR, while children with hemihypertrophy or the Beckwith-Wiedemann syndrome have predominantly PLNR [12]. The presence of multiple or diffuse nephrogenic rests is termed nephroblastomatosis.

The frequency of nephrogenic rests was established in an autopsy series of infants under 3 months of age. Nine of 1,035 infants (0.87%) had PLNRs, and ILNRs occurred in only two of 2,000 cases (0.1%) [14]. Most nephrogenic rests when identified are sclerosing, an apparently indolent or involutional phase. The vast majority will spontaneously resolve without the appearance of a tumor as the incidence of nephrogenic rests is about 100 times greater than that of Wilms' tumor (1/10,000 infants).

Nephrogenic rests are classified histologically as incipient or dormant nephrogenic rests, regressing or sclerosing nephrogenic rests, and hyperplastic nephrogenic rests [13]. Incipient or dormant rests are composed predominantly of blastemal or primitive epithelial cells resembling those in embryonic kidney and Wilms' tumor, but are microscopic with sharp margins from adjacent renal parenchyma. In infants and young children the term incipient is used while dormant is used in older children. Regressing or sclerosing rests demonstrate maturation of the cellular elements and progress to obsolescent rests which are composed primarily of hyalinized stromal elements. Hyperplastic nephrogenic rests are problematic in that they are often difficult to distinguish histologically or radiographically from small Wilms' tumors. They contain diffuse or synchronous proliferation of components throughout the rest. This uniform growth leads to preservation of the original shape of the rest in contrast with neoplastic proliferation of a single cell, which produces a more spherical expanding nodule within the rest. It is almost impossible for even the most sophisticated pediatric pathologist to distinguish a hyperplastic nephrogenic rest from a Wilms' tumor based on an incisional or needle biopsy which does not include the margin between the rest and the remaining kidney. "Preservation of the shape of the original rest is the most obvious clue that one is dealing with a hyperplastic, rather than a neoplastic change." [13] Most hyperplastic nodules lack a pseudocapsule at their periphery, while most Wilms' tumors have one. This is often the most helpful histologic finding in distinguishing these two lesions. Hence, biopsies which do not contain the lesion and its margin will rarely adequately differentiate between these two entities.

Nephrogenic rests are frequently found in association with Wilms' tumors despite their relatively rare occurrence. In a review of cases of Wilms' tumors reported in the National Wilms' Tumor Study-4 (NWTS-4), 41% of the unilateral Wilms' tumors were associated with nephrogenic rests [12], while in children with synchronous bilateral Wilms' tumor the incidence of nephrogenic rests was 99%. These were primarily PLNRs – possibly due to the fact that these lesions are much more prevalent than the ILNRs. Similarly, an increased incidence of nephrogenic rests is seen in children with the syndromes associated with Wilms' tumor which were discussed above (Table 10.1) [13].

Gylys-Morin and colleagues have demonstrated that magnetic resonance imaging (MRI) scans can be particularly helpful in following children with nephroblastomatosis, and it was later confirmed by Rohrschneider and coauthors that MRI or contrast-enhanced computed tomography (CT) were preferable to ultrasound in this setting [75, 142]. Alterations in imaging characteristics of the lesions may suggest a transition from nephrogenic rests to Wilms' tumor as does growth of isolated lesions.

Diffuse hyperplastic perilobar nephroblastomatosis (DHPLN) is a distinct entity which must be distinguished clinically from Wilms' tumor. Infants with DHPLN often present with large unilateral or bilateral flank masses (Fig. 10.4 A,B). A characteristic radiographic finding is massively enlarged kidneys that maintain their normal configuration and lack evidence of necrosis. As with the isolated nephrogenic rests, proliferation of the thin rind of nephrogenic rests on the periphery of the kidney preserve its normal configuration, but produce marked enlargement of its size. This is in contrast to Wilms' tumor where the normal renal configuration and collecting system are generally distorted. Nephrectomy is *not* required in cases of DHPLN. Chemotherapy, however, has been employed to control the proliferative element of the nephrogenic rests and to accelerate the decrease in size of the kidney and secondary respiratory compromise. It has not, however, been established that treatment with chemotherapy will decrease the occurrence of Wilms' tumors. A recent review of 52 cases of DHPLN revealed

Table 10.1 Association of nephrogenic rests with Wilms' tumor and associated syndromes

Population	PLNR (%)	ILNR (%)
Unilateral Wilms' tumor	25	15
Bilateral Wilms' tumor (synchronous)	74–79	34–41
Bilateral Wilms' tumor (metachronous)	42	63–75
Beckwith-Wiedemann/hemihypertrophy & Wilms' tumor	70–77	47–57
Aniridia and Wilms' tumor	12–20	84–100
Denys-Drash and Wilms' tumor	11	78

PLNR, perilobar nephrogenic rests; ILNR, intralobar nephrogenic rests
Adapted from Beckwith JB, Med Pediatr Oncol 21:158–168, 1993)

a mean age of diagnosis of 16 months. Involvement was bilateral in 49 children. Thirty-three patients had biopsy and adjuvant therapy. Eighteen (55%) developed Wilms' tumors at a mean of 35 months. Sixteen patients had initial nephrectomy and adjuvant therapy and three (19%) developed a Wilms' tumor at a mean

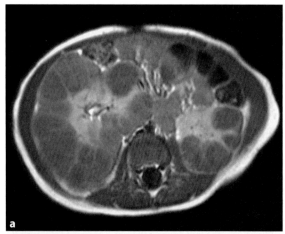

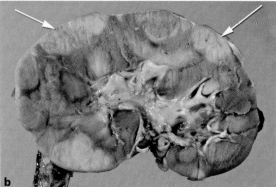

Fig. 10.4 (**a**) MRI of a 15-month-old male presenting with palpable bilateral flank masses revealed diffuse subcapsular lesions without necrosis most consistent with diffuse perilobar nephroblastomatosis. (**b**) Kidney removed from a similar child demonstrates diffuse lesions (*arrows*) in the perilobar region which histologically were nephrogenic rests.

of 36 months from diagnosis. All three patients who did not receive adjuvant therapy developed Wilms' tumors by 10 months after diagnosis. In total, 24 of 52 children developed Wilms' tumors; single in 13 and multiple in 11 children. Eight of the 24 children had anaplastic tumors, an extremely high proportion [121].

An increased risk of Wilms' tumors arising in multicystic dysplastic kidneys has been suggested and in the past many of these lesions were resected to prevent the occurrence of Wilms' tumor. Narchi summarized 1,041 infants and children with multicystic dysplastic kidneys reported in the world's literature in 26 series and found no cases of Wilms' tumors and concluded that nephrectomy was not required [115]. The frequency of nephrogenic rests in multicystic dysplastic kidneys has been estimated to be 4%, approximately five times the prevalence in a random autopsy population of infants under 3 months of age [7]. If one were to estimate the frequency of Wilms' tumor in these kidneys, the standard risk of one in 10,000 infants might be said to be increased to one in 2,000. Review of the NWTS pathology files, however, identified only three cases of dysplastic kidneys in over 7,000 children with Wilms' tumor over a 26-year interval, and only one case in more than 1,500 referral cases sent to Dr. Beckwith from around the world. Although it is impossible to estimate the number of children at risk from Wilms' tumors in remaining dysplastic kidneys, it must be concluded that the risk of development of Wilms' tumor in kidneys with multicystic dysplasia or congenital obstruction must be extremely low and does not justify nephrectomy to avoid the development of Wilms' tumors.

10.4 Pathology of Renal Tumors

The collection of large numbers of renal tumor specimens by the cooperative group trials has facilitated the development of accurate pathologic classifications in a much shorter period of time than would have been feasible without these trials. Early reports of Wilms' tumors and the initial cooperative group trials included essentially all renal sarcomas under this rubric. With time and experience, however, several subgroups of tumors have now been identified, which are at particularly high risk of recurrence and adverse outcome [10, 9]. In NWTS-1 anaplastic and sarcomatous variants comprised only 11.5% of the tumors, yet they accounted for 51.9% of the deaths due to tumor. Unfavorable histology proved to be the most important factor in outcome in NWTS-1 and that finding continues through the current trials. Wilms' tumors are currently divided into those with "favorable" histology and those with "unfavorable" histology (Table 10.2). The later group includes tumors with focal or diffuse anaplasia [49, 61]. Clear cell sarcoma of the kidney and malignant rhabdoid tumors of the kidney were initially grouped with the unfavorable histology Wilms' tumors although their adverse outcome was well recognized in NWTS-1 [9]. They are now considered as distinct entities from Wilms' tumor based on their pathologic appearance and response to quite different therapies [105, 173].

The staging system used by the NWTSG is a pretreatment surgical staging system (Table 10.3). It must be carefully distinguished when comparing treatment results with children treated with the SIOP protocols where the staging information is obtained *after* preliminary treatment of the tumors (Table 10.4). The intensity of adjuvant treatment in the NWTSG protocols is determined by such factors as regional lymph node involvement and penetration of the renal capsule by tumor, which cannot be accurately determined by radiographic studies. The staging criteria have been adjusted during the course of the NWTSG studies as the prognostic significance of criteria were established [48].

SIOP has developed a classification of renal tumors based on their postchemotherapy histology after resection. This was recently revised based on review of outcomes of children compared with the histologic appearance [170]. Tumors are now classified as completely necrotic (low-risk tumor), blastemal (high-risk tumor) and others (intermediate-risk tumors). The prognostic implications of this classification will be assessed on the current study as will the potential for decreasing extent of therapy of the more favorable groups.

Wilms' tumor is characterized as a triphasic embryonal neoplasm with blastemal, stromal, and epithelial components [10] (Fig. 10.5). Each of these components can express several patterns of differ-

Table 10.2 Pathologic classification of renal tumors

Histology
Favorable histology Wilms' tumor
Unfavorable histology Wilms' tumor
Diffuse anaplasia
Focal anaplasia
Clear cell sarcoma
Malignant rhabdoid tumor of the kidney
Renal cell sarcoma
Renal adenocarcinoma
Renal neurogenic tumors
Renal teratoma

Table 10.3 Staging system utilized by the National Wilms' Tumor Study Group

Stage	Description
I	Tumor limited to the kidney and completely excised without rupture or biopsy. Surface of the renal capsule is intact.
II	Tumor extends through the renal capsule, but is completely removed with no microscopic involvement of the margins. Vessels outside the kidney contain tumor. Also placed in Stage II are cases in which the kidney has been biopsied before resection or where there is "local" spillage of tumor (during resection) limited to the tumor bed.
III	Residual tumor is confined to the abdomen and not from hematogenous spread. Also included in Stage III are cases with tumor involvement of the abdominal lymph nodes, rupture of the tumor with "diffuse" peritoneal contamination extending beyond the tumor bed, peritoneal implants, and microscopic or grossly positive resection margins.
IV	Hematogenous metastases at any site.
V	Bilateral renal involvement.

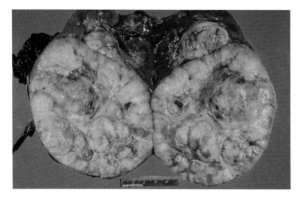

Fig. 10.5 Kidney with favorable histology Wilms' tumor reveals lesion arising from the renal parenchyma with normal renal tissue extending over the surface of the tumor. This finding radiographically helps establish the origin of the tumor from within the kidney as compared with neuroblastoma which can indent the renal tissue, but is rarely surrounded by it.

Table 10.4 Staging system utilized by the Societe Internationale d'Oncologie Pediatrique (Based on findings after preoperative therapy)

Stage	Description
I	Tumor limited to the kidney, complete excision
II	Tumor extending outside the kidney, complete excision – Invasion beyond the capsule, perirenal/perihilar – Invasion of the regional lymph nodes* (Stage IIN1) – Invasion of extra-renal vessels – Invasion of ureter
III	Invasion beyond the capsule with incomplete excision – Preoperative or perioperative biopsy – Preoperative/perioperative rupture – Peritoneal metastases – Invasion of para-aortic lymph nodes# – Incomplete excision
IV	Distant Metastases
V	Bilateral renal tumors

*Hilar nodes and/or periaortic nodes at the origin of the renal artery
Para-aortic nodes below the renal artery

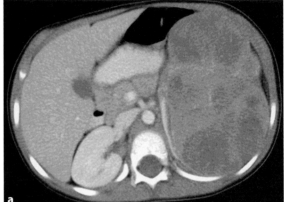

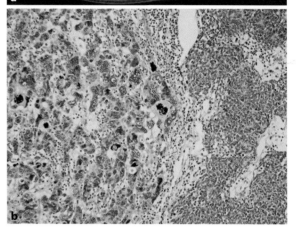

Fig. 10.6 (**a**) CT scan of a 2.5-year-old girl who presented with a large asymptomatic left abdominal mass. Child underwent primary resection which revealed a stage II tumor. (**b**) Histology of the tumor demonstrated areas of anaplasia on the *left* with remarkable nuclear atypia adjacent to areas of bland favorable histology tumor on the *right*.

entiation which define the histologic subgroups of Wilms' tumors. One particular subtype, the fetal rhabdomyomatous nephroblastoma, has been associated with poor response to chemotherapy, but a generally favorable prognosis [103]. In contrast, the diffuse blastemal subtype is associated with presentation at an advanced stage, but also with rapid response to chemotherapy. The anaplastic tumors are characterized by large, pleomorphic, and hyperchromatic nuclei with abnormal multipolar mitotic figures (Fig. 10.6 A,B). Anaplasia can occur in the epithelial, stromal, or blastemal populations or any combination of these three. Anaplasia occurs primarily in children over 2 years of age. In NWTS-1 66.7% of the patients with anaplasia relapsed and 58.3% succumbed to their tumor [9]. Even in this early report the distinct implications of the "diffuse" versus the "focal" pattern was appreciated with a higher frequency of relapse and death in the "diffuse" subgroup. This was confirmed in review of the NWTS-2 and NWTS-3 data. While children with stage I anaplastic tumors generally did well, children with stage II to IV tumors did poorly. The severity of dysplasia was not a predictive factor. However, anaplasia in extrarenal tumor sites and a predominantly

a   **FOCAL ANAPLASIA**
REVISED DEFINITION

> ANAPLASIA IS SHARPLY LOCALIZED WITHIN THE PRIMARY TUMOR, WITHOUT MARKED NUCLEAR OR MITOTIC ATYPIA IN THE REMAINDER OF THE LESION

EXTENSION
o r
METASTASIS

PRIMARY TUMOR

b   ## DIFFUSE ANAPLASIA

A   NON-LOCALIZED ANAPLASIA

B   LOCALIZED ANAPLASIA WITH SEVERE NUCLEAR UNREST ELSEWHERE

C   ANAPLASIA OUTSIDE TUMOR CAPSULE OR IN METASTASES

D   **?**   RANDOM BIOPSY REVEALS ANAPLASIA

Fig. 10.7 (**a**) Schematic diagrams of the current definitions of focal and (**b**) diffuse anaplasia. (Reprinted from Journal of Surgical Pathology, 20, Pablo Faria et al, "Focal versus diffuse anaplasia in Wilms' tumor – New definitions with prognostic significance: A report from the National Wilms' Tumor Study", 909–920, 1996, with permission from Lippincott Williams & Wilkins.)

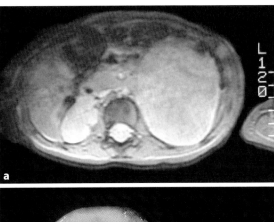
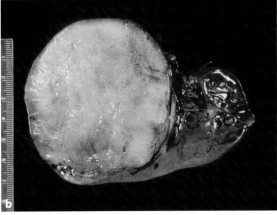

Fig. 10.8 (**a**) MRI scan of a 21-month-old female who presented with a palpable left flank mass. (**b**) Cut surface of the tumor reveals homogeneous texture of the tumor consistent with clear cell sarcoma of the kidney.

blastemal tumor pattern were both adverse prognostic factors [179]. The definitions of diffuse and focal anaplasia are now well established [49] (Fig. 10.7 A,B).

Approximately 1% of children presenting with a unilateral tumor will develop contralateral disease. Fifty-eight of 4,669 children registered in the first four NWTSG studies developed metachronous disease [37]. Analysis of this cohort by a matched case control study demonstrated that the children with nephrogenic rests had a significantly increased risk of metachronous disease, particularly those with PLNRs. This finding was especially true for young children where a Wilms' tumor occurred in 20 of 206 children under 12 months old in comparison to zero of 304 children over 12 months old. These young infants under 12 months of age with Wilms' tumor who also

have nephrogenic rests require regular surveillance for several years for the development of contralateral disease. This increased risk for metachronous tumors in children with Wilms' tumor and nephrogenic rests has been confirmed by others [15].

Clear cell sarcoma of the kidney (CCSK) is a highly malignant tumor with an unusual proclivity to produce bony metastasis. It generally presents as a large unifocal and unilateral tumor with homogeneous mucoid, tan or gray-tan cut surface but may have foci of necrosis or prominent cyst formation [4, 10] (Fig. 10.8 A,B). CCSK invades surrounding renal parenchyma rather than compressing the margin into a pseudocapsule as occurs with a Wilms' tumor. Its classic appearance is that of a deceptively bland tumor with uniform oval nuclei with a delicate chromatin pattern and a prominent nuclear membrane and sparse, poorly stained, vacuolated "water-clear" cytoplasm with indistinct cell membranes. While the cells often appear in cords or nests divided by an arborizing network of vessels and supporting spindle cell septa, nine major histologic patterns have been identified [5]. The cell of origin of

CCSK is not known. In addition to osseous metastasis, clear cell sarcoma also has a significant incidence of brain metastasis. Late recurrence is seen with this tumor, with 30% of the relapses occurring greater than 2 years after diagnosis [93]. For this reason clinical trials must consider results after an adequate interval of follow-up.

Malignant rhabdoid tumors of the kidney occur in young infants with a median age of 11 months, and 85% of the cases occur within the first 2 years of life [173]. A characteristic involvement of the perihilar renal parenchyma is seen. Histologically rhabdoid tumors are characterized by monomorphous, discohesive, rounded-to-polygonal cells with acidophilic cytoplasm and eccentric nuclei containing prominent large "owl eye" nucleoli reminiscent of skeletal muscle, but lacking its cytoplasmic striations, ultrastructural features, and immunochemical markers [10]. A large PAS-positive hyaline, cytoplasmic inclusion occurs in a variable population of tumor cells and is a hallmark of this tumor [76]. Ultrastructural examination reveals parallel cytoplasmic filamentous inclusions packed in concentric whorled arrays, a distinctive feature of this tumor that suggests a neuroectodermal origin. The tumor tends to infiltrate surrounding renal parenchyma rather than compress it. Rhabdoid tumors are notable for the occurrence of second primary neuroglial tumors in the midline of the brain resembling medulloblastoma [23]. A consistent deletion of 22q11-12 was described in both renal and extrarenal rhabdoid tumors [120, 147]. These deletions have now been demonstrated to delineate an area of overlap at the site of the *hSNF5/INI1* gene, and tumors have biallelic alternations or deletions of this gene [17, 168].

The occurrence of primitive neuroectodermal tumor (PNET) of the kidney is well documented [141]. It is clearly distinct from Wilms' tumor and the other variants previously discussed, and demonstrates spread to lymph nodes, lung, bone, liver, and bone marrow as is seen in PNET at other anatomic locations [118].

10.5 Clinical Presentation

The classic presentation of Wilms' tumor is the identification of an asymptomatic flank mass in an otherwise healthy toddler. It is often noted during a bath or by the pediatrician at a routine visit, and the mass may be considerable in size. This is in marked contrast with neuroblastoma, which is seen in the same age group, but frequently presents with pain, often from osseous metastasis. Wilms' tumor may also be associated with hematuria, but with a much lower frequency than is seen with renal cell carcinoma. Rarer presentations are with hypertension or fever. Occasionally a child may suffer abdominal trauma and present with pain and an abdominal mass out of proportion to that expected based on the severity of the injury. Radiographic examination will reveal a mass that cannot be attributed to the trauma alone.

10.6 Treatment

All children treated on protocols of the NWTSG, UKCCSG, and SIOP received adjuvant chemotherapy for Wilms' tumor based on the early work of Sidney Farber, which demonstrated the efficacy of this approach. Only in the last decade has a trial been performed in which adjuvant therapy was not used in a small proportion of children with extremely low-risk tumors. Optimal chemotherapy regimens have been established by a series of well-designed randomized studies primarily performed by the NWTSG in the USA and Canada and SIOP in Europe. Surgery continues to play a critical role in the treatment of Wilms' tumor despite advances in chemotherapy. Accurate staging and safe and complete resection of the tumor are key elements in achieving cure. Local control is rarely achieved by chemotherapy and radiotherapy alone.

10.6.1 Chemotherapy

Wilms' tumor was the first malignant pediatric solid tumor with a demonstrated response to dactinomycin [47]. Many additional effective agents have been subsequently identified: vincristine, doxorubicin, cyclophosphamide, ifosphamide, and etoposide.

Children with stage I tumors were treated on the third NWTSG protocol (NWTS-3) with an 11-week regimen of vincristine and dactinomycin without abdominal radiation based on the results of the initial two studies. The 4-year relapse-free survival (RFS) and overall survival (OS) were 89.0% and 95.6%, respectively [42]. The other three stages were treated on a regimen which involved randomization of two or four arms (Table 10.5). This study supported the addition of doxorubicin to the treatment of children with stage III tumors, but did not demonstrate any benefit to the addition of doxorubicin or radiotherapy for children with stage II tumors or benefit from the addition of cyclophosphamide to the treatment of children with stage IV tumors.

NWTS-4 built upon the lessons learned from the prior studies and addressed the issue of whether dose intensification could be safely utilized to decrease the number of visits for chemotherapy and yet maintain the favorable results previously achieved. Dactinomycin and doxorubicin were administered in single, moderately high doses compared with the traditional divided dose regimens for each drug. This study also evaluated the use of two time intervals for the administration of chemotherapy: a short course (18–26 weeks depending on the regimen and stage) versus a long course (54–66 weeks). The findings of this study were that the pulse-intensive regimens actually produced less hematologic toxicity than the standard regimens allowing greater dose intensity with comparable outcomes [66, 64]. The second randomization demonstrated no benefit in any of the stages to the long interval of therapy over the short interval [65].

A recent analysis of patients with favorable histology stage II and III Wilms' tumors treated on NWTS-3 and -4 assessed the efficacy of the addition of doxorubicin [27]. While no benefit was seen in the stage II patients, an increase in the 8-year EFS and OS of randomized patients was seen for those with stage III disease who received doxorubicin, actinomycin D, and vincristine (84% and 89%) compared with those who received actinomycin D and vincristine alone (74% and 83%). When a large group of nonrandomized patients were added to the analysis, the beneficial effect on OS was not seen. This addition of nonrandomized patients unfortunately added some question of bias.

The goal of NWTS-5 was to evaluate preliminary findings from pilot studies that loss of heterozygosity (LOH) for chromosomes 1p and 16q were associated with an adverse prognosis. To most efficiently address this question, it was the first study from NWTSG that did not involve randomization of treatment. This study demonstrated that LOH at either site in children with favorable histology stage I and II was predictive of decreased EFS, and in children with stage III and IV disease the presence of LOH at both sites was predictive [74]. A subsequent analysis has suggested that expression of telomerase RNA may also be an adverse prognostic factor for favorable histology Wilms' tumor, but confirmatory studies will be required [46].

Treatment of children with anaplastic tumors with standard therapy has resulted in a high rate of failure. Hence, in sequential studies therapy has been intensified. Review of the NWTS-3 and 4 studies demonstrated that children with focal anaplasia have an excellent outcome when treated with vincristine, doxorubicin, and dactinomycin [61]. The addition of cyclophosphamide to this regimen improved the 4-year relapse-free survival in children with diffuse anaplasia with stages II to IV disease from 27.2% to 54.8%. Subsequent studies in NWTS-5 have further intensified therapy with the use of doxorubicin, cyclophosphamide, vincristine, and etoposide. The 4-year EFS and OS of stage I patients were 69.5% and 82.6%, respectively, compared with the same survivals for stage I favorable histology of 92.4% and 98.3% [46]. The EFS progressively declined for increasing stage from 82.6% for stage II, 64.7% for stage III, and only 33.3% for stage IV. Clearly even with this intensification of therapy patients with anaplasia do not fare well.

Doxorubicin was found to be particularly effective in the treatment of clear cell sarcoma of the kidney [5, 63]. However, the results have remained below those of standard histology Wilms' tumors. No benefit was seen to pulse-intensive administration of the agents, and there was no difference in survival at 5 and 8 years

Table 10.5 Randomization for favorable histology Wilms' Tumors on NWTS-3

Stage	Treatment	Results	
		4-year DFS	4-year OS
II	Vcr, Dac	87.4%	91.1%
	Vcr, Dac + XRT (20 Gy abd)	NS	NS
	Vcr, Dac, Dox	NS	NS
	Vcr, Dac, Dox + XRT (20 Gy abd)	NS	NS
III	Vcr, Dac + XRT (10 Gy abd)	Improved survival with addition of doxorubicin	
	Vcr, Dac + XRT (20 Gy abd)	82.0%	90.9%
	Vcr, Dac, Dox + XRT (10 Gy abd)	No difference in local recurrence between 10 and 20 Gy	
	Vcr, Dac, Dox + XRT (20 Gy abd)		
VI	Vcr, Dac, Dox	79.0%	80.9%
	Vcr, Dac, Dox, Cyclo	NS improvement from the addition of cyclophosphamide	
	All abd XRT 20 Gy & Pulmonary XRT 12 Gy		

Vcr, vincristine; Dac, dactinomycin; XRT, radiotherapy; abd, abdomen; Dox, doxorubicin; Cyclo, cyclophosphamide; NS, not statistically significant
Data from D'Angio GJ et al Cancer 1989; 64:349)

between patients treated for 6 or 15 months [149]. Treatment on NWTS-5 consisted of vincristine, doxorubicin, cyclophosphamide alternating with cyclophosphamide, and etoposide for 24 weeks with local radiotherapy. An overall 5-year EFS and survival of 79% and 89% were achieved, but survival results remained very stage dependent: stage I, 100%; II, 87%; III, 74%; and IV, 36% [150]. The most frequent site of relapse was the brain in 11 of 21 cases.

Rhabdoid tumors have remained the most resistant to cure of all pediatric renal tumors. Analysis of 142 children treated on NWTS-1–5 showed an overall survival of 23.2% at 4 years [163]. Survival was stage dependent and children with stage I/II disease had a 41.8% 4-year survival while children with stage III, IV, or V tumors had a 15.9% 4-year survival. Survival was also clearly related to the age at presentation, with the 4-year survival worst for those 0–5 months of age at diagnosis (8.8%) and best for those over 2 years of age (41.1%). NWTS-5 used an intensive therapy with carboplatinum, etoposide, and cyclophosphamide. Unfortunately, no improvement in survival occurred with the series of treatments from NWTS-1–5 and no survival benefit was demonstrated with the use of doxorubicin.

10.6.2 Preoperative Chemotherapy

SIOP has promoted the use of preoperative treatment of children with Wilms' tumor with radiotherapy or chemotherapy since the early 1970s. Histologic confirmation of the diagnosis before therapy is not routinely recommended by SIOP. This approach has several risks. First, is the potential for administration of chemotherapy for benign disease. Second, modification of tumor histology by the chemotherapy may occur. Third, staging information may be lost. Fourth, a malignant rhabdoid tumor of the kidney or clear cell sarcoma may be present which will not respond to standard therapies. Treatment without an initial diagnosis is difficult to sustain when NWTSG and SIOP studies have demonstrated a 7.6–9.9% rate of benign or altered malignant diagnosis in children with a prenephrectomy diagnosis of Wilms' tumor [40, 178]. The United Kingdom Children's Cancer Study Group in a recent report identified 12% of cases that were clinically and radiographically consistent with Wilms' tumor, but had other diagnosis established by biopsy [171]. The histologic diagnosis following preoperative treatment in a group of children followed by NWTSG did not appear distorted by treatment, but it is less certain that staging is not altered [180].

The major driving force for the use of preoperative therapy by SIOP was the high rate of operative tumor rupture which occurred in their early series in which patients did not receive preliminary treatment. The rupture rate decreased from 33% (20 of 60) to 4% (3 of 72) with preoperative abdominal irradiation (20 Gy) in the first randomized SIOP study of renal tumors (SIOP-1) begun in 1971 [99]. It must be noted, however, that 33% is an extremely high frequency of rupture. Survival was not effected by the decrease in operative rupture and the incidence of local recurrence was not reported. In NWTS-1 and -2, operative rupture occurred in 22% and 12% of children, respectively [41, 40]. In a subsequent SIOP randomized study of Wilms' tumors begun in 1977 (SIOP- 5), the rate of rupture was essentially the same for children receiving abdominal irradiation (20 Gy) and dactinomycin (9%, 7 of 76) or a combination of vincristine and dactinomycin (6%, 5 of 88) [29, 100]. Radiotherapy after resection was based on the stage of the tumors, with stage I receiving no postoperative radiation and stage II and III patients receiving 15 Gy in the group treated initially with radiotherapy and 30 Gy in those treated initially with chemotherapy. In SIOP-6, begun in 1980, all patients received initial preoperative chemotherapy (vincristine and dactinomycin). Radiotherapy was administered after resection to those children with stage IIN1 and stage III disease. Children with stage IIN0 (lymph node negative) were randomized to receive either 20 Gy of radiotherapy versus no radiation to the tumor bed. All children received vincristine and dactinomycin for 38 weeks. After pretreatment 52% of cases were stage I and there was a low frequency of rupture (7%). The radiotherapy randomization was halted after 108 children were randomized, 58 to radiotherapy and chemotherapy and 50 to chemotherapy alone. Six local recurrences occurred in the 50 children who did not receive radiotherapy versus no recurrences in the group that did. These results suggested that prenephrectomy treatment altered the pathologic findings which would have led to a diagnosis of stage IIN1 or stage III disease (i.e., lymph node involvement or capsular penetration) and to the standard administration of local irradiation. Extended follow-up studies of these children showed ultimately no statistical difference in survival, as those with relapse had more treatment alternatives [88, 164]. The SIOP-6 protocol also extended chemotherapy to infants over 6 months of age [34]. The overall favorable outcome was not improved, and an unacceptable toxicity occurred in the young infants. In the SIOP-9 study, a reduced dose in infants was recommended.

In the SIOP-9 study initiated in 1987 there was a randomization between 4 and 8 weeks of preoperative therapy with actinomycin D and vincristine to determine if the additional 4 weeks of therapy produced a larger proportion of stage I tumors [165]. This study also replaced postoperative radiotherapy in stage II node negative children with administration of an an-

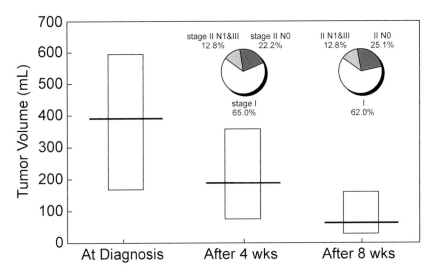

Fig. 10.9 Diagram of the results from the GPOH subgroup of SIOP-9 demonstrates the progressive decrease in the volume of the renal tumors after 4 and 8 weeks of preoperative chemotherapy. The *pie charts* demonstrate the distribution of tumor stages which reveal an increase in low stage I tumors compared with historical controls (not shown). (Reprinted from Urologic Clinics of North America, 27, Graff N et al, "The role of preoperative chemotherapy in the management of Wilms' tumor: The SIOP studies," 443–454, 2000 with permission from Elsevier.)

thracycline, epirubicin. Preoperative treatment consisted of 4 weekly courses of vincristine and 2 3-day courses of dactinomycin each 2 weeks versus 8 weeks of the identical therapy for patients without distant metastasis. No advantage was seen from the extended therapy in terms of staging at resection between the 4-week and 8-week courses: stage I 64 versus 62%, or of intraoperative tumor rupture: 1 versus 3% [56] (Fig. 10.09). Therapy after resection was based on the pathologic findings. Children with stage I disease and favorable or anaplastic histology received vincristine and dactinomycin for 17 weeks. Those with stage II and III tumors with favorable histology received vincristine, dactinomycin, and epirubicin (an anthracycline) for 27 weeks with no abdominal radiotherapy for stage II N0 disease or with 15 Gy of abdominal irradiation in cases of stages IIN1 and III disease. This therapy resulted in a 2-year event-free survival of 84% versus 83% for the 4- and 8-week therapies and overall-survivals of 92% and 87%, respectively. Children with metastatic disease received 6 weeks of therapy including weekly vincristine, three courses of dactinomycin, and two courses of epirubicin on weeks 1 and 6. The tumor size decreased by more than 50% in 52% of the cases and during the second 4 weeks of therapy there was another 50% reduction in 33% of the cases (Fig. 10.09). Inappropriate preoperative therapy was given to 5.5% of the cases including 1.6% who proved to have benign lesions or malignant lesions not expected to respond to the therapy including neuroblastoma, lymphoma, malignant rhabdoid tumors of the kidney, and renal carcinomas. In SIOP-9, the surgery related complications were reported to be 8% [55]. In this treatment regimen patients with posttherapy stage II disease receive an anthracycline while on the NWTS studies stage II disease receives vincristine and dactinomycin alone. In SIOP-9, an evaluation of

children with completely necrotic tumors at the time of resection demonstrated that they had an extremely favorable prognosis [20]. Complete necrosis was seen in 10% of 599 children enrolled in the study; 37 children with stages I to III disease and 22 with stage IV disease. Disease-free survival was 98% at 5 years for this cohort versus 90% for the other patients in SIOP-9. The only death in the stage I to III group was a toxic death and survival was 100% in the stage IV group.

The goal of both NWTSG and SIOP has been to decrease the intensity of therapy and yet achieve the maximum long-term survival. Both groups have decreased the amount of radiotherapy utilized during the course of their studies. Among the children with unilateral nonmetastatic favorable histology Wilms' tumors, 24% of those enrolled in NWTS (275 of 1,160) were given radiation therapy and 18% of those in SIOP (81 of 447) have received radiotherapy in the most recent studies [60]. SIOP has elected, however, to utilize an anthracycline rather than radiotherapy for their postchemotherapy stage IIN0 patients in whom excessive local relapse occurred without additional therapy. This results in around 48% of patients in SIOP studies with unilateral nonmetastatic, favorable histology patients receiving an anthracycline which is significantly greater than the 24% of comparable patients on NWTSG regimens.

10.6.3 Complications of Chemotherapy

Significant complications have occurred in some children treated with doxorubicin, particularly cardiomyopathy [68, 106]. The cumulative frequency of congestive heart failure in children treated on NWTS-1–4 was 4.4% at 20 years after diagnosis for those treated initially with doxorubicin, although recent estimates of the 20-year risk of congestive heart failure for children treated on NWTS-3 and 4 is now reported as 1.2% [27]. The relative risk was increased for females, by cumulative dose of doxorubicin, by use of pulmonary irradiation, and irradiation of the left renal fossa. Subclinical echocardiographic abnormalities have been demonstrated in children who received as little as 45 mg per square meter of doxorubicin [101]. Only long-term follow-up of children who have received doxorubicin will document what dose, if any, is free of long-term implications.

Second malignant neoplasms are also a concern. NWTSG has reported a 1.6% incidence of second malignant neoplasms occurring by 15 years after treatment [25]. The incidence correlated with prior treatment of relapsed tumor, the amount of abdominal radiation, and the use of doxorubicin. Acute myelogenous leukemia was seen in patients whose treatment included either doxorubicin or etoposide [154].

While renal failure is produced by bilateral nephrectomy, it also results from the nephropathy associated with several of the genetic syndromes. A significant incidence of renal failure results from FSGS in children with WAGR syndrome and from diffuse mesangial sclerosis in children with Denys-Drash syndrome. The cumulative incidence of end-stage renal failure at 20 years after diagnosis of unilateral Wilms' tumor was 74% for 17 patients with the Denys-Drash syndrome, 36% for 37 patients with WAGR, 7% for 125 males with hypospadias or cryptorchidism, and 0.6% for 5,347 patients without any of the other conditions [28] (Fig. 10.10A). In children with bilateral tumors, all of these incidences are increased: 50% for the Denys-Drash syndrome, 90% for WAGR, 25% for associated genitourinary abnormalities, and 12% for those without associated conditions (Fig. 10.10B).

Other complications identified in patients after treatment for Wilms' tumor include diffuse interstitial pneumonitis, loss of stature, and difficulties with pregnancy primarily related to abdominal and pelvic irradiation [57, 69, 79, 90].

10.6.4 Surgery

The NWTSG has advocated initial resection of the tumor in all of its protocols. Despite the fact that most Wilms' tumors present as a large mass, resection is generally feasible. Wilms' tumor, in contrast with neuroblastoma, is much less likely to invade surrounding organs and lymph nodes, which complicates the resection. Children undergoing initial nephrectomy in a NWTS-3 study published in 1992 demonstrated a complication rate of 19.8% in a group that was very closely followed [131]. The most frequent complication was intestinal obstruction occurring in 6.9% of

the children followed by extensive intraoperative hemorrhage (>50 ml/kg of body weight) occurring in 5.8% [133]. Injuries to other visceral organs (1%) and extensive vascular injuries (1.4%) were much less frequent. Nine deaths were attributed to surgical complications (0.5%), only one of which was intraoperative. The factors which were associated with an increased risk of surgical complications were advanced-stage local disease, intravascular extension of the tumor, and resection of other organs. "Adherent" organs were often found not to be invaded by the tumor, but rather compressed, distorted, or adherent without actual tumor infiltration. Extensive resection involving removal of other organs or procedures which are of a magnitude to be life threatening, should be aborted and a biopsy obtained of the tumor and regional lymph nodes, followed by administration of chemotherapy prior to a second attempt at resection. Following this algorithm, 93% of 131 children enrolled in NWTS-3 who were initially judged as "unresectable" at surgery or by imaging studies were successfully resected after initial chemotherapy and/or irradiation [135]. Only eight children with tumors that grew or failed to respond did not undergo subsequent nephrectomy.

Complications in the NWTS-4 study have also been assessed [139]. Surgeons were discouraged from performing extensive operations on children in this study involving resection of adjacent organs or massive tumors. Complications occurred in 12.7% of a random sample of 534 of the 3,335 patients treated on this study. Again, intestinal obstruction was the most frequent complication (5.1%) followed by extensive hemorrhage (1.9%), wound infection (1.9%), and vascular injury (1.5%). The factors associated with an increased risk of complications were again assessed. Intravascular extension into the inferior vena cava or atrium and nephrectomy performed through a flank or paramedian incision were both significant factors. Tumor diameter greater or equal to 10 cm was also associated with increased complications. Finally, the risk of complications was increased if the resection was performed by a general surgeon rather than a pediatric surgeon or pediatric urologist. SIOP reported a complication rate of 8% in a recent study involving 598 patients registered on SIOP-9. These patients were pretreated with vincristine, dactinomycin and epirubicine or doxorubicin prior to nephrectomy [55]. The most frequent events were small bowel obstruction (3.7%) and tumor ruptures (2.8%). The latter is not reported as a complication in the NWTS reviews. Other complications occurred in 2.0% of patients. A prospective study of surgical complications by SIOP and NWTSG has been completed and results are pending.

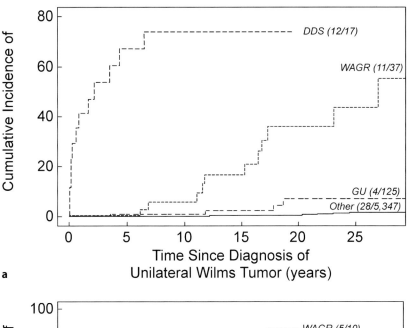

a

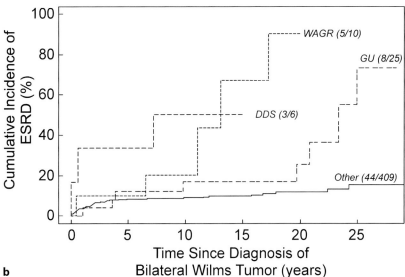

b

Fig. 10.10 (**a**) Cumulative incidence of end stage renal disease (ESRD) in children with unilateral Wilms' tumor with Denys-Drash syndrome (DDS), WAGR syndrome, associated genitourinary anomalies (GU) and other anomalies (Other) over time. (**b**) Similar plot of children with bilateral Wilms' tumors. In both groups of children a very significant incidence of ESRD is documented. (Reprinted from The Journal of Urology, 174, Norman E. Breslow, et al, "End stage renal disease in patients with Wilms' tumor: Results from the National Wilms' Tumor Study Group and The United States Renal Data System", 1972–1975, 2005, with permission from the American Urological Association.)

10.6.4.1 Surgical Details

Radiographic imaging is critical prior to resection of a renal tumor. The most important factors to assess in these studies are the presence of two functioning kidneys, contralateral tumor, and evidence of intravascular extension of the tumor. Intraoperative and not preoperative identification of intravascular extension has been associated with an increased incidence of surgical complications [114]. The organ of origin of the tumor can be determined in most cases with the differential diagnosis generally between neuroblastoma and Wilms' tumor. This can generally be determined by the configuration of the kidney and the mass. In neuroblastoma the mass will generally indent the kidney, while in Wilms' tumor the mass will arise from within the kidney and distort its internal configuration. Often a thin rim of renal parenchyma can be seen extending over the neoplasm in Wilms' tumor (Fig. 10.11). Intra-abdominal staging has been difficult to assess radiographically unless there is extensive lymph node involvement or intrahepatic metastasis. A radiograph of the chest and CT scan will determine the presence of pulmonary metastasis. If the lesions are seen on the radiograph, their malignant nature can generally be assumed. Smaller lesions seen only on the CT scan should generally be biopsied to confirm their malignant nature. Bone scans and brain scans are routinely performed only if the renal tumor proves to be a clear cell sarcoma or rhabdoid tumor.

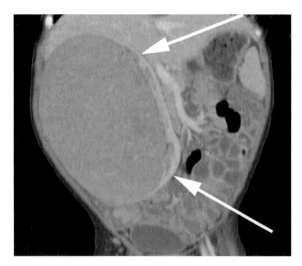

Fig. 10.11 CT scan of a 6-month-old infant with Wilms' tumor which demonstrates in the coronal reformats the classic finding of intrarenal tumors; a margin of renal parenchyma enveloping the tumor (*arrows*).

Renal tumors must be resected through an adequate subcostal or thoracoabdominal incision. Struggling through an inadequate incision will often result in rupture of the tumor, both increasing the stage of the tumor and the risk for intra-abdominal recurrence [152]. A flank incision should not be used for resection in pediatric renal tumors because of the limited exposure it provides.

The abdomen should be explored including inspection for hepatic metastasis and intraperitoneal spread. The vena cava, if it is accessible, should also be palpated to assess for intravascular extension of tumor. The contralateral kidney should be palpated for tumor, although it is not currently suggested that the kidney be completely exposed and visualized. Exploration of the contralateral kidney with opening of Gerota's fascia was recommended by the NWTSG based on the 5% occurrence of synchronous lesions. In NWTS-2 and -3 contralateral involvement was not detected before exploration by intravenous pyelography (IVP) or CT scan in approximately one-third of the children with bilateral tumors [19]. Review of children with bilateral tumors treated on NWTS-4 identified only nine of 122 children in whom the diagnosis of bilateral disease was missed by the preoperative imaging studies (CT scan, ultrasonography, or MRI) [137]. All but one of these lesions were small: five were less than 1 cm and three were 1–3 cm in diameter. Recent review of this material, however, has suggested that some of the small lesions on the contralateral kidney which were initially thought to be small Wilms' tumors would now be more correctly defined as hyperplastic nephrogenic rests [140]. The overall outcome of children with these small lesions was also extremely favorable

with no recurrences. Future studies by NWTSG and COG will not require examination of the contralateral side if there is no suggestion of involvement on the preoperative radiographic studies.

The colon is then mobilized off the anterior aspect of the kidney and the renal mass. Although early descriptions of resection recommended initial control of the renal hilum, this is often not feasible with extremely large tumors and must await mobilization of the mass to allow exposure of the hilum. Premature attempts at vascular control, particularly of left-sided tumors, may result in ligation of the superior mesenteric artery [132]. Biopsy of the renal mass should not be performed unless the decision is to not proceed with a complete resection. Biopsy will contaminate the peritoneum and increase the stage of the tumor.

Biopsy of lymph nodes in the renal hilum and along the vena cava or aorta is critical for adequate staging. Even in children with stage IV disease, local staging is critical as it will determine whether or not abdominal radiotherapy is utilized in most cooperative group protocols. Studies have demonstrated that the surgeon's gross inspection and assessment of lymph nodes does not reliably correspond with the pathologic involvement of tumor with false-negative and false-positive rates of 31.3% and 18.1%, respectively [117]. An increased incidence of local recurrence occurred in children enrolled in NWTS-4 in whom biopsy of lymph nodes was not performed, particularly stage I cases [152]. This suggested that under treatment of local disease in these children due to inadequate staging resulted in an increased frequency of local relapse. While grossly involved lymph nodes are generally resected, an extensive retroperitoneal lymph node resection has not been demonstrated to improve local control or survival [87].

As the tumor is mobilized the ureter is divided close to the bladder to avoid creating a "diverticulum" on the bladder which might produce recurrent urinary tract infection. This will also assure that any extension of tumor into the ureter is entirely resected. Gross hematuria in children with Wilms' tumor is infrequent, but its occurrence suggests extensive involvement of the renal pelvis with possible extension into the ureter. Cystoscopy should be considered in these children to identify extension of the tumor into the bladder and to avoid transection of the tumor thrombus during division of the ureter. Ureteral extension that is entirely resected does not increase the local stage of the tumor. If the tumor involves the upper pole, the adrenal gland is generally resected to achieve adequate margins around the tumor and also to obtain periaortic or pericaval lymph node tissue. In children with lower pole lesions, the adrenal gland may be preserved.

The factors associated with an increased risk of local recurrence are stage III disease, unfavorable histology (especially diffuse anaplasia), and tumor rupture during surgery [152]. The only factor over which the surgeon has control is rupture of the tumor. Multiple regression analysis adjusting for the combined effects of histology, lymph node involvement, and age reveal that tumor spillage remained significant and was greatest in children with stage II disease who received less intensive therapy. Most tumor ruptures occur during mobilization of the posterior aspect of the tumor where it is adherent to the diaphragm. An adequate incision and resection of a segment of the adherent diaphragm can often prevent rupture.

Resection of adjacent organs (liver, spleen, or pancreas) or resection of massive Wilms' tumors were discouraged in the recent NWTSG studies based on prior results. Such extensive resections are associated with a significant increase in surgical complications [131]. Only in this situation should the primary tumor be biopsied along with perihilar and periaortic/pericaval lymph nodes.

Preoperative evaluation of children with renal tumors must include studies of coagulation. "Acquired" von Willebrand disease has been seen in children with Wilms', tumor which can produce problems with hemostasis if it is not identified and treated appropriately prior to surgery [35].

10.6.4.2 Preoperative Therapy

Preoperative treatment of Wilms' tumor is generally accepted in certain circumstances in the North American studies: occurrence of Wilms' tumor in a solitary kidney, bilateral renal tumors, tumor in a horseshoe kidney, intravascular extension of the tumor above the intrahepatic vena cava, and respiratory distress from extensive metastatic tumor. Pretreatment biopsy should be obtained. Percutaneous biopsy is often utilized although needle tract seeding has been reported [97]. The aim of treatment (prior to surgical resection in the bilateral tumors and tumor in a horseshoe or solitary kidney) is to preserve maximum renal parenchyma and function. A horseshoe kidney is often not recognized prior to surgical exploration in many cases; the large size of the tumor often distorts the anatomy concealing its presence [116]. An increased incidence of urine leak and ureteral injury occur in this situation due to the aberrant anatomy of the collecting systems.

Although growth of the remaining kidney has been documented (achieving 180% volume augmentation), the occurrence of focal segmental glomerulosclerosis has been reported in children with a unilateral kidney [45, 162]. In the NWTSG-1–4 population, the incidence of renal failure following unilateral nephrectomy was only 0.25% [138]. Studies from Europe on pretreatment of unilateral Wilms' tumor have demonstrated that in most instances a nephrectomy is still required rather than a partial nephrectomy because of the extent of tumor involvement in the kidney at presentation [167].

The efficacy of preoperative chemotherapy in allowing the safe performance of partial nephrectomy for Wilms' tumor has been evaluated by several centers. McLouie and associates in Toronto obtained percutaneous biopsy in 37 children with Wilms' tumor and then administered multiagent chemotherapy for 4–6 weeks. A partial nephrectomy was then performed in nine children (four with unilateral and five with bilateral tumors) [108]. Two children suffered intra-abdominal relapse. Only four of the 30 unilateral tumors (13.3%) were amenable to a partial nephrectomy. Another analysis of the feasibility of partial nephrectomies was performed at St. Jude Children's Research Hospital [175]. Preoperative CT scans of 43 children with non-metastatic unilateral Wilms' tumor were reviewed retrospectively. Criteria utilized to determine if a partial nephrectomy would have been feasible were involvement by the tumor of one pole and less than one-third of the kidney, a functioning kidney, no involvement of the collecting system or renal vein, and clear margins between the tumor and surrounding structures. Utilizing these criteria, only two of 43 scans (4.7%) suggested partial nephrectomy was feasible. The primary concerns regarding use of preoperative chemotherapy to create "resectable" small tumors is that these children with small tumors at presentation may be curable by surgical resection alone [38, 110]. While the role of partial nephrectomy has been suggested in children with Beckwith-Wiedemann syndrome or hemihypertrophy in whom smaller tumors may be identified by prospective screening, the efficacy of this approach has not been established [109].

10.6.4.3 Bilateral Wilms' Tumor

Children with bilateral tumors are generally younger than those with unilateral lesions with a mean age of 25 versus 44 months [24]. Preservation of renal parenchyma is a critical issue for these children. In the NWTSG review of renal failure in 55 children from NWTS-1–4, 39 children had bilateral tumor involvement. Increasing efforts to preserve renal parenchyma in bilateral cases in the sequence of the NWTSG studies resulted in a decline in the incidence of renal failure from 16.4% in NWTS-1 and -2 to 9.9% in NWTS-3 and 3.8% in NWTS-4 [138]. Although the incidence may increase in the more recent studies as children age, this declining frequency is also due in part to increased attempts to save part of the kidneys by initial treatment of the tumor with chemotherapy. Preliminary treatment in most cases following biopsy and staging will produce shrinkage of the tumor and facilitate its resection with preservation of a portion of the kidney. It is important to biopsy all tumors as "discordant" pathology does occur with a favorable lesion on one side and unfavorable lesion (generally anaplastic) on the other. Bilateral lesions are rarely seen in association with clear cell sarcoma or rhabdoid tumors of the kidney. Ninety-eight children with bilateral Wilms' tumors underwent a partial nephrectomy of 134 kidneys during NWTS-4 [80]. Complete resection of gross disease was accomplished in 118 (88%) of the 134 kidneys. A higher incidence of positive surgical margins (16%, 19/134) and local tumor recurrence (8.2%, 11/134) was seen in this group of children. These were justified by the attempt to preserve renal tissue and avoid renal failure. Overall, portions of 72% of the kidneys were preserved and the 4-year survival rate was 81.7%.

The United Kingdom Children's Cancer Study Group (UKCCSG) has also reported attempts at maximal preservation of renal parenchyma with preoperative chemotherapy [92]. Survival was equivalent for those with initial resection versus preoperative chemotherapy, but greater preservation of renal parenchyma was seen in those treated with initial chemotherapy. Radiation has been advocated to prevent relapse in children with partial nephrectomy for bilateral disease, but irradiation will impair the ability of the kidney to grow [119, 155].

The presence of rhabdomyomatous histology has been associated with poor response to preoperative chemotherapy as defined by decrease in size on radiographic evaluation, but it has been found to be associated with favorable survival [2].

10.6.4.4 Intravascular Extension

Intravascular extension of a tumor thrombus occurs in 4% of children with Wilms' tumor. Identification of vascular extension by preoperative radiographic studies or early in the surgical exploration is critical to avoid a tumor embolus during mobilization of the kidney. Ultrasonography is probably more sensitive than is CT scan. The presence of intravascular extension does not affect the prognosis of the tumor as long as it is successfully resected [130]. Traditionally, intravascular extension has been managed by nephrectomy with resection of the tumor thrombus into the renal vein or vena cava. Cardiopulmonary bypass has been required for children with atrial extension of the tumor thrombus, but is associated with a significant incidence of complications (70%) [114].

In a NWTSG report of intravascular extension of Wilms' tumor, 30 children (15 with caval and 15 with atrial extension) were treated initially with chemo-

therapy after biopsy of the renal mass. After treatment, a decrease in the size of the intravascular extension was noted in 23 children and complete resolution of the tumor thrombus was seen in 7 children [134]. Of the 15 children with tumor initially extending into the atrium, a complete or marked response occurred and the tumor was removed transabdominally without bypass. Tumor embolism did not occur during chemotherapy. Fibrous adherence of tumor to the caval wall developed in some children and, in two, occlusion of the inferior vena cava (IVC) occurred postoperatively. A similar study of Wilms' tumor with intracaval thrombus in the UK Children's Cancer Study Group UKW3 trial showed that 59 patients of 730 registered had intracaval extension. The authors concluded that preoperative therapy is a useful adjunct to shrink the tumor and thrombus [112].

More recently, a review of all of the children treated on NWTS-4 identified 165 of 2,731 patients with intravascular extension into the IVC (134 patients) or atrium (31 patients) [153]. Sixty-nine of these patients received preoperative chemotherapy (55 with IVC extension and 14 with atrial extension). Five complications were encountered during preoperative chemotherapy including tumor embolism and tumor progression in one patient each, and three patients with adult respiratory distress syndrome, one of which was fatal. Intravascular extension of the tumor regressed in 39 of 49 children with comparable pre- and post-therapy radiographic studies, including regression in seven of twelve in whom the tumor regressed from an atrial location, avoiding the need for cardiopulmonary bypass. A high frequency of surgical complications occurred in these patients, 36.7% in the children with atrial extension and 17.2% in those with IVC extension. The frequency of surgical complications was 26% in the primary resection group versus 13.2% in children with preoperative therapy. When all the complications were considered including those which occurred during preoperative chemotherapy (one of those five also had a surgical complication), the incidence of complications among those receiving preoperative therapy was not statistically different from the incidence among those who underwent primary resection, although most of the severe complications occurred in the primary resection group. Preoperative therapy clearly facilitated surgical resection by decreasing the extent of the tumor thrombus.

10.6.4.5 Surgery Alone for Select Favorable Wilms' Tumors

A small group of children with Wilms' tumor may require only resection of the primary tumor and kidney without adjuvant treatment. The outcome of children less than 2 years of age with stage I tumors weighing under 550 gm registered in the NWTSG studies were reviewed [59]. The 4-year relapse-free survival for children meeting these criteria exceeded 90%, suggesting that they could be selected for treatment with surgery alone. A similar review by the United Kingdom Children's Cancer Study Group in which children with stage I tumors received only vincristine "monotherapy", also demonstrated that infants under 2 years of age had particularly favorable 4-year EFS and OS of 93.2% and 98.1%, respectively [123].

A pathologic review of children treated on NWTS-4 published in 1994 also demonstrated that age under 2 years of age and specimen weight of less than 550 gm was highly associated with the absence of adverse microsubstaging variables [62]. A prospective pilot study of this question was performed at Children's Hospital in Boston. Eight children with stage I disease who were under 2 years of age with unilateral, favorable histology tumors with a combined tumor and kidney weight under 550 gm were resected and followed without adjuvant therapy [96]. One child developed a metachronous tumor cured by resection and chemotherapy. Continued evaluation of this series showed no episodes of local recurrence [151].

One component of NWTS-5 was a trial of surgery only for children under 2 years of age with small (<550 gm tumor and kidney) stage I favorable histology tumors. Seventy-five infants were enrolled in this study [67]. Three infants developed metachronous, contralateral Wilms' tumors and eight relapsed 0.3–1.05 years after diagnosis. The sites of relapse were pulmonary (5 cases) and operative bed (3 cases). The 2-year disease-free survival including both relapse and metachronous tumors was 86.5%. The 2-year survival rate was 100% with a median follow-up of 2.84 years. The 2-year disease-free survival excluding metachronous tumors was 89.2%, and the 2-year cumulative risk of metachronous contralateral Wilms' tumor was 3.1%. The stopping rule for the study required closure after these 75 infants were enrolled, but continuing evaluation of this cohort has demonstrated that they have done very well with a high rate of salvage for recurrence as they were previously untreated with chemotherapy. Further studies of these infants will be required to establish their optimal therapy and observation without therapy should not be considered unless the patients are on a therapeutic trial.

10.6.4.6 Neonatal Wilms' Tumor

Wilms' tumor occurs rarely in the neonate. A review of the 3,340 children entered into the NWTS studies from 1969 to 1984 revealed only 27 neonates (≤30 days old) with renal tumors (0.8%) [82]. Over half of the neonates (18) had mesoblastic nephroma and four others had nonneoplastic lesions. One infant had a malignant rhabdoid tumor and four had Wilms' tumors. All of these children with Wilms' tumor had favorable histology tumors without metastasis. They did well, receiving a variety of treatments ranging from surgery alone to 15 months of three-drug therapy. A subsequent report of 15 cases of Wilms' tumor occurring in neonates in the first 30 days of life again demonstrated favorable histology tumors and absence of metastatic disease [136]. Ten of these infants received postoperative chemotherapy and five were followed without additional treatment. Only one of these five children recurred in the renal fossa and lungs and ultimately succumbed to her disease at 16 months of age. The other children are all disease-free at a median follow-up of 31 months.

10.6.4.7 Extra-Renal Wilms' Tumor

An extra-renal site of primary Wilms' tumor is uncommon. These extra-renal tumors behave identically to tumors arising within the kidney and should be treated both locally and systemically based on the same criteria [3, 33]. Common sites of occurrence of extra-renal Wilms' include the retroperitoneum, inguinal canal, scrotum, and vagina. Rare sites are the uterus, cervix, ovary, mediastinum, and the presacral space.

10.7 Renal Cell Carcinoma

Children with renal cell carcinoma are generally older than those with Wilms' tumor, and frequently present with symptoms of flank pain and gross hematuria (Fig. 10.2) [94]. Radiographically they are indistinguishable from Wilms' tumor. Renal cell carcinoma in children displays gross and microscopic pathologic features similar to those seen in tumors occurring in adults (Fig. 10.12 A,B,C). Clinical stage at the time of diagnosis is the most important prognostic factor and the identification of renal vascular invasion did not appear to be an adverse predictor. Radical nephrectomy and regional lymphadenectomy remain the primary modality for cure and children with distant spread have a grave prognosis. The mean age for presentation with renal cell carcinoma in a pediatric population was 14 years. Overall survival is much worse than for Wilms' tumor with a 5-year survival in a recent series of only 30%. Analysis of multiple factors including age, tumor size, location, and histology failed to demonstrate they were predictors of survival. Only stage and achieving complete tumor resection were meaningful prognostic factors. Survival was 60% in chil-

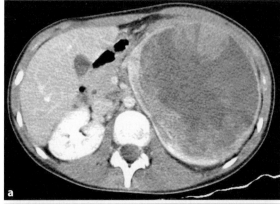

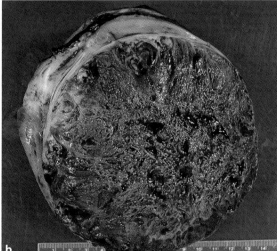

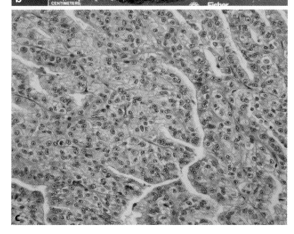

Fig. 10.12 (**a**) CT scan of a 13-year-old female who presented with a palpable left flank mass. Wilms' tumor and renal cell carcinoma cannot be distinguished based on the appearance of the tumor on radiographic studies. (**b**) Cut surface demonstrates a large renal tumor with areas of focal necrosis surrounded by an attenuated renal tissue. (**c**) Microscopic findings of this tumor were consistent with renal cell carcinoma.

dren with complete resection of the primary tumor and zero in those with only partial resection. While

survival by stage was well documented with 92.5% for stage I, 84.5% for II, 72.7% for III, and 12.7% for IV, it should be noted that those with positive nodes but no distant metastasis had survival rates three times that of adult historical controls [53]. Renal cell carcinoma is remarkably resistant to chemotherapy preventing cure in most children who present with metastatic disease [111]. Ten to twenty percent of patients have nodal involvement identified at surgery, but lack evidence of distant metastatic disease. In a review of children receiving adjuvant therapy, no benefit could be defined for its use [53].

Nephron-sparing surgery has been utilized in patients with small polar lesions in whom there is no evidence of a multicentric tumor. In these selected cases with tumors less than 4 cm and a normal contralateral kidney, the risk of local recurrence is reported to be 2% or less, which is comparable to the frequency of metachronous recurrence in the contralateral kidney after a unilateral radical nephrectomy.

The occurrence of late relapses long after nephrectomy, prolonged stability of disease in the absence of systemic therapy, and rare cases of spontaneous regression of tumors have stimulated an interest in immunotherapy comparable to that utilized in melanoma. Trials of immuno-modulating therapy with interferon-alpha and interleukin-2 (IL-2) have demonstrated some efficacy, but maintenance of a durable cure has been elusive [52]. One trial randomized 294 patients with advanced stage renal cell carcinoma to receive placebo or 9 months of subcutaneous lymphoblastoid interferon. Regrettably, similar recurrence rates occurred in the two groups and worse survival was seen in those randomized to interferon [166]. With the significant toxicity involved with immunotherapy, demonstration of improved survival in randomized trials will be required before this can be adopted as standard therapy.

10.8 Mesoblastic Nephroma

Congenital mesoblastic nephroma, also referred to as fetal renal hamartoma or leiomyomatous hamartoma, is the most common renal tumor identified in the neonatal period. Although it was initially diagnosed and treated as a congenital Wilms' tumor, mesoblastic nephroma was defined as a distinct entity in 1967 [21]. Mesoblastic nephromas present most frequently in the neonatal period as a palpable flank mass that can be massive in size (Fig. 10.13A). Additional symptoms seen at presentation include hematuria, hypertension, vomiting, and jaundice [81].

Mesoblastic nephroma accounted for 2.8% of 1,905 renal tumors submitted to the early NWTSG studies. Grossly, these tumors generally have a homogeneous rubbery appearance resembling a uterine fibroid in color and consistency although cystic variants are seen (Fig. 10.13B). Microscopically they are composed of sheets of fibrous or mesenchymal stroma within which bizarre and dysplastic tubules and glomeruli are irregularly scattered [22]. The tumor can invade intact renal parenchyma, and extra-renal infiltration into the perihilar connective tissues is common. The histologic subtypes of this tumor include: the classic type (24% of cases), the cellular type (66%), and the mixed type (10%). The pluripotency of these tumors is revealed by their differentiation into angiomatoid patterns, cartilaginous nests, and their elicitation of intratumoral hematopoiesis in addition to the tiny nephroblastic epithelial foci.

A characteristic chromosomal translocation, t(12;15)(p13;q25), has been described which results in fusion of the *ETV6* (also known as *TEL*) gene from 12p13 with the *NRTK3* neurotrophin-3 receptor gene (also known as *TRKC*) from 15q25 [157, 158]. This results in a chimeric RNA which is characteristic of both infantile fibrosarcoma and the cellular variant of congenital mesoblastic nephroma. This may be of assistance in differentiating the cellular variant from other lesions which must be considered in the differential diagnosis including clear cell sarcoma and rhabdoid tumors of the kidney. It also suggests a close relation between infantile fibrosarcoma and the cellular variant of mesoblastic nephroma [4].

Nephrectomy alone usually cures this tumor. Resection should include generous margins around all gross tumor to avoid local recurrence. Particular attention should be paid to the medial aspect of the kidney including the hilum and great vessels because of this tumor's proclivity to extend into the perirenal soft tissues. Several children have been reported with local recurrence [8] or metastasis to the brain, bones, lungs, and heart [6, 77, 146, 169]. In some of these cases, the histology has revealed an unusual degree of mesenchymal cell immaturity and hypercellularity, suggesting a more aggressive tumor [22]. These rare occurrences, however, support the concept that mesoblastic nephroma cannot be considered as a simple hamartoma and that complete nephrectomy with negative pathologic margins for tumor is critical in all cases.

In a series of 51 children with mesoblastic nephroma identified in the NWTSG series, adequate operative excision was achieved in 43 of 51 children while eight had local extension and ten had tumor spillage during resection [81]. The use of adjuvant therapy in these cases depended upon the era in which the children were treated. Twenty-three infants treated primarily after 1978 had surgical resection alone. Prior to 1978, 24 had surgery plus chemotherapy and, before 1976, four children also received irradiation. Survival was excellent in this entire group and only one child succumbed to sepsis during chemotherapy. One child

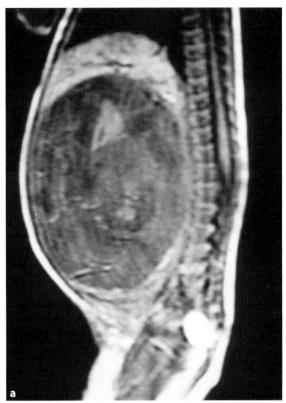

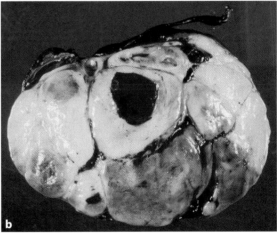

Fig. 10.13 (**a**) Sagittal views of an MRI scan of a newborn infant with a massive renal tumor. (**b**) Cut surface of the tumor shows the classic appearance of rubbery tissue without necrosis consistent with a mesoblastic nephroma.

recurred at 6 months despite receiving dactinomycin and vincristine. The tumor was surgically re-excised and the child was treated with cyclophosphamide and doxorubicin, and remained without disease 18 months later.

A SIOP study of 29 children with mesoblastic nephroma confirmed the early age at which this tumor is seen. There were only five infants older than 4 months at presentation in the series [145]. Five infants with the cellular type of tumor received some chemotherapy. Two infants in this series died from sepsis following surgery, but the remainder are alive and free of disease 4 years following surgery. Again this tumor was noted to infiltrate the renal hilum or perirenal tissue.

A neonate with an extensively infiltrating tumor was treated with 8 weekly courses of vincristine prior to resection [30]. The tumor regression occurred with treatment, facilitating its resection and cure.

Beckwith has reported the largest cohort of children with recurrent or metastatic lesions from his large collected series [6]. Twenty-four cases of aggressive tumor were seen in a series of 330 mesoblastic nephromas. Of these cases, eight had metastatic disease, 17 had relapse in the peritoneum or retroperitoneum, and six of the infants have succumbed with persistent disease. Recurrences occurred in children following initial chemotherapy or irradiation, which suggests that conventional adjuvant therapy may not decrease the incidence of relapse. Histologic criteria were not helpful in predicting outcome. Beckwith supports aggressive surgical attempts to remove all gross tumor and stresses the need for close monitoring for 1 year following surgery. Relapse was apparent in 23 of the 24 cases within 11 months of resection. Ultrasonography of the local site is adequate and scans for metastatic disease are unrewarding.

10.9 Cystic Nephroma

Cystic nephroma is indistinguishable grossly and radiographically from its malignant neoplastic cousins, cystic partially-differentiated nephroblastoma (CPDN) and cystic nephroblastoma. All lesions are composed of purely cystic masses characterized by multiple thin-walled septations. In cystic nephroma, the septations are lined by flattened, cuboidal or hobnail epithelium and are composed entirely of differentiated tissues without blastemal or other embryonal elements which are the distinguishing characteristic of CPDN [89]. While the term "multilocular cyst of the kidney" has been employed, "cystic nephroma" is preferred because the lesion appears to be neoplastic and not congenital. In the cystic nephroblastoma or cystic Wilms' tumor there are solid nodules on the septae of blastemal or embryonal elements characteristic of Wilms' tumor. An unexplained synchronous occurrence has been reported of cystic nephroma and pleuropulmonary blastoma [44, 85].

These lesions should not be confused with cystic clear cell sarcoma, cystic mesoblastic nephroma, or multicystic dysplastic kidney [1]. Cystic nephroma, CPND, and cystic nephroblastoma can be distinguished from multicystic dysplastic kidney because they are confined only to a portion of the kidney with normal renal parenchyma being identified while the cystic changes of multicystic dysplastic kidney almost always involve the entire kidney (its etiology is early in utero urinary tract obstruction). Contralateral renal anomalies are frequent in dysplastic kidneys including ureteropelvic junction obstruction and reflux. Multicystic dysplastic kidney is often identified antenatally or in the newborn period while the other lesions occur later.

Generally, nephrectomy will be curative in both cystic nephroma and CPDN [89]. Twenty-three children with these cystic lesions were identified in the NWTSG series: five with cystic nephroma and 18 with CPDN. Only one case of CPDN had local recurrence and there were no distant metastases. A more recent review of the NWTSG files of the CPDN cases has again confirmed that primary resection appears to be adequate for all lesions removed intact [18]. In cases where the lesion is isolated to one pole of the kidney, a partial nephrectomy may be considered; however, it must be remembered that these tumors can resemble cystic variants of clear cell sarcoma of the kidney which carry an entirely different prognosis [11, 160] This is the major concern regarding the use of nephron-sparing surgery as suggested by some for these cystic lesions [143].

Teratoid Wilms' tumor, a rare variant of nephroblastoma, has a predominance of teratoid elements in more than 50% of the tumor. Sixteen cases have been reported in the world literature. Treatment has not yet been established; however, a 4-month-old with localized disease was treated with surgery alone successfully [181].

References

1. Agrons GA, Wagner BJ, Davidson AJ, Suarez ES (1995) Multilocular cystic renal tumor in children: Radiologic-pathologic correlation. Radiographics 15:653–669
2. Anderson J, Slater O, McHugh K, Duffy P, Pritchard J (2002) Response without shrinkage in bilateral Wilms' tumor: Significance of rhabdomyomatous histology. J Pediatr Hematol Oncol 24:31–34
3. Andrews PE, Kelalis PP, Haase GM (1992) Extrarenal Wilms' tumor: Results of the National Wilms' Tumor Study. J Pediatr Surg 27:1181–1184
4. Argani P, Fritsch M, Kadkol SS, Schuster A, Beckwith JB, Perlman EJ (2000) Detection of the ETV6-NTRK3 chimeric RNA of infantile fibrosarcoma/cellular congenital mesoblastic nephroma in paraffin-embedded tissue: Application to challenging pediatric renal stromal tumors. Mod Pathol 13:29–36

5. Argani P, Perlman EJ, Breslow NE, Browning NG, Green DM, D'Angio GJ, Beckwith JB (2000) Clear cell sarcoma of the kidney: A review of 351 cases from the National Wilms' Tumor Study Group Pathology Center. Am J Surg Pathol 24:4–18

6. Beckwith J (1993) Reply. Pediatr Pathol 13:886–887

7. Beckwith J (1996) Wilms' tumor in multicystic dysplastic kidneys: What is the risk? Dialogues in Pediatric Urology 78:1P

8. Beckwith JB (1974) Mesenchymal renal neoplasms of infancy revisited. J Pediatr Surg 9:803–805

9. Beckwith JB, Palmer NF (1978) Histopathology and prognosis of Wilms' tumors: Results from the First National Wilms' Tumor Study. Cancer 41:1937–1948

10. Beckwith JB (1983) Wilms' tumor and other renal tumors of childhood: A selective review from the National Wilms' Tumor Study Pathology Center. Hum Pathol 14:481–492

11. Beckwith JB (1986) The John Lattimer lecture. Wilms' tumor and other renal tumors of childhood: An update. J Urol 136:320–324

12. Beckwith JB, Kiviat NB, Bonadio JF (1990) Nephrogenic rests, nephroblastomatosis, and the pathogenesis of Wilms' tumor. Pediatr Pathol 10:1–36

13. Beckwith JB (1993) Precursor lesions of Wilms' tumor: Clinical and biological implications. Med Pediatr Oncol 21:158–168

14. Bennington J, Beckwith J (1975) Tumor of the kidney, renal pelvis, and ureter. Atlas of Tumor Pathology, 2nd Series. Armed Forces Institute of Pathology, Bethesda, MD, pp 31–91

15. Bergeron C, Iliescu C, Thiesse P, Bouvier R, Dijoud F, Ranchere-Vince D, Basset T, Chappuis JP, Buclon M, Frappaz D, et al. (2001) Does nephroblastomatosis influence the natural history and relapse rate in Wilms' tumour? A single centre experience over 11 years. Eur J Cancer 37:385–391

16. Bernstein L, Linet M, Smith MA, Olshan A (1999). Renal tumors. In: Ries L, Smith MA, Gurney J (eds) Cancer incidence and survival among children and adolescents: United States SEER Program 1975–1995. National Cancer Institute, Bethesda, MD, pp 79–90

17. Biegel JA, Zhou JY, Rorke LB, Stenstrom C, Wainwright LM, Fogelgren B (1999) Germ-line and acquired mutations of INI1 in atypical teratoid and rhabdoid tumors. Cancer Res 59:74–79

18. Blakeley M, Shamberger RC, Norkool P (2003) Outcome of children with cystic partially-differentiated nephroblastoma treated with or without chemotherapy. J Pediatr Surg

19. Blute ML, Kelalis PP, Offord KP, Breslow N, Beckwith JB, D'Angio GJ (1987) Bilateral Wilms' tumor. J Urol 138:968–973

20. Boccon-Gibod L, Rey A, Sandstedt B, Delemarre J, Harms D, Vujanic G, De Kraker J, Weirich A, Tournade MF (2000) Complete necrosis induced by preoperative chemotherapy in Wilms' tumor as an indicator of low risk: Report of the international society of paediatric oncology (SIOP) nephroblastoma trial and study 9. Med Pediatr Oncol 34:183–190

21. Bolande RP, Brough AJ, Izant RJ Jr (1967) Congenital mesoblastic nephroma of infancy. A report of eight cases and the relationship to Wilms' tumor. Pediatrics 40:272–278

22. Bolande RP (1974) Congenital and infantile neoplasia of the kidney. Lancet 2:1497–1499

23. Bonnin JM, Rubinstein LJ, Palmer NF, Beckwith JB (1984) The association of embryonal tumors originating in the kidney and in the brain. A report of seven cases. Cancer 54:2137–2146

24. Breslow N, Beckwith JB, Ciol M, Sharples K (1988) Age distribution of Wilms' tumor: Report from the National Wilms' Tumor Study. Cancer Res 48:1653–1657

25. Breslow NE, Takashima JR, Whitton JA, Moksness J, D'Angio GJ, Green DM (1995) Second malignant neoplasms following treatment for Wilm's tumor: A report from the National Wilms' Tumor Study Group. J Clin Oncol 13:1851–1859

26. Breslow NE, Norris R, Norkool PA, Kang T, Beckwith JB, Perlman EJ, Ritchey ML, Green DM, Nichols KE (2003) Characteristics and outcomes of children with the Wilms' tumor-Aniridia syndrome: A report from the National Wilms' Tumor Study Group. J Clin Oncol 21:4579–4585

27. Breslow NE, Ou SS, Beckwith JB, Haase GM, Kalapurakal JA, Ritchey ML, Shamberger RC, Thomas PR, D'Angio GJ, Green DM (2004) Doxorubicin for favorable histology, Stage II-III Wilms' tumor: Results from the National Wilms' Tumor Studies. Cancer 101:1072–1080

28. Breslow NE, Collins AJ, Ritchey ML, Grigoriev YA, Peterson SM, Green DM (2005) End stage renal disease in patients with Wilms' tumor: Results from the National Wilms' Tumor Study Group and the United States Renal Data System. J Urol 174:1972–1975

29. Burger D, Moorman-Voestermans CG, Mildenberger H, Lemerle J, Voute PA, Tournade MF, Rodary C, Delemarre JF, Sandstedt B, Sarrazin D, et al. (1985) The advantages of preoperative therapy in Wilms' tumour. A summarised report on clinical trials conducted by the International Society of Paediatric Oncology (SIOP). Z Kinderchir 40:170–175

30. Chan KL, Chan KW, Lee CW, Saing H (1995) Preoperative chemotherapy for mesoblastic nephroma. Med Pediatr Oncol 24:271–273

31. Choyke PL, Siegel MJ, Craft AW, Green DM, DeBaun MR (1999) Screening for Wilms' tumor in children with Beckwith-Wiedemann syndrome or idiopathic hemihypertrophy. Med Pediatr Oncol 32:196–200

32. Clericuzio CL (1993) Clinical phenotypes and Wilms' tumor. Med Pediatr Oncol 21:182–187

33. Coppes MJ, Wilson PC, Weitzman S (1991) Extrarenal Wilms' tumor: Staging, treatment, and prognosis. J Clin Oncol 9:167–174

34. Coppes MJ, Tournade MF, Lemerle J, Weitzman S, Rey A, Burger D, Carli M, Voute PA (1992) Preoperative care of infants with nephroblastoma. The International Society of Pediatric Oncology 6 experience. Cancer 69:2721–2725

35. Coppes MJ, Zandvoort SW, Sparling CR, Poon AO, Weitzman S, Blanchette VS (1992) Acquired von Willebrand disease in Wilms' tumor patients. J Clin Oncol 10:422–427

36. Coppes MJ, Haber DA, Grundy PE (1994) Genetic events in the development of Wilms' tumor. N Engl J Med 331:586–590

37. Coppes MJ, Arnold M, Beckwith JB, Ritchey ML, D'Angio GJ, Green DM, Breslow NE (1999) Factors affecting the risk of contralateral Wilms' tumor development: A report from the National Wilms' Tumor Study Group. Cancer 85:1616–1625

38. Cozzi F, Schiavetti A, Bonanni M, Cozzi DA, Matrunola M, Castello MA (1996) Enucleative surgery for stage I nephroblastoma with a normal contralateral kidney. J Urol 156:1788–1791; discussion 1791–1783

39. Craft AW (1995) Screening for Wilms' Tumor in patients with aniridia, Beckwith syndrome, or hemihypertrophy. Med Pediatr Oncol 24:231–234

40. D'Angio GJ, Evans AE, Breslow N, Beckwith B, Bishop H, Feigl P, Goodwin W, Leape LL, Sinks LF, Sutow W, et al. (1976) The treatment of Wilms' tumor: Results of the national Wilms' tumor study. Cancer 38:633–646

41. D'Angio GJ, Evans A, Breslow N, Beckwith B, Bishop H, Farewell V, Goodwin W, Leape L, Palmer N, Sinks L, et al. (1981) The treatment of Wilms' tumor: Results of the Second National Wilms' Tumor Study. Cancer 47:2302–2311

42. D'Angio GJ, Breslow N, Beckwith JB, Evans A, Baum H, deLorimier A, Fernbach D, Hrabovsky E, Jones B, Kelalis P, et al. (1989) Treatment of Wilms' tumor. Results of the Third National Wilms' Tumor Study. Cancer 64:349–360

43. DeChiara TM, Robertson EJ, Efstratiadis A (1991) Parental imprinting of the mouse insulin-like growth factor II gene. Cell 64:849–859

44. Delahunt B, Thomson KJ, Ferguson AF, Neale TJ, Meffan PJ, Nacey JN (1993) Familial cystic nephroma and pleuropulmonary blastoma. Cancer 71:1338–1342

45. Dinkel E, Britscho J, Dittrich M, Schulte-Wissermann H, Ertel M (1988) Renal growth in patients nephrectomized for Wilms' tumour as compared to renal agenesis. Eur J Pediatr 147:54–58

46. Dome JS, Bockhold CA, Li SM, Baker SD, Green DM, Perlman EJ, Hill DA, Breslow NE (2005) High telomerase RNA expression level is an adverse prognostic factor for favorable-histology Wilms' tumor. J Clin Oncol 23:9138–9145

47. Farber S (1966) Chemotherapy in the treatment of leukemia and Wilms' tumor. JAMA 198:826–836

48. Farewell VT, D'Angio GJ, Breslow N, Norkool P (1981) Retrospective validation of a new staging system for Wilms' tumor. Cancer Clin Trials 4:167–171

49. Faria P, Beckwith JB, Mishra K, Zuppan C, Weeks DA, Breslow N, Green DM (1996) Focal versus diffuse anaplasia in Wilms' tumor – New definitions with prognostic significance: A report from the National Wilms' Tumor Study Group. Am J Surg Pathol 20:909–920

50. Fischbach BV, Trout KL, Lewis J, Luis CA, Sika M (2005) WAGR syndrome: A clinical review of 54 cases. Pediatrics 116:984–988

51. Francke U, George DL, Brown MG, Riccardi VM (1977) Gene dose effect: Intraband mapping of the $LDH A$ locus using cells from four individuals with different interstitial deletions of 11p. Cytogenet Cell Genet 19:197–207

52. Fyfe G, Fisher RI, Rosenberg SA, Sznol M, Parkinson DR, Louie AC (1995) Results of treatment of 255 patients with metastatic renal cell carcinoma who received high-dose recombinant interleukin-2 therapy. J Clin Oncol 13:688–696

53. Geller JI, Dome JS (2004) Local lymph node involvement does not predict poor outcome in pediatric renal cell carcinoma. Cancer 101:1575–1583

54. Gillan TL, Hughes R, Godbout R, Grundy PE (2003) The Simpson-Golabi-Behmel gene, GPC3, is not involved in sporadic Wilms' tumorigenesis. Am J Med Genet A 122:30–36

55. Godzinski J, Tournade MF, deKraker J, Lemerle J, Voute PA, Weirich A, Ludwig R, Rapala M, Skotnicka G, Gauthier F, et al. (1998) Rarity of surgical complications after postchemotherapy nephrectomy for nephroblastoma. Experience of the International Society of Paediatric Oncology-Trial and Study "SIOP-9". International Society of Paediatric Oncology Nephroblastoma Trial and Study Committee. Eur J Pediatr Surg 8:83–86

56. Graf N, Tournade MF, De Kraker J (2000) The role of preoperative chemotherapy in the management of Wilms' tumor. The SIOP studies. Urol Clin N Amer 27:443–454

57. Green DM, Finklestein JZ, Tefft ME, Norkool P (1989) Diffuse interstitial pneumonitis after pulmonary irradiation for metastatic Wilms' tumor. A report from the National Wilms' Tumor Study. Cancer 63:450–453

58. Green DM, Breslow NE, Beckwith JB, Norkool P (1993) Screening of children with hemihypertrophy, aniridia, and Beckwith-Wiedemann syndrome in patients with Wilms' tumor: A report from the National Wilms' Tumor Study. Med Pediatr Oncol 21:188–192

59. Green DM, Breslow NE, Beckwith JB, Takashima J, Kelalis P, D'Angio GJ (1993) Treatment outcomes in patients less than 2 years of age with small, stage I, favorable-histology Wilms' tumors: A report from the National Wilms' Tumor Study. J Clin Oncol 11:91–95

60. Green DM, Breslow NE, D'Angio GJ (1993) The treatment of children with unilateral Wilms' tumor. J Clin Oncol 11:1009–1010

61. Green DM, Beckwith JB, Breslow NE, Faria P, Moksness J, Finklestein JZ, Grundy P, Thomas PR, Kim T, Shochat S, et al. (1994) Treatment of children with stages II to IV anaplastic Wilms' tumor: A report from the National Wilms' Tumor Study Group. J Clin Oncol 12:2126–2131

62. Green DM, Beckwith JB, Weeks DA, Moksness J, Breslow NE, D'Angio GJ (1994) The relationship between microsubstaging variables, age at diagnosis, and tumor weight of children with stage I/favorable histology Wilms' tumor. A report from the National Wilms' Tumor study. Cancer 74:1817–1820

63. Green DM, Breslow NE, Beckwith JB, Moksness J, Finklestein JZ, D'Angio GJ (1994) Treatment of children with clear-cell sarcoma of the kidney: A report from the National Wilms' Tumor Study Group. J Clin Oncol 12:2132–2137

64. Green DM, Breslow NE, Evans I, Moksness J, Finklestein JZ, Evans AE, D'Angio GJ (1994) The effect of chemotherapy dose intensity on the hematological toxicity of the treatment for Wilms' tumor. A report from the National Wilms' Tumor Study. Am J Pediatr Hematol Oncol 16:207–212

65. Green DM, Breslow NE, Beckwith JB, Finklestein JZ, Grundy P, Thomas PR, Kim T, Shochat S, Haase G, Ritchey M, et al. (1998) Effect of duration of treatment on treatment outcome and cost of treatment for Wilms' tumor: A report from the National Wilms' Tumor Study Group. J Clin Oncol 16:3744–3751

66. Green DM, Breslow NE, Beckwith JB, Finklestein JZ, Grundy PE, Thomas PR, Kim T, Shochat SJ, Haase GM, Ritchey ML, et al. (1998) Comparison between single-dose and divided-dose administration of dactinomycin and doxorubicin for patients with Wilms' tumor: A report from the National Wilms' Tumor Study Group. J Clin Oncol 16:237–245

67. Green DM, Breslow NE, Beckwith JB, Ritchey ML, Shamberger RC, Haase GM, D'Angio GJ, Perlman E, Donaldson M, Grundy PE, et al. (2001) Treatment with nephrectomy only for small, stage I/favorable histology Wilms' tumor: A report from the National Wilms' Tumor Study Group. J Clin Oncol 19:3719–3724

68. Green DM, Grigoriev YA, Nan B, Takashima JR, Norkool PA, D'Angio GJ, Breslow NE (2001) Congestive heart failure after treatment for Wilms' tumor: A report from the National Wilms' Tumor Study group. J Clin Oncol 19:1926–1934

69. Green DM, Peabody EM, Nan B, Peterson S, Kalapurakal JA, Breslow NE (2002) Pregnancy outcome after treatment for Wilms' tumor: A report from the National Wilms' Tumor Study Group. J Clin Oncol 20:2506–2513

70. Gronskov K, Olsen JH, Sand A, Pedersen W, Carlsen N, Bak Jylling AM, Lyngbye T, Brondum-Nielsen K, Rosenberg T (2001) Population-based risk estimates of Wilms' tumor in sporadic aniridia. A comprehensive mutation screening procedure of PAX6 identifies 80% of mutations in aniridia. Hum Genet 109:11–18

71. Gross R (1950) Treatment of mixed tumors of the kidney in childhood. Pediatrics 6:843–852

72. Grundy P, Telzerow P, Paterson MC, Haber D, Berman B, Li F, Garber J (1991) Chromosome 11 uniparental isodisomy predisposing to embryonal neoplasms. Lancet 338:1079–1080

73. Grundy PE, Telzerow PE, Breslow N, Moksness J, Huff V, Paterson MC (1994) Loss of heterozygosity for chromosomes 16q and 1p in Wilms' tumors predicts an adverse outcome. Cancer Res 54:2331–2333

74. Grundy PE, Breslow NE, Li S, Perlman E, Beckwith JB, Ritchey ML, Shamberger RC, Haase GM, D'Angio GJ, Donaldson M, et al. (2005) Loss of heterozygosity for chromosomes 1p and 16q is an adverse prognostic factor in favorable-histology Wilms' tumor: A report from the National Wilms' Tumor Study Group. J Clin Oncol 23:7312–7321

75. Gylys-Morin V, Hoffer FA, Kozakewich H, Shamberger RC (1993) Wilms' tumor and nephroblastomatosis: Imaging characteristics at gadolinium-enhanced MR imaging. Radiology 188:517–521

76. Haas JE, Palmer NF, Weinberg AG, Beckwith JB (1981) Ultrastructure of malignant rhabdoid tumor of the kidney. A distinctive renal tumor of children. Hum Pathol 12:646–657

77. Heidelberger KP, Ritchey ML, Dauser RC, McKeever PE, Beckwith JB (1993) Congenital mesoblastic nephroma metastatic to the brain. Cancer 72:2499–2502

78. Henry I, Bonaiti-Pellie C, Chehensse V, Beldjord C, Schwartz C, Utermann G, Junien C (1991) Uniparental paternal disomy in a genetic cancer-predisposing syndrome. Nature 351:665–667

79. Hogeboom CJ, Grosser SC, Guthrie KA, Thomas PR, D'Angio GJ, Breslow NE (2001) Stature loss following treatment for Wilms' tumor. Med Pediatr Oncol 36:295–304

80. Horwitz JR, Ritchey ML, Moksness J, Breslow NE, Smith GR, Thomas PR, Haase G, Shamberger RC, Beckwith JB (1996) Renal salvage procedures in patients with synchronous bilateral Wilms' tumors: A report from the National Wilms' Tumor Study Group. J Pediatr Surg 31:1020–1025

81. Howell CG, Othersen HB, Kiviat NE, Norkool P, Beckwith JB, D'Angio GJ (1982) Therapy and outcome in 51 children with mesoblastic nephroma: A report of the National Wilms' Tumor Study. J Pediatr Surg 17:826–831

82. Hrabovsky EE, Othersen HB Jr, deLorimier A, Kelalis P, Beckwith JB, Takashima J (1986) Wilms' tumor in the neonate: A report from the National Wilms' Tumor Study. J Pediatr Surg 21:385–387

83. Hughes-Benzie RM, Hunter AG, Allanson JE, Mackenzie AE (1992) Simpson-Golabi-Behmel syndrome associated with renal dysplasia and embryonal tumor: Localization of the gene to Xqcen-q21. Am J Med Genet 43:428–435

84. Hughes-Benzie RM, Pilia G, Xuan JY, Hunter AG, Chen E, Golabi M, Hurst JA, Kobori J, Marymee K, Pagon RA, et al. (1996) Simpson-Golabi-Behmel syndrome: Genotype/phenotype analysis of 18 affected males from 7 unrelated families. Am J Med Genet 66:227–234

85. Ishida Y, Kato K, Kigasawa H, Ohama Y, Ijiri R, Tanaka Y (2000) Synchronous occurrence of pleuropulmonary blastoma and cystic nephroma: Possible genetic link in cystic lesions of the lung and the kidney. Med Pediatr Oncol 35:85–87

86. Jadresic L, Leake J, Gordon I, Dillon MJ, Grant DB, Pritchard J, Risdon RA, Barratt TM (1990) Clinicopathologic review of twelve children with nephropathy, Wilms' tumor, and genital abnormalities (Drash syndrome). J Pediatr 117:717–725

87. Jereb B, Tournade MF, Lemerle J, Voute PA, Delemarre JF, Ahstrom L, Flamant R, Gerard-Marchant R, Sandstedt B (1980) Lymph node invasion and prognosis in nephroblastoma. Cancer 45:1632–1636

88. Jereb B, Burgers JM, Tournade MF, Lemerle J, Bey P, Delemarre J, Habrand JL, Voute PA (1994) Radiotherapy in the SIOP (International Society of Pediatric Oncology) nephroblastoma studies: A review. Med Pediatr Oncol 22:221–227

89. Joshi VV, Beckwith JB (1989) Multilocular cyst of the kidney (cystic nephroma) and cystic, partially differentiated nephroblastoma. Terminology and criteria for diagnosis. Cancer 64:466–479

90. Kalapurakal JA, Peterson S, Peabody EM, Thomas PR, Green DM, D'Angio G J, Breslow NE (2004) Pregnancy outcomes after abdominal irradiation that included or excluded the pelvis in childhood Wilms' tumor survivors: A report from the National Wilms' Tumor Study. Int J Radiat Oncol Biol Phys 58:1364–1368

91. Koufos A, Grundy P, Morgan K, Aleck KA, Hadro T, Lampkin BC, Kalbakji A, Cavenee WK (1989) Familial Wiedemann-Beckwith syndrome and a second Wilms' tumor locus both map to 11p15.5. Am J Hum Genet 44:711–719

92. Kumar R, Fitzgerald R, Breatnach F (1998) Conservative surgical management of bilateral Wilms' tumor: Results of the United Kingdom Children's Cancer Study Group. J Urol 160:1450–1453

93. Kusumakumary P, Chellam VG, Rojymon J, Hariharan S, Krishnan NM (1997) Late recurrence of clear cell sarcoma of the kidney. Med Pediatr Oncol 28:355–357

94. Lack EE, Cassady JR, Sallan SE (1985) Renal cell carcinoma in childhood and adolescence: A clinical and pathological study of 17 cases. J Urol 133:822–828

95. Ladd W (1938) Embryoma of the kidney (Wilms' Tumor). Ann Surg 108:885–902

96. Larsen E, Perez-Atayde A, Green DM, Retik A, Clavell LA, Sallan SE (1990) Surgery only for the treatment of patients with stage I (Cassady) Wilms' tumor. Cancer 66:264–266

97. Lee IS, Nguyen S, Shanberg AM (1995) Needle tract seeding after percutaneous biopsy of Wilms' tumor. J Urol 153:1074–1076

98. Lee SB, Haber DA (2001) Wilms' tumor and the WT1 gene. Exp Cell Res 264:74–99

99. Lemerle J, Voute PA, Tournade MF, Delemarre JF, Jereb B, Ahstrom L, Flamant R, Gerard-Marchant R (1976) Preoperative versus postoperative radiotherapy, single versus multiple courses of actinomycin D, in the treatment of Wilms' tumor. Preliminary results of a controlled clinical trial conducted by the International Society of Paediatric Oncology (S.I.O.P.). Cancer 38:647–654

100. Lemerle J, Voute PA, Tournade MF, Rodary C, Delemarre JF, Sarrazin D, Burgers JM, Sandstedt B, Mildenberger H, Carli M, et al. (1983) Effectiveness of preoperative chemotherapy in Wilms' tumor: Results of an International Society of Paediatric Oncology (SIOP) clinical trial. J Clin Oncol 1:604–609

101. Lipshultz SE, Colan SD, Gelber RD, Perez-Atayde AR, Sallan SE, Sanders SP (1991) Late cardiac effects of doxorubicin therapy for acute lymphoblastic leukemia in childhood. N Engl J Med 324:808–815

102. Little MH, Williamson KA, Mannens M, Kelsey A, Gosden C, Hastie ND, van Heyningen V (1993) Evidence that WT1 mutations in Denys-Drash syndrome patients may act in a dominant-negative fashion. Hum Mol Genet 2:259–264

103. Maes P, Delemarre J, de Kraker J, Ninane J (1999) Fetal rhabdomyomatous nephroblastoma: A tumour of good prognosis but resistant to chemotherapy. Eur J Cancer 35:1356–1360

104. Maheswaran S, Park S, Bernard A, Morris JF, Rauscher FJ 3rd, Hill DE, Haber DA (1993) Physical and functional interaction between WT1 and p53 proteins. Proc Natl Acad Sci 90:5100–5104

105. Marsden HB, Lawler W, Kumar PM (1978) Bone metastasizing renal tumor of childhood: Morphological and clinical features, and differences from Wilms' tumor. Cancer 42:1922–1928

106. Marx M, Langer T, Graf N, Hausdorf G, Stohr W, Ludwig R, Beck JD (2002) Multicentre analysis of anthracycline-induced cardiotoxicity in children following treatment according to the nephroblastoma studies SIOP No.9/GPOH and SIOP 93–01/GPOH. Med Pediatr Oncol 39:18–24

107. McDonald JM, Douglass EC, Fisher R, Geiser CF, Krill CE, Strong LC, Virshup D, Huff V (1998) Linkage of familial Wilms' tumor predisposition to chromosome 19 and a two-locus model for the etiology of familial tumors. Cancer Res 58:1387–1390

108. McLorie GA, McKenna PH, Greenberg M, Babyn P, Thorner P, Churchill BM, Weitzman S, Filler R, Khoury AE (1991) Reduction in tumor burden allowing partial nephrectomy following preoperative chemotherapy in biopsy proved Wilms' tumor. J Urol 146:509–513

109. McNeil DE, Langer JC, Choyke P, DeBaun MR (2002) Feasibility of partial nephrectomy for Wilms' tumor in children with Beckwith-Wiedemann syndrome who have been screened with abdominal ultrasonography. J Pediatr Surg 37:57–60

110. Moorman-Voestermans CG, Aronson DC, Staalman CR, Delemarre JF, de Kraker J (1998) Is partial nephrectomy appropriate treatment for unilateral Wilms' tumor? J Pediatr Surg 33:165–170

111. Motzer RJ, Bander NH, Nanus DM (1996) Renal-cell carcinoma. N Engl J Med 335:865–875

112. Lall, A, Pritchard-Jones K, Walker J, Jutton C, Stevens S, Azmy A, Carachi R (2006) Wilms' tumor with intracaval thrombus in the UK Children's Cancer Study Group UKW3 trial. J Ped Surg 41:382–387

113. Muto R, Yamamori S, Ohashi H, Osawa M (2002) Prediction by FISH analysis of the occurrence of Wilms' tumor in aniridia patients. Am J Med Genet 108:285–289

114. Nakayama DK, Norkool P, deLorimier AA, O'Neill JA Jr, D'Angio GJ (1986) Intracardiac extension of Wilms' tumor. A report of the National Wilms' Tumor Study. Ann Surg 204:693–697

115. Narchi H (2005) Risk of Wilms' tumour with multicystic kidney disease: A systematic review. Arch Dis Child 90:147–149

116. Neville H, Ritchey ML, Shamberger RC, Haase G, Perlman S, Yoshioka T (2002) The occurrence of Wilms' tumor in horseshoe kidneys: A report from the National Wilms' Tumor Study Group (NWTSG). J Pediatr Surg 37:1134–1137

117. Othersen HB Jr, DeLorimer A, Hrabovsky E, Kelalis P, Breslow N, D'Angio GJ (1990) Surgical evaluation of lymph node metastases in Wilms' tumor. J Pediatr Surg 25:330–331

118. Parham DM, Roloson GJ, Feely M, Green DM, Bridge JA, Beckwith JB (2001) Primary malignant neuroepithelial tumors of the kidney: A clinicopathologic analysis of 146 adult and pediatric cases from the National Wilms' Tumor Study Group Pathology Center. Am J Surg Pathol 25:133–146

119. Paulino AC, Wilimas J, Marina N, Jones D, Kumar M, Greenwald C, Chen G, Kun LE (1996) Local control in synchronous bilateral Wilms' tumor. Int J Radiat Oncol Biol Phys 36:541–548

120. Perlman EJ, Ali SZ, Robinson R, Lindato R, Griffin CA (1998) Infantile extrarenal rhabdoid tumor. Pediatr Dev Pathol 1:149–152

121. Perlman EJ, Faria P, Soares A, Hoffer F, Sredni S, Ritchey M, Shamberger RC, Green D, Beckwith JB (2006) Hyperplastic perilobar nephroblastomatosis: Long-term survival of 52 patients. Pediatr Blood Cancer 46:203–221

122. Ping AJ, Reeve AE, Law DJ, Young MR, Boehnke M, Feinberg AP (1989) Genetic linkage of Beckwith-Wiedemann syndrome to 11p15. Am J Hum Genet 44:720–723

123. Pritchard-Jones K, Kelsey A, Vujanic G, Imeson J, Hutton C, Mitchell C (2003) Older age is an adverse prognostic factor in stage I, favorable histology Wilms' tumor treated with vincristine monochemotherapy: A study by the United Kingdom Children's Cancer Study Group, Wilm's Tumor Working Group. J Clin Oncol 21:3269–3275

124. Rahman N, Arbour L, Tonin P, Renshaw J, Pelletier J, Baruchel S, Pritchard-Jones K, Stratton MR, Narod SA (1996) Evidence for a familial Wilms' tumour gene (FWT1) on chromosome 17q12-q21. Nat Genet 13:461–463

125. Rance T (1814) Case of fungus hematodes of the kidneys. Med Phys J 32:19

126. Rauscher FJ 3rd, Morris JF, Tournay OE, Cook DM, Curran T (1990) Binding of the Wilms' tumor locus zinc finger protein to the EGR-1 consensus sequence. Science 250:1259–1262

127. Rauscher FJ, 3rd (1993) The WT1 Wilms' tumor gene product: A developmentally regulated transcription factor in the kidney that functions as a tumor suppressor. FASEB J 7:896–903

128. Reeve AE, Sih SA, Raizis AM, Feinberg AP (1989) Loss of allelic heterozygosity at a second locus on chromosome 11 in sporadic Wilms' tumor cells. Mol Cell Biol 9:1799–1803

129. Riccardi VM, Sujansky E, Smith AC, Francke U (1978) Chromosomal imbalance in the Aniridia-Wilms' tumor association: 11p interstitial deletion. Pediatrics 61:604–610

130. Ritchey ML, Kelalis PP, Breslow N, Offord KP, Shochat SJ, D'Angio GJ (1988) Intracaval and atrial involvement with nephroblastoma: Review of National Wilms' Tumor Study-3. J Urol 140:1113–1118

131. Ritchey ML, Kelalis PP, Breslow N, Etzioni R, Evans I, Haase GM, D'Angio GJ (1992) Surgical complications after nephrectomy for Wilms' tumor. Surg Gynecol Obstet 175:507–514

132. Ritchey ML, Lally KP, Haase GM, Shochat SJ, Kelalis PP (1992) Superior mesenteric artery injury during nephrectomy for Wilms' tumor. J Pediatr Surg 27:612–615

133. Ritchey ML, Kelalis PP, Etzioni R, Breslow N, Shochat S, Haase GM (1993) Small bowel obstruction after nephrectomy for Wilms' tumor. A report of the National Wilms' Tumor Study-3. Ann Surg 218:654–659

134. Ritchey ML, Kelalis PP, Haase GM, Shochat SJ, Green DM, D'Angio G (1993) Preoperative therapy for intracaval and atrial extension of Wilms' tumor. Cancer 71:4104–4110

135. Ritchey ML, Pringle KC, Breslow NE, Takashima J, Moksness J, Zuppan CW, Beckwith JB, Thomas PR, Kelalis PP (1994) Management and outcome of inoperable Wilms' tumor. A report of National Wilms' Tumor Study-3. Ann Surg 220:683–690

136. Ritchey ML, Azizkhan RG, Beckwith JB, Hrabovsky EE, Haase GM (1995) Neonatal Wilms' tumor. J Pediatr Surg 30:856–859

137. Ritchey ML, Green DM, Breslow NB, Moksness J, Norkool P (1995) Accuracy of current imaging modalities in the diagnosis of synchronous bilateral Wilms' tumor. A report from the National Wilms' Tumor Study Group. Cancer 75:600–604

138. Ritchey ML, Green DM, Thomas PR, Smith GR, Haase G, Shochat S, Moksness J, Breslow NE (1996) Renal failure in Wilms' tumor patients: A report from the National Wilms' Tumor Study Group. Med Pediatr Oncol 26:75–80

139. Ritchey ML, Shamberger RC, Haase G, Horwitz J, Bergemann T, Breslow NE (2001) Surgical complications after primary nephrectomy for Wilms' tumor: Report from the National Wilms' Tumor Study Group. J Am Coll Surg 192:63–68; quiz 146

140. Ritchey ML (2005) Renal sparing surgery for Wilms' tumor. J Urol 174:1172–1173

141. Rodriguez-Galindo C, Marina NM, Fletcher BD, Parham DM, Bodner SM, Meyer WH (1997) Is primitive neuroectodermal tumor of the kidney a distinct entity? Cancer 79:2243–2250

142. Rohrschneider WK, Weirich A, Rieden K, Darge K, Troger J, Graf N (1998) US, CT and MR imaging characteristics of nephroblastomatosis. Pediatr Radiol 28:435–443

143. Sacher P, Willi UV, Niggli F, Stallmach T (1998) Cystic nephroma: A rare benign renal tumor. Pediatr Surg Int 13:197–199

144. Safford S, Goyeau D, Freemerman A, Bentley R, Everett M, Grundy P, Skinner M (2003) Fine mapping of Wilms' tumors with 16q loss of heterozygosity localizes the putative tumor suppressor gene to a region of 6.7 megabases. Ann Surg Oncol 10:136–143

145. Sandstedt B, Delemarre JF, Krul EJ, Tournade MF (1985) Mesoblastic nephromas: A study of 29 tumours from the SIOP nephroblastoma file. Histopathology 9:741–750

146. Schlesinger A (1995) Congenital mesoblastic nephroma metastatic to the brain: A report of two cases. Pediatr Radiol 25:S73–S75

147. Schofield DE, Beckwith JB, Sklar J (1996) Loss of heterozygosity at chromosome regions 22q11–12 and 11p15.5 in renal rhabdoid tumors. Genes Chromosomes Cancer 15:10–17

148. Schweisguth O, Bamberger J (1963) Le Nephroblastome de l'enfant. Ann Chir Infant 4:335–354

149. Seibel N, Li S, Breslow N, Beckwith J, Green D, D'Angio G, Ritchey M, PR T, Grundy P, Finklestin J (2003) Effect of duration of treatment on treatment outcome for patients with clear cell sarcoma of the kidney (CCSK): A report from the National Wilms' Tumor Study Group. Proc Am Soc Clin Oncol 22:800

150. Seibel N (2005) Outcome of Clear Cell Sarcoma of the kidney (CCSK) treated on the National Wilms' Tumor 5 Study (NWTS). American Surgical Clinical Oncology

151. Shamberger RC, Macklis RM, Sallan SE (1994) Recent experience with Wilms' tumor: 1978–1991. Ann Surg Oncol 1:59–65

152. Shamberger RC, Guthrie KA, Ritchey ML, Haase GM, Takashima J, Beckwith JB, D'Angio GJ, Green DM, Breslow NE (1999) Surgery-related factors and local recurrence of Wilms' tumor in National Wilms' Tumor Study 4. Ann Surg 229:292–297

153. Shamberger RC, Ritchey ML, Haase GM, Bergemann TL, Loechelt-Yoshioka T, Breslow NE, Green DM (2001) Intravascular extension of Wilms' tumor. Ann Surg 234:116–121

154. Shearer P, Kapoor G, Beckwith JB, Takashima J, Breslow N, Green DM (2001) Secondary acute myelogenous leukemia in patients previously treated for childhood renal tumors: A report from the National Wilms' Tumor Study Group. J Pediatr Hematol Oncol 23:109–111

155. Smith GR, Thomas PR, Ritchey M, Norkool P (1998) Long-term renal function in patients with irradiated bilateral Wilms' tumor. National Wilms' Tumor Study Group. Am J Clin Oncol 21:58–63

156. Sredni ST, de Camargo B, Lopes LF, Teixeira R, Simpson A (2001) Immunohistochemical detection of p53 protein expression as a prognostic indicator in Wilms' tumor. Med Pediatr Oncol 37:455–458

157. Steenman M, Westerveld A, Mannens M (2000) Genetics of Beckwith-Wiedemann syndrome-associated tumors: Common genetic pathways. Genes Chromosomes Cancer 28:1–13

158. Steenman MJ, Rainier S, Dobry CJ, Grundy P, Horon IL, Feinberg AP (1994) Loss of imprinting of IGF2 is linked to reduced expression and abnormal methylation of H19 in Wilms' tumour. Nat Genet 7:433–439

159. Stiller CA, Parkin DM (1990) International variations in the incidence of childhood lymphomas. Paediatr Perinat Epidemiol 4:303–324

160. Streif W, Gassner I, Janetschek G, Kreczy A, Judmaier W, Fink FM (1997) Partial nephrectomy in a cystic partially differentiated nephroblastoma. Med Pediatr Oncol 28:416–419

161. Sutow W (1963) Vincristine (Leurocristine) sulfate in the treatment of children with metastatic Wilms' Tumor. Pediatrics 32:880–887

162. Thorner PS, Arbus GS, Celermajer DS, Baumal R (1984) Focal segmental glomerulosclerosis and progressive renal failure associated with a unilateral kidney. Pediatrics 73:806–810

163. Tomlinson GE, Breslow NE, Dome J, Guthrie KA, Norkool P, Li S, Thomas PR, Perlman E, Beckwith JB, D'Angio GJ, Green DM (2005) Rhabdoid tumor of the kidney in the National Wilms' Tumor Study: Age at diagnosis as a prognostic factor. J Clin Oncol 23:7641–7645

164. Tournade MF, Com-Nougue C, Voute PA, Lemerle J, de Kraker J, Delemarre JF, Burgers M, Habrand JL, Moorman CG, Burger D, et al. (1993) Results of the Sixth International Society of Pediatric Oncology Wilms' Tumor Trial and Study: A risk-adapted therapeutic approach in Wilms' tumor. J Clin Oncol 11:1014–1023

165. Tournade MF, Com-Nougue C, de Kraker J, Ludwig R, Rey A, Burgers JM, Sandstedt B, Godzinski J, Carli M, Potter R, et al. (2001) Optimal duration of preoperative therapy in unilateral and nonmetastatic Wilms' tumor in children older than 6 months: Results of the Ninth International Society of Pediatric Oncology Wilms' Tumor Trial and Study. J Clin Oncol 19:488–500

166. Trump D, Elson P, Propert K (1996) Randomized controlled trial of adjuvant therapy with lymphoblastoid interferon. Proc Am Soc Clin Oncol 15:353

167. Urban CE, Lackner H, Schwinger W, Klos I, Hollwarth M, Sauer H, Ring E, Gadner H, Zoubek A (1995) Partial nephrectomy in well-responding stage I Wilms' tumors: Report of three cases. Pediatr Hematol Oncol 12:143–152

168. Versteege I, Sevenet N, Lange J, Rousseau-Merck MF, Ambros P, Handgretinger R, Aurias A, Delattre O (1998) Truncating mutations of hSNF5/INI1 in aggressive paediatric cancer. Nature 394:203–206

169. Vujanic GM, Delemarre JF, Moeslichan S, Lam J, Harms D, Sandstedt B, Voute PA (1993) Mesoblastic nephroma metastatic to the lungs and heart – Another face of this peculiar lesion: Case report and review of the literature. Pediatr Pathol 13:143–153

170. Vujanic GM, Sandstedt B, Harms D, Kelsey A, Leuschner I, de Kraker J (2002) Revised International Society of Paediatric Oncology (SIOP) working classification of renal tumors of childhood. Med Pediatr Oncol 38:79–82

171. Vujanic GM, Kelsey A, Mitchell C, Shannon RS, Gornall P (2003) The role of biopsy in the diagnosis of renal tumors of childhood: Results of the UKCCSG Wilms' tumor study 3. Med Pediatr Oncol 40:18–22

172. Waziri M, Patil SR, Hanson JW, Bartley JA (1983) Abnormality of chromosome 11 in patients with features of Beckwith-Wiedemann syndrome. J Pediatr 102:873–876

173. Weeks DA, Beckwith JB, Mierau GW, Luckey DW (1989) Rhabdoid tumor of kidney. A report of 111 cases from the National Wilms' Tumor Study Pathology Center. Am J Surg Pathol 13:439–458

174. Wiedemann R (1983) Tumours and hemihypertrophy associated with Wiedemann-Beckwith syndrome. Eur J Pediatri 141:129

175. Wilimas JA, Magill L, Parham DM, Jerkins G, Kumar M, Douglass EC (1990) Is renal salvage feasible in unilateral Wilms' tumor? Proposed computed tomographic criteria and their relation to surgicopathologic findings. Am J Pediatr Hematol Oncol 12:164–167

176. Willetts IE (2003) Jessop and the Wilms' tumor. J Pediatr Surg 38:1496–1498

177. Wilms M (1899) Die Mischgeschwulste der Niere. Die Mischgeschwulste, Arthur Georgi, Leipzig, 1:143

178. Zoeller G, Pekrun A, Lakomek M, Ringert RH (1994) Wilms' tumor: The problem of diagnostic accuracy in children undergoing preoperative chemotherapy without histological tumor verification. J Urol 151:169–171

179. Zuppan CW, Beckwith JB, Luckey DW (1988) Anaplasia in unilateral Wilms' tumor: A report from the National Wilms' Tumor Study Pathology Center. Hum Pathol 19:1199–1209

180. Zuppan CW, Beckwith JB, Weeks DA, Luckey DW, Pringle KC (1991) The effect of preoperative therapy on the histologic features of Wilms' tumor. An analysis of cases from the Third National Wilms' Tumor Study. Cancer 68:385–394

181. Inoue, M, Uchida K, Kohei O, Nahida Y, Deguchi T, Komada Y, Kusunoki M (2006) Teratoid Wilms' tumor: A case report with literature review. J Pediatr Surg 41:1759–1763

Neuroblastoma and Other Adrenal Tumors

11

Michael P. La Quaglia, Daniel N. Rutigliano

Contents

11.1 Neuroblastoma

11.1.1 History

Neuroblastoma is a malignancy of childhood derived from neural crest cells appearing anywhere along the distribution of the sympathetic nervous system. It is the most common extra-cranial solid tumor of infancy, with most cases occurring under 1 year of age. The term neuroblastoma first originated in 1910 and was used by Dr. James Wright to describe a new group of tumors [1]. These neuroblastic tumors run a spectrum from poorly differentiated and malignant (neuroblastoma), to partially differentiated (ganglioneuroblastoma), and ending with completely differentiated and benign ganglioneuroma [2].

Outcomes in these patients were poor in the early 1900s as surgery was the only modality available for treatment. In the 1960s the introduction of chemotherapy in the treatment of these patients began and with it came improvement in survival rates. However, certain groups of these patients continued to do poorly despite aggressive treatment leading to the development of specific risk factors for determining disease aggressiveness and subsequently the type of therapies used. Today most children under 1 year of age or with low-risk tumors continue to have a good prognosis with successful treatments, but over 40% of patients will present with metastatic disease. Of those with metastatic disease most will not survive more than 5 years [3].

This chapter will cover the incidence, pathology, and treatment of neuroblastoma as well as other tumors of adrenal origin in the pediatric patient.

11.1.2 Embryology

The adrenal glands (suprarenal glands) develop from cells of two different origins. The adrenal cortex is formed from cells originating from the mesoderm while the adrenal medulla develops from neural crest cells. Neural crest cells form from ventrolateral migration of neuro-ectodermal cells originating within the neural tube at approximately 3 weeks of development. These neural crest cells divide into two cell groups that give rise to sensory ganglia of cranial and spinal nerves as well as migrating to various other positions in the body to give rise to melanocytes and sympathetic ganglia (Fig. 11.1). The adrenal cortex is formed first, usually during the sixth week of development. By the seventh week neural crest cells from sympathetic ganglia migrate to form a mass on the medial side of the developing cortex. Over the next few months un-

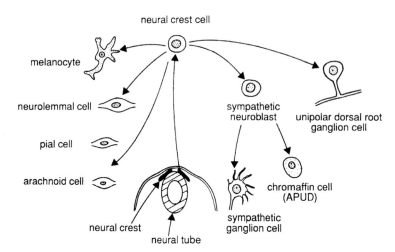

Fig. 11.1 Pathways of neural crest cell differentiation.

til birth the fetal cortex will grow and differentiate as it encapsulates itself around the mass of neural crest cells. As they are surrounded, these cells differentiate into the secretory cells of the adrenal medulla. At about 1 year of age the final architecture of the adrenal gland is present with 3 layers of adrenal cortex surrounding the mature cells of the adrenal medulla [4].

11.1.3 Incidence

Sympathetic nervous system tumors account for 7.8% of all pediatric cancer in children less than 15 years of age, of which over 97% are neuroblastomas. Neuroblastomas are the most common cancer of infancy, with an incidence rate approximately double that of leukemia. Approximately 650 children are diagnosed with neuroblastoma each year with an annual incidence rate of 9.5 per million children. This incidence rate appears to be stable over a 21-year observation period. Rates among infants, however, may be increasing somewhat in recent years [5].

Age plays a significant role in neuroblastoma, with infants and children under 1 year of age having twice the incidence rate of children in their second year of life. Sixteen percent of infant neuroblastomas are diagnosed during the first month of life and 41% are found by 3 months of age [5]. These perinatal neuroblastomas typically have a clinical course that is generally benign with regression in the size of the mass over time [6].

11.1.3.1 Risk Factors

There have been many reports of environmental factors and/or medical conditions associated with the development of neuroblastoma. Most of these studies,

however, do not have enough statistical power or data collection to conclusively establish a definitive link. A few reports have demonstrated a dose-response relationship with alcohol use as well as the development of fetal alcohol syndrome [7, 8]. Paternal exposures to occupational hazards such as pesticides and electromagnetic fields have also been implicated [9, 10]. Maternal smoking does not appear to be a risk in early studies, but increased medical use of drugs such as amphetamines, phenytoin for seizures, diuretics, or treatments for vaginal infections, and use of recreational drugs appear to have an increased risk [7, 8, 11].

Birth characteristics do not appear to incur any risk factors. Use of sex hormones and fertility drugs, however, has been superficially linked with the development of neuroblastoma [12]. A report evaluating a history of breast-feeding in neuroblastoma patients found that there was an inverse relationship between the two. Children who were breast-fed were less likely to develop neuroblastoma and this relationship increased with longer periods of breast-feeding duration [13]. Folic acid has long been known to protect against neural tube defects but it has also been linked to a 60% reduction in incidence rates of neuroblastoma in one Canadian study after folic acid fortification of flour was initiated [14].

All of these studies lack sufficient patient populations and/or statistical power to unequivocally be associated with an increased risk of neuroblastoma. This does not preclude a possible role of environmental factors, but to date no strong environmental exposure or factor has been identified.

11.1.3.2 Associated Syndromes and Heredity

No strong familial inheritance patterns for neuroblastoma have been well established. About 1–2% of children diagnosed have a history of another family member with neuroblastoma, suggesting a possible dominant pattern with incomplete penetrance [15]. The appearance of neuroblastoma in monozygotic twins has been reported in 7 cases in the literature. These cases most likely represent twin–twin placental metastasis rather than any true type of genetic syndrome [16, 17]. It should be emphasized to parents that siblings and future offspring are only at minimal risk for future development of disease [15].

Associated congenital abnormalities occur rarely with neuroblastoma but there may be an association with other syndromes of neural crest origin such as Hirschsprung's disease, central hypoventilation syndrome (Ondine's curse), neurofibromatosis (von Recklinghausen's disease), and hypomelanosis of Ito [18–21]. These syndromes are part of the so-called neurocristopathies and may have common genetic mutations that contribute to tumorigenesis.

11.1.4 Histopathology

Histological and molecular analysis of neuroblastoma cells has become an important factor in the evaluation of patients and in treatment planning. An open biopsy is usually recommended to obtain an adequate amount of tissue sampling and to preserve histological architecture, rather than fine needle biopsy. In some centers multiple needle biopsies have provided adequate diagnostic tissue.

11.1.4.1 Histology

Neuroblastoma cells are typically small round blue cells with hyperchromatic nuclei and a scant amount of cytoplasm. Neuritic processes or neuropil are seen as well as Homer-Wright pseudo rosettes (Fig. 11.2a–c). Histologically the tumor must be differentiated from similar small, round blue cell tumors such as Ewing's sarcoma, lymphoma, and rhabdomyosarcoma (Fig. 11.2d). As these cells are of sympathetic neural origin they will stain for various neural proteins and filaments that help to aid in the diagnosis. The stage of differentiation of these neuroblastoma cells varies from immature to mature and presents a spectrum that may be found within one tumor specimen. The amount of Schwann cells present appears to correlate with the degree of maturation found.

Various methods of histological classification have been proposed over the years, but the Shimada system has become the most widely used and accepted. This system of evaluation categorizes neuroblastoma into two histological groupings, favorable and unfavorable. These groupings are based upon the age of the patient, the mitotic-karyorrhexis index, the amount of Schwann cells, and the degree of cellular differentiation [22]. Numerous studies have shown that this classification correlates significantly with disease prognosis and outcome [23–26]. A new International Neuroblastoma Pathology Classification has been developed and is outlined in Chap. 6.

Recently, a new subtype of undifferentiated neuroblastoma has been identified. This subtype has been labeled as large cell neuroblastoma due to the fact that it is composed of predominantly larger-than-normal appearing cells with sharply outlined nuclear membranes and 1–4 prominent nucleoli [27]. Enlargement and a greater number of prominent nucleoli in neuroblastoma has been reported to correlate with amplification of the N-myc oncogene [28]. When compared with patients with traditional undifferentiated neuroblastoma, these patients were noted to present with disease at an older age, with a higher rate of metastatic disease, and to have a much poorer outcome. Due to its rare nature and the limited information available within the literature, more work is needed to further characterize and differentiate this subtype from traditional neuroblastoma before any other recommendations can be made.

11.1.4.2 Biological Features

In an attempt to further study the mechanism of neuroblastoma tumor development, numerous molecular and cell biology assays have been performed on these cells. These studies have found associations between biologic features and disease aggressiveness, response to chemotherapy, survival, and relapse rates.

The DNA index (DNA ploidy) has become an important indicator of disease responsiveness. The DNA index refers to the amount of DNA within the nucleus of the cell compared to expected amounts. This is usually measured via flow cytometry or cytogenetic analysis. Hyperdiploidy (DNA index >1) has been found to correlate with a better response to chemotherapy, lower disease stage at presentation, and improved overall outcome [29–31]. This improvement in outcome is especially noted in the infant population [29]. Conversely, the opposite is true for diploid tumor specimens.

N-myc is an oncogene found on chromosome 2p and the discovery of its potential for amplification in neuroblastoma has led it to become one of the most important biological factors for prognosis [31, 32]. N-myc is a transcription factor which binds with another protein called Max to activate its targets for transcription. It is suspected that overexpression of N-myc may activate angiogenesis pathways that increase tumor growth and metastasis [33]. Detection of amplification can be accomplished by a variety of techniques

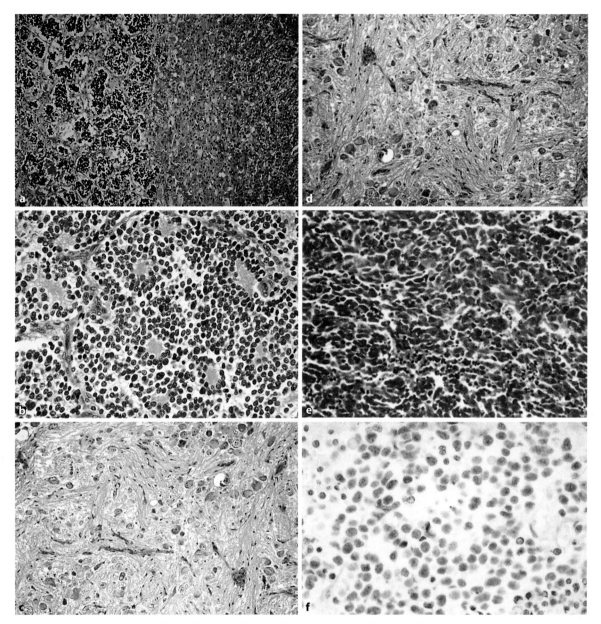

Fig. 11.2 a Photomicrograph of neuroblastoma showing the small uniform cells with dense, darkly staining nuclei and scant cytoplasm. Homer–Wright pseudorosettes are also seen. **b** Photomicrograph of ganglioneuroblastoma showing islands of neu- roblastoma cells surrounded by ganglioneuroma. **c** Photomicrograph comprised of mature ganglion cells, Schwann's cells and neuropil. **d** Unidifferentiated small round cell tumor

including PCR, Southern blot, fluorescent in situ hybridization (FISH), and immunohistochemistry. Most centers and cooperative groups consider 10 or more copies of N-myc detected by FISH to be consistent with genomic amplification (Fig. 11.3). Mice models that have been induced to overexpress N-myc develop neuroblastoma, providing further evidence of a direct link of this gene with tumorigenesis [34]. The excess number of N-myc genes usually leads to a higher level of expression of N-myc protein but it appears that the amplification itself rather than the overexpression is the predominant adverse factor [23, 35–37].

Approximately 30% of neuroblastoma cases are found to be N-myc amplified. Amplification is much more likely in cases of advanced stage (40–45%) versus low stage neuroblastoma (5–10%). When present in low stage disease, however, it may predict poorer survival and outcome. Overall patients with N-myc amplification have rapid disease progression and 90% will die of disease progression regardless of therapy

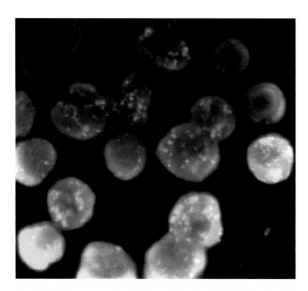

Fig. 11.3 Fluorescent in situ hybridization (FISH) showing N-myc amplification in tumors cells.

provided. Shimada classification, DNA Index, and N-myc amplification have all been found to be independent prognostic variables in disease progression and outcome [23, 31, 38–40]. Hyperdiploidy has been found to rarely occur with N-myc amplification, but when it does it appears that the effects of amplification outweigh the more favorable prognosis of the DNA hyperploidy [39].

Nerve growth factor (NGF) and its receptor tyrosine kinase (TRK) have also been found to correlate with disease and progression. TRK is a transmembrane protein and appears to be involved in cellular differentiation and apoptosis [41, 42]. There are three subtypes of receptors found, TRK-A, TRK-B, and TRK-C. Expression of TRK-A on the cells of neuroblastoma has been found to correlate with a good prognosis, younger age, and tumor regression. Lack of TRK-A is seen with overexpression of N-myc and consequently carriers a poorer prognosis [41, 43–45]. These data suggest that the TRK-A/NGF pathway plays a role in the neuroblastoma differentiation and programmed cell death seen in the regression of tumors among infants. The presence of TRK-B is associated with chromosomal abnormalities such as gain of 17q and loss of heterozygosity for 14q. TRK-B expression is seen in many tumors that have a poor outcome and may correlate with N-myc amplification [42, 46]. Reports have also shown that TRK-B activation can have a role in chemotherapeutic resistance within these tumors [47, 48]. TRK-C is seen in tumors with favorable prognosis and no N-myc amplification [49]. The balance of expression of these three tyrosine kinase receptors may be what is important in maintaining a favorable prognosis and disease regression [50].

Chromosomal aberrations in neuroblastoma are frequently present. Loss of heterozygosity and deletion of chromosome 1p has been found in 30–50% of neuroblastoma, more commonly in tumors of diploid karyotype [51, 52]. This finding has been found to correlate strongly with N-myc amplification and poor prognosis [53–57]. This segment may be the site of a suppressor gene of N-myc function or amplification [58]. Loss of 1p is a risk factor for disease progression and is seen in very few low-stage tumors. Identification of this abnormality should promote an upstaging of a low-risk tumor to a higher grouping for more intensive therapy [54, 56].

Gain on chromosome 17, specifically the 17q region, is another abnormality commonly found on genetic analysis. This region is considered to house the Survivin gene; this gene is a family member of inhibitor of apoptosis proteins. It has been reported to occur in as many as 50% of neuroblastoma cases and is an adverse prognostic factor correlating with advanced age at diagnosis, N-myc amplification with 1p deletion, and increased relapse rates [59–61]. Similar to N-myc, it is gene amplification of this region rather than gene expression that appears to be correlated to poor prognosis and higher stage [62].

Various other genes and chromosomal abnormalities have been reported in the literature as well with varying degrees of impact. These include loss of heterozygosity for 14q, bcl-2 overexpression, ras expression, ret expression, and telomerase activity. Based upon these analyses three biological groups of neuroblastoma have been proposed. The first subgroup is found in patients younger than 1 year of age with hyperdiploidy and TRK-A expression and tends to regress spontaneously. The second subgroup begins to show some evidence of cytogenetic instability with 17q gain, TRK-B expression, and a near-diploid karyotype. This group of tumors tends to occur in older patients with more advance disease and progression. The third subgroup has loss of chromosome 1p, N-myc amplification, and diploid DNA karyotype. Tumor growth is rapid and aggressive within this group with most children presenting with advance disease and an expected survival of <5% [63, 64] (Table 11.1).

11.1.5 Clinical Presentation

Tumor symptoms are variable and depend upon the age of the patient at diagnosis, the site of origin, and the presence of metastatic involvement. Most neuroblastomas are found in children less than 1 year of age and can be seen on fetal ultrasound in rare cases of perinatal neuroblastoma by about 33 weeks of gestation [6]. Sixty-five percent of neuroblastomas originate within the abdomen in the adrenal gland, though this number raises

Table 11.1 Biologic subtypes of neuroblastoma

Features	Type 1	Type 2	Type 3
Age	<1 yr	>1 yr	>1 yr
DNA Ploidy	Hyperdiploid	Near diploid	Near diploid
TRK expression	High TRK-A	TRK-B	High TRK-B
N-myc amplification	None	Low	High
Chromosomal Aberrations	None	17q gain	1p LOH, 17q gain
Outcomes	Good, tumor regression often	Advance stage of disease, 40–50% survival	Rapid tumor growth and metastasis, Poor survival

to 90% for tumors diagnosed within the first month after birth [6]. The organ of Zuckerkandl in the pelvis near the aortic bifurcation is the second most common location for tumors of abdominal origin. Outside of the abdomen, thoracic and cervical paraspinal tumors are the next most common locations of origin.

Symptoms vary with location of the primary mass. An abdominal primary can present with abdominal pain, increasing abdominal girth/distention or changes in bowel or dietary habits. Patients with severe distention may even present with respiratory distress secondary to massive liver involvement, impaired diaphragm movement, and abdominal cavity volume loss (Fig. 11.4). Tumors arising within the organ of Zuckerkandl may involve the small bowel and/or the bladder resulting in dysfunction and possible urinary or gastrointestinal obstruction [65]. Paraspinal tumors can invade neural foramina and/or nerve plexus resulting in paresthesias and possible paralysis. Dural involvement can cause spinal cord compression and

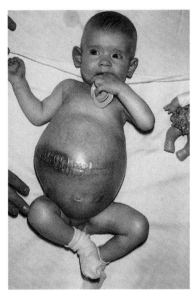

Fig. 11.4 Patient with marked abdominal distention from Stage 4S neuroblastoma.

requiring emergent steroid and chemotherapy treatments. Multifocal neuroblastoma is rare and usually presents in infants where it surprisingly has a good prognosis [66].

Fetal neuroblastomas are frequently noted as incidental findings on ultrasound as noted above but there can be associated maternal signs and symptoms correlating with disease. Signs of catecholamine excess such as excessive sweating, headaches, flushing, or anxiety may be seen in the mother [67, 68]. Pre-eclampsia has been associated with widely disseminated fetal neuroblastoma. Large tumor size or metastatic involvement of the placenta is associated with the development of fetal hydrops [6, 69]. Treatment algorithms involve serial ultrasounds for stable pregnancies to tocolytics and steroids in cases of pre-eclampsia and fetal hydrops [69].

In neuroblastoma presenting postnatally, metastatic disease infiltrating bone and bone marrow may result in a presentation of generalized bone pain and limping. Marrow involvement can lead to anemia, leukopenia, and thrombocytosis with resultant weakness, infection, and abnormal bleeding or bruising [65]. Patients with Stage 4S disease characteristically present with nontender subcutaneous nodules that have a purple/blue or gray color to them. These represent metastatic deposits of neuroblastoma cells. Spread of metastases to the periorbital and retro-bulbar areas of the eyes may present with the appearance of "raccoon eyes" and give the impression of facial trauma to the child (Fig. 11.5).

Rarely, children with neuroblastoma can present with a paraneoplastic syndrome consisting of symptoms related to opsoclonus/myoclonus and/or ataxia. This syndrome often results in rapid bursts of chaotic eye movements, irregular jerking movements of the muscles, and ataxia. The mechanism for this syndrome has not been fully elucidated but it appears to be an immunologic mechanism related to antineuronal antibodies and a primary tumor that is usually densely infiltrated with lymphocytes [70–72]. Although opso-

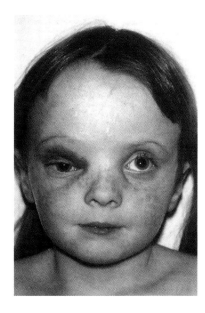

Fig. 11.5 "Raccoon eyes" resulting from neuroblastoma metastatic to both orbits.

clonus is uncommon among neuroblastoma patients, approximately 50% of patients who present with opsoclonus will have neuroblastoma [73]. Most patients with this syndrome tend to have localized disease and favorable outcome [74]. Neurologic function remains poor, however, as this syndrome tends to be pervasive despite tumor removal and can be associated with neurologic and cognitive deficits as well as psychomotor retardation [70, 72]. Treatment with adrenocorticotropic hormone (ACTH) is effective in some cases in reduction of symptoms; otherwise plasmapheresis and intravenous gamma-globulin have been reported to be effective in refractory cases [74, 75]. Currently, there is an ongoing randomized prospective COG trial (ANBL00P3) that is attempting to evaluate the effectiveness of immunosuppressive therapy combined with cyclophosphamide use. In addition, the study will look at how the addition of intravenous gamma-globulin improves response rates as well as long-term outcomes from this syndrome.

11.1.6 Diagnostic Work-up

The diagnosis of neuroblastoma requires a pathologist familiar with these tumors and other small, round, blue cell tumors such as lymphomas, neuro-ectodermal tumors and rhabdomyosarcoma. The minimum international criteria for the establishment of diagnosis is either a tissue biopsy with histological confirmation or the presence of unequivocal tumor cells within a bone marrow biopsy/aspirate AND increased levels of urinary catecholamine metabolites [31]. Immunohistochemistry and genetic analysis have become increasing important procedures performed upon the

diagnosis of these tissues as discussed earlier in this chapter.

Ninety to ninety-five percent of all neuroblastomas will have elevated urinary catecholamines. The two most common metabolites found are vanillylmandelic acid (VMA) and homovanillic acid (HVA); these are the metabolites of dopamine and norepinephrine, respectively [65]. Levels of these metabolites are age specific and can be altered with renal function impairment or excessive dietary intake of amines such as bananas in infants [76]. There have been many attempts internationally at mass screening of the pediatric population based upon VMA and HVA levels [77–79]. All have resulted in increased incidence of neuroblastoma, especially among the perinatal and infant populations, but there have been no reductions in overall mortality despite early favorable reports from Japan [77, 80, 81]. There has also been no reduction in the incidence of advanced stage disease among those countries which have performed screening [82]. As a result, screening the mass population for neuroblastoma has proven to be neither cost effective nor useful in lowering mortality from advance disease and is not recommended. Screening programs have been discontinued in most countries, including Japan.

Approximately 70% of patients with neuroblastoma have been found to have metastatic disease at diagnosis. As a result of this, all newly diagnosed patients must undergo bilateral bone marrow aspirates and biopsies to determine the extent of disease. Imagining studies of the primary tumor site via CT or MRI are valuable in establishing baseline measurement of tumor size as well as evaluating for metastatic disease within the chest or abdomen (Figs. 11.6–11.10). CT scans are the preferred method for evaluation of chest and abdominal tumors while MRI has its greatest usefulness in the evaluation of paraspinal tumors. I131 metaio-

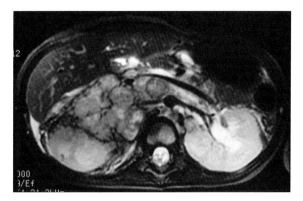

Fig. 11.6 Axial T2-weighted image demonstrates a large right adrenal mass and conglomerate adenopathy which encases the aorta and bilateral renal arteries. The IVC and left renal vein are displaced. Irregular marrow involvement of the vertebral body is seen.

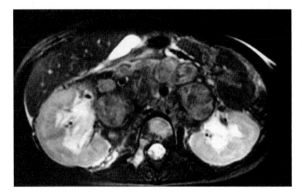

Fig. 11.7 Axial T2-weighted image shows extensive adenopathy extending across the midline. The aorta and IVC are encased by tumor. Marrow involvement is seen in the right posterior element and vertebral body.

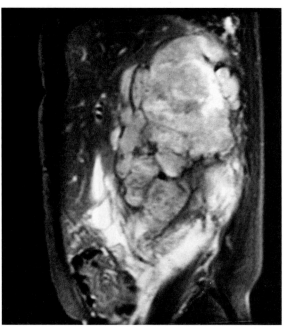

Fig. 11.9 Sagittal T2-weighted image demonstrates extensive nodal masses.

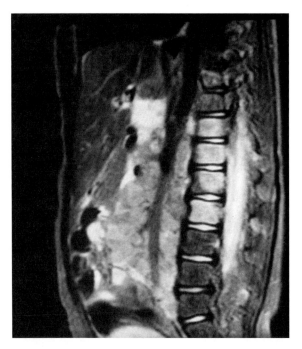

Fig. 11.8 Displacement of the aorta which is encased by mass and adenopathy is seen on sagittal T2-weighted image. Several vertebral bodies are involved.

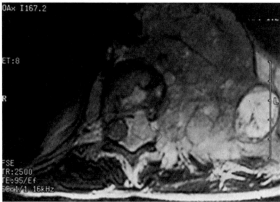

Fig. 11.10 Axial T2-weighted image shows a displaced spinal cord by tumor extension through the neural foramen. The aorta is encased.

dobenzylguanidine (MIBG) scan or bone scans are needed to evaluate for bony disease. MIBG scans use a labeled isotope derivative of norepinephrine to view for areas of increased uptake and activity (Fig. 11.11). This whole body scan is very accurate and specific for the detection of metastasis and occult disease. In addition, MIBG scan can be used to evaluate the effectiveness of therapy in high-risk patients and may be able to detect residual bone marrow or cortical disease not otherwise discovered by other imaging modalities [83]. Recently, there has been use of PET scanning for

the detection of non-MIBG avid disease or in the follow-up of high risk patients after resection [84].

Complete blood count as well as serum chemistries are also needed during the initial work-up. Elevated levels of serum lactate dehydrogenase (LDH) >1,000 and ferritin levels >150 have been associated with adverse outcomes of disease, most likely representing increased tumor burden [23]. Lumbar puncture is not necessary as central nervous system (CNS) metastasis is rare and puncture may be associated with increased risk of CNS metastasis development [85]. See Chap. 4.

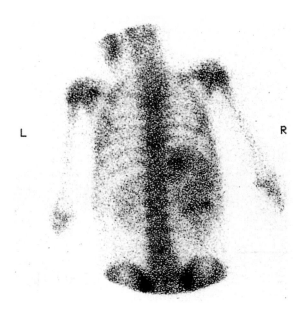

Fig. 11.11 MIGB Scan showing increased uptake within the tumor.

11.1.7 Staging

The use of staging criteria to accurately describe the extent of disease present in these patients has been of great importance to helping physicians map out and organize treatment plans. Four systems have evolved over time: the Evans classification [86], the St. Jude system [87], the TNM (Tumor-Nodal-Metastasis) system, and the International Neuroblastoma Staging System (INSS) [31].

The INSS was established in 1989 and is currently the most accepted and widely used system (Fig. 11.12). Similarities exist among the staging systems, with most agreeing that completely resected localized tumor constitutes Stage 1 disease. Stage 2 disease is divided into 2A and 2B based upon the incomplete resection and/or the presence of positive ipsilateral lymph nodes. Stage 3 disease describes the presence of the primary tumor crossing the midline or a unilateral tumor with positive contralateral lymph nodes, also any tumor originating from the midline with bilateral lymph node involvement. All classifications describe Stage 4 disease with the presence of tumor dissemination to other organs, bone, or distant lymph nodes. Also common to all systems is a subtype of Stage 4 disease term Stage 4-S. This subtype is reserved for infants and children less than 1 year of age with localized primary tumors, minimal marrow involvement, and spread limited to the skin and liver. This pattern of disease spread has been associated with a better outcome than other Stage 4 patients [88–90].

A recent European study attempted to establish guidelines for stage I patients for initial surgery or no surgery based upon predetermined radiological surgical risk factors schema [91]. The idea was to avoid surgery and its complications in those patients in whom a complete resection was not appropriate. Though this study was hindered by a lack of compliance to the protocol, in the future a staging system may be developed that is not dependant upon the current need for surgical intervention.

11.1.8 Risk Groupings

To guide physicians in treatment planning, a risk stratification system has been developed in which patients are assigned to one of three groupings: low, intermediate, and high risk. These groupings are based upon the success of treatment given and survival rates. The benefit of risk grouping is to provide the patient with the best possible treatment plan while minimizing the need for toxic therapies.

In North America, risk grouping is based upon recommendations of the Children's Oncology Group (COG) schema (Table 11.2). Three groups consisting of low, intermediate, or high risk were created and based upon overall survival rates of >90%, 70%–90%, and <30% 3 years after diagnosis. Determination of a patient's risk assignment is based upon INSS stage, age, N-myc status, Shimada histologic classification, and DNA ploidy.

11.1.8.1 Low Risk

All patients with INSS Stage 1 disease are low-risk patients regardless of age, N-myc status, Shimada class, or DNA ploidy. All INSS Stage 2A/2B patients are also in this group with the exception of those who are >1 year old, that have N-myc amplification AND unfavorable Shimada class. Stage 4S patients (who by definition are <1 year of age) that are without N-myc amplification have a favorable Shimada histology and are hyperdiploid are also in this group.

11.1.8.2 Intermediate Risk

All INSS Stage 3 and 4 patients who are <1 year of age AND without N-myc amplification are intermediate risk regardless of other tumor biology features. Patients with INSS Stage 3 disease who are >1 year old without N-myc amplification AND a favorable Shimada histology are also in this grouping. INSS Stage 4S patients are upgraded to intermediate risk if they are without N-myc amplification but have either

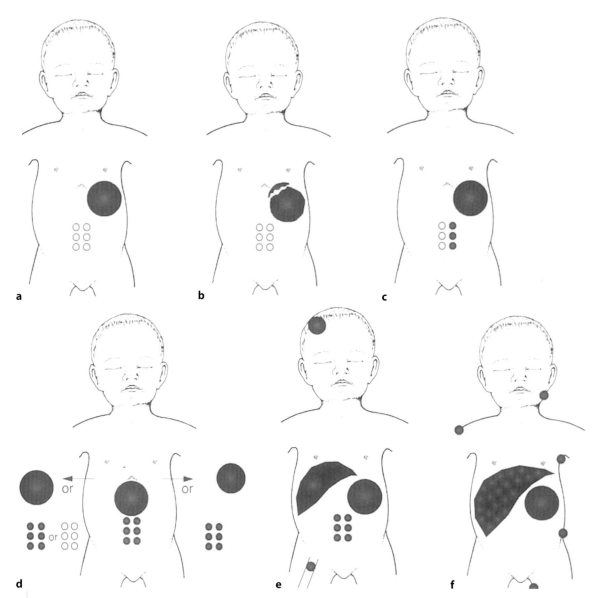

Fig. 11.12 International neuroblastoma staging system (INSS). Stage 1: Completely resected localized tumor confined to the area of origin with negative lymph nodes. Stage 2A: Incompletely resected localized tumor with negative lymph nodes. Stage 2B: Unilateral tumor with complete or incomplete resection; positive ipsilateral lymph nodes, *contralateral* lymph nodes negative. Stage 3: Large ipsilateral tumor crossing the midline with or without positive regional lymph node involvement; or a unilateral tumor with positive contralateral lymph nodes; or a midline tumor with bilateral regional lymph node involvement. Stage 4: Metastatic tumor spread to distant organs, lymph nodes, and bone marrow. Stage 4S: Subset of Stage 4 patients who are less than 1 year of age and present with a localized tumor with limited tumor dissemination to the liver, skin, and/or bone marrow.

unfavorable Shimada histology OR near diploid DNA status.

11.1.8.3 High Risk

All INSS Stage 4 patients >1 year of age fall into this grouping as well as Stage 4 patients <1 year with N-myc amplification. Stage 3 patients of any age with N-myc amplification are defined as high risk as well. Stage 3 patients >1 year old without N-myc amplification but who have an unfavorable Shimada histology are upgraded to high risk. Patients with INSS Stage 2A/2B are upgraded to high risk if they are >1 year old and possess BOTH N-myc amplification and an unfavorable Shimada histology. Any Stage 4S

Table 11.2 Children's Oncology Group Neuroblastoma Risk Group Assignment Schema

INSS Stage	Age	MYCN Status	Shimada Classification	DNA Ploidy	Risk Group
1	0–21y	Any	Any	Any	Low
2A/2B	<365d	Any	Any	Any	Low
	≥365d–21y	NonAmp	Any	–	Low
	≥365d–21y	Amp	Fav	–	Low
	≥ 365d–21y	Amp	Unfav	–	High
3	<365d	NonAmp	Any	Any	Intermediate
	<365d	Amp	Any	Any	High
	≥365d–21y	NonAmp	Fav	–	Intermediate
	≥365d–21y	NonAmp	Unfav	–	High
	≥365d–21y	Amp	Any	–	High
4	<548d	NonAmp	Any	Any	Intermediate
	<548d	Amp	Any	Any	High
	≥548d–21y	Any	Any	–	High
4S	<365d	NonAmp	Fav	>1	Low
	<365d	NonAmp	Any	=1	Intermediate
	<365d	NonAmp	Unfav	Any	Intermediate
	<365d	Amp	Any	Any	High
Biology Defined By:	MYCN Status: Amplified (Amp) versus NonAmplified (NonAmp) Shimada Classification: Favorable (Fav) versus Unfavorable (Unfav) DNA Ploidy: DNA Index (DI) >1 is favorable, =1 is unfavorable; hypodiploid tumors (with DI <1) will be treated as a tumor with a DI >1 (DNA index <1 [hypodiploid] to be considered favorable ploidy).				

patient with N-myc amplification is upgraded to high risk.

The discovery of new biological and genetic markers provides constant pressure to adjust these groupings to include new data. As a result some controversy exists over how to handle small subgroups of patients within these larger groups. Some studies out of Europe advocate the inclusion of chromosome 1p status to the risk-grouping scheme. These data use 1p status along with age, stage, and N-myc status to define a new group of low-risk patients who have improved survival over those with 1p abnormalities [57]. The benefit to such a grouping may be the reduction of chemotherapy given to patients with localized disease and normal chromosome 1p.

11.1.9 Treatment

The planning and treatment of neuroblastoma is intimately linked with the stage and prognosis of the patients' disease. Treatment of neuroblastoma is a multi-modality effort using surgery, chemotherapy, radiation and bone marrow/stem cell transplantation. The use of each therapy will be discussed below as needed. All patients should have baseline urinary catecholamine metabolites (VMA, HVA) measured prior to the onset of therapy. These metabolites can function as a marker for treatment success and if elevated can mean the presence of persistent disease or recurrence.

11.1.9.1 Spinal Cord Compression

Immediate treatment should be undertaken for neuroblastoma with symptomatic spinal cord compression. Symptoms can include paralysis or parasthesia, incontinence, and bladder dysfunction. Recovery appears to be improved with a shorter duration of compression and less intensity of symptoms. Decompression of the cord is warranted and may be accomplished via laminotomy, radiation, or chemotherapy. All appear to have similar outcomes but surgery may result in scoliosis later in life [92, 93]. Since most patients will probably require chemotherapy with or without surgery, current COG recommendations are for chemotherapy first with surgery reserved for patients who do not improve [94–96]. The risk of scoliosis is directly related to the use of laminectomy and the dose of radiation.

11.1.9.2 Fetal and Perinatal Tumors

The diagnosis of neuroblastoma within the fetal and perinatal population has increased dramatically over the past few decades with improvements in obstetrical ultrasound technology. Over 90% are located within the adrenal gland [69, 97], with most being localized INSS Stage 1 or 2 tumors [97–99]. The health and well-being of the mother are of paramount importance and pregnancies can be carried to term as long as no complications from pre-eclampsia or fetal hydrops occur. Monitoring the growth of detected masses can be achieved with serial ultrasounds at scheduled visits. Maternal or fetal distress after 28 weeks of gestation should prompt the use of tocolytics as well as steroids for fetal lung maturity and delivery as soon as possible [69]. Published data on these patients have shown that the vast majority of these tumors have favorable biologic profiles with no N-myc amplification [97–99]. Treatment for these patients should be based upon COG risk grouping, with the majority falling into the low risk group. These patients do very well with surgery alone and have an associated survival of 96% and an event-free survival of 91% [6].

Because of the low biological aggressiveness of these tumors as well as the good long-term outcome, observation has also been recommended for these patients. The presumption is that these tumors will regress and newborns will be spared the invasiveness and potential complications of surgery. Tumors less than 5 cm are very likely to be of low stage and can be followed via serial ultrasound to monitor for increased growth and spread [6]. VMA and HVA levels can also be monitored as a relative indicator for increased size and spread. Studies have shown that patients monitored with this approach continue to have good survival rates with two thirds of patients avoiding surgery secondary to tumor regression. In those patients where tumor growth continued to increase on ultrasound, these patients underwent successful surgical resection without any upstaging of disease. Chemotherapy is still effective as salvage if needed [6, 100, 101]. The COG is currently investigating observation as a viable management option in perinatal neuroblastoma patients with a prospective single arm clinical trial.

11.1.9.3 Low-Risk Group

Patients in this group have a survival rate of >90%. Patients with INSS Stage 1 disease can be treated with surgery alone without the need for adjuvant chemotherapy [102, 103]. Relapse following excision can be successfully treated with chemotherapy at that time to induce remission. As discussed above, small, localized tumors discovered at birth or during the prenatal period can potentially be observed as they tend to spontaneously regress [104].

Stage 2A/2B low-risk tumors are also treated with initial surgery without the need for preoperative chemotherapy. Overall survival in these patients is >90% with surgery alone [105, 106]. The application of chemotherapy is reserved for patients in whom <50% of tumor was resected or in patients who possess severe organ/life threatening symptoms [107]. Chemotherapy consists of a platin agent (usually carboplatin), cyclophosphamide, doxorubicin, and etoposide. This is given for 6–24 weeks with doses dependant upon the extent of disease and patient age/weight. Radiation therapy is rarely given in this group and is reserved only for tumors presenting with life-threatening symptoms or spinal cord compression.

Treatment of children with low-risk Stage 4S disease has been controversial in the past and is dependant upon the clinical presentation of the patient. These tumors have favorable biologic features and survival rates of 80–95%. Children who are asymptomatic with disease appear to have a good outcome when treated with supportive care alone as some of these tumors can undergo spontaneous regression [90, 108–110]. Of the patients who do present with symptoms, these can be managed with minimal low-dose chemotherapy; resection of the primary tumor does not appear to improve outcome or survival. Some infants with Stage 4S disease may present with extensive and diffuse liver involvement that can cause respiratory compromise and symptoms of abdominal compartment syndrome with decreased venous return and renal impairment. These patients may require ventilator support and abdominal decompression surgery in addition to systemic chemotherapy and radiation therapy to the liver.

11.1.9.4 Intermediate-Risk Group

Patients in this risk grouping have a survival rate of 70–90%. All patients in this group receive surgery and chemotherapy as the primary modalities of treatment. Goals of surgery should be to establish the diagnosis, obtain adequate tissue for histologic and biologic testing, resect as much primary tumor as possible, and perform adequate lymph node sampling for staging. Variations in survival in this group appear to be related to patient age and tumor biology, with patients less than 1 year of age, or tumors with more favorable characteristics, having higher rates of treatment success [105, 111, 112].

Chemotherapy for these patients consists of 12–24 weeks of carboplatin, cyclophosphamide, doxorubicin, and etoposide. Infants and children with tumors of favorable biology are treated with 12 weeks of low-dose chemotherapy in an attempt to reduce long-term complications and injury. Following this scheme overall survival for INSS Stage 3 patients is 95%, 90% for Stage 4S patients, and 70% for Stage 4 patients. Tumor ploidy has a particular impact on Stage 4 patients with near DNA diploidy predicting early treatment failures [113]. Chemotherapy should be given to patients to avoid any potential need for nephrectomy to treat abdominal neuroblastoma [114] and radiation therapy is reserved for residual disease after a full course of chemotherapy is received. Current COG national phase 3 trials are looking at the outcome of reduced chemotherapy treatments for patients with favorable biology to four cycles of chemotherapy and to eight cycles of chemotherapy for patients with diploid tumors or unfavorable biology [65]. A recent study by Kushner, et al. has also shown that a subset of Stage 4 patients without N-myc amplification and without extensive bone marrow involvement may do well without cytotoxic therapy [110].

11.1.9.5 High-Risk Group

This group consists of any INSS Stage 4 patients older than 1 year or those N-myc amplification, Stage 4S patients with N-myc amplification, and Stage 3 patients with N-myc amplification or unfavorable Shimada class. Stage 2A/2B patients with unfavorable tumor biology are also within the grouping. Survival in this group continues to be poor despite aggressive therapies with long-term survival between 10–30%. Survival for Stage 3 patients, however, with current intensive therapy has been improved to approximately 60% [65].

Therapy for these patients consists of intensive chemotherapy (induction and myeloablative) with surgery and radiation for local tumor control followed by maintenance therapy.

Induction Chemotherapy: The goal of induction chemotherapy is to induce tumor remission, decrease tumor growth, and improve tumor resectability if possible. Response rates vary from 60–90% with the most common drugs used being cyclophosphamide, ifosfamide, cis/carboplatin, vincristine, doxorubicin, and etoposide. One study by Kushne [115] demonstrated a highly effective protocol of cyclophosphamide, vincristine, doxorubicin alternating with cycles of cispla-

tin, and etoposide. Additional benefits of intensive induction chemotherapy include the clearing of the bone marrow of tumor cells allowing for safer harvesting of cells for autologous transplantation. The response rate of tumor to induction therapy appears to correlate with outcome and chances for long-term disease-free survival. One European study of 549 high-risk patients showed that persistent cortical bone lesions and bone marrow involvement were independent adverse prognostic factors [116]. In addition, the response of MIBG scintigraphy following therapy has been shown to highly correlate with treatment outcome [83, 117, 118].

Myeloablative Consolidation Therapy: The purpose of this round of chemotherapy is to destroy any remaining tumors cells that have survived. This stage of treatment takes place after surgery has been attempted to remove the primary tumor. The use of consolidation therapy has significantly improved progression-free survival in these patients. The European Neuroblastoma Group showed a dramatic increase in survival in patients who received consolidation therapy for 23 months versus 6 months for patients with no additional therapy [119]. A study performed by Matthay, et al. compared high-dose myeloablative consolidation therapy with autologous transplant versus nonmyeloablative consolidation therapy (Fig. 11.13). The 3-year, event-free survival rate was significantly better for the group that received more intensive chemotherapy and transplantation (34% versus 18%) [3]. Myeloablative consolidation therapy is now recommended for all high-risk patients except for those undergoing specialized protocols.

Bone Marrow/Stem Cell Transplantation: The ability to transplant stem cells for reconstitution of a patient's bone marrow has allowed for higher doses of

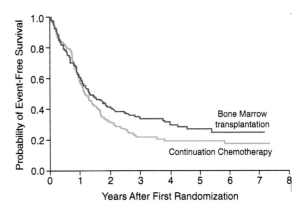

Fig. 11.13 Probability of event-free survival among patients assigned to bone marrow transplantation or continuation chemotherapy. Follow-up began at the time of the first randomization (8 weeks after diagnosis). The difference in survival between the two groups was significant at 3 years (P=0.034). Reprinted from Ref. [3].

myeloablative chemotherapy to be given to these patients. The type of bone marrow transplant received, autologous vs. allogeneic, appears to have no difference on tumor-free survival or relapse rates [120]. Advances in transplant methodology, however, have made autologous transplant the safer and more feasible method and this can be obtained through peripheral blood stem cell collection instead of traditional bone marrow harvest. Allogenic transplant has been associated with higher toxicity rates, death, and rejection, and is no longer recommended [121].

Recently there has been debate on the need for autologous stem cells collected to undergo purging of any possible neuroblastoma cells before re-infusion into patients. Neuroblastoma cells can be detected within blood samples of patients via PCR analysis in concentrations of 1 per million [122, 123]. In addition, the majority of high-risk neuroblastoma patients have metastatic disease to the bone marrow at diagnosis [124]. However, as most bone marrow and stem cell harvesting occurs after 2–4 cycles of chemotherapy, the number of viable tumor cells harvested may be at a minimum [125]. A current COG study is looking at outcomes in patients who receive purged or unpurged autologous stem cell transplant following myeloablative therapy and its effect on relapse-free survival.

Surgery: The mainstay of therapy in the treatment of local neuroblastoma, surgical intervention also has a role in both diagnosis and treatment of advanced stage neuroblastoma. Biopsy of a suspected neuroblastoma should be undertaken if needed before initial chemotherapy and can be approached by open or minimally-invasive techniques, especially in the thoracic cavity. After initial induction chemotherapy has been given and a response noted, resection of the primary tumor and local disease should be undertaken. The goal of any surgical intervention should be the removal of all gross visible disease. Surgical approach will depend upon the location of the primary tumor with a thoracoabdominal incision recommended for adrenal primaries, midline incision for pelvic tumors, open thoracotomy for thoracic tumors, and modified radical neck for cervical chain tumors (Fig. 11.14a–d). Laparoscopic adrenalectomy has been reported in the literature for small, localized, well-encapsulated tumors [126]. However, no studies have compared this approach to open resection or its effectiveness on long-term survival and local recurrence rates. Resection and staging of retroperitoneal lymph nodes are limited by this approach as well.

In the past, aggressive surgical resection of high-risk patients, especially those with Stage 4 disease, has been highly debated. Recent studies, however, have showed an improvement in survival rates with more extensive surgery and better response to chemotherapy [127–130]. La Quaglia, et al. showed that in 141 patients with Stage 4 disease, who present with a majority of metastasis to the bone, overall survival was increased to 50% and local recurrence decreased to 10% in patients who had gross total resection compared to those who did not. Other studies have shown that failure to control the primary site of disease is a leading cause of disease progression and can lead to further systemic spread [131, 132]. As a result of these findings, aggressive surgical removal of all primary tumor should be the goal of surgery in all neuroblastoma patients older than 1 year of age.

Radiotherapy: Neuroblastoma is a radiosensitive tumor and as such radiotherapy should be used in all high-risk patients after surgery regardless of the presence of gross or microscopic residual disease to reduce the incidence of primary local relapse [133]. In addition, radiotherapy has been shown to be of benefit to select 4S patients and patients with symptomatic spinal cord compression. A typical dose of 2000–2010 cGy is given to the abdomen or thoracic cavities. Total body irradiation has been used in the past prior to bone marrow transplant to ablate the marrow but is now not currently part of any protocols. The use of intraoperative radiotherapy is now being explored with increasing frequency as a means to deliver higher doses of radiation to the tumor bed with less toxicity [134–136]. Though the optimal dose response curve has yet to be finalized, these studies have shown improved local control.

Maintenance Therapy: Efforts have been made to develop therapies that will improve progression-free survival after treatment. Retinoic acid has been shown to induce neuroblastoma cells to differentiate into benign cells in culture [137, 138]. The study by Matthay et al. randomized patients to either receive 6 months of 13-cis-retinoic acid following completion of chemotherapy or no further therapy (Fig. 11.15). The patients who received retinoic acid had a significant improvement in the 3-year event-free survival [3, 139]. Furthermore it appears that high-dose pulse therapy is more efficacious than low-dose continuous infusions [140]. Side effects from extended treatment with retinoids are generally mild and include dry skin, oral fissures, cheilitis, and headaches. Currently it is recommended that all high-risk patients receive 6 months of treatment with 13-cis-retinoic acid following chemo and myeloablative therapies.

11.1.9.6 Recurrent Neuroblastoma

Recurrence of neuroblastoma is highly dependant upon the patient's initial stage of disease and tumor biology as well as upon the extent of resection and previous treatment received. Treatment of recurrent disease is determined by risk group assessment at the time of

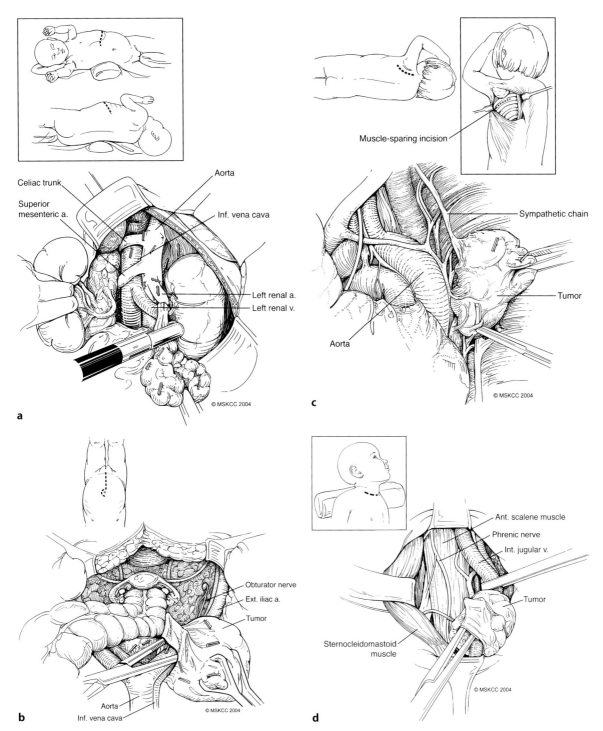

Fig. 11.14 (**a**) Patient positioning for a thoracoabdominal incision for an abdominal neuroblastoma. Identification of the inferior vena cava, aorta, celiac trunk, superior mesenteric artery, and renal vasculature is essential during dissection of tumor off surrounding tissues. (**b**) Incision for a pelvic neuroblastoma. Identification of the inferior vena cava, aorta, iliac vessels, ureter, and obturator nerve is necessary during dissection of the tumor. (**c**) Incision for a muscle-sparing thoracotomy for a thoracic neuroblastoma. Carefully dissection of tumor off the sympathetic chain should be attempted. (**d**) Modified neck incision for cervical neuroblastoma. Careful identification of underlying vascular and neurological structures, i.e., phrenic nerve, is necessary during dissection.

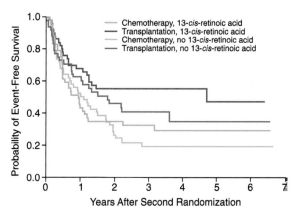

Fig. 11.15 Probability of event-free survival among patients who were randomly assigned to receive a bone marrow transplant plus 13-cis-retinoic acid, transplant without 13-cis-retinoic acid, continuation chemotherapy plus 13-cis-retinoic acid, or continuation chemotherapy without 13-cis-retinoic acid. Follow-up began at the time of the second randomization (34 weeks after diagnosis). Overall event-free survival was significantly better in the group treated with transplantation plus 13-cis-retinoic acid than in the group assigned to continuation chemotherapy without 13-cis-retinoic acid (P=0.02). Reprinted from Ref. [3].

diagnosis in addition to the patient's age and tumor biology at time of recurrence. Attempts should be made to obtain new tissue samples for biological analysis of the recurrence and comparison to the initial tumor. Widespread recurrence has a poor prognosis despite aggressive therapy [142, 143]. Central nervous system disease is more common with recurrence and may be seen in 5–10% of cases [85, 144].

Low-risk Disease: Low-risk patients with local-regional recurrence are treated with resection if possible. If a gross total resection is done, then no further treatment is needed. If less than a total resection is obtained, then 12 weeks of chemotherapy is warranted. If the tumor pathology revels unfavorable biological markers and a total resection cannot be obtained, then 24 weeks of chemotherapy is given. Local recurrence with unfavorable Shimada classification or N-myc amplification has a poor prognosis and requires aggressive high-dose chemotherapy. Any child initially classified as low-risk who is older than 1 year at the time of recurrence has a poor prognosis and needs aggressive therapy; myeloablative protocols with retinoic acid may improve outcome [3].

Metastatic recurrence of low-risk patients is treated according to the pattern of disease spread, tumor biology, and age of the patient. Patients who are under 1 year of age with favorable tumor biology and a 4S pattern of disease spread are observed if the recurrence occurs within 3 months of initial diagnosis. If metastatic disease increases after 3 months or if the initial

recurrence was not in a 4S pattern, then the primary tumor is resected and patients receive 12–24 weeks of chemotherapy. If the metastatic tumor is found to have any unfavorable tumor biology, then initial resection if followed by 24 weeks of chemotherapy.

Intermediate-risk Disease: Intermediate-risk patients who have a recurrence are also treated based upon the time to recurrence and tumor biology. If the local-regional recurrence occurs more than 3 months after completion of chemotherapy and has favorable biology, then resection is the primary method of treatment. If a total resection of all gross disease is not possible, 12 weeks of additional chemotherapy is given. If the recurrence is metastatic or has occurred less than 3 months following completion of the primary treatment or has unfavorable biology, patient outcome is poor. These patients should be treated with aggressive high-dose chemotherapy, myeloablative therapy, and retinoic acid.

High-risk Disease: Any recurrence in a high-risk patient is associated with a very poor prognosis. Conventional therapy protocols have been unsuccessful in these patients and they should be considered for phase 1 or 2 clinical trials.

11.1.9.7 Experimental Treatments

New techniques and treatments are under development to improve survival in high-risk patients as well as to deliver treatments more effectively with fewer side effects. One such treatment is the use of [133] labeled MIBG to deliver treatments specifically to the neuroblastoma cells and avoid toxicity to surrounding organs and tissues. Recent studies have been done using this radiolabeled MIBG prior to surgery, in combination with chemotherapy, for residual disease [145–147]. Newer chemotherapeutic agents, such as topotecan and irinotecan, have been shown to have activity against neuroblastoma refractory to other treatments [148–150]. A COG study is currently looking at the combination of irinotecan plus temozolomide as salvage therapy [151]. Another agent being used at some centers is etoposide. This is an oral topoisomerase II inhibitor that has shown some effect in refractory and relapsed patients [152]. Immunologic therapies are also currently under investigation. These include the use of monoclonal antibodies, cytokine therapies, and vaccines. One such antibody being used is the anti-G (D2) monoclonal antibody 3F8 [153, 154]. The limitations of these therapies right now appear to be the risk of allergic reactions as well as severe signs and symptoms of an immune reaction such as fever, pain, and skin irritation. Research is also being performed on the value of anti-angiogenic therapy in the treatment of neuroblastomas as these tumors are frequently well vascularized. Other potential targets of therapy include tyrosine kinase inhibitors to affect the TRK-NGF pathway, direct targeting of N-myc amplified cells, and the creation of chimeric antibodies to deliver cytotoxic drugs.

11.2   Other Adrenal Tumors

Other masses of the adrenal gland are rare during childhood and often result in endocrinologic hyperactivity disorders. Pheochromocytomas typically over secrete catecholamines while tumors of the adrenal cortex may result in Cushing's syndrome from excess steroid production.

11.2.1   Pheochromocytoma

Pheochromocytomas arise from chromaffin cells, most commonly within the adrenal medulla. The incidence of right-sided adrenal gland tumors is higher than for the left. They account for approximately 1% of the cases of childhood hypertension due to their potential for oversecretion of the catecholamines epinephrine and norepinephrine [155]. Most commonly these tumors are benign (90%), with 10% malignant, 10% bilateral, and 10% extra-adrenal cases noted to occur. This pattern leads to the creation of the "rule of 10" [156]. While this rule holds true in adults it appears that among the pediatric population there may be a higher incidence of extra-adrenal locations of approximately 30% [157–159]. These extra-adrenal tumors are called paragangliomas and are most likely to be located within the abdominal cavity, with the organ of Zuckerkandl at the aortic bifurcation being one of the more common sites [160]. Extra-adrenal tumors appear to have a worse prognosis than primary adrenal tumors; however, no difference has been found in the metastatic potential between the two types [161–163].

The presenting symptoms of a child with pheochromocytoma can vary and mimic other disease processes. Signs and symptoms include headaches, palpitations, weight loss, nervousness, tachycardia, and hypertension. This hypertension can be sustained or paroxysmal. It has also been shown to be more severe in children than in adults and is associated with retinopathy (40%) and cardiomyopathy (40%) [155, 160, 164]. The mainstay of diagnosis is the finding of elevated urinary catecholamines detected over a 24-h period. In addition, measurement of catecholamine metabolites vanillylmandelic acid, normetanephrine, and metanephrine should also be performed from the urine. The ratio of epinephrine to norepinephrine can also have an important use in the diagnosis of extra-adrenal pheochromocytomas as these tumors lack the enzyme to convert norepinephrine to epinephrine. Once a diagnosis is confirmed, a CT scan of the chest/abdomen/pelvis should be performed to evaluate the location and extent of disease. The use of iodine-131 metaiodobenzylguanidine (MIBG) scans can be useful to confirm adrenal uptake as well as to help identify additional sites of extra-adrenal disease [160].

Pheochromocytomas most commonly occur as a sporadic tumor. However, they can be associated with some well-defined hereditary disorders in approximately 10% of all cases. These include multiple endocrine neoplasias (MEN) 2A and 2B, von Hippel-Lindau disease, Sturge-Weber syndrome, and von Recklinghausen's disease (neurofibromatosis Type 1) [165]. Among patients with MEN type 2 bilaterality is much more common and the risk of developing a contralateral tumor following a unilateral adrenalectomy is approximately 50% [166]. Mutations within the RET proto-oncogene of MEN patients appears to be the basis for the increased susceptibility to tumor development. Unlike the adult version of this tumor, in children it has begun to appear that even cases of sporadic tumors may have an underlying genetic origin. A recent report looking at 270 sporadic pheochromocytomas identified germline mutations of known susceptibility genes in approximately 24% of cases. This value rose to 70% in children under 10 years of age [167]. Carefully genetic screening should be considered for all patients diagnosed with pheochromocytoma under 10 years of age.

Surgical treatment of pheochromocytoma is curative in all localized cases. There is currently no accepted staging system for pheochromocytoma. If the histology following resection is benign, no further treatment is necessary and repeat biochemical assays are performed at follow-up to document the removal of all functioning pheochromocytoma. Historically, open adrenalectomy was the procedure of choice for this disease. However, consideration to the small size of these tumors in children as well as their frequent benign nature has led most surgeons to opt for performing a laparoscopic resection [160, 168–170]. Documented benefits of the laparoscopic approach include fewer complications, less OR time, less pain, and shorter hospital stays. Both transperitoneal and retroperitoneal approaches have been described, with the lateral transperitoneal approach appearing to be the most popular [160].

No matter which approach is chosen, all children with pheochromocytoma must undergo preparation for resection with a 2- to 3-week course of alpha-blockade, most commonly phenoxybenzamine or prazosin. (See Table 11.3) Usually 0.2–0.5 mg/kg of phenoxybenzamine is given in a divided dose twice a day until surgery. This is increased gradually until blood pressure is controlled or a maximum dose of 3 mg/kg

Table 11.3 Pheochromocytoma

Preoperative preparation for 10–14 days
Alpha-adrenoceptor blockade:
phenoxybenzamine 0.5 mg/kg orally 12-hourly, increasing gradually to 3 mg/kg orally 12-hourly
plus
Beta-adrenoceptor blockade: propranolol 0.2 mg/kg orally 6-hourly, increasing gradually to 1.5 mg/kg 6-hourly
Other drugs which have been used: labetolol (combined alpha and beta blocker) or magnesium sulfate
Perioperative management
Meticulous fluid balance with continuous invasive hemodynamic monitoring (IABP, CVP, PCWP)
Epidural blockade plus general anesthesia
Vasodilator infusion titrated to effect (use either phentolamine, nitroprusside, or magnesium sulfate)
Beta blockade by continuous infusion of esmolol (500 bg/kg then 100–300 pg/kg/min) or labetolol infusion
Vasopressors available for actite hypotension (either phenylephrine or dopamine)
Intensive care postop for analgesia, monitoring, and weaning from hemodynamic support drugs

IABP, intra-arterial blood pressure; CVP, central venous pressure; PCWP, pulmonary artery capillary wedge pressure

is reached. This aids in the correction of the child's underlying hypertension prior to surgery as well as more importantly blocking against the effects of catecholamine release secondary to tumor manipulation during resection. During surgery, invasive hemodynamic monitoring is essential, as well an adequate supply of fluids and volume expanders to correct for fluctuations in blood pressure. In addition, rapidly acting vasodilating agents such as sodium nitroprusside and vasopressive agents should be available within the OR and ready for infusion at their proper concentrations according to the patient's size and weight.

11.2.2 Adrenal Cortical Tumors

Tumors of the adrenal cortex are rare within the pediatric population, comprising less than 0.5% of all childhood neoplasm [171] and 6% of all pediatric adrenal tumors [172]. These tumors can present with a wide range of symptoms dependant upon their level of hormonal activity and from which zone of the cortex the tumor arises from. The adrenal cortex is comprised of three zones each of which produce a hormone or steroid: the zona glomerulosa (outer) produces aldosterone, the zona fasciculata (middle) produces glucocorticoid, and the zona reticularis (inner) produces sex hormones as well as some glucocorticoids.

The majority of pediatric patients who present with tumors of the adrenal cortex are female and under 5 years of age [173, 174]. These tumors can be benign adenomas or malignant carcinomas. The survival rate for carcinomas 5 years after treatment tends to be more favorable than in adults, where it is approximately 40%. Because of the high percentage of adrenal masses that are diagnosed as neuroblastoma it is felt that any in-

cidental masses discovered should undergo resection [160]. An exception to this rule, however, would be a small perinatally detected mass that fails to grow after close follow-up via repeated ultrasonography.

11.2.2.1 Adrenal Adenoma

Adenomas are benign masses that are likely to be responsible for oversecretion of endogenous steroids (Cushing's Syndrome) [175] as well as rare cases of aldosterone over-secretion (Conn's Syndrome) [176, 177]. Symptoms from these tumors are associated with excessive hormonal secretion such as virilization, hypertension, and hypercortisolism. High concentrations of plasma and urinary cortisol levels are detected along with low levels of adrenocorticotropic hormone levels consistent with a functional adrenal mass. Diagnosis can be confirmed with CT or MRI scanning of the abdomen and pelvis to determine the location and size of the mass. There are no clear differentiating radiologic features to establish benign versus malignant disease, though larger size masses tend towards malignancy [178]. As such all adrenal adenomas should be resected and may be performed via laparoscopic techniques based upon the success of these procedures in adults.

11.2.2.2 Adrenal Cortical Carcinoma

Carcinoma of the adrenal cortex may present as a functioning or nonfunctioning adrenal mass. Most cases, however, are associated with excessive androgen production and symptoms of virilization [179–181]. In addition, Cushing's syndrome may also be present with the characteristic signs of hypertension, central obesity, moon face, and buffalo hump. Diagnostic testing also includes evaluation of cortisol, sex hormone levels, and metabolites in both the plasma and urine. CT scan or MRI of the abdomen and pelvis should be performed in all children in whom the diagnosis is suspected to identify the location and size of the primary tumor. In addition, CT scan of the chest is helpful to locate any sites of metastasis [179]. The most common sites of metastatic disease include the lung, liver, and lymph nodes.

Adrenal cortical carcinoma has been noted to have an association with Li-Fraumeni syndrome, Beckwith-Wiedemann syndrome, and congenital hemi-hypertrophy [182–184]. This association suggests an underlying genetic basis to this tumor, possibly related to p53 mutations of the germline. Brazilian studies have reported on a specific mutation of p53, termed R337H, which they noted was associated with a higher incidence of adrenal carcinoma [185]. Because of these noted associations, genetic screening of children with adrenal cortical carcinoma for the above syndromes should be considered.

Treatment of all adrenal cortical carcinomas is dependant upon complete surgical resection [181, 186, 187]. Perioperative replacement of steroids is necessary due to the suppressed hypothalamic-pituitary-adrenal axis and the abrupt removal of the endogenous source of excess steroid production. Gross removal of all tumor should be the goal of surgery even at the expense of nearby structures as patients with incomplete resections have been shown to have a poorer prognosis [188]. Tumor size (>200c3), age at diagnosis greater than 3.5 years, and onset of symptoms within 6 months of diagnosis all have been associated with a worse outcome [188, 189]. Aneuploid tumors, identified by flow cytometric analysis of DNA content, have been discovered to be more aggressive and have a poorer prognosis [190, 191].

Staging of adrenal cortical carcinoma is based on the TNM classification determined by the size of the primary tumor, degree of local invasion, and spread to lymph nodes or distant sites. Stage 1 and 2 patients have localized disease to the adrenal gland without evidence of invasion or regional/distant spread. These patients are treated primarily with complete resection without the need for additional adjuvant therapies. Stage 3 disease consists of tumors that have invaded the surrounding adrenal fat or those which have positive local regional lymph nodes. Complete surgical resection is again the treatment of choice with adjuvant therapy reserved for patients with residual disease. Stage 4 patients are those with local invasion of tumor into adjacent structures with positive lymph nodes or those patients with distant metastatic spread of disease. These patients should undergo removal of all localized disease if possible in addition to any functional metastatic lesions [192]. Systemic chemotherapy with mitotane is frequently used as adjuvant therapy. It can achieve a clinical response in approximately 30% of patients with a durable complete remission possible [193–195]. Cisplatin has also been reported to be effective in some cases [196–198], alone and in combination with carboplatin/etoposide [199, 200]. Radiation therapy may also be useful for patients that have bony metastasis or areas with localized unresectable tumor [201].

A current Phase 3 COG trial (ARAR0332) is evaluating patient outcomes in the treatment of adrenal cortical carcinoma with surgery plus regional lymph node dissection and multi-agent chemotherapy. All Stage 1 and 2 patients will receive treatment with surgery alone. Stage 2 patients will also undergo an extended regional lymph node dissection. Stage 3 and 4 patients will undergo surgery with the addition of multiagent chemotherapy consisting of cisplatin (50 mg/m2), etoposide (100 mg/m2), and doxorubicin (25 mg/m2) for 8 cycles as well as mitotane administration daily for 8 months. Endpoints of this study will look at outcomes, success of surgery, toxicity from chemotherapy, and the incidence of germline/genetic mutations.

References

1. Wright J (1910) Neurocytoma or neuroblastoma, a kind of tumor not generally recognized. J Exp Med (12):556–561
2. Everson TC (1958) Spontaneous regression of cancer. Conn Med 22(9):637–643
3. Matthay KK, Villablanca JG, Seeger RC, et al. (1999) Treatment of high-risk neuroblastoma with intensive chemotherapy, radiotherapy, autologous bone marrow transplantation, and 13-cis-retinoic acid. Children's Cancer Group. N Engl J Med 341(16):1165–1173
4. Moore K, Persaud T (1993) The developing human: Clinically oriented embryology, 5th edn. W.B. Saunders, Philadelphia
5. Goodman M GJ, Smith M, Olshan A Symapathetic Nervous System Tumors (ICCC IV). National Cancer Insitute, SEER Program 1999
6. Nuchtern JG (2006) Perinatal neuroblastoma. Semin Pediatr Surg 15(1):10–16
7. Kramer S, Ward E, Meadows AT, et al. (1987) Medical and drug risk factors associated with neuroblastoma: A case-control study. J Natl Cancer Inst 78(5):797–804
8. Schwartzbaum JA (1992) Influence of the mother's prenatal drug consumption on risk of neuroblastoma in the child. Am J Epidemiol 135(12):1358–1367
9. Spitz MR, Johnson CC (1985) Neuroblastoma and paternal occupation. A case-control analysis. Am J Epidemiol 121(6):924–929
10. Wilkins JR, 3rd, Hundley VD (1990) Paternal occupational exposure to electromagnetic fields and neuroblastoma in offspring. Am J Epidemiol 131(6):995–1008

11. Bluhn EC, Daniels J, Pollock BH, Olshan AF (2006) Maternal use of recreational drugs and neuroblastoma in offspring: A report from the Children's Oncology Group (United States). Cancer Causes Control 17 663–669

12. Michalek AM, Buck GM, Nasca PC, et al. (1996) Gravid health status, medication use, and risk of neuroblastoma. Am J Epidemiol 143(10):996–1001

13. Daniels JL, Olshan AF, Pollock BH, et al. (2002) Breast-feeding and neuroblastoma, USA and Canada. Cancer Causes Control 13(5):401–405

14. French AE, Grant R, Weitzman S, et al. (2003) Folic acid food fortification is associated with a decline in neuroblastoma. Clin Pharmacol Ther 74(3):288–294

15. Kushner BH, Gilbert F, Helson L (1986) Familial neuroblastoma. Case reports, literature review, and etiologic considerations. Cancer 57(9):1887–1893

16. Anderson J, Kempski H, Hill L, et al. (2001) Neuroblastoma in monozygotic twins – A case of probable twin-to-twin metastasis. Br J Cancer 85(4):493–496

17. Boyd TK, Schofield DE (1995) Monozygotic twins concordant for congenital neuroblastoma: Case report and review of the literature. Pediatr Pathol Lab Med 15(6):931–940

18. Bolande RP, Towler WF (1970) A possible relationship of neuroblastoma to Von Recklinghausen's disease. Cancer 26(1):162–175

19. Kushner BH, Hajdu SI, Helson L (1985) Synchronous neuroblastoma and von Recklinghausen's disease: A review of the literature. J Clin Oncol 3(1):117–120

20. Stovroff M, Dykes F, Teague WG (1995) The complete spectrum of neurocristopathy in an infant with congenital hypoventilation, Hirschsprung's disease, and neuroblastoma. J Pediatr Surg 30(8):1218–1221

21. Oguma E, Aihara T, Shimanuki Y, et al. (1996) Hypomelanosis of Ito associated with neuroblastoma. Pediatr Radiol 26(4):273–275

22. Shimada H, Ambros IM, Dehner LP, et al. (1999) The International Neuroblastoma Pathology Classification (the Shimada system). Cancer 86(2):364–372

23. Lau L (2002) Neuroblastoma: A single institution's experience with 128 children and an evaluation of clinical and biological prognostic factors. Pediatr Hematol Oncol 19(2):79–89

24. Sano H, Bonadio J, Gerbing RB, et al. (2006) International neuroblastoma pathology classification adds independent prognostic information beyond the prognostic contribution of age. Eur J Cancer 42(8):1113–1119

25. Goto S, Umehara S, Gerbing RB, et al. (2001) Histopathology (International Neuroblastoma Pathology Classification) and MYCN status in patients with peripheral neuroblastic tumors: A report from the Children's Cancer Group. Cancer 92(10):2699–2708

26. Chatten J, Shimada H, Sather HN, et al. (1988) Prognostic value of histopathology in advanced neuroblastoma: A report from the Childrens Cancer Study Group. Hum Pathol 19(10):1187–1198

27. Tornoczky T, Kalman E, Kajtar PG, et al. (2004) Large cell neuroblastoma: A distinct phenotype of neuroblastoma with aggressive clinical behavior. Cancer 100(2):390–397

28. Kobayashi C, Monforte-Munoz HL, Gerbing RB, et al. (2005) Enlarged and prominent nucleoli may be indicative of MYCN amplification: A study of neuroblastoma (Schwannian stroma-poor), undifferentiated/poorly differentiated subtype with high mitosis-karyorrhexis index. Cancer 103(1):174–180

29. Look AT, Hayes FA, Nitschke R, et al. (1984) Cellular DNA content as a predictor of response to chemotherapy in infants with unresectable neuroblastoma. N Engl J Med 311(4):231–235

30. Taylor SR, Blatt J, Costantino JP, et al. (1988) Flow cytometric DNA analysis of neuroblastoma and ganglioneuroma. A 10-year retrospective study. Cancer 62(4):749–754

31. Brodeur GM, Pritchard J, Berthold F, et al. (1993) Revisions of the international criteria for neuroblastoma diagnosis, staging, and response to treatment. J Clin Oncol 11(8):1466–1477

32. Brodeur GM, Seeger RC, Schwab M, et al. (1984) Amplification of N-myc in untreated human neuroblastomas correlates with advanced disease stage. Science 224(4653):1121–1124

33. Benard J (1995) Genetic alterations associated with metastatic dissemination and chemoresistance in neuroblastoma. Eur J Cancer 31A(4):560–564

34. Weiss WA, Aldape K, Mohapatra G, et al. (1997) Targeted expression of MYCN causes neuroblastoma in transgenic mice. EMBO J 16(11):2985–2995

35. Cohn SL, London WB, Huang D, et al. (2000) MYCN expression is not prognostic of adverse outcome in advanced-stage neuroblastoma with nonamplified MYCN. J Clin Oncol 18(21):3604–3613

36. Seeger RC, Brodeur GM, Sather H, et al. (1985) Association of multiple copies of the N-myc oncogene with rapid progression of neuroblastomas. N Engl J Med 313(18):1111–1116

37. Seeger RC, Wada R, Brodeur GM, et al. (1988) Expression of N-myc by neuroblastomas with one or multiple copies of the oncogene. Prog Clin Biol Res 271:41–49

38. Bagatell R, Rumcheva P, London WB, et al. (2005) Outcomes of children with intermediate-risk neuroblastoma after treatment stratified by MYCN status and tumor cell ploidy. J Clin Oncol 23(34):8819–8827

39. George RE, London WB, Cohn SL, et al. (2005) Hyperdiploidy plus nonamplified MYCN confers a favorable prognosis in children 12 to 18 months old with disseminated neuroblastoma: A Pediatric Oncology Group study. J Clin Oncol 23(27):6466–6473

40. Iehara T, Hosoi H, Akazawa K, Matsumoto Y et al. (2006) MYCN gene amplification is a powerful prognostic factor even in infantile neuroblastoma detected by mass screening. Br J Cancer 94 1510–1515

41. Azar CG, Scavarda NJ, Nakagawara A, et al. (1994) Expression and function of the nerve growth factor receptor (TRK-A) in human neuroblastoma cell lines. Prog Clin Biol Res 385:169–175

42. Brodeur GM, Nakagawara A, Yamashiro DJ, et al. (1997) Expression of TrkA, TrkB and TrkC in human neuroblastomas. J Neurooncol 31(1–2):49–55

43. Nakagawara A, Arima-Nakagawara M, Scavarda NJ, et al. (1993) Association between high levels of expression of the TRK gene and favorable outcome in human neuroblastoma. N Engl J Med 328(12):847–854

44. Schramm A, Schulte JH, Klein-Hitpass L, et al. (2005) Prediction of clinical outcome and biological characterization of neuroblastoma by expression profiling. Oncogene 24(53):7902–7912

45. Suzuki T, Bogenmann E, Shimada H, et al. (1993) Lack of high-affinity nerve growth factor receptors in aggressive neuroblastomas. J Natl Cancer Inst 85(5):377–384

46. Nakagawara A, Azar CG, Scavarda NJ, et al. (1994) Expression and function of TRK-B and BDNF in human neuroblastomas. Mol Cell Biol 14(1):759–767

47. Ho R, Eggert A, Hishiki T, et al. (2002) Resistance to chemotherapy mediated by TrkB in neuroblastomas. Cancer Res 62(22):6462–6466

48. Jaboin J, Hong A, Kim CJ, et al. (2003) Cisplatin-induced cytotoxicity is blocked by brain-derived neurotrophic factor activation of TrkB signal transduction path in neuroblastoma. Cancer Lett 193(1):109–114

49. Yamashiro DJ, Liu XG, Lee CP, et al. (1997) Expression and function of Trk-C in favourable human neuroblastomas. Eur J Cancer 33(12):2054–2057

50. Lucarelli E, Kaplan D, Thiele CJ (1997) Activation of trk-A but not trk-B signal transduction pathway inhibits growth of neuroblastoma cells. Eur J Cancer 33(12):2068–2070

51. Brodeur GM, Fong CT (1989) Molecular biology and genetics of human neuroblastoma. Cancer Genet Cytogenet 41(2):153–174

52. Gilbert F, Balaban G, Moorhead P, et al. (1982) Abnormalities of chromosome 1p in human neuroblastoma tumors and cell lines. Cancer Genet Cytogenet 7(1):33–42

53. Fong CT, Dracopoli NC, White PS, et al. (1989) Loss of heterozygosity for the short arm of chromosome 1 in human neuroblastomas: Correlation with N-myc amplification. Proc Natl Acad Sci 86(10):3753–3757

54. Caron H, van Sluis P, de Kraker J, et al. (1996) Allelic loss of chromosome 1p as a predictor of unfavorable outcome in patients with neuroblastoma. N Engl J Med 334(4):225–230

55. Caron H, van Sluis P, van Hoeve M, et al. (1993) Allelic loss of chromosome 1p36 in neuroblastoma is of preferential maternal origin and correlates with N-myc amplification. Nat Genet 4(2):187–190

56. Maris JM, White PS, Beltinger CP, et al. (1995) Significance of chromosome 1p loss of heterozygosity in neuroblastoma. Cancer Res 55(20):4664–4669

57. Simon T, Spitz R, Faldum A, et al. (2004) New definition of low-risk neuroblastoma using stage, age, and 1p and MYCN status. J Pediatr Hematol Oncol 26(12):791–796

58. Oren M (1992) The involvement of oncogenes and tumor suppressor genes in the control of apoptosis. Cancer Metastasis Rev 11(2):141–148

59. Bown N, Cotterill S, Lastowska M, et al. (1999) Gain of chromosome arm 17q and adverse outcome in patients with neuroblastoma. N Engl J Med 340(25):1954–1961

60. Bown N, Lastowska M, Cotterill S, et al. (2001) 17q gain in neuroblastoma predicts adverse clinical outcome. U.K. Cancer Cytogenetics Group and the U.K. Children's Cancer Study Group. Med Pediatr Oncol 36(1):14–19

61. Lastowska M, Cotterill S, Pearson AD, et al. (1997) Gain of chromosome arm 17q predicts unfavourable outcome in neuroblastoma patients. U.K. Children's Cancer Study Group and the U.K. Cancer Cytogenetics Group. Eur J Cancer 33(10):1627–1633

62. Tajiri T, Tanaka S, Higashi M, et al. (2006) Biological diagnosis for neuroblastoma using the combination of highly sensitive analysis of prognostic factors. J Pediatr Surg 41(3):560–566

63. Lastowska M, Cullinane C, Variend S, et al. (2001) Comprehensive genetic and histopathologic study reveals three types of neuroblastoma tumors. J Clin Oncol 19(12):3080–3090

64. Maris JM, Matthay KK (1999) Molecular biology of neuroblastoma. J Clin Oncol 17(7):2264–2279

65. Goldsby RE, Matthay KK (2004) Neuroblastoma: Evolving therapies for a disease with many faces. Paediatr Drugs 6(2):107–122

66. Hiyama E, Yokoyama T, Hiyama K, et al. (2000) Multifocal neuroblastoma: Biologic behavior and surgical aspects. Cancer 88(8):1955–1963

67. Newton ER, Louis F, Dalton ME, et al. (1985) Fetal neuroblastoma and catecholamine-induced maternal hypertension. Obstet Gynecol 6(Suppl):49S–52S

68. Voute PA, Jr, Wadman SK, van Putten WJ. Congenital neuroblastoma (1970) Symptoms in the mother during pregnancy. Clin Pediatr 9(4):206–207

69. Jennings RW, LaQuaglia MP, Leong K, et al. (1993) Fetal neuroblastoma: Prenatal diagnosis and natural history. J Pediatr Surg 28(9):1168–1174

70. Antunes NL, Khakoo Y, Matthay KK, et al. (2000) Antineuronal antibodies in patients with neuroblastoma and paraneoplastic opsoclonus-myoclonus. J Pediatr Hematol Oncol 22(4):315–320

71. Cooper R, Khakoo Y, Matthay KK, et al. (2001) Opsoclonus-myoclonus-ataxia syndrome in neuroblastoma: Histopathologic features-a report from the Children's Cancer Group. Med Pediatr Oncol 36(6):623–629

72. Rudnick E, Khakoo Y, Antunes NL, et al. (2001) Opsoclonus-myoclonus-ataxia syndrome in neuroblastoma: Clinical outcome and antineuronal antibodies-a report from the Children's Cancer Group Study. Med Pediatr Oncol 36(6):612–622

73. Boltshauser E, Deonna T, Hirt HR (1979) Myoclonic encephalopathy of infants or "dancing eyes syndrome". Report of 7 cases with long-term follow-up and review of the literature (cases with and without neuroblastoma). Helv Paediatr Acta 34(2):119–133

74. Koh PS, Raffensperger JG, Berry S, et al. (1994) Long-term outcome in children with opsoclonus-myoclonus and ataxia and coincident neuroblastoma. J Pediatr 125(5 Pt 1):712–716

75. Russo C, Cohn SL, Petruzzi MJ, et al. (1997) Long-term neurologic outcome in children with opsoclonus-myoclonus associated with neuroblastoma: A report from the Pediatric Oncology Group. Med Pediatr Oncol 28(4):284–288

76. Numata K, Kusui H, Kawakatsu H, et al. (1997) Increased urinary HVA levels in neuroblastoma screens related to diet, not tumor. Pediatr Hematol Oncol 14(6):569–576

77. Asami T, Otabe N, Wakabayashi M, et al. (1995) Screening for neuroblastoma: A 9-year birth cohort-based study in Niigata, Japan. Acta Paediatr 84(10):1173–1176

78. Woods WG, Lemieux B, Leclerc JM, et al. (1994) Screening for neuroblastoma (NB) in North America: The Quebec Project. Prog Clin Biol Res 385:377–382

79. Woods WG, Tuchman M (1987) Neuroblastoma: The case for screening infants in North America. Pediatrics 79(6):869–873

80. Hanawa Y, Sawada T, Tsunoda A (1990) Decrease in childhood neuroblastoma death in Japan. Med Pediatr Oncol 18(6):472–475

81. Yamamoto K, Ohta S, Ito E, et al. (2002) Marginal decrease in mortality and marked increase in incidence as a result of neuroblastoma screening at 6 months of age: Cohort study in seven prefectures in Japan. J Clin Oncol 20(5):1209–1214

82. Woods WG, Tuchman M, Robison LL, et al. (1997) Screening for neuroblastoma is ineffective in reducing the incidence of unfavourable advanced stage disease in older children. Eur J Cancer 33(12):2106–2112

83. Kushner BH, Yeh SD, Kramer K, et al. (2003) Impact of metaiodobenzylguanidine scintigraphy on assessing response of high-risk neuroblastoma to dose-intensive induction chemotherapy. J Clin Oncol 21(6):1082–1086

84. Kushner BH, Yeung HW, Larson SM, et al. (2001) Extending positron emission tomography scan utility to high-risk neuroblastoma: Fluorine-18 fluorodeoxyglucose positron emission tomography as sole imaging modality in follow-up of patients. J Clin Oncol 19(14):3397–3405

85. Kramer K, Kushner B, Heller G, et al. (2001) Neuroblastoma metastatic to the central nervous system. The Memorial Sloan-Kettering Cancer Center Experience and A Literature Review. Cancer 91(8):1510–1519

86. Evans AE, D'Angio GJ, Randolph J (1971) A proposed staging for children with neuroblastoma. Children's cancer study group A. Cancer 27(2):374–378

87. Hayes FA, Green A, Hustu HO, et al. (1983) Surgicopathologic staging of neuroblastoma: Prognostic significance of regional lymph node metastases. J Pediatr 102(1):59–62

88. D'Angio GJ, Evans AE, Koop CE (1971) Special pattern of widespread neuroblastoma with a favourable prognosis. Lancet 1(7708):1046–1049

89. Evans AE, Chatten J, D'Angio GJ, et al. (1980) A review of 17 IV-S neuroblastoma patients at the Children's Hospital of Philadelphia. Cancer 45(5):833–839

90. Nickerson HJ, Nesbit ME, Grosfeld JL, et al. (1985) Comparison of stage IV and IV-S neuroblastoma in the first year of life. Med Pediatr Oncol 13(5):261–268

91. Cecchetto G, Mosseri V, De Bernardi B, et al. (2005) Surgical risk factors in primary surgery for localized neuroblastoma: The LNESG1 study of the European International Society of Pediatric Oncology Neuroblastoma Group. J Clin Oncol 23(33):8483–8489

92. De Bernardi B, Pianca C, Pistamiglio P, et al. (2001) Neuroblastoma with symptomatic spinal cord compression at diagnosis: Treatment and results with 76 cases. J Clin Oncol 19(1):183–190

93. Katzenstein HM, Kent PM, London WB, et al. (2001) Treatment and outcome of 83 children with intaspinal neuroblastoma: The Pediatric Oncology Group experience. J Clin Oncol 19(4):1047–1055

94. Hayes FA, Thompson E, Hvizdala E (1984) Chemotherapy as an alternative to laminectomy and radiation in the management of epidural tumor. J Pediatr (104):221–224

95. Hayes FA, Green M, O'Connor DM (1989) Chemotherapeutic management of epidural neuroblastoma. Med Pediatr Oncol (17):6–8

96. Hoover ML, Crawford S, Cohn SL (1995) Long-term outcome of patients with neuroblastoma and spinal compression. J Investig Med 43(Suppl 3):438A

97. Acharya S, Jayabose S, Kogan SJ, et al. (1997) Prenatally diagnosed neuroblastoma. Cancer 80:304–310

98. Sauvat F, Sarnacki S, Brisse H, et al. (2002) Outcome of suprarenal localized masses diagnosed during the perinatal period: A retrospective multi-center study. Cancer 94:2474–2480

99. Granata C, Fagnani AM, Gambini C, et al. (2000) Features and outcome of neuroblastoma detected before birth. J Pediatr Surg 35:88–91

100. Nishihira H, Toyoda Y, Tanaka Y, et al. (2000) Natural course of neuroblastoma detected by mass screening: 5-year prospective study at a single institution. J Clin Oncol 18(16):3012–3017

101. Holgersen LO, Subramanain S, Kripekar M, et al. (1996) Spontaneous resolution of antenatally diagnosed adrenal masses. J Pediatr Surg 31(1):153–155

102. Kushner B, Cheung NK, La Quaglia MP, et al. (1996) International neuroblastoma staging system stage 1 neuroblastoma: A prospective study and literature review. J Clin Oncol 14:2174–2180

103. Nitschke R, Smith EI, Shochat S, et al. (1988) Localized neuroblastoma treated by surgery: A Pediatric Oncology Group study. J Clin Oncol 6(8):1271–1279

104. Fritsch P, Kerbl R, Lackner H, et al. (2004) "Wait and see" strategy in localized neuroblastoma in infants: An option not only for cases detected by mass screening. Pediatr Blood Cancer 43(6):679–682

105. Perez CA, Matthay KK, Atkinson JB, et al. (2000) Biologic variables in the outcome of stages I and II neuroblastoma treated with surgery as primary therapy: A Children's Cancer Group study. J Clin Oncol 18(1):18–26

106. Strother DR, Children's Oncology Group Phase III Study of Primary Surgical Therapy in Children With Low-Risk Neuroblastoma. COG-P9641

107. Strother DR, van Hoff J, Rao PV, et al. (1997) Event-free survival of children with biologically favourable neuroblastoma based on the degree of initial tumor resection: Results from the Pediatric Oncology Group. Eur J Cancer 33(12):2121–2125

108. Nickerson HJ, Matthay KK, Seeger RC, et al. (2000) Favorable biology and outcome of stage IV-S neuroblastoma with supportive care or minimal therapy: A Children's Cancer Group study. J Clin Oncol 18(3):477–486

109. Guglielmi M, De Bernardi B, Rizzo A, et al. (1996) Resection of primary tumor at diagnosis in stage IV-S neuroblastoma: Does it affect the clinical course? J Clin Oncol 14(5):1537–1544

110. Kushner BH, Kramer K, Laquaglia MP, et al. (2006) Liver involvement in neuroblastoma: The memorial Sloan-Kettering experience supports treatment reduction in young patients. Pediatr Blood Cancer 46(3):278–284

111. Matthay KK, Perez C, Seeger RC, et al. (1998) Successful treatment of stage III neuroblastoma based on prospective biologic staging: A Children's Cancer Group study. J Clin Oncol 16(4):1256–1264

112. West DC, Shamberger RC, Macklis RM, et al. (1993) Stage III neuroblastoma over 1 year of age at diagnosis: Improved survival with intensive multimodality therapy including multiple alkylating agents. J Clin Oncol 11(1):84–90

113. Look AT, Hayes FA, Shuster J, et al. (1991) Clinical relevance of tumor cell ploidy and N-myc gene amplification in childhood neuroblastoma: A Pediatric Oncology Group study. J Clin Oncol 9(4):581–591

114. Shamberger RC, Smith EI, Joshi V, et al. (1998) The risk of nephrectomy during local control in abdominal neuroblastoma. J Pediatr Surg 33(2):161–164

115. Kushner B, La Quaglia MP, Bonilla MA, et al. (1994) Highly effective induction therapy for stage 4 neuroblastoma in children over 1 year of age. J Clin Oncol 12(12):2607–2613

116. Ladenstein R, Philip T, Lasset C, et al. (1998) Multivariate analysis of risk factors in stage 4 neuroblastoma patients over the age of one year treated with megatherapy and stem-cell transplantation: A report from the European Bone Marrow Transplantation Solid Tumor Registry. J Clin Oncol 16(3):953–965

117. Katzenstein HM, Cohn SL, Shore RM, et al. (2004) Scintigraphic response by 123I-metaiodobenzylguanidine scan correlates with event-free survival in high-risk neuroblastoma. J Clin Oncol 22(19):3909–3915

118. Matthay KK, Edeline V, Lumbroso J, et al. (2003) Correlation of early metastatic response by 123I-metaiodobenzylguanidine scintigraphy with overall response and event-free survival in stage IV neuroblastoma. J Clin Oncol 21(13):2486–491

119. Pinkerton CR (1991) ENSG 1-randomised study of high-dose melphalan in neuroblastoma. Bone Marrow Transplant 7(Suppl 3):112–113

120. Matthay KK, O'Leary MC, Ramsay NK, et al. (1995) Role of myeloablative therapy in improved outcome for high risk neuroblastoma: Review of recent Children's Cancer Group results. Eur J Cancer 31A(4):572–575

121. Matthay KK, Seeger RC, Reynolds CP, et al. (1994) Comparison of autologous and allogeneic bone marrow transplantation for neuroblastoma. Prog Clin Biol Res 385:301–307

122. Seeger RC, Reynolds CP, Gallego R, et al. (2000) Quantitative tumor cell content of bone marrow and blood as a predictor of outcome in stage IV neuroblastoma: A Children's Cancer Group Study. J Clin Oncol 18(24):4067–4076

123. Burchill SA, Lewis IJ, Abrams KR, et al. (2001) Circulating neuroblastoma cells detected by reverse transcriptase polymerase chain reaction for tyrosine hydroxylase mRNA are an independent poor prognostic indicator in stage 4 neuroblastoma in children over 1 year. J Clin Oncol 19(6):1795–1801

124. DuBois SG, Kalika Y, Lukens JN, et al. (1999) Metastatic sites in stage IV and IVS neuroblastoma correlate with age, tumor biology, and survival. J Pediatr Hematol Oncol 21(3):181–189

125. Saarinen UM, Wikstrom S, Makipernaa A, et al. (1996) In vivo purging of bone marrow in children with poor-risk neuroblastoma for marrow collection and autologous bone marrow transplantation. J Clin Oncol 14(10):2791–2802

126. de Lagausie P, Berrebi D, Michon J, et al. (2003) Laparoscopic adrenal surgery for neuroblastomas in children. J Urol 170(3):932–935

127. La Quaglia MP, Kushner BH, Su W, et al. (2004) The impact of gross total resection on local control and survival in high-risk neuroblastoma. J Pediatr Surg 39(3):412–417; discussion 412–417

128. Shorter NA, Davidoff AM, Evans AE, et al. (1995) The role of surgery in the management of stage IV neuroblastoma: A single institution study. Med Pediatr Oncol 24(5):287–291

129. Castel V, Tovar JA, Costa E, et al. (2002) The role of surgery in stage IV neuroblastoma. J Pediatr Surg 37(11):1574–1578

130. Koh CC, Sheu JC, Liang DC, et al. (2005) Complete surgical resection plus chemotherapy prolongs survival in children with stage 4 neuroblastoma. Pediatr Surg Int 21(2):69–72

131. Cheung NK, Kushner BH, LaQuaglia M, et al. (2001) N7: A novel multi-modality therapy of high risk neuroblastoma (NB) in children diagnosed over 1 year of age. Med Pediatr Oncol 36(1):227–230

132. Kuroda T, Saeki M, Nakano M, et al. (2000) Surgical treatment of neuroblastoma with micrometastasis. J Pediatr Surg 35(11):1638–1642

133. Wolden SL, Gollamudi SV, Kushner BH, et al. (2000) Local control with multimodality therapy for stage 4 neuroblastoma. Int J Radiat Oncol Biol Phys 46(4):969–974

134. Haas-Kogan DA, Swift PS, Selch M, et al. (2003) Impact of radiotherapy for high-risk neuroblastoma: A Children's Cancer Group study. Int J Radiat Oncol Biol Phys 56(1):28–39

135. Haase GM, Meagher DP, Jr, McNeely LK, et al. (1994) Electron beam intraoperative radiation therapy for pediatric neoplasms. Cancer 74(2):740–747

136. Leavey PJ, Odom LF, Poole M, et al. (1997) Intra-operative radiation therapy in pediatric neuroblastoma. Med Pediatr Oncol 28(6):424–428

137. Abemayor E, Chang B, Sidell N (1990) Effects of retinoic acid on the in vivo growth of human neuroblastoma cells. Cancer Lett 55(1):1–5

138. Redfern CP, Lovat PE, Malcolm AJ, et al. (1995) Gene expression and neuroblastoma cell differentiation in response to retinoic acid: Differential effects of 9-cis and all-trans retinoic acid. Eur J Cancer 31A(4):486–494

139. Reynolds CP, Matthay KK, Villablanca JG, et al. (2003) Retinoid therapy of high-risk neuroblastoma. Cancer Lett 197(1–2):185–192

140. Kohler JA, Imeson J, Ellershaw C, et al. (2000) A randomized trial of 13-Cis retinoic acid in children with advanced neuroblastoma after high-dose therapy. Br J Cancer 83(9):1124–1127

141. George RE, Li S, Medeiros-Nancarrow C, Neuberg D et al. (2006) High-risk neuroblastoma treated with tandem autologous peripheral-blood stem cell-supported transplantation: Long-term survival update. J Clin Oncol 24:2891–2896

142. Pole JG, Casper J, Elfenbein G, et al. (1991) High-dose chemoradiotherapy supported by marrow infusions for advanced neuroblastoma: A Pediatric Oncology Group study. J Clin Oncol 9(1):152–158

143. Castel V, Canete A, Melero C, et al. (2000) Results of the cooperative protocol (N-III-95) for metastatic relapses and refractory neuroblastoma. Med Pediatr Oncol 35(6):724–726

144. Blatt J, Fitz C, Mirro J, Jr (1997) Recognition of central nervous system metastases in children with metastatic primary extracranial neuroblastoma. Pediatr Hematol Oncol 14(3):233–241

145. Mastrangelo S, Tornesello A, Diociaiuti L, et al. (2001) Treatment of advanced neuroblastoma: Feasibility and therapeutic potential of a novel approach combining 131-I-MIBG and multiple drug chemotherapy. Br J Cancer 84(4):460–464

146. Troncone L, Rufini V, Luzi S, et al. (1995) The treatment of neuroblastoma with [131I]MIBG at diagnosis. Q J Nucl Med 39(Suppl 1):65–68

147. Garaventa A, Bellagamba O, Lo Piccolo MS, et al. (1999) 131I-metaiodobenzylguanidine (131I-MIBG) therapy for residual neuroblastoma: A mono-institutional experience with 43 patients. Br J Cancer 81(8):1378–1384

148. Langler A, Christaras A, Abshagen K, et al. (2002) Topotecan in the treatment of refractory neuroblastoma and other malignant tumors in childhood – A phase-II-study. Klin Padiatr 214(4):153–156

149. Saylors RL, 3rd, Stine KC, Sullivan J, et al. (2001) Cyclophosphamide plus topotecan in children with recurrent or refractory solid tumors: A Pediatric Oncology Group phase II study. J Clin Oncol 19(15):3463–3469

150. Vassal G, Doz F, Frappaz D, et al. (2003) A phase I study of irinotecan as a 3-week schedule in children with refractory or recurrent solid tumors. J Clin Oncol 21(20):3844–3852

151. Wagner LM, Crews KR, Iacono LC, et al. (2004) Phase I trial of temozolomide and protracted irinotecan in pediatric patients with refractory solid tumors. Clin Cancer Res 10(3):840–848

152. Kushner BH, Kramer K, Cheung NK (1999) Oral etoposide for refractory and relapsed neuroblastoma. J Clin Oncol 17(10):3221–3225

153. Cheung NK, Kushner BH, Cheung IY, et al. (1998) Anti-G(D2) antibody treatment of minimal residual stage 4 neuroblastoma diagnosed at more than 1 year of age. J Clin Oncol 16(9):3053–3060

154. Kushner BH, Kramer K, Cheung NK (2001) Phase II trial of the anti-G(D2) monoclonal antibody 3F8 and granulocyte-macrophage colony-stimulating factor for neuroblastoma. J Clin Oncol 19(22):4189–4194

155. Revillon Y, Daher P, Jan D, et al. (1992) Pheochromocytoma in children: 15 cases. J Pediatr Surg 27(7):910–911

156. Bravo EL (1983) Pheochromocytoma. Current concepts in diagnosis, localization, and management. Prim Care 10(1):75–86

157. Fonkalsrud EW (1991) Pheochromocytoma in childhood. Prog Pediatr Surg 26:103–111

158. Goldfarb DA, Novick AC, Bravo EL, et al. (1989) Experience with extra-adrenal pheochromocytoma. J Urol 142(4):931–936

159. Hodgkinson DJ, Telander RL, Sheps SG, et al. (1980) Extra-adrenal intrathoracic functioning paraganglioma (pheochromocytoma) in childhood. Mayo Clin Proc 55(4):271–276

160. Rescorla FJ (2006) Malignant adrenal tumors. Semin Pediatr Surg 15(1):48

161. Pommier RF, Vetto JT, Billingsly K, et al. (1993) Comparison of adrenal and extraadrenal pheochromocytomas. Surgery 114(6):1160–1165; discussion 1165–1166

162. Sclafani LM, Woodruff JM, Brennan MF (1990) Extraadrenal retroperitoneal paragangliomas: Natural history and response to treatment. Surgery 108(6):1124–1129; discussion 1129–1130

163. Whalen RK, Althausen AF, Daniels GH (1992) Extra-adrenal pheochromocytoma. J Urol 147(1):1–10

164. Sawin RS (1997) Functioning adrenal neoplasms. Semin Pediatr Surg 6(3):156–163

165. Neumann HP, Berger DP, Sigmund G, et al. (1993) Pheochromocytomas, multiple endocrine neoplasia type 2, and von Hippel-Lindau disease. N Engl J Med 329(21):1531–1538

166. Lairmore TC, Ball DW, Baylin SB, et al. (1993) Management of pheochromocytomas in patients with multiple endocrine neoplasia type 2 syndromes. Ann Surg 217(6):595–601; discussion 601–603

167. Neumann HP, Bausch B, McWhinney SR, et al. (2002) Germ-line mutations in nonsyndromic pheochromocytoma. N Engl J Med 346(19):1459–1466

168. Clements RH, Goldstein RE, Holcomb GW, 3rd (1999) Laparoscopic left adrenalectomy for pheochromocytoma in a child. J Pediatr Surg 34(9):1408–1409

169. Miller KA, Albanese C, Harrison M, et al. (2002) Experience with laparoscopic adrenalectomy in pediatric patients. J Pediatr Surg 37(7):979–982; discussion 979–982

170. Vargas HI, Kavoussi LR, Bartlett DL, et al. (1997) Laparoscopic adrenalectomy: A new standard of care. Urology 49(5):673–678

171. Bergada I, Venara M, Maglio S, et al. (1996) Functional adrenal cortical tumors in pediatric patients: A clinicopathologic and immunohistochemical study of a long term follow-up series. Cancer 77(4):771–777

172. Chudler RM, Kay R (1989) Adrenocortical carcinoma in children. Urol Clin North Am 16(3):469–479

173. Lack EE, Mulvihill JJ, Travis WD, et al. (1992) Adrenal cortical neoplasms in the pediatric and adolescent age group. Clinicopathologic study of 30 cases with emphasis on epidemiological and prognostic factors. Pathol Annu 27 Pt 1:1–53

174. Ribeiro RC, Michalkiewicz EL, Figueiredo BC, et al. (2000) Adrenocortical tumors in children. Braz J Med Biol Res 33(10):1225–1234

175. Lee PD, Winter RJ, Green OC (1985) Virilizing adrenocortical tumors in childhood: Eight cases and a review of the literature. Pediatrics 76(3):437–444

176. Decsi T, Soltesz G (1995) Aldosteronoma in children: A partial review of the literature. Eur J Pediatr 154(3):247

177. Etker S (1995) Aldosteronoma in childhood. J Pediatr Surg 30(7):1113

178. Cagle PT, Hough AJ, Pysher TJ, et al. (1986) Comparison of adrenal cortical tumors in children and adults. Cancer 57(11):2235–2237

179. Ciftci AO, Senocak ME, Tanyel FC, et al. (2001) Adrenocortical tumors in children. J Pediatr Surg 36(4):549–554

180. Sabbaga CC, Avilla SG, Schulz C, et al. (1993) Adrenocortical carcinoma in children: Clinical aspects and prognosis. J Pediatr Surg 28(6):841–843

181. Michalkiewicz E, Sandrini R, Figueiredo B, et al. (2004) Clinical and outcome characteristics of children with adrenocortical tumors: A report from the International Pediatric Adrenocortical Tumor Registry. J Clin Oncol 22(5):838–845

182. Engstrom W, Lindham S, Schofield P (1988) Wiedemann-Beckwith syndrome. Eur J Pediatr 147(5):450–457

183. Sbragia-Neto L, Melo-Filho AA, Guerra-Junior G, et al. (2000) Beckwith-Wiedemann syndrome and virilizing cortical adrenal tumor in a child. J Pediatr Surg 35(8):1269–1271

184. Varley JM, Evans DG, Birch JM (1997) Li-Fraumeni syndrome – A molecular and clinical review. Br J Cancer 76(1):1–14

185. Ribeiro RC, Sandrini F, Figueiredo B, et al. (2001) An inherited p53 mutation that contributes in a tissue-specific manner to pediatric adrenal cortical carcinoma. Proc Natl Acad Sci 98(16):9330–9335

186. Stewart JN, Flageole H, Kavan P (2004) A surgical approach to adrenocortical tumors in children: The mainstay of treatment. J Pediatr Surg 39(5):759–763

187. Meyer A, Niemann U, Behrend M (2004) Experience with the surgical treatment of adrenal cortical carcinoma. Eur J Surg Oncol 30(4):444–449

188. Ribeiro RC, Sandrini Neto RS, Schell MJ, et al. (1990) Adrenocortical carcinoma in children: A study of 40 cases. J Clin Oncol 8(1):67–74

189. Ribeiro RC, Sandrini R (1994) Adrenocortical carcinoma in children: Clinical aspects and prognosis. J Pediatr Surg 29(1):122

190. Taylor SR, Roederer M, Murphy RF (1987) Flow cytometric DNA analysis of adrenocortical tumors in children. Cancer 59(12):2059–2063

191. Venara M, Sanchez Marull R, Bergada I, et al. (1998) Functional adrenal cortical tumors in childhood: A study of ploidy, p53-protein and nucleolar organizer regions (AgNORs) as prognostic markers. J Pediatr Endocrinol Metab 11(5):597–605

192. Pommier RF, Brennan MF (1992) An eleven-year experience with adrenocortical carcinoma. Surgery 112(6):963–970; discussion 970–971

193. Karakousis CP, Uribe J, Moore R (1981) Adrenal adenocarcinomas: Diagnosis and management. J Surg Oncol 16(4):385–389

194. Lubitz JA, Freeman L, Okun R (1973) Mitotane use in inoperable adrenal cortical carcinoma. JAMA 223(10):1109–1112

195. Luton JP, Cerdas S, Billaud L, et al. (1990) Clinical features of adrenocortical carcinoma, prognostic factors, and the effect of mitotane therapy. N Engl J Med 322(17):1195–1201

196. Chun HG, Yagoda A, Kemeny N, et al. (1983) Cisplatin for adrenal cortical carcinoma. Cancer Treat Rep 67(5):513–514

197. Hesketh PJ, McCaffrey RP, Finkel HE, et al. (1987) Cisplatin-based treatment of adrenocortical carcinoma. Cancer Treat Rep 71(2):222–224

198. Tattersall MH, Lander H, Bain B, et al. (1980) Cis-platinum treatment of metastatic adrenal carcinoma. Med J Aust 1(9):419–421

199. Ayass M, Gross S, Harper J (1991) High-dose carboplatinum and VP-16 in treatment of metastatic adrenal carcinoma. Am J Pediatr Hematol Oncol 13(4):470–472

200. Bukowski RM, Wolfe M, Levine HS, et al. (1993) Phase II trial of mitotane and cisplatin in patients with adrenal carcinoma: A Southwest Oncology Group study. J Clin Oncol 11(1):161–165

201. Percarpio B, Knowlton AH (1976) Radiation therapy of adrenal cortical carcinoma. Acta Radiol Ther Phys Biol 15(4):288–292

Liver Tumors in Children

12

Jay L. Grosfeld, Jean-Bernard Otte

Contents

12.1 Introduction

Liver tumors in children are relatively uncommon when compared with other malignant conditions in the pediatric age group. This chapter deals with the three most common malignant liver tumors in childhood; hepatoblastoma (HB), hepatocellular carcinoma (HCC), and embryonal undifferentiated sarcoma.

12.2 Hepatoblastoma

Hepatoblastoma (HB) is the most frequent liver tumor in children, representing approximately 80% of all malignant liver neoplasms and 1% of all pediatric malignancies, with a peak incidence in the first 3 years of life [1–3]. Epidemiological studies from the National Center for Health Statistics in the USA describe an incidence of 0.7 cases per one million per year [1]. Hepatoblastoma rates have increased from 0.6 to 1.2 per million in the past two decades [2]. Ninety-one percent of children less than 5 years of age have hepatoblastoma whereas 87% of those between 15 and 19 years have hepatocellular carcinoma (HCC). For all children less than 20 years of age, 67% have HB and 31% have HCC. HB is an embryonic tumor that probably arises from a pluripotent stem cell occurring in the liver during embryonal life [3].

12.2.1 Associated Genetic Alterations

A number of genetic alterations are seen in association with hepatoblastoma. They include the Beckwith-Wiedemann syndrome, characterized by an overgrowth syndrome, an umbilical defect (either an umbilical hernia or omphalocele) and macroglossia [4, 5]. Children with the Beckwith-Wiedemann syndrome have an increased incidence of HB, Wilms' tumor, rhabdomyosarcoma, neuroblastoma, and pancreatoblastoma [5]. There is a loss of heterozygosity at the 11p15.5 locus [3,6]. A relatively high incidence of trisomy 20, trisomy 2, and rarely trisomy 18, gains in chromosome

8q and 17q, and chromosomal loss in 1p have been associated with HB [7–9]. Chromosomal imbalances of Xp and Xq detected by genomic hybridization have also been noted in HB [10]. Nuclear and cytoplasmic accumulations of beta-catenin mutations associated with chromosomal instability and abnormalities of the Wnt/beta-catenin signaling pathway are seen in patients with HB and may contribute to tumorigenesis [11, 12]. p53 gene mutations and overexpression are infrequent [13]. A significant increase in the risk of HB has been noted in families with familial adenomatous polyposis [4, 14, 15] and Gardner's syndrome, which is related to APC gene mutations affecting chromosome 5q [16]. Survivors of HB who have this particular syndrome are at risk for developing familial adenomatous polyposis at a young age [14, 15]. Cases of HB have been associated with hemihypertrophy, total parenteral nutrition (TPN) related cholestasis, and Type 1 glycogen storage disease [3, 17]. Environmental factors that may play a role in the occurrence of hepatic tumors include maternal use of oral contraceptives [18]. HB has also been observed in patients with familial intrahepatic cholestasis, renal or adrenal agenesis, fetal alcohol syndrome, and Prader-Willi syndrome [19, 20, 21].

In 1997, Ikeda, et al. reported data from the Japanese Pediatric Cancer Registry that indicated HB accounted for 58% of the diagnosed malignancies among extremely low-birth-weight (VLBW <1000 g) infants [22]. Since these babies have many problems associated with prematurity that require various treatments including TPN, phototherapy, and administration of numerous drugs, they may be more vulnerable to certain toxic affects of these substances, suggesting that it is possible that certain postnatal exposures might be tumor promoting [23]. More recently, McLaughlin, et al. confirmed that VLBW babies have a significantly increased risk of developing HB [2]. Low birth weight was a factor independent of gestational age. The odds ratio (OR) of the occurrence of HB was 56.9 for babies weighing less than 1000 g compared to an OR of 5 for those weighing 1000–1400 g and 1.6 for those weighing 1500–2499 g with a 95% confidence interval [2]. Associated factors included male sex (2:1), young maternal age, high maternal prepregnancy weight, maternal hypertension, maternal smoking while pregnant, and presumptive use of fertility drugs [2, 24, 25]. The Children's Oncology Group (COG) in the USA is currently conducting a case-controlled study evaluating this relationship by interviewing mothers and collecting DNA from 600 HB cases and 720 controls.

12.2.2 Clinical Presentation

Hepatoblastoma is more common in boys [3, 7]. It usually presents as an abdominal mass often detected by a parent while bathing the child or is visibly apparent when changing or dressing the child. This is observed in more than 60% of the cases. Most of the patients are less than 3 years of age. Rarely, HB has been observed in the newborn [26, 27]. Other frequent presenting findings include anorexia, failure to thrive, abdominal pain, and abdominal distension. Diarrhea is less commonly observed. Some patients present with fever; however, jaundice is rarely seen since the liver function is otherwise normal. Other common findings include anemia and thrombocytosis. Hepatoblastoma can occasionally rupture and cause intra-abdominal bleeding and present with findings of an acute abdomen [27].

12.2.3 Laboratory Investigations

Most liver function studies in instances of HB are usually normal, in contrast with HCC, which may be associated with underlying liver disease. The most useful test is the measurement of the serum alpha-fetoprotein (AFP) level, which is elevated in at least 70% of children with HB. When elevated at diagnosis, this serum tumor marker is an excellent aid in diagnosis, monitoring response to therapy and, importantly, in the early detection of tumor recurrence [29]. A low serum AFP level (<100 ng/ml) at presentation is a poor prognostic factor [30]. In infants under 6 months of age at diagnosis, the serum AFP level must be corrected for residual fetal AFP. A child presenting with a liver mass between 6 months and 3 years of age, a very high serum AFP level, and typical findings on imaging most often has HB. Elevation of the serum AFP level may also be seen in infants with yolk-sac tumors, sarcomas, hamartomas, and occasionally hemangioendothelioma, suggesting that a diagnostic tissue biopsy should be obtained prior to initiating treatment. Serum beta human chorionic gonadotrophin (β-HCG) level should be obtained in children who demonstrate isosexual precocity [3].

12.2.4 Diagnostic Imaging

The best initial, not invasive, and least expensive imaging investigation of a child with a liver mass is ultrasonography of the abdomen. The abdominal ultrasonogram identifies the origin of the mass, determines the extent of the lesion, and discerns whether the lesion is solid or cystic and whether it is a solitary or a multifocal tumor. Abdominal ultrasound can detect the presence of tumor extension into major vessels, namely the hepatic veins, the vena cava, and the portal vein, which is essential for precise surgical staging and assessing preoperative resectability. Some investigators suggest that to avoid a diagnostic pitfall in differentiating between the various liver malignancies, a diagnostic biopsy is justified [30]. Our practice is to recommend a biopsy to exclude other tumor types in children less than 6 months (e.g., mesenchymal hamartoma) or older than 3 years (e.g., hepatocellular carcinoma), especially in children with modestly raised serum AFP levels. Biopsy can be done with open surgical technique or preferably percutaneously using ultrasound guidance [31]. To prevent tumor seeding, the needle should be advanced through a short depth of normal liver tissue (a portion that will be resected at future surgery). Wang, et al., demonstrated the utility of transthoracic echocardiography for early detection of subclinical cardiac metastases [32]. Lung metastases were more common in children with detectable cardiac involvement. For assessing the relationship of the tumor to the surrounding vital structures such as bile ducts and vessels, computed tomography (CT) and magnetic resonance imaging (MRI), utilizing appropriate vascular enhancement, are essential to determine resectability and exclude intra-abdominal tumor extension beyond the liver (Fig. 12.1 a,b). Lymph node involvement is exceptional in hepatoblastoma. Since HB spreads by vascular invasion, typically to the lungs, CT of the chest should be obtained.

Recent advances in technology including helical (spiral) CT scanning with three-dimensional reconstruction and magnetic resonance angiography have eliminated the necessity of performing hepatic arteriography to determine resectability of HB (Figs. 12.2a–d, 12.3). Currently, we believe that hepatic angiograms are reserved for therapeutic measures including regional drug infusion and transhepatic chemoembolization (TACE).

12.2.5 Histopathology

Hepatoblastoma most commonly appears as a single bulky mass surrounded by a pseudocapsule. Because the capsule is indistinct, microscopic invasion may be found beyond the main lesion. Occasionally, HB may present as a multifocal lesion. During the last two decades, histological subtypes have been described .The fetal/embryonal subtypes were the first to be identified, while the macrotrabecular subtype was the last. The description of these morphotypes resulted in the now widely used HB classification system, which is currently employed in SIOPEL studies (International Liver Tumors Strategy Group of the International Society of Pediatric Oncology, ISPO/SIOP) [33]. Apart

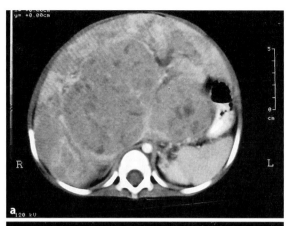
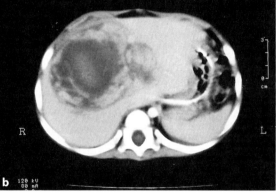

Fig. 12.1 a, b (**a**) Abdominal CT scan shows HB involving both lobes of the liver. (**b**) CT scan from the same patient after 6 courses of chemotherapy prior to surgical resection.

from separating HB from HCC, this classification recognizes that the histopathology of HB reflects distinct phases of liver cell development and maturation. Hepatoblastomas may be of the pure epithelial type that contains either fetal or embryonal cells or a mixture of the two histologic subtypes (Table 12.1, Fig. 12.4a,b). Other epithelial subtypes include the macrotrabecular subtype and the small cell undifferentiated subtype

Table 12.1 Classification of hepatoblastoma (HB) according to the SIOPEL Liver Tumor Strategy Group

Wholly epithelial type
Fetal ("purely fetal") subtype
Embryonal/mixed fetal and embryonal subtype
Macrotrabecular subtype
Small cell undifferentiated subtype (SCUD; formerly anaplastic)
Mixed epithelial and mesenchymal type
Without teratoid features
With teratoid features
Hepatoblastoma, not otherwise specified (HBL-NOS)

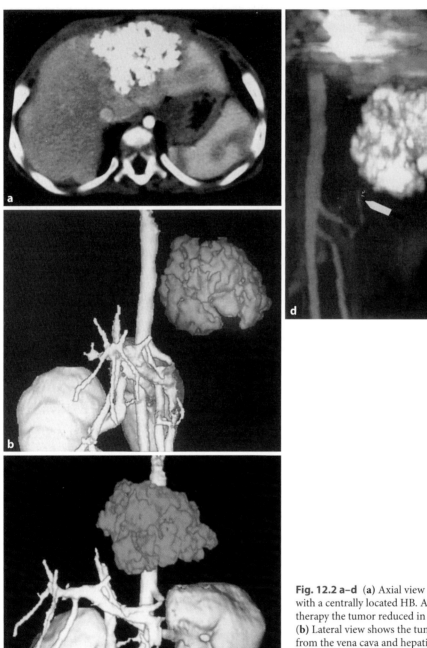

Fig. 12.2 a–d (**a**) Axial view image of CT scan of an infant with a centrally located HB. After four courses of chemotherapy the tumor reduced in size and became calcified. (**b**) Lateral view shows the tumor (*gray–upper right*) separated from the vena cava and hepatic veins. (**c**) 3-D image shows the relationship of the tumor (*green*) and portal vein. (**d**) Oblique view shows the relationship of the hepatic artery (*arrow*) and the tumor.

(formerly anaplastic). A mixed form of HB contains mesenchymal tissue in addition to epithelial components (Fig. 12.4c). The mesenchymal component can present with or without teratoid features. The impact of histopathology on prognosis of HB is not entirely clear. The small cell undifferentiated subtype is generally regarded as high-risk morphology [34]. In a North American study reported by Haas, et al., Stage I children with purely fetal subtype had the most favorable prognosis [34]. Fetal tumor histology resembles the liver of the embryo and consists of uniform trabeculae of small, round cells with abundant cytoplasm and distinct cytoplasmic membranes. Portal tracts and biliary ducts are not seen. The favorable status of fetal histology observed in the US Intergroup study was not confirmed by the SIOPEL study [29].

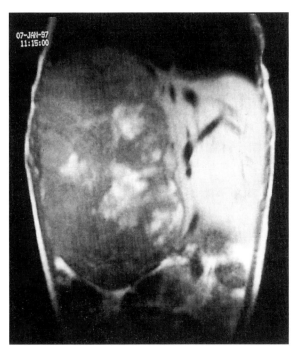

Fig. 12.3 Example of an MR image showing the tumor in relationship to the major vessels.

Table 12.2 Intergroup (Children's Cancer Group/Pediatric Oncology Group) staging system for hepatoblastoma/hepatocellular carcinoma

Stage	Descriptive Criteria
I	Complete tumor resection at diagnosis (segmentectomy, lobectomy, extended lobectomy)
II	Total resection of gross tumor but with evidence of microscopic residual disesase
IIa	Intrahepatic
IIb	Extrahepatic
IIIa	Gross residual tumor following resection at initial operation *or* complete resection with significant tumor spill and/or positive lymph nodes
IIIb	Localized primary tumor not resected; biopsy only
IV	Distant metastases with the primary tumor either (IVa) completely or (IVb) incompletely resected

12.2.6 Staging

The extent of the disease at diagnosis is variable, and since this directly influences outcome, a reproducible staging system is essential. It facilitates comparison

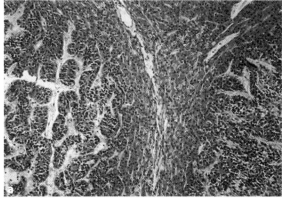

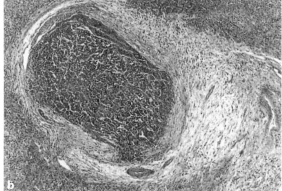

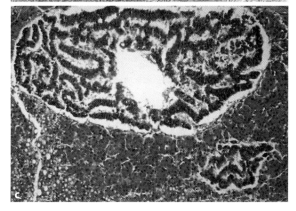

Fig. 12.4 a–c (**a**) Photomicrograph (×72) of an infant with HB sowing both fetal (*left*) and embryonal (*right*) histology. (**b**) Photomicrograph (×4.7) with embryonal tumor in a portal vessel. (**c**) Histological example of a mixed mesenchymal tumor type containing osteoid.

of patients between series, accurate interpretation of data from clinical trials, and should ideally have prognostic value. In the past, a number of staging systems existed for liver tumors in children including the US Intergroup Hepatoblastoma/Hepatocarcinoma Study based on tumor extent, operative findings, and tumor histology [35] (Table 12.2). In Asia and parts of Europe, the International Union Against Cancer used a TNM staging system (tumor size, nodal status, and

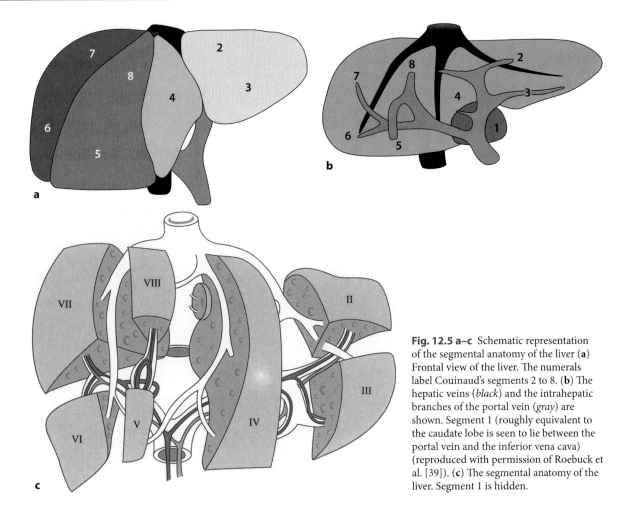

Fig. 12.5 a–c Schematic representation of the segmental anatomy of the liver (**a**) Frontal view of the liver. The numerals label Couinaud's segments 2 to 8. (**b**) The hepatic veins (*black*) and the intrahepatic branches of the portal vein (*gray*) are shown. Segment 1 (roughly equivalent to the caudate lobe is seen to lie between the portal vein and the inferior vena cava) (reproduced with permission of Roebuck et al. [39]). (**c**) The segmental anatomy of the liver. Segment 1 is hidden.

presence or absence of metastases). The German Co-operative Liver tumor study had an alternate staging system similar to the USA [36]. Also in Europe, the International Society of Pediatric Oncology (SIOP) developed a prechemotherapy treatment, presurgical staging system evaluating the extent of disease (PRE-TEXT) based on imaging findings. In the SIOPEL-l prospective trial, a preoperative surgical staging system, based on Couinaud's segmentation of the liver [37], was developed and adopted for subsequent SI-OPEL prospective trials [29]. The PRETEXT system (Fig. 12.5a,b), (based exclusively on imaging obtained at diagnosis) divides the liver into four sections: the left lobe of the liver consists of a lateral (Couinaud's segments II and III) and a medial section (segment IV, quadrate lobe), whereas the right lobe is divided into an anterior (segments V and VIII) and a poste-rior section (segments VI and VII). Couinaud's seg-ment I (caudate lobe) is not included in this division. The tumor is classified into one of the four categories depending on the number of sections free of tumor (Table 12.3, Fig. 12.6). Patients are staged according

Table 12.3 Definitions of PRETEXT number

PRETEXT I:	One section is involved and three adjoining sections are free
PRETEXT II:	One or two sections are involved, but two adjoining sections are free
PRETEXT III:	Two or three sections are involved, and not two adjoining sections are free
PRETEXT IV:	All four sections are involved

to the PRETEXT system at diagnosis, during neoad-juvant chemotherapy and before surgery [29]. This staging system, which is, very roughly, an estimate of the extent of tumor and difficulty of the expected surgical resection, aims to identify patients in whom complete tumor resection could be performed by means of a partial hepatectomy or who would require total hepatectomy and liver transplantation. This sys-tem has been validated in the SIOPEL-1 study where

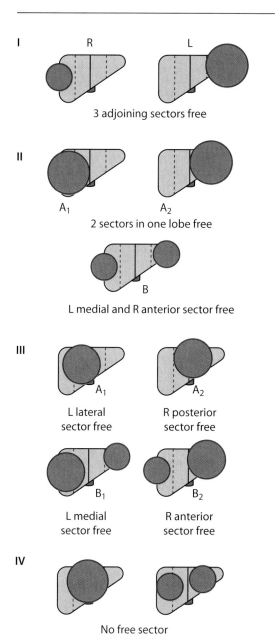

I   R   L

3 adjoining sectors free

II
A₁   A₂

2 sectors in one lobe free

B

L medial and R anterior sector free

III
A₁   A₂

L lateral   R posterior
sector free   sector free

B₁   B₂

L medial   R anterior
sector free   sector free

IV

No free sector

Fig. 12.6 PRETEXT grouping system according to SIOPEL (Liver Tumor Strategy Group of the International Society of Pediatric Oncology-SIOP/ISPO) (From de Ville de Goyet J, Otte JB. Liver tumors and resections. In: Pediatric surgery and urology: Long-term outcomes. Stringer MD, Oldham KT, Moribund PD (eds). Cambridge University Press, Cambridge (in press).

the PRETEXT grouping at presentation was the only significant prognostic factor in a multivariate analysis [29]. The PRETEXT system is quite different from other well-known liver tumor staging systems. The PRETEXT system was specifically developed to stage the tumor before surgical treatment, whereas the other systems stage the tumor postoperatively. The predictive value of the PRETEXT system was fur-

ther analyzed and validated by Aronson, et al. [38]. These authors concluded that this staging system: (1) has moderate accuracy with a tendency to overstage patients, (2) shows good interobserver agreement regarding reproducibility, (3) shows superior predictive value for survival compared to other staging systems, and (4) offers the opportunity to monitor the effect of preoperative therapy.

The PRETEXT grouping system was revised in 2005 to improve the original definition, to clarify the definitions of criteria for extrahepatic extension of tumor and to add new criteria for patients with caudate lobe involvement, tumor rupture, ascites, direct extension of tumor to the stomach or diaphragm, tumor focality, lymph node involvement, distant metastases, and vascular involvement [39]. Although the PRETEXT system is principally used for HB, the 2005 revision may be applicable to all primary malignant liver tumors of childhood, including HCC and epithelioid hemangioendothelioma. The inclusion of additional criteria (Table 12.4) allows for risk stratification in the current SIOPEL studies. Patients are considered high risk with any of the following: serum AFP level <100 mg/L, PRETEXT IV, extension beyond the liver in the abdomen, distant metastases, intraperitoneal hemorrhage, and involvement of hepatic veins, vena cava or portal vein (Table 12.5).

Aronson, et al. recently questioned the predictive accuracy of the Children's Oncology Group (COG) staging system and suggested that the PRETEXT system showed superior predictive value for survival [38]. Both COG and the Japanese Liver Tumor Group trials plan to employ the PRETEXT staging system in future protocols [40]. In the planned COG studies, the defined surgical guidelines indicate that patients with PRETEXT I and any unifocal PRETEXT 2 tumors that have at least a 1.0 cm margin on diagnostic imaging will be resected at diagnosis. All other patients will receive preoperative chemotherapy.

12.2.7 Treatment Guidelines

12.2.7.1 Chemotherapy

During the past 30 years, there has been an improved survival for patients with HB based on refinements in surgical techniques, a better understanding of the hepatic segmental anatomy, advances in chemotherapy, and the advent of liver transplantation as a therapeutic modality for patients with unresectable disease. HB is a surgical neoplasm and only complete tumor resection results in a realistic hope for cure. Long-term disappearance of tumor with complete remission with chemotherapy alone has been anecdotally observed. However, chemotherapy is a cornerstone in the man-

Table 12.4 2005 PRETEXT criteria for «extrahepatic» extension of tumor

C
Caudate lobe involvement
C1 Tumor involving the caudate lobe
C0 All other patients
Al(i)l C1 patients are at least PRETEXT II

E
Extrahepatic abdominal disease
E0 No evidence of tumor spread in the abdomen (except N)
E1 Direct extension of tumor into adjacent organs or diaphragm
E2 Peritoneal nodules
Add suffix „a" if ascites is present, e.g., E0a

F
Tumor focality
F0 Patient with solitary tumor
F1 Patient with two or more discrete tumors

H
Tumor rupture or intraperitoneal hemorrhage
H1 Imaging and clinical findings of intraperitoneal hemorrhage
H0 Al(i)l other patients

M
Distant metastases
M0 No metastases
M1 Any metastasis
Add suffix or suffixes to indicate location

N
Lymph node metastases
N0 No nodal metastases
N1 Abdominal lymph node metastases only
N2 Extra-abdominal lymph node metastases (with or without abdominal lymph node metastases)

P
Portal vein involvement
P0 No involvement of the portal vein or its left or right branches
P1 Involvement of either the left or the right branch of the portal vein
P2 Involvement of the main portal vein
Add suffix "a" if intravascular tumor is present, e.g., P1a

V
Involvement of the IVC and/or hepatic veins
V0 No involvement of the hepatic veins or inferior vena cava (IVC)
V1 Involvement of one hepatic vein but not the IVC
V2 Involvement of two hepatic veins but not the IVC
V3 Involvement of all three hepatic veins and/or the IVC
Add suffix "a" if intravascular tumor is present, e.g., V3a

Table 12.5 Risk stratification in hepatoblastoma for current SIOPEL studies

High risk (HR) = patients with any of the following:
Serum alpha-fetoprotein <100 microgram/L
PRETEXT IV
Additional PRETEXT criteria
E1, E1a, E2, E2a
H1
M1 (any site)
N1, N2
P2, P2a
V3, V3a
Standard risk (SR) = all other patients

agement of HB. Although chemosensitivity varies between patients, it is an essential component of the management and complementary to radical surgical resection to affect a cure. In general, surgeons agree that preoperative chemotherapy helps to reduce the size of most tumors and obtains better demarcation between the tumor and surrounding liver tissue [31, 41, 42]. Consequently, tumors are more likely to be completely resected without increasing perioperative morbidity or mortality. It is also speculated that residual microscopic disease may behave more aggressively under the influence of hepatotrophic factors stimulating liver regeneration if preoperative chemotherapy has not been used [42]. On the other hand, von Schweinitz and coworkers [44] have shown that there is little to be gained from prolonging chemotherapy beyond the planned treatment regimen, which incurs the risk of developing chemoresistance.

In the USA, primary laparotomy has been a traditional practice with either tumor resection followed (or not) [45] by adjuvant chemotherapy or a tumor biopsy followed by chemotherapy and delayed secondary resection [46, 47]. In the Intergroup Hepatoblastoma/Hepatocellular Carcinoma Study, 28% of HB tumors were completely resected at diagnosis (Stage I) and 4% (Stage II) were incompletely excised. These patients had a 91% and 100% 5-year survival, respectively. However, the surgical guidelines of the protocol lacked clear recommendations regarding which tumor should or should not be resected at diagnosis. The decision to biopsy and use preoperative chemotherapy would shift a patient to Stage III status. Lack of a uniform surgical approach was identified as a weakness in the study protocol [40]. The study compared the use of cisplatin and doxorubicin in one treatment arm to cisplatin, vincristine, and 5-fluorouracil (5-FU) in the other arm. The overall 3-year survival rates were 63% and 71%, respectively [48]. Although the difference between the groups was not significant, the cisplatin/doxorubicin group had a higher toxicity rate. All eight deaths related to drug toxicity occurred in the doxorubicin group. In addition, children receiving doxorubicin had longer hospital stays, an increased requirement for supportive TPN, and an increased rate of drug-related complications [49]. A significant response to preoperative chemotherapy was observed in Stage III patients allowing complete tumor resection in 70–80% of these cases [17, 49, 50, 52]. Preoperative chemotherapy had no effect on operative mortality; however, increased transfusion requirement and a higher operative morbidity was observed in patients that received chemotherapy preoperatively [52]. Phase III studies comparing cisplatin and carboplatin vs. cisplatin, vincristine, and 5-FU were stopped when an increased risk of adverse events were observed in patients receiving cisplatin/carboplatin. In addition, the use of a cytoprotective drug, amifostine to reduce cisplatin ototoxicity was not beneficial [40].

The German Cooperative Pediatric Liver Tumor Study also recommended primary surgery for patients with resectable hepatoblastoma. In Study HB-89 [44], patients with HB restricted to one liver lobe underwent primary surgery; larger tumors were initially treated with chemotherapy and resected at second-look surgery. All patients received three drugs (ifosfamide, cisplatin, and doxorubicin) either as adjuvant or neoadjuvant therapy. The results supported the use of preoperative chemotherapy in all patients with HB and that was implemented in the subsequent HB-99 study [42]. In the 2003 LT HB-98 study, patients were divided into risk groups. Standard-risk (SR) patients with a localized potentially resectable tumor received ifosfamide, cisplatin, and doxorubicin, and surgical resection [53]. Thirty-four of 35 (94%) Stage I–III patients survived. High-risk (HR) patients were defined as those with either multifocal tumors, or vascular invasion, extrahepatic spread and metastases [53, 55]. They were treated with carboplatin and etoposide (VP-16). Responders underwent resection of the primary tumor and metastectomy. Five of 9 (55%) achieved remission status [55].

In contrast, the studies coordinated by the SIOPEL group have concentrated on using preoperative chemotherapy [31, 56]. In SIOPEL-1, all patients were treated preoperatively with four courses of cisplatin and doxorubicin (PLADO); surgical resection was followed by two more courses of chemotherapy. If the tumor was judged unresectable by imaging after four courses of chemotherapy, attempting surgical resection was delayed until after the sixth course. If the tumor remained localized to the liver but was still unresectable, liver transplantation was recommended as the primary operative procedure if some response to chemotherapy had been obtained in the absence of extrahepatic tumor extent or metastatic disease. The

SIOPEL-2 pilot study [28] was designed to test the efficacy and toxicity of two chemotherapy regimens, one for patients with HB confined to the liver and involving no more then three hepatic sections "standard–risk (SR) HB," and one for instances of HB extending into all four sections and/or with lung metastases or intra-abdominal extrahepatic spread "high-risk (HR) HB." Those with SR-HB were treated with four courses of cisplatin monotherapy, delayed surgery, and then two more courses of cisplatin. Patients with HR-HB were given cisplatin alternating with carboplatin and doxorubicin, pre- and postoperatively. For SR-HB patients (n = 77), and HR-HB patients (n = 58), the 3-year progression-free survival rates were 89% and 48%, respectively. For SR-HB patients, the efficacy of cisplatin monotherapy and the cisplatin/doxorubicin combination are now being compared in a prospective randomized trial (SIOPEL-3 study). For HR-HB patients, intensified chemotherapy with cisplatin, doxorubicin, and carboplatin is being investigated in a SIOPEL-4 study.

In unifocal HB, PRETEXT grouping based on imaging studies at diagnosis in some cases may lead to overstaging the tumor from PRETEXT III to PRETEXT IV when the anatomic border separating a lateral section from the sections of the liver harboring the bulging mass is simply displaced (due to compression) but not invaded [39]. Indeed, repeat imaging studies after chemotherapy, when the tumor has shrunken, can demonstrate that the anatomic border is free from invasion and allow for correct staging and performance of a partial hepatectomy (right or left trisegmentectomy). In multifocal HB with lesions scattered in the different sections of the liver, clearance of one section, (e.g., the left lateral section) [54] can apparently be achieved by chemotherapy in some cases, tempting the surgeon to perform a partial rather than a total hepatectomy. However, this strategy is not recommended because of the high risk of leaving viable malignant tumor cells in the remaining section. Therefore, in multifocal hepatoblastoma, liver transplantation is the best treatment option, whatever the apparent result of chemotherapy. Further intensification of chemotherapy when the response to completion of full courses of chemotherapy according to protocol is considered unsatisfactory, and hazardous attempts at partial liver resection in order to avoid liver transplantation "at any cost" are no longer justified since the efficacy of primary liver transplantation for unresectable HB has been validated during the last decade.

12.2.7.2 Surgical Resection

Careful preoperative assessment of children with liver tumors is essential to establish whether the tumor is

Right hemihepatectomy (segments 5–8±1)   Left hemihepatectomy (segments 2–4)

Fig. 12.7 Liver anatomy and types of partial liver resection (reproduced with permission from Stringer [41]).

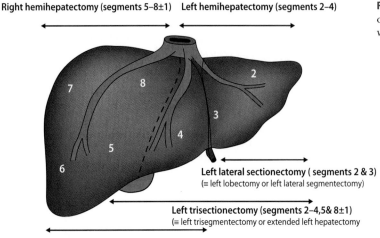

Left lateral sectionectomy (segments 2 & 3)
(≡ left lobectomy or left lateral segmentectomy)

Left trisectionectomy (segments 2–4,5& 8±1)
(≡ left trisegmentectomy or extended left hepatectomy)

Right trisectionectomy (segments 4–8±1)
(≡ right trisegmentectomy or extended right hepatectomy)

Other resections: Segmental or non-anatomical

N.B. The caudate lobe (segment 1) is not visible

resectable and determine the hepatic functional reserve of the patient if they have cirrhosis [49]. The procedure is performed under general endotracheal anesthesia. Large-bore venous access is obtained in the upper extremities. A percutaneous arterial line is placed to monitor blood pressure and blood gas tensions. Urine output is monitored through an indwelling bladder catheter. The objective of the surgical procedure is to obtain a complete resection of the tumor, both macro- and microscopically, which is paramount for cure of HB (and other liver cancers). The surgical strategy should be based on a sound knowledge of segmental liver anatomy as espoused by Couinaud [57], vascular occlusion techniques and expertise in performing the different types of liver resections, including the most extensive procedures (left or right trisegmentectomies) (Fig. 12.7). Intraoperative ultrasound is useful in confirming the location of major vessels and other structures. The reader is referred to previous reports describing the operative procedures in detail [3, 17, 59, 50]. Nonanatomical, atypical resections are best avoided, except in rare cases (i.e., pedunculated tumor), because of an increased risk of incomplete tumor removal and a higher incidence of postoperative complications [42]. Very extensive liver resections (up to 80% of the liver mass) can be tolerated by young children with HB and hepatic regeneration can be complete within 3 months, despite the administration of toxic agents since they usually have no underlying liver disease and excellent hepatic reserve [58]. Liver function rapidly returns to normal without long-term sequelae. Complete tumor resection can be easily achieved with a partial hepatectomy when the intrahepatic extent is limited to one or two sections (PRETEXT I and II). When the tumor involves three sections (PRETEXT III), preoperative neoadjuvant chemotherapy can make lesions initially considered "unresectable" become resectable with a trisegmentectomy [32, 53–55].

12.2.7.3 Liver Transplantation

Previous studies have validated the concept of total hepatectomy and primary transplantation for unresectable HB. In SIOPEL-1 [59], 12 patients (8% of all patients enrolled from 1990–1994) underwent liver transplantation as the primary surgical option (after appropriate preoperative chemotherapy) in seven children and as a rescue procedure in five children because of incomplete partial resection or tumor relapse after partial hepatectomy. The long-term, disease-free patient survival was 66% for the entire series and 85% and 40% for primary transplants and rescue transplants, respectively. Current follow up is >10 years for all patients. All eight patients with PRETEXT IV tumors and all six patients with multifocal HB were cured of their disease. Of the seven patients with macroscopic extension into the portal vein and/or the hepatic veins/vena cava, 71% became long-term, disease-free survivors, as well as four of five (80%) children who had lung metastases at presentation with complete clearance of lung lesions after chemotherapy. If no more than seven patients received a primary trans-

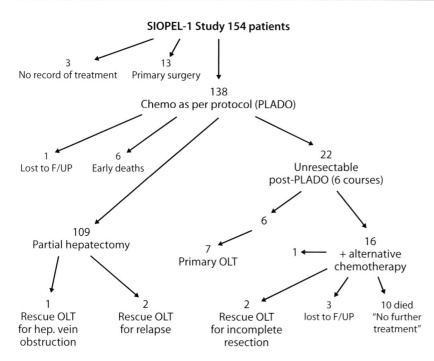

Fig. 12.8 Flowchart of SIOPEL-1 study (reproduced with permission from Otte [61]).

plant (5% of the 138 patients treated with chemotherapy as per protocol), the full potential could have been higher (around 15%) [60] (Fig. 12.8).

An extensive review of the world experience collected 147 cases of liver transplantation for HB [59]. Data were contributed by 24 centers (12 in North America, 10 in Europe, 1 in Japan and Australia each). Their experience, gained mostly during the preceding decade, comprised 10 to 16 cases per center in 6 instances and between 1 and 9 cases in 16 instances. Twenty-eight (19% of the total) patients presented with macroscopic venous extension and 12 (8%) with lung metastases. A total of 106 patients (72%) underwent a primary transplant and 41 (28%) received a rescue transplant, either for incomplete resection with partial hepatectomy or for tumor relapse after previous partial hepatectomy. Twenty-eight (19%) received a live, donor-related liver transplant, and 119 (81%) received a postmortem liver graft. Median follow-up since diagnosis for surviving patients was 38 months (range 1 to 121 months). Overall disease-free survival at 6 years posttransplant was 82% and 30% for primary transplants and for rescue transplants, respectively. It was 82% and 71% after living related donor liver transplantation and postmortem liver transplantation, respectively. Multivariate statistical analysis showed no difference in regard to gender, age, and lung metastases at presentation or type of transplant. For primary transplants, the only parameter significantly related to overall survival was macroscopic venous invasion (P = 0.045). Remarkably, the 6-year, disease-free survival (82%) for the 106 patients who received a primary

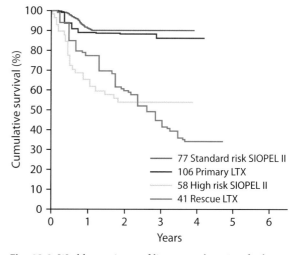

Fig. 12.9 World experience of liver transplantation for hepatoblastoma: patient survival curves after primary and rescue transplants [61], compared with progression-free survivals of patients treated for "high-risk and "low-risk" hepatoblastomas in SIOPEL-2 study [57].

transplant was similar to the 3-year, progression-free survival (89%) for the 77 HB patients with standard-risk hepatoblastoma confined to the liver and involving no more than 3 hepatic sections that were enrolled in the SIOPEL-2 study [28] (Fig. 12.9). In a recent review of the UNOS database in the USA concerning liver transplantation in 135 children with unresectable or recurrent HB, the one, five, and 10 year survival was 79%, 69%, and 66% respectively [61]. The median age at transplantation was 2.9 ± 2.5 years. Sixteen percent received a graft from a live donor. Fifty-five percent of the deaths were due to metastases or recurrent disease [61].

12.2.8 Outcomes

12.2.9 Surgical Morbidity and Mortality

In experienced surgical units, major intraoperative complications of liver resection for HB such as severe bleeding, air embolism, and unrecognized bile duct injury are infrequent and operative mortality is very low, even after extended hepatectomies, since children with HB have no underlying liver disease. As an example, Table 12.6 summarizes the 25 years (1978–2003) of experience gained at Cliniques Saint-Luc, Brussels [60] with 53 children treated for HB. There were 39 partial hepatectomies, including 23 right or left trisegmentectomies, and 13 primary liver transplants (two

from deceased donors and 11 from living related donors). Only one child died from surgical complications (extensive portal vein thrombosis present at diagnosis). Postoperative bleeding requiring reoperation was encountered in 2 patients (3.5%). The incidence of biliary complications was 7.6% after partial hepatectomy and 23% following liver transplantation (Table 12.7). Actuarial disease-free survival was 89% and 79% in transplant patients and in children treated with partial hepatectomy, respectively (Fig. 12.10). Although individual centers treat relatively small numbers of patients with liver cancer, the best overall survival rates are obtained in experienced units that include liver transplantation in their surgical armamentarium [61]. Some centers have reported their overall experience while others have reported their experience with transplanted patients only. Apart from the SIOPEL group, cooperative study groups have not included transplantation in their strategy. Table 12.8 summarizes relevant reports published during the last decade. It suggests that the modern strategy of combining che-

Table 12.6 Experience at Cliniques Saint-Luc, Brussels (1978-2003) (53 patients)

Types of resection	
No resection (biopsies only, all negative)	1
Nonanatomic resection	1
Partial hepatectomy	38
Left lateral segmentectomy	2
Left hepatectomy	1
Left trisegmentectomy	5 (1 rescue OLT for technical failure of ex-situ resection)
Right hepatectomy	12 (1 rescue OLT for tumor relapse)
Right trisegmentectomy	18 (2 rescue OLT for technical failure)
Primary OLT	13

OLT, orthotopic liver transplantation

Table 12.7 Cliniques Saint-Luc Brussels experience (1978–2003)

Surgical complications after resection for hepatoblastoma after partial hepatectomy (n=39)		
Postoperative bleeding requiring surgery	2	Surgical correction
Bile duct stricture	2	Roux-en-Y loop
Bile duct section	1	Roux-en-Y loop
Liver necrosis after ex-situ surgery	1	Rescue transplant
Small bowel obstruction	2	Surgical revision
Portal vein thrombosis	1*	Rescue transplant
Budd-Chiari syndrome (late)	1	Rescue transplant
After liver transplantation (n=17)		
Bile leak	1	Surgical revision
Anastomotic stricture	3	Surgical revision
Small bowel obstruction	3	Surgical revision
Portal vein thrombosis	1*	Liver failure/death*

* (same patient)

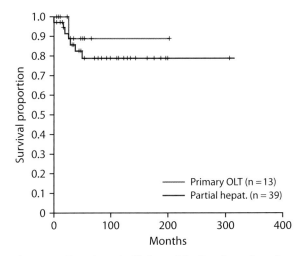

Fig. 12.10 Experience in Cliniques Saint-Luc, Brussels: patient survival curves after primary transplantation (OLT) and partial hepatectomy (reproduced with permission from Otte [60]).

motherapy and radical tumor resection enables the majority of children with HB to be cured. The results of treating high-risk HB (involving all four hepatic sections and/or presenting with evidence of extrahepatic disease) are still less than satisfactory. Better results are achieved when patients are managed within a specialist pediatric center performing both major liver resection and liver transplantation surgery [63].

In the USA, protocol " AHEP 0531: Treatment of Children with all stages of Hepatoblastoma" is currently under review by the National Cancer Institute. This is a risk-based protocol in which patients are stratified into low-, intermediate-, and high-risk categories. The low-risk category includes Stage I patients resected at diagnosis defined as PRETEXT I and unifocal PRETEXT II patients with at least a 1.0 cm resection margin on imaging. Stage I patients with favorable histology that are highly curable will receive reduced chemotherapy in an attempt to limit morbid-

Table 12.8 Hepatoblastoma: survival rates in pediatric series

	Reference	Interval	Center	N	Transplant	Survival
A. Single center experiences	Stringer [69]	1981–1993	London, UK	41	2%	67%
	Srinivasan [70]	1992–2001	London, UK	13	100%	85%
	Pimpalwar [62]	1991–2002	Birmingham, UK	34	41%	91%
	Molmenti [71]	1984–2002	Dallas, USA	9	100%	66%
	McDiarmid a	1984–2001	UCLA,USA	16	100%	75%
	Mejia [72]	1986–1999	Omaha, USA	10	100%	70%
	Gauthier a	1985–2004	Paris, France	64	5%	68%
	Otte [60]	1978–2003	Brussels, Belgium	53	32%	87%
B. Multicenter studies	Sasaki [73]	1991–1999	JPLT-1 b	134	0%	73%
	von Schweinitz [36]	<1994	HB-89 c	72	0%	75%
	Fuchs [44]	1994–1998	HB-94 c	69	3%	77%
	Ortega [35]	1989–1992	COG d	182	0%	57–69%
	Pritchard [55]	1990–1994	SIOPEL-1 e	154	8%	75%
	Perilongo [34]	1995–1998	SIOPEL-2 e	SR (f):77	0%	91%
				HR (g):58	12%	53%
	Austin [61]	1987–2004	UNOS (USA)	135	100%	1 yr 79% 5 yr 69% 10 yr 66%

a unpublished data, personal communications
b JPL T-1:Japan Study Group for Pediatric Liver Tumors
c HB-89 & HB-94: GermanCooperative Pediatric Liver Tumor studies
d COG: Children's Oncology Group, USA
e SIOPEL: Liver Tumor Strategy Group of International Society of Pediatric Oncology
f SR = standard risk
g HR= high risk

ity without altering event-free survival (EFS). Patients with a resected Stage I tumor with fetal histology will not receive chemotherapy. Intermediate-risk patients include those with Stage I small cell undifferentiated histology, and Stage II and III. The PRETEXT grouping assisted by central review of imaging will be investigated to evaluate if it helps to determine resectability. A lower dose of doxorubicin will be added to cisplatin, 5-FU, and vincristine in an effort to diminish excessive toxicity. A mandatory surgical consultation is required to determine resectability at the onset of the third chemotherapy cycle allowing time to plan surgical resection as soon as blood cell counts recover following the fourth cycle. The effect of microscopic positive margins on the risk of relapse will also be studied [40]. High risk patients are those with metastases (Stage IV tumors) that currently represent 25% of the HB cases and have less than a 25% survival. These children will receive an upfront window of chemotherapy using vincristine and irinotecan in hopes of achieving an increased tumor response rate. The efficacy of surgical resection of lung metastases that are resistant to chemotherapy will also be evaluated.

The Liver Tumor Subcommittee of the Children's Oncology Group Rare Tumor Committee has developed a feasibility study, "COG AHEP-04P1: Early referral of patients with potentially unresectable hepatoblastoma for evaluation by centers with surgical expertise in major liver resection and liver transplantation" [40, 63, 64]. This transplant referral feasibility study is also currently undergoing review by the National Cancer Institute. This study examines the role of liver transplantation in unresectable HB PRETEXT III patients with either vena cava (V) or portal vein (P) involvement or those with PRETEXT IV tumors. The goal of the study is to achieve complete surgical resection of all tumor after four cycles of chemotherapy even if it requires complete hepatectomy and liver transplantation.

All patients enrolled in the American COG feasibility study who undergoes liver transplantation will be enrolled in the international PLUTO registry [64]. PLUTO stands for *Pediatric Liver Unresectable Tumor Observatory* and was developed by the SIOPEL strategy group. This will allow online registration of children undergoing liver transplantation for a malignant liver tumor. The aim is to establish an international multicenter database with prospective registration of children (<18 years) presenting with unresectable tumor (HB, HCC, epithelioid hemangioendothelioma) undergoing primary or rescue liver transplantation. A remote data entry system will be accessible online, worldwide, and free of charge. This prospective database was launched in July, 2006 (https://pluto.cineca.org) [64]. It is expected that when sufficient numbers of patients are accrued, the PLUTO database will allow

us to address several issues that remain unclear when evaluating retrospective HB studies, including the prognostic significance of vascular invasion, optimal timing of transplantation, optimal amount and timing of pretransplant (neoadjuvant) and posttransplant (adjuvant) chemotherapy, the value of liver transplantation in children presenting with a relapse after partial liver resection, the potential role of transplantation in children who initially present with metastatic disease that resolves on neoadjuvant chemotherapy, and the amount of immunosuppression needed following transplantation. A prospective evaluation is also necessary to assess the role of liver transplantation for HCC and epithelioid hemangioendothelioma, which may behave differently in children than in adults.

12.2.10 Guidelines for Early Referral of Patients with Hepatoblastoma to a Transplant Unit

According to the results of published studies, the following guidelines have been developed for early consultation with a transplant surgeon [31]:

1. Multifocal PRETEXT IV HB is a clear and undisputed indication for primary liver transplantation, whatever the result of chemotherapy. Apparent clearance of one liver lobe should not distract from this guideline because of the high probability of persistent microscopic viable neoplastic cells. Pediatric oncologists should resist the temptation to intensify chemotherapy in a vain effort to avoid transplantation. These patients should be treated within the same protocol as patients with localized tumors amenable to partial hepatectomy, with as many cycles of chemotherapy before and after transplantation as patients submitted to partial hepatectomy for a localized HB.

2. Primary liver transplantation may be the best option for large, solitary PRETEXT IV HB, involving all four sections of the liver, unless tumor downstaging is demonstrated after initial chemotherapy. If this is the case, a clear retraction of the tumor from the anatomic border of one lateral sector would allow performance of a radical trisegmentectomy.

3. Unifocal, centrally located PRETEXT II and III tumors involving main hilar structures or all three main hepatic veins should be considered for primary liver transplantation because these venous structures would presumably not become free of tumor after chemotherapy. Heroic attempts at partial hepatectomy would be best avoided because of the risk of incomplete resection of malignant tissue.

12.2.10.1 Contraindications

Persistence of viable extrahepatic tumor deposits after chemotherapy, not amenable to surgical resection, is the only absolute contraindication for liver transplantation. Macroscopic venous invasion (portal vein, hepatic veins, vena cava) is not a contraindication if complete resection of the invaded venous structures can be accomplished. When there is evidence or suspicion of invasion of the retrohepatic vena cava, it should be resected «en-bloc» and reconstructed [65]. Review of the world experience showed that venous extent was associated with a significantly shorter survival (P = 0.045) [59]. In contrast, 71% of these patients were alive and disease-free >10 years after liver transplantation in the SIOPEL-l study. Of the nine TNM IV A/IVB patients (eight with major intrahepatic venous invasion) reported by Reyes and associates, seven were alive and disease-free 21–146 months after transplantation [66]. Patients with lung metastases at presentation should not be excluded from liver transplantation if the metastases clear completely after chemotherapy. Long-term, disease-free survival was obtained in 80% of such patients in the SIOPEL-l study and 58% in the world experience. Complete eradication of metastatic lesions by chemotherapy and surgical resection of any suspicious remnant after chemotherapy is a paramount prerequisite for transplantation [67]. When tumor resection by partial hepatectomy is incomplete or when intrahepatic relapse is observed after a previous partial hepatectomy, performing a rescue liver transplantation may be a relative contraindication because of the disappointing results observed in the SIOPEL-l study and in the reported world experience.

12.2.10.2 Timing of Transplantation

Timing of liver transplantation should not be delayed in excess of a few weeks after the last course of chemotherapy (as per protocol). An expeditious access to organ donors is required to meet this requirement. If this is not possible with postmortem organ donation (including split liver grafts), a live-related donor is a valuable option [68].

12.2.11 Surveillance

Preoperative chemotherapy and the availability of liver transplantation have improved the outcome of children with HB [3, 59, 61, 66, 69–74]. Patients with conditions associated with an increased risk of HB may benefit from early detection as a result of surveillance programs using periodic measurement of the serum AFP level and abdominal sonography. These may include patients with Beckwith-Wiedemann syndrome, glycogen storage disease, hemihypertrophy and a family history of familial adenomatous polyposis or Gardner's syndrome [53]. Whether surveillance for HB will become an option for very low-birth-weight infants in the future is still not clear.

12.3 Hepatocellular Carcinoma

12.3.1 Epidemiology and Incidence

Approximately one million new cases of HCC are observed worldwide annually [75]. Most cases are noted in adult patients. Hepatocellular carcinoma HCC in children has a different incidence and epidemiologic background and responds differently to treatment than HB. HCC in children behaves somewhat similar to HCC in the adult. The incidence of HCC has remained rather consistent for the past decade occurring in 0.5–1.0 cases per million children [1]. The epidemiology of HCC varies with the global region and exhibits wide geographic variations [77, 78]. The incidence of HCC in Eastern Asia and sub-Saharan Africa is significantly higher than in Western countries (Europe, Australia, and New Zealand) and Caucasian populations in North and South America [77–81]. In contrast to HB (usually occurring in children less than 3 years of age), the median age for children with HCC is 10–11.2 years [3]. The male to female ratio is 2:1 in young children, but increases with age. Liver disease as a result of alcohol consumption is a major factor in the development of adult HCC that does not affect the incidence in children. While most cases of HCC in adults and 70% in children from Asia and Africa occur in patients with pre-existing liver disease or inflammation, only 33% of children with HCC in Western countries have cirrhosis [79–82]. HCC in patients with liver disease often occurs in areas where viral hepatitis B is endemic [7, 8, 79, 80]. The seropositive rate for the hepatitis B surface antigen approaches 100% in children with HCC in Taiwan and mainland China [83, 84]. Studies of the DNA in HCC tissue indicate that hepatitis B viral sequences have been incorporated [85]. A nationwide hepatitis B vaccination program in Taiwan reduced the incidence of HCC in children less than 10 years of age [83]. HCC has also been observed in patients with liver disease related to chronic active hepatitis C. This is associated with an RNA virus for which there is no vaccine available. Hepatitis C has been identified in almost 80% of HCC cases in Japan, 38% in France, and 20% in the USA [86]. The incidence of HCC increases with time (two to four decades) suggesting that chronic active hepatitis C is a slowly progressing premalignant condition. The age-adjusted incidence rates of HCC in the USA have doubled over the past two decades [87, 88].

Half of the cases are related to hepatitis C virus and the rate is expected to increase during the next decade in the 45–65 year age group.

HCC has also been observed in children with other types of congenital metabolic and inflammatory diseases including tyrosinemia [89], glycogen storage disease-I [90, 91], PiZZ alpha-1 antitrypsin deficiency [92], Alagille syndrome [93, 94], Neiman-Pick disease [95], Fanconi's anemia, liver cell dysplasia [96], liver cell adenoma [97], agenesis of the portal vein [98], Gardner's syndrome [99], and chronic hepatic congestion after Fontan repair for congenital heart disease [100]. Children with severe cholestasis and liver disease related to neonatal hepatitis [101], biliary atresia [102], progressive familial intrahepatic cholestasis (PFIC) [103, 104], and liver mitochondrial respiratory chain disease [105] are at an increased risk of developing HCC. Long-term administration of total parenteral nutrition (TPN) complicated by liver disease and subsequent cirrhosis has also been associated with development of HCC. The simultaneous occurrence of HCC and Wilms' tumor has been reported [106] as has the association of HCC with Wilms' tumor in siblings with Bloom syndrome [107]. HCC has also been observed 9–16 years after successful treatment of Wilms' tumor [108, 109]. These latter patients were managed by chemotherapy and irradiation that included the liver in the radiation portal. HCC has been reported as a late rare event in children with acute lymphocytic leukemia that acquired transfusion-related HCV [110, 111]. A number of environmental exposures have been identified that may increase the risk of HCC, including exposure to aflatoxin, nitrosamines, polyvinyl chloride, hormonal therapy for sterility, pesticides, paint metal pigment, and in association with dietary iron overload in Black Africans [8, 112–114]. Chromosomal aberrations have been observed in patients with HCC including gains in 1q, 8q, and 17q, and loss of 4q, 8p [10]. p53 and beta-catenin mutations have been noted in HCC and may influence tumorigenesis [12, 115, 116].

12.3.2 Clinical Findings

The findings on physical examination are similar to those noted for patients with HB, namely, abdominal mass, right-upper quadrant fullness or pain, weight loss, anorexia, and rarely vomiting [3, 49, 117]. Jaundice may be a presenting finding in a small number of children with cirrhosis due to cholestatic conditions (biliary atresia, neonatal hepatitis, etc.). In cirrhotic children, splenomegaly and cutaneous spider angiomas may be observed. Some cases may present with the onset of acute abdominal pain due to tumor rupture. Ascites may be associated with underlying liver disease in children with cirrhosis but rarely may also be a manifestation of extrahepatic tumor spread in noncirrhotic patients. Gastrointestinal bleeding from esophageal varices caused by hepatic artery-portal vein fistula as a manifestation of HCC has rarely been observed [118]. Gynecomastia has occasionally been noted in patients with the fibrolamellar variant of HCC [81, 119]. Twenty-five percent of children with HCC have metastases at the time of diagnosis, most frequently to the lungs, which may result in respiratory symptoms. Other sites of metastases include the brain and bone marrow.

12.3.3 Laboratory Findings

Although most children with HB have an elevated serum AFP level, this marker is elevated in only 50–70% of patients with HCC. The serum ferritin level may be elevated in 50% of cases and the carcinoembryonic antigen (CEA) level is elevated in 30%. High serum vitamin B-12 and transcobalamin levels may be seen in children with the fibrolamellar variant of HCC [81, 120, 121]. All children with HCC should be screened for exposure to viral hepatitis B and C. Similar to HB, some children with HCC may be anemic and others may demonstrate thrombocytosis. One-third of the HCC cases in the USA occur in children with cirrhosis and may present with elevated serum liver enzyme levels (AST) and those with splenomegaly may show pancytopenia. Careful assessment of hepatic functional reserve in children with cirrhosis is important prior to embarking on major hepatic resection. Iodocyanine-green (ICG) dye clearance has been used as a predictor of successful hepatic resection in adult patients with HCC and cirrhosis [122]. The dye is cleared by hepatocytes and excreted in unconjugated bile. Ninety percent should be cleared from the blood stream 15 min after intravenous dye administration. Fifteen to 20% ICG retention suggests resection of two segments will be well tolerated; 20–30% retention will permit a single segment to be safely resected; however, greater than 40% dye retention is associated with liver failure following even a minimal resection [123]. Preoperative galactose elimination capacity has also been used to predict complications and survival after hepatic resection in cirrhotic patients but the authors have no personal experience with this test [124]. Determining the Child-Pugh status of cirrhotic patients may also be useful in selecting the most appropriate treatment. Child-Pugh class A and B patients tolerate therapeutic interventions (i.e., hepatic resection, transarterial catheter embolization, liver transplantation) much better than Child-Pugh class C children who have short life expectancy [123]. Therefore, the serum albumin, bilirubin, prothrombin time, and sodium level (evaluating hyponatremia as an indicator of ascites) should be measured preoperatively.

12.3.4 Imaging

Plain abdominal radiographs may demonstrate a right-upper abdominal mass. Less than 10% of the tumors are calcified. Abdominal ultrasonography can discern between a cystic and solid lesion and often detect tumor in vascular and biliary structures. In HCC, contemporary high resolution triple phase computed tomography (CT), CT angioportography, magnetic resonance imaging (MRI) and MR-angiography (MRA) have been increasingly useful in determining tumor extent and involvement of vascular and biliary structures [123]. HCC is often multifocal and may present with a variable number and distribution of tumor nodules. While identifying larger nodules is not difficult, recognizing lesions less than 1.0 cm is still a challenge. Positron emission tomography (PET) using 18-fluorodeoxyglucose may be useful in identifying unsuspected extrahepatic disease [125, 126]. Three-dimensional CT image analysis techniques are now available to estimate tumor volume and provide detailed intrahepatic anatomy that resembles the actual intraoperative findings [123]. CT volumetry may permit calculation of resected tumor volume and anticipated size of the remnant liver in planning resection [86, 127]. Diagnostic laparoscopy has been used in adults with HCC in instances with uncertain imaging studies to determine if extrahepatic disease is present and may upstage the patient and avoid unnecessary attempts at resection [128]. Plain radiograph and CT of the chest should be obtained to rule out lung metastases. As in instances of HB, hepatic arteriography is currently limited to instances of HCC managed by hepatic artery infusion or transcatheter chemoembolization.

12.3.5 Histopathology

HCC is an epithelial malignancy that often has the same histological appearance noted in adults characterized by large pleomorphic cells with prominent nucleoli that resemble mature hepatocytes and have a compact or trabecular growth pattern [85, 129]. HCC often presents with bilobar involvement with either multicentric tumor nodules or diffuse intrahepatic spread. They commonly show absence of a fibrous tumor capsule and evidence of hemorrhage, necrosis, and vascular invasion [81]. In adults with HCC, nuclear grade and microvascular invasion are multivariate risk factors predictive of a poor outcome [130].

This observation has not been established in any pediatric tumor studies.

The fibrolamellar variant of HCC (FL-HCC) occurs more often in older children and adolescents representing 30% of HCC cases less than 20 years of age [81]. It is usually not associated with cirrhosis or viral hepatitis and occurs more commonly in American Caucasians than in Asians. FL-HCC is characterized by a well-circumscribed single mass composed of tumor cells with a hyaline eosinophilic cytoplasm and broad bands of collagen-rich fibrous tissue. CT of the abdomen may demonstrate a heterogeneous solitary mass with a central scar that may be calcified. Thirty percent have metastases at the time of diagnosis. Of interest, is that serum AFP levels may be normal, but serum vitamin B-12, transcobalamin, neurotensin levels, and aromatase expression may be elevated [81, 119, 120]. Cytogenetic alterations noted in FL-HCC include chromosomal loss at 9p, 16p, and Xq and gain at 4q [10], and may be different in primary and recurrent disease [131]. A third subtype of liver cell tumor with aggressive behavior and histology intermediate between HB and HCC has been recently reported [132]. The lesion termed transitional cell liver tumor (TLCT) is observed in older children that have high serum AFP-levels and beta-catenin mutations associated with increased tumorigenicity [132, 133].

Tumor biopsy is essential in suspected HCC cases to confirm the diagnosis prior to initiating treatment. The differential diagnosis includes HCC, HB, epithelial sarcoma, rhabdoid tumors, and a variety of benign tumors including adenomas, focal nodular hyperplasia, hemangioendothelioma, teratoma, and mesenchymal hamartoma. Different biopsy techniques have been used including fine needle aspiration (FNA), tru-cut needle core acquisition, laparoscopic acquired biopsy, and open biopsy. FNA may miss tumor nodules and provides limited material for study. Despite the small size of the needle, local dissemination of HCC has been reported in children after use of FNA [134, 135]. Tru-cut biopsies have been more useful in our experience with multiple entry when necessary providing adequate tissue for study [55]. Acquiring a biopsy with ultrasound guidance is useful. Traditional open biopsy is still favored by many surgeons and allows a better assessment of the liver involvement and acquisition of adequate tissue for histological and biological/genetic studies under direct vision. More recently, diagnostic laparoscopy has been employed to evaluate for tumor resectability and acquire biopsy material under direct vision. Identification of unsuspected extrahepatic extension of disease or involvement of lymph nodes may avoid a formal laparotomy in some instances [123,128].

Table 12.9 Classification of hepatocellular carcinoma. Current AJCC/UICC TNM, Histologic grade, and fibrosis score*

Tumor (T)			
TX cannot be assessed			
T0 no evidence of primary			
T1 solitary tumor – no vascular invasion			
T2 solitary tumor – vascular invasion or multiple tumors all <5.0 cm			
T3 multiple tumors >5.0 cm or tumor involving portal or hepatic veins			
T4 tumor with direct invasion of adjacent organs or perforation of visceral peritoneum			
Lymph nodes (N) – regional	**Metastases (M) – distant**		
NX cannot be assessed	MX – cannot be assessed		
N1 no nodal metastases	M0 none		
N2 nodal metastases	M1 distant metastases		
Staging (by group)	**T**	**N**	**M**
I	T1	N0	M0
II			
IIIA	T2	N0	M0
IIIB	T3	N0	M0
IIIC			
IV	T4	N0	M0
	any T	N1	M0
	any T	any N	M1
Histologic grading	**Fibrosis Score (F)**		
Gx cannot be assessed	F0 0–4 (none to moderate fibrosis)		
G1 well differentiated	F1 5–6 (severe fibrosis to cirrhosis)		
G2 moderately differentiated			
G3 poorly differentiated			
G4 undifferentiated			

*Green F et al. [144]

12.3.6 Staging

While tumor staging has been an important consideration in determining the plan of treatment and prognosis, no single staging system for HCC has been universally accepted. This is related to the fact that two-thirds of childhood cases have no underlying liver disease as a confounding factor. Most childhood cases of HCC have been staged and treated according to COG (in the USA) and SIOP in Europe (PRETEXT) systems and protocols employed for HB despite the fact that the two tumors are biologically different. The TNM system had traditionally been used in adults; however, it does not take into account hepatic function which influences outcome since the majority of adult patients with HCC have liver disease. A number of staging systems have subsequently been developed (mainly in adults) evaluating liver function and tumor extent based on clinical and radiographic findings as a guideline for treatment [136–140]. The most popular

are the Okuda system [136] in Japan (evaluating tumor size, ascites, bilirubin, and albumin) and Cancer of the Liver Italian Program (CLIP) system [138] (includes risk scores for Child-Pugh classification, tumor morphology and extent, serum AFP level, and portal vein thrombosis) [141–143]. Neither of these systems include pathological findings making them more useful for patients with more advanced liver disease and they may not predict prognosis after resection [86]. Recently, a new American Joint Commission for Cancer (AJCC)/International Union Against Cancer (UICC) staging system for HCC was developed that incorporates TNM, histologic grade, stage grouping, and liver fibrosis score [86, 144] (Table 12.9). This has not been employed in childhood cases, but is an attractive alternative in patients that undergo primary tumor resection as it would be applicable to the 33% of cases of HCC with pre-existing liver disease as well as the majority (67%) of children without cirrhosis. Since this system utilizes information acquired after tumor resection and is in part pathology based, it may not be as useful for patients receiving other nonresectional treatments or preoperative neoadjuvant chemotherapy [123].

12.3.7 HCC Studies in Children

Since HCC is a relatively uncommon tumor in children, information concerning the management and outcomes in these cases is dependent upon the results of larger series from group studies in the USA, Germany, Europe (SIOP), and Asia. Many patients in these studies were managed in a similar manner to younger patients with HB. Katzenstein, et al. [145] described the outcomes of 46 children with HCC treated in the POG and CCG Intergroup Hepatoma study (INT-0098). Ten of the 46 children had the FL-HCC variant. At the time of diagnosis, only eight children were amenable to complete primary tumor resection (Stage I), 25 had an unresectable tumor (Stage III), and 13 had metastases (Stage IV) and had a biopsy followed by chemotherapy. There were no Stage II patients in the study. Twenty patients were randomized to receive cisplatin, vincristine, and 5-FU while 26 were treated with cisplatin and continuous infusion of doxorubicin. Tumor resection was possible in only two Stage III patients after chemotherapy and they eventually died from recurrent disease. There was no difference in response or survival between the two chemotherapy regimens. Although seven of eight Stage I patients (88%) survived following complete resection and chemotherapy, the overall EFS at 5 years was a dismal 17% [145]. None of the Stage IV patients survived. Although the median length of survival in FL-HCC patients was longer, there was no difference in the rate of tumor resectability, incidence of advanced disease, and response to treatment when compared to other HCC patients, indicating that children with FL-HCC do not have a more favorable prognosis [145, 146].

Von Schweinitz described the findings in 42 patients in the German Cooperative Liver Tumor Study HB-99 [147]. Eighteen of 20 Stage I patients with HCC remained in remission after complete primary tumor resection. Two of three Stage II patients and seven of eight Stage IIIA patients with tumor spill or lymph node involvement remained in remission after resection and treatment with carboplatin and etoposide. Only one of 22 patients with unresectable tumors (Stage IIIB) or metastases (Stage IV) survived. Altering chemotherapy by adding topotecan and doxorubicin or combining cisplatin, alpha-interferon, doxorubicin, and 5-fluouracil was unsuccessful in inducing a response in cases that progressed [55].

Czauderna, et al. reported the findings in 39 patients in the SIOPEL-1 study [82]. The median age

was 12 years and 13 (33%) had cirrhosis. Two children underwent primary tumor resection at diagnosis and received adjuvant chemotherapy (PLADO). Preoperative PLADO neoadjuvant chemotherapy was employed in 37 children that were staged by PRETEXT imaging. Only one child was classified as PRETEXT I while 14 were PRETEXT II. In the entire group, 24 of 39 (62%) had advanced disease (extrahepatic spread in seven and vascular invasion in eight) and were considered PRETEXT III (n = 11) and IV (n = 13). The tumor was multifocal in 56%, and 31% had metastases at diagnosis. A partial response to neoadjuvant chemotherapy was noted in 18 of 37 children (49%) and only 12 of these patients (32%) had subsequent complete tumor resection. Adding these patients to the two children that had upfront primary resection, the overall resection rate was 36%. The overall 5-year survival was 28% and the 5-year EFS for the entire study group was 17%. Then only long-term survivors had complete tumor resection. Six patients in this group had FL-HCC and two survived. The length of survival in the four FL-HCC children that died was 25 months compared to 11 months for other HCC patients that succumbed. This difference was not significant, mirroring the experience of Katzenstein, et al. [146].

In SIOPEL-2, the chemotherapy was intensified by alternating cisplatin every 14 days with carboplatin and doxorubicin. In 17 evaluable patients, the tumor was multifocal in nine (53%), six (35%) had extrahepatic tumor or vascular invasion, and three (18%) had metastatic disease. One died after massive gastrointestinal bleeding without treatment. A partial response was observed in six of 13 (46%) children that received the intensified chemotherapy regimen. Complete tumor resection was possible in eight patients (47%); three at diagnosis, one with transplantation, and four following chemotherapy. More than half the cases (53%) never became operable. Twelve of the 17 patients died from progressive disease, one as a result of surgical complications and four were alive at a median follow-up of 53 months. The 3-year overall survival was 22% and was not improved by drug intensification [28]. Currently, the new SIOPEL-5 study and German group trial is evaluating noncirrhotic HCC patients staged according to the PRETEXT system and receiving neoadjuvant PLADO chemotherapy and thalidomide (an antiangiogenic agent) followed by surgery and postoperative metronomic chemotherapy [personal communication].

12.3.8 Factors Influencing Outcome

In adults, due to a high incidence of advanced disease and severe underlying liver disease, only 20–30% of patients are operative candidates for hepatic resection. Patient survival after hepatic resection for HCC varies somewhat according to selection criteria and the population studied. Despite improvements in operative mortality as a result of a better understanding of segmental liver anatomy, improved operative techniques, and intensive care, the overall survival for HCC remains dismal. This is often due to a high rate of intrahepatic tumor recurrence, or developing a second cancer in the remnant liver affected by an increased risk of carcinogenesis and continued marginal liver function. Poor prognostic indicators following resection in adult patients include: tumors size >5.0 cm, cirrhosis, vascular invasion, presence of tumor at the resection margin, advanced tumor grade, absence of a tumor capsule, preoperative serum AFP >10,000 ng/ml, preoperative AST level >2X normal, preoperative transcatheter arterial chemoembolization, and high volume intraoperative transfusion requirements [123]. Only 10% percent of adult patients with recurrence are candidates for a second resection. Recurrence within 12 months of the initial resection is a poor prognostic indicator of outcome [148]. There is little information available regarding reoperation for resection in children with recurrent HCC.

Another high risk group of HCC patients are those that initially present with an acute abdominal emergency due to spontaneous tumor rupture, which is a potentially fatal complication [149, 150]. These patients often have tumors >5.0 cm (70%), multiple tumors (68%) and cirrhosis [150]. Tumor rupture may occur in as many as 11% of cases in adults and is associated with a survival of 54% at 1 year and 21% at 5 years vs. 72% and 33.9% in nonruptured HCC [149]. In a recent study by Buczkowski, et al. [150], survival in ruptured HCC was improved with delayed hepatic resection following initial angiographic embolization when compared to those undergoing emergency surgery. This is another area where information is sparse concerning children. In contrast, noncirrhotic patients with a solitary tumor less than 5.0 cm without vascular invasion and surgical margins negative for tumor 1.0 cm or more, have had 5-year survival rates as high as 78% following complete tumor resection [123]. Fortunately, in Western countries, the majority of children with HCC have no underlying liver disease and if early detection of tumor was possible, the outlook for these patients might be improved following complete resection.

A poor response to systemic chemotherapy (20–30%) has been observed in adult patients with HCC [151]. This may be related to tumor heterogeneity, or the overexpression of a multidrug resistance gene or both [152]. Regional chemotherapy (hepatic artery infusion and transcatheter arteriographic chemoembolization techniques) is more effective; however, both techniques are ineffective for long-term tumor control.

In childhood HCC studies in the USA and Europe, 45–50% of patients have at least a partial response to chemotherapy and the two most important prognostic factors are extent of disease according to Stage and PRETEXT status and the presence of metastases at the time of diagnosis [82, 145]. Yu, et al. [117] reported on 16 patients with HCC from South Korea where the incidence of liver disease is higher. Sixty-eight percent were seropositive for hepatitis B, 50% had overt cirrhosis and eight of 16 were resectable. Four children had primary tumor resection and four underwent resection after chemotherapy. The 5-year EFS was 27%. Prognostic factors included stage, presence of metastases, and complete tumor resection.

Children with metastatic HCC rarely survive. Ahn, et al. described a 9-year-old boy with HCC and lung metastases that resolved with cisplatin and doxorubicin therapy. The child survived following trisegmentectomy [153].

12.3.9 Liver Transplantation for Hepatocellular Carcinoma

Experience with liver transplantation in children with HCC is somewhat limited. Early studies showed that survival at 5 years following transplantation in adults ranged from 15% to 30% for HCC developed in normal liver or associated with hepatitis B. In contrast, the posttransplant outcome does not seem to be influenced by incidental HCC associated with a chronic, nonviral liver disease [96]. Multifocal tumors and vascular invasion negatively impacts survival in adult patients [154]. For symptomatic HCC, guidelines regarding indications for liver transplantation are mainly derived from experience gained with adult patients using tumor size and the number of tumor nodules to determine outcome [155]. The most conventional criteria for transplantation are the so-called Milan criteria [155]: no more than three tumors, each not more than 3 cm in size, or a single tumor, not more than 5 cm in diameter, and no evidence of extrahepatic disease or vascular invasion. More recently, in adult patients, survival in the range of 70% to 94% has been observed in highly selected patients without vascular invasion [155–159]. In the USA, UNOS employs the Milan criteria for selection and allocates the organs according to the MELD (model of end-stage liver disease) scoring system [61, 160–162]. Recent studies suggest that, in an otherwise normal liver, the present cut-off for tumor size might be expanded to 6.5 cm or 7 cm [163, 164]. Some authors suggest that neoadjuvant chemotherapy and transcatheter arterial embolization (TACE) is useful as a bridge to transplantation while the patient is on the waiting list, may downstage the tumor, achieves local control, and improves survival

Table 12.10 Hepatocellular carcinoma: survival rates in pediatric series

Reference	Interval	Center	n	Survival	Transplant
Czauderna [82]	1990–1994	SIOPEL-l	39	28%	0%
Czauderna*	1994–1998	SIOPEL-2 b**	17	22%	6%
Von Schweinitz [20]	1989–1993	HB-89 ***	12	33%	0%
Fuchs [24]	1994–1998	HB-94 ***	25	25%	0%
Katzenstein [145]	n.a.	INT -0098 ****	46	19%	0%
Chen [254]	n.a.	Taipei	Median survival 23 months	55 *****	0%
Reyes [66]	1989–1998	Pittsburgh	19	63%	100%
		Multicenter (UNOS)	43	1 yr 86%	100%
Austin [61]	1987–2004			5 yr 63%	100%
				10 yr 58%	100%

* unpublished data, personal communication
** SIOPEL: Société Internationale d'Oncologie Pédiatrique
*** HB-89 & HB-94: German Cooperative Pediatric Liver Tumor studies
**** INT-0098: Paediatric Oncology and Children's Cancer Groups, USA
***** 68% with cirrhosis

after transplantation with a 1- and 5-year survival of 98% and 93%, respectively [165]. Roayaie, et al. [166] used preoperative chemotherapy and TACE followed by transplantation in 80 adult patients with HCC >5.0 cm. Doxorubicin was administered intraoperatively and postoperatively. The 5-year survival was 44%. HCC patients with viral infection may have a higher incidence of tumor recurrence following transplantation and a lower survival rate due to recurrence of viral hepatitis in the transplanted organ [167, 168]. Use of antiviral therapies postoperatively reduces the risk of graft loss by preventing HBV recurrence [169]. Patients with HCC related to HVC infection do not do as well and are at risk for tumor recurrence and the development of new tumors resulting from recurrent HCV in the graft [170].

Table 12.10 summarizes the world experience in children. A 5-year, disease-free survival rate of 63% has been obtained in the only reported experience of liver transplantation for HCC in childhood and adolescence with a significant number of patients [66]. Austin, et al. [61] described 41 children from the UNOS registry with HCC that had liver transplantation. The 1-, 3-, and 5-year survival was 86%, 63%, and 58%, respectively (Table 12.10). Broughan, et al. [171] suggested that preoperative chemotherapy prior to transplantation in children with HCC reduces tumor bulk, lowers the rate of metastases, and is associated

with fewer local recurrences following transplantation. While the median age of patients with HCC is approximately 11 years, Luks, et al. [172] described their experience with liver transplantation for tyrosinemia and noted that in 10% of cases, foci of HCC were present by 2 years of age. They suggested early transplantation in this group of patients. Similarly, HCC may occur early in children with biliary atresia and cirrhosis following a failed Kasai hepatoportoenterostomy. These patients should be under surveillance for the occurrence of HCC [173].

There is clear evidence of improved survival after liver transplantation for HCC in adult and pediatric patients during the last decade [61, 86 123, 158, 174]. Since the majority of children with HCC in western countries have no underlying liver disease, this suggests that liver transplantation may be quite useful treatment in carefully selected unresectable cases. The PLUTO registry may shed further light on the role of transplantation in HCC [64].

12.3.10 Alternative Nonresectional Therapy

Since many patients with HCC are not candidates for hepatic resection or liver transplantation, a number of palliative therapies have been developed to achieve local tumor control and manage recurrent disease. Left untreated, the median survival for HCC ranges from 1 to 8 months [75]. Overall 5-year survival is 3–5%.

Treatment techniques include hepatic artery infusion, transcatheter arterial chemoembolization (TACE), transcatheter targeted radioimmunotherapy, percutaneous chemical ablation (percutaneous alcohol injection-PEI), and thermal ablative treatments (cryotherapy, high intensity ultrasound, and radiofrequency ablation [RFA]) [86, 123]. Most of the information concerning these techniques is acquired from adult studies. With the exception of a few anecdotal reports, experience using these methods of treatment is somewhat limited in the pediatric age group. However, since HCC in children often behaves in a similar manner to HCC in adults, extrapolation of the data is likely to be useful in pediatric patients.

12.3.10.1 Hepatic Artery Infusion

Early on, hepatic artery ligation was attempted to cause tumor ischemia, infarction, and cell death. However, because of the dual blood supply to the liver both from the portal vein and hepatic artery, the peripheral areas of tumor remained perfused, allowing tumor regrowth [175]. Due to the poor response to systemic chemotherapy in HCC, regional treatment using hepatic artery infusion of chemotherapy agents was employed. The concept was to provide an increased local concentration of antitumor drugs and reduce potential systemic toxicity. While an improved tumor response to HA chemoinfusion was noted in sporadic cases of HB in children [176–178], it has not been beneficial long term in HCC.

12.3.10.2 Transcatheter Arterial Chemoembolization (TACE)

TACE is a combination of treatments applying targeted chemotherapy and embolization that has an ischemic and regional chemotherapeutic effect on HCC. A variety of cytotoxic agents have been used, including cisplatin, doxorubicin, and mitomycin-C, which are mixed with Lipiodol to form a covalent conjugate that is injected through the catheter into the hepatic artery branch feeding the tumor. Percutaneous placement of the catheter is guided by angiographic techniques. The conjugate remains in the tumor resulting in a slow release of agents to exert a maximum chemotherapeutic effect. Prechemotherapy embolization is used in instances of high blood flow to the tumor to increase the dwell time of the drugs. Postinfusion embolization to partially occlude the artery is accomplished by insertion of gelfoam pledgets further reducing the blood flow to the tumor. Partial embolization allows the

procedure to be repeated and is associated with better response rate than a single treatment [179]. In adult studies the response rate ranges widely from 24% to 55%; however, significant reduction in tumor size by 50% occurs in only 20% of cases. Llovet, et al. reported an improved 2-year survival in 36% of patients treated with TACE [180]. TACE is associated with complications including abdominal pain and fever, and rarely pancreatitis, sclerosing cholangitis, necrotizing cholecystitis, and renal insufficiency [181]. Patients with distant metastases, Child-Pugh class C cirrhosis and portal vein occlusion or portal hypertension and renal failure are not candidates for this treatment [86]. Although TACE as primary therapy for HCC is mainly palliative [181–184] and has generally not shown an improved survival, when used as a multimodal adjunct to surgical resection and prior to transplantation, it has been beneficial [165, 166, 179, 182]. Zhang, et al. [179] in a study concerning 120 patients with HCC, reported a 5-year disease-free rate of 51% with two preoperative TACE applications followed by hepatic resection, compared to 35.5% after a single TACE and 21% with resection alone. Mean disease-free length of survival was 66.4 months, 22.5 months, and 12.5 months, respectively.

There are few studies concerning the use of TACE in children. Kitahara, et al. [185] and Berthold, et al. [186] reported its use in cases of HB. Uemura, et al. described survival in a 12-year-old with an initially unresectable HCC that underwent a successful left hepatic lobectomy after TACE reduced the tumor size [187]. Malogolowkin, et al. described an experience with chemoembolization in 11 children with unresectable tumors (6 HB, 3 HCC, 2 sarcomas) using cisplatin, doxorubicin, and mitomycin followed by gelfoam embolization. Complete surgical resection was possible in five children after TACE including two with HCC [188]. One HCC patient was unresponsive to treatment and succumbed, another survived the resection but died of progressive cirrhosis, and the third HCC patient is a long-term survivor. Czauderna, et al. [189] reported a preliminary experience with TACE in five children; four with HB and one with HCC using cisplatin, doxorubicin, and mitomycin mixed with Lipiodol. The patient with HCC died as a result of a pulmonary embolus after the third chemoembolization treatment. The authors attributed the pulmonary embolus to the use of Lipiodol [190]. Arcement and colleagues described the use of TACE as an adjunct to liver transplantation in 14 children with unresectable liver tumors (7 HB, 7 HCC) [191]. Prechemotherapy embolization was used in hypervascular tumors to decrease flow. Patients then received cisplatin and/or doxorubicin followed by gelfoam embolization. The procedure was repeated every 3–4 weeks based on the status of hepatic function and patency of the hepatic artery. None of the patients were converted to a candidate for hepatic resection. Three of six patients that were subsequently transplanted had HCC and one survived. Further studies concerning chemoembolization in children are warranted.

12.3.10.3 Portal Venous Embolization

Introduced by Shimamura in 1977 [192], portal venous embolization (PVE) has been utilized in adults with liver disease to induce hypertrophy of the remaining liver remnant. The portal venous branch on the side of the tumor is cannulated percutaneously and polyvinyl alcohol and coils are inserted to induce portal vein occlusion under fluoroscopic control [193–195]. This has a dual effect; the first is an antitumor effect of alcohol by causing thrombosis of the embolized tumor area and shrinkage, and second, this results in compensatory hypertrophy of the unperfused opposite liver lobe increasing the potential hepatic functional reserve in patients with cirrhosis in preparation for hepatic resection of the tumor. Matsumata, et al. [196] noted a reduction in intrahepatic recurrence of HCC by temporarily embolizing the ipsilateral portal vein with starch microspheres. Recent studies have demonstrated that PVE induces hypertrophy of the remnant liver in 86% of Childs-Pugh Class A patients and is associated with a lower complication rate and length of hospital stay than in patients not treated with PVE [194]. PVE may have utility in children with HCC and underlying liver disease with marginal hepatic function.

12.3.10.4 Ablative Therapies

Percutaneous ethanol injection. Percutaneous ethanol injection (PEI) has been employed in adults with HCC for more than two decades [197, 198]. The mechanism of action is twofold: first alcohol diffuses into cells producing immediate coagulation necrosis resulting from cellular dehydration and protein denaturation, and second, alcohol enters the tumor circulation which induces endothelial cell necrosis and platelet aggregation with small vessel thrombosis leading to tumor cell ischemia and cell death [49]. Percutaneous injection is usually carried out under ultrasound guidance. Ninety-five percent ethanol is delivered through 21- or 22-gauge needles of adequate length (15–20 cm). The needles have a conical tip and 2–3 side holes. Ethanol may not diffuse evenly through large tumors, leaving some areas unharmed. The upper limit of tumor size for this therapy is usually 4.0 cm. Efficacy of treatment is determined by needle biopsy of the periphery of the tumor to examine for cell necrosis. Multiple injections are performed over a 4-week period, often in an am-

bulatory facility. The length of survival following PEI is similar to resection in selected patients [199, 200]. Overall survival after PEI is 90% at 1 year and varies between 45% and 75% at 3 years. The best outcomes are observed in well-differentiated solitary tumors less than 4.0 cm in diameter [201]. Local intrahepatic recurrence is common (>60%) and may be related to multifocal tumors occurring at different sites rather than in the treated area. Recurrence in the treatment field may occur in 10–15% of cases. Contraindications to therapy include extrahepatic metastases and evidence of coagulopathy with an elevated prothrombin time and thrombocytopenia (platelet count <40,000/mm3). Complications have been observed including pain, fever, and transient elevation of liver enzymes (AST). Instances of neoplastic seeding of the peritoneal wall have been identified. Pleural tracking, pneumothorax, pleural effusion, and hemothorax have rarely been observed. Transient alcohol intoxication has been occasionally observed. Ohnishi, et al. [202] reported that in patients with small HCC, percutaneous acetic acid injection had better tissue penetration, a higher complete response rate, lower recurrence rate, and better 1- and 2-year survival than PEI. Sparse information is available concerning PEI in children [102]. It is unlikely that this form of treatment will have a significant role in the management of children with HCC.

Thermal ablation. Cryotherapy has been used to devitalize neoplastic tissue by freezing the tissue, resulting in necrosis. Cold injury is produced by liquid nitrogen at a temperature of -196oC delivered by a cryoprobe placed at laparotomy using intraoperative ultrasound guidance. The lesion undergoes a 15-min freeze and 5- to 7-min thawing period followed by a second freeze/thaw application. The aim is achieve complete tumor ablation with a 1.0-cm margin of normal tissue. The probe track is filled with gelfoam at the conclusion of the procedure. Most of the experience with this technique has been obtained in adult patients with colon cancer metastatic to the liver. Zhou, et al. [203] described the results of cryotherapy in 167 adults with HCC. As primary treatment, the 5-year survival rate was 23%. When used for tumor recurrence, the 5-year survival rate was 42% and increased to 57% if the frozen mass was resected. This technique is associated with a risk of liver fracture, bile leak, hemorrhage, and rarely acute respiratory distress syndrome [204]. A cryoshock syndrome characterized by disseminated intravascular coagulation and multisystem organ failure is a rare (1%) complication of hepatic cryotherapy [205]. This modality was designed for patients with limited hepatic reserve to treat multiple lesions and avoid resection. Cryotherapy has for the most part fallen out of favor in the adult setting and has not been popularized in children.

Radiofrequency ablation. Radiofrequency ablation (RFA) is currently the most commonly used technique employed to achieve local tumor control by thermal injury. Alternating electric current with radiofrequency waves (RF) of 460 kHz is provided by a radiofrequency generator and delivered by a needle electrode place directly into the tumor tissue at operation using ultrasound guidance [206]. Local frictional heating of liver tissue around the electrode results in thermal coagulation necrosis. The treatment may require 2–3 RF electrodes for larger lesions [207]. The major use of RFA is in instances of metastatic colon cancer. RFA is used to treat tumors that are unresectable by virtue of their number, location, or size in relation to the liver volume. The procedure is relatively safe and when used as primary therapy is associated with a 3-year survival from 36–59% and local recurrence rates of 3.6–30% [205, 207]. Recurrence rates at the RFA treatment site is less than 10% with most treatment failures noted in larger tumors >4.0 cm. The mortality rate is low (0.5–2.3%) and the complication rate is 7–9% [206, 208]. Complications include pain, fever, infection, local abscess, bile duct injury, and liver failure [209]. In a comparison study, Livragi, et al. showed that RFA was superior to ethanol injection in causing complete tumor necrosis with fewer treatments but had a higher complication rate [210]. Pearson, et al. noted a lower incidence of tumor recurrence and complications with RFA than cryoablation [211]. Kim, et al. [212] described 19 patients with HCC and decompensated cirrhosis treated with a 200W generator and cooled tip RFA electrodes. The tumor size ranged from 0.8 to 5.0 cm. Complete tumor necrosis without marginal recurrence was achieved in 88% of patients according to contrast CT scans. Median survival was 12 ±1.7 months. There was one remote recurrence and two patients died of posttreatment liver failure. RFA has also been used in conjunction with TACE for unresectable HCC. Vettri, et al. [213] reported that 34 of 51 patients with HCC had complete tumor devascularization following combined treatment. Lesion size less than 5.0 cm was associated with a good result. The 1- and 2-year survival was 89% and 67%, respectively. RFA has also been used as an adjunct to surgery and a bridge to liver transplantation [206, 214]. Combining RFA with hepatic resection permits removal of a large tumor in one sector and ablation of multiple smaller lesions while still preserving an adequate volume of remnant liver [206]. Lu, et al. described the use of RFA in 52 patients with unresectable HCC awaiting liver transplantation. Forty-two patients subsequently went on to transplantation with a 76% 3-year tumor-free survival [214]. To our knowledge, RFA has not been applied in pediatric HCC studies.

12.3.11 Novel Therapies

Since many children with HCC have unresectable disease at times complicated by underlying liver disease (33%), and have a relatively poor response to systemic chemotherapy (45%), alternative types of less invasive systemic treatment have been sought.

12.3.11.1 Hormonal Treatment

Jonas, et al. noted that 39% of patients with HCC were estrogen receptor positive, a finding that was associated with a poor prognosis following hepatic resection [215]. Similarly, androgenic receptors have been associated with a worse outcome. Therapeutic trials with tamoxifen, a drug frequently used in breast cancer patients with estrogen-positive receptors have been employed in HCC. Tamoxifen suppresses insulin-like growth factor (IGF-1), downregulates transforming growth factor alpha (TGF-a), and inhibits angiogenesis. Boix, et al. showed that tamoxifen was of slight benefit but only in female patients with HCC [216]. However, in a study of nearly 1,000 patients with HCC in the Italian randomized multicenter CLIP study, Perrone and colleagues reported that tamoxifen provided no benefit when compared to placebo controls [217]. Trials using high-dose tamoxifen similarly did not provide a survival benefit to HCC patients [218, 219].

In an experimental rodent model, Schindel and Grosfeld demonstrated that hepatic resection significantly enhanced growth of residual intrahepatic tumor implants as well as remote subcutaneous hepatoma implants [220]. Octreotide (a synthetic somatostatin analog) inhibited the dramatic tumor growth rate observed following liver resection [220]. Frizelle confirmed that octreotide inhibits experimental liver metastases [221]. Somatostatin receptors have been identified in normal liver and liver tumor cells. Although Kouroumalis, et al. showed an improved median survival in patients with HCC treated with octreotide vs. untreated controls, this was not confirmed by others in similar subsequent studies [222, 223].

12.3.11.2 Angiogenesis and Antiangiogenesis

It has been well established that tumor growth is dependent on influx of neocapillary formation, a process known as angiogenesis. A number of growth factors influence the extent of endothelial proliferation and migration, among them VEGF (vascular endothelial growth factor). Sun, et al. noted that VEGF expression and microvascular density was greater in children with HCC than adults with HCC or children with other liver malignancies [224]. All the children with

HCC and increased VEGF expression in that study were dead within 2 years. The authors suggested that children with HCC have extensive angiogenesis that may influence rapid tumor growth and a poor prognosis [224]. Use of antiangiogenic compounds to prevent the tumor from acquiring new blood vessels is an attractive treatment concept. Teicher and associates demonstrated antiangiogenic and antitumor effects using a protein-kinase C-beta inhibitor additive to cisplatin, interferon, and gemcitabine that resulted in decreased tumor vessels and growth delay in HCC xenografts [225]. Recognizing that antiangiogenic therapies alone may reduce vascularity and inhibit tumor growth but may not result in tumor cell death, suggests that this form of treatment is best added to other cytotoxic agents. Antiangiogenic therapy using TNP-470 and interferon alpha 2a has shown promise in adult HCC studies [226, 227]. Thalidomide, a well-established antiangiogenic agent used in adults with HCC [228] is currently being used in combination with combined chemotherapy in liver tumor protocols in children [55, 81].

12.3.11.3 Other Treatments

Zeng, et al. described improved long-term survival in patients with unresectable HCC after intrahepatic arterial infusion of a 131I-anti HCC monoclonal antibody [229]. This method was used for cytoreduction prior to tumor resection. The posttreatment resection rate was 53% compared to 9% for hepatic artery infusion of chemotherapy alone. The 5-year survival was 28% in antibody-treated patients vs. 9% in controls. Hata and associates described using conjugates of anti-AFP antibody for immunotargeting AFP producing pediatric liver cancer [230]. While tumor response to hepatic artery infusion of tumor necrosis factor alpha and interferon gamma is improved in the experimental setting [231], activation of cytotoxic T-lymphocytes using antigenic stimulating cells (dendritic cells), employing cytokines (IL-2) or subcutaneous recombinant interferon-alpha in association with chemotherapy has been associated with poor clinical response rates [123, 232]. Leung, et al. suggested that combined treatment with cisplatin, interferon-alpha, doxorubicin, and 5-fluorouracil (PIAF) resulted in an improved response rate (50%) in unresectable patients with HCC and favorable prognostic factors [233]. The use of interferon and retinoids have reduced the rate of recurrence of HCC after tumor ablation by other methods, particularly in adult patients with viral (hepatitis C) induced liver disease [234].

12.3.11.4 Gene Therapy

Treatment of liver cancer with gene therapy has been attempted but is in the early stages of development [76, 123, 235, 236]. Retroviral and adenoviral vectors mediate gene transfer methods and partial hepatectomy may increase the efficiency of retrovirus delivery into hepatocytes. Gene therapy might be a useful method of limiting the progression of liver cancer by altering the biology of the tumor and surrounding normal liver tissue.

A suicide gene is defined as transfer of a gene encoding a metabolically active enzyme into the genome of the cancer cell. The enzyme metabolizes and converts a nontoxic prodrug to a highly cytotoxic compound which can selectively kill a genetically modified cancer cell. In addition to facilitating cell suicide, transfection of tumor cells with gene-encoded viruses may enhance expression of tumor-specific antigens and cytokines and alter oncogene and tumor suppressor activity [123, 235]. Beta-catenin gene mutations have been identified in both HBL and HCC, and overexpression of this gene is associated with increased tumorigenesis. Transfected RNA interference against beta-catenin in vitro inhibits liver tumor proliferation suggesting that beta-catenin may be a future target for in vivo gene therapy [12]. A number of difficulties have been identified that limit the current utility of gene therapy, including tumor heterogeneity, variable tumor cell uptake, and limiting injury to normal surrounding hepatic tissue. Improved methods of gene delivery, better tumor specificity, and prolonging transgene expression are needed [123].

12.3.12 Public Health Intervention, Prevention, and Surveillance

Early detection of HCC and partial hepatic resection in noncirrhotic patients when possible and liver transplantation in unresectable patients and those with cirrhosis are the best current treatments. Unfortunately, many patients with HCC are unresectable at diagnosis and transplantation is hindered by donor shortage. Despite successful resection, in those with underlying liver disease the highly oncogenic nature of the remnant cirrhotic liver frequently results in the development of new HCC lesions, impacting negatively on long-term survival [237]. Efforts are being directed to preventing HCC, by implementing vaccination programs (for HBV), safe transfusion methodology, use of universal precautions among hospital employees and other health care providers, and employing antiviral agents to keep acute hepatitis from becoming chronic and chronic hepatitis from progressing to cirrhosis.

As previously noted, distinct geographic variation in the occurrence of HCC is observed. In Asia and sub-Saharan Africa, most cases are related to exposure to hepatitis B virus. In Europe and North America, most adult cases of HCC occur in patients with alcoholic cirrhosis and hepatitis C infection. Most childhood cases of HCC in Western countries occur in an otherwise normal liver, whereas children in Africa and Asia have a high incidence of liver disease due to hepatitis B infection. Transfusion transmission of hepatitis viruses has for the most part been eliminated.

Hepatitis B vaccination became available in 1982. Infants that acquire HBV prenatally have a 90% risk of developing HBV infection. Many HBV-infected children have normal serum alanine transferase (AST) levels and minimal chronic hepatitis. Children with chronic HBV are usually asymptomatic but still may develop chronic liver disease and HCC [238]. Prior to HBV vaccination, there was an increased incidence of HBV-related HCC in Taiwan and China [83, 84]. A significant decrease in HCC occurrence was observed in children less than 10 years of age following institution of a universal HBV vaccination program in Taiwan [84]. The incidence of HCC was reduced from 0.54 to 0.2 cases per 100,000 children after the vaccination program was established. HBV-vaccine failure and failure to receive HBV immunoglobulin at birth are the main causes of HCC-prevention failure [239]. Of interest was the fact that HBV carrier children born after initiation of the vaccination program had a higher risk of developing HCC than those before the program was started [239]. Some underdeveloped countries in sub-Saharan Africa have not implemented vaccination programs and therefore many cases have not been eliminated. Both interferon-alpha and Lamivudine are used to treat chronic HBV infection but life-long treatment is required [238]. The Global Alliance for Vaccine and Immunizations and the Bill and Melinda Gates Foundation are aiding resource-limited countries by providing funding for HBV vaccination programs [78].

Hepatitis C was first identified in 1989. HCV is a RNA-related virus with various genotypes for which there is currently no vaccine available. Global prevalence is 1–3%. HCV infection is associated with high risk cultural practices including acupuncture, tattoos, body piercing, scarring, drugs, and contaminated blood products. Universal precautions and reduction in transfusion-related transmission have been useful precautionary measures. Antiviral treatment eliminates detectable HCV in 50–80% of clinically infected cases, which presumably should reduce the risk of HCC [78, 240]. Interferon therapy (IFN) alone has not resulted in a sustained response in chronic HCV. The combination of Ribaviran and IFN has been a major treatment advance and results in a sustained response

in 30–40% of chronic HCV patients. Patients with genotype 1 respond better. IFN + Ribaviran is useful first-line therapy in 60% of acute cases; however, adverse events occur in 23–27% of cases and often require discontinuation of therapy [240, 241]. These medications are expensive and for many are unaffordable. HCC survival rates remain poor, but early detection and antiviral treatment in developed countries has improved survival in selected patients [79]. Development of an HCV vaccine has been elusive and better methods of detection for HCC are needed.

The natural history of HCV in children is not well characterized [242]. The prevalence ranges from 0.05 to 0.4% and the main mode of transmission is vertical (maternal–infant). HCV appears to be a milder disease in children than adults and children may respond better to treatment [243]. HCV progresses slowly in children with only mild liver biopsy findings and no symptoms in most children. Therapy with IFN and Ribaviran is effective in 50% of children and significant inflammation and fibrosis can occur in childhood. Chronic infection can have serious long-term consequences including end stage liver disease (ESLD) and HCC [88, 111].

Surveillance programs have been established for high-risk patients with hepatitis C infection that suggest monitoring the serum AFP levels and obtaining an ultrasound study every 6 months may be helpful in identifying early stage tumors and improving outcomes [123, 244]. These studies imply that surveillance for HCC should be considered in patients with chronic hepatitis B or C, aflatoxin exposure, patients with cirrhosis being considered for liver transplantation, Fanconi's disease, and younger children with tyrosinemia and progressive familial intrahepatic cholestatic disorders and a failed Kasai procedure for biliary atresia [104, 172, 173].

12.4 Embryonal Sarcoma of the Liver

Embryonal sarcoma of the liver is a relatively uncommon pediatric hepatic neoplasm that occurs more frequently in older children and adolescents but has also been described in infancy [81, 245]. An increased incidence of undifferentiated sarcoma is noted in children in Southern Africa [79]. Clinical presentation includes abdominal pain, occasional fever, and the presence of a right-upper quadrant abdominal mass. Lakhdor, et al. described an instance of fatal parathyroid hormone-induced humoral hypercalcemia of malignancy in a 3-month-old infant with a poorly differentiated hepatic sarcoma [245]. The tumor may occasionally arise in a mesenchymal hamartoma or a solitary liver cyst [246, 247]. Stringer and Alizai described eight instances of undifferentiated embryonal sarcoma associated with mesenchymal hamartomas that were reported in the literature [246]. The fact that mesenchymal hamartomas usually occur in infants that may have an elevated serum AFP level suggests that biopsy of the lesion is advisable before contemplating administration of chemotherapy for a presumed HB or HCC. In addition to HB and HCC, other malignant tumors included in the differential diagnosis are rhabdomyosarcoma that may arise from bile duct structures (see Chap. 14), teratomas, angiosarcoma, and leiomyosarcoma [55,147]. Benign neoplasms include focal nodular hyperplasia, benign adenoma, and vascular lesions (see Chap. 9).

Histologically, embryonal sarcoma is an undifferentiated mesenchymal lesion with polygonal spindle cells, pleomorphic stromal elements with abundant mitotic figures, and occasional multinucleated giant cells [248–250]. Immunohistochemical analysis shows that the tumor stains positively for vimentin, alpha-1 antitrypsin, cytokeratin AE1/3, p53, and Bcl-2 [251]. Nonrandom mutations of the p53 gene have been identified in undifferentiated embryonal tumor tissue but not the surrounding normal liver parenchyma, suggesting the mutations are tumor specific and may play a role in tumorigenesis of this lesion [250]. Although mutations of the beta-catenin gene is noted in other malignant pediatric liver tumors (HB and HCC), they have not been identified in embryonal sarcoma tissue [250].

The treatment of choice for embryonal sarcoma is complete operative resection. The tumors are chemosensitive and may respond to variable protocols that are applied to children with rhabdomyosarcoma including vincristine, actinomycin-D, doxorubicin and cytoxan or ifosfamide, etoposide, and melphalan sometimes combined with adjuvant radiotherapy. In an Italian-German soft tissue sarcoma study, 12 of 17 children with hepatic embryonal sarcoma achieved remission following treatment with chemoradiation and surgery [252]. In some instances, the tumor became resectable after neoadjuvant treatment [247, 252]. Cure is usually possible following complete tumor resection. Survival has been achieved in unresectable cases without metastases following liver transplantation [253].

References

1. Darbari A, Sabin KM Shapiro CN, Schwarz KB (2003) Epidemiology of primary hepatic malignancies in US children. Hepatology 38:560–566
2. McLaughlin C, Baptiste MS, Schymura MJ, et al. (2006) Maternal and infant birth characteristics and hepatoblastoma. Am J Epidemiol 163:818–828
3. De Ugarte DA, Atkinson JB (2006) Liver tumors. In: Grosfeld, JL, O'Neill JA Jr, Fonkalsrud EW, Coran AG (eds) Pediatric surgery, 6th edn. Mosby-Elsevier, Philadelphia, pp 502–514
4. Ding SF, Michail NE, Habib NA (1994) Genetic changes in hepatoblastoma. J Hepatol 20:672–675
5. Vaughan WG, Sanders DW, Grosfeld JL, et al. (1995) Favorable outcome in children with Beckwith-Wiedemann syndrome and intra-abdominal malignant tumors. J Pediatr Surg 30:1042–1044
6. Albrecht S, von Schweinitz D, Waha A, et al. (1994) Loss of maternal alleles on chromosome arm 11p in hepatoblastoma. Cancer Res 54:5041–5044
7. Bowman LC, Riely CA (1996) Management of pediatric liver tumors. Surg Oncol Clin North Am 5:451–459
8. Greenberg M, Filler RM (1993) Hepatic tumors. In: Pizzo P, Poplack D (eds) Management of common cancers of childhood. Lippincott, Philadelphia, pp 697–711
9. Tanaka K, Vemoto S, Asonume K, et al. (1997) Hepatoblastoma in a two year old girl with trisomy 18. Eur J Pediatr Surg 2:298
10. Terracciano L, Tornillo L (2003) Cytogenetic alteration in liver cell tumors as detected by comparative genomic hybridization. Pathologica 95:71–82
11. Buendia MA (2002) Genetic alterations in hepatoblastoma and hepatocellular carcinoma: Common and distinct aspects. Med Pediatr Oncol 39:530–535
12. Sanghathat S, Kusafuka T, Miao J, et al. (2006) In vitro RNA interference against beta-catenin inhibits proliferation of pediatric hepatic tumors. Int J Oncol 28:715–722
13. Chen TC, Hsieh LL, Kuo TT (1995) Absence of p53 gene mutation and infrequent overexpression of p53 protein in hepatoblastoma. J Pathol 176:243–247
14. Hughes LI, Michels W (1992) Risk of hepatoblastoma in familial adenomatous polyposis. Am J Med Genet 43:1023–1025
15. Garber JE, Li FP, Kingston JE, et al. (1988) Hepatoblastoma and familial adenomatous polyposis. J Natl Cancer Inst 80:1626–1628
16. Thomas D, Pritchard J, Davidson R, et al. (2003) Familial hepatoblastoma and APC gene mutations: Renewed call for molecular research. Eur J Cancer 39:2200–2204
17. Geiger JD (1996) Surgery for hepatoblastoma in children. Curr Opin Pediatr 276–282
18. Otten J, Smets R, De Jager R, et al. (1977) Hepatoblastoma in an infant after contraceptive intake during pregnancy. New Engl J Med 297:222
19. Kahn A, Bader L, Hoy GR, Sinks LF (1979) Hepatoblastoma in a child with fetal alcohol syndrome. Lancet 1:1403–1404
20. Hashizumi K, Nakajo T, Kawarasaki H, et al. (1991) Prader-Willi syndrome with deletion of 15q11, q13 associated hepatoblastoma. Acta Pediatr Jpn 33:718–722
21. Richter A, Grabhorn E, Schulz A, et al. (2005) Hepatoblastoma in a child with progressive familial intrahepatic cholestasis. Pediatr Transplant 9:805–808
22. Ikeda H, Matsuyama S, Tanimura M (1997) Association between hepatoblastoma and very low birth weight: A trend or chance? J Pediatr 130:557–560

23. Ross J (1997) Hepatoblastoma and birth weight: Too little, too big, or just right? J Pediatr 130:516–517

24. Pang D, McNally R, Birch JM (2003) Parental smoking and childhood cancer: Results from the United Kingdom Childhood Cancer Study. Br J Cancer 88:373–381

25. Sorahan T, Lancashire RJ (2004) Parental cigarette smoking and childhood risk of hepatoblastoma: OSCC data. Br J Cancer 90:1016–1018

26. Ammann RA, Plaschkes J, Leibundgut K (1999) Congenital hepatoblastoma: A distinct entity? Med Pediatr Oncol 32:466–468

27. Sinta L, Freud N, Dulitzki F (1992) Hemoperitoneum as the presenting sign of hepatoblastoma in the newborn. Pediatr Surg Int 7:131–133

28. Perilongo G, Shafford E, Maibach R, et al. (2004) Risk-adapted treatment for childhood hepatoblastoma. Final report of the second study of the International Society of Pediatric Oncology-SIOPEL 2. Eur J Cancer 40:411–421

29. Brown J, Perilongo G, Shafford E, et al. (2000) Pretreatment prognostic factors for children with hepatoblastoma-results from the International Society of Paediatric Oncology (SIOP) study SIOPEL 1. Eur J Cancer 36:1418–425

30. Schnater JM, Aronson DC, Plaschkes J, et al. (2002) Surgical view of the treatment of patients with hepatoblastoma: Results from the first prospective trial of the International Society of Pediatric Oncology Liver Tumor Study Group. Cancer 94:1111–1120

31. Czauderna P, Otte JB, Pritchard J, et al. (2005) Guidelines for surgical treatment of hepatoblastoma in the modern era. Recommendations from the Childhood Liver Tumor Strategy Group (SIOPEL) of the International Society of Pediatric Oncology (SIOP). Eur J Cancer 41:1031–1036

32. Wang JN, Chen JS, Chung Y, et al. (2002) Invasion of the cardiovascular system in childhood malignant hepatic tumors. J Pediatr Hematol Oncol 24:436–439

33. Zimmermann A (2005) The emerging family of hepatoblastoma tumours: From ontogenesis to oncogenesis. A review. Eur J Cancer 1:1503–1514

34. Haas JE, Muzsynski KA, Krailo M, et al. (1989) Histopathology and prognosis in childhood hepatoblastoma and hepatocarcinoma. Cancer 4:1082–1095

35. Ortega JA, Douglass EC, Feusner JH, et al. (2000) Randomized comparison of cisplatin/vincristine/fluorouracil/cisplatin/continuous infusion doxorubicin for treatment of pediatric hepatoblastoma: A report from the Children's Cancer Group and the Pediatric Oncology Group. J Clin Oncol 18:2665–2675

36. von Schweinitz D, Byrd DJ, Hecker H, et al. (1997) Efficiency and toxicity of ifosfamide, cisplatin and doxorubicin in the treatment of childhood hepatoblastoma. Study Committee of the Cooperative Paediatric Liver Tumour Study HB89 of the German Society for Paediatric Oncology and Haematology. Eur J Cancer 33:1243–1249

37. Couinaud C (1954) Basis anatomiques des hepatectomies gauche et drought regles: Techniques qui en decoulent. J Chir (Paris) 70:933–936

38. Aronson D, Schnater JM, Staalman C, et al. (2005) The predictive value of the PRETreatment EXTent of disease (PRETEXT) system in hepatoblastoma: Results from the International Society of Pediatric Oncology Liver Tumor Study Group (SIOPEL-1). J Clin Oncol 23:1245–1252

39. Roebuck D, Aronson A, Clapuyt P, et al. (2005) PRETEXT: A revised staging system for primary malignant liver tumors of childhood. Pediatr Radiol 2007; 37:123-132

40. Meyers RL, Malogolowkin MH, Rowland JM, Krailo M (2006) Predictive value of the PRETEXT staging system in children with hepatoblastoma. Presented at the 37th annual meeting American Pediatric Surgical Association, Hilton Head, SC, May 27, 2006

41. Stringer M (2000) Liver tumors. Semin Pediatr Surg 9:196–208

42. Fuchs J, Rydzynski J, Hecker H, et al. (2002) The influence of preoperative chemotherapy and surgical technique in the treatment of hepatoblastoma—A report from the German Cooperative Liver Tumours Studies HB-89 and HB-94. Eur J Pediatr Surg 12:255–261

43. von Schweinitz D, Faundez A, Teichmann B, et al. (2000) Hepatocyte growth-factor-scatter-factor can stimulate postoperative tumor-cell proliferation in childhood hepatoblastoma. Int J Cancer 85:151–159

44. von Schweinitz D, Hecker H, Harms D, et al. (1995) Complete resection before development of drug resistance is essential for survival from advanced hepatoblastoma-a report from the German Cooperative Pediatric Liver Tumor Study HB-89. J Pediatr Surg 30:845–852

45. Finegold M (2002) Chemotherapy for suspected hepatoblastoma without effort at surgical resection is bad practice. Med Pediatr Oncol 39:484–486

46. Ortega JA, Krailo MD, Haas JE, et al. (1991) Effective treatment of unresectable or metastatic hepatoblastoma with cisplatin and continuous infusion doxorubicin chemotherapy: A report from the Children Cancer Study Group. J Clin Oncol 9:2167–2176

47. Douglass EC, Reynolds M, Finegold M, Cantor AB, Glycksman A (1993) Cisplatin, vincristine, and fluorouracil therapy for hepatoblastoma: A Pediatric Oncology Group study. J Clin Oncol 11:96–99

48. Ortega JA, Douglass E, Feusner J, et al. (1994) A randomized trial of cisplatin/vincristine/5-fluorouracil vs. CCP/doxorubicin continuous infusion for the treatment of hepatoblastoma: Results from the Pediatric Inter-Group Hepatoma Study (abstr). Proc Am Soc Clin Oncol (ASCO) 13:416

49. Grosfeld, JL (1998) Hepatoblastoma and hepatocellular carcinoma. In: Carachi R, Azmy A, Grosfeld, JL (eds) Surgery of childhood tumors. Arnold, London, pp 178–198

50. LaQuaglia MP, Shorter NM, Blumgart LH (2002) Central hepatic resection for pediatric tumors. J Pediatr Surg 37:986–989

51. Reynolds M (1995) Conversion of unresectable to resectable hepatoblastoma and long term follow up. World J Surg 19:814–816

52. King DR, Ortega J, Campbell J, et al. (1991) Surgical management of children with incompletely resected hepatic cancer facilitated by intensive chemotherapy. J Pediatr Surg 26:1074–1081

53. Haberle B, Bode U, von Schweinitz D (2003) Differentiated treatment protocols for high and standard risk hepatoblastoma-an interim report of the German Liver Tumor Study HB99. Klin Pediatr 215:159–165

54. Dall'Igna P, Cecchetto G, Toffolutti T, et al. (2003) Multifocal hepatoblastoma is there a place for partial hepatectomy? Med Pediatr Oncol 40:113–116

55. von Schweinitz D (2006) Management of liver tumors in childhood. Semin Pediatr Surg 15:17–24

56. Pritchard J, Brown J, Shafford E, et al. (2000) Cisplatin, doxorubicin and delayed surgery for childhood hepatoblastoma: A successful approach -results of the first prospective study of the International Society of Pediatric Oncology. J Clin Oncol 18:3819–3828

57. Couinaud C (1992) The anatomy of the liver. Ann Ital Chir 63:693–697

58. Wheatley JM, Rosenfield NS, Berger L, LaQuaglia MP (1996) Liver regeneration in children after major hepatectomy for malignancy-evaluation using a computer-aided technique of volume measurement. J Surg Res 61:183–189

59. Otte JB, Pritchard J, Aronson DC, et al. (2004) Liver transplantation for hepatoblastoma: Results from the International Society of Pediatric Oncology (SIOP) study SIOPEL-1 and review of the world experience. Pediatr Blood Cancer 42:74–83

60. Otte JB, de Ville de Goyet J, Reding R (2005) Liver transplantation for hepatoblastoma: Indications and contraindications in the modern era. Pediatr Transplant 9:557–565

61. Austin MT, Leys CM, Feurer ID, et al. (2006) Liver transplantation for childhood hepatic malignancy: A review of the United Network for Organ Sharing (UNOS) database. J Pediatr Surg 41:182–186

62. Pimpalwar AP, Sharif K, Ramani P, et al. (2002) Strategy for hepatoblastoma management: Transplant versus nontransplant surgery. J Pediatr Surg 37:240–245

63. Otte JB, de Ville de Goyet J (2005) The contribution of transplantation to the treatment of liver tumors in children. Semin Pediatr Surg 14:233–238

64. Otte JB, Meyers R (2006) Correspondence. J Pediatr Surg 41:607–608

65. Chardot C, Saint-Martin C, Gilles A, et al. (2002) Living-related liver transplantation and vena cava reconstruction after total hepatectomy including the vena cava for hepatoblastoma. Transplantation 73:90–92

66. Reyes JD, Carr B, Dvorchik I, et al. (2000) Liver transplantation and chemotherapy for hepatoblastoma and hepatocellular carcinoma in childhood and adolescence. J Pediatr 136:795–804

67. Perilongo G, Brown J, Shafford E, et al. (2000) Hepatoblastoma presenting with lung metastases: Treatment results of the first cooperative, prospective study of the International Society of Pediatric Oncology on childhood liver tumors. Cancer 89:1845–1853

68. Otte JB, Rosati R, Janssen M (2004) Parental experience with life-related donor liver transplantation. Pediatr Transplant 8:317–321

69. Stringer MD, Hennayake S, Howard ER, et al. (1995) Improved outcome for children with hepatoblastoma. Brit J Surg 82:386–391

70. Srinivasan P, McCall J, Pritchard J, et al. (2002) Orthotopic liver transplantation for unresectable hepatoblastoma. Transplantation 74:652–655

71. Molmenti EP, Wilkinson K, Moment H, et al. (2002) Treatment of unresectable hepatoblastoma with liver transplantation in the pediatric population. Am J Transplant 2:535–538

72. Mejia A, Lagans A, Shaw BW, et al. (2005) Living and deceased donor liver transplantation for unresectable hepatoblastoma at a single centre. Clin Transplant 19:721–725

73. Sasaki F, Matsunaga T, Iwafuchi M, et al. (2003) Outcome of hepatoblastoma treated with the JPLT-1 (Japanese Study Group for Pediatric Liver Tumor) Protocol-1:A report from the Japanese Study Group for Pediatric Liver Tumor. J Pediatr Surg 37:851–856

74. Fuchs J, Rydzynski J, von Schweinitz D, et al. (2002) Pretreatment prognostic factors and treatment results in children with hepatoblastoma: A report from the German Cooperative Pediatric Liver Tumor Study HB-94. Cancer 95:172–182

75. Parker SL, Tong T, Bolden S, Wingo PA (1996) Cancer statistics 1996. CA Cancer J Clin 46:5–27

76. Cusnir M, Patt YZ (2004) Novel systemic therapy options for hepatocellular carcinoma. Cancer J 10:97–103

77. El-Serag HB (2001) Epidemiology of hepatocellular carcinoma. Clin Liver Dis 5:87–107

78. O'Brien TR, Kirk G, Zhang M (2004) Hepatocellular carcinoma: A paradigm of preventive oncology. Cancer J 10:67–73

79. Moore SW, Millar AJ, Hadley GP, et al. (2004) Hepatocellular carcinoma and liver tumors in South African children: A case for increased prevalence. Cancer 101:642–649

80. Hadley GP, Govender D, Landres G, et al. (2004) Primary tumors of the liver in children: An African perspective. Pediatr Surg Int 20:314–318E

81. Malogolowkin MH, Zimmerman A, Plashkes J. Liver tumors in adolescents and young adults. (in press)

82. Czauderna P, MacKinley G, Perilongo G, et al. (2002) Hepatocellular carcinoma in children: Results of the first prospective study of the International Society of Pediatric Oncology Group. J Clin Oncol 20:2798–2804

83. Chang MH, Chen CJ, Lai MS, et al. (1997) Universal Hepatitis B vaccination in Taiwan and the incidence of hepatocellular carcinoma in children. Taiwan Childhood Hepatoma Study group. N Engl J Med 336:1855–1859

84. Tsai HL, Liu CS, Chin TW, et al. (2004) Hepatoblastoma and hepatocellular carcinoma in children. J Chin Med Assoc 67:83–88

85. LaBerge JM (2003) Liver tumors. In: O'Neill JA Jr, Grosfeld, JL, Fonkalsrud EW, et al. (eds) Principles of pediatric surgery, 2nd edn. Mosby, St Louis, pp 239–247

86. Pawlik TM, Scroggins CR, Thomas MB, Vauthey J-N (2004) Advances in the surgical management of liver malignancies. Cancer J 10:74–87

87. El-Serag, HB, Mason MC (1999) Rising incidence of hepatocellular carcinoma in the United States. N Engl J Med 340:743–750

88. El-Serag HB (2004) Hepatocellular carcinoma: Recent trends in the United States. Gastroenterology 127(Suppl 1): S27–S34

89. Van Spronson FJ, Bijleveldem M, van Maldegem BT, Wijburg IA (2005) Hepatocellular carcinoma in hereditary tyrosinemia type 1 despite 2(-2 nitro 4–3 trifluoro-methylbenzenyl)1–3 cyclohexanedione therapy. J Pediatr Gastroenterol Nutr 40:90–93

90. Bianchi L (1993) Glycogen storage disease I and hepatocellular tumors. Eur J Pediatr 152(Suppl 1):S63–S70

91. Franco LM, Krishnamurthy V, Bali D, et al. (2005) Hepatocellular carcinoma in Glycogen storage disease type 1a: A case series. J Inherit Metab Dis 28:153–162

92. Hadzic N, Quaglia A, Mieli-Vergani G (2006) Hepatocellular carcinoma in a 12 year old child with PiZZ alpha-1-antityrpsin deficiency. Hepatology 43:194–196

93. Halvorsen RA J, Garrity S, Kun C, et al. (1995) Coexisting hepatocellular carcinoma in a patient with arteriohepatic dysplasia. Abdom Imaging 20:191–196

94. Bhadri VA, Storman MO, Arbuckle S, et al. (2005) Hepatocellular carcinoma in children with Alagille's syndrome. J Pediatr Gastroenterol Nutr 51:676–678

95. Pennington DJ, Sivit CJ, Chandra RS (1996) Hepatocellular carcinoma in a child with Niemann-Pick disease: Imaging findings. Pediatr Radiol 26:220–221

96. Esquivel CO, Gutierrez C, Cox KL, et al. (1999) Hepatocellular carcinoma and liver cell dysplasia in children with chronic liver disease. J Pediatr Surg 29:1465–1469

97. Janes CH, McGill DB, Ludwig J, Krom RA (1993) Liver adenoma at age three years and transplantation later after development of carcinoma. Hepatology 17:583–585

98. Pichon N, Maisonette F, Pichon-Lefievre F, et al. (2003) Hepatocellular carcinoma with congenital agenesis of the portal vein. Jpn J Clin Oncol 33:314–316

99. Gruner BA, DeNapoli TS, Andrews W, et al. (2000) Hepatocellular carcinoma in children associated with Gardner's syndrome or familial adenomatous polyposis. J Pediatr Hematol Oncol 22:90–91

100. Ghaferi AA, Hutchins GM (2005) Progression of liver pathology in patients undergoing the Fontan procedure: Chronic passive congestion, cardiac cirrhosis, hepatic adenoma and hepatocellular carcinoma. J Thorac Cardiovasc Surg 129:1348–1352

101. Moore L, Bourne AJ, Preston H, Byard RW (1997) Hepatocellular carcinoma following neonatal hepatitis. Pediatr Pathol Lab Med 17:601–610

102. Kohno N, Kitatani H, Wada H, et al. (1995) Hepatocellular carcinoma complicating biliary cirrhosis caused by biliary atresia. J Pediatr Surg 30:1713–1716

103. Whitington PF, Freese DK, Alonso EM, et al. (1994) Clinical and biochemical findings in progressive familial intrahepatic cholestasis. J Pediatr Gastroenterol Nutr 18:134–141

104. Knisley AS, Strautnieks SS, Meier Y, et al. (2006) Hepatocellular carcinoma in 10 children under 5 years of age with bile salt export pump deficiency. Hepatology 44:478–486

105. Scheers I, Badry V, Stephenne X, Sokal EM (2005) Risk of hepatocellular carcinoma in liver mitochondrial respiratory chain disorders. J Pediatr 141:414–417

106. Maitra A, Ramnanai DM, Margraf LR, Gazdar AF (2000) Synchronous Wilms' tumor and fibrolamellar hepatocellular carcinoma in a four year old boy. Pediatr Dev Pathol 3:492–496

107. Jain D, Hui P, McNamara J, Schwartz D (2001) Bloom syndrome in siblings: First reports of hepatocellular carcinoma and Wilms' tumor with documented anaplasia and nephrogenic rests. Pediatr Dev Pathol 4:585–589

108. Kovalik JJ, Thomas PRM, Thomas MB, et al. (1991) Hepatocellular carcinoma as second malignant neoplasms in successfully treated Wilms' tumor patients. Cancer 67:342–344

109. Hartley AL, Dirch JM, Blair V, et al. (1994) Second primary neoplasms in a population based series of patients diagnosed with renal tumors in childhood. Med Pediatr Oncol 22:318–322

110. Kumari TP, Shanvas A, Mathews A, Kusumackomary P (2000) Hepatocellular carcinoma: A rare late event in childhood acute lymphocytic leukaemia. J Pediatr Hematol Oncol 22:289–290

111. Strickland DK, Jenkins JJ, Hudson MM (2001) Hepatitis C infection and hepatocellular carcinoma after treatment of childhood cancer. J Pediatr Hematol Oncol 23:527–529

112. Saurin JC, Taniere P, Mion F, et al. (1997) Primary hepatocellular carcinoma in workers exposed to vinyl chloride: Report of two cases. Cancer 79:1671–1677

113. Mays ET, Christopherson W (1984) Hepatic tumors induced by sex steroids. Semin Liver Dis 4:147–157

114. Mendishona E, MacPhail AP, Gordeyk VR, et al. (1998) Dietary iron overload as a risk factor for hepatocellular carcinoma in Black Africans. Hepatology 27:1563–1566

115. Pang A, Ng, IO, Fan ST, Kwong YL (2003) Clinicopathologic significance of genetic alterations in hepatocellular carcinoma. Cancer Genet Cytogenet 146:8–15

116. Kusafuka T, Fukuzawa M, Oue T, et al. (1997) Mutation analysis of p53 gene in childhood malignant solid tumor. J Pediatr Surg 32:1175–1180

117. Yu SB, Kim HY, Eo H, et al. (2006) Clinical characteristics and prognosis of pediatric hepatocellular carcinoma. World J Surg 30:43–50

118. Sachdeva R. Yapor M, Schwersenz A, et al. (1993) Massive variceal bleeding caused by a hepatic artery-portal vein fistula: A manifestation of hepatocellular carcinoma in a 12 year old. J Pediatr Gastroenterol Nutr 16:468–471

119. Hany MA, Betts DR, Schmugge M, et al. (1997) A childhood fibrolamellar hepatocellular carcinoma with increased aromatase activity and a near triploid karyotype. Med Pediatr Oncol 28:136–138

120. Kane SP, Murray-Lyon IM, Paradinas FJ, et al. (1978) Vitamin B12 binding protein as a tumor marker for hepatocellular carcinoma. Gut 19:1105–1109

121. Paradinas FJ, Melia WM, Wilkinson ML, et al. (1982) High serum vitamin B12 binding capacity as a marker of fibrolamellar variant of hepatocellular carcinoma. Br Med J 25:840–842

122. Hemming AW, Scudamore OH, Shackledon CR, et al. (1992) Iodocyanine green clearance as a predictor of successful hepatic resection in cirrhotic patients. Am J Surg 163:515–518

123. Cormier JN, Thomas KT, Chari RS, Pinson CW (2006) Management of hepatocellular carcinoma. J Gastrointest Surg 10:761–780

124. Redaelli CA, Dufour JF, Wagner M, et al. (2002) Preoperative galactose elimination capacity predicts complications and survival after hepatic resection. Ann Surg 235:77–85

125. Wudel LJ Jr, Delbeke D, Morris D, et al. (2003) The role of [18F] fluorodeoxyglucose positron emission tomography imaging in the evaluation of hepatocellular carcinoma. Am J Surg 69:117–124

126. Hain SF, Fogelman I (2004) Recent advances in imaging hepatocellular carcinoma: Diagnosis, staging and response assessment functional imaging. Cancer J 10:121–127

127. Shoup M, Gonen M, D'Angelica M, et al. (2003) Volumetric analysis predicts hepatic dysfunction in patients undergoing major liver resection. J Gastrointest Surg 7:325–330

128. Weitz J, D'Angelica M, Jernagen W, et al. (2004) Selective use of diagnostic laparoscopy before planned hepatectomy for patients with hepatocellular carcinoma. Surgery 135:273–281

129. Klein MM, Molmenti EP, Colombani PM, et al. (2005) Primary liver carcinoma in people younger than 30 years. Am J Clin Pathol 124:512–518

130. Lauwers GY, Terris B, Balis VJ, et al. (2002) Prognostic histologic indicators of curatively resected hepatocellular carcinomas: A multi-institutional analysis of 425 patients with definition of a histologic prognostic index. Am J Surg Pathol 26:25–34

131. Wilkens L, Bredt M, Flemming P, et al. (2000) Cytogenetic aberrations in primary and recurrent fibrolamellar hepatocellular carcinoma detected by comparative genomic hybridization. Am J Clin Pathol 114:867–874

132. Prokurat A, Kluge P, Kosciesza A, et al. (2002) Transitional liver cell tumors (TLCT) in older children and adolescents: A novel group of aggressive hepatic tumors expressing beta-catenin. Med Pediatr Oncol 39:510–518

133. Peng SY, Chin WJ, Lai PL, et al. (2005) High alpha fetoprotein level correlates with high stage, early recurrence and poor prognosis of hepatocellular carcinoma: Significance of hepatitis virus infection, age, p53 and beta-catenin mutations. Int J Cancer 112:44–50

134. Postovsky S, Elapid R, Otte GB, et al. (2001) Late recurrence of combined hepatocellular carcinoma and hepatoblastoma in a child: Case report and review of the literature. Eur J Pediatr Surg 11:61–65

135. Postovsky S, Elapid R, Ben-Rush MW, et al. (2001) Local dissemination of hepatocellular carcinoma in a child after fine needle aspiration. Med Pediatr Oncol 36:667–668

136. Okuda K, Ohtsuki T, Obata H, et al. (1985) Natural history of hepatocellular carcinoma and prognosis in relation to treatment: Study of 850 patients. Cancer 56:918–928

137. Llovet JM, Bru C, Bruix J (1999) Prognosis of hepatocellular carcinoma: The BCLC staging classification. Semin Liver Dis 19:329–338

138. The Cancer of the Liver Italian Program (CLIP) Investigators (2000) Prospective validation of the CLIP score: A new prognostic system for patients with cirrhosis and hepatocellular carcinoma. Hepatology 31:840–845

139. Vauthey JN, Lauwers GY, Esnaola NF, et al. (2002) Simplified staging for hepatocellular carcinoma. J Clin Oncol 20:1527–1536

140. Levy I, Sherman M (2002) Staging of hepatocellular carcinoma: Assessment of CLIP, Okuda, and Child-Pugh staging systems in a cohort of 257 patients in Toronto. Gut 50:881–885

141. Helton WS, Strasberg SM: AHPBA/AJCC Consensus Conference on staging of hepatocellular carcinoma: Rationale and overview of the conference. HPB 2003;5:230–242

142. Henderson JM, Sherman M, Tavill A, et al. (2003) AHPBA/AJCC Consensus Conference on staging hepatocellular carcinoma: Consensus statement. HPB 5:243–250

143. Zhao WH, Ma ZM, Zhou XC, et al. (2002) Prediction of recurrence and prognosis in patients with hepatocellular carcinoma after resection by use of the CLIP score. World J Gastroenterol 8:237–242

144. Green F, Page D, Fleming I, et al. (2002) Cancer staging handbook, 6th edn. Springer-Verlag, New York, pp 131–144

145. Katzenstein H, Krailo MD, Malogolowkin MH, et al. (2002) Hepatocellular carcinoma in children and adolescents: Results from the Pediatric Oncology Group and the Children's Cancer Group Intergroup Study. J Clin Oncol 20:2789–2797

146. Katzenstein HM, Krailo MD, Malogolowkin MH, et al. (2003) Fibrolamellar hepatocellular carcinoma in children and adolescents. Cancer 97:2006–2012

147. von Schweinitz D (2004) Treatment of liver tumors in children. In: Clavian PA, Fong Y, Lyerly H, et al. (eds) Liver tumors: Current and emerging therapies. Jones and Bartlett, Boston, pp 409–426

148. Shimada M, Takenada K, Gion T, et al. (1996) Prognosis of recurrent hepatocellular carcinoma: A 10-year surgical experience in Japan. Gastroenterol 111:720–726

149. Yeh CN, Lee WC, Jena LB, et al. (2002) Spontaneous tumor rupture and prognosis in patients with hepatocellular carcinoma. Br J Surg 89:1125–1129

150. Buczkowski AK, Kim PT, Ho SD, et al. (2006) Multidisciplinary management of ruptured hepatocellular carcinoma. J Gastrointest Surg 10:379–386

151. Mathurin P, Raynard B, Dharancy S, et al. (2003) Meta-analysis evaluation of adjuvant therapy after curative liver resection for hepatocellular carcinoma. Ailment Pharmacol Ther 17:1247–1261

152. Shen DW, Lu YG, Chin KV, et al. (1991) Human hepatocellular carcinoma cell lines exhibiting multidrug resistance unrelated to MRD-1 gene expression. J Cell Sci 98:317–322

153. Ahn SI, Seo JM, Shim SH, et al. (2001) Hepatocellular carcinoma and lung metastases in a nine year old boy. J Pediatr Surg 36:1599–1601

154. Klintmalm GB (1998) Liver transplantation for hepatocellular carcinoma: A registry report of the impact of tumor characteristics on outcome. Ann Surg 228:479–490

155. Mazzaferro V, Regalia E, Doci R, et al. (1996) Liver transplantation for the treatment of small hepatocellular carcinoma in patients with cirrhosis. New Engl J Med 334:693–699

156. Llovet JM, Fuster J, Bruix J (1999) Intention-to-treat analysis of surgical treatment for early hepatocellular carcinoma: Resection versus transplantation. Hepatology 30:1434–1440

157. Wudel L, Chapman W (2003) Indications and limitations of liver transplantation for hepatocellular carcinoma. Surg Oncol Clin North Am 12:77–90

158. Bismuth H, Majno PE, Adam R (1999) Liver transplantation for hepatocellular carcinoma. Semin Liver Dis 19:311–322

159. Jonas S, Bechstein WO, Steinmuller T, et al. (2001) Vascular invasion and histopathologic grading determine outcome after liver transplantation for hepatocellular carcinoma in cirrhosis. Hepatology 33:1080–1086

160. Kamath PS, Wiesner RH, Malinchoc M, et al. (2001) A model to predict survival in patients with end-stage liver disease. Hepatology 33:464–470

161. Cholongitas E, Papatheodoris GV, Vangeli M (2005) Systemic review: The model for end-stage liver disease—Should it replace Child-Pugh classification for assessing prognosis in cirrhosis. Ailment Pharmacol Ther 22:1079–1089

162. Patt CH, Thuluvath PJ (2002) Role of liver transplantation in the management of hepatocellular carcinoma. J Vasc Interv Radiol 13:S205–S210

163. Yao FY, Ferrell L, Bass NM, et al. (2001) Liver transplantation for hepatocellular carcinoma: Expansion of the tumor size limits does not adversely impact survival. Hepatology 33:1394–1403

164. Roayaie S, Frischer JS, Emre SH, et al. (2002) Long-term results with multimodal adjuvant therapy and liver transplantation for the treatment of hepatocellular carcinoma larger than 5 centimetres. Ann Surg 235:533–539

165. Graziadai IW, Sandmueller H, Waldenberger P, et al. (2003) Chemoembolization followed by liver transplantation for hepatocellular carcinoma impedes tumor progression while on the waiting list and leads to excellent outcomes. Liver Transpl 9:557–563

166. Roayaie S, Frischewr JS, Emre SH, et al. (2002) Long-term results with multimodal adjuvant therapy and liver transplantation for the teatment of hepatocellular carcinoma greater than 5.0 cm. Ann Surg 235:533–539

167. Philosophe B, Greig PP, Hemming AW, et al. (1998) Surgical management of hepatocellular carcinoma: Resection or transplantation? J Gastrointest Surg 2:2–27

168. Chung SW, Toth JL, Rezeig M, et al. (1994) Liver transplantation for hepatocellular carcinoma. Am J Surg 167:317–321

169. Hemming AW, Cattral MS, Reed AI, et al. (2001) Liver transplantation for hepatocellular carcinoma. Ann Surg 233:652–659

170. Saxena R, Ye MQ, Emre S, et al. (1999) Denovo hepatocellular carcinoma in an hepatic allograft with remnant hepatitis C cirrhosis. Liver Transpl Surg 5:81–82

171. Broughan TA, Esquivel CO, Vogt DP, et al. (1994) Pretransplant chemotherapy in pediatric hepatocellular carcinoma. J Pediatr Surg 29:1319–1322

172. Luks FT, St Vil D, Hancock BJ, et al. (1993) Surgical and metabolic aspects of liver transplantation for tyrosinemia. Transplantation 56:1376–1380

173. Tatekawa Y, Asonuma K, Uemoto S, et al. (2001) Liver transplantation for biliary atresia associated with malignant hepatic tumors. J Pediatr Surg 36:436–489

174. Yoo HY, Opatt CH, Geschwind JF, et al. (2003) The outcome of liver transplantation in patients with hepatocellular carcinoma in the United States between 1988–2001: 5-year survival has improved significantly with time. J Clin Oncol 21:4329–4335

175. Yang R, Liu Q, Rescorla FJ, Grosfeld JL (1995) Experimental liver cancer: Improved response after hepatic artery ligation and infusion of tumor necrosis factor alpha, and interferon gamma. Surgery 118:768–774

176. Golladay ES, Mollitt DL, Osteen PK, et al. (1985) Conversion to respectability by intra-arterial infusion chemotherapy after failure of systemic chemotherapy. J Pediatr Surg 20:715–717

177. Yokomari Y, Hari T, Asoh S, et al. (1991) Complete disappearance of unresectable hepatoblastoma by continuous infusion therapy through the hepatic artery. J Pediatr Surg 26:844–846

178. Sue K, Ikeda K, Nakagawara A, et al. (1989) Intrahepatic arterial injections of cisplatin-phosphatidylcholine-Lipiodol suspension in two unresectable hepatoblastoma cases. Med Pediatr Oncol 17:496–500

179. Zhang Z, Liu Q, Ho J, et al. (2000) The effect of preoperative transcatheter hepatic artery chemoembolization on disease free survival after hepatectomy. Cancer 89:2606–2612

180. Llovet JM, Real MI, Montana X, et al. (2002) Arterial embolization or chemoembolization versus symptomatic treatment inpatients with unresectable hepatocellular carcinoma: A randomized controlled trial. Lancet 359:1734–1739

181. Bismuth H, Morino M, Sherlock D, et al. (1992) Primary treatment of hepatocellular carcinoma by arterial embolization. Am J Surg 163:387–394

182. Haider Z, Hag T, Munir K, et al. (2006) Median survival time of patients after transcatheter chemoembolization for hepatocellular carcinoma. J Coll Physicians Surg Pak 16:265–269

183. Hiraoko A, Kumagi T, Hirooka M, et al. (2006) Prognosis following transcatheter arterial embolization for 121 patients with unresectable hepatocellular carcinoma with or without a history of treatment. World J Gastroenterol 12:2075–2079

184. Majno PE, Adam R, Bismuth H, et al. (1997) Influence of preoperative intraarterial Lipiodol chemoembolization on resection and transplantation for hepatocellular carcinoma in patients with cirrhosis. Ann Surg 236:688–701

185. Kitahara S, Makuuchi M, Ishizone S, et al. (1995) Successful left trisegmentectomy for ruptured hepatoblastoma using intra-operative transarterial embolization. J Pediatr Surg 30:1709–1712

186. Berthold F, Schultheis KH, Aigner K, et al. (1986) Combination chemotherapy and chemoembolization in the treatment of primary inoperable hepatoblastoma. Klin Pediatr 198:257–261

187. Uemura S, Todani T, Watanabe Y, et al. (1993) Successful left hepatectomy for hepatocellular carcinoma in a child after transcatheter embolization: Report of a survival. Eur J Pediatr Surg 3:54–56

188. Malogolowkin MH, Stanley P, Steele DA, Ortega JA (2000) Feasibility and toxicity of chemoembolization for children with liver tumors. J Clin Oncol 18:1279–1284

189. Czauderna P, Zbrzezniak G, Narozanski W, et al. (2006) Preliminary experience with arterial chemoembolization for hepatoblastoma/hepatocellular carcinoma in children. Pediatr Blood Cancer 46:825–828

190. Czauderna P, Zbrzezniak G, Narozanski W, et al. (2005) Pulmonary embolism: A fatal complication of arterial chemoembolization for advanced hepatocellular carcinoma. J Pediatr Surg 40:1647–1650

191. Arcement CM, Towbin RB, Gerber DA, et al. (2000) Intrahepatic chemoembolization in unresectable pediatric liver malignancies. Pediatr Radiol 30:779–785

192. Shimamura T, Nakajima Y, Une Y, et al. (1977) Efficacy and safety of preoperative percutaneous transhepatic portal embolization with absolute alcohol: A clinical study. Surgery 121:135–141

193. Abdalla EK, Hicks ME, Vauthey JN (2001) Portal vein embolization: Rationale, technique and future prospects. Br J Surg 88:165–175

194. Madoff DC, Hicks ME, Abdalla EK, et al. (2003) Portal vein embolization with polyvinyl alcohol particles and coils in preparation for major liver resection for hepatic malignancy: Safety and effectiveness—Study in 26 patients. Radiology 227:251–260

195. Farges O, Belghiti J, Kianmanesh R, et al. (2003) Portal vein embolization before right hepatectomy: Prospective clinical trial. Ann Surg 237:208–217

196. Matsumata T, Kanematsu K, Takenaka T, et al. (1989) Lack of intrahepatic recurrence of hepatocellular carcinoma by temporary portal venous embolization with starch microspheres. Surgery 105:188–191

197. Sugiura N, Takara K, Ohto M, et al. (1983) Percutaneous intratumoral injection of ethanol under ultrasound imaging for treatment of small hepatocellular carcinoma. Acta Hepatol Jpn 24:920–923

198. Livraghi T, Festi D, Monti F, et al. (1986) Ultrasound guided percutaneous alcohol injection of small hepatic and abdominal tumors. Radiology 161:309–312

199. Castels A, Bruix J, Bru C, et al. (1993) Treatment of small hepatocellular carcinoma in cirrhotic patients: A cohort study comparing surgical resection and percutaneous ethanol injection. Hepatology 18:1121–1126

200. Chen MS, Li SQ, Zheng V, et al. (2006) A prospective randomized trial comparing percutaneous local ablative therapy and partial hepatectomy for small hepatocellular carcinoma. Ann Surg 243:321–328

201. Orlando A, D'Antoni A, Camma C, et al. (2000) Treatment of small hepatocellular carcinoma with percutaneous ethanol injection: A validated prognostic model. Am J Gastroenterol 95:2921–2927

202. Ohnishi K, Yashioka H, Ito S, Fujiwara K (1998) Prospective randomized control trial comparing percutaneous acetic acid and percutaneous ethanol injection for small hepatocellular carcinoma. Hepatology 27:67–72

203. Zhou XD, Tang ZY (1998) Cryotherapy for primary liver cancer. Semin Surg Oncol 14:171–174

204. Chapman WC, Debelak JP, Pinson CW, et al. (2000) Hepatic cryoablation but not radiofrequency ablation results in lung inflammation. Ann Surg 231:752–761

205. Weber SM, Lee FT Jr (2005) Expanded treatment of hepatic tumors with radiofrequency ablation and cryotherapy. Oncology 19:27–32

206. Pawlik TM, Izzo F, Cohen DS, et al. (2003) Combined resection and radiofrequency ablation for advanced hepatic malignancies: Results in 172 patients. Ann Surg Oncol 10:1059–1069

207. Curley SA, Marra P, Beaty K, et al. (2004) Early and late complications after radiofrequency ablation of malignant liver tumors in 608 patients. Ann Surg 239:430–468

208. Curley SA, Izzo F, Ellis LM, et al. (2000) Radiofrequency ablation of hepatocellular cancer in 110 patients with cirrhosis. Ann Surg 232:381–391

209. Bleicher RJ, Allegra DP, Nora DT, et al. (2003) Radiofrequency ablation of 447 complex unresectable liver tumors: Lessons learned. Ann Surg Oncol 10:53–58

210. Livraghi T, Goldberg SN, Lazzaroni S, et al. (1999) Small hepatocellular carcinoma: Treatment with radiofrequency ablation vs. ethanol injection. Radiology 210:655–661

211. Pearson AS, Izzo F, Hemming RY, et al. (1999) Intraoperative radiofrequency ablation or cryoablation for hepatic malignancies. Am J Surg 178:592–599

212. Kim YK, Kim CS, Chung GH, et al. (2006) Radiofrequency ablation of hepatocellular carcinoma with decompensated cirrhosis: Evaluation of therapeutic efficacy and safety. AJR Am J Roentgenol 116(5 Suppl):S261–268

213. Vettri A, Moreto P, Doriguzzi A, et al. (2006) Radiofrequency ablation after transcatheter chemoembolization for unresectable non-early hepatocellular carcinoma. Eur Radiol 16:661–669

214. Lu DS, Yu NL, Raman CS, et al. (2005) Percutaneous radiofrequency ablation of hepatocellular carcinoma as a bridge to liver transplantation. Hepatology 41:1130–1137

215. Jonas S, Bechstein WO, Heinze T, et al. (1997) Female sex hormone receptor status in advanced hepatocellular carcinoma and outcome after surgical resection. Surgery 121:456–461

216. Boix L, Bruix J, Castells A, et al. (1993) Sex hormone receptors in hepatocellular carcinoma: Is there a rationale for hormonal treatment? J Hepatol 17:187–191

217. Perrone E, Gallo C, Daniele, et al. (2002) Tamoxifen in the treatment of hepatocellular carcinoma: 5-year results of the CLIP-1 multicentre randomized controlled trial. Curr Pharm Des 8:1013–1019

218. Riestra S, Rodriguez M, Delgado M, et al. (1998) Tamoxifen does not improve survival of patients with advanced hepatocellular carcinoma. J Clin Gastroenterol 26:200–203

219. Chow PK, Tai BC, Tan CK, et al. (2002) High-dose tamoxifen in the treatment of inoperable hepatocellular carcinoma: A multi-centre randomized controlled trial. Hepatology 36:1221–1226

220. Schindel DT, Grosfeld JL (1997) Hepatic resection enhances growth of residual intrahepatic and subcutaneous hepatoma which is inhibited by octreotide. J Pediatr Surg 32:995–998

221. Frizelle FA (1995) Octreotide inhibits the growth and development of three types of experimental liver metastases. Br J Surg 82:1577

222. Kouroumalis E, Skordilis P, Thermos K, et al. (1998) Treatment of hepatocellular carcinoma with octreotide: A randomized controlled study. Gut 42:442–447

223. Yuen ME, Poon RT, Lai CL, et al. (2002) A randomized placebo-controlled study of long acting octreotide for the treatment of advanced hepatocellular carcinoma. Hepatology 36:687–691

224. Sun XY, Wu SD, Liao XF, Yuan JY (2005) Tumor angiogenesis and its clinical significance in pediatric malignant liver tumor. World J Gastroenterol 11:741–743

225. Teicher BA, Menon K, Alvarez E, et al. (2001) Antiangiogenic and antitumor effects of a protein kinase C beta inhibitor in human hepatocellular carcinoma and gastric cancer xenografts. In vivo 15:185–193

226. Leung TW, Patt YZ, Lau WY, et al. (1999) Compete pathological remission is possible with systemic combination chemotherapy for inoperable hepatocellular carcinoma. Clin Cancer Res 5:1676–1681

227. Minischetti M, Vacca A, Ribatti D, et al. (2000) TNP-470 and recombinant human interferon-alpha 2a inhibit angiogenesis synergistically. Br J Cancer 109:829–837

228. Patt YZ, Hassan MM, Lozano RD, et al. (2000) Durable clinical response of refractory hepatocellular carcinoma to orally administered thalidomide. Am J Clin Oncol 23:319–321

229. Zeng ZC, Tang ZY, Liu KD, et al. (1998) Improved long-term survival for unresectable hepatocellular carcinoma with a combination of surgery, and intrahepatic arterial infusion of 131I-anti HCC monoclonal antibody. Phase I/II clinical trials. J Cancer Res Clin Oncol 124:275–280

230. Hata Y, Takada N, Sasaki F, et al. (1992) Immunotargeting chemotherapy for alpha fetoprotein producing pediatric liver cancer using conjugates of anti-AFP antibody. J Pediatr Surg 27:724–727

231. Yang R, Liu Q, Rescorla FJ, Grosfeld JL (1995) Experimental liver cancer: Improved response after hepatic artery ligation and infusion of tumor necrosis factor and alpha interferon gamma. Surgery 118:768–774

232. Patt YZ, Hassan MM, Lozano RD, et al. (2003) Phase II trial of systemic continuous fluorouracil and subcutaneous recombinant interferon alpha-2b for treatment of hepatocellular carcinoma. J Clin Oncol 21:421–427

233. Leung TW, Tang AM, Zee B, et al. (2002) Factors predicting response and survival in 149 patients with unresectable hepatocellular carcinoma treated by combination cisplatin, interferon-alpha, doxorubicin, and 5 fluorouracil chemotherapy. Cancer 94:421–427

234. Kubo S, Nishiguchi S, Hirohashi K, et al. (2002) Randomized clinical trial of long-term outcome after resection of hepatitis C virus—Related hepatocellular carcinoma by postoperative interferon therapy. Br J Surg 89:418–422

235. Panis Y, Rad ARK, Boyer O, et al. (1996) Gene therapy for liver tumors. Oncol Clin North Am 5:461–473

236. Kanai F, Shiratori Y, Yoshida Y, et al. (1996) Gene therapy for alpha feto-protein producing human hepatoma cells by adenovirus mediated transfer of herpes simplex virus thymidine-kinase gene. Hepatology 231:1359–1368

237. Sasaki Y, Imaoka S, Masutani S, et al. (1992) Influence of co-existing cirrhosis on long-term prognosis after surgery in patients with hepatocellular carcinoma. Surgery 112:515–521

238. Broderick AL, Jonas MM (2003) Hepatitis B in children. Semin Liver Dis 23:59–68

239. Chang MH, Chen TH, Hsu HM, et al. (2005) Taiwan Hepatocellular Carcinoma Study group—Prevention of hepatocellular carcinoma by universal vaccination against hepatitis B virus: The effect and problems. Clin Cancer Res 11:7953–7957

240. Leung NW (2002) Management of viral hepatitis C. J Gastroenterol Hepatol 17(Suppl 1):S146–S154

241. Ikeda M, Fujiyama S, Tanaka M, et al. (2005) Risk factors for development of hepatocellular carcinoma in patients with chronic hepatitis C after sustained response to interferon. J Gastroenterol 40:220–222

242. Schwimmer JB, Balistreri WF (2000) Transmission, natural history and treatment of hepatitis C virus infection in the pediatric population. Semin Liver Dis 20:37–46

243. Rao GS, Molleston JP (2005) Children with hepatitis C. Curr Gastroenterol Rep 7:37–44

244. Tanaka H, Nouso K, Kobashi H, et al. (2006) Surveillance of hepatocellular carcinoma in patients with hepatitis C virus infection may improve patient survival. Liver Int 26:543–551

245. Lakhdor F, Lawson D, Schatz DA (1994) Fatal parathyroid hormone related protein induced humoral hypercalcemia of malignancy in a three month old infant. Eur J Pediatr 153:718–720

246. Stringer MD, Alizai NK (2005) Mesenchymal hamartomas of the liver: A systemic review. J Pediatr Surg 40:1681–1690

247. Chowdhary SK, Trehan A, Das A, et al. (2004) Undifferentiated embryonal sarcoma in children: Beware of the solitary liver cyst. J Pediatr Surg 39:E9–12

248. Garcia-Bonafe M, Allende H, Fantova MJ, Tarragona J (1997) Fine needle aspiration cytology of undiffrenetiated embryonal sarcoma of the liver. A case report. Acta Cytol 41(4 Suppl):1273–1278

249. deChadarevian JP, Pawel BR, Faerber EN, Weintraub WH (1994) Undifferentiated embryonal sarcoma arising in conjunction with mesenchymal hamartoma of the liver. Mod Pathol 7:490–493

250. Sangkhathat S, Kusafuka T, Nara K, et al. (2006) Non-random p53 mutations in pediatric undifferentiated (embryonal) sarcoma of the liver. Hematol Res 35:229–234

251. Kiani B, Ferrell LD, Qualman S, Frankel WL (2006) Immunohistochemical analysis of embryonal sarcoma of the liver. Appl Immunohistochem Mol Morphol 14:193–197

252. Bisogno G, Pilz T, Perilongo G, et al. (2000) Undifferentiated sarcoma of the liver in childhood: A curable disease. Cancer 94:252–257

253. Dower NA, Smith LJ, Lees G, et al. (2000) Experience with aggressive therapy in three children with unresectable malignant liver tumors. Med Pediatr Oncol 34:132–135

254. Chen JC, Chen CC, Chen W, et al. (1998) Hepatocellular carcinoma in children: Clinical review and comparison with adult cases. J Pediatr Surg 33:1350–1354

Malignant Germ Cell Tumors

13

Frederick J. Rescorla

Contents

13.1 Introduction

Germ cell tumors are a relatively uncommon group of neoplasms which can have a variety of presentations affecting the fetus, infant, child, and adolescent. They are interesting for several reasons: in children the extragonadal site predominates compared with gonadal locations; the most common malignant histology is yolk sac tumor which has alpha fetoprotein as a sensitive marker; although in the past these tumors have had a poor prognosis they have been noted with excellent survival in the era of cooperative group trials utilizing cisplatin, etoposide, and bleomycin; and, based on the effectiveness of chemotherapy, neoadjuvant therapy followed by surgery is indicated to avoid excision of normal structures in unresectable cases.

The location of the tumor often determines the timing of presentation. For instance, with vaginal lesions, bleeding often occurs relatively early in the disease progression and these tumors rarely have metastases at diagnosis [44]. In comparison, sacrococcygeal and retroperitoneal abdominal tumors often achieve a large size prior to the onset of symptoms and the rate of metastases in these tumors is over 50% [9, 43]. The histologic variants also differ by site and age. Among the extragonadal sites, yolk sac histology predominates in the younger children, which include all of the sacrococcygeal and genital tumors. In mediastinal tumors a significant proportion are older children and the histology is more varied including germinoma, choriocarcinoma, and mixed tumors with either benign and malignant or multiple malignant components.

13.2 Embryology and Classification

Germ cell tumors are thought to arise from arrested or aberrant migration of common progenitor cells. These primordial cells originate near the allantois of the embryonic yolk sac endoderm and migrate to the genital ridge at 4–5 weeks gestation. Abnormal deposition can give rise to tumors in extragonadal locations including the central nervous system, neck, mediastinum, retroperitoneum, and sacrococcygeal region. Most childhood germ cell tumors are benign, comprising mature and immature teratomas. Teratomas contain elements from one or more of the embryonic germ layers and contain tissue foreign to the site of origin [17, 34]. Immature teratomas contain primitive neuroepithelium and are graded between I and III [39]. The Pediatric Oncology Group (POG)/Children's Cancer Group (COG) intergroup studies have confirmed the role of complete surgical excision alone as treatment for pediatric immature teratoma regardless of histologic grade [15, 37].

Yolk sac tumor (also called endodermal sinus tumor) is the most common malignant histologic variant in infancy and childhood and can develop metastases to lymph nodes or lungs. Other malignant histologic types include choriocarcinoma and embryonal carcinoma. Germinoma (seminoma and dysgerminoma) are unusual in infancy and childhood and occur commonly in the central nervous system and mediastinum as well as at the gonadal sites in the adolescent age group. Malignant elements coexist in approximately

25% of pediatric germ cell tumors [24] and benign elements (teratoma) are often present with malignant tumors particularly in the mediastinum [8] and ovary [10].

13.3 Genetics and Risk Factors

Children with intersex disorders, undescended testes, and Klinefelter's syndrome associated with thoracic teratoma have an increased risk of germ cell tumors. Children with intersex disorders have an increased risk of developing gonadoblastoma, an in situ lesion with the capability of transforming into dysgerminoma, yolk sac tumor, immature teratoma, or choriocarcinoma [46]. The presence of a Y chromosome is thought to be the risk factor and thus includes male pseudohermaphrodites (under-androgenized males) with testosterone deficiency, androgen insensitivity syndrome, or 5α reductase deficiency as well as mixed gonadal dysgenesis [46]. The risk of malignancy in complete androgen insensitivity is approximately 3.6% at age 20 and 22% at age 30 [36]. Gonadectomy is recommended in these children.

The occurrence of testicular cancer is also increased in boys with undescended testes. Approximately 0.4% of the general population has undescended testes; however, the incidence among males with testicular cancer is 3.5–12% [22]. In addition, the risk appears even higher with intra-abdominal testes as Campbell [12] notes that this site accounts for only 14.3% of undescended testes but 48.5% of the tumors in undescended testes. In addition, the contralateral testes are also at increased risk as 20% of tumors in patients with undescended testes occur in the contralateral scrotal testes [29]. Seminomas occur with an increased frequency in the undescended testes compared with descended testes [51]. Although some have noted a decreased rate of seminoma after orchiopexy [30], the effect of orchiopexy on the rate of testicular cancer is not known.

13.4 Tumor Markers

Yolk sac tumors are the most common histologic type of malignant germ cell tumor in childhood and serum alpha-fetoprotein (AFP) levels should be obtained at the time of presentation. Choriocarcinoma, although less common, has human chorionic gonadotropin (hCG) as an easily identifiable serum marker. Persistently elevated levels after surgery are suggestive of residual disease whereas elevations after an initial drop can indicate progressive or recurrent disease.

AFP is normally elevated in fetal life and as synthesis does not stop completely at birth, the half-life, which is usually considered to be 5 days, may vary during the first few months of life [53]. AFP levels should drop to normal by 9 months of age [52]. The half-life of hCG is 16 h. Lactate dehydrogenase is elevated in many germ cell tumors; however, this is a nonspecific marker.

13.5 Extragonadal Germ Cell Tumors

Extragonadal tumors account for approximately two-thirds of pediatric germ cell tumors compared to only 5–10% in adults [41]. The sacrococcygeal site is the most common, followed by the anterior mediastinum, pineal, retroperitoneum, and less commonly the neck, stomach, and vagina. The current staging system utilized by the Children's Oncology Group (COG) for extragonadal tumors is listed in Table 13.1. The overall risk-based treatment scheme utilized by COG is listed in Table 13.2.

Table 13.1 Children's Oncology Group staging system for malignant extragonadal tumors in childhood

Stage I	Complete resection at any site, coccygectomy for sacrococcygeal site, negative tumor margins
Stage II	Microscopic residual; lymph nodes negative
Stage III	Lymph node involvement with metastatic disease. Gross residual or biopsy only; retroperitoneal nodes negative or positive.
Stage IV	Distant metastases, including liver

Table 13.2 Current risk-based treatment of childhood malignant germ cell tumors. Patients with initial biopsy or incomplete resection will have surgical resection of residual disease after completion of initial therapy. Patients who are complete responders (no viable tumor) receive no further therapy, and those with partial response receive additional chemotherapy. Patients with progressive disease receive alternative chemotherapy.

Group	Treatment

Low-risk
    Stage I gonadal
    All immature teratomas
	Surgery and observation

Intermediate-risk
    Stage II-IV testes
    Stage II-III ovary
    Stage I-II extragonadal
	Surgery and PEB x 3 cycles

High-risk
    Stage IV ovary
    Stage III-IV extragonadal
	Surgery and PEB x 4 cycles

P, cisplatin; E, etoposide; B, bleomycin

13.6 Sacrococcygeal Tumors

Sacrococcygeal tumors are relatively rare, affecting approximately 1:35,000 live births [47]. They occur more commonly in girls (70–80%) and they usually present in one of two clinical patterns: neonates with large predominately benign tumors (mature and immature teratomas) (Fig. 13.1); or, infants and children between birth and 4 years of age with primarily pelvic, malignant (yolk sac) tumors (Fig. 13.2).

Sacrococcygeal teratomas can also be noted in utero and if the lesion is greater than 5 cm in size abdominal delivery should be considered in order to avoid dystocia and tumor rupture [21]. High output cardiac failure can also occur due to shunting leading to fetal hydrops [11]. Detection early in gestation (<30 weeks) and hydrops are ominous and properly selected fetuses less than 30 weeks may benefit from fetal resection or intervention. Adzick, et al. [1] reported the first successful fetal resection. Makin, et al. [33] reported 41 antenatally diagnosed SCTs and performed fetal intervention in 12, including cyst drainage to facilitate delivery or relieve bladder obstruction and laser ablation or alcohol sclerosis for hydrops. Although the overall survival for antenatally diagnosed lesions was 77%, the survival for fetal intervention was 50% and only 14% for fetal intervention for hydrops. One recent study noted that the survival for prenatally detected lesions was highest for small lesions (<10 cm) or larger predominantly cystic tumors (100%), whereas the survival was lowest (48%) in the large (>10 cm) lesions with increased vascularity, vascular steal syndrome, or rapid growth [5].

Altman, et al. (in a survey of the Surgical Section of the American Academy of Pediatrics) developed a classification system which is widely utilized today (Fig. 13.3) [2]. In this survey the rate of malignancy was higher in older infants (<2 months, 7% girls and 10% boys malignant; >2 months, 48% girls and 67% boys malignant). Malignancy rates in children presenting after the newborn period in many series is as high as 90% [18, 42]. The higher malignancy rate with the less apparent lesions may be due to an error in the initial diagnosis, which is most commonly confused with a neural defect. In addition, many older infants may have no external mass and symptoms may develop later as the mass enlarges, frequently leading to constipation and urinary tract dysfunction.

An interesting group of children first reported by Ashcraft and Holder present with an autosomal dominant condition consisting of the triad of presacral teratomas, anal stenosis, and sacral defects [3]. Currarino [14] suggested that adhesions between endoderm and neural ectoderm form, causing a split notochord resulting in this association of defects.

Prior to surgical resection of a neonatal tumor, the degree of pelvic and abdominal extension should be

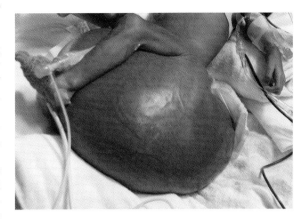

Fig. 13.1 A large Type I sacrococcygeal teratoma.

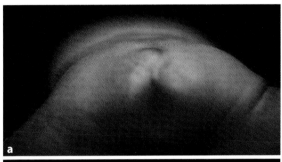

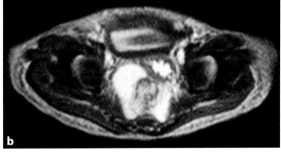

Fig. 13.2 a, b A 2-month-old boy with a malignant sacrococcygeal tumor (**a**) Photograph of small external portion (**b**) MRI scan demonstrating a pelvic tumor.

determined by ultrasound, CT, or MRI. In cases with significant pelvic extension, an abdominal approach (open or laparoscopic) may be needed to mobilize the pelvic component and divide the middle sacral artery. In addition, in high vascular flow lesions it may be useful to gain control of the distal aorta in order to allow temporary vascular occlusion if bleeding is encountered [25]. The lesion can be excised with the child in the prone position (Fig. 13.4). Excision of the coccyx is an essential part of the procedure as Gross, et al. [26] initially reported a 37% recurrence rate when the coccyx was not removed. Closure of the wound can be accomplished by bringing the apex of

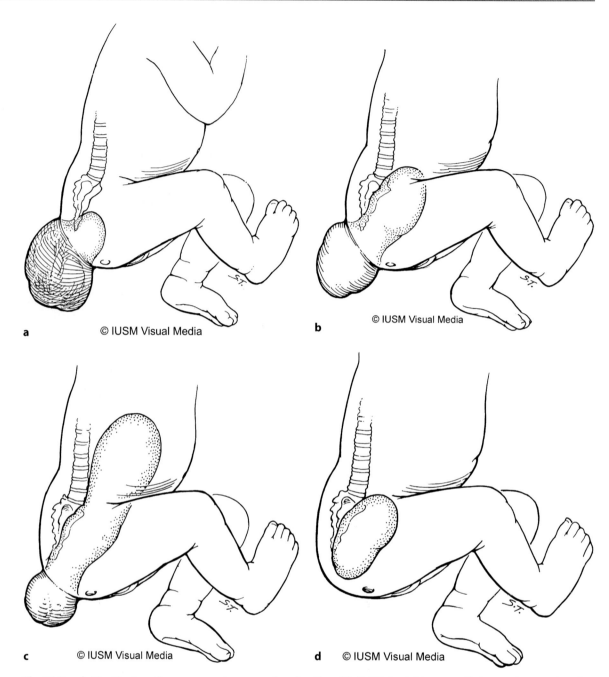

Fig. 13.3 a–d Classification of sacrococcygeal teratomas based on Altman's study (**a**) Type I (46.7%) is predominantly external (**b**) Type II (34.7%) is external with intrapelvic extension (**c**) Type III (8.8%) is visible externally but predominantly pelvic and abdominal (**d**) Type IV (9.8%) is entirely presacral.

the anterior inverted "V" incision to the open of the posterior portion as demonstrated in Figure 13.5. This brings the rectum back to a more posterior location from its original displaced position. Sometimes this closure leaves unsightly protruding tissue laterally, and an alternative closure reported by Fishman, et al.

[20] involved closure bringing the ventral portion of the lateral flaps to a more central posterior.

Most neonates have mature or immature teratomas and are managed with observation during the first few days of life. Operative resection is usually carried out in the first week of life. Recurrent tumors are noted in

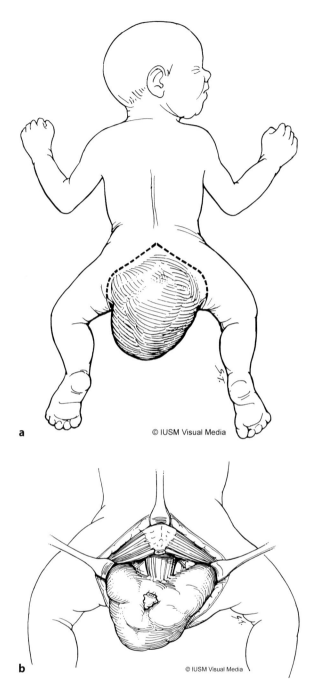

Fig. 13.4 a, b Operative excision of (**a**) Sacrococcygeal teratoma in a neonate with an inverted "V" incision (**b**) The tumor along with the coccyx is excised, taking care to avoid injury to the rectum.

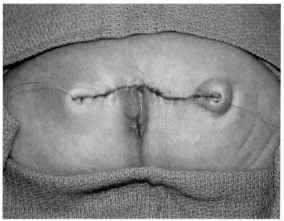

Fig. 13.5 Transverse closure.

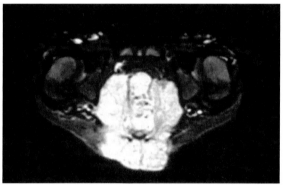

Fig. 13.6 Appearance of a large unresectable sacrococcygeal yolk sac tumor treated successfully with biopsy, neoadjuvant chemotherapy and subsequent excision.

4–21% of these cases [6, 42] and 50% of these are malignant. The development of malignancy may be the result of a pathologic sampling error which missed an initial malignancy or incomplete resection that leaves a small malignant focus. Follow-up should include serial serum AFP levels to ensure return to normal by

9 months of age as well as follow-up serum AFP levels and rectal examination every 3 months to 3 years of age.

Older infants and children with primarily malignant presacral tumors can be approached in a similar fashion; however, due to extensive abdominal extension, initial resection is often not possible and biopsy and neoadjuvant chemotherapy with cisplatin, etoposide, and bleomycin are utilized (Fig. 13.6). The introduction of platinum-based therapy in the late 1970s has significantly improved the survival of these malignant tumors. Schropp, et al. [47] noted an 11% survival prior to 1978 and 86% after 1978 with the use of platinum-containing therapy.

The POG/CCG intergroup study of 74 infants with malignant sacrococcygeal tumors comprised 62 girls and 12 boys with a median age of 21 months [43]. Fifty-nine percent had metastatic disease at diagnosis and the initial procedure was biopsy in 45 and resection in 29. All patients received chemotherapy with etoposide, bleomycin, and either standard or high-dose cisplatin. The overall 4-year event-free survival (EFS) and survival were 84 ±6% and 90 ±4%, respectively. There was no difference in survival based on presence or absence of metastases, initial or delayed resection, or dose of cisplatin. This study confirmed the effective role of neoadjuvant chemotherapy in initially unresectable cases. Long-term follow-up of the newborn and older children is necessary as neuropathic bladder or bowel abnormalities have been reported in 35–41% of patients [23, 35].

13.7 Abdominal/Retroperitoneal

Abdominal and retroperitoneal sites account for approximately 4% of pediatric germ cell tumors [9]. Most tumors at these sites are benign with malignancy occurring in 15% of cases. The recent POG/CCG study included 25 children with 80% less than 5 years of age [9]. The most common symptoms were abdominal or back pain followed by fever, weight loss, constipation, or an acute abdomen. Elevated AFP was the most common marker abnormality as yolk sac tumor was identified in 19, and in four with components of choriocarcinoma, serum beta HCG was elevated. Most had advanced unresectable disease and seventeen had metastatic disease at diagnosis.

Although the majority of patients could only undergo debulking or biopsy, the postchemotherapy outcome was excellent. Four children with initial biopsy only had no residual tumor after chemotherapy and 13, with subsequent surgery, had complete resection. A few had progressive disease or chemotherapy-associated mortality. The 6-year EFS was 82.8 ±10.9% and overall survival 87.6 ±9.3%. This is compared to a mortality of over 80% prior to the advent of cisplatin-based chemotherapy [25]. Based on this study primary excision should be performed if a complete resection can be accomplished without removing normal structures. Otherwise, initial biopsy with neoadjuvant chemotherapy will usually allow a secondary resection.

An interesting subgroup of these tumors is the infantile choriocarcinoma syndrome in which infants present in the first 7 months of life with anemia and hepatomegaly. Tumor production of ß-HCG in these infants can lead to precocious puberty. These tumors are thought to arise as primary placental tumors with metastasis to the fetal liver. The mother must also be followed as metastatic disease has occurred in the mother [9].

13.8 Mediastinal

The mediastinal site for germ cell tumors accounts for approximately 6–18% of all pediatric mediastinal

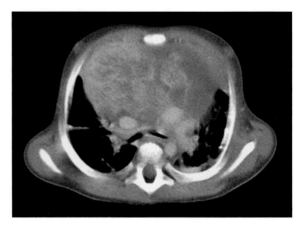

Fig. 13.7 CT scan of a large mediastinal germ cell tumor with airway compromise.

tumors and of these 86% are benign [7, 25]. Many of these tumors achieve a large size prior to detection probably due to the lack of confining boundaries (Fig. 13.7). The clinical presentation is usually respiratory distress in younger children whereas older patients present with chest pain, precocious puberty or facial fullness reflective of venous obstruction. Malignant mediastinal germ cell tumors are more commonly in males and an association with Klinefelter's syndrome has been noted. The presence of hypogonadism, relative increase in leg length compared with overall stature and mild developmental delay should lead to the consideration of Klinefelter's syndrome [8, 32]. Mediastinal germ cell tumors are also associated with hematologic malignancies including leukemia and erythrophagocytic syndrome.

There were 36 patients with mediastinal lesions in the recent POG/CCG study [8]. Tumor marker elevations included 29 with increased serum AFP and 16 with elevated serum ß-hCG. The histology was more heterogeneous than other extragonadal sites with yolk sac tumor found among the children less than 5 years of age whereas older patients had yolk sac tumors as well as germinoma, choriocarcinoma, and mixed tumors.

Fourteen children underwent resection at diagnosis followed by chemotherapy with twelve survivors. Eighteen children underwent biopsy followed by neoadjuvant chemotherapy and subsequent resection with thirteen survivors.

Biopsy technique options include image-guided or open technique using the Chamberlain anterior approach or standard thoracotomy. Eight of ten image-guided biopsies in the POG/CCG study were successful. In this study both resection at diagnosis and post chemotherapy was frequently difficult due to adherence to the thymus, pericardium, superior vena cava, innominate vein, subclavian artery, aorta, vagus and phrenic nerves, as well as lung. Occasional sacrifice of these structures is needed to accomplish a complete resection. Resections were accomplished most frequently (20/31) by median sternotomy followed by thoracotomy (11/31).

Anterior mediastinal tumors pose unique anesthetic risks and careful preoperative assessment should be performed to determine the form of anesthetic. There is a risk for cardiopulmonary arrest with induction of anesthesia due to tracheal compression [27, 40]. Greater than 35–50% tracheal compression is associated with increased morbidity [4, 49]. If significant airway compression is present, a percutaneous image-guided biopsy with local anesthesia with or without sedation may allow confirmation of malignancy and administration of neoadjuvant chemotherapy to decrease tumor size prior to resection.

The survival on the POG/CCG study was 71 ±10% with all deaths occurring in boys over 15 years of age. Interestingly, no death occurred in patients with yolk sac tumors. In some patients with mixed tumors, the benign elements (teratoma) may persist or enlarge as the malignant elements shrink with chemotherapy. Logothetis, et al. [32] described this as the "Growing Teratoma Syndrome." In the POG/CCG study over half of the postchemotherapy specimens contained mature and immature teratoma [8]. In view of the high rate of viable germ cell tumors, complete resection of any residual tumor present after completion of chemotherapy should be performed.

13.9 Genital

Primary germ cell tumors of the genital region are rare, primarily occurring in girls less than 3 years of age [13, 38]. Presenting signs and symptoms include most commonly vaginal bleeding followed by a pelvic mass or urinary obstruction (Fig. 13.8) [44]. This lesion can be confused with the botryoides type of embryonal rhabdomyosarcoma. Older reports utilizing surgery and VAC (vincristine, dactinomycin, and cyclophosphamide) reported a 67% survival but only a 25% vaginal preservation rate [13]. A report from POG/CCG concerning 13 children (12 vaginal, 1 penile) utilizing a neoadjuvant approach with etoposide, bleomycin, and either standard or high-dose cisplatin reported a 4-year survival of 91.7% [44]. Genital preservation was possible in 11 of 12 survivors. In view of this data the initial procedure should be a biopsy only unless an initial complete excision can result in a normal vagina. After initial biopsy, neoadjuvant therapy consisting of cisplatin, etoposide, and bleomycin is administered. Postchemotherapy evaluation usually demonstrates significant shrinkage and at this point a second procedure can often achieve complete resec-

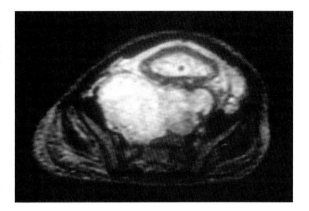

Fig. 13.8 CT scan demonstrating a pelvic mass associated with a vaginal germ cell tumor.

tion of the residual mass. In the POG/CCG study, 9 of 11 treated with neoadjuvant therapy had residual masses including one with progression, one had residual yolk sac tumor, and seven had no identifiable residual tumor [44].

13.10 Testes

Most boys present with a testicular mass allowing preoperative evaluation; however, some present with an acute scrotum with signs and symptoms of torsion, hydrocele, or hernia leading to intraoperative diagnosis and evaluation. A scrotal ultrasound may demonstrate a solitary mass in a child presenting with testicular swelling or mass. If a discrete mass is noted along with normal-appearing testes, this may represent a testicular teratoma and enucleation is considered adequate therapy. These would not be associated with an elevated serum AFP level. Diagnostic work-up should include determination of serum markers and an abdominal and chest CT. The initial diagnostic procedure is a transinguinal exploration with occlusion of the spermatic vessels at the internal ring prior to mobilization of the testes. If a solitary mass is noted, it should be excised with ligation of the entire spermatic cord at the level of the internal ring. Children with no other evidence of disease are followed with serum AFP levels and if these decline to normal appropriately, are considered Stage I (Table 13.3). The role of observation alone in the management of Stage I testes was confirmed in the CCG/POG study of 63 Stage I tumors [48]. This study excluded boys older than 10 years and therefore consisted entirely of patients with yolk sac tumors. The 6-year survival rate was 100% and EFS 78.5% ±7.0%. Most recurrences occurred within 6 months and all were salvaged with chemotherapy. Of interest, transcrotal violation was

Table 13.3 Children's Oncology Group staging system for testes tumors

Stage I	Limited to testis (testes), completely resected by high inguinal orchiectomy; no clinical, radiographic, or histologic evidence of disease beyond testes. Patients with normal or unknown tumor markers at diagnosis must have a negative ipsilateral retroperitoneal node sampling to confirm Stage I disease if radiographic studies demonstrate lymph nodes >2 cm.
Stage II	Transscrotal orchiectomy; microscopic disease in scrotum or high in spermatic cord (≤5 cm from proximal end).
Stage III	Retroperitoneal lymph node involvement, but no visceral or extra-abdominal involvement. Lymph nodes >4 cm by CT or >2 cm and <4 cm with biopsy proof.
Stage IV	Distant metastases, including liver.

associated with a significantly increased rate of recurrence. Most (85%) of children will present with Stage I disease compared to only 35% of adult patients [19, 28]. The predominant histology in prepubertal children is yolk sac tumor and thus the serum AFP levels are elevated.

If preoperative evaluation reveals retroperitoneal disease (Stage III) or pulmonary metastases (Stage IV), an initial inguinal orchiectomy is still performed followed by chemotherapy (Table 13.2). Residual disease should be excised and if viable tumor is present, additional chemotherapy administered. The survival of Stage II tumors in the recent study treated with postoperative chemotherapy although small (n=17) was 100% [45]. The survival of Stage III and IV patients treated with chemotherapy was still very high with a 6-year overall survival and EFS of 100 and 94.1% for Stage III and 90.6 and 88.3% for Stage IV [16].

13.11 Ovary

Ovarian tumors are one of the more common germ cell tumors in female children and adolescents. Of all ovarian masses, most (80%) are benign (epithelial cysts, teratomas, immature teratomas) often with predominantly cystic components (Fig. 13.9). Symptoms include pain, distention, or the presence of a mass. Less common presentations include acute abdomen secondary to torsion or tumor rupture and precocious puberty.

Billmire, et al. [10] reported the CCG/POG experience with 131 childhood and adolescent girls which is the largest series in the era of modern chemotherapy. In this report 57% of the tumors had cystic components, thus highlighting the difficulty of determining malignancy preoperatively. The mean age was 11.9 years. In addition, the histology showed mixed tumors in most, with teratoma coexisting with malignant elements in 60 girls.

The 6-year EFS and survival by Stage in the POG/CCG study were: Stage I 95%, 95.1%; Stage II 87.5%, 93.8%; Stage III 96.6%, 97.3%; and Stage IV 86.7%, 93.3%. Based on this study as well as the excellent results observed in Stage I patients, the current recommendation is to treat Stage I patients with observation alone. It is imperative for the surgeon to accurately stage the patient as inappropriate low staging of the patient would result in under treatment of the child. In addition, in the removal of presumed benign tumors, care should be exercised to avoid tumor spill as this would result in upstaging (I to II) if a malignancy was present in the lesion. There were several other interesting observations in this study: five of 58 Stage III patients were Stage III based on positive ascitic fluid alone; and, the surgeon's determination of negative lymph nodes by inspection and palpation were confirmed by histologic examination of the involved nodes.

Based on the findings of this study there were several minor changes in the surgical staging procedure to include omental inspection and lymph node inspection but not biopsy (Table 13.4). The staging system is listed in Table 13.5. Tumors with extensive involvement of other structures may be initially managed with biopsy and postchemotherapy excision. Radical removal of the uterus is not recommended. On the recent study 11 tumors were bilateral with four benign

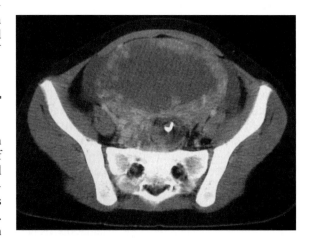

Fig. 13.9 CT scan of a large malignant ovarian mixed yolk sac tumor and teratoma with solid and cystic components.

Table 13.4 Children's Oncology Group operative guideline for ovary tumors

1.	Collect ascites or peritoneal washings for cytology
2.	Examine entire peritoneal surface and liver; excise suspicious lesions
3.	Unilateral oophorectomy
4.	Wedge biopsy of contralateral ovary, only if suspicious
5.	Omental inspection and excision if adherent or contains nodules
6.	Biopsy of suspicious or enlarged retroperitoneal or pelvic lymph nodes

Table 13.5 Children's Oncology Group staging system for ovary tumors

Stage I	Limited to ovary (peritoneal evaluation should be negative). No clinical, radiographic, or histologic evidence of disease beyond the ovaries.
Stage II	Microscopic residual; peritoneal evaluation negative.
Stage III	Lymph node involvement; gross residual or biopsy only; contiguous visceral involvement (omentum, intestine, bladder); peritoneal evaluation positive for malignancy.
Stage IV	Distant metastases, including liver.

teratomas on the contralateral side. The current recommendation for bilateral tumors is to attempt ovarian preservation if possible on the least involved side, particularly if a plane of demarcation exists between the tumor and normal ovarian tissue. These findings and conclusions are consistent with other germ cell tumors reflective of effective chemotherapy to increase the success of conservative surgery.

Many adolescents present with primarily cystic lesions and most of these are benign. Laparoscopy has been widely utilized in the management of ovarian lesions in childhood, adolescents, and adults. The main controversy surrounds the ability to perform a cancer type procedure in cases where the exact tumor histology (benign vs. malignant) cannot be determined preoperatively. If the lesion is primarily solid or if the serum markers are elevated, an open procedure is indicated. If the serum markers are normal and the lesion is primarily cystic, particularly if there is a very large cystic component, a less invasive technique may be considered; however, avoidance of tumor spill must be assured. One minimal access procedure involves laparoscopic excision of the tumor from its attachments, placement in a retrieval bag, and delivering the neck of the bag outside of the abdominal cavity through the umbilical opening. The cyst is then punctured, the fluid removed and the cystic lesion, contained within the bag removed without spill and sent for pathologic examination. In the second technique, useful for giant cysts, the cyst is exposed through an approximate 5-cm incision, and a bag glued to the cyst with cyanoacrylate adhesive as described by Shozu, et al. [50]. The cyst is then incised by cutting through the center of the bag–cyst interface, the fluid removed without spill, and the decompressed cyst then removed from the abdominal cavity (Fig. 13.10). The remainder of the

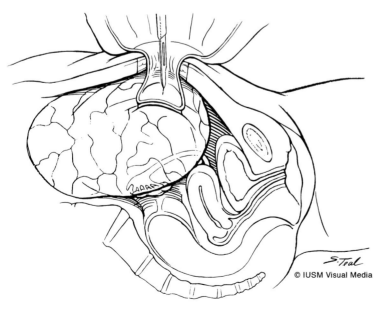

© IUSM Visual Media

Fig. 13.10 Illustration of technique involving fixation of a plastic sheet to a large benign cystic ovarian tumor with decompression without spill.

standard procedure, peritoneal/ascitic fluid sampling, omental inspection, and excision and evaluation of the peritoneal surface can be performed laparoscopically. The only aspect which cannot be accomplished is palpation of retroperitoneal nodes, although depending on the size and habitus of the child or adolescent, a small incision may allow this to be accomplished.

13.12 Conclusion

The survival for pediatric germ cell tumors has dramatically improved since the introduction of platinum-based therapy in the 1970s. The survival for Stage I gonadal tumors and all immature teratomas at any site is excellent and these are managed by surgical excision alone and subsequent observation. The survival for intermediate-risk tumors including Stage II-IV testes, Stage II-III ovarian, and Stage I-II extragonadal is also very high and reductions in therapy have been possible based on cooperative pediatric trials conducted in the 1990s. The survival for high-risk tumors, Stage III-IV extragonadal, and Stage IV ovarian is lower and these currently are managed with longer courses of chemotherapy.

References

1. Adzick NS, Crombleholme RM, Morgan MA, et al. (1997) A rapidly growing fetal teratoma. Lancet 349:538–539
2. Altman RP, Randolph JG, Lilly JR (1974) Sacrococcygeal teratoma: American Academy of Pediatrics Surgical Section Survey – 1973. J Pediatr Surg 9:389–398
3. Ashcraft KW, Holder TM (1974) Hereditary presacral teratoma. J Pediatr Surg 9:691–697
4. Azizkhan RG, Dudgeon DL, Buck JR, et al. (1985) Life-threatening airway obstruction as a complication to the management of mediastinal masses in children. J Pediatr Surg 20:816–822
5. Benachi A, Durin L, Maurer SV, et al. (2006) Prenatally diagnosed sacrococcygeal teratoma: A prognostic classification. J Pediatr Surg 41:1517–1521
6. Bilik R, Shandling B, Pope M, et al. (1993) Malignant benign neonatal sacrococcygeal teratoma. J Pediatr Surg 28:1158–1160
7. Billmire DF (1999) Germ cell, mesenchymal, and thymic tumors of the mediastinum. Semin Pediatr Surg 8:85–91
8. Billmire D, Vinocur C, Rescorla F, et al. (2001) Malignant mediastinal germ cell tumors: An intergroup study. J Pediatr Surg 36:18–24
9. Billmire D, Vinocur C, Rescorla F, et al. (2003) Malignant retroperitoneal and abdominal germ cell tumors: An intergroup study. J Pediatr Surg 38:315–318
10. Billmire D, Vinocur C, Rescorla F, et al. (2004) Outcome and staging evaluation in malignant germ cell tumors of the ovary in children and adolescents: An intergroup study. J Pediatr Surg 39:424–429
11. Bond SJ, Harrison MR, Schmidt KG, et al. (1990) Death due to high-output cardiac failure in fetal sacrococcygeal teratoma [Review]. J Pediatr Surg 25:1287–1291
12. Campbell HE (1942) Incidence of malignant growth of the undescended testicle. Arch Surg 44:353–369
13. Copeland LJ, Sneige N, Ordonez NG, et al. (1985) Endodermal sinus tumor of the vagina and cervix. Cancer 5:2258–2565
14. Currarino G, Coln D, Votteler T (1981) triad of anorectal, sacral, and presacral anomalies. AJR. Am J Roentgenol 137:395–398
15. Cushing B, Giller R, Ablin A, et al. (1999) Surgical resection alone is effective treatment for ovarian immature teratoma in children and adolescents: A report of the Pediatric Oncology Group and Children's Cancer Group. Am J Obstet Gynecol 181:353–358
16. Cushing B, Giller R, Cullen JW, et al. (2004) Randomized comparison of combination chemotherapy with etoposide, bleomycin, and either high-dose or standard-dose cisplatin in children and adolescents with high-risk malignant germ cell rumors: A Pediatric Intergroup Study – Pediatric Oncology Group 9049 and Children's Cancer Group 8882. J Clin Oncol 22:2691–2700
17. Dehner LP (1983) Gonadal and extragonadal germ cell neoplasia of childhood [Review]. Hum Pathol 14:493–511
18. Ein SH, Mancer K, Adeyemi SD (1985) Malignant sacrococcygeal teratoma – Endodermal sinus, yolk sac tumor – In infants and children: A 32 year review. J Pediatr Surg 20:473–477
19. Einhorn LH, Donahue JP (1979) Combination chemotherapy in disseminated testicular cancer: The Indiana University experience. Semin Oncol 6:87
20. Fishman SJ, Jennings RW, Johnson SM, et al. (2004) Contouring buttock reconstruction after sacrococcygeal teratoma resection. J Pediatr Surg 39:439–441
21. Flake AW (1993) Fetal sacrococcygeal teratoma [Review]. J Pediatr Surg 2:113–120
22. Fonkalsrud EW (1978) The undescended testis [Review]. Curr Prob Surg 15:1–56
23. Gabra HO, Jesudason EC, McDowell HP, et al. (2006) Sacrococcygeal teratoma – A 25-year experience in a UK regional center. J Pediatr Surg 41:1513–1516
24. Göbel U, Schneider DT, Calaminus G, et al. (2000) Germ-cell tumors in childhood and adolescence. Ann Oncol 11:263–271
25. Grosfeld JL, Billmire DF (1985) Teratomas in infancy and childhood. Curr Probl Cancer 9:1–53
26. Gross Re, Clatworthy HW, Meeker IA (1951) Sacrococcygeal teratoma in infants and children. Surg Gynecol Obstet 92:341–354
27. Halpern S, Chatten J, Meadows AT, et al. (1983) Anterior mediastinal masses: Anesthesia hazards and other problems. J Pediatr 102:407–410
28. Hopkins TB, Jaffe N, Colody A, et al. (1978) The management of testicular tumors in children. J Urol 12:96
29. Johnson DE, Woodhead DM, Pohl DR, et al. (1968) Cryptorchidism and testicular tumorigenesis. Surgery 63:919–922

30. Jones BJ, Thornhill JA, O'Donnell B, et al. (1991) influence of prior orchiopexy on stage and prognosis of testicular cancer. Eur Urol 19:201–203

31. Lindahl H (1988) Giant sacrococcygeal teratoma: A method of simple intraoperative control of hemorrhage. J Pediatr Surg 23:1068–1069

32. Logothetis CJ, Samuels ML, Trindade A, et al. (1982) The growing teratoma syndrome. Cancer 50:1629–1635

33. Makin EC, Hyett J, Ade-Ajay N, et al. (2006) Outcome of antenatally diagnosed sacrococcygeal teratomas: A single-center experience (1993–2004). J Pediatr Surg 41:388–393

34. Malogolowkin MH, Ortega JA, Krailo M, et al. (1989) Immature teratomas: Identification of patients at risk for malignant recurrence. J Natl Cancer Inst 81:870–874

35. Malone PS, Spitz L, Kiely EM, et al. (1990) The functional sequelae of sacrococcygeal teratoma. J Pediatr Surg 25:679–680

36. Manuel M, Katayama PK, Jones HW Jr (1976) The age of occurrence of gonadal tumors in intersex patients with a Y chromosome. Am J Obstet Gynecol 124:293–300

37. Marina N, Cushing B, Giller R, et al. (1999) Complete surgical excision is effective treatment for children with immature teratomas with or without malignant elements: A Pediatric Oncology Group/Children's Cancer Group intergroup study. J Clin Oncol 17:2137–2143

38. Norris HJ, Bagley GP, Taylor HB (1970) Carcinoma of the infant vagina: A distinctive tumor. Arch Pathol 90:473–479

39. Norris HJ, Zirkin HJ, Benson WL (1976) Immature (malignant) teratoma of the ovary: A clinical and pathological study of 58 cases. Cancer 37:2359–2372

40. Northrip DR, Bohman BK, Tsueda K (1986) Total airway occlusion and superior vena cava syndrome in a child with an anterior mediastinal tumor. Anesth Analg 65:1079–1082

41. Pantoja E, Llobet R, Gonzales-Flores B (1976) Retroperitoneal teratoma: Historical review. J Urol 115:520–523

42. Rescorla FJ, Sawin RS, Coran AG, et al. (1998) Long-term outcome for infants and children with sacrococcygeal teratoma: A report from the Children's Cancer Group. J Pediatr Surg 33:171–176

43. Rescorla F, Billmire B, Stolar C, et al. (2001) The effect of cisplatin dose and surgical resection in children with malignant germ cell tumors at the sacrococcygeal region: A pediatric intergroup trial (POG 9049/CCG 8882). J Pediatr Surg 36:12–17

44. Rescorla F, Billmire D, Vinocur C, et al. (2003) The effect of neoadjuvant chemotherapy and surgery in children with malignant germ cell tumors of the genital region: A pediatric intergroup trial. J Pediatr Surg 38:910–912

45. Rogers PC, Olson TA, Cullen JW, et al. (2004) Treatment of children and adolescents with Stage II testicular and Stages I and II ovarian malignant germ cell tumors: A pediatric intergroup study – Pediatric Oncology Group 9048 and Children's Cancer Group 8891. J Clin Oncol 22:3563–3569

46. Rutgers JL, Scully RE (1992) Pathology of the testes in intersex syndromes [Review]. Semin Diagn Pathol 4:275–291

47. Schropp KP, Lobe TE, Rao B, et al. (1992) Sacrococcygeal teratoma: The experience of four decades. J Pediatr Surg 27:1075–1079

48. Schlatter M, Rescorla F, Giller R, et al. (2003) Excellent outcome in patients with Stage I germ cell tumors of the testes: A study of the Children's Cancer Group/Pediatric Oncology Group. J Pediatr Surg 38:319–324

49. Shamberger RC, Holzman RS, Griscom NT, et al. (1991) CT quantitation of tracheal cross-sectional area as a guide to the surgical and anesthetic management of children with anterior mediastinal masses. J Pediatr Surg 26:138–142

50. Shozu M, Segawa T, Sumitani H, et al. (2001) Leak-proof puncture of ovarian cysts: Instant mounting of plastic bag using cyanoacrylate adhesive. Obstet Gynecol 97:1007–1010

51. Sohval AR (1954) Testicular dysgenesis as an etiologic factor in cryptorchidism. J Urol 72:693–702

52. Tsuchida Y, Endo Y, Saito S, et al. (1978) Evaluation of alpha-fetoprotein in early infancy. J Pediatr Surg 13:155–162

53. Wu JT, Book L, Sudar K (1981) Serum alpha-fetoprotein (AFP) levels in normal infants. Pediatr Res 15:50–52

Soft Tissue Sarcoma

14

Richard J. Andrassy

Contents

14.1 Introduction

The soft-tissue sarcomas (STS) of childhood are a relatively rare and heterogeneous group of tumors that may occur anywhere in the body and respond quite differently to therapy. STSs account for 7.4% of all cancers in children younger than 20 years [1]. These soft tissue sarcomas are divided almost equally between rhabdomyosarcomas originating from striated muscle and nonrhabdomyosarcoma soft tissue sarcomas (NRSTS). Sarcomas are malignant tumors of mesenchymal cell origin. They are named according to the normal tissue they resemble – for example, rhabdomyosarcoma (skeletal muscle), leiomyosarcoma (smooth muscle), and fibrosarcoma and malignant fibrous histiocytoma (connective tissue), neurofibrosarcoma or malignant peripheral nerve sheath tumor (neurofibrosarcomas, as seen in patients with neurofibromatosis), liposarcoma (adipose), synovial sarcoma (synovium), peripheral nerve sheath tumors (peripheral nerve), and angiosarcoma (blood and/or lymphatic vessels). Other sarcomas include rare entities such as alveolar soft-part sarcoma, extraosseous Ewing's sarcoma, peripheral neuroectodermal tumors, epitheloid sarcoma, and hemangiopericytoma.

Rhabdomyosarcoma (Greek for rhabdos, "rod," mys "muscle," sarkos "flesh") is a primary malignancy in children and adolescents that arises from embryonic mesenchyme with the potential to differentiate into skeletal muscle. The original distinction of soft tissue sarcomas and bone sarcomas from epithelial and hematopoietic tumors is attributed to Virchow who, in the middle 1850s propounded his theory of "cellular pathology" which ascribed the origin of tumors to specific types of cells [2]. Since we now know that STS differs widely in their response to therapy, this chapter will separate the NRSTS from the RSTS in discussion. Much of the data about RSTS comes from pediatric studies since RSTS is rare in adults. Much of our knowledge about pediatric NRSTS comes from adult patients since NRSTS is more common in adults than children.

14.2 Section 1

14.2.1 Nonrhabdomyosarcoma Soft Tissue Sarcomas

14.2.2 Epidemiology

It was estimated that, in 2004, 8,680 new patients with STS would be diagnosed in the USA with approximately 850 in patients less than 20 years [1]. The distribution of patient age at diagnosis varies among the histologic subtypes. Fibrosarcoma, for example, is more common in infants, whereas synovial sarcoma and malignant peripheral nerve sheath tumor (MPNST) are more frequently encountered in older children and adults [1, 3]. There is a slight male predominance of NRSTS (male-to-female ratio 1.2:1) in both adults and children [1]. There is no evidence that the incidence of NRSTS is increasing in either children or adults. Epidemiologic data suggesting an etiology are present in less than 5% of patients diagnosed with NRSTS. Therapeutic radiation doses result in a cumulative incidence of in-field sarcomas in 1–2% of long-term cancer survivors 10–15 years after therapy [4, 5], with pleomorphic high-grade sarcoma (also known as malignant fibrous histiocytoma) being most common. Patients with Li-Fraumeni syndrome, a rare autosomal dominant disease characterized by germ line p53 mutations, have an increased risk for development of RMS as well as NRSTS [6, 7]. Approximately half of all patients with MPNST are diagnosed in patients with neurofibromatosis-1 (NF-1, Von-Recklinghausen's disease) [8], and 2–13% of patients with NF-1 will develop a MPNST [8–12]. Desmoid tumors occur in 4–20% of all patients with familial Gardner syndrome [13–15].

14.2.3 Molecular and Biopathology of Soft Tissue Tumors

The pathologist plays a key role in the diagnosis and thus future management of the patient with NRSTS. The optimal biopathologic evaluation includes the morphologic immunocytochemical ultrastructural, cytogenetic, molecular, and biochemical factors that influence response to oncologic management and overall survival. Adequate tissue must be provided for a complete diagnosis since accurate diagnosis is frequently complex and will require histologic, cytogenetic, molecular, and other studies. Submission of tissue for cytogenetics and retention of the frozen section tissue blocks at -70° for molecular, reverse transcriptase polymerase chain reaction (RT-PCR), biochemical, and microarray gene product analyses will aid in diagnosis. Cytogenetic imprints allow for fluorescent in situ hybridization (FISH) evaluation of mutated genes, tumor defining translocations, and other cytogenetic abnormalities.

Specific chromosomal translocations define several STSs in children. For example, t(x;18) (p11;q11) occurs in about 90% of synovial sarcomas [16, 17]. Molecular studies identified two novel genes that are arranged in synovial sarcoma: SS18 (formerly S4T) at 18q11 and SSX at Xpll [18]. In addition, two predominant forms of the SS18–SSX fusion transcript, SS18–SSXI and SSI8–SSX2, have been described and are related to histopathologic and clinical features. SSXI is associated with both biphasic and monophasic tumors, whereas SSX2 is identified with monophasic tumors exclusively [19, 20].

The SS1 transcript is associated with a higher proliferation rate, metastatic disease occurrence, and shortened survival compared with the SSX2 transcript [20, 21].

Myxoid liposarcoma, which is most commonly seen in children and adolescents, is similarly characterized by tumor defining translocations t(12;16) (q13;pII) (FUS/TLS-CHOP) and t(12;22) (q13; q12) (EWS-CHOP). These translocations lead to fusion of transcription factors participating in adipocytic differentiation [22, 23]. The EWS gene is also fused with other genes associated with several childhood sarcomas, including Ewing's sarcoma, desmoplastic small round cell tumor clear cell sarcoma (malignant melanoma of soft parts), and extraskeletal myxoid chondrosarcoma [24, 25]. Many NRSTSs are associated with loss of heterozygosity (LOH) of tumor suppressor genes. The role of LOH of the tumor suppressor gene p53 in tumor development with the familial cancer syndrome was first described by Li and Fraumeni [26–29]. As many as 10% of STSs in children may be associated with the autosomal dominant Li-Fraumeni syndrome. Further supporting this LOH effect is the strong association between MPNST and NF-1, a common autosomal dominant disorder associated with chromosomal abnormalities at 17q11.2 (NF1 tumor suppressor gene locus) [24].

Interestingly, MPNSTs tend to arise in NF-1 patients with neurofibromatosis at an earlier age than in patients without neurofibromatosis [30–34].

NRSTS, most commonly pleomorphic undifferentiated sarcoma (MFH), may be associated with prior radiotherapy for a primary tumor. Genetic abnormalities following radiation are well recognized in tumorigenesis [4, 5]. In particular, soft tissue tumor development following radiotherapy in children with Li-Fraumeni family cancer syndrome and hereditary retinoblastoma are noted more frequently in nonsyndromatic cancer patients [6].

The association of benign and malignant smooth muscle tumors with Epstein-Barr virus (EBV) in children infected with the human immunodeficiency virus (HIV), immune suppression (organ transplantation, leukemia), and immune compromise (ataxia-telangiectasia syndrome is well documented [35–38].

Although certain childhood tumors may resemble an adult counterpart with respect to histopathologic appearance, there are significant biologic differences between these childhood and adult tumors that alter diagnosis, management, prognosis, and survival. This is truer for young children and infants than for older adolescents.

In my own experience, synovial sarcoma, malignant fibrous histiocytoma, neurofibrosarcoma and extraossseous Ewing's sarcoma have been the most common NRSTSs to need surgical intervention. Also, fibrosarcomas and undifferentiated sarcomas occur to a reasonable degree. The synovial sarcomas metastasize to regional lymph nodes and lung more frequently than the others [39, 40].

14.2.4 Clinical Presentation

NRSTSs may arise in any part of the body; however, most are seen in the extremities and trunk. Most are painless, enlarging masses. Symptoms generally are related to compression of nerves or vessels. Systemic symptoms are rare.

14.2.5 Staging

Pediatric NRSTSs have traditionally been staged according to the Intergroup Rhabdomyosarcoma Study group surgicopathologic grouping system (to be described in greater detail in the Rhabdomyosarcoma section of this chapter) (Table 14.1) [41]. The International Union Against Cancer Staging Systems incorporates size (a or b), nodal status (No or N1), invasiveness (T1 or T2), and the presence or absence of metastases (Table 14.2) [42].

For the adult with NRSTS, the most commonly employed system is the one developed by the American Joint Committee on Cancer (AJCC) [43]. This system recognizes four distinct histologic grades and this attribute in combination with size are the primary determinants of clinical stage. This system combines

Table 14.1 Intergroup RMS Study Group Surgicopathologic Staging System and Clinical Outcome According to Clinical Group [41]

Group	Description	5-yr. event-free survival (%)	5-yr. survival (%)
I	Localized disease, completely resected	72–83	84–90
II	Microscopic residual, completely resected with nodes, nodes involved with microscopic residual	65–72	84–88
III	Incomplete resection	–	35–54
IV	Distant metastases	15 (2 yrs)	34 (2 yrs)

Table 14.2 Clinical International Union Against Cancer Staging System for Pediatric Soft Tissue Tumors [42]

Stage	Tumor, Node	Metastasis
1	T1a–T1b, NO	MO
2	T2a–T2b, NO	MO
3	Any T, N 1	MO
4	Any T, Any N	M1

<a, ≤5 cm; b, >5 cm; M1, distant metastases; NO, no nodal disease; N1, regional node metastases; T1, tumor limited to organ or tissue of origin; T2, tumor invades contiguous organs or tissues and/or with malignant effusion

low-grade tumors regardless of size and depth into one category and recognizes two subsets of nonmetastatic high-grade tumors based on size and depth.

Histologic grading has been used in both adult and pediatric studies as an adjunct to clinical staging because it is highly predictive of clinical outcome [43–45]. The system developed by the National Cancer Institute of the United States (NCI) by Costa and colleagues stratifies STS into three different grades based on histologic subtype and a composite of histopathologic parameters that includes tumor necrosis, cellularity, pleomorphism, and mitotic activity [42]. The grading system used by the French Federation of Cancer Centers Sarcoma Group is based on tumor differentiation, mitotic count, and necrosis and appears to better predict the risk of metastases and mortality when compared to the NCI grading system [44, 46].

The Pediatric Oncology Group (POG) developed and prospectively tested a pediatric grading system for

NRSTS [47] based on the histologic system developed by Costa, et al. [42]. This grading system identified three different grades to tumor based on histopathologic subtype: amount of necrosis, number of mitoses, and cellular pleomorphism. Infantile tumors such as hemangiopericytoma and fibrosarcoma are considered grade 1 in this classification given their relatively benign clinical course despite their aggressive appearance on histologic examination [48, 49].

14.2.6 Prognostic Factors

Tumor respectability and presence or absence are the most important prognostic factors. The clinical outcome for completely resected NRSTSs is quite good, but over 20% of these children eventually develop disease recurrence and ultimately die from their disease [50–52]. Risk factors for recurrence are important in determining prognosis, therapy, and intensity of therapy. The most significant adverse prognostic factors for survival are tumor size, histologic grade, and microscopic resection margin. Size and grade predict early relapse, where as surgical margin status is associated with late relapses [53].

There are relatively few trials, mostly retrospective, in children predicting clinical outcome in patients with surgically resected disease [53–56]. In the St. Jude Children's Research retrospective review, clinical group, lack of radiotherapy use, large tumor size, and intra-abdominal primary site predicted local recurrence, whereas tumor size, invasiveness, and high histologic grade predicted distant failure.

14.2.7 Summary of Prognostic Factors

Factors associated with increased risk of recurrence:
a) Microscopic positive margins
b) Intra-abdominal primary tumors
c) No radiotherapy
d) Tumor size >5 cm

Factors associated with increased risk of distant recurrence:
a) Tumor size >5 cm
b) Invasive tumors
c) High histologic grade

Factors associated with decreased survival:
a) Microscopic positive margins
b) Tumor size >5 cm
c) High histologic grade
d) Intra-abdominal primary tumor site

Metastatic disease at the time of initial presentation occurs in approximately 15% of children with NRSTS

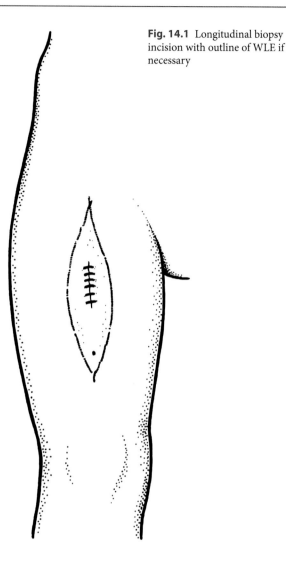

Fig. 14.1 Longitudinal biopsy incision with outline of WLE if necessary

[54]. The lung is the most common site of distant metastases, although metastases to bone, liver, and mesentery have also been reported. Regional lymph node spread is rare with most histologic subtypes; however, it can occur in high-grade lesions, synovial sarcoma, angiosarcoma, and epithelioid sarcoma. The prognosis of patients with lymphatic metastases is similar to patients with metastatic disease at other sites.

14.2.8 General Treatment Considerations

Multimodal therapy in a coordinated fashion offers the best chance for a successful outcome. Although the evaluation and treatment of NRSTSs in children is similar to adult therapy, some important differences need to be considered. In some young patients the biology of the tumor seems to be less aggressive, while the complications of adjuvant therapy may be greater (i.e., radiation-induced injury). The long-term effects on growth and second malignancies need to be weighed against the potential benefits [57–64]. First, adequate tissue for diagnosis must be obtained. This may be by excisional or incisional biopsy. Determination of resectability is done by clinical judgment and review of imaging studies. For unresectable tumors, consideration of neoadjuvant irradiation or chemotherapy must be entertained, although results in children haven't been overly encouraging. Complete surgical resection remains the mainstay of treatment and should be attempted whenever feasible without causing undue loss of tissue or function.

14.2.9 Surgery

Surgery is the essential component of the management of NRSTSs and the approach is site specific. Although wide local excision is the optimal approach, the amount of tumor-free margin necessary is not precisely known. It is generally better to have close margins near neurovascular bundles than to primarily resect these vital structures. Some tumors, such as hemangiopericytoma, infantile fibrosarcoma and the angiomatoid variant of MFH are less biologically aggressive and can be treated more conservatively [65].

Proper treatment begins with proper biopsy. Some tumors can be diagnosed by fine needle aspiration (FNA) or core biopsy. In our own experience, FNA biopsy in children was quite reliable in making a diagnosis in selected patients [66]. However, since the classification of NRSTSs is now dependent on cytogenetic and molecular studies, open biopsy more reliably provides adequate tissue. Longitudinal incisions are preferred in the extremity to allow for excision of the biopsy tract at the time of definitive resection (Fig. 14.1). Inappropriately placed incisions at any location makes resection or flap closure more difficult. If wide local excision with adequate margins can't be obtained easily at initial biopsy, it is better to wait for the diagnosis and plan definitive resection at a later time. Controversy remains on what constitutes an adequate margin. Although some adult studies have suggested a 2-cm margin, this is largely empirical and would be impractical if not impossible in most children. It appears in my own practice that narrow margins near neurovascular bundles may not be as significant as narrow or thin margins in muscular planes. Recurrence is less common nearer the neurovascular bundle than in other tissue planes. In a study concerning margins resection of NRSTS, Blakely, et al. [67] noted that a margin less that 1 cm had a higher local recurrence rate. An adequate wide resection includes the tumor, its pseudocapsule, and a margin of normal tissue removed in all directions en bloc. Cure can be obtained without removal of the entire muscle compartment and proper resection may obviate the need for postoperative radiation or at least decrease the intensity of radiation.

Because some tumors have a pseudocapsule (such as synovial sarcoma), they may be inappropriately shelled out with the operating surgeon believing that he/she has completely removed the tumor, although microscopic, if not gross disease, was left behind. Local recurrence rates are extremely high in these circumstances. High-grade tumors that are larger than 5 cm or extend beneath the fascia may require a much more aggressive approach, because their potential for local recurrence is significant. Pathologic examination or postoperative imaging studies suggesting that there is residual tumor or very thin margins should prompt the surgeon to recommend re-excision of the primary site to ensure local control. Overall, the most important surgical aspect for local control and decreasing recurrence is wide local excision (WLE) with clear margins.

14.2.10 Lymph Node Dissection

In general, because lymph node involvement for most NRSTSs is rare, nodal evaluation has not been a routine. Regional lymph node involvement may be as high as 15% in some NRSTSs such as synovial sarcoma and high-grade lesions, such as angiosarcoma or epithelioid sarcoma [39, 40]. Therefore, in some centers, including our own, sentinel lymph node mapping and biopsy for synovial sarcoma of the extremity or trunk is routinely performed. This may best be done at the time of WLE and is done with the injection of a combination of technetium-labeled sulfur colloid and isosulfan blue dye (Lymphazurim) [68]. A radioisotope detector is used to localize the sentinel node and an incision is made over the localized area to then identify the blue nodes with high radioisotope count that represent the nodal basin. Formal lymph node dissection may be performed or radiation considered if the sentinel node is positive.

14.2.11 Surgical Re-resections

Many patients referred to our center have gross or microscopic residual disease left at the primary site despite the best efforts of the referring physician. Frequently the surgeon biopsying the lesion does not suspect a malignancy. Even when the surgeon believes he/she has done a complete dissection, as many as 50% of patients may have gross or microscopic residual disease. We routinely recommend re-excision to establish clear margins and lymph node status.

14.2.12 Synovial Sarcomas

Synovial sarcomas are malignant, high-grade, soft tissue neoplasms that account for 7–8% of all malignant soft tissue sarcomas and are the most common NRSTS in pediatric patients [39, 40]. The most common location is the lower extremity, followed by the upper extremity, trunk, abdomen, and head and neck. Approximately 30% of patients with synovial sarcoma are younger than 20 years of age, yet this remains an uncommon tumor in most centers. The most common site for metastases is the lung and survival with metastatic disease is rare. Regional lymph node metastases can occur in as many as 15% of patients and is a more common occurrence in synovial sarcoma than other NRSTS. Initial biopsy should be incisional unless the lesion is small and can be excised safely with negative margins. All extremity incisions should be longitudinal, when possible, to allow easy WLE. Many of these tumors have a pseudocapsule that allows the tumor to shell out fairly easily, giving the surgeon a false sense of security that the tumor has been totally excised. Microscopic and even gross residual disease may be overlooked. Early re-excision for gross or microscopic disease appears to have a positive effect on recurrence and survival. In our own experience, the risk of recurrence and subsequent metastases and death are increased when tumors are greater than 5 cm. Surgical resection and re-resection with adequate but not necessarily large margins are the key to successful management. Although all synovial sarcomas are considered high-grade at our institution, chemotherapy does not appear to be effective. Pappo, et al. [69] reported the only prospective pediatric trial addressing the value of adjuvant chemotherapy in NRSTS by the Pediatric Oncology Group (POG). Seventy-five children with completely resected lesions were assigned to receive observation vs. adjuvant chemotherapy with vincristine, actinomycin D, cyclophosphamide (VAC), and doxorubicin.

The 3-year disease-free survival rates for these two groups did not differ (74% vs. 76%). Outcome for children with metastatic NRSTS continues to be poor; fewer than 20% of patients are disease free at 3 years [69]. Radiation therapy, either external beam or brachytherapy, is considered in all patients with microscopic residual disease or positive lymph nodes. It appears that radiation therapy might be of value even in patients with complete resection, because local recurrence may be reduced in completely resected patients given radiation. In our series [40], although small and retrospective, patients who received radiation therapy in addition to operation and chemotherapy experienced fewer failures than those treated by operation and chemotherapy only. Brennan (70) has reported that local recurrence was the same for adult patients with a positive margin, whether or not they had radiation. But if the margins were negative, local recurrence was decreased if radiation was given. We have used sentinel lymph node mapping in a small number of patients to determine lymph node status of these patients [68].

Tumor size greater than 5 cm has also been reported to herald local recurrence and distant relapse. In our study, patients with tumor size less than 5 cm and with monophasic histology had better progression-free survival outcomes than those with tumors 5 cm or greater and biphasic histology (p=0.09 and p=0.14, respectively). Brennan [70] noted that patients with a lesion larger than 5 cm had a 40% greater chance of local recurrence than those with a lesion less than 5 cm. Mullen and Zagars [11] recommended that adjuvant chemotherapy be considered for patients with tumors greater than 5 cm or with metastatic disease. There was some indication from their study that chemotherapy might be of value for extremity lesions, although this has not been confirmed. Spunt and coworkers [50] reported that distant recurrence was associated with tumor size larger than 5 cm, high-grade histologic lesions, and invasiveness. Pappo and colleagues (69) reported specifically on 37 children with synovial sarcoma and found that tumor size significantly impacted progression-free survival. They concluded that the mainstay of treatment is complete surgical resection. They also found that local control rates for patients with negative surgical margins were not dependent on the extent (depth) of the surgical margin.

The role of postoperative adjuvant therapy remains controversial. Fontanesi and associates [72] reported 37 patients with synovial sarcoma at St. Jude Children's Research Hospital and concluded that irradiation is of limited value for patients with adequate surgical margins, but recommended radiation therapy for patients with incomplete resection or partial response to chemotherapy. Brennan [70] reported that local recurrence was the same for adult patients with a positive margin, whether or not they had radiation. However, if margins were negative, then local recurrence was decreased if radiation was given. Blakely and coworkers [67] described 26 patients with synovial sarcoma, six of whom (23.1%) had a local recurrence. None of these six received radiation therapy and they concluded that radiation may be of benefit if the margin is less than 1 cm.

Adjuvant chemotherapy was used in our series in selected patients and included various regimens including vincristine, doxorubicin, cyclophosphamide, actinomycin D, dacarbazine, ifosfamide, etoposide, methotrexate, and cisplatin. None appeared effective, although no conclusions can be made based on this nonrandomized and varied approach. Pappo and associates [73] reported the only prospective pediatric trial addressing the value of adjuvant chemotherapy in NRSTS by the Pediatric Oncology Group (POG). Seventy-five children with completely resected lesions were assigned to receive observation vs. adjuvant chemotherapy with vincristine actinomycin D cyclophosphamide (VAC) and doxorubicin. The 3-year disease-free survival rates for these two groups were similar (74% vs. 76%). However, patients with high-grade, completely resected tumors fared worse than those with lower-grade, completely resected tumors, and they suggested that a prospective trial of adjuvant chemotherapy in high-grade, completely resected NRSTS may be warranted. Outcome for children with metastatic NRSTS continues to be poor; fewer than 20% of patients are disease-free at 3 years [73]. There are current trials evaluating ifosfamide, doxorubicin, and vincristine in children with unresectable or metastatic NRSTS.

What lessons have we learned from our own patients and review of other series? Primary re-resection of the tumor should be considered in all patients. Many will have gross or microscopic residual, and re-resection seems to decrease the risk of local recurrence and improve survival. Attempts at a clear margin is warranted if this can be done without mutilation. There are no conclusive data that a 1-cm margin is any better than a 5-mm or even smaller margin, but if there is enough surrounding tissue to get a 1 cm margin safely, then it may be worth the attempt. When resecting tumors in the groin, it may be of value to resect the round ligament and canal of Nuck in females, because recurrence may occur in the labia or canal. We have had two such patients in the last 4 years. This is frequently outside the radiated field, and recurrence was noted in the canal near the labia. Lymph nodes may be positive in more than 10–15% of patients and may be histologically positive even when clinically negative. Consider sentinel node mapping and biopsy of regional nodes. Our limited experience with sentinel node mapping in NRSTS indicates that this is an effective technique to sample the regional lymph nodes.

Chemotherapy has not proved to be of value to date, and prospective trials to define active agents are needed. Metastatic and gross residual disease is treated, however, with combinations of ifosfamide, doxorubicin, and vincristine, but without much improvement in patient survival.

Radiation therapy, either external beam or brachytherapy, is considered in all patients with microscopic residual or positive nodes. It appears that is should also be considered in patients with complete resection, because local control and relapse are reduced in the completely resected patients given radiation. Whether this is evidence of residual disease or the biologic aggressiveness of the tumor is unknown. Follow-up should consist of physical exam, CT or MRI, and chest radiography or CT. We have had patients experience local recurrence many years after initial resection and adjuvant therapy. Therefore we have suggested follow-up evaluations every 2 months for 1 year, then every 6 months for 2 years and every year thereafter.

Because these tumors are rare, no single institution has a large experience and only by multicenter prospective studies will further answers to the many questions posed be answered.

14.2.13 Infantile Fibrosarcoma and Adult-Type Fibrosarcoma

Fibrosarcoma is one of the common NRSTSs that occur in the pediatric population accounting for approximately 13% of fibroblastic-myofibroblastic tumors in children and adolescents and 12% of soft tissue malignancies in children younger that 1 year [74]. Infantile fibrosarcoma (IFS) is histologically similar to its adult counterpart. The diagnosis is made based on the presence of characteristic t(12;15) translocation and age at diagnosis.

Adult-type fibrosarcoma (ATS) is estimated to comprise at most 1–3% of all sarcomas [75]. IFS affects predominantly young infants and it rarely occurs after 2 years of age [76]. The second incidence peak is observed in patients 10–15 years of age with AFS. Our experience has been that of pediatric patients who are usually over 8 years of age, have extremity lesions, and recurrence is local.

Despite the name fibrosarcoma, in infants this tumor does commonly metastasize, even though there may be local recurrences [77]. In a review of the literature detailing the experience with 52 cases of IFS, 37 (71%) had their primary tumor on an extremity and 15 (29)% on the trunk [78]. Head and neck and abdominal primaries have been reported [77]. The presentation is usually with a rapidly growing localized mass. Metastases, when they do occur, are mainly to lung or bone.

WLE is the primary treatment and almost always results in long-term cure in children with IFS. Of the patients with extremity primaries described previously, 92% were free of metastatic disease and 95% were alive despite a 32% local recurrence rate; only six have died (11.5%) [78]. Because late local recurrences do not appear to affect overall survival of patients with IFS, conservative surgical management aimed at maintaining as much function as possible and avoiding amputation is often the preferred approach.

Because of the long-term effects of radiation and/or chemotherapy, these modalities are rarely used in this tumor. Spontaneous regression of incompletely resected cases has been reported.

14.2.14 Malignant Fibrous Histiocytoma

Malignant fibrous histiocytoma (MFH) is most commonly reported NRSTS in adults. In our experience, it has been the second most common NRSTS in children, although overall, it is quite rare [65]. The most common site was the extremity, and early re-excision appeared to be beneficial. Tumor size greater than 5 cm had a worse prognosis. Local recurrence led to metastases and death. The angiomatoid variant histology had a 100% survival. Our overall 5-year survival rate was 71%; significant prognostic factors included the ability to resect with adequate margins, tumor size, and recurrence. The use of chemotherapy and radiation did not improve survival although this may be affected by patient selection with larger and more aggressive lesions receiving chemotherapy and radiation. Prospective trials of preoperative and postoperation radiation as well as adjunctive chemotherapy for high-grade lesions are ongoing.

14.2.15 Malignant Peripheral Nerve Sheath Tumor (MPNST) (Malignant Schwannoma, Neurofibrosarcoma)

MPNSTs primarily occur in adults. They account for only 5–10% of STSs in children and most commonly in children with neurofibromatosis [11, 12]. Children with NF-1 may develop neurofibrosarcoma at any time in their life. They may arise from neurofibromas, but at present there are no markers or other clinical aspects indicating a higher risk or malignant potential. Neurofibromatosis is a relatively common inherited disorder, approaching a frequency of 1 in 3,000 live births. Often thought of as a one-disease process, it is actually two different genetic disorders with some common features. Neurofibromatosis I (NF-1), or Von Reckinghausen's disease, is transmitted in an autosomal dominant pattern with the gene localized to the long arm of chromosome 17 [80]. The much-less-common neurofibromatosis 2 (NF2) also is inherited via an autosomal dominant fashion; however, it approaches a frequency of only 1 in 50,000 live births. The responsible gene is on the long arm of chromosome 22 [81].

Children with NF have a lifetime risk for malignancy related to NF1 of 5% [82] and have been shown in one series to have a 4,600-fold increased risk to develop malignant peripheral nerve sheath tumors [83, 84]. In our own review of children with neurofibrosarcoma treated at M. D. Anderson Cancer Center [12], the average age at diagnosis was 13.8 years (range, 3 to 19.9 years). Nineteen patients (50%) had neurofibromatosis. The tumor site was most frequently extremity and trunk, followed by head and neck and retroperitoneum. Survival is poor unless local control is obtained.

Recurrence and distant metastases are difficult to treat since neurofibrosarcoma does not respond well to adjuvant therapy at present.

In the past, the most commonly used regimen included combinations of vincristine, cyclophosphamide, dactinomycin, and doxorubicin [85]. Currently, there is no optimal regimen and the patients are treated similarly to standard NRSTS. Recently topoisomerase II-alpha gene and protein were found to be overexpressed in MPNST specimens and furthermore were related to poor survival [86]. This suggests that newer regimens combining agents inhibiting topoisomerase II-alpha and ifosfamide should be considered in treatment. Although there are limited data, the outcome of sporadic and NF-1-associated MPNSTs is considered similar [87].

14.2.16 Alveolar Soft Part Sarcoma

Alveolar soft part sarcoma (ASPS) is a rare sarcoma that usually arises in persons between 15 and 35 years of age [88]. ASPS is considered to be a tumor of uncertain differentiation with no specific cell lineage identified to date [89]. In adults, almost half of the patients present with an extremity mass, the thigh being the most common location, and 65% of patients had distant metastases at diagnosis [90]. In the children, ten (53%) of the patients had their primary tumors in the extremity [91]. Only four (21%) of the 19 patients had distant metastases. The most common metastatic site is the lung, followed by brain, bone, and lymph nodes [92]. In pediatric series [91], with a median follow-up of 74 months, the 5-year overall survival was 91%. Surgical excision is the primary therapy and radiation is employed for residual tumor. Chemotherapy has not proven effective to date.

14.2.17 Leiomyosarcoma

This tumor is very rare in children and only three leiomyosarcomas were reported in a large series of 135 soft tissue tumors in infants and children from the Mayo Clinic [93]. There have been reports of a link between EBV and leiomyosarcoma in children with acquired immunodeficiency syndrome [35–37]. The tumor has been reported to arise in the orbit, perineum, saphenous vein, bladder, cecum, colon, and ovary in children. The most common primary site in children is the gastrointestinal tract, especially the stomach [94].

14.2.18 Liposarcoma

Although one of the more common STSs in adults, liposarcoma is rare in children. Myxoid liposarcoma is the most common histologic type in children [95]. The two most common primary sites are the lower extremity and trunk. The most common lower extremity site is the thigh-knee region; the most common truncal site is the retroperitoneum. Metastases are rare. Treatment is WLE and total resection if possible, even if the retroperitoneum offers the best chance of cure [95]. Retroperitoneal sarcomas may not be completely resected and radiation therapy has been considered.

14.3 Section 2

14.3.1 Rhabdomyosarcoma

Rhabdomyosarcoma (Greek for *rhabdos*, "rod," mys, "muscle;" sarkos, "flesh") is a primary malignancy in children and adolescents that arises from embryonic mesenchyme with the potential to differentiate into skeletal muscle. Rhabdomyosarcoma (RMS) comprises over 50% of all soft tissue sarcomas in children, and is thus the most common soft tissue sarcoma. Sarcomas in adults arise mostly in the extremities, while RMS in children occurs in any anatomical location of the body where there is skeletal muscle, as well as in sites where there is no skeletal muscle, (e.g., urinary bladder, bile ducts, etc.). The most common sites are the head and neck region and the genitourinary tract, with only 20% in the extremities. The disease can arise at any site and in any tissue in the body except bone.

The original distinction of soft-tissue sarcomas and bone sarcomas from epithelial and hematopoietic tumors is attributed to Virchow who, in the middle 1850s, propounded his theory of "cellular pathology" which ascribed the origin of tumors to specific types of cells [2]. The first case of RMS was described by Webner in 1854 and was a 21 year-old patient with a tongue tumor [96]. In 1946, Stout [97] described a series of case reports of adults with a malignant condition of the trunk and limbs. In 1954, Pack, et al. [98] described a group of children with RMS of the skeletal muscle. In 1958, Horn and Enterline [99] proposed a classification of this tumor into the following four subgroups: embryonal, alveolar, botryoid, and pleomorphic. During those early years, surgery was the only therapy available, and radical excision was the standard. Survival rates were overall poor, except in selected sites that could have total excision by radical surgery such as amputation or pelvic exenteration. Survival rates of 7–70% were seen depending on site [96].

In 1950, Stobbe [100] demonstrated improvement in outcome in head and neck sites when radiation therapy was added after incompletely resected RMS. In 1961, Pinkel and Pinkren [101] advocated adjuvant chemotherapy after complete surgical excision and postoperative radiation therapy, which was the beginning of the multimodal approach to solid tumors.

Recognizing the value of this multimodal approach as well as the relative rarity of these tumors, the leadership of the three US cooperative pediatric cancer research groups, (The Children's Cancer Study Group, the pediatric sections of Cancer and Leukemia Group B, and the Southwest Oncology Group) in concert with the National Cancer Institute (NCI) formed the Intergroup Rhabdomyosarcoma Study Group (IRS) in 1972 to investigate the therapy and biology of RMS and undifferentiated sarcoma (UDS) in previously untreated patients less than 21 years of age. Since then, five successive clinical protocols involving almost 5,000 patients have been completed: IRS-I, 1972–1978; IRS-II, 1978–1984; IRS-III, 1984–1991; IRS-IV Pilot (for patients with advanced disease only), 1987–1991; and IRS IV, 1991–1997 [1, 2, 4–6, 11, 18]. Based on lessons learned from these studies, IRS-V was opened in 1997 for patients with low-risk disease (i.e., with a good prognosis for survival), and subsequently in 1999 for the other patients.

Although the trend has been toward far less mutilating surgery, the surgeon plays an even greater role in initial biopsy and staging, as well as primary re-excision, appropriate wide local resections, and second-look operations. The surgeon should be involved early in the multimodal approach to treatment.

14.3.2 Epidemiology

RMS is the third most common solid tumor in infants and children, behind neuroblastoma and Wilms' tumor. There are approximately 250–300 new cases per year in the USA. There is a slightly increased incidence in males compared to females, (3:2), and in Caucasians compared to non-Caucasians, (12:5). The peak age at presentation is bimodal, with the primary peak occurring between 2 and 5 years of age and the secondary peak between 15 and 19 years of age.

Patients with RMS appear to have a higher incidence of other congenital anomalies [102]. Both RMS and Wilms' tumor have an increased incidence of genitourinary anomalies. RMS has an association with anomalies of the central nervous system [102]. Patients with Von Recklinghausen neurofibromatosis (NF-1) have an increased risk of RMS [103, 104].

The Li-Fraumeni familial cancer syndrome, first reported in 1969, includes soft tissue sarcomas occurring in siblings and cousins, with parents and other relatives having a variety of malignancies including RMS, adrenocortical carcinoma, glioblastoma, breast cancer, and lung cancer [105, 106]. This syndrome is an autosomal dominant disorder and is frequently associated with a germline mutation of p53 [107]. Breast cancer in mothers has been shown to be the major associated malignancy in families of children with soft tissue malignancy [108]. A review of the mothers of 13 children with RMS showed a 3- to 13.5-fold increased risk for breast cancer over controls [109].

Other somewhat weaker associations with fetal alcohol syndrome, maternal exposure to marijuana or cocaine, X-rays, and employment as a healthcare worker have been suggested [110–112].

RMS has also been observed in association with Beckwith-Wiedemann syndrome, a fetal overgrowth syndrome associated with abnormalities on chromosome 11p15, where the gene for insulin-like growth factor II (IGF-II) is located [113].

The two histologic subtypes of RMS, embryonal and alveolar, have been found to have distinct genetic alterations that may play a role in the pathogenesis of these tumors. Alveolar RMS has been demonstrated to have a characteristic translocation between the long arm of chromosome 2 and the long arm of chromosome 13, referred to as t(2;13) (q35;q14). This translocation fuses the PAX3 gene (believed to regulate transcription during early neuromuscular development) with the FKHR gene (a member of the forkhead family of transcription factors). It is believed that this fusion transcription factor may inappropriately activate transcription of genes that contribute to a transformed phenotype. The variant t(1;13) (p36;q14) fuses the PAX7 gene located on chromosome 1 with FKHR. Patients with tumors expressing the PAX-FKHR fusion tend to be younger and more likely to present with an extremity lesion, suggesting a distinct clinical phenotype. Polymerase chain reaction (PCR) assays are now available that allow for confirmation of the diagnosis of alveolar RMS based on the presence of these fusion genes [113–116].

Embryonal RMS is known to have loss of heterozygosity (LOH) at the 11p15 locus with loss of maternal genetic information and duplication of paternal genetic information. This is the location of the IGF-II gene. IGF-II has been demonstrated to stimulate the growth of rhabdomyosarcoma cells, whereas the blockade of this factor using monoclonal antibodies will inhibit tumor growth both in vitro and in vivo [117]. Several other solid neoplasms are associated with genomic deletions on the short arm of chromosome 11, including Wilms' tumor, hepatoblastoma, and neuroblastoma.

The Myo D family of genes code for DNA-binding proteins that regulate the transcription of DNA sequences encoding myogenic proteins such as desmin, creatine kinase, and myosin [118, 119]. In rhabdomyosarcoma, the downregulation of this gene does not occur, so that MyoD1 expressions stay at high levels in tumor cells [120]. The biologic significance of this overexpression is not clear; however, the detection of high levels of the MyoD1 gene product has been considered in making the diagnosis of rhabdomyosarcoma [121].

The change in DNA content of a cell has been described in a variety of tumors and may have some prognosis significance. Embryonal RMS tumors have been found to have DNA contents ranging between diploid and hyperdiploid (1.1–1.8 times the normal amount of DNA). It has been reported that diploid embryonal RMS tumors may have a worse prognosis than hyperdiploid tumors. Near-tetraploidy was associated with alveolar histology [113, 122].

RAS oncogene mutations have been described in RMS cell lines and tumor specimens. It is not known whether these alterations are involved in RMS tumor pathogenesis or reflect secondary abnormalities that occur during tumor progression [113].

Aberrant expression of the MET oncogene in embryonal and alveolar RMS tumor samples and established cell lines has been described. MET encodes the receptor for HGF/scatter factor, which is known to control cell motility and invasion in epithelial cells. It is hypothesized that the overexpression of MET may provide RMS cells with the same property as embryonal myoblasts to migrate into surrounding connective tissues [123].

14.3.3 Pathology

RMS cells arise from undifferentiated mesodermal tissue and fall into the broader category of the small, round, blue-cell tumors of childhood. Differentiation of specific tumor type is made by a combination of light microscopy, immunohistochemical techniques, electron microscopy, and molecular genetic techniques. The characteristic feature that permits a tumor to be classified as RMS is the identification of myogenic lineage. Typically, this consists of the light microscopic identification of cross-striations characteristic of skeletal muscle or characteristic rhabdomyoblasts [117, 124]. Skeletal muscle or muscle-specific proteins can be identified by immunohistochemical staining.

Histologically, RMS is classified with the category of small, round, blue-cell tumors of childhood, a category that also includes neuroblastoma, Ewing's sarcoma, small-cell osteogenic sarcoma, non-Hodgkin's lymphoma, and leukemia. Each of the two major subtypes of RMS, embryonal and alveolar, has a characteristic histological appearance. The embryonal subtype, particularly the botryoid and spindle-cell variants, were thought to have a much better prognosis. There is now controversy as to whether the histological subtype or the site of the tumor most strongly influences prognosis. Embryonal RMS is the most common histological

Table 14.3 Histologic variants of childhood rhabdomyosarcoma: International Rhabdomyosarcoma Pathologic Classification [125]

I.	Favorable prognosis
	a. Botryoid
	b. Spindle-cell
II.	**Intermediate prognosis**
	a. Embryonal
	b. Pleomorphic (rare)
III.	**Poor prognosis**
	a. Alveolar (including solid variant)
	b. Undifferentiated

Table 14.4 Histologic distribution of patients with RMS in IRS-III [126]

Embryonal	53%
Alveolar	19%
Undetermined	18%
Undifferentiated	7%
Botryoid	5%
Extraosseous Ewing's	3%

subtype comprising more than 30% of all newly diagnosed tumors.

Botryoid RMS, described as a "cluster of grapes," is seen in cavitary structures and has a good prognosis. The spindle-cell variants arise disproportionately in the paratesticular region but may also be seen in the head and neck, especially the orbit, and the extremities [126, 127]. They are almost always associated with limited disease and have a less aggressive pattern of behavior than do the classic embryonal tumors, and an extremely good prognosis; however, both types account for only 5–6% of all rhabdomyosarcomas [127].

The pathologic description of RMS as a tumor of myogenic lineage was first advanced in 1958 by Horn and Enterline [99]. These investigators proposed the first classification scheme, one that divided rhabdomyosarcoma into four different pathologic types – embryonal, botryoid, alveolar, and pleomorphic. This system has been used for decades and has been modified into a "universal" system by a collaborative effort of a group of international pediatric pathologists in 1994. This system ascribes prognostic significance to each histologic subtype by classifying them into favorable-, intermediate-, and poor-prognosis groups [125] (see Table 14.3).

The alveolar variant is seen in approximately 20% of tumors and frequently arises from the extremities, trunk, or perineum. These are classified as unfavorable-prognosis tumors [125]. The alveolar variant is characterized by a prominent alveolar arrangement of stroma and dense, small, round tumor cells resembling those of lung tissue. A subtype of alveolar RMS is the "solid" alveolar rhabdomyosarcoma, characterized by an architecture of dense cellular sheets lacking any intercellular stroma but with cytologic features identical to those found in the classic alveolar

tumors. Undifferentiated sarcoma is a poorly defined category of sarcomatous tumors whose cells show no evidence of myogenesis or other differentiation [126, 127]. The distribution of histologic subtypes is shown in Table 14.4.

A number of monoclonal antibodies have been shown to react with elements of rhabdomyosarcomas and have been useful in their diagnosis. These include antibodies to desmin, muscle-specific actin, sarcomeric actin, and myoglobin. All have been used to confirm the myogenous lineage of cells, and when used in combination have very good specificity and sensitivity [128]. MyoD1 has been mentioned earlier in this chapter. Other nonmyogenous protein products that can be identified in these tumors include cytokeratin, neuron-specific enolase, S-100 protein, and Leu-7.

14.3.4 Clinical Presentation

The clinical presentation of RMS will depend on the site or origin of the primary tumor, the age of the patient, and the presence or absence of metastatic disease. The majority of symptoms will be related to compression of local structures and occasionally mild pain. There are no classic paraneoplastic syndromes associated with RMS.

The head and neck region is the most common site of presentation and accounts for about 35% of the patients in the IRS studies [129]. The head and neck sites are divided into the orbits (10%), parameningeal tissues (middle ear, nasal cavity and Paranasal sinuses, Nasopharynx, and Infratemporal fossa; 15%), and nonparameningeal tissues (scalp, face, oral cavity, oropharynx, hypopharynx, and neck; 10%). These tumors are most commonly of the embryonal subtype and rarely spread to regional lymph nodes [129–131]. Orbital tumors produce proptosis, and occasionally, ophthalmoplegia. Those arising from parameningeal sites often produce nasal, aural, or sinus obstruction with or without a mucopurulent or sanguinous discharge. Head and neck RMS arising from sites other than the orbit or parameningeal sites often present as a pain-less, enlarging mass which tends to remain localized [132]. Parameningeal tumors may extend into the cranium with resultant cranial nerve palsy and meningeal symptoms.

Genitourinary RMS accounted for 26% of all primary tumors in the IRS-III study [129]. These tumors are considered as two distinct entities: bladder/prostate tumors (10%) and non-bladder/prostate tumors, the latter occurring in paratesticular sites, perineum, vulva, vagina, and uterus (16%). Paratesticular RMS may present as a painless swelling in the scrotum or inguinal canal and may initially be thought to be a hernia, hydrocele, or varicocele. Bladder tumors produce hematuria and urinary obstruction. Prostate tumors can produce large pelvic masses resulting in urinary frequency or constipation if significant compression of the bladder or intestinal tract occurs. RMS can also arise in the male or female genital tracts. Vaginal tumors tend to occur in very young children and present with a mass or vaginal bleeding and discharge. The uterine tumors generally present in older girls and are quite extensive by the time of diagnosis. Paratesticular RMS has a high predilection of lymph node spread to the retroperitoneum, especially in boys over 10 years of age [128]. The vaginal tumors rarely spread to regional lymph nodes.

Extremity RMS occurs in approximately 20% of patients [133, 134]. These tumors present with a mass and have a high incidence of regional lymph nodes (50%) [133, 134]. The majority of these tumors are of the alveolar subtype, and because of site and possibly histology, are more aggressive.

Approximately 15% of children with RMS present with metastatic (Group IV) disease and their prognosis has not improved significantly over the last 15 years, despite changes in therapy [129, 135]. Isolated lung metastases appear to be rare and should be biopsied to prove disease.

Neonatal presentation of RMS is extremely rare with only 14 cases (0.4% of patients in IRS I-IV) being reported [136]. They tend to be embryonal/botryoid or undifferentiated in histology.

14.3.5 Diagnosis

The diagnosis of rhabdomyosarcoma usually is made by direct open biopsy. There are no helpful markers or specific imaging studies. The pathologist is expected to identify the histologic subgroups of RMS to allow adequate staging and direct therapy. For this purpose, several grams of tissue are needed. Biopsies of GU RMS frequently are performed using the endoscope. Needle biopsies that are performed to establish the diagnosis of prostatic RMS are difficult to interpret and must in-

Table 14.5 Preoperative/treatment evaluation

History/physical (ht. wt.)
Measure lesion (Physical or imaging)
CBC/Diff/plts.
Urine analysis
Electrolytes, creatinine, Ca/Phos
Alk. Phos./LDH/bilirubin, SGPT
Bone marrow biopsy/aspirate
Chest x-ray
MRI or CT of primary
CT Chest
MRI or CT head (for head tumors)
Bone scan
CSF cytology (for parameningeal)
EKG or echocardiogram (selective)

The most important part of the diagnostic process is obtaining adequate tissue for histologic and cytologic diagnosis and classification. This procedure is generally accomplished by open incisional biopsy under general anesthesia.

clude several cores. Trunk and extremity RMS should have excisional or incisional biopsy, with the incision placed so that it will not interfere with the incision required for subsequent WLE. This usually means an axial incision in extremities. WLE with clear margins is the ultimate goal. Regional lymph nodes are evaluated depending on location of the primary. Trunk and extremity lesions have a high incidence of lymph node involvement and sentinel lymph node mapping is advised [134, 137].

Patients with RMS require a complete workup before definitive surgery. The preoperative evaluation includes imaging, blood work, and bone marrow evaluation. Complete preoperative or pretreatment evaluation is shown in Table 14.5.

14.3.6 Staging and Clinical Grouping

Pretreatment staging for RMS is performed to stratify the extent of the disease for different treatment regimens as well as to compare outcome. This classification is a modification of the TNM staging system and is based on primary tumor site, primary tumor size, clinical regional node status, and distant spread [134, 138] (Table 14.6).

Table 14.6 Pretreatment staging classification

Stage	Sites	T	Size	N	M
1	Orbit	T_1 or T_2	a or b	N_0 or N_x	M_0
	Head and neck (excluding parameningeal)				
	Bladder/non-prostate				
2	Bladder/prostate	T_1 or T_2	a	N_0 or N_x	M_0
	Extremity				
	Cranial parameningeal				
	Other (includes trunk, retroperitoneum, perineal, biliary, intrathoracic)				
3	Bladder/prostate	T_1 or T_2	a	N_1	
	Extremity		b	$N_0/N_1/N_x$	M_0
	Cranial parameningeal				
	Other (as in Stage 2)				
4	All	T_1 or T_2	a or b	$N_0/N_1/N_x$	M_1

Definitions			
Tumor			
	T_1		Confined to anatomic site of origin
		a)	≤5 cm diameter in size
		(b)	>5 cm diameter in size
	T_2		Extension and/or fixation to surrounding tissue
		(a)	≤5 cm diameter in size
		(b)	>5 cm diameter in size
Regional nodes			
	N_0		Regional nodes not clinically involved
	N_1		Regional nodes clinically involved by neoplasm
	N_x		Clinical status of regional nodes unknown (especially sites that preclude lymph node evaluation)
Metastasis			
	M_0		No distant metastasis
	M_1		Metastasis present

Pretreatment size is determined by external measurement or MRI or CT, depending on the anatomic location. The staging is "clinical" and should be done by the responsible surgeon based on preoperative imaging and physical findings. Intraoperative and/or pathologic results should not affect the stage (but will effect clinical group).

14.3.7 Clinical Grouping

The clinical grouping system developed by the Intergroup Rhabdomyosarcoma Group (IRS), is based on the pretreatment and operative outcome (Table 14.7). Its basic premise is that total tumor extirpation at the original site is the best hope for cure and stratifies patients according to their resectability. This had led, in the past, to aggressive and often mutilating procedures. This system does not take into account the biological nature or natural history of the tumor, nor does it account for the experience and the aggressiveness of the operating surgeon.

With the advent of more frequent use of biopsy and neoadjuvant chemotherapy, there has been a "Group Shift" from Group I or II to Group III, where biopsy was followed by neoadjuvant therapy. Group assignment is based on intraoperative findings and postoperative pathologic status and most include final pathologic verification of margins, residual tumor, node involvement, and cytological examination of pleural and peritoneal fluid, when applicable.

Table 14.7 The clinical grouping system developed by the Intergroup Rhabdomyosarcoma Group (IRS)

Group I:	**Localized disease, completely resected**
	(Regional nodes not involved – lymph node biopsy or sampling is highly advised [9602]/required [9803, 9802], except for head and neck lesions
	(a) Confined to muscle or organ of origin
	(b) Contiguous involvement – infiltration outside the muscle or organ of origin, as through fascial planes
	Notation: This includes both gross inspection and microscopic confirmation of complete resection. Any nodes that may be inadvertently taken with the specimen must be negative. If the latter should be involved microscopically, then the patient is placed in Group IIb or IIC (See below).
Group II:	**Total gross resection with evidence of regional spread**
	(a) Grossly resected tumor with microscopic residual disease (surgeon believes that he has removed all of the tumor, but the pathologist finds tumor at the margin of and additional resection to achieve clean margin is not feasible [9602]/reasonable[9803, 9802]). No evidence of gross residual tumor. No evidence of regional node involvement. Once radiotherapy and chemotherapy have been started, re-exploration and removal of the area of microscopic residual does not change the patient's group.
	(b) Regional disease with involved nodes, completely resected with microscopic residual.
	Notation: Complete resection with microscopic confirmation of no residual disease makes this different from Groups IIa and IIc. Additionally, in contrast to Group IIa, regional nodes (which are completely resected, however) are involved, but the most distal node is histologically negative.
	(c) Regional disease with involved nodes, grossly resected, but with evidence of microscopic residual and/or histologic involvement of the most distal regional node (from the primary site) in the dissection.
	Notation [9602 only]: The presence of microscopic residual disease makes this group different from Group IIb, and nodal involvement makes this group different from Group IIa.
Group III:	**Incomplete resection with gross residual disease**
	(a) After biopsy only
	(b) After gross or major resection of the primary (>50%)
Group IV:	**Distant metastatic disease present at onset** **(lung, liver, bones, bone marrow, brain, and distant muscle and nodes)**
	Notation: [9602 only] The above excludes regional lymph nodes and adjacent organ infiltration, which places the patient in a more favorable grouping. (As noted above in Group II).
	The presence of positive cytology in CSF, pleural or abdominal fluids as implants on pleural or peritoneal surfaces or in the omentum are regarded as indications for placing the patient in Group IV.

Numbers provided are the specific study number under the IRS protocols.

Both clinical grouping and pretreatment staging have been shown to correlate with outcome [134, 139, 140].

Based on the findings from IRS I-IV, risk groups have been established for treatment in IRS-V. The IRS-V Study combines group, stage, and histology subtype to allocate patients to three different therapeutic protocols according to risk of recurrence. Low-risk patients have an estimated 3-year failure-free survival (FFS) rate of 88%; intermediate-risk patients have an estimated 3-year FFS rate of 55–76%, and high-risk patients have a 3-year FFS rate of <30%. Multidisciplinary treatment is recommended as defined by histologic subtype and primary site, as well as the extent of disease at diagnosis and response to treatment. The goal is to achieve local control with preservation of form and function [141]. See Table 14.8 for IRS-V Groups.

14.3.8 Treatment

The approach to the treatment of RMS has been multimodal for greater than 30 years. The advances in understanding the biology and treatment of this disease can largely be attributed to the IRS Study Groups (IRS I-V). The specific surgical treatment for RMS has progressively been less mutilating or surgically aggressive while maintaining the excellent survival statistics of earlier studies.

The surgical treatment of RMS is site-specific, and will be discussed by individual site. The general principles include complete wide excision of the primary tumor and surrounding uninvolved margins while preserving cosmesis and function.

Initial biopsy is generally incisional except in small lesions, where excisional biopsy is possible. Some lesions will have a pseudocapsule which may allow the lesion to be shelled out, giving the surgeon the false notion that he/she has removed the entire lesion. Many of the sites will have gross or microscopic residual, and a pretreatment re-excision is warranted if this can be done without mutilation [142].

Biopsy of any lesion may involve the need for reoperation and wide excision. Longitudinal incisions are frequently better than horizontal incisions on areas such as an extremity. A biopsy to confirm malignancy requires that the biopsy tract be excised at the time of reoperation; if the biopsy site is inappropriately placed, this excision may require much larger incisions or resections than would be necessary.

Solid-tumor biopsies are traditionally divided into excisional biopsies, in which the entire tumor is included in the specimen, and incisional biopsies in which only a portion of the tumor is included. In an excisional biopsy, margins should be carefully marked to allow re-resection should the biopsy reveal a positive margin on review. Ideally, excisional biopsies are planned to allow resections that will leave behind only negative margins. If such an excisional biopsy results in too large a resection, then incisional biopsy is more appropriate.

If biopsy margins are not carefully marked on both the specimen and the operative field (usually by sutures or clips), the ability of the surgeon to subsequently obtain negative margins is severely compromised. For example, an inappropriate approach to biopsy may lead to further difficulties in the case of testicular masses. Any testicular mass should be approached through an inguinal rather than a scrotal incision so that proximal control of the cord can be obtained and a WLE performed without seeding the scrotum with tumor. The proximal spermatic cord should be examined for free margins. Higher excision may be necessary if tumor is still present. Biopsy of the tumor through the scrotum may lead to further need of scrotal resection and increased risk of local recurrence.

Table 14.8 IRS V Risk Groups

Low risk	Stage 1	Clinical Groups I and II, N_0, All favorable sites (orbit and head/neck, nonparameningeal, genitourinary tract, non-bladder prostate
	Stage 1	Clinical Group III, N_0, N_x, orbit only
	Stage 2	Clinical Group I, N_0, N_x, All other (unfavorable) sites, tumor ≤5 cm in widest diameter
Intermediate risk	Stage 1	Clinical Group II, N_1, all favorable sites (See above)
	Stage 1	Clinical Group III, N_0, N_x. N_1, all favorable sites except orbit
	Stage 2	Clinical Groups II and III, N_0, N_x, or N_1, all other sites
	Stage 3	Clinical Groups II and III, N_0, N_x, or N_1. all other sites
High risk protocol	Stage 4	Clinical Group IV, N_0, N_x, or N_1, any site with metastatic disease, including tumor cells in CSF, pleural, or peritoneal fluid or omental implants.

Secondary excision after initial biopsy and neoadjuvant therapy has a better outcome than do partial or incomplete excision. There has been a shift of more patients into clinical group III, but chemotherapy followed by delayed or second-look surgery has allowed for better prognosis with less mutilating surgery. Biopsy of regional nodes, or sentinel lymph node mapping to evaluate nodes is warranted in selected sites such as the extremity.

In some patients with extremity or trunk RMS, initial tumor resection is thought to be complete, but then histopathologic review reveals microscopic residual disease corresponding to clinical Group IIa in the surgical margins. In many of these patients, primary re-excision (PRE) is possible, achieving wider disease-free margins. Hays, et al. [44] demonstrated the benefits of PRE. In IRS-I and IRS-II, 154 patients with extremity or trunk RMS were initially placed in clinical Group IIa; then 41 patients underwent successful PRE and were converted to clinical Group I prior to the onset of adjuvant therapy. These patients were compared with 113 patients who had microscopic residual disease and did not undergo PRE and with 73 patients who were free of disease after the initial resection (clinical Group I). Among the 41 PRE patients, the 3-year Kaplan-Meier survival estimate was 91%, compared with 74% for Group IIa patients not undergoing PRE and 74% for Clinical Group I patients. This approach may be applicable to tumors of other locations as well. PRE should be considered, even if the margins are apparently normal, if the initial resection was not a "cancer" operation (i.e., malignancy was not suspected at initial excision) [142, 143].

Second look operation (SLO) has been used for several pediatric tumors to evaluate therapeutic response and to remove any residual tumor after completing initial therapy. The use of SLO was evaluated in IRS-III and shown to be beneficial in clinical Group II RMS patients [144–147]. The performance of SLO changed the response status in a significant number of patients; 12% of presumed CR patients were found to harbor residual tumor, while 74% of both PR and NR patients were recategorized as CR after operation. The survival rate of these recategorized PR and NR patients was similar to that of patients confirmed to be CR at re-exploration [146, 147].

The general surgical principles learned from IRS I to IRS IV and thus considered in IRS V include:

1. Patients with localized, completely resected disease (Group I) generally have the best prognosis for 5-year FFS and overall survival. Patients with metastases at diagnosis (Group IV) have the worst outlook, and those with Group II and III disease have an intermediate prognosis. Thus, it has been preferable to try to remove all visible tumor, if feasible without excessive morbidity.

2. When a lesion has been resected, primary re-resection is indicated if the primary operation was not a cancer operation for malignancy. Any question of margin status should warrant re-resection. Group I (totally resected) patients with embryonal RMS won't be subjected to postoperative external-beam radiotherapy (XRT) [148].

3. It is desirable to preserve organ function and thus spare such structures as the eye, vagina, and bladder. Also, patients with tumor at or near these sites have a good prognosis. Primary chemotherapy followed by radiation therapy is the recommended approach. Delayed excision of initially unresected tumor may improve prognosis by changing a partial response into a complete response after initial shrinkage of the tumor by chemotherapy, with or without XRT [146].

4. There is a relationship between age at diagnosis and likelihood of regional lymph node involvement in boys with nonmetastatic paratesticular rhabdomyosarcoma. EFS in IRS IV was better for boys younger than 10 years of age, as the nodal relapse rate was lower than in those 10 years of age and older. We now recommend performing a modified ipsilateral retroperitoneal lymph-node dissection in older boys who have no clinical evidence of regional node involvement. If the nodes are uninvolved, cyclophosphamide and XRT are withheld; if tumor is present in the nodes, cyclophosphamide and XRT are given in addition to vincristine and actinomycin D [128, 149].

Other considerations for IRS V include a more aggressive approach to evaluating lymph nodes. In earlier IRS studies [129, 150] lymph node involvement was thought to be rare at most sites, since the nodes were rarely evaluated. More recent studies have suggested that the incidence of involved lymph nodes in patients with primary tumors of the extremity may be higher than initially suspected [151]. Sentinel lymph-node mapping, using a vital dye such as Lymphazurin blue along with radio-labeled technetium sulfur colloid, can localize the regional node most likely to contain tumor cells [137]. The surgeon removes the indicated sentinel node and the pathologist can investigate thoroughly the presence or absence of tumor in that node. The sentinel node reflects the status of the nodal basin. If the node is positive, then the nodal basin is irradiated. The utility of sentinel-lymph node mapping is being evaluated in IRS V.

For patients whose tumors are initially deemed unresectable, a second-look procedure should be considered after initial chemotherapy. Imaging studies have not been consistently reliable in determining actual response to treatment. In IRS III, 75% of children with Group III tumors with evidence of partial or no response on imaging studies had either a patho-logically complete response (CR) or were converted to such a response by resection of all remaining tumor. However, most (but not all) patients who have shown a CR on imaging studies are confirmed as having such a response by secondary surgery. Survival was better on those patients who converted to CR. Secondary surgery is less beneficial in children with Stage IV dis-ease. Second-look surgery is least useful for tumors in the head and neck sites but is appropriate for tumors in the trunk and limb sites. A trend toward improved survival in patients converted to CR by means of sec-ond-look operations has been enduring [146, 147].

14.3.9 Chemotherapy

Prior to multimodal therapy, surgery alone for RMS resulted in survival rates of <20%. Local micrometa-static disease, nodal disease, or unrecognized/un-treated distant disease frequently led to early recur-rence and subsequent death due mainly to advanced metastatic disease.

The development of adjuvant and later neoadjuvant chemotherapy has led to a marked increase in sur-vival. The IRS studies have shown progressively bet-ter survival rates with less mutilating surgery and less chemotoxicity [101, 129, 152–154].

Agents with known activity in the treatment of RMS include vincristine (V), actinomycin D (A), doxorubi-cin (Dox), cyclophosphamide (C), ifosfamide (I), and etoposide (E). Melphalan and cisplatin were evaluated for their potential role in combination chemotherapy for patients with locally extensive or metastatic disease and did not improve outcome compared with other options in the randomized trials involving patients with clinical group III or IV disease [129, 155].

VAC has been the gold standard for combination chemotherapy in the treatment of most cases of RMS. Consecutive large randomized trials have allowed for modifications of this combination tailored to specific subgroups according to clinical group and site of dis-ease. In patients with clinical group I embryonal his-tology tumors, results of IRS-III showed equivalent survival for patients treated with VA only vs. VAC [129]. In IRS-IV, patients with clinical group I para-testicular or orbital disease were treated with VA alone for 2 years. In an IRS-V pilot study, VA chemotherapy alone is given to patients with "low-risk" disease, in-cluding: (a) Stage 1 clinical group I/II (N0) orbital, head and neck (nonparameningeal), GU tract (non-bladder/prostate); (b) Stage 2 clinical group I, and (c) Stage 1, clinical group-III (orbit only N0) [113, 141].

When evidence of the efficacy of etoposide and if-osfamide for RMS was recognized [156], this was in-corporated into a randomized treatment protocol in IRS-IV. Randomization of VAC vs. VAI vs. VIE was done for nonmetastatic RMS. Data from IRS-IV in-dicate that the current standard combination of VAC, with cyclophosphamide at 2.2g/m2 per dose with GCSF is equally efficacious with regard to failure-free and overall survival as are VAI and VIE [157].

Improving therapy for patients with intermediate-risk disease may be accomplished by the introduction of new agents. Dose intensification using known active chemotherapeutic agents should also be considered. Preliminary IRS-IV results have shown an improve-ment in FFS for intermediate-risk embryonal RMS, probably related to an increased cyclophosphamide dose [158]. Escalation of cyclophosphamide from 0.9g/m2 in IRS-III to 2.2g/m2 in IRS-IV has improved the FFS of patients with embryonal RMS but not those with alveolar RMS or undifferentiated RMS [158].

Data from IRS-I, IRS-II, and IRS-III in 1,431 pa-tients indicate that there is no benefit from adding doxorubicin (DOX) to the combination of vincristine, actinomycin D, and cyclophosphamide (VAC) in pa-tients with group III and group IV disease, whether analyzed together or within group III and group IV categories individually [129, 141, 153, 154]. The addi-tion of DOX and cisplatin with or without etoposide to the VAC regimen has not improved outcome for patients with advanced disease in IRS-III [129, 153, 154].

Patients with metastatic disease have a poor prog-nosis despite aggressive therapy. Intensive, multiagent combinations have been utilized in an attempt to im-prove survival. The SIOP has reported a 53% response rate to carboplatin/epirubicin/vincristine in previously untreated patients with metastatic RMS [159].

The use of methotrexate in front-line treatment reg-imens offers the potential advantages of relative lack of additive myelosuppression and a different mechanism of action. In a phase II trial, Pappo, et al. have reported a 33% response rate to high-dose methotrexate in pa-tients with previously untreated, advanced-stage RMS [160].

Topotecan, a campotothecin analog which acts as an inhibitor of topoisomerase I, is being examined for its potential role in RMS. (Inhibition of topoisomerase I will thereby inhibit DNA repletion). The IRSG has re-cently reported a 45% response rate to topotecan used in a window setting in newly diagnosed patients with nonparameningeal metastatic RMS [161, 162]. An IRS-V pilot for metastatic RMS is currently evaluating topotecan in combination with cyclophosphamide in an upfront window prior to VAC/radiation therapy. It appears to be active in newly diagnosed patients with metastatic RMS and can be given in combination with VAC [161].

Autologous bone marrow transplantation (ABMT) has been utilized in several of the childhood solid tu-

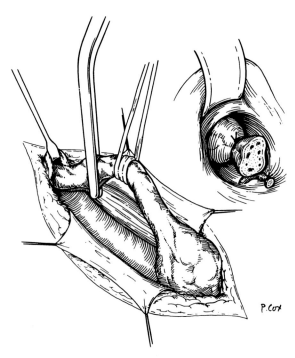

Fig. 14.2 Proximal control of the spermatic cord and orchiectomy through an inguinal incision

mors. To date, the use of ABMT has not been of value in patients with metastatic RMS [163, 164].

Thus, the recommendations for IRS-V which is presently ongoing are:

1. Low-risk patients have localized embryonal RMS in favorable sites (Stage 1) or in unfavorable sites (Stages 2 and 3) that has been grossly removed; the patients with the best prognosis are placed in subgroup A and receive VA with or without XRT. The others, placed in subgroup B, receive VAC ±XRT.
2. Intermediate-risk patients have localized alveolar RMS or undifferentiated sarcoma (Stages 1–3) or embryonal RMS (Stages 2 and 3) with gross residual disease (Group III), or embryonal RMS with metastases (Group IV) at <10 years of age at diagnosis. They are randomized to receive VAC or VAC alternating with vincristine and cyclophosphamide plus topotecan, along with XRT.
3. High-risk patients have embryonal RMS at ≥10 years of age, or alveolar RMS or undifferentiated sarcoma at any age <21 years, with metastases at diagnosis (Group IV). They receive a trial of irinotecan [165] over 6 weeks followed by VAC. Irinotecan is continued at intervals for those who have responded to it initially, but is omitted for nonresponders. High-risk patients with cranial parameningeal tumors and meningeal impingement at diagnosis receive VAC without irinotecan.

14.3.10 Radiotherapy

Radiotherapy is tailored for specific sites and extent of disease. In some sites, such as head and neck or pelvis, tumors often cannot be completely removed surgically. Radiation therapy may be used in conjunction with chemotherapy to eradicate residual tumor cells. The guidelines for radiation doses have changed over successive IRS studies. The dosage is now tailored to the amount of residual disease (gross or microscopic) and tumor response.

In IRS-IV, radiation therapy was defined by clinical group. Patients with completely resected clinical group I, (CG-I), TNM Stage 1 and 2 tumors received no radiotherapy. Patients with completely resected CG-I, TNM Stage 3 and patients with CG-II tumors received conventional XRT to a total dose of 4,140 cGy. Clinical Group-III patients were randomized to receive 5,040-cGy external-beam radiation or hyperfractionated radiotherapy to a dose of 5,940 cGy. The results of IRS-IV suggested that, at least so far, there is no indication that giving hyperfractionated XRT to 59.4 Gy in two daily fractions of 1.1 Gy, with a 6-h interfractional interval, will result in a better local-regional control rate among children with Group III tumors than that obtained with 50.4 Gy in 1.8 fractions daily [166, 167].

There is no evidence to show benefit from giving radiation to patients with completely resected, local lesions (Group I), provided that the histologic subtype is embryonal RMS [148]. Graded doses of irradiation are appropriate for all other patients, based on the patient's group at the time of the study entry. Volumes to be irradiated include the pretreatment primary tumor and regional lymph-nodal area, if involved. Patients with group IV disease receive XRT to both the primary site and to the sites of metastases, within the limits of bone-marrow tolerance.

A recent analysis of patients with group II disease in IRS-I to IRS-IV has shown improved outcome in IRS-III and IRS-IV, perhaps due to intensified therapy [168].

Local failure rates for patients with group III disease in the IRS-III and IRS-IV studies have recently been reviewed. The rates have remained stable or improved. In IRS-IV, local failure rates were 2% in orbit primary sites, 16% in cranial parameningeal sites, and 12% in other head/neck sites. Local failure rates were 7% in extremity sites, 19% in genitourinary sites, and 14% in other sites [168].

Current IRSG results suggest that most patients with cranial parameningeal sarcoma, including those with localized intracranial extension in contiguity with the primary tumor at diagnosis, can be successfully managed with systemic chemotherapy and XRT. Radiation therapy is directed to the primary tumor, including any extension, along with a 2-cm margin, to include the adjacent meninges. Whole-brain XRT and intrathecal anticancer agents are not necessary in the absence of diffuse meningeal involvement as multiple intracranial metastases [131, 169].

A rapid summary of the recommendations for radiation therapy in IRS-V include: patients with completely excised embryonal RMS (i.e., group I) receive no XRT. However, patients with completely excised (group I) alveolar RMS and undifferentiated sarcoma receive XRT to the primary site [148]. Other patients receive XRT as a function of group, histologic subtype, and status of regional lymph nodes and/or distant metastases. Patients with metastases receive XRT to the primary tumor and to sites of metastases within the limits of bone marrow tolerance [141].

14.3.11 Management by Site

14.3.12 Head and Neck

Head and neck lesions include superficial head and neck, orbit, parotid, buccal, laryngeal, and oropharyngeal locations. The multidisciplinary approach to therapy has allowed less-aggressive surgical procedures while maintaining an excellent prognosis at this site. Wide excision is appropriate when feasible, but the possibility of achieving wide margins is restricted to small superficial lesions [170].

The orbit has had excellent results from therapy because the tumor is usually confined to the bony orbit and there is a paucity of lymphatics.

Parameningeal tumors are associated with a poor prognosis because of the propensity for extension and the presence of abundant lymphatics [129, 171–173]. Abramson, et al. [174] demonstrated that radiation therapy plus chemotherapy was the most effective treatment for orbital rhabdomyosarcoma; this type of therapy ended the need for orbital exenteration. Survival of more than 90% of patients is standard with combined vincristine, actinomycin-D, and radiation therapy [129, 132, 175].

Metastatic spread to regional nodes is seen in less than 3% of patients [129]. Cervical lymph node biopsy or sentinel lymph node mapping does not appear warranted unless nodes are clinically involved. Patients with nodal involvement should be treated according to the IRS Intermediate-risk protocol.

Thus, except for small lid lesions, the role of surgery for orbital primaries is limited to biopsy alone [132, 173, 175, 176]. Orbital exenteration has been used selectively in recurrent disease.

Nonorbital, nonparameningeal sites include superficial and deep tumors that do not impinge on the meninges. For some tumors, such as parotid, laryngeal, oropharyngeal, and other deep tumors, surgery is lim-

ited to biopsy followed by chemotherapy and XRT for tumor eradication [173]. This treatment regime has led to survival rates of 83% [177, 178].

The need for alkylating agents in orbital and nonorbital head and neck sites has been previously questioned [132, 133, 173, 176]. In IRS III, patients with orbital and nonparameningeal head and neck tumors who received intensive VA and radiation therapy had the same rate of survival (90%) as did patients in IRS-II who received those therapies in conjunction with alkylating agents [129, 152]. The current recommendation for this low-risk group is to receive VA with or without XRT [140].

Parameningeal RMS often occurs in hidden sites; this frequently results in delayed diagnosis and a relatively poor prognosis [132, 173, 175]. Fifteen percent of patients with parameningeal RMS present with metastatic disease [129]. Bone erosion is a predictor of local relapse [179]. More intensive treatment of parameningeal RMS has resulted in increased survival [180]. This regimen has included VAC therapy, intrathecal chemotherapy, and radiation therapy to the entire cranial neuraxis. Patients receiving intensified therapy had a rate of tumor-free survival that increased from 33% to 57% and a reduction in failure of local tumor control from 28% to 6% [180]. The value of prophylactic XRT to the central nervous system has been questioned [181]. In IRS-III, radiation therapy and intrathecal chemotherapy were based on the degree of meningeal involvement and most patients received an amount of radiation therapy less than that used in IRS II. There was no decrease in PFS in patients in IRS-III compared to those in IRS-II [129, 152].

Craniofacial resection for anterior skull-based tumors of the nasal areas, paranasal sinuses, temporal fossa, and other such sites should be reserved to those surgical teams expert in its performance and to secondary procedures when tumor persists after initial chemo- and radiation therapy. In some reports, no viable tumor could be found in the resected specimens despite a residual mass effect on imaging studies [146, 147, 182]. Other studies have suggested a good correlation between evidence of stable residual disease on computed tomography (CT) and subsequent local relapse and death [183]. This is being investigated further.

14.3.13 Genitourinary Sites

The genitourinary sites include the bladder, prostate, paratesticular areas, vagina, uterus, vulva, and rarely, the kidneys or ureter. Rhabdomyosarcoma is the most common malignancy of the pelvic structures in children. Tumors in these locations are considered in two different categories on account of their different prognoses according to site: bladder/prostate vs. vulvo-vagina, uterus, and paratesticular. These sites accounted for approximately 25% of cases in the IRS-III report [129]. In 6% of those patients with pelvic tumors in the IRS-I and IRS-II studies, the exact site of origin within the pelvis could not be defined. Tumors in the vagina and testicular areas have a good prognosis and are more commonly of embryonal histology, often with the botryoid (vaginal) or the spindle cell (paratesticular) variant.

Bladder and prostate rhabdomyosarcomas can be difficult to distinguish from one another because of their anatomical proximity and tendency to grow to large size prior to diagnosis. When this determination is possible, it becomes evident that patients with bladder primaries have a better prognosis than those with tumors arising from the prostate [145]. The majority of tumors in these areas are of embryonal (71%) or botryoid (20%) variants; 2% are of alveolar histology [126].

In IRS-III, it was found that children with tumors of the bladder or prostate who received more intensive chemotherapy and earlier radiation therapy had a survival rate only slightly lower than patients with head and neck tumors. This finding contrasts with that of IRS-II [129, 152–154, 184].

Bladder/prostate tumors commonly arise near the area of the trigone and produce symptoms of bladder outlet obstruction or hematuria. Diagnosis is usually made by cystoscopic evaluation and biopsy as well as CT or MRI scanning. Previously, the initial management of these tumors in children was usually anterior or total pelvic exenteration followed by chemotherapy and radiation; this treatment produced very good long-term survival rates, approaching 85% in some series, but it also necessitated the morbidity of permanent urinary conduit and in some cases, colostomy [184, 185]. Today, bladder salvage is an important goal and less aggressive surgical means are common [186–189]. Neoadjuvant chemotherapy and radiation have decreased the rate of exenterative cystectomy from greater than 50% to approximately 30% [186–188]. In IRS-III, 50% of patients with bladder RMS received cisplatin in addition to VAdrC-VAC and irradiation. Of 171 children with primary bladder lesions enrolled in the IRS-I through IRS-III studies, 40 underwent partial cystectomy after receiving neoadjuvant chemotherapy and radiation. Relapse occurred in nine patients (seven locally). The Kaplan-Meier estimate of survival rate with a functioning bladder among all children with bladder/prostate tumors in IRS-III was 60%. Long-term survival was in excess of 80% [186–188].

Exenteration is not primary treatment any longer for RMS of the prostate. This site comprised about 5% of newly diagnosed cases in IRS-III. The mean age at the time of diagnosis was 5.3 years. Most tumors were relatively large, had embryonal histology, and were clinically localized but unresectable without major loss of organ function. The 44 patients with group III tumors (gross residual disease) were treated according to the IRS-III protocol. Forty-three of them underwent biopsy only, and one patient had subtotal resection as the initial procedure. The average number of surgical procedures per patient was two (range, one to five). Six of the 44 patients had no additional surgery. The second-look procedures performed in the other 38 patients included exenteration (14), prostatectomy (7), cystoscopic/perineal needle biopsy (8), laparotomy with biopsy (6), and subtotal excision with bladder salvage (3). Additional surgery was required for four patients, for evaluation of residual mass, postoperative fistula, ureteral stricture, or small bowel obstruction. Six patients with relapse or residual disease underwent additional chemotherapy and late exenteration (3), prostatectomy (1), or biopsy (2). Four of the six have been cured, one in treatment for a second malignancy, and the other had residual disease after exenteration. Thus, 36 of the 44 patients with Group III tumors were cured (minimum follow-up 6 years; range 6 to 11 years), compared with 23 of 47 patients in IRS-II. The bladder salvage rate for those cured of their disease also was better (64% vs. 57% of IRS-II). Conservative, delayed surgery, performed after intensive chemotherapy with or without radiotherapy, yields a better cure rate while maintaining a high rate of bladder salvage in children with group III prostatic RMS [190].

14.3.14 Paratesticular RMS

Paratesticular RMS represents 7% of all childhood rhabdomyosarcomas and 12% of childhood scrotal tumors [149]. Most paratesticular RMS are embryonal, nonmetastatic, and highly curable with multimodal therapy including surgery, multiagent chemotherapy, and, for patients with retroperitoneal lymph node (RPLN) involvement or incompletely resected disease, radiation therapy [191].

Most tumors present as a painless scrotal mass and are frequently easily resected (Group I). Survival rates exceed 90% for Group I and II patients [127, 135]. Lesions adjacent to the testis or spermatic cord should be removed by orchiectomy and resection of the entire spermatic cord through an inguinal incision with proximal control of the spermatic cord (Fig. 14.2). The contralateral testis may be transposed to the adjacent thigh, temporarily, when scrotal radiotherapy is required. Open scrotal biopsy or tumor spillage should be avoided because inguinal recurrence may follow and spillage or open biopsy requires scrotectomy and/or radiation. If biopsy is warranted before orchidectomy, the following steps should be followed: (1) atraumatic high control of the spermatic cord; (2) mobilize the testis and cord carefully isolated from the operative field; (3) biopsy site closed and testes covered while awaiting frozen section report; (4) instruments used for biopsy, gowns, and gloves changed; (5) if biopsy report is positive, testes and the entire cord including the atraumatic clamp should be removed together; (6) the field should be thoroughly irrigated. Patients with spillage are considered Clinical Group IIa regardless of the completeness of resection [192].

The incidence of nodal metastatic disease for paratesticular RMS has been reported to be as high as 26–43% of patients [149, 180, 193, 194]. During IRS-III, all patients were required to undergo ipsilateral retroperitoneal lymph node dissection (IRPLND). During IRS-IV, clinical evaluation of the RPLNs using CT was utilized. In this study, only those patients with lymph node involvement on CT required surgical evaluation of the RPLNs. This led to "down-grouping" about 15% of patients from group II (lymph nodes positive) to group I (total resection, no nodal disease). This effect was higher in adolescents (>30%). This change led to less patients receiving radiation to the retroperitoneum, but also a poorer FFS in IRS-IV and a higher relapse rate. For younger patients (<10 years of age), long-term survival rate did not differ between IRS-III and IRS-IV, and was excellent, (IRS-III, 100%; IRS-IV, 98%). However, treatment in about 30% of adolescents assigned to Group I tumor status in IRS-IV failed, and the patients required retreatment with poor salvage. In IRS-IV, patients given RPLN radiation and intensive three-agent chemotherapy including alkylating agents, survival at 3 years was 100%. Based on these data, the IRSG returned to recommending RLND for all patients over 10 years of age.

This still remains controversial since the International Society of Pediatric Oncology (SIOP) no longer recommends RPLND for any patients. Olive, et al. [194] concluded that chemotherapy was effective in eradicating occult micrometastases, which may have been missed if RPLND was not performed. Thus, they concluded the RPLND was not necessary in completely resected paratesticular RMS treated with multiagent chemotherapy.

RPLND is associated with significant long-term complications. Heyn, et al. [195] found RPLND to be associated with intestinal obstruction, loss of ejaculatory function, and lower extremity lymphedema.

There are risks associated with using the more intensive chemotherapy protocol as well. Cyclophosphamide is an N-phosphorylated cyclic derivative of nitrogen mustard. Side effects of cyclophosphamide include immunosuppression, pulmonary fibrosis, sterility, and testicular atrophy in men [196].

Present recommendations are that all patients with paratesticular RMS should have thin-cut abdominal and pelvic CT scans with double contrast to evaluate for evidence of nodal involvement. Patients ≥10 years of age receive ipsilateral retroperitoneal nerve-sparing template node dissection. Patients with Group II disease receive intensified treatment (e.g., VAC and RPLN radiation) [197]; disease in children (ages <10 years) can be staged with abdominal thin-cut (i.e., 5-mm slices) CT scan reserving IRLND for patients with a positive CT scan. Patients with group I disease should receive VA without radiation. Inguinal nodes are rarely involved and are biopsied only if clinically positive or if the scrotum is invaded by tumor. Inguinal nodes are not considered regional, and when positive, places the patient in Stage 4 (Clinical Group IV).

14.3.15 Vulva, Vaginal and Uterus

Vulvo-vaginal and uterine RMS is the most common malignancy of the pediatric female genital system. This tumor generally presents in the first few years of life, with vaginal bleeding, discharge, and/or a vaginal mass. If the tumor arises from the vulva, it consists of a firm nodule embedded in the labial folds, or it may be periclitoric in location. Diagnosis is made by incisional or excisional biopsy. Vaginal lesions generally have embryonal or botryoid embryonal histology and have an excellent prognosis [124, 139, 198]. Vulvar lesions may have alveolar histology, but because most are localized, they also have a good prognosis. The vaginal lesions usually arise from the anterior vaginal wall in the area of the embryonic vesico-vaginal septum (urogenital sinus). The bladder, prostatic utricle, prostate, and lower vagina all arise from the urogenital sinus. Because these are common sites for RMS in both sexes, one might speculate regarding the common occurrence in this location.

Before 1972, pelvic exenteration was the accepted surgical approach for vaginal RMS. Beginning in 1972, the IRS Group began to enter patients on prospective clinical trials. The first eight patients entered with nonmetastatic vaginal RMS all underwent primary surgical intervention followed by postoperative chemotherapy with VAC. Three patients also received radiotherapy. Because vaginal RMS appeared to be responsive to chemotherapy, IRS-II (1978–1984) consisted of a primary chemotherapy regimen followed by delayed surgical intervention ± radiation. Fourteen of 20 patients (70%) eventually underwent surgical resection [124].

During IRS-III (1984–1988) these patients were given primary chemotherapy consisting of VAC plus DOX and cisplatin after initial biopsy (clinical group III). Only seven of 23 patients (30%) underwent surgical resection after primary chemotherapy. Six of the seven patients had no viable tumor in the resected specimen and one had maturing rhabdomyoblasts. The presence of rhabdomyoblasts may not signify persistent active disease [49]. At M. D. Anderson Cancer Center, we have continued chemotherapy without resection when rhabdomyoblasts are found. No viable tumor or rhabdomyoblasts were found after further chemotherapy or subsequent biopsy in these patients. Only six patients in IRS-III underwent radiotherapy [198].

During IRS-IV (1988–1996) only three of 21 patients (13%) underwent surgical resection after primary chemotherapy. Three patients had rhabdomyoblasts only, whereas one patient who underwent early second-look surgery had rhabdomyoblasts and a small amount of viable tumor. No patient in IRS-IV had a cystectomy, and all but one patient are alive with no evidence of disease.

Early IRS studies suggested that patients with primary tumors of the uterus were a distinct group, distinguished from those with primary tumors arising in the vagina by older age, propensity to local recurrence, and poorer prognosis. Early surgical treatment was radical. Beginning in 1984 (IRS-III), these patients were treated with neoadjuvant chemotherapy consisting of adriamycin (ADR), cisplatin (CPDD), vincristine (VCR), dactinomycin (AMD), and cyclophosphamide. These therapies allowed for less extensive resection and less irradiation with excellent local and distant control of disease. Survival continues to improve with less radical surgical intervention [199].

The general principles for tumors of the vagina, vulva, and uterus in IRS-V include biopsy and staging followed by chemotherapy as directed by stage and group (i.e., risk category). Second- and third-look operation with biopsy and cystoscopy are common. Distal vaginal lesions may be polypoid or localized and amenable to primary resection or delayed resection. Rarely is vaginectomy or hysterectomy indicated except for recurrent or persistent viable tumor. Lymph node involvement is very rare. Oophorectomy is not done except for direct involvement with advanced or recurrent disease.

A primary chemotherapy approach with the gold-standard of VAC, followed by local resectional therapy and occasional use of radiotherapy where indicated has produced excellent results [200]. Patients ages 1–9 years fared the best (5-year survival of 98%) and patients outside of this age range especially benefited from the intensified therapy used in IRS-III or IRS-IV. (5-year survival of 67% on the IRS-I/II vs. 90% in IRS III/IV) [200].

14.3.16 Trunk

Trunk as primary site for RMS includes paraspinal, thoracic or chest wall, abdominal wall, intra-abdominal, and pelvic/retroperitoneum. They tend to have a higher incidence of alveolar histology and a somewhat worse prognosis in some sites [201, 202]. These lesions present differently depending on site and will be discussed separately.

14.3.17 Paraspinal

Paraspinal RMS presents as an enlarging mass in the paravertebral muscle area. This is usually diagnosed by incisional biopsy and must be distinguished from extraosseous Ewing's sarcoma, which is more common in this site in my experience. For all truncal tumors, the biopsy should be performed in the long axis of the tumor (i.e., parallel to the ribs), to allow for WLE and rib resection as necessary.

Most patients with paraspinal lesions will require preresectional chemotherapy. Many will require postoperative radiation therapy. WLE is frequently done in conjunction with plastic surgeons, who can assist in flap closure of the defect. In small children, it may be wise to eliminate radiation therapy close to the spine whenever feasible.

14.3.18 Abdominal Wall

This location is also relatively rare (<1% of all patients) and requires excisional or incisional biopsy followed by wide local complete resection or neoadjuvant chemotherapy followed by second-look surgery. In a review of IRS patients, FFS at 5 years was 65% [203]. Older patients with alveolar histology and larger tumors had a worse prognosis.

14.3.19 Chest Wall

Chest-wall and intrathoracic tumors are rare sites of pediatric sarcomas. Of 2,747 patients registered in IRS I, II, and III, only 105 had chest wall, pleura, lung, or heart as a primary site. It had been suggested that these sites have a poorer prognosis. Factors attributed to this include histology, advanced stage at presentation, and difficulties in local resection. Early studies showed high rates of local and distant relapse [90]. A review of IRS II and III [201] showed 84 patients with thoracic sarcomas. Seventy-six were chest-wall tumors, three were lung tumors, four were pleural tumors, and one arose from the heart. Sixty (71%) of the patients had achieved a complete response. Thirty-nine patients had a local relapse, and 22 patients had a distant relapse. Forty-two percent of patients survived. PFS was not significantly associated with histology, site, clinical group, or IRS Study. Overall survival was significantly associated with clinical group, size, and local or distant recurrence, but not histology or IRS Study by univariate analysis. In a multivariate analysis, only clinical group, local, and distant recurrence showed statistical significance. Thus, if survival is to be improved, local tumor control with negative margins must be achieved. Because clinical group II patients were treated with XRT and had a better survival rate than did those in clinical group I (totally resected and thus no XRT), the resection may have left microscopic or even gross residual disease. Either second-look surgery or consideration of local XRT for possible residual disease in clinical group I may be indicated to improve survival [201].

Specific surgical management of chest wall RMS includes initial biopsy and staging (biopsy longitudinal to ribs). Following neoadjuvant chemotherapy, the tumor is resected to clear margins and attached pleura or lung is removed as necessary. If needed, wide local resection can be followed by chest wall reconstruction usually with a synthetic material covered by a myocutaneous flap. Frequently, tumor size reduction will allow resection with primary closure.

14.3.20 Retroperitoneal/Pelvic

RMS of the retroperitoneum and pelvis usually presents as a large bulking tumor with the exact site of origin difficult to determine [204]. Frequently, these tumors invade or involve vital organs or vessels and only biopsy can be performed at initial exploration. Previous reports from earlier IRS studies have indicated a poor prognosis for these sites [25]. Blakely, et al. [205] reported on 94 patients with Group III disease from IRS-III and IRS-IV pilot and found a 57% FFS rate at 4 years. They found that age <10 years at diagnosis and embryonal histology were favorable prognostic factors, as was the performance of a debulking procedure prior to instituting chemotherapy and radiation therapy [205]. Recently Raney, et al. [206] reported on the results of 56 patients with localized retroperitoneal and pelvic RMS. Fifty-four of these patients had gross residual disease (clinical group III) at the completion of the initial diagnostic procedure. Two patients underwent grossly complete surgical excision with microscopic involved margins without (Group IIA) or with (Group IIC) tumor-involved regional lymph nodes that were removed prior to beginning chemotherapy. Only 15 patients (27%) had 50% or more of the tumor removed before beginning chemotherapy and were classified as debulked, while the other 41

patients were classified as having biopsy only. In the 15 patients who underwent excision of 50% or more of the tumor prior to initiation of chemotherapy/radiotherapy, thus far there have been no failures after treatment. By contrast, 15 of the 41 patients who underwent biopsy only developed recurrent sarcoma. Thus, it would appear that debulking prior to chemotherapy/radiotherapy may be of value when it can be achieved safely and with minimum morbidity. Otherwise, an alternative would be delayed primary excision after shrinkage with chemotherapy.

14.3.21 Biliary

Patients with biliary RMS do relatively well with chemotherapy and radiotherapy without aggressive surgical resection [207, 208]. Most patients have the botryoid variant of embryonal RMS, which responds well to chemotherapy. Although these tumors present with significant obstructive jaundice, biopsy followed by neoadjuvant chemotherapy will commonly reduce the jaundice without the need for resection, internal, or external biliary drainage. Surgical resection or bypass are fraught with significant complications. Spunt, et al. [208] reported on 25 patients treated in IRSG Studies I through IV and found that total resection was rarely possible, external biliary drains were frequently associated with infection, and tumors responded well to combination chemotherapy without aggressive surgical intervention.

14.3.22 Perineum/Perianal

Rhabdomyosarcoma (RMS) of the perineum or anus is a rare sarcoma of childhood with a relatively poor prognosis. Blakely, et al. [209] reported 71 patients treated by IRS studies I through IV (1972–1997). The majority (64%) were at an advanced stage (clinical group III and IV) at initial presentation and 50% had positive regional lymph nodes (LN) involvement. The 5-year FFS rate for all patients was 45% and the overall survival rate was 49%. Characteristics that were associated with significantly improved survival rate were primary tumor size less than 5 cm, lower (less advanced) clinical group and stage, negative lymph node status, and age less than 10 years. When the extent of disease was controlled for multivariate analysis, only age less than 10 predicted an improved outcome. The 5-year overall survival rate for patients less than 10 years of age was 71% vs. 20% in older patients (p<.001). Because of the high incidence of regional LN involvement, biopsy of clinically suspicious nodes should be done and sentinel lymph node mapping for nonclinically suspicious nodes should be entertained.

14.3.23 Extremity

Primary tumors of the extremity accounted for 19% of RMS in IRS-III [133], and 20% of patients in IRS-IV [210]. Despite the intensive efforts of the IRSG, outcome for children with extremity RMS remains suboptimal compared with that of children with RMS in more favorable sites. Improvements in survival have been seen with subsequent studies, but estimated 5-year survival has been at about 74% for patients without distant metastatic disease [133]. Analysis of these studies has suggested that the improvement is attributed to the intensification of therapy directed at patients identified to have a poorer prognosis, while allowing a decrease in therapy for those with a good prognosis. Various prognostic factors have been suggested for extremity RMS in children. The elements of the Lawrence/Gehan [138] staging system used in IRS-IV are local tissue invasiveness, tumor size, presence of nodal and distant metastases, and site. Since extremities are relatively unfavorable sites, no extremity tumors are classified as Stage I by this system. A total of 139 patients were entered in IRS-IV with extremity-site RMS and were assigned a preoperative stage. Preoperative staging was Stage 2, n=34; Stage 3, n=73; Stage 4, n=32. Clinical Grouping was Group I, n=31; Group II, n=21; Group III, n=54; and Group IV, n=33. Three-year FFS was 55%, and the overall survival rate was 70%. FFS was significantly worse for patients with advanced disease. Totally resected patients (Group I) had a 3-years FFS of 91% [210].

Initial treatment consists of biopsy either incisional or excisional. This should be done in a longitudinal or axial direction to allow for wide local excision. If wide local excision can be done without mutilation, this should be considered. The standard 2-cm margins are arbitrary and not practical in children. There is little evidence that a clear margin of a few millimeters is at any higher risk for recurrence than larger margins. Amputation is rarely indicated except for larger recurrent or persistent disease. Excision of the entire muscle from origin to insertion, as once recommended, is no longer necessary or recommended. The importance of complete resection is emphasized since survival is markedly improved with total excision or microscopic residual only. Careful determination of margin status is extremely important and re-resection at initial or subsequent operation is warranted. Hays, et al. [142] demonstrated that patients with node negative extremity and trunk sarcomas who underwent re-excision for microscopic residual tumor had a significant survival rate that was higher than those who did not have re-excision or were reported to have no residual tumor after initial resection. It has been our policy to recommend re-excision for all patients referred to our institution after previous resection no matter what was previously reported. We have found residual and even gross disease in patients reported to have complete resection (probably due to the surgeon being unaware of cancer being present).

Lymph node involvement with extremity RMS in IRS I and II was considered to be only 12% [12, 150, 133, 211]. This was because few patients actually had lymph node biopsy. LaQuaglia, et al. [212] reported an incidence of 40% positive nodes. In a review of IRS-IV, Andrassy, et al. [133] demonstrated that 39% of patients who underwent evaluation of their lymph nodes had histologic confirmation of disease. Neville, et al. [210] in a review of IRS-IV data, found that 50% of biopsied lymph nodes contain disease. Of the patients whose lymph nodes were clinically negative but were biopsied anyway, 17% were found to have microscopic disease. Histologically positive lymph nodes is a statistically significant predictor of FFS. Although lymph node dissection has not proven to improve survival rate, positive regional nodes should be irradiated to prevent local recurrence. We have used and recommended lymphatic mapping with sentinel node biopsy to evaluate the regional nodes [137, 210]. If sentinel lymph node mapping is not available, aggressive sampling is warranted.

14.3.24 Complications

Complications of treatment for RMS are varied and extensive. These include chemotherapy toxicity and death, radiation related acute and long-term complications, and standard surgical complications of biopsy and resection. For a more in-depth review of the complications in pediatric surgical oncology see Miller, et al. [64]. Long-term follow-up of all patients is warranted for delayed complications and second malignancies [213].

14.3.25 Treatment of Metastatic Disease

Metastatic disease most commonly involves the lung (58%), bone (33%), regional lymph nodes (33%), liver (22%), and brain (20%) [143]. Of patients enrolled in the IRS-III [24], 14% were clinical group IV at the time of diagnosis. Primary sites more likely to have metastases include the extremities (23%), parameningeal (13%), retroperitoneal, trunk, gastrointestinal, and Intrathoracic sites. Primary sites with a low incidence of metastases include the orbit (1.8%), nonparameningeal or nonorbital head and neck (4.5%), and genitourinary sites [96]. Metastatic disease is the single most important predictor of clinical outcome in patients with RMS. The 3-year FFS is only 25% in patients with metastatic disease [129, 154]. As mentioned previously, regional node metastases vary with the site of the primary (extremity the highest) and also affects survival.

The lung is the most common site of metastatic disease. Patients with lung-only metastases appear to have a somewhat better prognosis than multiple sites or metastases to bone or liver [135]. Patients with lung-only metastases have a greater incidence of favorable histology and a smaller number of extremity primaries [135]. Since RMS is highly chemosensitive, resection of numerous metastases for RMS does not appear indicated. In my own experience, isolated single metastases to the lung have a better prognosis than multiple metastases. For this reason, I believe it is of value to biopsy a single metastasis to confirm histology. The better prognosis may well be related to treatment of nonmetastatic lung lesions other than RMS. Persistent or recurrent disease after chemotherapy may warrant resection both for diagnosis and possibly decreasing tumor burden. Overall, there has been little improvement in survival for patients with metastatic disease. These are presently in Stage IV, group IV and are considered high risk. Aggressive chemotherapy and radiation in an attempt to improve survival is being studied. During IRS-IV, 127 eligible patients were treated for metastatic disease with one of two regimens that incorporated a window of either ifosfamide and etoposide with vincristine, dactinomycin, and cyclophosphamide or vincristine, melphalan and VAC. The estimated overall survival and FFS was 39% and 25% at 3 years. Overall survival at 3 years was influenced by histology (47% for embryonal vs. 34% for all others), and increasing number of metastatic sites. By multivariate analysis, the presence of two or fewer metastatic sites was the only significant predictor [214].

14.3.26 Outcomes

The overall trend has been an increase in survival for each subsequent IRS study. The survival rate depends on clinical group, stage, and primary site. The overall 5-year survival rate in IRS-III Study was 71%; 90% for clinical group I, 80% for clinical group II, 70% for clinical group III, and 30% for clinical group IV [154]. The survival rate by pretreatment staging classification was 80% for Stage I, 68% for Stage II, 49% for Stage III, 21% for Stage IV [214].

Overall, FFS rates for the patients treated on IRS-IV did not differ from those seen for similar patients treated on IRS-III; estimated 3-year FFS rate was 76% on IRS-III and 77% on IRS-IV. FFS rates were improved for patients with embryonal rhabdomyosarcoma treated on IRS-IV compared to those of similar patients treated on IRS-III (3-year FFS rates, 83% vs. 74%). The improvement seemed to be restricted to pa-

tients with Stage II or Stage II/III, group I/II embryonal RMS. The sites of treatment failure were local only in 93 patients (51%), regional in 30 (17%), and distant in 58 (32%). Salvage therapy after relapse differed by group. Forty-one percent of the patients with group I/II tumors, compared with 22% of those with group III tumors, were alive 3 years after relapse [140]. The overall survival for recurrent RMS is very poor. In the Intergroup Rhabdomyosarcoma Study Group (IRS) III, IV, and IV pilot, the 5-year survival for 605 patients who experienced relapse after treatment was less than 20%. At 5 years, patients with botryoid RMS had a survival rate of 64%; embryonal, 26%; and alveolar or undifferentiated, 5% [191, 215]. Surgical resection was not an independent prognostic variable, which impacted survival in these studies. In the review by Hayes-Jordan, et al. [216] from M. D. Anderson Cancer Center, there was a trend toward improved survival in patients who have aggressive resections for recurrent RMS compared to those who have nonoperative therapy. These results are hard to interpret since recurrence at unresectable sites such as multiple bony sites did poorly. It is also known that patients with multiple sites of metastases do worse the patients with a single metastasis. In a review by the German cooperative group on recurrent soft tissue sarcomas in children [24, 216], 17 patients underwent surgery, and the investigators found no statistically significant difference in FFS for patients with alveolar vs. embryonal histology (P=.058). However, embryonal patients demonstrated superior overall survival when compared to those with alveolar histology (P=.027). Aggressive operative therapy vs. local therapy did not correlate with improved overall survival [216]. We still offer resection on recurrent disease, particularly if there is a chance of complete resection.

References

1. Gurney JG, Young JL, Roffers SD, et al. (1999) Soft tissue sarcomas. In: Gloecker Ries IA, Smith MA, Gurney JG, et al. (eds) SEER Pediatric Monograph: Cancer incidence and survival among children and adolescents, United States SEER program 1975–1995. National Cancer Institute, Bethesda, pp 111–124
2. Ruymann FB, et al. (1991) Epidemiology of soft tissue sarcomas. In: Maurer HM, Ruymann FB, Pochedly C (eds) Rhabdomyosarcoma and related tumors in children and adolescents. CRC Press, Boca Raton
3. Hayes-Jordan AA, Spunt SL, Poquette CA, et al. (2000) Nonrhabdomosarcoma soft tissue sarcomas in children: Is age at diagnosis an important variable? J Pediat Surg 35:948–953
4. Laskin WH, Silverman IA, Enzinger JM (1988) Postradiation soft tissue sarcomas. An analysis of 53 cases. Cancer 62:2330–2340

5. Cha C, Antonescu CR, Quan MI, et al. (2004) Long-term results with resection of radiation-induced soft tissue sarcomas. Ann Surg 239:903–909

6. Malkin D (1993) p53 and the Li-Fraumeni syndrome. Cancer Genet Cytogent 66:83–92

7. Malkin D, Li FP, Strong LC (1990) Germ line p53 mutations in a familial syndrome of breast cancer sarcomas, and other neoplasms. Science 250:1233–1238

8. Glover IW, Stein CK, Legius F, et al. (1991) Molecular and cytogenetic analysis of tumors in von Recklinghausen neurofibromatosis. Genes Chromosomes Cancer 3:62–70

9. Ducatman BS, Scheithauer BW, Piepgras DG, et al. (1986) Malignant peripheral nerve sheath tumors. A clinicopathologic study of 120 cases. Cancer 57:2006–2021

10. Evans DG, Baser ME, McGaughran J, et al. (2002) Malignant peripheral nerve sheath tumours in neurofibromatosis 1. J Med Genet 39:311–314

11. Neville HL, Seymour-Dempsey K, Slopis J, et al. (2001) The role of surgery in children with neurofibromatois. J Pediat Surg 36:25–29

12. Neville H, Lorpron C, Blakely M, Andrassy RJ (2003) Pediatric neurofibrosarcoma. J Pediat Surg 38:343–346

13. Clark SK, Neale KF, Landgrebe JC, et al. (1999) Desmoid tumours complicating familial adenomatous polyposis. Br J Surg 86:1185–1189

14. Heiskanen I, Jarvinen HJ (1996) Occurrence of desmoid tumours in familial adenomatous polyposis and results of treat. Int J Colorectal Dis 11:157–162

15. Gurbuz AK, Giardiello FM, Petersen GM, et al. (1994) Desmoid tumours in familiar adenomatour polyposis. Gut 35:377–381

16. Sreekantaiah C, Ladanyi M, Rodriguez E, et al. (1994) Chromosomal aberrations in soft tissue tumors. Relevance to diagnosis, classification, and molecular mechanisms. Am J Pathol 144:1121–1134

17. Limon J, Mrozek K, Mandahl N, et al. (1991) Cytogenetics of synovial sarcoma: Presentation of ten new cases and review of the literature. Genes Chromosomes Cancer 3:338–45

18. Clark J, Rocques PI, Crew AJ, et al. (1995) Identification of novel genes, SYT to tow genes, SSX1 and SSX2, encoding proteins with homology to the Kruppel-associated box in human synovial sarcoma. EMBO J 14:2333–2340

19. Crew AJ, Clark J, Fisher C, et al. (1995) Fusion of SYT to two genes, SSX1 and SSX2, encoding proteins with homology to the Kruppel-associated box in human synovial sarcoma. EMBO J 14:2333–2340

20. Kawai A, Woodruff J, Healey JH, et al. (1998) SYT-SSX gene fusion as a determinant of morphology and prognosis in synovial sarcoma. N Engl J Med 338:153–160

21. Nilsson G, Skytting B, Xie Y, et al. (1999) The SYT-SSX1 variant of synovial sarcoma is associated with a high rate of tumor cell proliferation and poor clinical outcome. Cancer Res 59:3180–3184

22. Aman P, Ron D, Mandahl N, et al. (1992) Rearrangement of the transcription factor gene CHOP in myxoid kiposarcomas with t(12; 16) (q13; p11). Genes Chromosomes Cancer 5:278–285

23. Crozat A, Aman P, Mandahl N, et al. (1993) Fusion of CHOP to a novel RNA-binding protein in human myxoid liposarcoma. Nature 363:640–644

24. Barr FG, Chatten J, D'Cruz CM, et al. (1995) Molecular assays for chromosomal translocations in the diagnosis of pediatric soft tissue sarcomas. JAMA 273:553–557.

25. Ohno T, Ouchida M, Lee Il, et al. (1944) The EWS gene, involved in Ewing family of tumors, malignant melanoma of soft parts and desmoplastic small round cell tumors, codes for an RNA binding protein with novel regulatory domains. Oncogene 9:3087–3097

26. Li FP, Fraumeni JF Jr (1969) Rhabdomyosarcoma in children: Epidemiologic study and identification of a familial cancer syndrome. J Natl Cancer Inst 43:1365–1373

27. Li FP, Fraumeni JF Jr (1982) Prospective study of a family cancer syndrome. JAMA 247:2692–2694

28. Knudson AG Jr (1985) Hereditary cancer, oncogenes, and antioncogenes. Cancer Res 45:1437–1443

29. Orkin S (1986) Reverse genetics and human disease. Cell 47:845–850

30. D'agostino An, Soule EH, Miller RH (1963) Primary malignant neoplasms of nerves (malignant neurilemomas) in patients without manifestations of multiple neurofibromatosis (von Recklinghausen's disease). Cancer 16:1003–1014

31. Diagostino An, Soule EH, Miller RH (1963) Sarcomas of the peripheral nerves and somatic soft tissues associated with multiple neurofibromatosis (von Recklinghausen's disease). Cancer 16:1015–1027

32. Storm FK, Eilber IR, Mirra J, et al. (1980) Neurofibrosarcoma. Cancer 45:126–129

33. Guccion JG, Enzinger JM (1979) Malignant schwannoma associated with von Recklinghausen's neurofibromatosis. Virchows Arch A Pathol Anat Histol 383:43–57

34. Fienman Nil, Yakovac WC (1970) Neurofibromatosis in childhood. J Pediatr 76:339–346

35. McLoughlin LC, Nord KS, Joshi VV, et al. (1991) Disseminated leiomyosarcoma in a child with acquired immune deficiency syndrome. Cancer 67:2618–2621

36. McClain KI, Leach CT, Jenson IIB, et al. (1995) Association of Epstein-Barr virus with leiomyosarcomas in children with AIDS. N Engl Med 332:12–18

37. Shen SC, Yunis FJ (1976) Leiomyosarcoma developing in a child during remission of leukemia. J Pediatr 89:780–782

38. Swanson PF, Dehner IP (1991) Pathology of soft tissue sarcomas in children and adolescents. In: Maurer HM, Ruymann IB, (eds) Rhabdomyosarcoma and related tumors in children and adolescents. CRC Press, Boca Raton, 385–420

39. Andrassy RJ (2002) Advances in the surgical management of sarcomas in children. Amer J Surg 184:484–491

40. Andrassy RJ, Okeu MF, Despa S, Raney RB (2001) Synovial sarcoma in children: Surgical lesions from a single institution and review of the literature. J Am Coll Surg 192:305–313

41. Mauer HM, Beltangady M, Gerhan EA, et al. (1988) The Intergroup Rhabdomyosarcoma Study-1. A final report. Cancer 61:209–220

42. Costa J, Westley RA, Glatstein E, et al. (1984) The grading of soft tissue sarcomas. Results of a clinicohistopathologic correlation in a series of 163 cases. Cancer 53:530–541

43. Fleming ID, Cooper SJ, Henson DE, et al. (1998) AJCC cancer staging handbook. Lippincott-Raven, Philadelphia

44. Guillou I, Coindre JM, Bonichon F, et al. (1997) Comparative study of the National Cancer Institute and French Federation of cancer Centers Sarcoma Group grading systems in a population of 410 adult patients with soft tissue sarcoma. J Clin Oncol 15:350–362

45. van Unnik JA, Coindre JM, Contesso C, et al. (1993) Grading of soft tissue sarcomas: Experience of the EORtTC Soft Tissue and Bone Sarcoma Group. Eur J Cancer 29A:2089–2093

46. Coindre JM, Trojani M, Contesso G, et al. (1986) Reproducibility of a histopathologic grading system for adult soft tissue sarcoma. Cancer 58:306–309

47. Parham DM, Webber BI, Jenkins JJ III, et al. Nonrhabdomyosarcomatous soft tissue sarcomas of childhood: Formulation of a simplified system for grading. Mod Pathol 8(7):705–710

48. Rodriguez-Galindo C, Ramsey K, Jenkins JJ, et al. (2000) Hermangiopericytoma in children and infants. Cancer 88:198–204

49. Loh MI, Ahn P, Perez-Atayde AR, et al. (2002) Treatment of infantile fibrosarcoma with chemotherapy and surgery: Results from the Dana-Farber Cancer Institute and children's Hospital, Boston. J Pediatr Hematol Oncol 24:722–726

50. Spunt SI, Poquette CA, Hurt YS, et al. (1999) Prognostic factors for children and adolescents with surgically resected nonrhabdomyosarcoma soft tissue sarcoma: An analysis of 121 patients treated at St. Jude Children's Research Hospital. J Clin Oncol 17:3697–3705

51. Marcus KC, Grier HE, Shamberger RC, et al. (1997) Childhood soft tissue sarcoma: A 20-year experience. J Pediatr 131:603–607

52. Pratt CB, Pappo AS, Gieser P, et al. (1999) Role of adjuvant chemotherapy in the treatment of surgically resected pediatric nonrhabdomyosarcomatous soft tissue sarcomas: A Pediatric Oncology Group Study. J Clin Oncol 17:1219–1226

53. Stojadinovic A, Leung DH, Allen P, et al. (2002) Primary adult soft tissue sarcoma: Time-dependent influence of prognostic variables. J Clin Oncol 20:4344–4352

54. Pappo AS, Rao BN, Jenkins JI, et al. (1999) Metastatic non-rhabdomyosarcomatous soft-tissue sarcomas in children and adolescents: The St. Jude Children's Research Hospital experience. Med Pediatr Oncol 33:76–82

55. Spunt SI, Hill DA, Motosue AM, et al. (2000) Clinical features and outcome of children with unresected non-rhabdomyosarcoma soft tissue sarcoma (NRSTS). Med Pediatr Oncol 35:279 (abst)

56. Spunt SI, Hill DA, Motosue AM, et al. (2002) Clinical features and outcome of initially unresected nonmetastatic pediatric nonrhabdomyosarcoma soft tissue sarcoma. J Clin Oncol 20:3225–3235

57. Butler MS, Robertson WW Jr, Rate W, et al. (1990) Skeletal sequelae of radiation therapy for malignant childhood tumors. Clin Orthop 25:235–240

58. Smith MD, Xue H, Strong L, et al. (1993) Forty-year experience with second malignancies after treatment of childhood cancer: Analysis of outcome following the development of the second malignancy. J Pediatr Surg 28:1342–1349

59. Humpl T, Fritsche M, Bartels U, et al. (2001) survivors of childhood cancer for more than twenty years. Acta Oncol 40:44–49

60. Feig SA (2001) Second malignant neoplasms after successful treatment of childhood cancers. Blood Cells Mol Dis 27:662–666

61. Rich DC, Corpron CA, Smith MB, et al. (1997) Second malignant neoplasms in children after treatment of soft tissue sarcoma. J Pediatr Surg 32:369–372

62. Moller TR, Garwicz S, Barlow L, et al. (2001) Decreasing late mortality among five year survivors of cancer in childhood and adolescence: A population-based study in the Nordic counties. J Clin Oncol 19:3173–3181

63. Corpron CA, Black TC, Ross MI, et al. (1996) Melanoma as a second malignant neoplasm after childhood cancer. Am J Surg 171:459–462

64. Miller SD, Adrassy RJ (2003) Complications in pediatric surgical oncology. J Amer Col Surg 197:832–837

65. Corpron CA, Black CT, Raney RB, et al. (1996) Malignant fibrous histiocytoma in children. J Pediatr Surg 31:1080–1083

66. Smith MB, Katz R, Black CT, et al. (1993) A rational approach to the use of fine-needle aspiration biopsy in the evaluation of primary and recurrent neoplasms in children. J Pediatr Surg 28:1245–1247

67. Blakely ML, Spurbeck WW, Pappo AS, et al. (1999) The impact of marginson? Outcome in pediatric nonrhabdomyosarcoma soft tissue sarcoma. J Pediatr Surg 34:672–675

68. Neville HL, Andrassy RJ, Lally KP, et al. (2000) Lymphatic mapping with sentinel node biopsy in pediatric patients. J Pediatr Surg 35:961–964

69. Pappo AS, Fontanesi J, Luo X, et al. (1994) Synovial sarcoma in children and adolescents: The St. Jude Children's Research Hospital experience. J Clin Oncol 12:2660–2666

70. Brennan MF (1997) The enigma of local recurrence. Am Surg Oncol 2:1–12

71. Muller JR, Zagars CK (1994) Synovial sarcoma outcome following conservation surgery and radiotherapy. Radiother Oncol 33:23–30

72. Fontanesi J, Pappo AS, Parham DW, et al. (1996) Role of irradiation in management of synovial sarcoma: St. Judes Children's Research Hospital experience. Med Pediatr Oncol 26:264–267

73. Pappo AS, Parham DM, Rao BM, et al. (1999) Soft tissue sarcomas in children. Semin Surg Oncol 16:121–143

74. Coffin CM, Dehner LP (1993) Vascular tumors in children and adolescents: A clinicopathologic study of 228 tumors in 222 patients. Pathol Ann 28:97–120

75. Fisher C (1990) The value of electromicroscopy and immunohistochemistry in the diagnosis of soft tissue sarcomas: A study of 200 cases. Histopathology 16:441–454

76. Coffin CM, Jaszez W, O'Shea PA, et al. (1994) So-called congenital infantile fibrosarcoma: Does it exist and what is it. Pediat Pathol 14:133–150

77. Soule EH, Pritchard DJ (1977) Fibrosarcoma in infants and children: A review of 110 cases. Cancer 40:1711–1721

78. Blocker S, Koenig J, Ternberg J (1987) Longenital fibrosarcoma. J Pediatr Surg 22:665–670

79. Dobson I, Dickey LB (1956) Spontaneous regression of malignant tumors: Report of a twelve year spontaneous complete regression of an extensive fibrosarcoma with speculations about regression and dormancy. Am J Surg 92:162–173

80. Barker D, Wright E, Nguyen L, et al. (1987) Gene for von Recklinghausen neurofibromatosis in the pericentromeric region of chromosome 17. Science 236:1100–1102

81. Roulean GA, Wertelecki W, Haines JF, et al. (1987) Genetic linkage of bilateral acoustic neurofibromatosis to a DNA marker on chromosome 22. Nature 329:246–248

82. Riccardi VM (1981) Von Reckinghausen neurofibromatosis. N Engl J Med 305:1617

83. Ducatman BS, Scheitnauer BW, Peipgras DG, et al. (1986) Malignant peripheral nerve sheath tumors: A clinicopathologic study of 120 cases. Cancer 57:2006–20021

84. DeCou JM, Rao BN, Parham DM, et al. (1995) Malignant peripheral nerve sheath tumors: The St. Jude Children's Research Hospital experience 2:524–529

85. Raney R, Schnaufer I, Ziegler M, et al. (1987) Treatment of children with neurogenic sarcoma. Experience at the Children's Hospital of Philadelphia, 1958–1984. Cancer 59:1–5

86. Skotheim RI, Kallioniemi A, Bjerkhagen B, et al. (2003) Topoisomerase-11 alpha is upregulated in malignant peripheral nerve sheath tumors and associated with clinical outcome. J Clin Oncol 21:4586–4591

87. Doorn PE, Molenaar WM, Buter J, et al. (1995) Malignant peripheral nerve sheath tumors in patients with and without neurofibromatosis. Eur J Surg Oncol 21:78–82

88. Christopherson WM, Foote FW, Stewart FW (1952) Alveolar soft-part sarcoma: Structurally characteristic tumors of uncertain histogenesis. Cancer 5:100–111

89. Yagihashi S (1992) Alveolar soft part sarcoma: Are we approaching the goal of determining its histogenesis? Acta Pathol Jpn 42:466–468

90. Portera CA Jr, Ho V, Patel SR, et al. (2001) Alveolar soft part sarcoma: Clinical course and patterns of metastasis in 70 patients treated at a single institution. Cancer 91:585–591

91. Casanova M, Ferrar A, Bisogno G, et al. (2000) Alvelar soft part sarcoma in children and adolescents: A report from the soft-tissue sarcoma Italian Cooperative Group. Ann Oncol 11:1445–1449

92. Raney RB (1979) Alveolar soft-part sarcoma. Med Pediatr Oncol 6:367–370

93. Soule EH, Mahour GH, Mills SD, et al. (1968) Soft-tissue sarcomas of infants and children: A clinicopathologic study of 135 cases. Mayo Clin. Proc 43:313–326

94. Johnson H, Hutter H Jr, Paplanus SH (1980) Leiomyosarcoma of the stomach: Results of surgery and chemotherapy in an eleven-year old girl with liver metastasis. Med Pediatr Oncol 8:137–142

95. LaQuaglia MP, Spiro SA, Ghovimi L, et al. (1993) Liprosarcoma in patients younger than or equal to 22 years of age. Cancer 72:3114–3119

96. Ruymann FB (1987) Rhabdomyosarcoma in children and adolescents: A review. Hematol Oncol Clin North Am 1:621–654

97. Stout AP (1946) Rhabdomyosarcoma of the skeletal muscle. Ann Surg 123:447

98. Pack GT, et al. Rhabdomyosarcoma of the skeletal muscle: Report of 100 cases. Surgery 32:1023–1952

99. Horn RC, et al. (1958) Rhabdomyosarcoma: A clinicopathological study and classification of 39 cases. Cancer 11:181–199

100. Stobbe GC, et al. (1950) Embryonal rhabdomyosarcoma of the head and neck in children and adolescents. Cancer 3:826

101. Pinkel D, et al. (1961) Rhabdomyosarcoma in children. JAMA 175:293–298

102. Ruymann F, et al. (1988) Congenital anomalies associated with rhabdomyosarcoma: A report from the Intergroup Rhabdomyosarcoam Study. Med Pedatr Oncol 16:13

103. Hartley AN, et al. (1993) Patterns of cancer in the families of children with soft tissue sarcoma. Cancer 72:923–930

104. Seymour-Dempsey K, et al. (2002) Neurofibromatosis: Implications for the general surgeon. J Am Coll Surg 195(4):553–561

105. Li FP, et al. (1969) Soft tissue sarcomas, breast cancer and other neoplasms: A familial syndrome? Ann Intern Med 71:747–752

106. Li FP, et al. (1988) A cancer family syndrome in twenty-four kindreds. Cancer Res 48:5358–5362

107. Mandell LR, et al. (1989) The influence of extensive bone erosion on local control in non-orbital rhabdomyosarcoma of the head and neck. Int J Radiat Oncol Biol Phys 17:649–653

108. Strong LC, et al. (1992) The Li-Fraumeni Syndrome: From clinical epidemiology to molecular genetics. Am J Epidemiol 135:190–199

109. Birch JM, et al. (1984) Excess risk of breast cancer in the mothers of children with soft tissue sarcomas. Br J Cancer 49:325–331

110. Grufferman A, et al. In utero X-ray exposure and risk of childhood rhabdomyosarcoma. Society for Epidemiologic Research 4th Annual Meeting, Buffalo, New York, June 11, 1991

111. Grufferman S, et al. (1993) Parents use of recreational drugs and risk of rhabdomyosarcoma in their children. Cancer Causes Control 4:217–224

112. Rodeberg DA, et al. (2002) Surgical principles for children? Adolescents with newly diagnosed rhabdomyosarcoma: A report from the Soft Tissue Sarcoma Committee of the Children's Oncology Group. Sarcoma 6:111–122

113. Dagher R, et al. (1999) Rhabdomyosarcoma: An overview. Oncologist 4:34–44

114. Li M, et al. (1997) Molecular genetics of Beckwith-Wiedemann Syndrome. Curr Opin Pediatr 9:623–629

115. Morison IM, et al. (1998) Insulin-like growth factor 2 and overgrowth: Molecular biology and clinical implications. Mol Med Today 4:110–115

116. Turc Carel C, et al. (1986) Consistent chromosomal translocation in alveolar rhabdomyosarcoma. Cancer Genet CytoGenet 19:361–362

117. Wexler LH, et al. (1994) Pediatric soft tissue sarcomas. Ca Cancer J Clin 44:211–247

118. Leader M, et al. (1989) Myoglobin: An evaluation of its role as a marker of rhabdomyosarcomas. Br J Cancer 59:106–109

119. Weintraub H, et al. (1991) The myoD gene family: Nodal point during specification of the muscle cell lineage. Science 251:761–166

120. Tapscott SJ, et al. (1993) Deficiency in rhabdomyosarcomas of a factor required for MyoD activity and myogenesis. Science 259:1450–1453

121. Shapiro DN, et al. (1991) Relationship of tumor-cell ploidy to histologic subtype and treatment of outcome in children and adolescents with unresectable rhabdomyosarcoma. J Clin Oncol 9:159–166

122. Kilpatrick SE, et al. (1994) Relationship of DNA ploidy to histology and prognosis in rhabdomyosarcoma. Cancer 74:3227–3233

123. Ferracini R, et al. (1996) Retrogenic expression of the MET proto oncogene correlates with the invasive phenotype of human rhabdomyosarcomas. Oncogene 12:1697–1705

124. Andrassy RJ, et al. (1999) Progress in the surgical management of vaginal rhabdomyosarcoma: A 25-Year Review From the Intergroup Rhabdomyosarcoma Study Group. J Pediatr Surg 34:731–735

125. Asmar L, et al. (1994) Agreement among and within groups of pathologists in the classification of rhabdomyosarcoma and related childhood sarcomas: Report of an international study of four pathology classifications. Cancer 74:2579–2588

126. Newton WA, et al. (1991) Pathology of rhabdomyosarcoma and related tumors. In: Maurer HM, Ruyman FB, Pochedly C (eds) Rhabdomyosarcoma and related tumors in children and adolescents. CRC Press, Boca Raton

127. Newton WA, et al. (1995) Classification of rhabdomyosarcomas and related sarcomas. Pathologic aspects and proposal for a new classification. An intergroup rhabdomyosarcoma study. Cancer 76:1073–1085

128. Wiener ES, et al. (2001) Controversies in the management of paratesticular rhabdomyosarcoma: Is staging retroperitoneal lymph node dissection necessary for adolescents with resected paratesticular rhabdomyosarcoma? Semin Pediat Surg 10:146–152

129. Crist W, et al. (1995) Intergroup rhabdomyosarcoma study (IRS) III. J Clin Oncol 13:610–630

130. Raney RB Jr (1991) Rhabdomyosarcoma and related tumors of the head and neck in childhood. In: Maurer HM, Ruymann FB, Pochedly C (eds) Rhabdomyosarcoma and related tumors in children and adolescents. CRC, Boca Raton

131. Raney RB Jr, et al. (1987) Improved prognosis with intensive treatment of children with cranial soft tissue sarcomas arising in nonorbital parameningeal sites: A report from the intergroup rhabdomyosarcoma study. Cancer 59:147–155

132. Wharam M, et al. (1987) Management of orbital rhabdomyosarcoma. In Jacob C (ed) Cancers of the head and neck. Martinus Niijhoff, Boston

133. Andrassy RJ, et al. (1996) Extremity sarcomas: An analysis of prognostic factors from the intergroup rhabdomyosarcoma study (IRS) III. J Pediatr Surg 31:191–196

134. Neville HL, et al. (2000) Preoperative staging, prognostic factors, and outcome for extremity rhabdomyosarcoma: A preliminary report from the Intergroup Rhabdomyosarcoma Study IV (1991–1997.) J Pediatr Surg 35:317–321

135. Rodeberg D, et al. (2005) Characteristics and outcomes of rhabdomyosarcoma patients with isolated lung metastases from IRS-IV. J Pediatr Surg 40(1):256–262

136. Lobe TE, et al. (1994) Neonatal rhabdomyosarcoma: The IRS experience. J Pediatr Surg 29:1167–1170

137. Neville HL, et al. (2000) Lymphatic mapping with sentinel node biopsy in pediatric patients. J Pediatr Surg 35:961–964

138. Lawrence W Jr, et al. (1988) Surgical lessions from the intergroup rhabdomyosarcoma study (IRS) pertaining to extremity tumors. World J Surg 12:676–684

139. Andrassy RJ (1997) Rhabdomyosarcoma. Semin Pediatr Surg 6:17–23

140. Crist WM, et al. (2001) Intergroup rhabdomyosarcoma study-IV: Results for patients with nonmetastatic disease. J Clin Oncol 19:3091–3012

141. Raney RB, et al. (2001) The Intergroup Rhabdomyosarcoma Study Group (IRSG): Major lessons from the IRS-I through IRS-IV studies as background for the current IRS-IV treatment protocols. Sarcoma 5:9–15

142. Hays DM, et al. (1989) Primary re-excision for patients with "microscopic residual" following initial excision of sarcomas of trunk and extremity sites. J Pediatr Surg 24:5–10

143. Cofer BR, et al. (1998) Rhabdomyosarcoma. In: Andrassy RJ (ed). Pediatric surgical oncology. WB Saunders, Philadelphia

144. Wiener ES, et al. (1991) Rhabdomyosarcoma in extremity and trunk sites. In: Maurer HM, Ruymann FB, Pochedly C (eds) Rhabdomyosarcoma and related tumors in children and adolescents. CRC Press, Boca Raton

145. Wiener ES (1993) Rhabdomyosarcoma: New dimensions in management. Semin Pediatr Surg 2:47–58

146. Wiener ES, et al. (for the IRS Committee of CCSG, POG, UKCCSG) (1990) Second look operations in children in group III and IV rhabdomyosarcoma (RMS). SIOP XXII Meeting, October, Rome. Med Pediatr Oncol 18:408

147. Wiener E, et al. (for the IRS Committee of CCSG and POG) (1991) Complete response or not complete response? Second look operations are the answer in children with rhabdomyosarcoma. ASCO Annual Meeting, May 19–21, 1991, Houston, Texas. Proc Am Soc Clin Oncol 10:316

148. Wolden SL, et al. (1999) Indications for radiotherapy and chemotherapy after complete resection in rhabdomyosarcoma: A report from the Intergroup Rhabdomyosarcoma Studies (IRS) I to III. J Clin Oncol 17:3468–3475

149. Wiener ES, et al. (1994) Retroperitoneal node biopsy in paratesticular rhabdomyosarcoma. J Pediatr Surg 29:171–178

150. Lawrence W Jr, et al. (1988) Surgical lessions from the intergroup rhabdomyosarcoma study (IRS) pertaining to extremity tumors. World J Surg 12:676–684

151. Mandell L, et al. (1990) Prognostic significance of regional lymph node involvement in childhood extremity rhabdomyosarcoma. Med Pediatr Oncol 18:466–471

152. Crist W, et al. (For the IRS Committee) (1990) Prognosis in children with rhabdomyosarcoma – A report of IRS-I and IRS-II. J Clin Oncol 8:443–452

153. Maurer HM, et al. (1988) The intergroup rhabdomyosarcoma study-I: A final report. Cancer 61:209–220

154. Maurer HM, et al. (1993) The intergroup rhabdomyosarcoma study-II. Cancer 71:1904–1922

155. Ruymann F, et al. (1997) Comparison of two doublet chemotherapy regimes and conventional radiotherapy in metastatic rhabdomyosarcoma: Improved overall survival using ifosfamide/etoposide compared to vincristine/melphalan in IRSG-IV. Proc Am Soc Clin Oncol 16:521a

156. Miser JS, et al. (1987) Ifosfamide with mesna uroprotection and etoposide: An effective regimen in the treatment of recurrent sarcomas and other tumors of children and young adults. J Clin Oncol 5:1191–1198

157. Crist W, et al. (1999) Preliminary results for patients with local/regional tumors treated on the Intergroup Rhabdomyosarcoma Study-IV (1991–1997). Pro Am Soc Clin Oncol 18:18

158. Anderson GJ, et al. (1990) Rhabdomyosarcoma of the head and neck in children. Arch Otolaryngol Head Neck Surg 116:428–431

159. Gross M, et al. (1988) Therapy of rhabdomyosarcoma of the larynx. Int J Pediatr Otorhinolaryngol 15:93–97

160. Pappo AS, et al. (1997) A phase II trial of high-dose methotrexate in previously untreated children and adolescents with high-risk unresectable or metastatic rhabdomyosarcoma. J Pediatr Hematol Oncol 19:438–442

161. Pappo AS, et al. (2001) Up-front window trial of topotecan in previously untreated children and adolescents with metastatic rhabdomyosarcoma: An Intergroup Rhabdomyosarcoma Study (IRSG). J Clin Oncol 19:213–219

162. Vietti T, et al. (1997) Topotecan window in patients with rhabdomyosarcoma (RMS): An IRSG study. Proc Am Soc Clin Oncol 16:510a

163. Horowitz ME, et al. (1993) Total-body irradiation and autologous bone marrow transplant in the treatment of high-risk Ewing's sarcoma and rhabdomyosarcoma. J Clin Oncol 11:1911–1918

164. Koscielniak E, et al. (1997) Do patients with metastatic and recurrent rhabdomyosarcoma benefit from high-dose therapy with hematopoietic rescue? Report of the German/Austrian Pediatric Bone Marrow Transplantation Group. Bone Marrow Transplan 19:227–231

165. Furman W, et al. (1998) A Phase I study of irinotecan (CPT-11) in children with relapsed solid tumors. Proc Am Soc Clin Oncol 17:187a

166. Donaldson S, et al. (1995) Hyperfractionated radiation in children with rhabdomyosarcoma – Results of an intergroup rhabdomyosarcoma pilot study. Int J Radiat Oncol Biol Phys 32:903–911

167. Donaldson SS, et al. (2000) Results from the Intergroup Rhabdomyosarcoma Study-IV randomized trial of hyperfractionated radiation in children with rhabdomyosarcoma. Int J Radiat Oncol Biol Phys 48:178

168. Smith LM, et al. (2000) Which patients with rhabdomyosarcoma (RMS) and microscopic residual tumor (Group II) fail therapy? A report from the Intergroup Rhabdomyosarcoma Study Group (IRSG). Proc Am Soc Clin Oncol 19:577a

169. Raney RB, et al. (2000) Results of treating localized cranial parameningeal sarcoma on Intergroup Rhabdomyosarcoma (RMS) Studies (IRS)-II through IV. Med Pediatric Oncol 35:178

170. Healy GB, et al. (1991) The role of surgery in rhabdomyosarcoma of the head and neck in children. Arch Otolaryngol Head Neck Surg 117:1185–1188

171. Lawrence W Jr, et al. (1987) Lymphatic metastasis with childhood rhabdomyosarcoma. Cancer 60:910–915

172. Coene IMJH, et al. (1992) Rhabdomyosarcoma of the head and neck in children. Clin Otolaryngol 17:291–296

173. Wiener ES (1994) Head and neck rhabdomyosarcoma. Semin Pediatr Surg 3:203–206

174. Abramson DH, et al. (1979) The treatment of orbital rhabdomyosarcoma with irradiation and chemotherapy. Opthalmology 86:1330–1335

175. Fiorillo A, et al. (1991) Multidisciplinary treatment of primary orbital rhabdomyosarcoma: A single institution experience. Cancer 67:560–563

176. Kao GD, et al. (1993) The sequellae of chemoradiation therapy for head and neck cancer in children: Managing impaired growth, development and other side effects. Med Pediatr Oncol 21:60–66

177. Anderson JR, et al. (1998) Improved outcome for patients with embryonal histology but not alveolar histology rhabdomyosarcoma: Results from Intergroup Rhabdomyosarcoma Study IV (IRS-IV). Proc Soc Clin Oncol 17:526a

178. Gross M, et al. (1988) Therapy of rhabdomyosarcoma of the larynx. Int J Pediatr Otorhinolaryngol 15:93–97

179. Malkin D, et al. (1990) Germ line p53 mutations in a familial syndrome of breast cancer, sarcomas, and other neoplasms. Science 250:1233–1238

180. Raney RB Jr, et al. (1978) Paratesticular rhabdomyosarcoma in children. Cancer 42:729–736

181. Gasparini M, et al. (1990) Questionable role of CNS radioprophylaxis in the therapeutic management of childhood rhabdomyosarcoma with meningeal extension. J Clin Oncol 8:1854–1857

182. Tefft M, et al. (1981) Radiation therapy combined with systemic chemotherapy of rhabdomyosarcoma in children: Local control in patients enrolled into the intergroup rhabdomyosarcoma study. Natl Cancer Inst Monogr 56:75–81

183. Gilles R, et al. (1994) Head and neck rhabdomyosarcomas in children: Value of clinical and CT findings in the detection of local regional relapses. Clin Radiol 49:412–415

184. Raney RB, et al. (For the IRS Committee) (1980) Primary chemotherapy with or without radiation therapy and/or surgery for children with localized sarcoma of the bladder, prostate, vagina, uterus and cervix. A comparison of the results in intergroup rhabdomyosarcoma studies I and II. Cancer 66:2072–2081

185. Raney B, et al. (1993) Sequelae of treatment in 109 patients followed from five to fifteen years after diagnosis of sarcoma of the bladder and prostate: A report from the intergroup rhabdomyosarcoma study (IRS) committee. Cancer 71:2387–2394

186. Hays DM, et al. (1990) Partial cystectomy in the management of rhabdomyosarcoma of the bladder: A report from the intergroup rhabdomyosarcoma study. J Pediatr Surg 25:719–723

187. Hays DM, et al. (1991) Retention of functional bladders among patients with vesicle/prostatic sarcomas in the intergroup rhabdomyosarcoma studies (IRS) (1978–1990). Med Pediatr Oncol 19:423 (abstr)

188. Hays D, et al. (1995) Children with vesical rhabdomyosarcoma (RMS) treated by partial cystectomy, with neoadjuvant or adjuvant chemotherapy with or without radiotherapy. J Pediatr Hematol Oncol 17:46–52

189. Heyn R, et al. (1997) Preservation of the Bladder in patients with rhabdomyosarcoma. J Clin Oncol 15:69–75

190. Lobe TE, et al. (1996) The argument for conservative, delayed surgery in the management of prostatic rhabdomyosarcoma. J Pediatr Surg 31:1084–1087

191. Leuschner I, et al. (1993) Spindle cell variants of embryonal rhabdomyosarcoma in the paratesticular region: A report of the Inergroup Rhabdomyosarcoma Study. Am J Surg Pathol 17:221–230

192. Hamilton CR, et al. (1989) The management of paratesticular rhabdomyosarcoma. Clin Radiol 40:314–317

193. Goldfarb B, et al. (1994) The role of retroperitoneal lymphadenectomy in localized paratesticular rhabdomyosarcoma. J Urol 152:785–787

194. Olive D, et al. (1984) Paraaortic lymphadenectomy is not necessary in the treatment of localized paratesticular rhabdomyosarcoma. Cancer 54:1283–1287

195. Heyn R, et al. (for the IRS Study Committee) (1992) Late effects of therapy in patients with paratesticular rhabdomyosarcoma. J Clin Oncol 10:614–623

196. Wiener ES, et al. What is optimal management for children or adolescents with localized paratesticular rhabdomyosarcoma? Results in IRS-III and IRS-IV. J Pediatr Surg (in press)

197. Breneman JC, et al. (1996) The management of pediatric genitourinary rhabdomyosarcoma. In: Vogelzang NJ, et al (eds) The comprehensive textbook of genitourinary oncology. Williams & Wilkins, Baltimore

198. Andrassy RJ, et al. (1995) Conservative surgical management of vaginal and vulvar pediatric rhabdomyosarcoma: A report from the intergroup rhabdomyosarcoma study-III. J Pediatr Surg 30:1034–1036

199. Corpron CA, et al. (1995) Conservative management of uterine pediatric rhabdomyosarcoma: A report from the Intergroup Rhabdomyosarcoma Study III and IV Pilot. J Pediatr Surg 30:942–944

200. Arndt CA, et al. (2001) What constitutes optimal therapy for patients with rhabdomyosarcoma of the female genital tract? Cancer 91:2454–2468

201. Andrassy R, et al. (1998) Thoracic sarcomas in children. Ann Surg 227:170–173

202. Raney B, et al. (for the IRS Committee) (1982) Soft-tissue sarcoma for the trunk in childhood: Results of the intergroup rhabdomyosarcoma study (IRS), 1972–1976. Cancer 49:2612–2616

203. Beech TR, et al. (1999) What comprises appropriate therapy for children/adolescents with rhabdomyosarcoma arising in the abdominal wall? A report from the Intergroup Rhabdomyosarcoma Study Group. J Pediatr Surg 34:668–671

204. Crist WM, et al. (1985) Soft tissue sarcomas arising in the retroperitoneal space in children. A report from the intergroup rhabdo-myosarcoma study. Cancer 56:2125–2132

205. Blakely ML, et al. (1999) Does debulking improve survival rate in advanced-stage retroperitoneal embryonal rhabdomyosarcoma? J Pediatr Surg 5:736–741

206. Raney RB, et al. (2004) Results of treatment of 56 patients with localized retroperitoneal and Pelvic Rhabdomyosarcoma: A report from the Intergroup Rhabdomyosarcoma Study-IV, 1991–1997. Pediatr Blood Cancer 42:618–625

207. Pollono DG, et al. (1998) Rhabdomyosarcoma of extrahepatic biliary tree: Initial treatment with chemotherapy and conservative surgery. Med Pediatr Oncol 30:290–293

208. Spunt SL, et al. (2000) Aggressive surgery is unwarranted for biliary tract rhabdomyosarcoma. J Pediatr Surg 35:309–316

209. Blakely ML, et al. (2003) Prognostic factors and surgical treatment guidelines for children with rhabdomyosarcoma of the perineum or anus: A report of Intergroup Rhabdomyosarcoma Studies I through IV, 1972 through 1997. J Pediatr Surg 38:347–353

210. Neville HL, et al. (2000) Preoperative staging, prognostic factors, and outcome for extremity rhabdomyosarcoma: A preliminary report from the Intergroup Rhabdomyosarcoma Study IV (1991–1997). J Pediatr Surg 35:317–321

211. Andrassy RJ (2002) Advances in the surgical management of sarcomas in children. Am J Surg 184:484–491

212. La Quaglia MP, et al. (1990) Factors predictive of mortality in pediatric extremity rhabdomyosarcoma. J Pediatr Surg 25:238–243

213. Rich DC, et al. (1997) Second malignant neoplasms in children after treatment of soft tissue sarcoma. J Pediatr Surg 32:369–372

214. Breneman JC, et al. (2003) Prognostic factors and clinical outcomes in children and adolescents with metastatic rhabdomyosarcoma – A report from the Intergroup Rhabdomyosarcoma Study IV. J Clin Oncol 21:78–84

215. Hayes-Jordan A, Doherty DK, West SD, et al. (2006) Outcome after surgical resection of recurrent rhabdomyosarcoma. J Pediatr Surg 41:633–638

216. Klingbiel T, Pertl U, Hess CF, et al. (1998) Treatment of children with relapsed soft tissue sarcoma: Report of the german CESS/CWS REZ 91 trial. Med Pediatr Oncol 30:269–275

Lymphoma

15

Deborah F. Billmire

Contents

15.1 Introduction

Although treatment of lymphoma in children is primarily medical in nature, the pediatric surgeon plays an important role in establishing the diagnosis and also has an impact on the timely initiation of chemotherapy for these rapidly growing tumors. The surgeon's contributions are crucial to successful management. He or she must be aware of the clinical presentations of lymphoma so that the diagnosis is considered and tissue is appropriately handled. Fresh specimens should be submitted to the pathologist so that all testing can be accomplished to properly assign subtype and staging. The appropriate decision regarding biopsy versus resection must be made. Resection of major organs is generally unnecessary and major procedures may also entail morbidity that would delay initiation of chemotherapy. On the other hand, resection of localized tumors in some cases may reduce the amount of chemo-

therapy with its associated organ toxicity. The potential hazards of anesthesia should be recognized in certain situations and the possible use of less invasive diagnostic tools such as examination of pleural and ascitic fluids should be considered. Proper handling of tissue and prompt initiation of chemotherapy will allow for optimal response to therapy for these children.

Childhood lymphoma is divided into two major categories, Hodgkin's disease (HD) and non-Hodgkin's lymphoma (NHL). Although there is some overlap in presentation, the clinical features of non-Hodgkin's lymphoma are much more varied. The management and prognosis of these two categories are also different and each will be discussed separately.

15.2 Hodgkin's Disease

Hodgkin's disease accounts for approximately 6% of childhood cancer and 40% of pediatric lymphoma. The incidence varies from 0.3 to 3 per 100,000 person years [28]. The incidence of Hodgkin's disease increases with age and most pediatric cases occur in adolescents (Fig. 15.1). Hodgkin's disease is uncommon in children less than 10 years of age in the USA

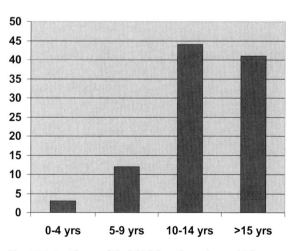

Fig. 15.1 Incidence of Hodgkin's lymphoma by age [42]

[58]. It occurs more frequently in males, particularly at younger ages. The histologic subtype also varies with age. Younger children are more likely to have lymphocyte-predominant or mixed cellularity. Adolescents most often have nodular sclerosing histology.

15.2.1 Histology/Tumor Markers

Hodgkin's disease is characterized on histologic examination by the Reed-Sternberg cell. This is a multinucleated giant cell with two prominent nucleoli that have a characteristic appearance said to resemble "owl eyes." These neoplastic cells are found in an inflammatory milieu including infiltrating lymphoid cells, plasma cells, and fibrous stroma that constitute the bulk of the enlarged node. There are four major subtypes of Hodgkin's disease that are defined by the relative proportions of normal lymphocytes to Reed-Sternberg cells. These subtypes are lymphocyte predominant, mixed cellularity, lymphocyte depleted and nodular sclerosing. Prognosis worsens with decrease in the proportion of lymphocytes.

The Reed-Sternberg cell has its origin from preapoptotic germinal center B cells. Similar to those non-Hodgkin's lymphomas that arise from B cell origin, there is an association of Hodgkin's disease with Epstein-Barr virus (EBV). EBV genetic material is found in up to 40% of children with Hodgkin's disease. It is most common in children less than 10 years and is usually seen in those with the mixed cellularity subtype. It is seldom found in those with nodular sclerosing histology.

15.2.2 Diagnostic Evaluation and Staging System

Children with Hodgkin's disease most often present with enlarged, rubbery nodes in the cervical or supraclavicular region. A complete physical examination with attention to all nodal areas as well as a careful examination of the abdomen should be performed. Blood work should include complete blood count, erythrocyte sedimentation rate, renal and hepatic function studies, and alkaline phosphatase. Imaging studies should include chest radiography and CT scans of the chest, abdomen, and pelvis. Bone scan should be performed in those with elevated alkaline phosphatase. Current protocols also employ gallium or positron emission tomography (PET) scans (Fig. 15.2). The fluorodeoxyglucose (FDG) PET scan has become the preferred modality for both initial diagnosis and follow-up scans because of its higher resolution, 1-day scan time and improved detection of disease below the diaphragm [13]. One study of combined PET/CT

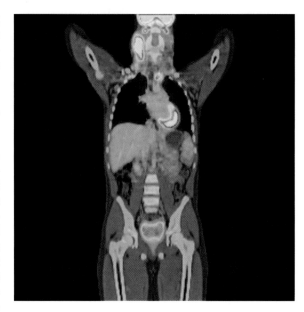

Fig. 15.2 PET-CT scan of mediastinal non-Hodgkin's lymphoma

scanning in childhood lymphoma (both Hodgkin's and non-Hodgkin's) noted better predictive value of negative scans than positive scans when used for follow-up imaging and recommended caution in interpretation of equivocal and positive scans [50]. In patients with stage III or IV disease and those with symptoms of fever or night sweats, bone marrow aspiration and biopsy are also needed. Staging laparotomy is no longer used in pediatric Hodgkin's lymphoma since all current pediatric protocols employ systemic chemotherapy.

The staging system for Hodgkin's disease is based on the revised Ann Arbor system [33] (Table 15.1). Patients are also given a designation of A or B based on symptomatic criteria. Patients with unexplained weight loss of greater than 10% of body weight in the 6 months preceding diagnosis, unexplained fevers greater than 38°C for greater than 3 days, or drenching night sweats are assigned to category B. All others are assigned to category A.

15.2.3 Clinical Presentation/Surgical Issues

In contrast to non-Hodgkin's lymphoma, Hodgkin's disease occurs primarily in nodal anatomic sites and tends to follow an orderly anatomic progression. There are 20 defined areas of nodal groupings (Table 15.2). Painless, rubbery enlargement of cervical or supraclavicular nodes is the most common presenting complaint and is seen in 80% of patients. Primary presentation as axillary or groin adenopathy is far less common and occurs in less than 3% of children (Fig. 15.3). The

Table 15.1 Cotswold modification of the Ann Arbor staging system for Hodgkin's Lymphoma [33]

Stage I	Involvement of single lymph node region (I) or localized involvement of a single extralymphatic organ or site (IE).
Stage II	Involvement of two or more lymph node regions on the same side of the diaphragm (II) or localized contiguous involvement of a single extralymphatic organ or site and its regional lymph node(s) with involvement of one or more lymph node regions on the same side of the diaphragm (IIE).
Stage III	Involvement of lymph node regions on both sides of the diaphragm (III), which may also be accompanied by localized contiguous involvement of an extralymphatic organ or site (IIIE), by involvement of the spleen (IIIS), or both (IIIE+S)
Stage IV	Disseminated (multifocal) involvement of one or more extralymphatic organs or tissues, with or without associated lymph node involvement, or isolated extralymphatic organ involvement with distant (nonregional) nodal involvement

Table 15.2 Defined nodal groupings for Hodgkin's lymphoma

Peripheral regions
Right neck; cervical, supraclavicular occipital, and preauricular
Left neck; cervical, supraclavicular occipital, and pre-auricular
Right infraclavicular
Left infraclavicular
Right axilla and pectoral
Left axilla and pectoral
Right epitrochlear and brachial
Left epitrochlear and brachial
Central regions
Waldeyer's ring (including base of tongue)
Mediastinum (including paratracheal)
Hilar
Mesenteric
Para-aortic (including retrocrural, portal and celiac)
Splenic/splenic hilar
Lower regions
Right iliac
Left iliac
Right inguinal and femoral
Left inguinal and femoral
Right popliteal
Left popliteal

release of lymphocytokines by the Reed-Sternberg cells produces systemic symptoms in up to one third of patients. These symptoms include fever, night sweats, and weight loss as described above.

The surgeon's role is to provide adequate tissue for diagnostic studies with minimal morbidity, and to provide staging information in selected subgroups. In general, an incisional or excisional biopsy of involved nodes is preferred. Use of cautery should be avoided on the tissue to be submitted to minimize coagulation artifact. Needle biopsies do not provide sufficient tissue for histologic and biologic studies.

Mediastinal involvement occurs in two thirds of patients at presentation and is relevant to prognosis.

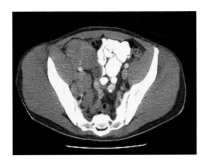

Fig. 15.3 CT scan demonstrating primary iliac nodal presentation of Hodgkin's lymphoma

A ratio of maximal diameter of the mass to the thoracic cavity greater than 1:3 on posterior-anterior chest radiography is associated with worsened prognosis [28]. The possibility of a mediastinal mass is a particularly important factor for the surgeon to be aware of in patients with lymphoma. In patients presenting with cervical or supraclavicular adenopathy, the status of the mediastinum must be assessed prior to anesthesia for biopsy. For those patients that present with an isolated mediastinal mass, a search should be made for more accessible disease outside the mediastinum for biopsy under local anesthesia. If a pleural effusion is present, the fluid may be aspirated for cytology but this is usually more successful in non-Hodgkin's lymphoma. The potential hazards of anesthesia must be considered prior to biopsy. It is well recognized that anterior mediastinal masses of all types pose a risk for respiratory or hemodynamic collapse under general anesthesia and multiple fatal cases have been reported. Loss of ventilation occurs at several levels. This may include severe narrowing of the trachea and bronchi and is further compromised under anesthesia by loss of smooth muscle airway tone causing distal collapse well beyond reach of a mechanical airway [51]. Encasement of the pulmonary arteries may also occur leading to mortality despite adequate airway control. Clinical symptomatology does not provide a reliable assessment of risk, but the presence of orthopnea is considered to be of particular concern [54]. Objective parameters such as peak expiratory flow rate (PEFR) less than 50% and tracheal cross section less than 50% of predicted are felt to be predictors of high risk as described by Shamberger [56, 57]. PEFR is easily done at the bedside and should be measured in the supine position as well as upright. The tracheal cross section should be calculated from the CT scan using an imaging window level of 450 and compared to the graph of normal values provided by Shamberger. Significant variance occurs when different CT window levels are used and calculations become unreliable [51]. In patients considered to be at high risk for general anesthesia, consideration should be given to biopsy in the upright position under local anesthesia or to prebiopsy radiation with shielding of selected nodes. Fine needle biopsy provided adequate tissue for diagnosis of lymphoma in up to 83% of pediatric patients in one series, but subtyping to determine therapy cannot be done with this type of tissue sample [61]. Once diagnosis is definitive and therapy is initiated, clinical response is rapid. Chemotherapy can be initiated through a peripherally inserted central catheter and within one or two cycles, general anesthesia can be safely undertaken to provide a more convenient central access with subcutaneous reservoir (Fig. 15.4a, 4b).

Although staging laparotomy is no longer performed for pediatric Hodgkin's disease, the concept of oophoropexy may still be relevant in certain patients. Radiation of the pelvic nodes (inverted Y field) or central pelvis may be employed in select cases. It is well known that pelvic radiation may result in premature ovarian failure with loss of fertility and endocrine function. This risk is directly related to radiation dose with consistent loss of ovarian function from single doses of 8 Gy or fractionated doses of 15 Gy [65]. The risk is inversely proportional to age at the time of treatment, thus putting younger patients at the highest concern for sterility and impact of loss of hormonal function.

Radiation doses for treatment of Hodgkin's disease typically involve 20–35 Gy. Prior to the development of oophoropexy for this problem, loss of ovarian function was almost universal. Oophoropexy, usually per-

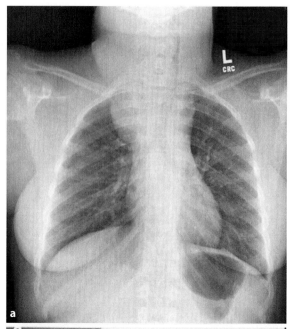

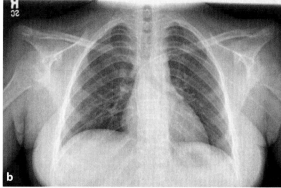

Fig. 15.4 Mediastinal Hodgkin's lymphoma demonstrating tracheal compression at diagnosis (**a**) relieved after one cycle of chemotherapy (**b**)

formed at the time of staging laparotomy, resulted in preservation of ovarian function in 0–66% of women [14, 30, 60]. Limited data on efficacy of oophoropexy is available in the pediatric age group. In 1992, Hays' report on staging procedures for advanced pediatric Hodgkin's disease included seven girls that had pelvic radiation to 21 Gy. Two had no oophoropexy and had delayed or no menarche. All five who had oophoropexy had normal menses [18]. In 1992, Williams and Mendenhall reported a laparoscopic technique for oophoropexy in patients planned to undergo inverted Y pelvic radiation for Hodgkin's disease [65]. Helpful operative details and illustrations are provided in the report. An umbilical camera port is placed initially and two additional working ports are placed 4 cm above the pubic symphysis. One port is in the midline and one is in the left lower quadrant. A 2-0 silk on a straight Keith needle is used to pass through the utero-ovarian ligament immediately adjacent to the ovary, then passed through the posterior uterine serosa overlying the lower uterine segment, and then through the contra-lateral utero-ovarian ligament. When this suture is tied intra-corporeally, the ovaries are brought together in the midline posterior to the uterus. The medial and lateral borders of each ovary are marked with clips for assistance in defining the radiation field by imaging. These authors provided a follow-up review of 12 patients in 1999 and stressed several points [64]. They cited reports by other authors of clip separation and recommended ultrasound imaging shortly before radiation to confirm that the clips remain associated with the ovaries [17]. They also described two patients in their series that had previously undergone open oophoropexy at the time of initial staging laparotomy. Laparoscopy was done as a second procedure 5 and 6 months later, respectively (just prior to radiation), and demonstrated that the ovaries had migrated back to their original positions. It was recommended that the oophoropexy be done in close proximity to the planned radiation to minimize time for migration of the ovaries. Finally, they also noted ovarian failure despite oophoropexy in four of five patients that had received six or more cycles of chemotherapy. Females that are to undergo radiation therapy to the central pelvis would need to have the ovaries pexed laterally to the pelvic sidewalls.

15.2.4 Treatment

Although primary treatment for Hodgkin's disease has been highly successful (90–95% survival) since the 1980s, the therapeutic strategies have been in constant evolution. Initial successful treatment for localized Hodgkin's lymphoma involved targeted radiation therapy in both adults and children with doses ranging from 35 to 40 Gy [63]. This management strategy required accurate assessment of spread of disease at diagnosis for success. The concept of staging laparotomy was developed to confirm extent of disease in the abdomen. The staging procedure itself was not of therapeutic benefit. From this body of experience, it was learned that staging laparotomy resulted in restaging (up or down) in 25–40% of patients that had been clinically staged by CT scan and lymphangiography [6, 63]. Approximately 80–90% of positive staging laparotomies for Hodgkin's disease in the pediatric population involve the spleen. The pattern of abdominal spread follows an orderly sequence similar to adults with nodal spread to the splenic hilum, then to the para-aortic region and finally to distal nodal groups [6]. Involvement of portahepatic nodes varies among pediatric reviews [6, 18]. Hays, et al. reviewed

49 pediatric staging laparotomies in a Children's Cancer Study Group protocol [18]. They noted poor compliance with complete staging guidelines and also analyzed the patterns of abdominal involvement. In this review, positive splenic hilar nodes were highly predictive of splenic involvement. They also confirmed that when para-aortic nodes were negative, the yield of more distal inferior nodes was very unlikely. Based of their data, they proposed a modified staging procedure in children with fewer required components. Follow-up data on these patients revealed no therapeutic benefit to staging laparotomy and a complication rate of 2.8–6% [6, 19]. In addition, there was a long-term risk of postsplenectomy sepsis.

The recognition that high-dose radiation in the growing child resulted in unacceptable musculoskeletal and cardiac toxicity and led to the adoption of chemotherapy for all stages of disease and provided systemic treatment impact. Staging laparotomy became unnecessary and treatment protocols were based on other parameters defining extent of disease. Risk factors such as tumor burden, presence of B symptoms, male gender, and sedimentation rate were included in risk stratification. The early chemotherapy regimens consisted of either nitrogen mustard, vincristine, procarbazine, and prednisone (MOPP), or doxorubicin, bleomycin, vinblastine, and dacarbazine (ABVD).

Further studies looked at combinations of these regimens in alternating cycles to allow greater efficacy from nonoverlapping mechanisms and to minimize toxicity. Radiation protocols were modified to consist of low-dose involved field radiation therapy (LD-IFRT) using 15–25 Gy.

Long-term follow-up has continued to reveal toxicities of the various chemotherapy agents as well as a significant incidence of second malignancies. The alkylating agent nitrogen mustard has been replaced by cyclophosphamide (combination therapy known as COPP) due to the more leukemogenic properties of the mustard.

Current trials are evaluating the success and comparative morbidity of various regimens with or without LD-IFRT [22, 26]. It has been observed in some trials that early responders to chemotherapy have better outcome and this has been incorporated as a decision factor to randomize whether or not to use radiation therapy.

Unlike many other pediatric tumors, the salvage rate for relapsed HD is quite high. This provides another area for controversy and discussion. Second courses of therapy carry an additional risk of toxicity and late second malignancy. Outcome goals must include not only short-term success but also long-term survival and quality of life.

15.2.5 Prognosis and Long Term Effects

Survival rates for pediatric Hodgkin's disease have been greater than 90% since the mid 1980s and provide a growing population of long-term cancer survivors. Long-term follow-up has revealed an increased risk for a spectrum of second malignancies with variable survival. In 1989, Meadows estimated the cumulative probability of any second neoplasm after treatment of pediatric Hodgkin's disease to be 20% after 20 years of follow-up [37]. A more recent follow-up study from Bhatia, et al. on behalf of the Late Effects Study Group looked at 1,380 children who had been treated for Hodgkin's disease and noted 88 second neoplasms with an actuarial incidence of 7% at 15 years after diagnosis [5]. Many of these neoplasms can be linked to specific treatment components and the risk of second neoplasm appears to be greater in children than adults. Recognition of these associations has stimulated the ongoing modifications of treatment protocols for pediatric Hodgkin's disease in an effort to balance short-term success with long-term outcome. The long latency for secondary solid tumors in particular makes this a challenging task with continued need for ongoing long-term follow-up.

Secondary leukemia, myelodysplastic syndrome, and non-Hodgkin's lymphoma all occur with increased risk after treatment of pediatric HD and carry a poor prognosis. The use of alkylating agents is strongly liked to secondary leukemia and has been variably liked to myelodysplastic syndrome and NHL in some studies [32].

Most solid tumors have a latency period of greater than 10 years. Breast cancer is well recognized as a secondary neoplasm of increased risk after treatment of pediatric Hodgkin's disease [47]. It is most strongly linked to radiation therapy with greatest risk when dose is greater than 40 Gy. These malignancies are often bilateral and are in the radiation field in the medial breast or upper-outer quadrant. Radiation therapy during puberty or young adulthood appears to increase the relative risk, presumably due to the proliferative state of the hormonally sensitive tissue. Chemotherapy and splenectomy may also be risk factors [32]. It is recommended that girls treated for pediatric HD be followed with annual breast exams until 25 years. Surveillance should then increase to include breast examination every 6 months and yearly mammography for those that received radiation therapy [32]. Secondary thyroid cancer is also linked to radiation therapy and is the second most common solid secondary cancer. Solid tumors of the gastrointestinal tract also occur with increased risk, particularly colorectal and gastric. The latency period is 10–20 years and symptoms are generally absent until advanced stages. It is recommended that monitoring surveillance be done beginning

15 years after radiation or at age 35 years (whichever is later) [32]. Lung cancer also carries an increase in relative risk. This is markedly potentiated by smoking and increases the relative risk by an additional 20 fold [32]. Secondary sarcomas have a relative increase in risk by 10 to 14.9 fold. Radiation and alkylating agents are both liked to bone tumors in particular, and these tumors are most likely to occur during the adolescent growth spurt.

15.3 Non-Hodgkin's Lymphoma

Non-Hodgkin's lymphoma accounts for approximately 60% of pediatric lymphomas [52]. The vast majority are high-grade tumors with rapid growth. The incidence of these tumors increases steadily with age. There has been a 30% increase in the annual incidence of pediatric lymphoma in the USA during the period from 1973 to 1991. European data also show an annual increase in incidence of childhood non-Hodgkin's lymphoma over the period from 1988 through 1997 [23].

15.3.1 Histology/Tumor Markers

Non-Hodgkin's lymphomas are classified pathologically by a combination of morphologic and immunophenotypic features. The main subcategories are undifferentiated, lymphoblastic, and large cell lymphomas. These three groups account for the vast majority of pediatric cases. Follicular lymphoma is a rare category with a more favorable prognosis.

15.3.1.1 Undifferentiated

Undifferentiated lymphomas account for 40–50% of cases of pediatric NHL. These are also called small, noncleaved cell lymphomas based on their histologic appearance. Burkitt's lymphoma typically has what has been called a "starry sky" appearance due to the presence of interspersed benign histiocytes among the neoplastic cells. The undifferentiated lymphomas are of B cell origin and include both Burkitt's and non-Burkitt's tumors. Most of the abdominal non-Hodgkin's lymphomas in children are in this subgroup. Immunophenotypically these tumors are distinguished by positive staining for the markers CD19 and CD 20. They are negative for the enzyme TdT.

15.3.1.2 Lymphoblastic

Lymphoblastic lymphomas account for 30–40% of childhood NHL. These tumors are of T cell origin and account for the majority of tumors presenting in the mediastinum. They may also demonstrate a starry sky appearance on histologic examination and the neoplastic cells have smaller nuclei. Immunophenotypically, these tumors are characterized by positive staining for the enzyme TdT, a known T cell characteristic.

15.3.1.3 Large Cell

Large cell lymphomas account for 15% of childhood NHL. These tumors are very aggressive in their behavior and are seen at all sites. They may be of B or T cell origin and are distinguished histologically by the presence of large nuclei.

15.3.1.4 Follicular

Follicular lymphomas are rare and account for less than 2% of pediatric non-Hodgkin's lymphoma [3]. They are of B cell origin and are characterized by follicular architecture on histologic examination. Immunophenotypic features include positive staining for CD20 and bcl-6. Most also show CD10 positivity. The most common anatomic primary site for these lymphomas is the head and neck region. Follicular lymphoma in children is usually low stage and has a favorable prognosis with complete excision. In contrast to adults, Bcl-2 expression is noted in a minority of cases. One pediatric series has shown that Bcl-2 expression is associated with disseminated disease and poor prognosis [34].

15.3.2 Diagnostic Evaluation/Staging System

Evaluation of the child with suspected or confirmed non-Hodgkin's lymphoma begins with a complete physical examination with particular attention to nodal areas. Involved peripheral nodes may provide a preferred means of tissue diagnosis with extensive chest or abdominal primary tumors. Laboratory evaluation should include complete blood count with differential, electrolytes, renal panel, and urinalysis and liver function studies. Lactic dehydrogenase (LDH) and uric acid are helpful as indices of metabolic turnover and LDH is recognized as a marker of tumor burden and prognosis [52]. Disease should be sought in diffuse sites including bilateral bone marrow aspirates, spinal fluid examination, chest x-ray and CT scan of the neck, chest, abdomen and pelvis. Bone scan should

Table 15.3 Murphy staging system for non-Hodgkin's lymphoma [41]

Stage	Criteria for extent of disease
Localized	
I	A single tumor (extranodal) or single anatomic area (nodal) with the exclusion of mediastinum or abdomen
II	A single tumor (extranodal) with regional node involvement
	Two or more nodal areas on the same side of the diaphragm
	Two single (extranodal) tumors with or without regional node involvement on the same side of the diaphragm
	A primary gastrointestinal tumor, usually in the ileocecal area, with or without involvement of associated mesenteria nodes only, grossly completely resected
Disseminated	
III	Two single tumors (extranodal) on opposite sides of the diaphragm
	Two or more nodal areas above and below the diaphragm
	All primary intra-thoracic tumors (mediastinal, pleural, thymic)
	All extensive primary intra-abdominal disease
	All parasipnal or epidural tumors, regardless of other tumor site(s)
IV	Any of the above with initial CNS and/or bone marrow involvement

also be performed. As in Hodgkin's disease, FDG-PET scans are also employed for staging and follow-up in some pediatric non-Hodgkin's lymphoma protocols [21]. Immune deficiency states are known to increase the risk of lymphoma and testing for human immunodeficiency virus should also be done.

The staging system employed for non-Hodgkin's lymphoma is shown in Table 15.3.

Although staging is undertaken at diagnosis, these should all be considered widespread tumors at diagnosis with an aggressive potential for rapid growth.

15.3.3 Clinical Presentation and Surgical Issues

The majority of childhood non-Hodgkin's lymphoma presents in extranodal sites. A review of 80 consecutive cases of pediatric NHL from St. Bartholomew's Hospital in London noted a primary site in peripheral

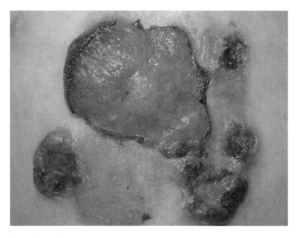

Fig. 15.5 Isolated cutaneous lymphoma

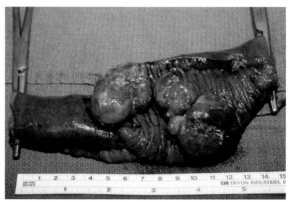

Fig. 15.6 Non-Hodgkin's lymphoma presenting as intestinal obstruction

lymph nodes in only 19% of cases [44]. The abdomen was the most common site presenting in 26% of children followed by extranodal head and neck (23%), and mediastinum (20%). Rare sites including gonads, genitals, skin, and bone accounted for 13% of cases (Fig. 15.5). All four cases of cutaneous lymphoma in Ng's series had localized disease only. Central nervous system disease may be asymptomatic or present with cranial nerve palsy. Involvement of the tonsils may also occur presenting with asymmetric enlargement or with other areas of disease. On rare occasions, isolated tonsillar involvement may be an unexpected finding. A review of routine tonsillectomy specimens by Garavello revealed 2 cases of non-Hodgkin's lymphoma in 1,123 specimens (.18%) from routine pediatric tonsillectomy without clinical suspicion [16].

15.3.3.1 Mediastinum

Mediastinal involvement occurs in about 20% of pediatric cases of non-Hodgkin's lymphoma. These are mainly lymphoblastic lymphomas of T cell origin. Clinical complaints may include symptoms of upper respiratory infection, chest pain, cough, shortness of breath, or signs of superior vena cava syndrome. These masses occur in the anterior mediastinum and carry the same anesthetic risks as described in the section on mediastinal Hodgkin's. Careful physical examination should be done to search for extrathoracic involvement for diagnosis. Pleural effusions are frequently seen (11% of Ng's series) and thoracentesis may provide adequate material for diagnosis [8, 44, 52]. Pericardial effusions may also occur and sometimes result in cardiac tamponade. In contrast to adult malignancy-associated tamponade, pediatric tamponade is effectively treated with percutaneous drainage [35]. Adult malignant effusions are usually a manifes-

tation of end stage disease and tend to loculate unless treated by pericardial window. Pediatric malignancy-associated tamponade usually has negative cytology and responds well to percutaneous drainage alone. In Medary's study, catheters remained in place for a mean of 5 days and were successfully discontinued without recurrence [35].

15.3.3.2 Abdomen

Non-Hodgkin's lymphoma presents as an abdominal primary site in 30% of children [44, 52]. The most common complaint is abdominal pain that has been present for several weeks before diagnosis [12]. Weight loss occurs in nearly half of patients and nausea and vomiting are common. A palpable mass is found in one third of cases. Those children that present with colicky abdominal pain and heme positive stools may have intussusception from an intramural mass in the distal ileum or cecum (Fig. 15.6). Fever is seen in 26% of children and an initial diagnosis of appendicitis may be made. In Fleming's consecutive series of 58 children with NHL of the abdomen, a preoperative diagnosis of lymphoma was made in only one child [12]. Most patients had a preoperative diagnosis of periappendiceal abscess or idiopathic intussusception. The multicenter Children's Cancer Study Group experience reported by LaQuaglia, et al. revealed a similar pattern with correct preoperative diagnosis in 15% of patients [29]. In this series, more than half of children had an urgent operation and most of those were felt to have appendicitis or intussusception.

The surgeon's approach to non-Hodgkin's lymphoma in the abdomen will be dictated by the clinical scenario and anatomic findings. Approximately half of the cases will involve the gastrointestinal tract and the vast majority of those will arise in the distal ileum or the right colon [12]. Most of the gastrointestinal lymphomas will present as an acute abdomen due to tenderness or obstruction and many are focal lesions that are amenable to straightforward resection with anastomosis. It is important for the surgeon to consider the possibility of lymphoma so that the tissue will be properly handled for histopathology and biologic studies. The remaining abdominal lymphomas will usually involve diffuse retroperitoneal spread or include direct infiltration of intra-abdominal viscera precluding a complete resection (Fig. 15.7). When this finding is discovered intraoperatively, a limited biopsy should be undertaken to allow accurate diagnosis and prompt initiation of chemotherapy. Subtotal resection and debulking procedures should be discouraged. Previous recommendations for debulking in the 1980s based on limited retrospective reviews were not confirmed in pediatric studies reported in the 1990s [15, 35, 56, 59, 67]. Surgical complications that lead to a delay in initiation of chemotherapy are felt to contribute to increased mortality risk [59]. Perforation of the bowel is also associated with a poor prognosis and may occur either spontaneously or secondary to surgical biopsy [66]. Second look procedures after induction chemotherapy should also be discouraged with studies showing either continued unresectability of the mass or necrotic tumor only [24, 56].

If an abdominal mass is discovered prior to laparotomy, the possibility of lymphoma should be considered and a search made for extra-abdominal tissue for biopsy. If ascites is present consideration should be given to paracentesis if possible. The diagnosis of NHL has been made by examination of peritoneal cytology, in several cases avoiding the need for more invasive procedures and potential complications [62].

Other abdominal presentations of non-Hodgkin's lymphoma are seen in a small number of cases. Primary involvement of the stomach is common in adults but was found in only one of 58 children in the St. Jude series [12]. There is usually diffuse infiltration of the gastric wall and thickened folds may be seen [27] (Fig. 15.8).

Jaundice often accompanies abdominal lymphoma, but is the presenting symptom in a minority of cases [49]. The liver itself may be the primary site with multiple parenchymal nodules [48]. Most cases are due to obstructive jaundice either from pancreatic involvement causing ampullary obstruction or from peri-portal adenopathy causing extrinsic compression of the common duct. Diagnosis has been made using peritoneal cytology, endoscopic biopsy, needle biopsy, and open biopsy. Percutaneous transhepatic drainage has been associated with complication of persistent biliary fistula causing delay in chemotherapy and is not recommended [62]. As in adults, the rapid response of

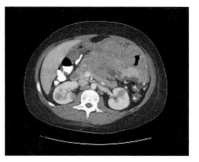

Fig. 15.7 CT scan demonstrating diffuse abdominal non-Hodgkin's lymphoma

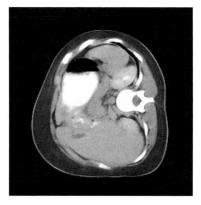

Fig. 15.8 CT scan demonstrating thickened gastric wall due to diffuse infiltration with non-Hodgkin's lymphoma

the tumor bulk to chemotherapy will allow early relief of obstruction [11].

Renal involvement with lymphoma is seen in approximately 4–27% of children and may consist of diffuse involvement or focal lesions [44]. Isolated involvement of the kidney may occur with clinical complaints of flank pain and hematuria. Asymptomatic hypertension has been reported as a presentation of renal lymphoma in children [4, 10].

Other rare abdominal sites include the female pelvic viscera. Primary ovarian lymphomas may present with ovarian enlargement [1]. They have generally been treated by excision and chemotherapy. Although some have questioned the ovary as a primary site, the ovaries have been shown to have small foci of lymphatic tissue in 54% of females in an autopsy series [39]. Well-documented cases of isolated ovarian involvement with follow-up have been reported [39]. In a series of 101 pediatric ovarian neoplasms from New Guinea, 3% were due to Burkitt's lymphoma [53]. Diffuse uterine enlargement from lymphoma has also been reported presenting as an abdominal mass in two young children [36, 40]. Both had additional sites of involvement (renal, CNS). In each case, diagnosis was

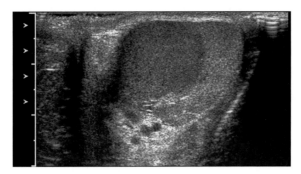

Fig. 15.9 Ultrasound imaging of testicular infiltration due to non-Hodgkin's lymphoma that manifested as testicular enlargement

made by uterine biopsy and the lymphoma was of B cell origin.

15.3.3.3 Testis

Infiltration of the testis by lymphoma is seen in 3–12% of children with non-Hodgkin's lymphoma at diagnosis and may be treated by systemic chemotherapy [9] (Fig. 15.9). Radiation therapy has been used in some protocols due to the concern of the testis as a "sanctuary site" less accessible to chemotherapy. A report by Dalle, et al. in 2001 summarized the French experience with testicular involvement in childhood B cell lymphoma and acute lymphocytic leukemia [9]. Testicular involvement at diagnosis was noted in 30 boys (5.3% of males). Involvement of other anatomic sites was present in all but one boy. Testicular enlargement was the presenting complaint in five of the boys and all underwent diagnostic orchiectomy. The remaining boys were noted to have testicular involvement, but presented with other complaints and underwent testicular biopsy or clinical confirmation only. All were treated with chemotherapy and none received radiation. Clinical regression of testicular involvement was seen in all patients and there were no episodes of testicular relapse. Survival was not influenced by the presence of testicular involvement. The authors concluded that systemic chemotherapy is sufficient for B cell non-Hodgkin's lymphoma in boys and that a careful search should be made for additional sites of disease in boys that present with testicular masses. In rare cases, primary lymphoma arising in the testis will present as testicular enlargement and diagnosis will be made at the time of biopsy or orchiectomy. Both follicular and Burkitt's lymphomas have been reported in children as a primary site [20, 25]. In general, these tumors are treated by orchiectomy and chemotherapy. Successful treatment by orchiectomy alone has been reported in a 3-year-old boy with stage I follicular lymphoma of the testis [20].

15.3.4 Treatment

Non-Hodgkin's lymphoma is considered a systemic disease in all patients and chemotherapy is the cornerstone of successful treatment. As in many other childhood cancers, there has been a remarkable evolution in treatment regimens since the 1960s with continued improvement due to multicenter, cooperative trials. Increasing knowledge of tumor biology has allowed recognition of differential sensitivity to chemotherapeutic agents among various phenotypic subgroups and risk group stratification. As survival improves for certain subgroups, attention may be refocused on reduction of treatment morbidity and long-term consequences. The surgeon's role in providing adequate tissue for accurate diagnosis and biologic studies is crucial in determining the appropriate chemotherapy regimen. It is important to minimize surgical morbidity so that chemotherapy can begin promptly for these tumors since they have such a rapid growth fraction.

The early era of chemotherapy with single agents and radiation produced a survival rate of only 20–30% for childhood NHL. The adoption of multiagent protocols in the 1970s increased survival to 60–70%. A CCG trial was undertaken in the 1970s to compare the two most successful regimens, the LSA2-L2 (cyclophosphamide, vincristine, prednisone, daunomycin, methotrexate, cytarabine, thioguanine, asparaginase, and carmustine) regimen of Wollner based on therapy for acute leukemia, and the COMP regimen (cyclophosphamide, vincristine, methotrexate, prednisone) of Ziegler [67]. This cooperative randomized trial revealed biologic differences in treatment response among the histologic subtypes. It was noted that the LSA2-L2 regimen was more effective for lymphoblastic lymphomas, while undifferentiated lymphomas did better with COMP [2].

Current chemotherapy for NHL is based on the principles of systemic therapy for all patients with attention to histology, immunophenotype, extent of disease, and central nervous system prophylaxis.

Children with low stage (I-II) disease receive multiagent chemotherapy with cyclophosphamide, vincristine, and prednisone. Those with Burkitt's and large cell histology may also receive doxorubicin or methotrexate. Those with lymphoblastic lymphoma may also receive doxorubicin, methotrexate, mercaptopurine, asparaginase, thioguanine cytarabine, or carmustine. In general, number of cycles and length of treatment is longer for the lymphoblastic lymphomas.

Children with advanced stage (III-IV) disease are treated with longer multiagent regimens. Those with Burkitt's histology receive cyclophosphamide, vincristine, prednisone, and high-dose methotrexate. They may also receive etoposide, ifosfamide, doxorubicin, cytarabine, or cisplatin. Those with lymphoblastic lymphoma receive vincristine, prednisone, daunorubicin, or doxorubicin and asparaginase. They may also receive methotrexate, cytarabine, cyclophosphamide, mercaptopurine, thioguanine, teniposide (SP), hydroxyurea, or carmustine. Those with large-cell lymphoma receive vincristine, prednisone, and methotrexate. They may also receive cyclophosphamide, mercaptopurine, thioguanine, hydroxyurea, asparaginase, daunorubicin, doxorubicin, carmustine, or bleomycin.

Central nervous system prophylaxis with intrathecal chemotherapy is given to most patients. If CNS involvement is present at diagnosis, cranial irradiation is usually administered.

The role of radiation therapy outside the central nervous system is limited to only a few situations for childhood NHL. It is occasionally used as emergent therapy for critical airway compression due to mediastinal tumors with shielding of nodal areas planned for biopsy and for massive testicular involvement.

The use of bone marrow transplantation for some types of non-Hodgkin's lymphoma is also under investigation in some centers [17, 31].

15.3.5 Prognosis and Long-term Issues

Children with limited Stage I and II non-Hodgkin's lymphoma have an excellent prognosis for all histologic subtypes with 85–95% 5-year survival. Current cooperative trials for these patients are focused on reductions of chemotherapy to reduce treatment-related morbidity.

Treatment of advanced Stage III and IV disease is more challenging and varies with histologic subtypes. Small cell and Burkitt's lymphomas have a 75% overall survival with current therapy and a recent French trial that included high-dose chemotherapy and etoposide had an 85% success rate [52]. Lymphoblastic lymphoma requires a more prolonged treatment regimen and has a survival of 65–75%. Large cell lymphoma is a more heterogeneous group and the survival for this subgroup is approximately 50–70%.

Unlike Hodgkin's disease, the salvage rate for relapse in non-Hodgkin's lymphoma is poor. Current treatment regimens include a variety of high-dose chemotherapy combinations and may also include bone marrow transplant [43].

References

1. Ambulkar I, Nair R (2003) Primary ovarian lymphoma: Report of cases and review of literature. Leuk Lymphoma 44:825–827

2. Anderson JR, Wilson JF, Jenkin DT, et al. (1983) Childhood non-Hodgkin's lymphoma: The results of a randomized therapeutic trial comparing a 4-drug regimen (COMP) with a 10-drug regimen (LSA2-L2). N Engl J Med 308:559–565

3. Atra A, Meller ST, Stevens RS, et al. (1998) Conservative management of follicular non-Hodgkin's lymphoma in childhood. Br J Haematol 103:220–223

4. Becker AM, Bowers DC, Margraf LR, et al. (2007) Primary renal lymphoma presenting with hypertension. Pediatr Blood Cancer 48(7):711–713

5. Bhatia S, Robison LL, Oberlin O, et al. (1996) Breast cancer and other second neoplasms after childhood Hodgkin's disease. N Engl J Med 334:745–751

6. Breuer CK, Tarbell NJ, Mauch PM, et al. (1994) The importance of staging laparotomy in pediatric Hodgkin's disease. J Pediatr Surg 29:1085–1089

7. Cesaro S, Pillon M, Visintin G, et al. (2005) Unrelated bone marrow transplantation for high-risk anaplastic large cell lymphoma in pediatric patients: a single center case series. Eur J Haematol 75:22–26

8. Chaignaud BE, Bonsack TA, Kozakewich HP, et al. (1998) Pleural effusions in lymphoblastic lymphoma: A diagnostic alternative. J Pediatr Surg 33:1355–1357

9. Dalle J-H, Mechinaud F, Michon J, et al. (2001) Testicular disease in childhood B-cell non-Hodgkin's lymphoma: The French Society of Pediatric Oncology experience. J Clin Oncol 19:2397–2403

10. Donadieu J, Patte C, Kalifa C, et al. (1992) Diagnostic and therapeutic problems posed by malignant non Hodgkin lymphoma of renal origin in children: Apropos of 7 cases. Arch Fr Pediatr 49:699–704

11. Fidias P, Carey RW, Grossbard ML (1995) Non-Hodgkin's lymphoma presenting with biliary tract obstruction. Cancer 75:1669–1677

12. Fleming ID, Turk PS, Murphy SB, et al. (1990) Surgical implications of primary gastrointestinal lymphoma of childhood. Arch Surg 125:252–256

13. Friedberg JW, Fischman A, Neuberg D, et al. (2004) FDG-PET is superior to Gallium scintigraphy in staging and more sensitive in the follow-up of patients with de novo Hodgkin lymphoma: A blinded comparison. Leuk Lymphoma 45:85–92

14. Gabriel DA, Bernard SA, Lambert J, et al. (1986) Oophoropexy and the management of Hodgkin's disease. Arch Surg 121:1083–1085

15. Gahukamble DB, Khamage AS (1995) Limitations of surgery in intra-abdominal Burkitt's lymphoma in children. J Pediatr Surg 30:519–522

16. Garavello W, Romagnoli M, Sordo L, et al. (2004) Incidence of unexpected malignancies in routine tonsillectomy specimens in children. Laryngoscope 114:1103–1105

17. Guglielmi R, Calzauna F, Pizzi, et al. (1980) Ovarian function after pelvic lymph node irradiation. Eur J Gynaecol Oncol 2:99–107

18. Hays DM, Fryer CJ, Pringle KC, et al. (1992) An evaluation of abdominal staging procedures performed in pediatric patients with advance Hodgkin's disease: A report from the Children's Cancer Study Group. J Pediatri Surg 27:1175–1180

19. Hays DM, Ternberg JL, Chen TT, et al. (1986) Postsplenectomy sepsis and other complications following staging laparotomy for Hodgkin's disease in childhood. J Pediatr Surg 21:628–632

20. Heller KN, Teruya-Feldstein J, LaQuaglia MP, et al. (2004) Primary follicular lymphoma of the testis: Excellent outcome following surgical resection without adjuvant chemotherapy. J Pediatr Hematol Oncol 26:104–107

21. Hernandez-Pampaloni M, Takalkar A, Yu JQ, et al. (2006) F-18 FDG-PET imaging and correlation with CT in staging and follow-up of pediatric lymphomas. Pediatr Radiol 36:524–531

22. Hudson MM (2002) Pediatric Hodgkin's therapy: Time for a paradigm shift. J Clin Oncol 20:3755–3757

23. Izarzugaza MI, Steliarova-Foucher E, Carmen Martos M, et al. (2006) Non-Hodgkin's lymphoma incidence and survival in European children and adolescents (1978–1997): Report from the Automated Childhood Cancer Information System project. Eur J Cancer 42:2050–2063

24. Kemeng MM, Magrath IT, Brennan MF (1982) The role of surgery in the management of American Burkitt's lymphoma and its treatment. Ann Surg 196:82–86

25. Koksal Y, Yalcin B, Uner A, et al. (2005) Primary testicular Burkitt lymphoma in a child. Pediatr Hematol Oncol 22:705–709

26. Kung FH, Schwartz CL, Ferree CR, et al. (2006) POG 8625: A randomized trial comparing chemotherapy with chemoradiotherapy for children and adolescents with Stages I, IIA, IIIA1 Hodgkin disease; a report from the Children's Oncology Group. J Pediatr Hematol Oncol 28:362–368

27. Kurosawa J, Matsunaga T, Shimaoka H, et al. (2002) Burkitt lymphoma associated with large gastric folds, pancreatic involvement, and biliary tract obstruction. J Pediatr Hematol Oncol 24:310–312

28. LaQuaglia MP (1999) Lymphoma. In: Carachi R, Azmy A, Grosfeld JL (eds) Surgery of childhood tumors. Arnold, London

29. LaQuaglia MP, Stolar CJH, Krailo M, et al. (1992) The role of surgery in abdominal non-Hodgkin's lymphoma: Experience from the Children's Cancer Study Group. J Pediatr Surg 27:230–235

30. Lefloch O, Donaldson DD, Kaplan HS (1976) Pregnancy following oophoropexy and total nodal irradiation in women with Hodgkin's disease. Cancer 38:2263–2268

31. Levine JE, Harris RE, Loberiza FR Jr, et al. (2003) A comparison of allogeneic and autologous bone marrow transplantation for lymphoblastic lymphoma. Blood 101:2476–2482

32. Lin H-MJ, Teitell MA (2005) Second malignancy after treatment of pediatric Hodgkin disease. J Pediatr Hematol Oncol 27:28–36

33. Lister TA, Crowther D, Sutcliffe SB, et al. (1989) Report of a committee convened to discuss the evaluation and staging of patients with Hodgkin's disease: Cotswolds Meeting. J Clin Oncol 7:1630–1636

34. Lorsbach RB, Shay-Seymore D, Moore J, et al. (2002) Clinicopathologic analysis of follicular lymphoma occurring in children. Blood 99:1959–1963

35. Magrath IT, Lwarga S, Carswell W, et al. (1974) Surgical reduction of tumor bulk in management of abdominal Burkitt's lymphoma. Br J Med 2:308–312

36. Marjanović B, Vujanić GM, Zamurović D, et al. (2000) Non-Hodgkin's lymphoma of the uterus and CNS. Pediatr Neurol 23:69–71

37. Meadows AT, Obringer AC, Marrero O, et al. (1989) Second malignant neoplasms following childhood Hodgkin's disease: Treatment and splenectomy as risk factors. Med Pediatr Oncol 17:477–484

38. Medary I, Steinherz LJ, Aronson DC, et al. (1996) Cardiac tamponade in the pediatric oncology population: Treatment by percutaneous catheter drainage. J Pediatr Surg 1996:197–200

39. Monterroso V, Jaffe ES, Merino MJ, et al. (1993) Malignant lymphomas involving the ovary: A clinicopathologic analysis of 39 cases. Am J Surg Pathol 17:154–170

40. Moon LD, Brenner C, Ancliff P, et al. (2004) Non-Hodgkin's lymphoma presenting with uterine and renal enlargement in a young girl. Pediatr Radiol 34:277–279

41. Murphy SB (1980) Classification, staging and end results of treatment of childhood non-Hodgkin's lymphomas: Dissimilarities from lymphomas in adults. Semin Oncol 7:332–339

42. Nachman JB, Sposto R, Herzog P, et al. (2002) Randomized comparison of low-dose involved-field radiotherapy and no radiotherapy for children with Hodgkin's disease who achieve a complete response to chemotherapy. J Clin Oncol 20:3765–3771

43. Nademanee A, Molina A, Dagis A, et al. (2000) Autologous stem-cell transplantation for poor-risk and relapsed intermediate- and high-grade non-Hodgkin's lymphoma. Clin Lymphoma 1:46–54

44. Ng YY, Healy JC, Vincent JM, et al. (1994) The radiology of non-Hodgkin's lymphoma in childhood: A review of 80 cases. Clin Radiol 49:594–600

45. Patte C, Leverger G, Michon J, et al. (1993) High survival rate of childhood B-cell lymphoma and leukemia (ALL) as a result of the LMB89 protocol of the SFOP. In: Proceedings of the fifth international conference on malignant lymphoma, Lugano, Switzerland, p 52

46. Pietsch JB, Shankar S, Ford C, et al. (2001) Obstructive jaundice secondary to lymphoma in childhood. J Pediatr Surg 36:1792–1795

47. Raj KA, Marks LB, Prosnitz RG (2005–2006) Late effects of breast radiotherapy in young women. Breast Dis 23:53–65

48. Ramos G, Murao M, de Oliveira BM, et al. (1997) Primary hepatic non-Hodgkin's lymphoma in children: A case report and review of the literature. Med Pediatr Oncol 28:370–372

49. Ravindra KV, Stringer MD, Prasad KR, et al. (2003) Non-Hodgkin lymphoma presenting with obstructive jaundice. Br J Surg 90:845–849

50. Rhodes MM, Delbeke D, Whitlock JA, et al. (2006) Utility of FDG-PET/CT in follow-up of children treated for Hodgkin and non-Hodgkin lymphoma. J Pediatr Hematol Oncol 28:300–306

51. Ricketts RR (2001) Clinical management of anterior mediastinal tumors in children. Semin Pediatr Surg 10:161–168

52. Sandlund JT, Downing JR, Crist WM (1996) Non-Hodgkin's lymphoma in childhood. N Engl J Med 334:1238–1248

53. Sengupta SK, Everett VJ (1987) Ovarian neoplasms in children and adolescents in Papua New Guinea. Aust N Z J Obstet Gynaecol 27:335–338

54. Shamberger RC (1999) Preanesthetic evaluation of children with anterior mediastinal masses. Semin Pediatr Surg 8:61–68

55. Shamberger RC, Weinstein HJ (1992) The role of surgery in abdominal Burkitt's lymphoma. J Pediatr Surg 27:236–240

56. Shamberger RC, Holzman RS, Griscom NT, et al. (1991) CT quantitation of tracheal cross-sectional area as a guide to the surgical and anesthetic management of children with anterior mediastinal masses. J Pediatr Surg 26:138–142

57. Shamberger RC, Holzman RS, Griscom NT, et al. (1995) Prospective evaluation by computed tomography and pulmonary function tests of children with mediastinal masses. Surgery 118:468–471

58. Spitz MR, Sider JG, Johnson CC, et al. (1986) Ethnic patterns of Hodgkin's disease incidence among children and adolescents in the United States, 1973–1982. J Natl Cancer Inst 76:235–239

59. Stein JE, Schwenn MR, Jacir NN, et al. (1991) Surgical restraint in Burkitt's lymphoma in children. J Pediatr Surg 26:1273–1275

60. Thomas PR, Wirstanly D, Peckamn MJ, Austin DE, et al. (1976) Reproductive and endocrine function in patients with Hodgkin's disease: Effects of oophorepexy and irradiation. Br J Cancer 33:226–231

61. van de Shoot L, Aronson DC, Behrendt H, et al. (2001) The role of fine-needle aspiration cytology in children with persistent or suspicious lymphadenopathy. J Pediatr Surg 36:7–11

62. Watanbe Y, Ito T, Horibe K, et al. (1997) Obstructive jaundice: An unusual initial manifestation of intra-abdominal non-Hodgkin's lymphoma in children: Complications of percutaneous transhepatic cholangial drainage. J Pediatr Surg 32:650–653

63. Whalen TV, LaQuaglia MP (1997) The lymphomas: An update for surgeons. Semin Pediatr Surg 6:50–55

64. Williams RS, Mendenhall N (1992) Laparoscopic oophoropexy for preservation of ovarian function before pelvic node irradiation. Obstet Gynecol 80:541–543

65. Williams RS, Littell RD, Mendenhall NP (1999) Laparoscopic oophoropexy and ovarian function in the treatment of Hodgkin disease. Cancer 86:2138–2141

66. Yanchar NL, Bass J (1999) Poor outcome of gastrointestinal perforations associated with childhood abdominal non-Hodgkin's lymphoma. J Pediatr Surg 34:1169–1174

67. Ziegler JL (1977) Treatment results of 54 American patients with Burkitt's lymphoma are similar to the African experience. N Engl J Med 297:75–80

Part C

Bone Tumors: Limb Salvage

16

Stephen R. Cannon

Contents

16.1 Introduction

Primary bone tumors in children are rare conditions, the upper limb being more rarely affected than the lower limb. The practicing general orthopedic surgeon may not see more than a single case of primary bone tumor per year. This rarity makes the recognition—particularly of malignant bone tumors—extremely difficult. Not surprisingly, this leads to difficulties and errors being made in specific treatment. With the establishment of bone tumor/cancer registries, the incidence of malignant primary disease of bone can be seen to be around six cases per million per year. The incidence of osteosarcoma, the most common primary malignant bone tumor, showing peak risks of incidence related to puberty is greatest between 10 and 14 years for girls and between 15 and 18 years for boys [1] (Fig. 16.1).

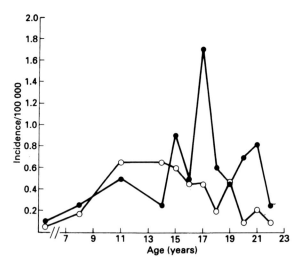

Fig. 16.1 Incidence of osteosarcoma in boys and girls related to age

The most common benign lesion of bone is undoubtedly the solitary osteocartilaginous exostosis (osteochondroma). This condition was first described by Sir Astley Cooper in 1918 [2]. Both solitary exostosis and multiple exostoses (diaphyseal aclasis) may lead to alteration of epiphyseal plate growth and joint subluxation [3]. Other common benign diseases affecting the skeleton include Ollier's disease [4] which, when associated with soft tissue hemangiomas is termed Maffucci's syndrome [5]. The true incidence of these conditions within the population is unknown, but it is well recognized that the enchondritic element of both syndromes may undergo malignant change [6]. The majority of giant cell tumors are found in the pelvis and lower limbs, although occasionally the distal and proximal radius may be involved. These lesions are, of course, exceedingly rare below the age of 15 years [7]. Of the primary malignant tumors of bone in childhood (Ewing's sarcoma and osteosarcoma), about 12–15% of cases occur in the upper limb, including the clavicle.

When considering the diagnosis of a bone tumor, it is probably wise to keep the above World Health Organization (WHO) classification in mind (Table 16.1). Lesions occurring predominantly in children are highlighted.

16.2 Presentation

The diagnosis is often missed simply because it is not considered. It is important to realize that no part of the anatomy is exempt from a bone tumor, and every bone, every muscle and every nerve in all anatomical areas have been recorded as being sites of primary musculoskeletal tumors.

Children often present with symptoms that can be confused with other musculoskeletal injuries. Most children seek medical attention because of pain. The clinician should have a high index of suspicion for pain that is constant, unrelated to activity, and is worse at night. The second most frequent complaint is of swelling. Of particular importance is the rate of tumor growth and whether there has been any relationship to trauma. The third more rare mode of presentation is the occurrence of a pathological fracture. Here, the presence of pain or swelling prior to the fracture is a most important clue to diagnosis. Constitutional symptoms of weight loss and occasionally fever are sinister observations, usually indicative of aggressive disease, often widespread. Examination of the area complained of is the responsibility of the physician, and the questions which should be asked are: first, is there tenderness and is there increase in the skin temperature? If there is a visible mass, how big is it? Has it changed in size since first noted? The physician should take appropriate measurements. Adjacent joints should be examined for the range of movement and the limb assessed for signs of muscle atrophy. The neurovascular status of the extremity involved should also be assessed. A complete physical examination should also be done, with particular reference to the regional lymph nodes and examination of the chest and abdomen where appropriate. Only after a very thorough history and careful examination should the next investigation, a plain radiograph, be performed.

16.3 Radiographic Investigations

The single most important investigation in a suspected bone tumor is the plain radiograph. This investigation may be diagnostic in itself and direct further treatment without additional investigation or indeed the radiograph may alert the surgeon to the possibility of a bone tumor being present. It is also important to emphasize that the radiologist is not a clinician in his own right and requires appropriate information of what the clinician suspects in order to give the best service. The radiograph should be taken in two views at right angles to each other, and when a lesion is recognized the following helpful diagnostic exercise should be undertaken.

1. What is the anatomical site of the lesion? Which bone is it in? Is it in the epiphysis, metaphysis, or diaphysis? Is it in the medullary canal or is it in the cortex, lying on the cortex or surrounding the cortex?
2. What effect is the lesion having on the bone? Is bone being destroyed? Is it a local destruction? Is it permeative or are there moth-eaten changes?

Table 16.1 WHO classification of common primary bone tumors

A Bone-forming tumors	
i) Benign	Osteoma
	Osteoid osteoma
	Osteoblastoma
ii) Intermediate	Aggressive (malignant) osteoblastoma
iii) Malignant	Osteosarcoma
	(a) Central (medullary)
	(b) Surface (peripheral)
	Parosteal osteosarcoma
	Periosteal osteosarcoma
	High-grade surface
B Cartilage-forming tumors	
i) Benign	Chondroma
	(a) Enchondroma
	(b) Periosteal (juxtacortical)
	Osteochondroma (osteocartilaginous exostosis)
	(a) Solitary
	(b) Multiple hereditary
	Chondroblastoma
	Chondromyxoid fibroma
ii) Malignant	Chondrosarcoma
	Dedifferentiated chondrosarcoma
	Mesenchymal chondrosarcoma
	Clear cell chondrosarcoma
C Giant cell tumor (osteoclastoma)	
D Marrow tumors (round cell tumors)	
	Ewing's sarcoma of bone
	Neuroectodermal tumor of bone
	Malignant lymphoma of bone
	Myeloma
E Vascular tumors	
i) Benign	Hemangioma
	Lymphangioma
	Glomus tumor
ii) Intermediate	Hemangioendothelioma
	Hemangiopericytoma
iii) Malignant	Angiosarcoma
	Malignant hemangiopericytoma
F Other connective tissue tumors	
i) Benign	Benign fibrous histiocytoma
	Lipoma
ii) Intermediate	Desmoplastic fibroma
iii) Malignant	Fibrosarcoma
	Malignant fibrous histiocytoma
	Liposarcoma
	Malignant mesenchymoma
	Leiomyosarcoma
	Undifferentiated sarcoma

Table 16.1 *(Continued)* WHO classification of common primary bone tumors

G Other tumors	
i) Benign	Neurilemmoma
	Neurofibroma
ii) Malignant	Chordoma
	Adamantinoma
H Simple bone cyst	
Aneurysmal bone cyst	
Classification of common primary bone tumors	

3. What is the bone doing in response to the lesion? Is there an endosteal reaction? Is there a periosteal reaction? Is a Codman's triangle, a sunburst pattern, or onion-skinning appearance present?
4. Is there anything about the lesion which is characteristic of a specific tumor? Is it forming new bone? Is there calcification? Does it have a ground glass appearance?

This approach is important, particularly in instances where the initial diagnosis can be safely made on the plain radiograph alone. Lesions which are inactive, i.e., those that have no symptoms and have a mature reaction around them, can often be observed. Biopsy is usually not necessary. Lesions which appear to be more aggressive, i.e., giant cell tumor or chondroblastoma, may require further evaluation with other radiographic techniques prior to discussing management. In deciding which radiological investigations to acquire, it is useful to communicate with the radiologist which question is being asked. The orthopedic surgeon requires information that answers four questions in order to stage the tumor within the limb.

First, what is the intraosseous extent of the tumor? Second, what is the extraosseous extent of the tumor and what proportion of the lesion is still subperiosteal? Third, is there any involvement of the adjacent intra-articular structures? Fourth, is the neuro-vascular bundle involved in the tumor process? If the tumor is malignant, then the clinician needs to know if there is any other bony lesion elsewhere and also if there is any metastatic spread to the lung.

Radioisotopic technetium 99m bone scintigraphy can be used both to determine the activity of a primary lesion and to search for other bony lesions. Occasionally the technetium bone scan can reveal the intraosseous extent of a lesion as well as computed tomography (CT) or magnetic resonance imaging (MRI) scanning [8] (Fig. 16.2). Lesions which do not have increased activity on the bone scan are usually benign. The two exceptions to this general rule are myeloma and Langerhans' histiocytosis. Lesions which have in-

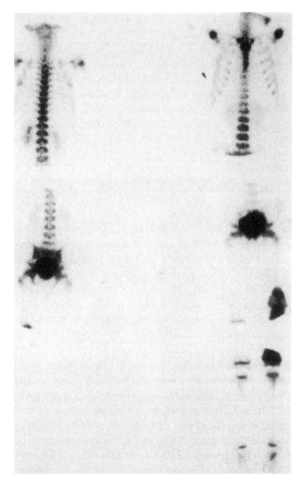

Fig. 16.2 Technetium bone scan of an osteosarcoma showing primary lesion and intraosseous extent.

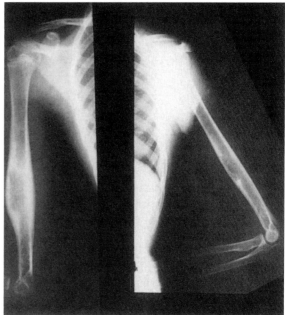

Fig. 16.3 Ewing's sarcoma showing cortical destruction.

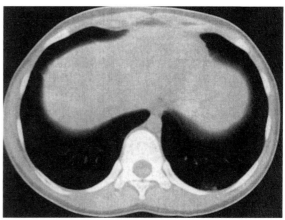

Fig. 16.4 CT scan chest showing multiple subpleural and parenchymal metastases.

creased activity may be benign or malignant. The intensity of uptake is not predictive as to the likelihood of malignancy. Classically, the bone scan appearances of osteosarcoma are of intense activity with an irregular outline [9]. Bone scintigraphy may also on occasion demonstrate pulmonary metastases in instances of osteosarcoma.

Computed tomography is a valuable noninvasive investigation which can determine not only the intramedullary extent of the tumor but also demonstrate extraosseous extension and the degree of cortical destruction (Fig. 16.3). It may also be used in conjunction with contrast medium to outline the relationship of the tumor to adjacent vascular structures or indeed to represent the vascularity of the lesion itself; CT scan of the lungs is important for accurate staging. Typically, metastases are found in the subpleural position (Fig. 16.4), but in spite of the greater sensitivity of this technique the proportion of patients with normal chest radiographs at presentation who are subse-

quently shown to have lung metastases by CT scan is only 10–15% [10].

Magnetic resonance imaging is now considered the most sensitive single method for assessing intramedullary involvement by tumor [11]. Although both CT and MRI can demonstrate the presence of extraosseous soft tissue extension, MRI is superior to CT in differentiating tumor from adjoining muscle [12, 13] (Fig. 16.5). However, MRI is not as accurate as CT in determining the relationship of a tumor to the cortex of a bone or in evaluating a lesion which is composed of dense bone [14]. In addition, there can be conside-

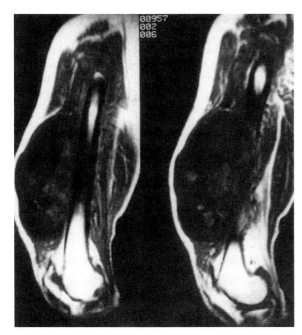

Fig. 16.5 MRI scan of Ewing's sarcoma showing large extraosseous mass.

rable difficulty in differentiating between tumor and peripheral edema in highly malignant tumors. It is also useful to use MRI in delineating the response to treatment by radiotherapy or chemotherapy by documenting reduction in tumoral mass and restoration of normal MRI signals [15].

Despite increasing sophistication of radiological investigations, the radiologist is at best usually only able to offer a differential diagnosis. Osteosarcoma, for example, may be confused with stress fracture, chronic osteomyelitis, ectopic ossification, and other highly malignant tumors that may induce active bone formation such as Ewing's sarcoma. The ultimate diagnosis, therefore, rests in the hands of the histopathologist and analysis of biopsy material.

16.4 Biopsy

Biopsy is the last but perhaps the most critical step in the evaluation of a bone tumor and should only be performed after extremely careful planning [16]. The surgeon who is responsible for the management of the patient with a primary bone tumor should be the individual to decide on the biopsy method and its approach. In a large series of patients with bone tumors, Mankin, et al. [17] concluded that the incidence of significant problems in patient management resulting in inappropriate biopsy techniques was 20% and that the incidence of wound healing complica-

tions related to a poorly planned biopsy was similarly high. They further noted that 8% of biopsies produced a significantly adverse effect on the patient's prognosis and in 5% led to an unnecessary amputation. Errors in diagnosis leading to inadequate treatment occurred twice as frequently when the initial biopsy was done at the referring hospital rather than a specialist center.

16.4.1 Fine Needle Aspiration (FNA)

This technique, which is generally used in the diagnosis of soft tissue tumors, has been popularized for initial diagnosis of primary bone tumors, particularly in Sweden [18]. A study of 300 consecutive patients not known to have a previous malignancy or suspected of having a local recurrence was analyzed. The FNA technique itself failed in 18% of patients. In those patients where material was obtained, 95% had correct diagnosis. It would appear that instances of chondrosarcoma presented the greatest difficulty in diagnosis and those with Ewing's sarcoma the least. The only real advantage of FNA is that it can be performed under simple analgesia as an outpatient procedure. It is also worthy of note that FNA in benign bone lesions had a very high incidence of inconclusive results.

16.4.2 Needle Biopsy

Targeted percutaneous needle biopsy using a Jamshidi or similar needle may often be sufficient to yield a diagnosis (Fig. 16.6). The technique is performed under radiological control and has 95% accuracy when dealing with lesions of the appendicular skeleton [19]. In malignant lesions, the needle biopsy tract should be subsequently removed en bloc with the tumor, and this requires a good rapport between surgeon and radiologist. Often, the tract can be marked with Indian ink following completion of the biopsy to facilitate removal. Failure to remove the tract may lead to local recurrence [20]. Although a rapid working diagnosis can often be achieved using frozen section or imprint techniques [21], it is important to emphasize that the analysis of small amounts of histological material requires pathological expertise of the highest caliber and is not, therefore, recommended if such expertise is not readily available.

16.4.3 Incisional Biopsy

Most commonly, biopsy is performed by an open technique, and ideally the biopsy tract should be as small as possible and go directly to bone. Postopera-

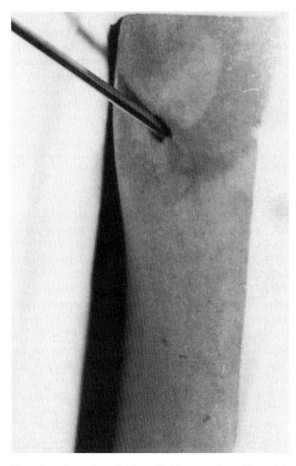

Fig. 16.6 Targeted Jamshidi needle biopsy under radiographic control.

tive hemostasis at the operation site is mandatory, and the wound should be closed using a subcuticular suture. It must be remembered that when definitive surgery is performed, the complete biopsy tract and all contaminated tissue must be removed en bloc with the tumor. Failure to do so will significantly increase the risk of local recurrence [22]. The surgeon who performs the open biopsy should keep in mind the definitive procedure that may be required and place the biopsy site accordingly. There is no objection to the use of a tourniquet providing it is released prior to closure and hemostasis obtained. Drains may be used, but they should be brought out close to the wound and in line with it so that excision of the drain tract can also be obtained. There are advocates for closing the biopsy defect in the tumor pseudocapsule with cement, but there is no proof that this lessens contamination and may, if placed under pressure, theoretically further spread the tumor by the intramedullary route.

16.4.4 Excisional Biopsy

Occasionally, an excisional biopsy will be more appropriate than either an incisional or needle biopsy. It is particularly indicated where the lesion is small and can easily be excised, often widely, without significant alteration in the patient's function. Lesions which are obviously applicable to excision biopsy are osteoid osteoma and osteochondroma, and it may also be appropriate in instances of low-grade chondrosarcoma affecting the medulla. It is often difficult to distinguish between active benign cartilage tumors and low-grade chondrosarcomas. When the entire lesion is removed allowing examination of the interface between the tumor, adjacent bone, and soft tissue, the pathologist is usually able to render a better opinion.

It cannot be overemphasized that in children osteomyelitis occurs more commonly than bone tumors. Material obtained, therefore, should also be sent for Gram staining and culture as well as histological analysis.

16.5 Staging Notations

The correlation of information gained from radiological imaging investigations and the biopsy allows classification of a malignant bone tumor into a staging system. The surgical staging system proposed by Enneking, et al. is easy to use clinically, and although it suffers from some significant oversimplification, it is generally acceptable [23]. The system is outlined in Table 16.2, and takes into account the three basic features that are recognized as having prognostic importance. These are, first, the histological grade of the tumor, second, its location and, third, the presence or absence of regional or distal metastases. The histological grade is classified as either low grade (G1) or high grade (G2). This grading system does not completely match purely histological grading systems but, in essence, low grade lesions will be the equivalent of Broders grade I and some II. The high-grade lesions would all be Broders II, III, and IV [24]. Regarding location, lesions are divided into those occurring in a specific compartment (T1) and those that are extracompartmental in nature (T2). The term "compartments" is defined as an anatomical structure bounded by natural barriers to tumor extension. Thus, a whole bone is considered a compartment as is a functional muscle group bounded by major fascial septa. Tumors spreading beyond these compartments or involving neurovascular structures are classified as extracompartmental. Some anatomical locations such as the axilla, antecubital fossa, periclavicular region, and midhand, are considered extracompartmental ab initio. In the lower limb the popliteal fossa and midfoot are similar problematic areas.

Table 16.2 Enneking's classification of surgical staging.

Stage		Grade	Site	Metastases
I	A	Low (G_1)	Intracompartmental (T_1)	None (M_0)
	B	Low (G_1)	Extracompartmental (T_2)	None (M_0)
II	A	High (G_2)	Intracompartmental (T_1)	None (M_0)
	B	High (G_2)	Extracompartmental (T_2)	None (M_0)
III	A	Low (G_1)	Intra- or extra- (T_1–T_2)	Regional or distant (M_1)
	B	High (G_2)	Intra- or extra- (T_1–T_2)	Regional or distant (M_1)

In malignant tumors, metastases occur most frequently to the lungs and they may occasionally occur in bone but are rare in local lymph nodes. When multiple bony lesions are sometimes seen, they are considered examples of multicentric primary tumors, though usually one lesion has the radiological features of a primary lesion and the others have characteristics of secondary intramedullary deposits. Skip lesions of an isolated area of tumor in the same bone as the primary were previously thought to occur in approximately 25% of cases; more recent data suggests the true incidence is probably much lower [25].

Similar staging systems have been applied to benign disease, but unfortunately they rarely predict the clinical course of the problem. The most predictive element in the course of treatment of benign disease is, in fact, the surgical treatment which is given. For example, wide simple excision of a cartilaginous exostosis will lead to resolution of the problem providing that the cartilage cap is not broken, whereas curettage of a giant cell tumor may result in a local recurrence rate of approximately 20%. In the upper limb, giant cell tumor commonly affects the distal radius and proximal humerus but tends to occur in only the mature skeleton. On the basis of the radiological appearance, Campanacci, et al. [26] proposed four subtypes which redefine the previously proposed terms of latent, active, and aggressive. Unfortunately, grade I often represents a benign fibrous histiocytoma and the other grades do not necessarily predict their clinical behavior. The picture is further complicated by the histological pattern of the tumor. The osteoclasts which are present are now considered to be only markers of the tumor activity, the tumor itself being represented by the stromal background. This background can vary from being very inconspicuous to frankly malignant [27]. This appearance can, of course, profoundly affect the extent of treatment. Primary de novo malignant giant cell tumor is a rare but well-recognized entity. Care is required, particularly in the differentiation of an osteoclast-rich osteosarcoma. When diagnosed, the treatment of a malignant giant cell tumor is similar to managing a malignant fibrous tumor.

16.6 Treatment of Common Primary Bone Tumors

16.6.1 Benign Bone-Forming Tumors

16.6.1.1 Osteoma

These usually present as small, painless, slowly enlarging lumps. Although most commonly occurring around the skull, any bone may be affected. The radiological appearance of an osteoma is a dense well-circumscribed lesion. Treatment is by surgical excision if the patient is symptomatic.

16.6.1.2 Osteoid Osteoma

This condition usually presents with vague pain, often nocturnal, and relieved characteristically by aspirin and other nonsteroidal anti-inflammatory agents [28]. The pain may be associated with tenderness and vasomotor disturbance. Classically, the osteoblastic nidus is within the cortex or spongiosa of long bones. The nidus is less than 1 mm in diameter and induces intense surrounding reactive change (Fig. 16.7). If the nidus is in a subarticular location diagnosis can be difficult, as the reactive changes may not occur. Intracapsular osteoid osteomas around the elbow have been mistaken for tuberculous synovitis [29] and rheumatoid arthritis [30]. It is also well recognized that long-standing disease can induce degenerative change [31].

The radiological investigation consists initially of a plain radiograph. This may or may not reveal the characteristic nidus. When marked reactive bone is seen, the differential diagnosis includes bone abscess, sclerosing osteomyelitis of Garré, osteochondritis, and stress fracture [32]. Bone scintigraphy will usually help lo-

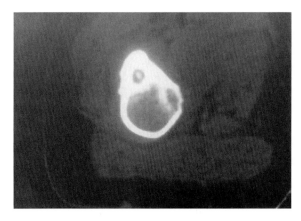

Fig. 16.7 CT radiograph of osteoid osteoma of the femur.

calize a nidus but is relatively nonspecific. Computed tomography, if applied in close 2-mm sections, will be successful in identifying accurate locations of the nidus prior to surgical resection [33].

The treatment of osteoid osteoma requires excision or ablation of the nidus. As the nidus is surrounded by dense reactive bone this can be difficult to achieve. The traditional approach requires wide exposure with radiological verification of the site. Szypryt, et al. [34] have described the use of intraoperative scintigraphy but this is rarely required. Excisional biopsy of the nidus under CT guidance is now performed with success [35] while electrothermal coagulation has also been explored and reported as successful.

The use of radioablation techniques has now become first-line management for the majority of osteoid osteomas, certainly all those occurring in the upper limb. Reported rates are of 90% success with one treatment of radioablation. Five percent of cases require a second attempt at treatment by this technique. Only 5% require surgical exploration and excision [35a.]

16.6.1.3 Osteoblastoma

This lesion has a similar appearance histologically to osteoid osteoma, but is larger and does not induce as much reactive surrounding change. It is an extremely rare lesion affecting mainly the axial skeleton, although any bone may be affected. Patients are predominantly male in their second or third decades [36].

The clinical presentation is of vague pain, less severe than osteoid osteoma, and not particularly relieved by salicylates. Occasionally there may be both swelling and joint dysfunction.

The radiological features classically show an expansile radiolucent lesion, with a thin shell of peripheral new bone.

Treatment consists of either curettage with or without bone grafting or local excision. Local excision results in good local control but reconstruction may be required. This recurrence rate may be as high as 20% following curettage, but the use of radiotherapy in extraspinal cases is rarely required [37].

16.6.2 Malignant Bone-Forming Tumors

16.6.2.1 Osteosarcoma

Osteosarcoma is the most common primary malignant bone tumor and can occur at any age, although most cases occur in the first two decades of life [38]. Most commonly affecting the two metaphyseal areas around the knee, the humerus is the third most common site, with tumors often arising at an earlier age than in the lower limb [39.]

Osteosarcomas are usually subtyped on the basis of their histological patterns as fibroblastic, chondroblastic, osteoblastic, telangiectatic, or mixed [40]. Although the subtype classification was originally thought to have a bearing on prognosis, carefully controlled studies now suggest that this is not the case. Histological grading is also an unreliable prognostic indication [41].

Patients present usually with a short history of pain followed by swelling, joint dysfunction, and occasionally pathological fracture. The many radiological advances which have occurred in the last decade have allowed very accurate staging of the tumor. The plain radiograph remains the initial diagnostic tool but tends to underestimate the local extent of the tumor. Accurate visualization of cortical destruction and soft tissue spread will be given by CT but this may miss skip lesions in the same bone. It is a useful technique in planning biopsy and local excision [42]. Today, CT of the chest is the accepted staging investigation to assess the potential presence of pulmonary metastases. Local staging of disease now depends heavily on MRI studies, particularly in the T2 mode, which will delineate accurately the intramedullary and soft tissue extent of the lesion; MRI will outline the relationship of the tumor to the adjacent joints and blood vessels (Fig. 16.8).

Preoperative bone scintigraphy using technetium isotopes is useful in identifying skip lesions and metachronous lesions in other bones. The radioisotope scan may also on occasions demonstrate pulmonary metastases [43].

Having performed the radiological staging procedures, it is necessary to establish the pathological diagnosis. At this stage a biopsy is performed. Many argue that an open biopsy is required. However, Stoker, et al. [44]. have shown the accuracy of Jamshidi needle

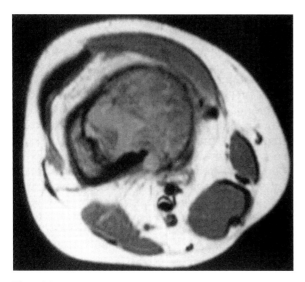

Fig. 16.8 MRI which outlines the relationship of the tumor to the adjacent joints and blood vessels.

biopsy cores obtained in a referral center under local anesthesia and image intensification. More recently similar accuracy has been shown in biopsying the soft tissue component of malignant tumors under ultrasound or MRI [44a.]

Historically, the early treatment of osteosarcoma was surgical ablation. In the upper limb this required either disarticulation of the shoulder for lesions in the distal humerus or forequarter amputation for more proximal growths. Survival, however, was poor with 5-year survival rates varying between 11% and 25% [45]. Cade [46] reported an alternative method of treatment employing preoperative radiation followed by surgical ablation only in those cases not developing pulmonary metastases. Many less amputations were performed but the survival rate was unaltered. This was subsequently confirmed by other series [47].

By the early 1970s, it became evident that this appalling survival rate might be improved by the use of adjuvant chemotherapy. Many different protocols were developed, some claiming a very high survival rate [48], but early on controlled trials of therapies were not performed. In the UK, the Medical Research Council combined with the European Organization for Research into Cancer Treatment (EORTC) set up controlled trials of adjuvant chemotherapy. More recently neoadjuvant chemotherapy has been employed and allows treatment of undetected micrometastases and causes necrosis of the tumor and may allow some shrinkage of the primary tumor. This latter effect may allow easier local resection and reconstruction of the limb. The initial trials compared the effect of Adriamycin (doxorubicin) and cisplatin with or without high-dose methotrexate. The two-drug arm performed better, resulting in a survival rate of 65% at 5 years. This two-drug arm has been compared with a Rosen T10 regime. The trial has accrued 400 cases. Analysis of them showed no material difference between the two regimes, therefore the two-drug regime is preferred because of less morbidity. A second trial attempting a dose intensification of the two-drug regime, the three courses of chemotherapy being given over 6 weeks as opposed to nine, using rescue by granulocyte cell stimulating factor, has also shown little difference in outcome. A further regime is now in progress which hopes to improve the curates of osteosarcoma. The trial is worldwide, involving both European and American oncologists and hopes to improve the outcomes which have been somewhat disappointing over the past 20 years. This randomized trial termed Euramos hopes to herald a new era of clinical investigation into osteosarcoma, which of course should always be treated under the guidance of a specialist team [48a].

Surgical intervention is now performed at around the tenth or eleventh week following commencement of chemotherapy and is continued in a randomized manner in the postoperative period. In most cases, a "wide excision" of the tumor is performed outside the tumor pseudocapsule with preservation of the neurovascular bundles, although often in tumors arising in the upper limb the circumflex nerve and the radial nerve may often be sacrificed to allow adequate clearance. Following wide excision functional reconstruction is only possible using either customized endoprostheses or allografts.

16.6.2.2 Parosteal Osteosarcoma

A recent multicentral pan-European trial has found no significant improvement in either local recurrence or survival in cases treated by chemotherapy. This is a low-grade malignant tumor developing on the external surface of large bones. The disease was first reported by Geschickter and Copeland in 1951 [49]. It has a long natural history and tends to affect patients in the second and third decades of life. Most patients present with a long-standing swelling associated with dull ache. The elbow is only rarely affected.

Treatment consists of wide local resection of the tumor with appropriate reconstruction. It is generally accepted that in most cases chemotherapy is not indicated. Review of the tumor may show high-grade changes in the fibrous elements. These tumors have a poorer prognosis [50], and chemotherapy may be indicated. Occasionally, the low-grade component may transform or dedifferentiate to a high-grade osteosarcoma [51]. Treatment for these latter cases is then as for an osteosarcoma (see Chap. 18).

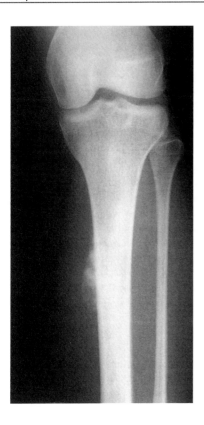

Fig. 16.9 X-ray osteosarcoma of tibia femur showing proximity of tumor to the popliteal vessels.

16.6.2.3 Periosteal Osteosarcoma

This is a very rare tumor; many still doubt its existence, although it probably is a variant of parosteal osteosarcoma with a prominent cartilaginous component [52, 53]. These tumors are usually small unicortical lesions (Fig. 16.9). Treatment is by wide resection and reconstruction where required. Whether chemotherapy is required in their management is still unclear [53a].

16.6.3 Benign Cartilage-Forming Tumors

16.6.3.1 Osteochondroma

These cartilage-capped bony protusions may develop in any bone derived from cartilage. They are usually discovered in childhood and many are found only as incidental findings on radiography (Fig. 16.10a,b). They are usually painless but pain can be invoked by mechanical irritation or nerve compression. Pseudoaneurysm has also been reported specifically in the popliteal regions [54].

If symptomatic, straightforward excision at the base is curative. If asymptomatic, they can be safely observed. Growth will continue until skeletal maturity. If growth appears to occur after skeletal maturity then malignant transformation must be considered even if the radiographic appearances do not alter. It is now considered that the size and thickness of the cartilage cap as assessed by MRI or CT is the critical factor. This is of course not visible on plain radiographs.

In diaphyseal aclasis the patient may also present with growth abnormality and subluxation at the radiohumeral joints. In this condition, removal of the lesions is rarely enough and the patients often require major reconstructions to correct the deformities [55]. The patient should be warned specifically of the possibility of malignant change associated with growth after maturity. Known lesions which cannot be palpated should be monitored by radiography. Unfortunately, bone isotope scanning cannot reliably differentiate benign from malignant cartilage lesions, but recent innovations such as PET scanning may be helpful in this regard [56].

16.6.3.2 Chondroblastoma

This is a rare bone tumor usually located in the epiphyseal plate which is essentially benign. Jaffe and Lichtenstein consider that it is a tumor developed from cartilaginous germ cells, although Higaki considers the cell of origin to be histiocytic [57, 58]. Typically, the patient is in the second decade and is more likely to be male. A long prodromal history is typical and there may be muscle wasting and joint restriction [59]. The most common site of occurrence is the upper humeral epiphyseal plate, although they can be associated with any primary or secondary site of ossification.

Typically, the lesion is radiolucent crossing the growth plate and intralesional calcification can be seen particularly with CT [60] (Fig. 16.10). CT may better illustrate the local invasive properties of the tumor. It is well recognized that chrondroblastoma may be associated with implantations in the lung. These "areas" if resected have a "benign" histological appearance and therefore represent implantation of vascularly transported tumor tissue rather than true metastases.

Treatment of the local lesion is by a combination of curettage and excision of any adjacent soft tissue extension. The outcome is very good but it may recur if not excised totally, and damage may be done to the growth plate. The application of autologous bone graft will lessen the recurrence rate but conversely makes local recurrence more difficult to detect by radiography. The recurrence rate is approximately 20%, but this may be further reduced by use of cryotherapy and other adjuvants [61].

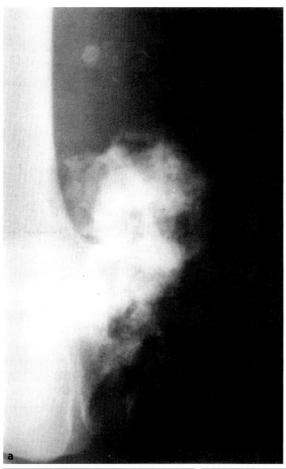

Fig. 16.10 a, b (**a**) Lateral radiograph showing osteochondroma of distal femur. (**b**) AP radiograph of proximal humerus showing chondroblastoma.

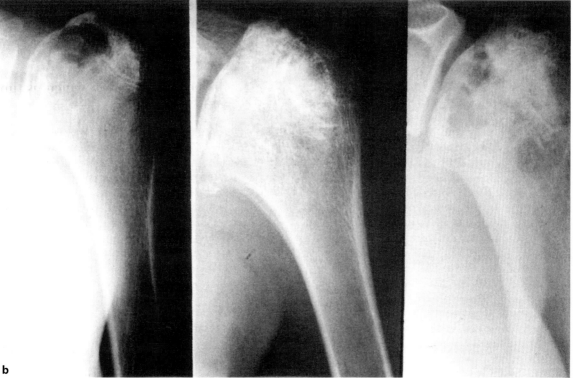

16.6.3.3 Chrondromyxoid Fibroma

This is a tumor which arises commonly in the upper tibia. It is most common in the second decade of life but may occur in any decade. There is a long prodromal history, often as long as 2 years [62]. With the exception of the clavicle, all bones can be involved, but it is much more common in the lower limb.

The radiological features are of an eccentric lesion in the metaphyseal area of a long bone. It is well defined but surrounding subperiosteal reaction may be slight [63].

As with chondroblastoma, treatment consists of an initial curettage and the recurrence rate can be reduced if the operation is supplemented with an autograft [64].

16.6.4 Malignant Cartilage-Forming Tumors

16.6.4.1 Chondrosarcoma

Chondrosarcoma is divided into two basic subgroups: primary chondrosarcoma which arises in normal bone, and secondary chondrosarcoma which arises in a pre-existing benign cartilage tumor, usually an enchondroma or cartilage cap of an exostosis. Primary lesions are twice as common. Chondrosarcoma occurs in 25–30% of adult tumors, secondary to enchondroma or an exostosis. Primary chondrosarcoma rarely occurs in childhood.

Although chondrosarcomas may occur in the young, they predominate after the third decade of life. Both sexes are equally afflicted. Most patients complain of pain but it is well recognized that a presenting mass may be painless [65]. The anatomical distribution favors the axial skeleton, but 10% of tumors occur in the humerus.

Classically, the radiological appearance is a thick-walled radiolucency with irregularly blotchy areas of calcification. On the medullary surfaces the cortex is scalloped and cortical penetration occurs late in the disease. It is frequently difficult to discern radiographically the presence of a pre-existing benign tumor (Fig. 16.11).

The only treatment effective in chondrosarcoma is excision, the adequacy of which is important in determining the outcome [66]. The survival outcome is also influenced by the degree of malignancy and the site, patients with pelvic lesions faring far worse than those with upper limb tumor [65]. Although most lesions require excision, preferably of a wide or radical nature, small corticated, low-grade lesions in the elderly may be best served by curettage and adjuvant therapy consisting of cryosurgery, phenolization or "cement" application.

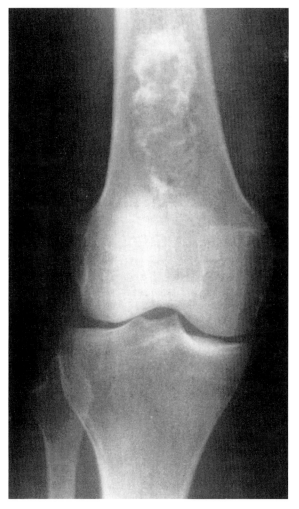

Fig. 16.11 AP radiograph of distal femur showing a chondrosarcoma arising in a pre-existing enchondroma.

16.6.4.2 Dedifferentiated Chondrosarcoma

This rare tumor was first described by Dahlin and Beabout in 1971 [67]. Additional mesenchymal elements are present in addition to the chondrosarcoma. The humerus is the second most common site. The radiological appearance may give a clue to the probability of this lesion, which may be represented by a purely lytic expansile area in an otherwise typical chondrosarcoma. The overall poor prognosis of patients with this tumor has led to attempts with the use of chemotherapy as a neo-adjuvant therapy in addition to surgery.

16.6.4.3 Mesenchymal Chondrosarcoma

This is a further subtype of chondrosarcoma which rarely affects the upper limb. It is characterized by a highly cellular primitive spindle cell stroma with focal chondroid differentiation [68]. The tumor occurs most frequently in the second decade of life.

In terms of radiography, it is extremely difficult to differentiate the lesion, which may resemble an osteosarcoma as soft tissue extension may be heavily calcified.

Treatment is similar to dedifferentiated chondrosarcoma, consisting of chemotherapy and resection. In Britain, the chemotherapy consists of the agents cisplatin, ifosfamide, and Adriamycin (doxorubicin).

16.6.4.4 Clear Cell Chondrosarcoma

This is an extremely rare tumor which is rather slow-growing, patients often having symptoms for up to 3 years. The most common site is the upper femur but the upper limb may also be affected [69]. The tumor appears as an osteolytic expansile lesion, usually at the proximal end of long bones. Treatment consists of complete surgical excision with reconstruction.

16.6.5 Benign Tumors of Histiocytic or Fibrohistiocytic Origin

16.6.5.1 Giant Cell Tumor

This is a locally aggressive but essentially benign bone tumor. It accounts for 5% of all primary bone tumors and afflicts the mature skeleton. There is a slight female predominance [70]. Although commonly affecting the knee, distal radius, and proximal humerus, the elbow region may be affected (Fig. 16.12) and indeed patients with multiple sites have been recorded [71]. All patients suspected of presenting with a giant cell tumor should have hyperparathyroidism excluded by biochemical testing.

Early lesions present radiographically as an expanding lytic lesion, eccentric to the long axis, often with fine trabeculae present. Most investigators believe that the tumor arises in the epiphysis (subarticular region) and extends to involve the metaphysis. Large lesions progress to cortical destruction and joint dysfunction.

On the basis of the radiological appearance, Campanacci, et al. [72] have proposed four subtypes which redefine the previously proposed terms of latent, active, and aggressive. Unfortunately, grade I probably often represents benign fibrous histiocytoma and the other grades do not necessarily predict their clinical behavior. The picture is further complicated by the histological pattern of the tumor. The osteoclasts which are present are now considered markers of the true tumor which is represented by the stromal background. This background can vary from being inconspicuous

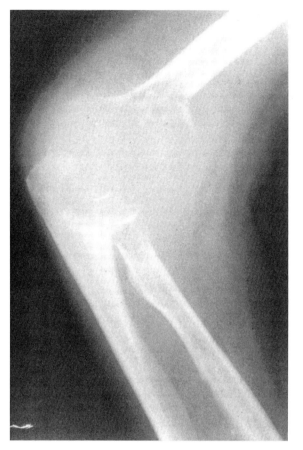

Fig. 16.12 Giant cell tumor: lateral x-ray of elbow joint.

to frankly malignant [73] and thus can profoundly affect treatment.

Another poorly understood phenomenon in these tumors is the likelihood of malignant transformation of a benign tumor either following multiple local recurrences or irradiation treatment [74], and care is required in establishing whether it is true malignant transformation of the giant cell tumor or sarcomatous induction by the radiotherapy when this modality of treatment has been used.

Primary de novo malignant giant cell tumor is a rare but well recognized entity, but care is required particularly in the subsequent differentiation of an osteoclast-rich osteosarcoma [75]. When diagnosed, their treatment is as for a malignant fibrous tumor (see below).

Given the multiplicity of combinations of local extent and histological appearance, it is difficult to be adamant regarding therapy. It is well recognized that curettage alone has a 20% or greater local recurrence rate [76]. Recent work by the European Musculoskeletal Oncology Society in a multicenter study suggests that the incidence of recurrence might be halved if adjuvant therapy (phenolization, cryotherapy, or po-lymethyl-methacrylate) is used in combination with intralesional techniques.

Curettage remains the mainstay of treatment; occasionally multiple attempts may be required. Reconstruction may not always be required after curettage and a number of patients have been treated by simple casting or cast-bracing until in-filling of the cavity [77]. If articular failure has occurred by fracture or tumor invasion, then reconstruction with a prosthesis or allograft will be required.

16.6.5.2 Nonossifying Fibroma/Benign Fibrous Histiocytoma

Nonossifying fibroma is generally the term given to a lesion which is larger than a fibrous cortical defect. The term metaphyseal fibrous defect may be used for both. The lesions are extremely common between the ages of 4 and 8 years and can affect any metaphysis [78]. They are rarely seen in adults, which probably reflects the natural history of the condition. Large lesions may be associated with pathological fractures [79].

The radiological features are characteristic, consisting of an eccentric lesion which may involve the cortex situated at the end of the diaphysis. A sclerotic rim is usually seen on the medullary border. Although the lesion does not usually require biopsy, unusual clinical or radiological features may justify the need for needle biopsy.

Treatment in the majority of cases is only observation. Enlargement or pathological fracture will demand curettage or block excision with or without bone grafting. Fractures occasionally lead to obliteration of the lesion [80].

Benign fibrous histiocytoma may have a similar histological picture to a nonossifying fibroma but tends to occur in older patients and is sited away from the metaphysis. Treatment requires either curettage or block excision.

16.6.6 Malignant Tumors of Histiocytic or Fibrohistiocytic Origin

16.6.6.1 Malignant Fibrous Histiocytoma

Malignant fibrous histiocytoma was first described by Feldman and Norman in 1972 [81]. It is a high-grade spindle cell lesion of bone which accounts for approximately 5% of all bone tumors. Although the peak incidence is in the fifth decade, it may occur at any age. Females seem to be preferentially affected in the second decade. Histologically, it resembles its soft tissue counterpart but must be differentiated from this and from fibroblastic subtype of osteosarcoma. The latter may be differentiated by osteoid or alkaline phosphatase production [82]. The clinical presentation is as for other bone tumors, with a usually fairly lengthy duration. The area affected is usually around the knee and the radiographic features are of a tumor with essentially a lytic component with ill-defined margins. Lymph node metastases may occur [83]. Unlike its soft tissue counterpart, malignant fibrous histiocytoma of bone has been shown to respond well to a number of chemotherapeutic agents, including Adriamycin (doxorubicin), ifosfamide, high-dose methotrexate, and cisplatin. Therefore, a combined approach using adjuvant or neoadjuvant chemotherapy, together with adequate surgery, seems the treatment of choice.

16.6.7 Bone Tumors of Vascular Origin

16.6.7.1 Hemangioendothelioma

Hemangioendothelioma is a locally aggressive nonmetastasizing tumor. All age groups can be affected and there is a male predilection. Radiographic appearances are of an osteolytic lesion which may occasionally produce a honeycomb pattern. Treatment is by adequate local surgery. Local recurrence is a problem.

16.6.7.2 Hemangiopericytoma

This is a low-grade malignant spindle cell tumor representing 0.1% of malignant bone tumors. It is also more common in males [84]. It again resembles its soft tissue counterpart and presents as an osteolytic bony lesion. The pelvis and lower limbs are more commonly affected. Wide surgical excision is the treatment of choice. The role of chemotherapy or radiotherapy is not yet established. Unfortunately, local recurrence is extremely common and metastases may occur extremely late.

16.6.7.3 Angiosarcoma

This is the high-grade counterpart of hemangioendothelioma. It is exceedingly rare. Again, wide surgery is the treatment of choice. Vascularity of the tumor may make limb salvage surgery extremely difficult. The tumor is radiosensitive [85]. The role for chemotherapy is not yet established.

16.6.8 Adamantinoma

Adamantinoma is an extremely rare bone tumor which occurs commonly in females, mainly in the second decade of life (Fig. 16.13). The bone which is commonly affected is the tibia [86]. Histologically, there is a mixture of spindle cells forming a fibrous stroma and islands of epithelial-like cells. It often arises in a background of fibrous dysplasia, and a differential diagnosis from metastatic carcinoma in the older patient may be difficult because of the expression of epithelial markers [21]. Occasionally, other long bones can be affected and multifocality has been recorded. Diagnosis may take many years because of the slow growth of the tumor. Radiologically, the lesion is lytic and well defined. Metastases are only found late in the disease. Treatment is excision, usually involving limb-saving techniques applied after diaphyseal resection and reconstruction.

16.6.9 Ewing's Sarcoma

Ewing's sarcoma is the second most common malignant bone tumor of children and adolescents. Although there is a wide histological spectrum, 10–15% of tumors fall into the category of malignant round blue cell tumor/Ewing's sarcoma [87]. The mean annual incidence approximates 0.6 per million of the total population [88]. It is rare below the age of 5 years, and the peak incidence is between 10 and 15 years. Male to female ratio is approximately 1.5:1, but this may vary with the age of the patient. Black and Chinese populations are less affected [89]. In addition to the standard presenting features, fever may occur, and this is more likely in patients with advanced or metastatic disease [90]. Pelvis, femur, tibia, and fibula account for 60% of all primary sites. Although the plain radiographic appearance may be characteristic with a moth-eaten central bony destruction having poorly defined margins and an associated parallel onion-skin periosteal lamination together with a large soft tissue extension, this picture is not always seen (Fig. 16.14). Further investigations are required to confirm the diagnosis. Approximately 20% of patients present with detectable metastases [91] which may be either pulmonary or be represented by multiple bone/bone marrow involvement. The serum lactate dehydrogenase (LDH) level may be elevated and this is associated with a poor prognostic outcome [92]. Other factors having a favorable influence on prognosis in Ewing's sarcoma are female gender [93], tumor volume at presentation [94], histological type [95], and proven histological response to chemotherapy [96].

Ewing's sarcoma represents a tumor where the utmost collaboration is required between surgeon, radi-

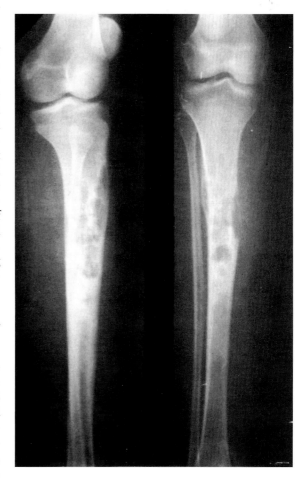

Fig. 16.13 AP and lateral view of adamantinoma of the tibia.

ologist and pathologist. The radiological appearance of osteomyelitis may be very similar, and this can be further complicated if the patient has a leucocytosis and/or fever. The pathologist must differentiate Ewing's tumor from primitive neuroectodermal tumor (PNET) and Askin's tumor, which can be done using neural specific immunohistochemistry. Similar problems may occur in distinguishing the tumor on histological grounds from rhabdomyosarcoma, neuroblastoma lymphoma, and small cell osteosarcoma. Rarely, primary malignant lymphoma of bone can present without disseminated lymph node or visceral disease. Again, immunohistochemistry using lymphoid markers is helpful in recognizing this category of tumor [97]. Ewing's sarcoma may also present as a extraskeletal lesion without a perceptible bony component. In this variant, there is a higher risk of lymphatic spread; this rare variant is usually treated using the principles employed in embryonal rhabdomyosarcoma [98]. There is no doubt that Ewing's sarcoma is a rapidly disseminating malignancy. Prior to the advent of effective chemotherapy, 90% of patients died within 5 years.

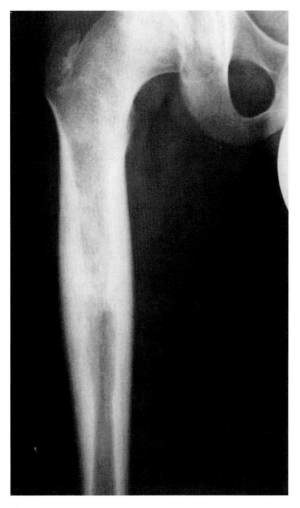

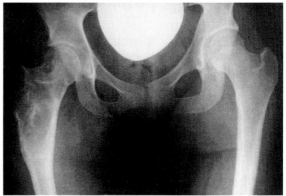

Fig. 16.15 Simple bone cyst proximal femur.

Fig. 16.14 Ewing's sarcoma of the femur exhibiting typical periosteal lamination (onion-skinning).

Conventionally, radiotherapy has had a major role in local treatment in Ewing's sarcoma [99]. Although the risk of local failure following radiation alone is difficult to assess, there is increasing evidence that the probability of cure with radiotherapy is related to limited tumor bulk and chemosensitivity as measured by tumor regression [100]. Radiotherapy also can affect growth if the epiphyses are treated leading to limb deformity and length inequality, and radiotherapy around the joints may lead to contracture formation. Radiotherapy in the pelvis may lead to visceral or gonadal damage, although excision alone may be similarly fraught with morbidity [101]. Although the debate continues, it is generally recognized that operative intervention is indicated for the local treatment in Ewing's sarcoma. In the axial skeleton, surgery is rarely indicated but in the pelvis considerable problems may be posed. Certainly, pelvic tumors are usually large and have extensive soft tissue extension invading the pelvic cavity when ini-

tially diagnosed. Their prognosis is particularly poor [102]. There is now good evidence that the prognosis of extensive pelvic lesion can be improved when the residual interosseous disease (following chemotherapy) is resected and reconstruction performed. Such resections are rarely "wide" and therefore are usually followed by postoperative radiotherapy. Whether radiotherapy can be omitted in patients who have had a particularly good chemotherapeutic response is the subject of on-going controlled trials [103]. (For management of Ewing's tumor affecting the chest wall see Chap. 18.)

16.6.9.1 Simple Bone Cyst (Unicameral Bone Cyst)

These fluid-filled cysts often arise in the metaphyseal region of long bones juxtaposed to the epiphyseal plate. They are usually brought to the patient's attention either by incidental X-ray or by pathological fracture. Fracture may lead to resolution of the cyst, but it is also well recognized that a traumatic episode may turn a cystic lesion into an aneurysmal bone cyst [104].

Cysts are commonly found in the proximal humerus and femur but may also occur in both the radius and ulna. They are commonly seen in childhood and adolescence, 90% of patients being younger than 20 years old. When they do occur in the adult, they tend to occur in either the ilium or os calcis.

Plain radiographs usually show a lesion which has a central medullary location and its length is usually greater than its width (Fig. 16.15). The transverse diameter of the cyst closest to the epiphysis is recognized as being as wide as the epiphysis. With age, the cyst grows towards the diaphysis. This appearance is contrary to an aneurysmal bone cyst (see below), which shows a centrifugal growth pattern. Where the cyst reacts with cancellous bone there is a bony reaction but periosteal reaction is extremely rare. There is no soft tissue component. Further radiological investigation is rarely performed, although it is possible to recognize fluid levels on a CT scan. Treatment can be difficult. Small cysts which are asymptomatic do not require any therapy. However, large cysts may require curettage, bone grafting, en bloc resection, or even nailing. It is now fairly universally accepted following the work of Campanacci, et al. [105] that these cysts will respond to an injection of methylprednisolone. If surgery is contemplated, incomplete removal of the cyst lining usually leads to local recurrence. The recurrence rate is much higher in children [106].

16.6.9.2 Aneurysmal Bone Cyst

These blood-filled expansile lesions present with pain and swelling and may follow a fracture. It is recognized that during pregnancy aneurysmal bone cysts may rapidly enlarge.

It is predominantly a disease of the first three decades of life and occurs equally in both sexes. It can affect any bone and 80% are recorded as occurring in the upper limb.

The radiological features are of a purely lytic expansile lesion which usually arises in the metaphysis. Extension may occur into the epiphysis when the growth plate has closed [107]. They may grow alarmingly and may mimic malignant tumors (Fig. 16.16). Again, if further radiological investigation is required, the multiple fluid levels seen on CT are practically diagnostic of an aneurysmal bone cyst [108].

The mainstay of treatment is a combination of curettage and bone grafting. Where the tumor arises in inaccessible sites or where excessive blood loss is feared, arterial embolization may be a helpful adjunct to treatment. In tumors that recur or remain inaccessible, small doses of radiation can be given [109].

16.6.10 Miscellaneous Tumors of Soft Tissue and Bone

16.6.10.1 Myositis Ossificans

This condition is particularly troublesome when it occurs around the elbow joint. Although it can occur following a single injury, it more usually follows chronic repetitive trauma. The most usual presentation is of a painless mass, although some patients may have considerable soft tissue inflammation and pain. The period of symptoms is usually short.

The radiographic features show no abnormality in the first 2–3 weeks and then speckled calcification

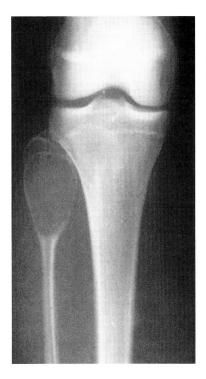

Fig. 16.16 Aneurysmal bone cyst proximal fibula showing large bone expansion.

becomes evident. A fully mature lesion can usually be seen at around 14 weeks. In general, the diagnosis should be made on clinical and radiological grounds as great care is required in the examination of a biopsy. Unfortunately, myositis ossificans can be easily mistaken for osteogenic sarcoma [110].

Treatment is usually by surgical excision, but this should not be performed until the lesions have matured. Surgical intervention prior to maturity leads to a high rate of local recurrence.

16.7 Surgical Management

16.7.1 Embolization

Though angiography is now rarely used in presurgical imaging protocols, it can be useful in helping the clinician decide whether a plane of dissection exists between the tumor and the local neurovascular structures and, therefore, allow some limb salvage procedure to be performed. Occasionally, in tumors such as aneurysmal bone cysts, hemangiomas, and vascular osteosarcomas, such as the telangiectatic variety, significant feeding vessels can be recognized. Use of embolization materials injected into these vessels may significantly decrease the vascularity and render excision either possible or more easily accomplished. Embolization may be accompanied by significant pain and discomfort in the affected limb and the procedure should really be timed to allow for surgery to follow within 24 h. Embolization used solely as a method of local treatment is not recommended.

16.7.2 Curettage Alone

Certain benign tumors, notably aneurysmal bone cyst and giant cell tumor, lend themselves to treatment by intralesional removal or curettage. The technique of curettage requires a direct approach to the most weakened part of the cortical bone in expansile lesions or the most anatomically easy access in true intramedullary lesions. A good window of cortical bone is removed to allow adequate visual access to all the various crevices within the medullary cavity. A thorough curettage is performed with a standard bone curette and the cavity is then further debrided using either an osteotome or dental burr. The whole cavity is then thoroughly lavaged with a pressurized pulsed lavage system. The technique leads to an acceptable rate of local recurrence which is variably reported. Giant cell tumor local recurrence rate as high as 40% can be recorded with this technique alone. Most surgeons now prefer to add some form of adjuvant therapy; the use of adjuvant therapy will decrease the local rate of recurrence to less than 15%. Local adjuvants which have been proposed include cryotherapy, phenolization, and the use of cement, the latter having a dual role; first, the hyperthermic reaction produced in the setting of cement causes local necrosis and further decreases the local recurrence rate, and, second, the cement itself may give immediate structural strength. For the younger patient, most authors prefer to remove the cement after an interval and substitute with bone graft. Lesions sited in the proximal humerus or distal radius are more suited to the simple curettage technique (Fig. 16.17).

16.7.3 Curettage and Bone Graft

When benign tumors occur in the subarticular position, the subchondral bone can be eroded and deformity of the articular surface can be encountered (Fig. 16.18). Treatment, therefore, must consist of gaining some mechanical support with either fresh autograft or allograft. The lesion is curettaged in the above manner and then morsellized cancellous autograft harvested from the iliac crest is inserted into the defect. This will allow reconstitution of the subchondral space and support the articular architecture of the joint (Fig. 16.19). Bone autograft is incorporated relatively quickly. The exact mechanism by which this incorporation occurs is not fully understood but has been previously investigated and reported by Burwell

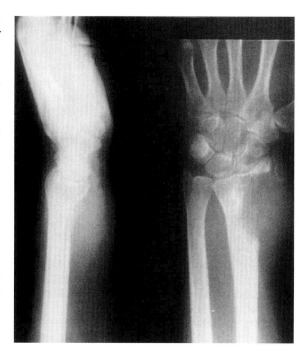

Fig. 16.17 Giant cell tumor of distal radius.

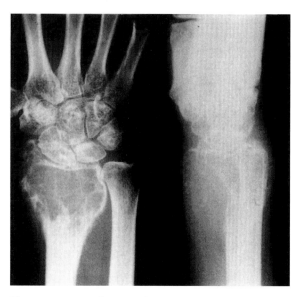

Fig. 16.18 Giant cell tumor of distal radius showing deformity of the articular surface.

[111]. The initial phase of incorporation in the first 2 weeks is analogous to fracture healing and is equally effective on both cancellous and cortical bone. Osteoblasts are laid down on the surface of the graft, and in the case of cancellous bone the osteoid seen laid down on top of the transplanted trabeculae of bone are rapidly absorbed. Eventually, all the graft of cancellous nature is resorbed. Where cortical fragments exist, the

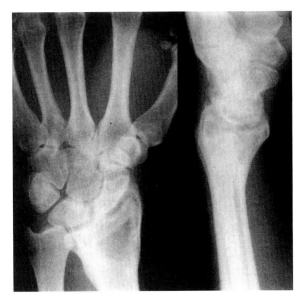

Fig. 16.19 Lesion of distal radius following curettage and bone grafting.

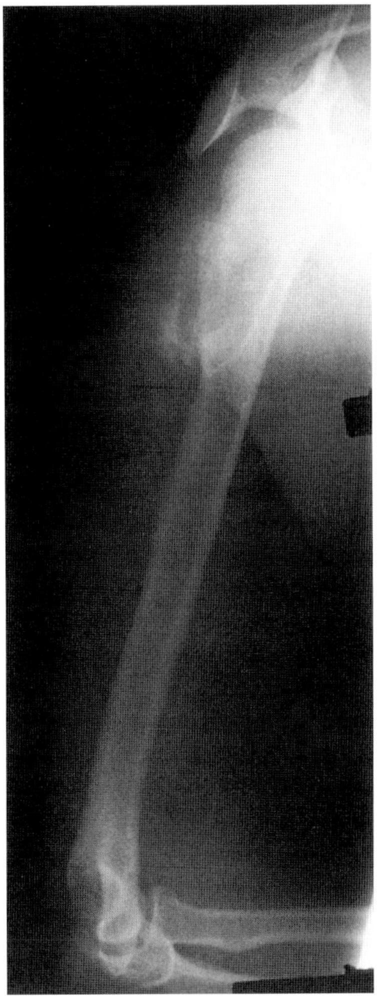

revascularization rate is slower and cortical fragments may be retained even following long-term incorporation. For this reason, cancellous grafting is preferred unless some mechanical strength is required, when cortical or fibular struts may be preferred. In recent years increasing use of bone graft substitute such as ApaPore, a synthetic hydroxy-appetite, have gained increasing amounts of popularity. They obviously avoid the morbidity of donor site harvest and usually incorporate within 6 months.

16.7.4 Excision Alone

Certain benign tumors which occur eccentrically on the bone surface are suitable for simple excision. The most classical variety is a osteochondroma or actively-growing exostosis (Fig. 16.20). Here, surgical therapy merely requires resection of the bony stalk of the exostosis at the junction with the host bone. Care must be taken, however, not to spill any of the cartilage fragments, which may lead to local recurrence. The technique of local excision can also be extended to lesions such as nonossifying fibroma, which occur eccentrically in the metaphysis of bone, and to certain low-grade malignant tumors, such as periosteal osteosarcoma, where the resulting defect in the diaphysis may not be great. However, care must always be taken to achieve an adequate surgical margin to prevent local recurrence, but most surgical oncologists now believe that the initially reported 5-cm margin is no longer required. Certainly, an adequate rim of normal host bone is all that is necessary, although occasionally this

Fig. 16.20 Preoperative illustrations of a proximal humeral osteochondroma.

may require grafting techniques to reconstitute the diaphysis (Fig. 16.21).

16.7.5 Osteoarticular Fibular Transplantation

This technique is suitable for fairly large defects which occur following resections of benign or aggressive tumors of the distal radius and proximal humerus. The proximal ipsilateral fibula is harvested and is generally used in a nonvascularized manner. Transplanted to the upper humerus, it will allow a rudimentary shoulder joint which is relatively pain-free, particularly in the younger child. There may also be some hypertrophy of the graft. When used to reconstitute the distal radius, the articular surface is placed adjacent to the scaphoid bone and acts as a structural support and articulation. The fibula is usually plated onto the residual radius and the radial collateral ligament of the wrist reconsti-

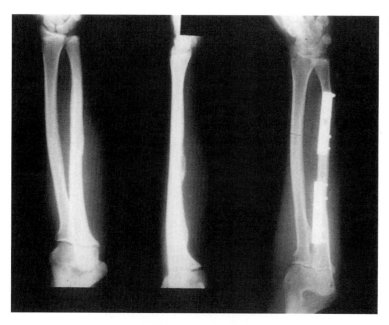

Fig. 16.21 Fibular grafting to reconstitute the diaphysis following tumor excision.

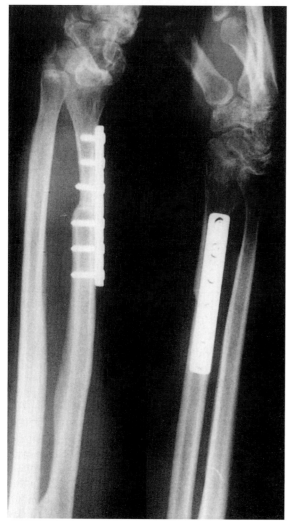

tuted by using a loop of extensor carpi radialis longus. An illustrative case is seen in Fig. 16.22.

16.7.6 Bone Transportation

This technique originally described by Ilizarov [112] was originally used in congenital deformity and post-traumatic situations which has been extended to the use of filling postsurgical defects following tumor surgery. The principle is to transport a bone cylinder over the length of the defect and achieve bony closure at the proximal end of the defect by callus distraction and at the distal end of the defect by contact of the cylinder with the host bone. It has significant problems in that it involves prolonged external fixation time of several months, although this is less so in the upper limb. All transport systems suffer from pin track infection and the incidence of this limits the technique to benign tumors. The technique is contraindicated, in my opinion, in malignant tumors where patients are undergoing chemotherapy. Extremely short defects can be managed by acute shortening of the limb followed by reconstitution of the length using a technique of callus distraction (Fig. 16.23). The regenerate bone is often difficult to visualize on plain radiography and the use of ultrasound techniques is indicated to measure the degree and quality of the bone regenerate. In the lower limb, rapid internal fixation and distal bone grafting is recommended, but in the upper limb this does not seem to be a prob-

Fig. 16.22 Osteoarticular fibular transplantation of the distal radius in giant cell tumor.

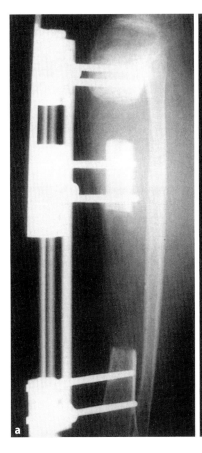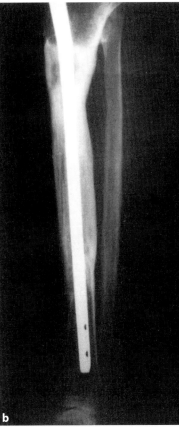

Fig. 23 a, b (**a**) Initial radiograph following bone transportation of the tibial diaphysis. (**b**) Final radiograph following bone transportation of the tibial diaphysis.

lem. Simple stabilization of the lengthening, which allows the regenerate to mature, appears to be all that is required. The technique is limited to diaphyseal defects. The rate of distraction is usually 1 mm per day, often in four quarter turns of the distracting device [113].

16.8 Surgery for Large Osteoarticular Defects

When considering whether limb salvage procedures are justified, it has been traditional to consider the long-term oncological result and compare that with results obtained historically with amputation. Subsequent comparisons can be made in four broad areas:

1. Is there any difference in overall survival by patients treated by the two methods?
2. What is the early and late morbidity for each type of reconstruction?
3. Is the function of the salvaged limb satisfactory and does it remain so over a period of prolonged follow-up?
4. Are there quality of life issues for patients undergoing limb salvage procedures as opposed to amputation?

16.8.1 Overall Survival

There have been a number of reports from single institutions [114, 115] which have concluded that the performance of limb salvage operations had no effect on the long-term survival of patients. These early reports have been confirmed by a number of multi-institutional reports [116–118]. Simon, et al. point out that the local recurrence rate of patients undergoing above-knee amputation for malignant bone tumors around the knee is about 10%, which is not dissimilar to patients undergoing limb salvage procedures. However, no patients who had a hip disarticulation suffered a local recurrence although at the cost of significant mutilation. Simon [119] reports a study from the Musculoskeletal Tumor Society, where the development of local recurrence was an extremely bad prognostic factor. Sixteen of seventeen people who developed local recurrence following limb salvage or amputation eventually died of their disease. Certainly, local recurrence usually requires amputation if there is no other metastatic disease. Even following amputation it would appear that survival is still unlikely. It is still, however, unclear whether the local recurrence represents poor response of the tumor to neoadjuvant chemotherapeutic agents and hence a poor prognosis or whether it is merely poor surgical decision-making. There are, of course, a large number of cases, particularly where local recurrence occurs late and is not associated with metastatic disease, where further limb salvage procedures may be considered.

16.8.2 Early Complications

Operations performed for limb salvage are fraught with complications. Acute vascular injury may occasionally occur, and venous thrombosis and pulmonary embolism may be encountered in the early postoperative period. Involvement of neural structures often leads to sacrifice of a nerve during resection of the tumor, but the most worrying complication in the early postoperative period is wound necrosis and subsequent infection. Loss of cutaneous cover requires urgent soft tissue coverage, often by a local skin flap or rarely by a myocutaneous free flap, so that the method of reconstruction can be covered. If infection ensues, then the complications, particularly where an endoprosthesis has been used, may be devastating. Often the limb requires amputation in the short or medium term. The onset of infection also delays the planned return of the patient to adjuvant chemotherapy.

It is important to emphasize that amputation itself is not without short- and long-term complications, and certainly local pressure sores from an external prosthesis, phantom pain, and overgrowth of the stump when amputation is performed in children are recognized complications.

Endoprostheses are now used in a variety of benign and malignant conditions. There is a greater tendency to use them in malignant conditions, often where the patient's survival may be in doubt and hence the patient's longevity limited. Complex reconstructions are rarely justified in this situation. Although techniques such as osteoarticular allografting and bone transportation may be considered in patients with benign or low-grade malignant disease, there are occasions when endoprostheses may be utilized. In our practice, this is usually in periarticular destructive lesions, the most common of which being recurrent giant cell tumor. The frequency of prosthetic utilization in various pathologies is outlined in Fig. 16.24. It can be seen that less than 20% of patients have a benign condition.

It is well known that most of the malignant bone and joint tumors have a predilection for the lower limb with a few cases occurring in the upper humeral metaphysis. It is therefore not surprising that if the distribution of prosthetic insertion throughout the body is studied, over 80% of the cases have insertion in the

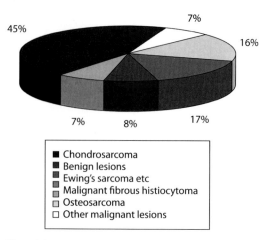

Fig. 16.24 Distribution of prosthetic utilization in various primary bone pathologies.

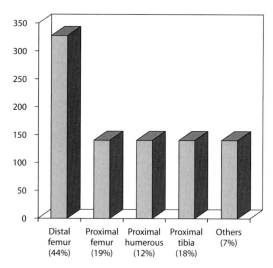

Fig. 16.25 Anatomical distribution of types of prostheses inserted.

lower limb. The proximal humerus remains the most common site replaced in the upper limb (Fig. 16.25). The foremost commonly replaced areas are therefore, in order of frequency, the distal femur and knee, the proximal femur and hip, the proximal tibia and knee and, last, the proximal humerus and shoulder. Occasionally, the diaphysis of femur, tibia, and humerus may be replaced, but these represent only a small fraction of the prostheses inserted. A similar low percentage exists for replacement of the whole bone and adjacent joints.

16.8.3 Allograft Techniques

Allografts suitable for osteoarticular reconstruction are usually only retrieved from deceased donors. This leads to a significant risk of human immunodeficiency virus (HIV) infection and secondary testing of the donor cannot be accomplished [120]. Such allografts are rarely used in a fresh situation and they must either be frozen with cartilage cryopreservation or freeze dried. Similarly, they must be sterilized by either ethylene oxide or gamma irradiation. Only frozen techniques will allow attempts at cartilage cryopreservation, but frozen and freeze-dried techniques tend to reduce the antigenicity of the allograft. When implanted, the biological response to a preserved allograft is, at first, similar to an autograft. However, secondarily, there is an immunological response which causes changes within the graft. The immunological response mounted by the host causes vascular necrosis, which is followed by a second peak of osteoblastic activity at the end of the first 4 weeks. There has been some experimental work by Musculo [121] that suggests tissue typing in allografts will lead to better incorporation. Union of the allograft usually occurs from creeping substitu-

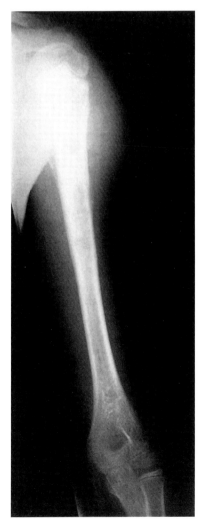

Fig. 16.26 Pathological fracture through osteosarcoma of the proximal humerus.

tion from the host bone, but there is usually excellent reconstruction of the soft tissues with the graft. The long-lasting presence of necrotic and revascularizing bone makes allografts more likely to fracture, but this is more of a problem in the lower limb. Strengthening of the allograft may be obtained by adding mechanical support or intramedullary cement. The overall fracture incidence is approximately 16% [122]. The overall complication rate and long-term function of proximal humeral allografts has been reported by O'Connor, et al. [123] and in a nonrandomized comparison of long-term function osteoarticular allograft functioned better than prostheses in the upper humeral position. This essentially has been due to better soft tissue reconstruction, and conforms with the previous work of Gebhardt, et al. [124]. Many of the complications of allograft use in the long term have resulted from the lack of vascularity. Capanna, et al. [125], have recently described a technique of using allograft shells combined with a vascularized fibular graft. This has not yet been used in an osteoarticular allograft, but may be of use where a scapulohumeral fusion is employed as the reconstructive method. While Mankin from the USA has popularized the use of cadaveric allografts, and although function in the upper limb is better than in the lower, there remain problems of sizing, stability, fracture, rejection, and degeneration [126, 127].

16.8.4 Endoprosthetic Techniques

Each area which is replaced has its own particular problems, and these are illustrated below.

16.8.4.1 Case 1

A 12-year-old boy presented with a 5-week history of pain and discomfort in the left shoulder which was ignored. While on holiday he fell from a donkey and sustained a pathological fracture. Staging investigations confirmed a pathological fracture through the left proximal humerus with no evidence of metastatic disease (Fig. 16.26). Biopsy confirmed high-grade osteosarcoma and the patient underwent neoadjuvant chemotherapy. The patient responded to chemotherapy and 6 weeks following the diagnosis underwent resection of the upper left humerus and endoprosthetic replacement (Fig. 16.27). The technical problems in performing upper humeral replacement in such a large tumor are twofold. The first is the proximity of the neurovascular bundle, part of which (the circumflex nerve) is particularly vulnerable as it winds round the surgical neck of the humerus. The second problem is the potential of intracapsular involvement of the glenohumeral joint. Fortunately, extra-articular

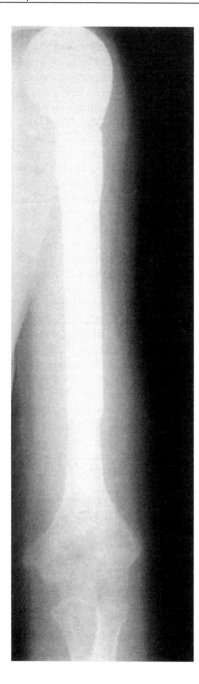

Fig. 16.27 Proximal humeral prosthetic replacement.

resection is rarely required and in this case intra-articular resection was performed. There remains considerable debate as to the method of reconstruction of the residual rotator cuff. Early attempts to preserve function by sewing the cuff to a terylene sleeve were met with considerable abrasion debris and sinus formation. Some surgeons still use such a cuff as an artificial capsule over which the rotator cuff is repaired. This technique may lead to considerable stiffness of the glenohumeral joint. Prosthetic replacement of the

upper humerus leads to excellent restoration of elbow and hand movement. Shoulder movement, however, remains quite limited. The usual outcome is that rotation is well controlled, although external rotation may be grossly exaggerated. Flexion and abduction are rarely better than 408 , and if the circumflex nerve is sacrificed may not be achieved at all. In manual workers where nerve sacrifice is anticipated, some form of biological or prosthetic arthrodesis of the glenohumeral joint may be a better alternative. Even where the circumflex nerve is preserved, rotator cuff function remains poor, and over time many prostheses sublax into the subacromial space. Early experience with bipolar prostheses where a reverse shoulder mechanism is utilized have shown much better functional movements without the risks of superior or inferior subluxation. The mechanism involves a hemisphere on a spiral component which is screwed into the glenoid with an HA collar. This snap fits into a concave surface inserted on to the upper humerus. Early 5-year results are now available and are encouraging [127].

16.8.4.2 Case 2

A 12-year-old boy presented with a 3-month history of pain and discomfort in the upper left femur. Initial investigation at another hospital showed an abnormal area on plain radiograph and this site underwent open biopsy, which showed Ewing's sarcoma. He was treated with chemotherapy and then underwent an intra-articular resection of the hip joint and upper third of the left femur. The prosthesis was inserted and a bipolar head placed on top of the prosthesis to give acetabular stability. The prosthesis was of an extendible variety (Fig. 16.28). The surgical technique involved detachment of the iliac psoas and all three gluteal muscles. It is usually possible to leave the tensor fascia lata intact which preserves innervation. The rest of the vastus muscles remained innervated although the vastus lateralis may be denervated and vastus intermedius is usually excised as a barrier to the tumor. Two methods of reconstruction of the abductor apparatus are possible. Usually the soft tissue is reconstructed using a nylon weave to connect the muscular structures to the tensor fascia lata. Abduction can be maintained but the altered lever arm means that many patients have a positive Trendelenburg gait. Another technique under investigation involves turning down part of the ilium attached to the anterior fibers of gluteus medius muscle to allow fibrosis of the muscle on to the prosthesis itself. The most frequent complication of this procedure is hip dislocation. The patient is advised to use a PoHo type brace for the first 2 months after operation.

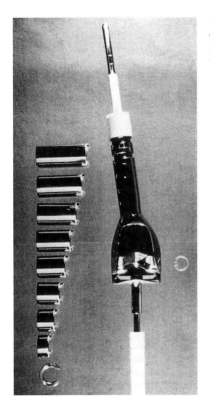

Fig. 16.28
Growing distal
femoral endopros-
thesis.

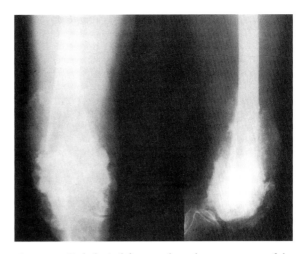

Fig. 16.29 Pathological fracture through osteosarcoma of the right distal femur.

16.8.4.3 Case 3

An 8-year-old girl presented with a 2-week history of pain in her right distal femur and awoke one morning following a tussle with her sibling in excruciating pain. Plain radiograph confirmed an undisplaced pathological fracture through an osteosarcoma of the distal right femur (Fig. 16.29). Percutaneous needle biopsy performed under general anesthesia confirmed a chondroblastic osteosarcoma. The patient received neoadjuvant chemotherapy and underwent resection of the tumor 6 weeks later. Analysis of the resected specimen confirmed 90% of the tumor had undergone complete necrosis. It was opted to reconstruct the limb using an uncemented expandable prosthesis (Fig. 16.30). The patient had an uneventful postoperative recovery and is now walking without a limp. Distal femoral replacement remains the most successful area in terms of early function following prosthetic insertion. The anatomy of the region means that the extensor apparatus is rarely severely damaged, and although the gastrocnemius is severely weakened by detachment of their origins, knee flexion can be fully compensated by the hamstrings. Therefore, it is often difficult to tell the operated side when observing gait in such patients. The mechanism used in this case to enable elongation of a prosthesis is termed minimally invasive. Elongation is achieved by insertion of an Allen key to turn a

low gear mechanism to achieve elongation of the body of the prosthesis. It is, however, likely that this young lady will require a revision of her prosthesis and perhaps surgical cessation of growth on the opposite limb in order to achieve limb balance at maturity. Over the last 2 years, increasing use of noninvasive magnetic endoprosthesis has been experienced. The prosthesis is similar to the prosthesis described above, but here the elongation is achieved by a motor placed within the body of the prosthesis. Placing the motor in a magnetic field produces a force of around 1,500 N, which allows very slow extension of the prosthesis. Some 4 mm of extension will be achieved in 16 min. The slow but strong elongation force is achieved by using an epicyclic gear box. To date the prosthesis is used mainly in the lower limb prosthesis where growth is more important, but experience is just beginning regarding the humerus [127].

16.8.4.4 Case 4

A 17-year-old boy presented with a rapidly enlarging swelling of the left proximal tibia. He denied any pain. Plain radiographs revealed a lytic area of the upper tibia through an area of abnormal bone. Jamshidi needle biopsy performed under local anesthetic confirmed an osteoblastic high-grade osteosarcoma; MRI showed a very large soft tissue mass extending into the anterior compartment (Fig. 16.31). Further staging investigations revealed no evidence of metastatic disease. The patient received neoadjuvant chemotherapy, which was uncomplicated, and 6 weeks later underwent prosthetic replacement of the right proximal tibia. The surgical resection of the proximal tibia is fraught with complications. The most important of

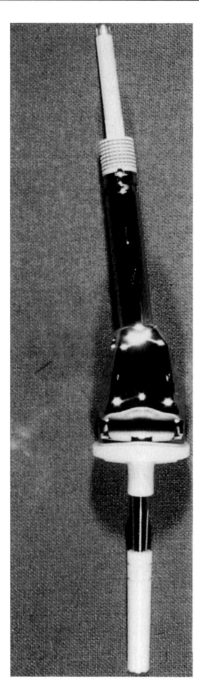

Fig. 16.30 Uncemented extendible distal femoral and knee prosthesis.

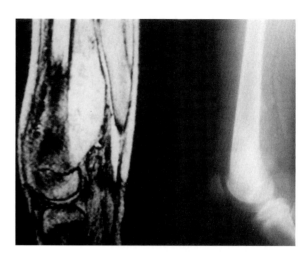

Fig. 16.31 Osteosarcoma of distal femur: MRI showing a large soft tissue mass extending into the posterior compartment.

rial ischemia, compartmental syndromes, and nerve palsy. Established neural palsy is, of course, treatable by use of an external ankle-foot orthosis (AFO), ankle arthrodesis or, where appropriate, tendon transfer. In the long term, the major functional disability lies in the weakness of the extensor mechanism. All upper tibial replacements undergo a medial gastrocnemius flap, and this further weakens the flexors of the knee, the long flexors having been previously detached. The extensor mechanism may be reconstructed by simple suture on to the transposed medial head of gastrocnemius, but others prefer a transposition of the upper fibula achieved by multiple osteotomy if this bone is still present or by turn-down of a portion of the distal patella (Fig. 16.32).

Postoperative rehabilitation is slow, and the patient is usually kept splinted in extension for a period of 6–8 weeks. The area of reconstruction of the extensor mechanism usually stretches, and the patient usually presents with patella alta and occasionally instability. Few can achieve a straight leg raise, although most achieve a normal walking pattern. This is achieved by throwing the tibia forward following hamstring relaxation and then locking the prosthesis in slight hyperextension.

16.8.5 Amputation and Disarticulation

Despite the current trend to perform limb salvage procedures in malignant disease following neoadjuvant chemotherapy, there are still a proportion of patients who are not suitable for this technique. The present primary amputation rate for musculoskeletal bone tumors at the Royal National Orthopaedic Hospital

these as regards long-term function is the detachment of the extensor mechanism. The next most common problem concerns the common peroneal nerve, which usually has to be mobilized and occasionally sacrificed in resection of the tumor. The vascular structures are closely applied to the posterior aspect of the knee and the anterior tibial artery is nearly always sacrificed, as it is grossly adherent to the tumor as it enters the anterior compartment. The early morbidity in these cases, therefore, usually is a combination of arte-

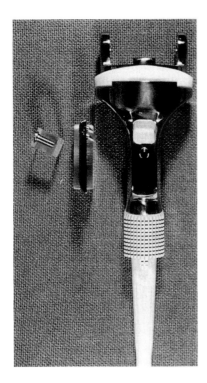

Fig. 16.32 Proximal tibial prosthetic replacement.

is 7%. The indications for primary amputation are as follows:

1. Late presenting tumors with widespread soft tissue contamination, including involvement of the neurovascular bundle, which do not respond to chemotherapy;
2. Difficult anatomical location where tumors surround the neurovascular bundle ab initio;
3. Advancement of tumors despite chemotherapy (poor response to chemotherapy);
4. Wide major displacement and pathological fracture at presentation.

The description of various techniques of amputation is not in the remit of this chapter. However, the most usual lesion which requires amputation is the proximal humeral osteosarcoma where there is widespread involvement of the axillary structures, often with encroachment onto the chest wall. Simple disarticulation of the glenohumeral joint is rarely sufficient in gaining tumor control. These patients unfortunately, require a forequarter amputation procedure.

16.9 Management of Local Recurrence

When the first meeting of the International Limb Salvage Association occurred at the Mayo Clinic in 1981, the goal of the symposium was to share experience and focus research into improved results of limb-sparing procedures. At that meeting, the local recurrence rate for all the reported series of limb salvage procedures was 4%. The society has continued to meet on a twice-yearly basis, and techniques of limb salvage have been popularized. The difficulty is that despite improved imaging techniques, the local recurrence rate for malignant tumors is now 10% (Enneking WF, personal communication). This seemingly detrimental step in terms of treatment of course results from a vast increase in the number of procedures performed and also a change in patient awareness and demands. Local recurrence usually occurs within 2 years from the primary procedure and the surgeon must be ever aware of its possibility. All limb salvage procedures have in common a very narrow resection margin at the level of the neurovascular bundle. It is not surprising that the majority of local recurrences tend to occur adjacent to this structure. To date, in the series at the Royal National Orthopaedic Hospital, London, we have had only one true recurrence within bone; 50% of local recurrences, because of involvement of neurovascular bundles, require either disarticulation or an ablative procedure in order to clear the problem. It is important that before undergoing such a procedure the patient is re-staged for the presence of metastatic disease. Where local recurrence occurs in tumors not adjacent to neurovascular structures but adjacent to bone, further resection and radiotherapy may be feasible.

16.10 Rehabilitation

The majority of limb salvage surgery procedures for primary bone tumors tends to occur in specialized units. Within those units are skilled physiotherapists and occupational therapists who have a wide experience in the rehabilitation of such difficult patients. The aim of biological reconstruction is not to use prolonged immobilization of joints and, therefore, removable splints rather than plaster fixation is generally preferred. Wherever possible, sound primary internal fixation of bone grafts is utilized. There is a continuing debate as to the effect of radiotherapy and chemotherapy upon biological fixation, and this appears to be greater if intra-arterial chemotherapy is considered [128]. Certainly in present regimes patients must be returned for further chemotherapy as rapidly as possible, and where a positive tumor margin is found in the tumor resection, radiotherapy must be considered in addition to attain local control. At present, radiotherapy can be administered in an interval between chemotherapy courses, and occasionally in a hyperfractionated manner. This is an extremely time-consuming and difficult technique, and more traditional approaches have been to delay radiotherapy until primary chemotherapy has been completed. Where patients have received an endoprosthesis, there is no concern regarding union of allograft to host or incorporation of graft, and therefore postoperative oncological management can begin as soon as the wound condition is satisfactory. With endoprosthesis of the proximal humerus, the lack of reliable reattachment of the rotator cuff or denervation or excision of the deltoid leads to significant problems with functional abduction and flexion of the shoulder joint. Although rapid mobilization of the elbow and distal limb is achieved, functional control of the shoulder is only slowly achieved, often not till approximately 6 months. At best, without a rotator cuff, only 40 degrees of flexion and abduction are achieved, although good rotational control of the limb is usually achieved by 6 months. Some early work is being performed on motorized abductor function by rotatory grafts of innervated latissimus dorsi. Whether this will achieve improved function in the long-term is still unclear. Careful evaluation of the patient is required in the presurgical period as arthrodesis of the shoulder is probably more suitable for a manual worker.

References

1. Souhami RL, Cannon SR (1995) Osteosarcoma. In: Peckham M, Pinedo H, Veronessi U (eds) Oxford textbook of oncology, vol II. Oxford University Press, Oxford, pp 1960–1976

2. Cooper A (1918) Exostosis. In: Cooper A, Travers B (eds) Surgical essays, 3rd edn. Cox & Son, London, pp 169–226

3. Solomon L (1961) Bone growth in diaphyseal aclasis. J Bone Joint Surg 43B:700–716

4. Ollier M (1900) Dyschondroplasie. Lyon Med 93:23–25

5. Maffucci A (1881) Di un caso di enchondroma ed angiome multiplo. Mov Med Chir 13:399–412

6. Ellmore SM, Cantrell WC (1966) Maffucci's syndrome—case report with a normal karyotype. J Bone Joint Surg 48A:1607–1613

7. McGeogh CM, Varian JP (1985) Osteoclastoma of the first metacarpal. J Hand Surg (Br) 10:129–130

8. Simon MA, Kirchner PT (1980) Scintigraphic evaluation of primary bone tumours. J Bone Joint Surg 62A:758–764

9. Murray IP (1980) Bone scanning in the child and young adult. Skeletal Radiol 5:1–14

10. Cohen M, et al. (1982) Lung CT of detection of metastases: Solid tissue neoplasms in children. Am J Radiol 139:895–898

11. Zimmer WD, Bergquist TH, McLeod RA, et al. (1985) Bone tumours: Magnetic resonance imaging versus computed tomography. Radiology 155:709–718

12. Aiser AM, Martel W, Braunstein EM, et al. (1986) MRI and CT evaluation of primary bone and soft tissue tumours. Am J Roentgenol 146:749–756

13. Bohndorf K, Reiser M, Lochner B, et al. (1986) Magnetic resonance imaging of primary tumours and tumour-like lesions of bone. Skeletal Radiol 15:511–517

14. Gillespy T III, et al. (1988) Staging of intraosseous extent of osteosarcoma. Radiology 167:765–767

15. Dooms GC, Hricak H, Sollitto RA, Higgins CB (1985) Lipomatous tumours and tumours with fatty component: MR imaging potential and comparison of MR and CT results. Radiology 157:479–483

16. Enneking WF (1982) Editorial: The issue of the biopsy. J Bone Joint Surg 64A:1119–1120

17. Mankin HJ, Lange TA Spanier SA (1982) The hazards of biopsy in patients with malignant primary bone and soft tissue tumours. J Bone Joint Surg 62A:1121–1127

18. Kreilbergs A, Bauer H, Brosjö O, et al. (1996) Cytological diagnosis of bone tumours. J Bone Joint Surg 78B:258–263

19. Stoker DJ, Cobb JP, Pringle JAS (1991) Needle biopsy of musculoskeletal lesions. J Bone Joint Surg 73B:498–500

20. Davies NM, Livesley PJ, Cannon SR (1993) Recurrence of osteosarcoma in a needle biopsy tract. J Bone Joint Surg 75B:977–978

21. Pringle JAS (1987) Pathology of bone tumours. Baillière's Clin Oncol 1:21–63

22. Cannon SR, Dyson PHP (1987) The relationship of the location of open biopsy of malignant bone tumours to local recurrence after resection and prosthetic replacement. J Bone Joint Surg 69B:492

23. Enneking WF, Spanier SS, Goodman MA (1980) A system for the surgical staging of musculoskeletal sarcomata. Clin Orthop 153:106–120

24. Broders AC (1964) The microscopic grading of cancer. In: Pack GT, Arrel IM (eds) Treatment of cancer and allied diseases. Hoeber, New York

25. Lewis RJ, Lotz MJ (1974) Medullary extension of osteosarcoma. Cancer 33:371–375

26. Campanacci M, Baldini N, Boriani S, et al. (1987) Giant cell tumour of bone. J Bone Joint Surg 69A:106–114

27. Hadders HN (1973) Some remarks on the histology of bone tumours. Year Book Cancer Res (Amsterdam) 22:7–10

28. Saville PD (1980) A medical option for the treatment of osteoid osteoma. Arth Rheum 23:1409–1411

29. Leonessa C, Savoni E (1971) Osteoma osteoide para articulare del gomito. Chir Organic Mov 59:487–492

30. Marcove RC, Freiberger RH (1966) Osteoid osteoma of the elbow - a diagnostic problem. J Bone Joint Surg 48A:1185–1190

31. Shifrin LZ, Reynolds WA (1971) Intra-articular osteoid osteoma of the elbow. Clin Orthop 81:126–129

32. Sim FH, Dahlin DC, Beabout JW (1975) Osteoid osteoma—diagnostic problems. J Bone Joint Surg 57A:154–159

33. Gamba JC, Martinez S, Apple J, et al. (1984) Computed tomography of axial skeletal osteoid osteomas. Am J Roentgenol 142:769–772

34. Szypryt EP, Hardy JG, Colton CL (1986) An improved technique of intra-operative bone scanning. J Bone Joint Surg 68B:643–646

35. Cannon SR, Briggs TWR, Johnson S, Remedios D (1998) Excision biopsy of osteoid osteoma under CT control. (in press)

35a. Rosenthal DI, Springfield DS, Gebhardt MC, Rosenberg AE, Mankin HJ (1995) Osteoid Osteoma: Percutaneous radio-frequency ablation radiology Nov 197(2)451–454

36. Lepage J, Rigault P, Nezelof C, et al. (1984) Benign osteoblastoma in children. Rev Clin Orthop 70:117–127

37. Canepa G, Defabiani F (1965) Osteoblastoma del radio. Minerva Ortop 16:645–648

38. Williams G, Barrett G, Pratt C (1977) Osteosarcoma in two very young children. Clin Paediat 16:548–551

39. Price CHG (1958) Primary bone-forming tumours and their relationship to skeletal growth. J Bone Joint Surg 40B:574–593

40. Simmons CC (1939) Bone sarcoma: Factors influencing prognosis. Surg Gycecol Obstet 68:67–75

41. Mankin HJ, Connor JF, Schiller AC, et al. (1985) Grading of bone tumours by analysis of nucleus DNA content using flow cytometry. J Bone Joint Surg 67A:404–413

42. Schreiman JS, Crass JR, Wick MR (1986) Osteosarcoma—role of CT in limb-sparing treatment. Radiology 161:485–488

43. Flowers JM Jr (1974) 99mTc-Polyphosphate up-take within pulmonary and soft tissue metastases from osteosarcoma. Radiology 112:377–378

44. Stoker DJ, Cobb JP, Pringle JAS (1991) Needle biopsy of musculoskeletal lesions. J Bone Joint Surg 73B:498–500

44a. Saifuddin A, Mann BS, Mahroof S, Pringle JA, Briggs TWR, Cannon SR (2005) Dedifferentiated Chondrosarcoma: Use of MRI to guide needle biopsy Clin Radiol 59(3)268–272

45. Sweetnam DR, Knowelden J, Seddon H (1971) Bone sarcoma—treatment by irradiation, amputation and a combination of the two. Brit Med J 2:363–367

46. Cade S (1955) Osteogenic sarcoma: A study based in 133 patients. J R Coll Surg Edin 1:79–111

47. Beck JC, Wara WM, Bovill EG Jr, et al. (1976) The role of radiation therapy in the treatment of osteosarcoma. Radiology 120:163–165

48. Rosen G, Tan C, Exelby P, et al. (1974) Vincristine, high-dose methotrexate with citrovorum factor rescue, cyclophosphamide and Adriamycin cyclic therapy following surgery in childhood osteogenic sarcoma. Proc Am Assoc Cancer Res 15:172

48a. Whelan J, Seddon B, Perisoglou M (2006) Management of Osteosarcoma. Curr Treat Options Oncol 7(6):444–455

49. Geschickter CF, Copeland MM (1951) Parosteal osteosarcoma of bone: A new entity. Ann Surg 133:790–807

50. Campanacci M, Picci P, Gherlinzoni F, et al. (1984) Parosteal osteosarcoma. J Bone Joint Surg 66B:313–321

51. Wold LE, Unni KK, Beabout JW, et al. (1984) Dedifferentiated parosteal osteosarcoma. J Bone Joint Surg 66A:53–59

52. Hall FM (1978) Periosteal sarcoma. Radiology 129:835–836

53. Campanacci M, Giunti A (1976) Periosteal osteosarcoma—Review of 41 cases. Ital J Orthop Trauma 2:23–35

53a. Grimer RJ, Bielack S, Flege S, Cannon SR, et al. (2005) Periosteal Osteosarcoma—A European review of outcome Eur J Cancer 41.2806–2811

54. Tomsu J, Procek J, Wagner K, et al. (1977) Vascular complications in osteochondromatosis. Rozhl Chir 56:696–699

55. Fogel GR, McElfresh EC, Peterson HA, et al. (1984) Management of deformities of the forearm in multiple heredity osteochondromas. J Bone Joint Surg 66A:670–680

56. Hudson TM, Chew FS, Manaster BJ (1983) Scintigraphy of benign exostoses and exostotic chondrosarcomas. Am J Roentgenol 140:581–586

57. Jaffe HL, Lichtenstein C (1942) Benign chondroblastoma of bone. Am J Path 18:969–983

58. Higaki S, Takeyama S, Tateishi A, et al. (1981) Clinical pathological study of twenty-two cases of benign chondroblastoma. Nippon Seikeigeha Gahhai Zasshi 55:647–664

59. Bloem JL, Mulder JD (1985) Chondroblastoma: A clinical and radiological study of 104 cases. Skeletal Radiol 14:1–19

60. Hudson TM, Hawkins IF Jr (1981) Radiological evaluation of chondroblastoma. Radiology 139:1–10

61. Huvos AG, Marcove RC (1973) Chondroblastoma of bone – a critical review. Clin Orthop 95:300–312

62. Rahimi A, Beabout JW, Ivins JC, et al. (1972) Chondromyxoid fibroma – a clinical pathological study of 76 cases. Cancer 30:726–736

63. Schajowicz F (1987) Chondromyxoid fibroma – a report of three cases with predominant cortical involvement. Radiology 164:783–786

64. Gherlinzoni F, Rock M, Picci P (1983) Chondromyxoid fibroma. J Bone Joint Surg 65A:198–204

65. Marcove RC, Miké V, Hutter RVP, et al. (1972) Chondrosarcoma of the pelvis and the upper end of the femur. J Bone Joint Surg 54A:561–572

66. Kaufman JH, Douglass HO Jr, Blake W, et al. (1977) The importance of initial presentation and treatment upon the survival of patients with chondrosarcoma. Surg Gyn Obstet 145:357–363

67. Dahlin DC, Beabout JW (1971) Dedifferentiation of low-grade chondrosarcoma. Cancer 28:461–466

68. Lichenstein L, Bernstein D (1959) Unusual benign and malignant chondroid tumour of bone. Cancer 12:1142–1157

69. Bjornsson J, Unni KK, Dahlin DC, et al. (1984) Clear cell chondrosarcoma of bone - observations in 47 cases. Am J Surg Path 8:223–230

70. Hutter RVP, Worcester JN Jr, Francis KC, et al. (1962) Benign and malignant giant cell tumours of bone. Cancer 15:653–610

71. Singson R, Feldman F (1983) Case report 229: Diagnosis of multiple (multicentric) giant cell tumours of bone. Skeletal Radiol 9:276–281

72. Campanacci M, Baldini N, Boriani S, et al. (1987) Giant cell tumour of bone. J Bone Joint Surg 69A:106–114

73. Hadders HN (1973) Some remarks on the histology of bone tumours. Year Book Cancer Res (Amsterdam) 22:7–10

74. Tudway RC (1959) Giant cell tumour of bone. Brit J Radiol 32:315–321

75. Nascimento AF, Huvos AG, Marcove RC (1979) Primary malignant giant cell tumour of bone. Cancer 44:1393–1402

76. Johnson EW Jr (1965) Adjacent and distal spread of giant cell tumours. Am J Surg 109:163–166

77. Kemp HBS, Cannon SR, Pringle J (1995) Shark-bite. A conservative surgical technique. British Orthopaedic Association, September, 1995

78. Caffey J (1955) On fibrous defects in cortical walls of growing tubular bones. Adv Pediatr 7:13–51

79. Arata MA, Peterson HA, Dahlin DC (1956) Pathological fractures through non-ossifying fibromas. J Bone Joint Surg 63A:797–808

80. Cunningham JB, Ackerman LV (1956) Metaphyseal fibrous defects. J Bone Joint Surg 38A:797–808

81. Feldman F, Norman D (1972) Intra- and extra-osseous malignant histiocytoma. Radiology 104:497–508

82. Ballance WA, et al. (1980) Osteogenic sarcoma. Malignant fibrous histiocytoma subtype. Cancer 62:763–771

83. Spanier SS, Enneking WF, Enriquez P (1975) Primary malignant fibrous histiocytoma of bone. Cancer 36:2084–2098

84. Tang JSH, et al. (1988) Haemangiopericytoma of bone. Cancer 62:848–859

85. Chow RW, Wilson CB, Olsen ER (1970) Angiosarcoma of the skull. Cancer 25:902–906

86. Unni KK, et al. (1974) Adamantinoma of long bones. Cancer 34:1796–1805

87. Huvos AG (1991) Ewing's sarcoma. In: Huvos AG (ed) Bone tumours: Diagnosis, treatment and prognosis. WB Saunders, Philadelphia, pp 523–52

88. Price CHG, Jeffree GM (1977) Incidence of bone sarcoma in South West England 1946–1974. Brit J Cancer 36:511–522

89. Glass AG, Fraimeni JFJR (1970) Epidemiology of bone cancer in children. J Natl Cancer Inst 44:187–199

90. Dahlin DC (1978) Bone Tumours; General Aspects and Data on 6221 Cases. CC Thomas, Springfield Ill 274–287

91. Hayes FA, et al. (1987) Metastatic Ewing's sarcoma remission, induction and survival. J Clin Oncol 5:1199–1204

92. Glaubiger DL, et al. (1980) Determination of prognostic factors and their influence on therapeutic results in patients with Ewing's sarcoma. Cancer 45:2213–2219

93. Gehan EA, et al. (1981) Prognostic factors in children with Ewing's sarcoma. Natl Cancer Inst Monogr 56:273–278

94. Gobel V, et al. (1987) Prognostic significance of tumour volume in localised Ewing's sarcoma of bone in children and adolescents. J Cancer Res Clin Oncol 113:187–191

95. Nascimento AG (1980) A clinicopathologic study of 20 cases of large cell (atypical) Ewing's sarcoma of bone. Am J Surg Pathol 4:29–36

96. Jurgens H, et al. (1988) Multidisciplinary treatment of primary Ewing's sarcoma of bone. Cancer 61:23–32

97. Miser JS, et al. (1988) Preliminary results of treatment of Ewing's sarcoma of bone in children and young adults. J Clin Oncol 6:484–490

98. Soule EH, Newton W Jr, Moon TE (1978) Extraskeletal Ewing's sarcoma: A preliminary review of 26 cases encountered in the Intergroup Rhabdomyosarcoma Study. Cancer 42:259–264

99. Donaldson SS (1981) A story of continuing success—Radiotherapy for Ewing's sarcoma. Int J Radiat Oncol Biol Phys 7:279–281

100. Sauer R, Jurgens H, Burgers JM (1987) Prognostic factors in the treatment of Ewing's sarcoma. Radiother Oncol 10:101–110

101. Kinsella TS, et al. (1984) Local treatment of Ewing's sarcoma: Radiation therapy versus surgery. Cancer Treat Rep 68:695–701

102. Li WK, et al. (1983) Pelvic Ewing's sarcoma: Advances in treatment. J Bone Joint Surg 65A:738–747

103. Dunst J, Sauer R, Burgers JM (1988) Radiotherapie beim Ewing's sarkom. Klin Pädiatr 200:261–266

104. Johnston CE II, Fletcher RR (1986) Traumatic transformation of unicameral bone cyst into aneurysmal bone cyst. Orthopedics 9:1441–1477

105. Campanacci M, Capanna R, Picci P (1986) Unicameral and aneurysmal bone cysts. Clin Orthop 204:35–36

106. Norman A, Schiffman M (1977) Simple bone cysts: Factors of age dependency. Radiology 124:779–782

107. Dyer R, Stelling CB, Fechner RE (1981) Epiphyseal extension of an aneurysmal bone cyst. Am J Roentgenol 137:153–168

108 Wang CC, Schulz MD (1953) Ewing's sarcoma. A study of fifty cases treated at the Massachusetts General Hospital, 1930–1952 inclusive. New Engl J Med 248:571–576

109. Biesecker JL, Marcove RC, Huvos AG, et al. (1970) Aneurysmal bone cysts. A clinicopathologic study of 66 cases. Cancer 26:615–625

110. Ackermann L, Ramamurthy S, Jablokow V, et al. (1988) Case report 488: Post-traumatic myositis ossificans mimicking a soft tissue neoplasm. Skeletal Radiol 17:310–314

111. Burwell RG (1964) Studies in the transplantation of bone: VII the fresh composite homograft/autograft of cancellous bone. An analysis of factors leading to osteogenesis in marrow transplants and in marrow containing bone grafts. J Bone Joint Surg 46B:110

112. Ilizarov GA, Ledidroev VI (1969) Replacement of defects of long tubular bones by means of one of their fragment. Vestn Klin 102:77–84

113. De Bastiani G, Aldegheri R, Renzo Brivio L, Trivella G (1987) Limb lengthening by callus distraction (callotasis). J Pediatr Orthop 7:129–134

114. Sim FH, Ivins JC, Taylor WF, Chao EYS (1985) Limb-sparing surgery for osteosarcoma: Mayo Clinic experience. Cancer Treat Sym 3:139–154

115. Lane JM, Glasser DB, Duane K, Healey JH, McCormack RR Jr, et al. (1987) Osteogenic sarcoma: Two hundred thirty-three consecutive patients treated with neoadjuvant chemotherapy. Orthop Trans 11:495

116. Winkler K, Beron G, Kotz R, Salzer-Kuntschik M, Beck J, et al. (1984) Neoadjuvant chemotherapy for osteogenic sarcoma. Results of a co-operative German/Austrian study. J Clin Oncol 2:617–624

117. Simon MA, Aschliman MA, Neal T, Mankin HJ (1986) Limb-salvage treatment versus amputation for osteosarcoma of the distal end of the femur. J Bone Joint Surg 68A:1331–1337

118. Bramwell VH, Burgers M, Sneath R, et al. (1992) A comparison of two short intensive adjuvant chemotherapy regimes in operable osteosarcoma of limbs in children and young adults. J Clin Oncol 10:1579–1591

119. Simon MA (1988) Current concepts review: Limb salvage for osteosarcoma. J Bone Joint Surg 70A:307–310

120. Buck BE, Malinin TI, Brown MD (1989) Bone transplantation and human immunodeficiency virus. An estimate of risk of acquired immunodeficiency syndrome (AIDS). Clin Orthop 240:129–136

121. Musculo DL, et al. (1987) Tissue typing in human massive allografts of frozen bone. J Bone Joint Surg 69A:583–595

122. Berry BH, Lord CF, Gebhardt MC, Mankin HJ (1990) Fractures of allografts. J Bone Joint Surg 72A:825–833

123. O'Connor MI, Rock MG, Sim FH, Chao EYS (1991) Limb salvage of the proximal humerus: Reconstruction with osteoarticular allograft versus endoprosthesis. In: Brown KLB (ed) Complications of limb salvage ISOCS, Montreal, pp 105–108

124. Gebhardt MC, Roth YF, Mankin HJ (1990) Osteoarticular allografts for reconstruction in the proximal part of the humerus after excision of a musculoskeletal tumour. J Bone Joint Surg 72A:334–345

125. Capanna R, Manfrini M, Ceruso M, Angeloni R, Lauris G, et al. (1991) A new reconstruction for metadiaphyseal resections: A combined graft (allograft shell plus vascularised fibula)—preliminary results. In: Brown KLB (ed) Complications of limb salvage. ISOCS, Montreal, pp 319–321

126. Mankin HJ, Dopperts S, Tomford W (1983) Clinical experience with allograft implantation: The first ten years. Clin Orthop 174:69–86

127. Urbaniak JR, Black KE Jr (1985) Cadaveric elbow allografts: A six year experience. Clin Orthop 197:131–140

127a.Cannon SR, Briggs TWR, Blunn G, Unwin P (2005) Endoprosthetic reconstruction of the proximal humerus using a constrained bi-articular prosthesis. Proceedings of the 13th International Symposium on Limb Salvage, Seoul, Korea, September 7–10, 2005

127b.Gupta A, Meswania J, Pollock R, Cannon SR, Briggs TWR, Taylor S, Blunn G (2006) Non-invasive distal femoral expandable endoprosthesis for limb salvage surgery in paediatric tumours. J Bone Joint Surg Br (5) 649–654

128. Marsden W, Stephens F, Waugh R, McCarthy S (1991) Soft tissue complications of intra-arterial chemotherapy: Definition, prevention and treatment. In: Brown KLB (ed) Complications of limb salvage. ISOCS Montreal, pp 313–317

Head and Neck Tumors

17

Diana L. Diesen, Michael A. Skinner

Contents

17.1 Introduction

Tumors of the head and neck present particular challenges for the pediatric surgeon asked to evaluate them. A working knowledge of the embryology, anatomy, physiology, and pathophysiology of the head and neck is needed. While the majority of these tumors are benign, an understanding of the fundamentals of surgical oncology is needed when approaching these tumors to ensure proper assessment and treatment.

The head and neck are formed from mesenchymal cells that develop from the paraxial and lateral plate mesoderm, neural crest, and ectodermal placodes in early fetal development. The paraxial mesoderm makes somites and somitomeres, which develop into part of the floor and meninges of the brain, the occipital lobe, and the muscle and connective tissue of the face. The lateral plate mesoderm develops into the laryngeal cartilage and connective tissue of the neck. The neural crest cells develop into the brain, the optic cup, the midface, and the pharyngeal arches.

The pharyngeal arches are separated by pharyngeal pouches and clefts. Each arch has a nerve and an artery, and develops into muscle, cartilage, and connective tissue. The arterial supply develops when the embryological heart is caudally displaced. Normal anatomy and its variants depend on selective fusion or atrophy of these arteries. In contrast to the arterial supply, the venous system is more variable in the size of the vessels and their course. The branches and connections of the internal, external, and anterior jugular veins provide the venous drainage for the head and neck.

The pharyngeal pouches develop into endocrine glands and the middle ear. Pouch 1 develops into the middle ear and the auditory tube. Pouch 2 develops into the palatine tonsil. Pouch 3 develops into the inferior parathyroid glands and the thymus. Pouches 4 and 5 develop into the superior parathyroid glands. The pharyngeal cleft develops into the external auditory meatus. The thyroid gland is not derived from a pouch but rather develops as an epithelial proliferation from the endoderm of the floor of the pharynx and descends along the thyroglossal tract to the level of the laryngeal primordium.

The thoracic duct and the right lymphatic duct drain lymph from the head and neck. The right side of the head and neck, right-upper extremity and the right thorax are drained by the right lymphatic duct which empties near the junction of the right subclavian and right internal jugular veins. The lower extremities, abdomen, and the left side of the head and neck are drained by the thoracic duct which passes posterior to the left common carotid artery and the left vagus nerve as it passes from the right to the left side of the body. The thoracic duct then arches anterosuperiorly and laterally between the left internal jugular vein and anterior scalene muscle to terminate near the junction of the left internal jugular and left subclavian veins. Valves present at the junction of each duct prevent reflux of venous blood. Small anastamotic connections between the two lymphatic ductal systems become important when obstruction or injury to one duct occurs.

The neck is divided based on anatomic triangles that are defined by the angle of the jaw, the clavicle, and the trapezius. Knowing the anatomical triangles of the neck is essential for both properly assessing and determining the prognosis of disease (Fig. 17.1, Table 17.1). The anterior and posterior triangles are separated by the sternocleidomastoid muscle. This muscle extends from medial clavicle to the mastoid bone. The anterior triangle is subdivided into four smaller triangles by the digastric, stylohyoid, and omohyoid muscles. These muscles then create the submandibular, carotid, submental, and inferior carotid triangles. The posterior triangle is divided into the superior occipital triangle and an inferior subclavian triangle by the omohyoid

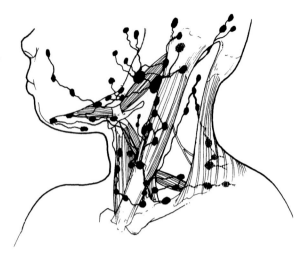

Fig. 17.1 Muscular triangles and associated lymphatics and lymph nodes of the head and neck.

muscle. The triangles with the most lymph nodes include submandibular, submental, anterior cervical, superficial cervical, and deep cervical node groups. Table 17.2 lists common developmental anomalies that present as masses in the head and neck.

17.2 Cervical Adenopathy

Cervical adenopathy is a common finding in pediatric patients and is usually the result of inflammatory processes. In one study, lymphadenopathy was noted in 44% of children under 5 presenting for a well child check and 64% of children presenting for a sick visit [121]. However, only 11–30% of biopsied lymph nodes

Table 17.1 Muscular triangles of the neck

	Muscular triangles of the neck	
Boundaries	**Posterior triangle**	**Anterior triangle**
Posterior	Trapezius muscle	Sternocleidomastoid muscle
Anterior	Stemocleidomastoid muscle	Midline of neck
Floor	Deep layer cervical fascia	Mylohyoid, hyoglossus, thyrohyoid, pharyngeal constrictor muscles
Roof	Superficial cervical fascia	Superficial cervical fascia, platysma muscle
Contents	Subclavian artery	Carotid artery
	Brachial plexus	Internal jugular vein
	Spinal accessory nerve	Submandibular gland
	Posterior cervical lymph nodes	Vagus nerve, recurrent laryngeal nerve, lymphatic tissue
Subtriangles	Occipital	Submandibular
	Subclavian	Carotid, submental, muscular

Table 17.2 Congenital anomalies presenting as head or neck mass

Anomaly	Origin
Cystic hygroma	Abnormal lymphatic drainage, abnormal lymphatic formation
Lymphangioma	Abnormal development of arterial, venous and lymphatic cannels
Second branchial cleft, cyst sinus, or fistula	Failure of obliteration of cervical sinus
Thyroglossal duct cyst	Failure of thyroglossal tract obliteration
Lingual thyroid	Failure of thyroid descent
Thymic cyst	Thymic remnant

harbor a malignant process [142, 157, 276, 299]. Self-limited, nonspecific adenitis from adenovirus, rhinovirus, and enterovirus infection of the upper respiratory tract is most common. Up to 3% of cases are due to cat scratch disease [133]. Measles, mumps, Epstein-Barr virus (EBV), cytomegalovirus (CMV), human immunodeficiency virus (HIV), herpes virus, parasitic, bacterial, and other viral infection may also cause cervical adenopathy. Noninfectious inflammatory disorders such as Kawasaki's disease, lupus, Langerhans cell histiocytosis, hemophagocytic lymphohistiocytosis, Castleman's disease, Rosai-Dorfman disease, Kihuchi disease, Churg-Strauss syndrome, and sardcoidosis may also cause adenopathy.

Lymphadenopathy is the initial finding in most malignancies of the head and neck in children [142, 200]. A thorough history and physical exam must be performed. Concerns in the history must include: location and duration of symptoms, associated systemic symptoms, sick contacts, animal exposure, trauma, immunization status, medications, recent travel, dental problems, and diet, including ingestion of unpasteurized animal products and undercooked meat. Often, there are no signs of inflammation, fevers, or upper respiratory symptoms. Malignancy should be suspected for all rapidly growing lymph nodes especially those occurring in the supraclavicular and posterior cervical triangle regions. Factors noted to be predictive of malignancy include nodes greater than 3 cm, supraclavicular or fixed nodes, and abnormal chest radiography [276].

Fine needle aspiration (FNA) is a tool often used in evaluating lymphadenopathy not responsive to antibiotic therapy. The data supporting FNA utilization is found mostly in the adult literature and its use in the pediatric population is limited [75, 196, 314]. To per-

form an FNA an experienced pathologist is needed not only for proper tissue procurement but also for appropriate tissue diagnosis. An 18- to 22-gauge needle with an attached syringe is inserted into the mass. Once the needle is in the mass, gentle aspiration is performed. The needle is then passed repeatedly through the mass from various angles while applying gentle suction. The tissue is then placed on a slide and stained. Ultrasound or CT guidance may be used for accurate mass localization, which is particularly helpful with deep masses of the neck.

Cervical lymphadenopathy is usually a result of acute adenitis. In up to two-thirds of these cases, an FNA can reveal the causative agent [41, 327]. The FNA tissue is usually sent for gram stain and cultures including aerobic, anaerobic, fungi, and mycobacteria. An acid-fast stain may also be used if clinically indicated. When malignancy is suspected, an FNA is not sufficient for analysis due to a substantial false negative rate [283]. Open surgical biopsy is indicated in the following cases: refractory systemic symptoms, hard or fixed lesions, supraclavicular nodes, abnormal chest radiography or CBC, or rapid growth or disease progression without evidence of inflammation.

When deciding which node should be excised it is generally best to remove the largest accessible node. In order to perform a lymph node excision, a small incision should be made over the suspicious nodule. Careful dissection with meticulous hemostasis should be performed, being careful to avoid capsule rupture (Fig. 17.2). If the tissues are matted or the node is fixed to surrounding vital structures, an incisional biopsy may be needed (Fig. 17.3). Keep in mind, the node may invade surrounding nerves and vessels, increasing the

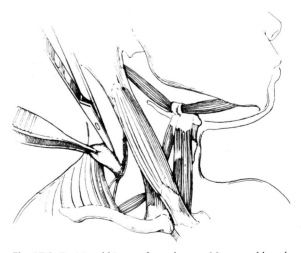

Fig. 17.2 Excisional biopsy of a neck mass. Masses and lymph nodes are completely removed without damaging vital structures. Illustration depicts a mass being dissected from the spinal accessory nerve.

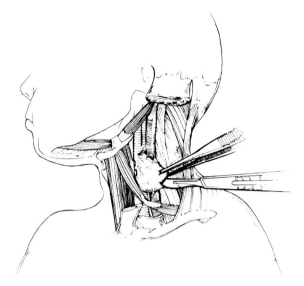

Fig. 17.3 Incisional biopsy of a neck mass. Illustration shows mass encasing the carotid sheath.

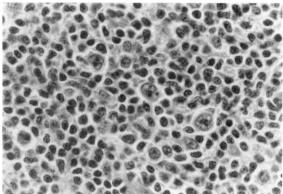

Fig. 17.4 Photomicrograph demonstrating multiple multinucleated Reed-Sternberg cells of Hodgkin's disease.

risk of iatrogenic injury. Since exposure may be difficult especially for deeper lymph nodes, a self-retaining retractor may be helpful. Care should also be taken to avoid damage to adjacent vital structures. Once the node is removed, the wound should be irrigated and the platysma reapproximated with interrupted absorbable suture. The skin is usually closed using an absorbable suture in a subcuticular pattern.

Once the lymph node is removed, it should be kept sterile and moist. The pathologist should be contacted to ensure proper stains and cultures are performed given the patient's clinical history. Part of the node should be sent for gram stain and aerobic, anaerobic, and fungal cultures. A fresh frozen sample may also be sent for histology and staining though a definitive diagnosis requires a permanent section. Proper communication with pathology will ensure that adequate tissue has been obtained for all infectious, immunologic, cytogenetic, and molecular studies requested.

17.3 Hodgkin's Disease

Hodgkin's disease (HD) or Hodgkin's lymphoma is a malignant lymphoma common in children and in adults over the age of 50. In 1932, Thomas Hodgkin first described seven of his patients who all had grossly abnormal lymph glands [125]. Following the description of the pathognomonic multinuclear giant cells by Sternberg in 1898 and subsequently illustrated by Reed in 1902, the cells have become known as Reed-Sternberg cells (Fig. 17.4) [237, 287].

Hodgkin's disease is the most common childhood cancer with an overall incidence of 7 per 100,000 in the USA [224]. The age at presentation has a bimodal distribution with a peak in adolescents and young adults and another in adults over the age of 50. In developing countries, children, especially boys, are affected at a younger age, but Hodgkin's disease is still uncommon before the age of 5 [63]. In childhood there is a male to female ratio of 0.9 (M/F) but this varies based on age with a male to female ratio of 5.3 in children less than five and a ratio of 0,8 in children 15–19 years of age [63, 224]. Relatives of patients with Hodgkin's disease are at a slightly increased risk for the disease, with familial forms accounting for 4.5% of all cases. Clusters of Hodgkin's disease have also been reported [63, 89, 170, 244]. Hodgkin's disease is more common in patients with impaired immune systems and/or a history of exposure to viruses such as EBV, CMV, or herpes virus 6 [110, 319].

17.3.1 Pathology and Genetics

On pathologic examination, Reed-Sternberg cells are pathognomonic for Hodgkin's disease though account for only 1% of the lymphoid tissue on examination. The lymph nodes also display reactive lymphocytes, macrophages, plasma cells, fibrous stroma, and collagen. Two common classification systems are the Rye classification and the WHO classification, both of which are based on the relative proportion of various cells on histologic examination. The Rye classification divides Hodgkin's disease into nodular sclerosis (50–60%), mixed cellularity (20–30%), lymphocyte predominant (10–15%), and lymphocyte depletion (10%) [168]. The WHO classification divides Hodgkin's into classical HD and nodular lymphocyte predominant HD [228]. In nodular lymphocyte predominant HD, most HRS cells express B-cell surface markers such as CD19 and CD20. Nodular lympho-

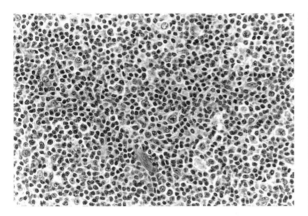

Fig. 17.5 Photomicrograph demonstrating nodular lymphocyte predominant Hodgkin's disease.

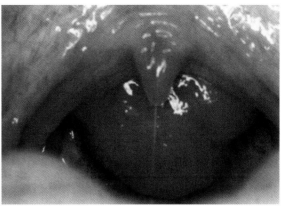

Fig. 17.6 Lymphoma of the nasopharynx.

cyte predominant HD accounts for only 5–10% of HD [228].

The most common histologic subtype in children is the nodular sclerosing variety representing ~70–80% of adolescent HD and 50% of HD in children under 10 years of age [224]. On histologic examination thick collagen bands divide the lymphoid tissue into nodules that are full of lacunar cells, a Reed-Sternberg variant, surrounded by clear space, lymphocytes, eosinophils, and histiocytes (Fig. 17.5). In the mixed cellularity subtype, there are a larger number of malignant cells with occasional necrosis. This mixed cellularity subtype is more common in younger children (30–35%) and less common in adolescents (10%). The lymphocyte predominant subtype, which is associated with early diagnosis and good prognosis, contains mature lymphocytes, benign histiocytes, and an occasional Reed-Sternberg cell. The lymphocyte depletion variant as the name implies has few lymphocytes and increased Reed-Sternberg cells. Although this variant is rare in children, it is usually diagnosed at an advanced stage and has a poor prognosis.

17.3.2 Clinical Presentation

More than 90% of Hodgkin's patients present with painless lymphadenopathy, and greater than 80% of these cases involve the cervical and supraclavicular lymph nodes. The nodes are firm, rubbery, and can be single or multiple. On physical examination, hepatic or splenic enlargement may be noted suggesting metastatic disease. Patients with mediastinal involvement may present with cough, stridor, dyspnea, dysphagia, or SVC syndrome due to compression of the airway, esophagus, or blood vessels. Children with mediastinal HD may occasionally present with hypertrophic osteoarthropathy, characterized by excessive skin and

bone on the distal parts of their etxtremities [11, 137]. Patients with retropharyngeal lymphoma may present with an acute airway obstruction (Fig. 17.6). If a transoral needle biopsy is attempted, rapid tumor enlargement may occur leading to airway obstruction. Up to one-third of all patients present with systemic symptoms of fever, night sweats, weight loss, fatigue, and pruritis. The pattern of fever is variable, and weeks of high fevers can be separated by afebrile periods. Only 20% of children have the fevers and night sweats common to many adult patients with HD [53, 261, 284]. Patients may present with various immunologic disorders such as treatment-resistant idiopathic thrombocytopenic purpura (ITP), Coombs'-positive hemolytic anemia , or rarely autoimmune neutropenia [53, 271]. In Hodgkin's patients, ITP may occur at any time including at diagnosis, during treatment, and even after splenectomy [32, 277].

17.3.3 Diagnostic Evaluation

The diagnosis of Hodgkin's disease can be made only after histologic examination of an affected lymph node. This node must show classic HRS cells or their variants for a diagnosis of HD, and further subclassification requires information about the architecture and proportions of various cells including HRS cells, lymphocytes, eosinophils, neutrophils, and collagen [285]. In order to obtain enough tissue with proper preservation of lymph node architecture, an open biopsy should be preformed. Fine needle aspiration does not provide an adequate sample. Some reports of successful diagnosis for lymphomas using core needle biopsies have emerged, although adequate sampling is difficult with core biopsies alone [22, 219]. Excisional biopsy should be performed if possible to give adequate tissue architecture. If the node cannot be removed without

Table 17.3 Ann Arbor staging classification for Hodgkin's disease [46]

Stage	Definition
I	Involvement of single lymph node region (I) or of a single extralymphatic organ or site (I_E)
II	Involvement of two or more lymph node regions on the same side of the diaphragm (II) or localized involvement of an extralymphatic organ or site and one or more lymph node regions on the same side of the diaphragm (II_E)
III	Involvement of lymph node regions on both sides of the diaphragm (III), which may also involve the spleen (III_s), an extralymphatic organ or site (III_E) or both (IIISE)
IV	Diffuse or disseminated involvement of one or more extralymphatic organs or tissues with or without associated lymph node involvement
A	No systemic symptoms
B	Presence of systemic symptoms prior to admission including unexplained fever, night sweats, or weight loss greater than 10% of body weight in 6 months prior to diagnosis

damage to surrounding vital structures, incisional biopsy is appropriate. If Reed-Sternberg cells are seen, a diagnosis may be made on frozen sections, although more tissue should be sent for routine staining, immunophenotyping, and cytogenetic analysis.

Laboratory studies include a complete blood cell count with white blood cell differential, erythrocyte sedimentation rate, serum alkaline phosphatase, renal and liver function tests, lactate dehydrogenase, urinalysis, and baseline thyroid function tests. Hodgkin's lymphoma spreads initially to contiguous lymph nodes and later can involve liver, lung, bone marrow, and the central nervous system, so further workup should focus on these areas. Imaging studies include anteroposterior (AP) and lateral chest radiographs; computed tomography (CT) scans of the high neck, chest, abdomen, and pelvis; CT of the primary site; and possibly a gallium-67 scintigraphy. A chest x-ray provides information on mediastinal involvement. Chest CT provides information about pulmonary as well as mediastinal involvement. In addition to pulmonary metastasis, HD can affect the chest wall, pleura, and pericardium [17, 247]. As an alternative or adjunct to CT scanning, MRI may be used [111]. Gallium-67 scintigraphy is especially useful to evaluate response to therapy since it can differentiate fibrosis from active disease [140, 318]. If this is to be done, a pretreatment gallium scan in needed. Both a bone marrow aspirate and biopsy are necessary for advanced stage disease

and in all stages with systemic symptoms, although its utility in early Hodgkin's is unclear.

17.3.4 Staging

Both children and adults with Hodgkin's disease are staged based on the Ann Arbor Classification system (Table 17.3) [46]. This classification system incorporates numbers of lymph nodes involved, location of affected lymph nodes, extranodal involvement, and systemic symptoms [46, 136]. Subclassification A indicates asymptomatic disease while subclassification B indicates symptoms including fever, night sweats, and unexplained weight loss of at least 10% of body weight over a 6-month period. Improved imaging and use of systemic chemotherapy in all HD patients has decreased the need for staging laparotomy. There is continued controversy over the role of staging laparotomy. Some oncologists now recommend staging laparotomy/laparoscopy in the following situations: intra-abdominal lymph node between 1 and 3 cm, splenomegaly, focal splenic abnormalities, focal hepatic abnormalities, and areas of abdominal uptake on gallium scan not otherwise explainable. Staging laparotomy may involve splenectomy, liver biopsy, and sampling of splenic hilar, celiac, porta hepatis, mesenteric, iliac and para-aortic lymph nodes. These criteria are not universal, and uniform indications for staging laparotomy do not currently exist.

17.3.5 Management

Hodgkin's disease should be managed with a multidisciplinary approach at a pediatric oncology center. Hodgkin's is sensitive to both chemotherapy and radiation. Previously, HD was treated with high-dose radiation therapy and later stage disease was treated with MAPP (mechlorethamine, vincristine, procarbazine, prednisone) and radiation [166]. Concerns existed over the long-term effects of this high dose radiation and chemotherapy on growth and development as well as the development of secondary malignancies.

Current recommendations for the treatment of HD include chemotherapy for all stages. Early stage Hodgkin's disease (clinical stage I and IIA) is well controlled by chemotherapy followed by field radiation. Multiple chemotherapeutic regimes have been used in early stage HD with good results. Cycles of VAMP (vinblastine, doxorubicin, methotrexate, prednisone) followed by field radiation between 15 and 25.5 Gy showed a 99% disease-free 5-year survival [78]. Treatment with OPPA (vincristine, procarbazine, prednisone, doxorubicin in males) and OEPA (vincristine, etoposide, prednisone, doxorubicin) followed by field radiation of

25–35 Gy has also been used with a 99% and 94% 5-year disease-free survival, respectively [256]. In adults ABVD (doxorubicin, bleomycin, vinblastine, dacarbazine) has been used successfully but concerns over toxicity has limited it use in children [129, 329].

Hodgkin's patients considered to have advanced disease include: patients with stage IIIa, IIIb, or IV; patients with B-symptoms; or patients with a mediastinal mass greater than one third the diameter of the chest. Treatment for these patients includes various chemotherapy combinations and various levels of field radiation. Traditionally, these patients were treated with MOPP and ABVD in addition to field radiation of 20–35 Gy with a 5-year disease-free survival of 87–93% [297]. Radiation dosing was based on response to chemotherapy. Other researchers have used OPPA and OEPA followed by COPP with field radiation with a 5-year event-free survival of 88% [256]. Other chemotherapeutic combinations are under investigation with the goal of decreasing drug toxicities and secondary malignancies.

The initial complete remission response rate for all stages of Hodgkin's disease is over 90%. For stage I or IIA Hodgkin's disease, 5-year disease-free survival for children is approximately 93–99% [78, 256]. For patients with advanced stage Hodgkin's disease the 5-year survival is 87–97% with a 5-year event-free survival of 88% [256, 297]. Factors that predict a poorer prognosis include male gender, disease stage IIb, IIIB, or IV, bulky mediastinal disease, WBC >13,500/microL, and hemoglobin <11.0 g/dl. Using a point system, giving one point for each of the above-mentioned criteria, 5-year disease-free survival is 94%, 85%, 71%, and 49% for 0–1, 2, 3, and 4–5 points, respectively [275].

After remission, patients need lifelong close follow-up for recurrent disease and long-term effects of chemotherapy and radiation. When relapse does occur, it is usually within the first 3 years and is associated with a poor prognosis [95]. Treatment for recurrent Hodgkin's disease includes another combination chemotherapy and/or autologous bone marrow or stem cell transplantation. Long-term complications of the radiation and chemotherapeutic interventions include impaired growth, thyroid dysfunction, gonadal dysfunction, cardiopulmonary toxicity, and strokes. Up to 7.6% of HD survivors will have a secondary malignancy at 20 years [206]. These secondary malignancies most often include thyroid cancer, breast cancer, and sarcomas.

17.4 Rhabdomyosarcoma

Rhabdomyosarcoma (RMS) is a soft tissue sarcoma that originates from immature mesenchymal cells destined to be striated skeletal muscle. It is the most common soft tissue sarcoma in children, accounting for up to 5% of all childhood cancer and 50–70% of all sarcomas. The annual incidence of rhabdomyosarcoma ranges from 5 to 8 per million children resulting in approximately 350 new cases each year [149, 242]. In the USA, rhabdomyosarcoma is more common in Caucasian children with a 2–3:1 ratio to African American children. The incidence of rhabdomyosarcoma throughout the world varies with increased incidences in Spain and decreased incidences in lower parts of Asia including China, Japan, India, and the Philippines [222, 288]. The incidence of rhabdomyosarcoma appears to be equal in Asian children as compared to Caucasian children in the USA [289]. The incidence is increased in males with a ratio of 1.4:1, but the incidence appears equal in cases of rhabdomyosarcoma of the head and neck [187]. Age of onset has two peak occurrences, the first in children 2–6 years of age and the second in adolescents 15–19 years old. Two-thirds of the patients are diagnosed younger than 6 years of age [288]. Age-related differences exist for the different sites of primary disease though tumors can arise in any region at any age. Younger children tend to have increased incidence of head, neck, and genitourinary rhabdomyosarcoma while older children have an increased incidence of tumors of the extremities, trunk, and male genital tract. For example, in patients with orbit RMS, 42% are aged 5–9 years and in these younger children tumors of the orbit tend to be of the embryonal type. Thirty-five percent of all rhabdomyosarcomas occur in the head and neck.

Most RMS are sporadic in occurrence, but some are known to be associated with familial syndromes such as neurofibromatosis, Li-Fraumeni syndrome, Rubinstein-Taybi syndrome, Gorlin basal cell nevus syndrome, Costello syndrome, and Beckwith-Wiedemann syndrome [72, 102, 113, 120, 163, 182, 272]. Many children with Li-Fraumeni syndrome in particular are noted to have mutations of p53 tumor suppressor gene, which has led some to speculate that children who develop RMS at a young age should be screened for a p53 mutation. Presence of a p53 mutation may lead one to reduce ionization and/or chemotherapeutic doses that may lead to secondary malignancy though there is no consensus on this topic [68]. Environmental factors that may be associated with the development of RMS include maternal use of marijuana and cocaine, intrauterine radiation exposure, low socioeconomic status, the use of antibiotics soon after birth, and exposure to alkylating agents [104, 105, 115, 171, 244]. Relatives of children with rhabdomyosarcoma may be at increased risk for the development of breast cancer, brain tumors, and adrenocortical carcinoma [25, 114, 163, 164].

17.4.1 Pathology and Genetics

RMS arise from immature mesenchyme cells that were destined to differentiate into muscle. Interestingly, these tumors arise in various locations including areas where striated muscle is not found, such as the bladder. On microscopic examination, the cells have immunohistochemical expression of actin, myosin, desmin, myoglobin, Z-band proteins, and/or MyoD with an eosinophilic cytoplasm [221]. Over 99% of RMS stain for polyclonal desmin, while actin, myogenin, and myoglobin are found in 95%, 95%, and 78% percent respectively [77]. Myogenin in particular is expressed more often by alveolar RMS. A DNA-binding protein expressed during early myogenesis, MYOD1, is also expressed in these tumors and can be identified by immunohistochemistry and Northern blot analysis [76, 258]. Other immunohistochemical stains may be helpful in identifying RMS. CD99 is a marker used in Ewing sarcoma but is positive in 15% of RMS patients [109]. Leukocyte common antigen, pan B lymphocyte antibodies, cytokeratin, epithelial membrane antigen, and neural markers such as neuron specific enolase and S-100 protein are positive in 5–20% of RMS cases. In addition to immunohistochemical staining, transmission electron microscopy (EM) is also useful in identifying myofilament, myotubular intermediate filaments, desmin, actin, and z-bands.

Four histological subtypes of RMS assist in both the categorization and prognosis of patients: embryonal (50%), botryoides and spindle cell (6%, 3%), alveolar (20–30%), and undifferentiated (10%). In addition to these four main histological groups, there are RMS tumors that are described as not otherwise specified and diffusely anaplastic (previously pleomorphic) which are associated with poor prognosis [143]. The botryoides and spindle class are less common but are asso-

ciated with the best prognosis. The embryonal RMS group has an intermediate prognosis while the alveolar group has a relatively poor prognosis.

The alveolar and embryonal RMS are distinguished based on the architecture of the tumor. Embryonal RMS appears as sheets of rhabdomyoblasts with occasional fusiform cells and no alveolar architecture (Fig. 17.7). The alveolar RMS is characterized by an alveolar architecture with rhabdomyoblasts interspersed among fibrovascular septae (Fig. 17.8) [127]. Botryoides RMS, whose name means "grape," has the gross appearance of a bunch of grapes. Histologically it is a mass beneath an epithelial layer and subepithelial layer of rhabdomyoblasts. Anaplastic RMS is characterized by atypical mitotic figures and large nuclear size [302, 303].

Cytogenetic and molecular markers have been found in rhabdomyosarcoma that can be useful for classification and prognostication. Most embryonal rhabdomyosarcoma have a loss of heterogeneity at the 11p15 locus near the IGF-II gene. This loss of heterogeneity is suggestive of the presence of a tumor suppressor gene in the region that is disrupted [86, 258, 259]. Overproduction of IGF-II, which is found in both embryonal and alveolar RMS, may then stimulate tumor growth [80]. The PAX3-FKHR translocation in alveolar RMS in particular is associated with overexpression of IGF-II [139]. Several other genetic mutations are associated with rhabdomyosarcoma including activation and/or mutations of the K-ras, N-ras, retinoblastoma, PTCH gene mutations, MDM2, CDK4, p53, and MYCN though the significance of these mutations has yet to been determined [6, 36, 290, 325] [87].

In alveolar RMS, the t(2;13)(g37;g14) translocation in which the long arms of chromosome 2 and 13 join to fuse PAX3 and FKHR is diagnostic of the alveo-

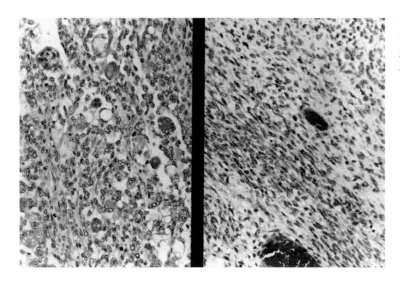

Fig. 17.7 Photomicrograph demonstrating embryonal rhabdomyosarcoma. *Left panel*, round cell rhabdomyosarcoma. *Right panel*, spindle cell rhabdomyosarcoma.

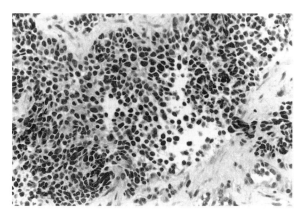

Fig. 17.8 Photomicrograph demonstrating alveolar rhabdomyosarcoma. Note clear areas with alveolar-like appearance.

lar subtype even in the absence of the characteristic histology (Fig. 17.8) [79, 305]. In particular, the solid alveolar variant may be histologically similar to the embryonal subtype but will possess this translocation. The mechanism by which this translocation produces RMS is unclear but it is postulated that it is due to increased upstream transcription of other genes during development [70, 92, 262]. Another translocation t(1;13)(p36;p14) fuses PAX7 and FKHR. This fusion is thought to increase upstream transcription but the mechanism is not fully understood [70]. These markers have been found to have prognostic value as well. For example, PAX7-FKHR patients tend to be younger patients with extremity lesions that tend to respond favorably to treatment [138, 236].

17.4.2 Clinical Presentation

Thirty-five to forty percent of rhabdomyosarcoma presents in the head and neck, usually as a nontender mass lesion with occasional overlying skin erythema [184, 185, 302]. These tumors tend to arise in the orbit (25%) and parameningeal sites (50%) with the remaining 25% arising in other locations including the scalp, parotid gland, oral cavity, pharynx, and neck [197]. An orbital tumor may present with proptosis, periorbital edema, ptosis, and/or opthalmoplegia. Parameningeal or nasopharyngeal tumors present with airway obstruction, local pain, chronic sinusitis and epistaxis. In the case of parameningeal lesions, cranial nerve palsies may result from direct extension. Middle ear tumors present as a polyploidy mass with earache, otitis media, and discharge which may be hemorrhagic.

Less than one quarter of patients have metastatic disease at diagnosis [146, 236]. When RMS does spread, it is either by direct extension or metastasis via the lymphatic and/or hematogenous route. Lymphatic

metastasis occur in less than 10% of the cases [123]. Hematogenous spread occurs in 10–20% of cases and is most often to the lungs (40–50%), bone marrow (20–30%), and bone (10%) [146, 160, 236].

17.4.3 Diagnostic Evaluation

After a thorough history and physical examination, further diagnostic evaluation should include the acquisition of laboratory data. A complete blood count (CBC) may show evidence of anemia due to inflammation and/or pancytopenia due to bone marrow involvement. Liver function tests are necessary to assess for possible metastatic disease to the liver and prior to administration of potentially hepatotoxic chemotherapy. Renal function tests, electrolytes, serum calcium, magnesium, phosphorous, and uric acid levels are also needed before the administration of potentially toxic chemotherapeutic agents. A urinalysis is also needed to assess for hematuria, which may indicate GU tract involvement.

Imaging studies are important tools to determine the presence of calcifications and boney involvement of the primary tumor and to search for metastatic disease. MRI or CT scans are important to fully assess tumor involvement of the head and neck and serve as a baseline when assessing response to therapy. For tumors of the head and neck in particular, MRI is superior for assessing involvement of adjacent structures and feasibility of resection thus should be performed when considering total resection. A chest radiograph and chest CT scan are necessary for evaluation of lung metastases. An abdominal US and/or CT is indicated to evaluate for liver metastasis. A radionuclide bone scan is indicated to assess for bony involvement. Bone marrow biopsies are also necessary to assess for metastatic disease even in patients with normal complete blood counts. In patients with parameningeal RMS a lumbar puncture is indicated to assess for leptomeningeal metastasis.

A biopsy of the tumor is necessary to definitively establish the diagnosis and guide treatment. In order to obtain enough tissue for diagnosis, an open biopsy is often performed, although core needle biopsy is also an alternative. Enough tissue is need for fluorescent in situ hybridization (FISH) and reverse transcriptase–polymerase chain reaction (RT-PCR) testing to assess for the molecular/genetic abnormalities already described.

17.4.4 Staging and Classification

The Intergroup Rhabdomyosarcoma (IRS) clinical staging system is shown in Table 17.4 [158, 159, 302].

It divides patients into clinical groups based on the localization of the primary tumor, the extent of surgical resection, and presence of residual disease/metastases [35, 159]. The Intergroup Rhabdomyosarcoma Study

divides patients based on the Tumor-Node-Metastasis system (TNM) which includes site of tumor, tissue invasion, tumor size, lymph node involvement, and metastatic disease (Table 17.5) [35, 158, 159]. Before treatment is begun, adequate staging must be complete which includes tissue conformation of RMS and TNM staging.

Table 17.4 Intergroup Rhabdomyosarcoma Clinical Staging System [64, 65, 158, 159, 302]

Clinical group	Extent of disease
I	A. Localized tumor, confined to site of origin, completely resected
	B. Localized tumor, infiltrating beyond site of origin, completely resected
II	A. Localized tumor, gross resection with microscopic residual disease
	B. Locally extensive tumor (positive regional lymph nodes), completely resected
	C. Locally extensive tumor (positive regional lymph nodes), gross resection with microscopic residual disease
III	A. Gross residual disease following surgical biopsy
	B. Gross residual disease after major resection
IV	Presence of distant metastases, any size primary tumor with or without regional lymph nodes

17.4.5 Treatment

Rhabdomyosarcoma of the head and neck is often treated with a combination of chemotherapy, radiation, and surgical resection if possible. Surgical resection of head and neck RMS should only be undertaken when the entire tumor can be removed without damage to vital structures and without major cosmetic or functional deformity. Occasionally superficial tumors of the scalp, ear, cheek, neck, or oropharynx may be completely excised. If complete surgical resection is not possible, chemotherapy and radiation should be administered to shrink the tumor if possible; a complete surgical resection may be possible after treatment. In these cases an incisional biopsy is needed for diagnosis. Random nodal sampling is not indicated. Suspicious lymph nodes should be biopsied for staging purposes, but extensive neck dissections are not indicated. There also does not appear to be a role for resection of metastatic lesions such as an isolated pulmonary nodule [296]. For patients with recurrent disease, surgical resection is warranted after repeated chemotherapy and radiation.

Table 17.5 TNM staging system of Intergroup Rhabdomyosarcoma Study IV [35, 158, 159]

Stage	Sites	T invasion	T-size	N	M
1	Orbit Head and neck excluding parameningeal Nonbladder, nonprostate genitourinary	T 1 or T2	a or b	NO, N1, Nx	MO
2	Bladder/prostate Extremity Cranial parameningeal Trunk/retroperitoneum	T1 or T2	a	NO or Nx	MO
3	Bladder/prostate Extremity Cranial parameningeal Trunk/retroperitoneum	TI or T2	a b	N1 N0 or N1 or Nx	M0
4	All sites	T1 or T2	a or b	NO or NI	M1

T tumor: TI confined to site of origin; T2 extension beyond site of origin.

a <5 cm in diameter; b >5 cm in diameter.

N, regional lymph nodes: NO, no involvement; N1, clinically involved; Nx, status unknown; M, metastases; MO, no distant metastases; M1, distant metastases present.

17.4.5.1 Chemotherapy and Radiation Therapy

For RMS tumors that are not completely surgically resectable, as is the case for most RMS of the head and neck, chemotherapy and radiation is the mainstay of treatment. The standard treatment is a combination of vincristine, dactinomycin, and cyclophosphamide as currently recommended by the Rhabdomyosarcoma Study Group [35, 64, 65, 184, 185]. The IRS-IV patients were divided into prognostic groups based on clinical and TNM staging. Based on the prognostic staging, they were assigned to chemotherapy regimes. Most treatment courses continue for approximately 45 weeks depending on the clinical stage at presentation. Additional agents such as doxorubicin, cisplatin, etoposide, and melphalan have not been shown to be beneficial though topotecan and irinotecan are under investigation for patients with resistant tumors and advanced or recurrent disease [34, 65, 91, 184, 185, 302, 220, 250, 317].

If residual and/or metastatic disease is present, radiation therapy may be added to the above chemotherapeutic regimen. Radiation is usually initiated after 2–3 cycles of chemotherapy except in those patients with parameningeal tumors or life-threatening tumors in which radiation is started immediately. Delay of radiation treatment beyond 4 months has been shown to impair local control [193]. Radiation doses vary based on tumor location, extent, and involvement of nodes. For the other clinical groups, local control was achieved with radiation to the primary tumor site in doses of 1.8–2 Gy daily depending on patient age and the size of tumor.

The IRS study group noted that radiation was unnecessary for clinical group I embryonal RMS and paratesticular tumors. All other clinical group 1 patients were recommended to have radiation for a total dose of 36 Gy. Those in clinical group II with residual disease after surgery received radiation doses 41.4–45 Gy which increased survival to 75–87% [273]. In clinical group III, IRS-IV recommends patients with gross residual disease receive 50.4 Gy except in orbital RMS in which 45 Gy is recommended. Patients with parameningeal tumors do benefit from higher radiation doses so the current recommendation is 50.4+ Gy to the site of the tumor with 2 cm margins of normal tissue [190, 193, 234]. For patients with metastatic disease radiation is recommended for the primary and metastatic tumors.

For patients with orbit tumors and clinical group I (completely excised) head and neck tumors, the 5-year survival is >85% [35, 65, 185]. For other tumors of the head and neck, the 5-year survival is about 75%. Relapse has been reported in approximately 1% of patients after 5 years [35, 65, 185]. When rhabdomyosarcoma recurs, it tends to be more resistant to chemotherapy and radiation and is associated with a poor prognosis. The treatment for recurrent RMS is again chemotherapy, radiation, and surgical resection if possible. There are no clear guidelines on chemotherapeutic regimens and radiation dosing in patients with recurrent rhabdomyosarcoma, but suggestions include vincristine, dactinomycin, and cyclophosphamide and also possibly doxorubicin, ifosfamide and etoposide, mesna, and actinomycin D [8, 29, 47, 147, 195, 316]. Further research is needed to identify better treatment protocols for this treatment-resistant group.

17.5 Non-Hodgkin's Lymphoma

Childhood non-Hodgkin's lymphoma (NHL) accounts for 10% of all pediatric malignancies and about 25% of all head and neck malignancies. The head and neck is the primary site for NHL 10–15% of the time, and is most commonly located in the lateral cervical lymphatic chain. Up to 30% of primary head and neck NHL are extranodal and include lymphoid tissue in Waldeyer's ring, the orbit, mandible, sinuses, salivary gland, and/or thyroid gland. The incidence of NHL is 10 per 100,000 accounting for approximately 500 new cases a year in the USA. The median age of presentation is 10 years with incidence increaseing with age [131, 202]. It is uncommon in children under the age of three. NHL is twice as common in Caucasians and 2–3 times more common in boys [173].

There is a form of endemic Burkitt's lymphoma in Equatorial African which is distinctive from the sporadic Burkitt's lymphoma noted in the rest of the world. In Africa, endemic Burkitt's lymphoma has an annual incidence of 10 per 100,000 and is associated with EBV in 95% of cases. It most commonly presents as a mass in the jaw, abdomen, orbit, central nervous system, or paranasal sinuses [176]. Sporadic Burkitt's has an annual incidence of 2 per 100,000 children, with only a 15% association with EBV and more commonly presents in the abdomen, bone marrow, and nasopharynx. In addition to EBV, other immunodeficiency syndromes such as ataxia-telengiectasia, Wiskott-Aldrich syndrome, and X-linked lymphoproliferative syndrome are associated with NHL [172]. There is also an increased incidence of NHL in children receiving immunosuppressive therapy and those with AIDS. Up to 1.6% of children with HIV will develop lymphoma, with Burkitt's or large cell being the most common [186]. HIV and other viral pathogens, immunosuppressive states, environmental toxins, and commercial products such as hair dyes have been associated with Burkitt's lymphoma.

17.5.1 Pathology and Genetics

Childhood NHL consists of three major subtypes: lymphoblastic lymphoma, large-cell lymphoma, and Burkitt's. The World Health Organization has developed a classification system that divides common pediatric lymphomas into B-cell and T-cell lymphomas and their subgroups. On histologic examination, lymphoma cells replace normal lymph node tissue. In the head and neck region, the most common lymphoma is B cell lymphoma, specifically small-cell noncleaved lymphoma. Histologically, the cells are undifferentiated, small, round lymphoid cells with detectable surface immunoglobulins. This uniform shape and size gives a "starry-sky" histology classic for Burkitt's lymphoma as shown in Fig. 17.9.

Both B and T cell lymphomas are associated with known chromosomal translocations affecting DNA binding transcription factors [60]. Up to 85% of Burkitt's patients have a t(8;14)(q24;q11) translocation resulting in transfer of the c-myc oncogene from chromosome 8 to the site of the immunoglobulin heavy chain locus on chromosome 14 [174]. This translocation causes activation of c-myc and increased proliferation of lymphoma cells. The location of the breakpoint on chromosome 8 is variable, suggesting different molecular subtypes of Burkitt's lymphoma based on different mechanisms of c-myc activation [9, 23, 106, 172].

In North American Burkitt's lymphoma the breakpoint is within the c-myc gene in more than 50% of tumors [107, 172, 266]. Less commonly t(8;22) and t(2;8) results in translocation of lambda and kappa immunologic light chain genes, respectively, to a region distal to the c-myc gene on chromosome 8 [177, 295]. Specific chromosomal abnormalities have been identified in T cell lymphoma patients. Approximately 25% of patients with T cell lymphoblastic lymphoma will have at least submicroscopic deletions of TAL1 with

3% of those cases associated with the t(1;14)(p32;q11) chromosomal abnormality [18, 191, 326]. Other chromosomal abnormalities have been noted in patients with T cell lymphoblastic lymphoma affecting the TCR, HOX11, and RHOMB genes [27, 118]. For B cell large cell lymphomas, an occasional translocation involving the c-myc gene has been demonstrated [307]. Some anaplastic large cell tumors inappropriately express a tyrosine kinase gene due to a t(2;5) translocation [199].

17.5.2 Clinical Presentation

Initially the NHL mass is painless but as rapid growth or compression of surrounding structures occurs, symptoms can develop. Symptoms are based on location of the primary tumor. Cervical NHL may produce neck pain, dysphagia, or dyspnea as tracheal or esophageal compression occurs. Rapidly enlarging tumors may produce mediastinal compression and associated respiratory distress or superior vena caval obstruction. Burkitt's lymphoma in Equatorial Africa most frequently presents with jaw involvement, especially in younger children. Jaw involvement is less common (~15%) in sporadic Burkitt's lymphoma and is not age-related [44, 254]. Children often have extranodal disease at the time of presentation which includes abdominal involvement (31%), mediastinal involvement (26%), or head and neck involvement (29%). Central nervous system (CNS) and bone marrow involvement may also occur [174, 177]. Systemic symptoms are not as common in NHL as in Hodgkin's disease but are a poor prognostic sign.

17.5.3 Diagnostic Evaluation

As with Hodgkin's lymphoma, an open biopsy should be performed to establish the diagnosis. An open excisional biopsy, or in the case of matted nodes, an incision biopsy, is usually needed to provide an adequate sample for histology, cytogenetics, flow cytometry, and molecular pathology. As with Hodgkin's disease, fine needle aspiration and core biopsy can be performed but often do not provide an adequate sample. Recommended laboratory studies include a complete blood cell count with white blood cell differential, erythrocyte sedimentation rate, serum alkaline phosphatase, renal and liver function tests, lactate dehydrogenase, urinalysis, uric acid levels, phosphate levels, and baseline thyroid function tests. Imaging studies should include anteroposterior (AP) and lateral chest radiographs, CT scans of the high neck, chest, abdomen and pelvis, bone scan, and CT/MRI of the primary site. A chest x-ray provides information on mediasti-

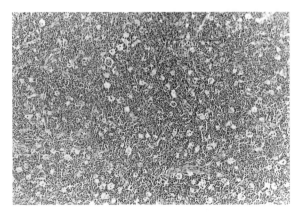

Fig. 17.9 Photomicrograph demonstrating Burkitt's lymphoma with classic "starry-sky" histology.

nal involvement. Chest CT also provides information about pulmonary as well as mediastinal involvement. Both a bone marrow aspirate and biopsy are necessary for staging of the disease. A lumbar puncture is also needed to evaluate for CNS involvement.

17.5.4 Staging and Classification

The St. Jude's Staging system is used to characterize NHL (Table 17.6) [202]. Tumor burden as measured by disease stage, serum LDH, and serum IL2 have all been shown to predict outcome [201, 230, 313].

17.5.5 Treatment

Treatment protocols for NHL are based on histologic subtype and disease stage as noted in Table 17.6. Chemotherapy remains the primary treatment for all histologic variants and stages of NHL. Radiation therapy is reserved for cases of relapse, CNS involvement, and emergency situations such as airway compromise due to mediastinal involvement. In general, surgery is used for diagnosis and perhaps in an emergent setting such as airway compromise. In the absence of surgical emergencies, there is no role for debulking procedures.

Table 17.6 St. Jude system for non-Hodgkin's lymphoma [202]

Stage	Definition
I	Single nodal or extranodal tumor site, excluding mediastinum or abdomen
II	Single extranodal tumor with regional lymph node involvement; two or more nodal areas on the same side of diaphragm; two single extranodal tumors with or without regional lymph node involvement on same side of the diaphragm
	Primary gastrointestinal tract tumor with or without associated mesenteric node involvement grossly resected
III	On both sides of the diaphragm: two single extranodal tumors; two or more nodal areas. All primary intrathoracic tumors
	All extensive, unresectable primary intra-abdominal disease
	All primary paraspinal or epidural tumors
IV	Any of the above with initial CNS and/or bone marrow involvement

Due to rapid turnover of lymphoblasts, patients often present with hyperuricemia, hyperphosphatemia, and renal dysfunction. As chemotherapy is initiated, tumor lysis syndrome may occur which is characterized by a rapid lysis of tumor cells resulting in increased uric acid, phosphate, potassium, and purines in the blood and renal tubules. This tumor lysis syndrome may result in increasing renal dysfunction. Patients must be aggressively hydrated before and during chemotherapy. Alkalization of the urine and allopurinol may be helpful in the treatment of hyperuricemia. In some cases, dialysis may be required to manage the renal failure associated with severe tumor lysis syndrome.

For limited disease (stage 1 and 2), treatment consists of three courses of CHOP (cyclophosphamide/doxorubicin/vincristine/prednisone) which results in a 5-year survival rate of 85–95% [2, 165, 189, 203, 223, 238, 240]. For advanced disease with high tumor burden, high dose regimens and the addition of ifosfamide, etoposide, and cytosine arabinoside (ara-C) have improved survival rates from 20% to around 80% in recent years [7, 30, 175, 238]. For patients with CNS involvement, intrathecal chemotherapy is added to the traditional chemotherapeutic regimen.

For Burkitt's lymphoma, patients receive 2–6 months of COMP and high-dose methotrexate, cytarabine and/or etoposide and ifosfamide [223, 238, 240]. Large cell lymphoma is treated with a CHOP combination resulting in a 50–70% event-free survival at 3 years [69, 132, 251, 252]. Research is underway examining the benefits of methotrexate, cytarabine, ifosfamide, and carboplatin.

Treatment for lymphoblastic lymphoma is the same as that for acute lymphocyte leukemia. The protocols consist of continuous therapy with 10- to 14-day rest periods; 15–32 months are required with multidrug regimes. Cure rates for limited disease are greater than 90% and range from 60% to 80% for advanced disease [7, 78, 239, 304]. These treatment protocols are also used for large cell lymphomas with good success. Anaplastic large cell lymphoma requires CNS prophylaxis. Current therapy for recurrent NHL includes chemotherapy and possible bone marrow transplantation, but overall prognosis is poor [23, 99, 107, 227].

17.6 Thyroid Tumors

Thyroid cancer represents about 3% of all childhood malignancies and 7% of cancers arising in the head and neck, with an incidence of 0.2 to 5 per million children annually [117]. The peak incidence of thyroid cancer in children occurs between 10–18 years of age, and females outnumber males 2:1 over the age of 10. In children under the age of 10, males tend to outnumber females.

The development of thyroid cancer is associated with radiation exposure. With decreasing use of radiation for benign disease, the incidence of thyroid cancer has decreased. Historically, up to 80% of all new cases of thyroid cancer were related to previous radiation to the neck for a variety of benign disorders including enlarged thymus, hypertrophied tonsils and adenoids, hemangiomas, nevi, eczema, and cervical adenitis [85]. The association of thyroid cancer and radiation exposure was again demonstrated in the Republic of Belarus after the 1986 Chernobyl nuclear power plant catastrophe [210, 218]. Within 4 years after the accident, a 62-fold increase in thyroid tumors was noted. These children were noted to have aggressive papillary carcinomas in younger children with an equal prevalence in males and females. Factors for the development of thyroid cancer following radiation exposure include higher radiation doses, young age at radiation initiation, and female sex.

Treatment for previous childhood malignancy is associated with an increased incidence of thyroid carcinoma. Most commonly these children had Hodgkin's lymphoma, whose treatment may lead to the development of thyroid nodules and thyroid cancer [1, 274]. Up to 50% of children receiving irradiation and chemotherapy for Hodgkin's disease, leukemia, and other head and neck malignancies develop elevated thyroid stimulating hormone (TSH) levels within 1 year of treatment [274, 309]. Not only radiation but also alkylating agents predispose to thyroid cancer. The latency between previous treatment and development of thyroid cancer is up to 25–30 years, which emphasizes the importance of continued follow-up in these patients [155, 209, 257].

17.6.1 Pathology and Genetics

The histologic subtypes of thyroid cancer include papillary or mixed (70–80%), follicular (20%), medullary (5–10%), and rarely, anaplastic [112, 130, 155, 257]. Histologically, papillary carcinoma will consist of papillae of epithelial cells arranged often with lymphocytic infiltrates and psammoma bodies (Fig. 17.10). In follicular carcinoma, malignant adenomatous cells form follicles with nuclear abnormalities, capsular invasion, or vascular invasion. Any tumor with papillary components is considered a papillary carcinoma. If follicular characteristics are also present, it is considered a papillary tumor with follicular architecture (Fig. 17.11). Approximately 5% of thyroid carcinomas are medullary thyroid carcinomas (MTC) that arises from the parafollicular C cells, derived from neural crest cells (Fig. 17.12). Histologically, these tumors have granular cytoplasm with islets of regular, undifferentiated cells.

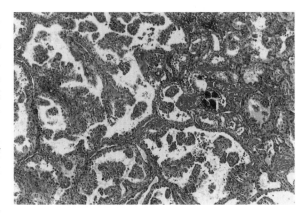

Fig. 17.10 Photomicrograph demonstrating papillary thyroid carcinoma with papillary architecture.

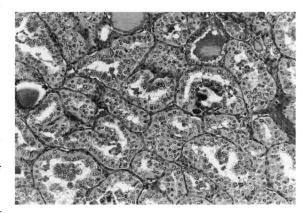

Fig. 17.11 Photomicrograph demonstrating follicular variant of papillary thyroid carcinoma.

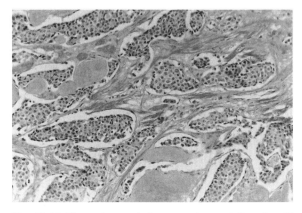

Fig. 17.12 Photomicrograph demonstrating medullary thyroid carcinoma with amyloid stroma and epithelial cytology.

The RET (REarranged during Transfection) gene appears to be play an important role in the development of thyroid cancer. The RET proto-oncogene is a receptor tyrosine kinase molecule located on chromosome ten and gene rearrangement is associated with papillary cancers. These rearrangements place RET adjacent to various ubiquitously expressed genes. The fusion genes are termed RET/PTC, and they exhibit increased expression of tyrosine kinase. This RET gene rearrangement is particularly common in radiation-induced thyroid tumors [28, 231, 253, 279]. Some studies suggest that particular RET fusion gene combinations are correlated with particular histologic subtypes. For example, one particular inversion of chromosome 10, PTC1, is more often associated with papillary carcinoma that tends to be more slow growing with clearer differentiation, while PTC3 is more often associated with follicular carcinoma which tends to grow more quickly, more aggressively, and with less differentiation [253].

Medullary thyroid carcinoma may occur sporadically, in patients having multiple endocrine neoplasia (MEN) type 2A or 2B, or in the familial medullary thyroid carcinoma (FMTC) syndrome. As in papillary thyroid cancer, the RET proto-oncogene also plays an important role in the development of medullary thyroid carcinoma as well as MEN syndromes in general [81, 126, 268]. These RET mutations affect the development of neural crest derived tissues. Various RET mutations may be found in as many as 40% of sporadic nonfamilial medullary thyroid carcinomas. Medullary thyroid carcinoma is usually the first tumor to develop in MEN 2B patients and is often the cause of death in these patients.

17.6.2 Clinical Presentation

Patients usually present with a thyroid mass, an enlarged cervical lymph node, or with both of these findings. Physical exam findings concerning for malignancy include firm nodules and nodules that are fixed to surrounding structures. Palpable cervical adenopathy is present in up to two-thirds of cases and adenopathy may be the only indication of thyroid cancer even in the absence of a thyroid nodule [112]. Other symptoms may include dysphagia, dyspnea, or dysphonia if tracheal or esophageal compression has occurred [10, 130, 209, 249]. Hoarseness indicates compression or invasion of the recurrent laryngeal nerve.

The lung is the most common site for metastases, aside from lymph nodes, with an incidence of about 6% at diagnosis [310, 330]. This is often accompanied by cervical lymph node metastases. Up to 50% of patients with papillary tumors have metastases to local cervical or mediastinal lymph nodes at the time of diagnosis [83]. Follicular tumors have less local lymph node disease but increased boney metastases. Cervical adenopathy and/or distant metastases is usually the first sign of medullary thyroid carcinoma.

17.6.3 Diagnostic Evaluation

Initial evaluation of a thyroid mass should begin with thyroid function tests, which are normal in the majority of cases. Imaging of a suspicious nodule may include an ultrasound study and a thyroid scan. An ultrasound can determine if a lesion is cystic solid or and may also serve as a guide during the surgery [208]. A thyroid scan with Tc 99m-Pertechnetate will determine if the mass contains functioning thyroid tissue and will classify the lesion. Carcinoma is identified in 30% of children who undergo surgical resection for cold nodules.

The pathologic diagnosis can either be established using thin-needle aspiration cytology or by frozen-section, although there is some controversy over the accuracy of frozen-sections in evaluating follicular lesions. The use of FNA in the adult population is well established and has decreased the incidence of thyroidectomy for benign conditions thus increasing the number of surgical patients with carcinoma [208]. Limitations of FNA include a false-negative rate from 1% to 6%, availability of an experienced cytopathologist, and an inability to differentiate benign from malignant follicular lesions. Since the pattern of thyroid disease in adolescents is similar to that in adults, it is likely that FNA is an acceptable way to evaluate thyroid nodules in this population [328]. In children younger than 13 years of age, aspiration is more difficult to perform and the pattern of benign disease is different than in adults. The natural history of these lesions and the safety of a nonoperative approach is unknown. Therefore, FNA should probably not be used in young children, and all children younger than 13 years of age should undergo surgical excision. A FNA may reveal cancer, a benign lesion, or a lesion suspicious for cancer. As with adults, benign nodules may be followed with serial physical and ultrasound examinations; resection is indicated if the nodule increases in size. Surgical resection is indicated for all malignant or suspicious nodules.

17.6.4 Surgical Management

Since there are no prospective clinical trials comparing surgical management of thyroid cancer in children, there is some controversy over the best surgical management of these patients. For differentiated thyroid carcinoma the most commonly recommended surgical options include either total or subtotal thyroidectomy. There is no difference in mortality or morbidity in patients having a total or subtotal thyroidectomy. The mortality rates ranges from 0% to 17% up to 28 years after treatment [112, 155, 249, 257]. Aggressive resection including total thyroidectomy, with lymph node dissection if the regional nodes are involved, has shown to increase local control of the tumor [54, 112, 155, 257]. Radioiodine ablative therapy is also most effective after total thyroidectomy since there is less thyroid tissue to absorb radionuclide. Also, if total thyroidectomy is performed, serum thyroglobulin levels may be used to monitor for tumor recurrence.

However, differentiated thyroid carcinoma in children is a relatively indolent disease and survival is apparently not related to the extent of gland removal, so total thyroidectomy is not necessarily required [112, 155, 209, 249, 257]. With total thyroidectomy, there is an increased incidence of major surgical complications, including injury to the recurrent laryngeal nerve 0–24% and hypoparathyroidism [71, 112, 155, 330]. Some surgeons suggest that a thyroid lobectomy with isthmus resection is acceptable for "minimal" differentiated carcinoma clearly isolated to one lobe. However, in one series 66% of patients had bilateral tumors and 81% of the tumors were multifocal [257]. Currently, a consensus is emerging that aggressive resection for differentiated thyroid cancer in children is the best surgical management. Currently, it is recommended that children with differentiated thyroid carcinoma undergo near total thyroidectomy and modified neck dissection to remove gross disease if necessary. After surgical resection, 131I remnant ablation and long-term suppressive thyroxin therapy are used to treat residual disease and prevent recurrence. Since residual tumor may be treated with radioiodine, tumors involving the recurrent laryngeal nerve need not be aggressively resected. The nerve may be spared and residual tumor treated.

Recurrent laryngeal nerve injury and permanent hypoparathyroidism are the two most concerning iatrogenic injuries following thyroid resection [112, 155, 209, 249, 257]. These risks increase with the extent of resection and younger age of the patient [155]. To prevent damage to the recurrent laryngeal nerve, the nerve should be identified along its entire course and be seen entering the larynx. Intraoperative nerve stimulation is often used in the adult population to trace the course of the nerve and a recent report demonstrated the usefulness of this technique in children. The parathyroid glands should also be protected. If there is any question as to the viability of the parathyroid glands, they should be autotransplanted into the sternocleidomastoid muscle or nondominant forearm. A near total thyroidectomy leaving a few grams of tissue adjacent to the recurrent laryngeal nerve and the superior parathyroid gland should help prevent damage to these structures.

The technique for thyroidectomy is demonstrated in Figs. 17.13a–g. The patient is placed in a supine position initially with the neck extended by placing towel rolls beneath the shoulders. An incision is made 2–3 cm above the sternal notch in a skin crease (Fig. 17.13a). Dissection is carried down through the platysma muscle. Subplatysmal flaps are elevated superiorly to the thyroid notch and inferiorly to the sternal notch (Fig. 17.13b). The strap muscles are separated, not divided, in the midline to expose the thyroid gland (Fig. 17.13c). Crossing branches of the anterior jugular vein may need to be divided. Exposure of the desired lobe is obtained by retracting the strap muscles laterally. If the tumor has invaded the surrounding strap muscle, the strap muscles should be removed en bloc with the thyroid nodule. Ligation of the middle thyroid veins on the anterolateral surface in the middle of the thyroid gland allows for proper mobilization (Fig. 17.13d). Prior to mobilizing the superior pole, the recurrent laryngeal nerve is identified. The thyroid gland is grasped with a Babcock clamp and retracted medially. The recurrent laryngeal nerve is identified by its relationship to the inferior thyroid artery. The right recurrent laryngeal nerve ascends laterally to the tracheal esophageal groove as it passes posteriorly to the inferior pole of the thyroid. The nerve then travels obliquely, closer toward the gland and crosses the inferior thyroid artery and ascends to enter the larynx. The left recurrent laryngeal nerve arises from the vagus and passes inferiorly and medially to the aorta and ascends to enter the larynx. The nerve usually travels in the tracheal-esophageal groove but may be more medial on the anterior aspect of the trachea. The nerve may pass over, under, or branch around the artery. With the exception of a right nonrecurrent laryngeal nerve, there is always a cross point. The nerve should be traced along its anterior plane until it can be seen entering the larynx. The terminal portion of the recurrent laryngeal nerve passes posteriorly to a lateral extension of thyroid tissue. A neurostimulator may be used to aid in recurrent laryngeal nerve localization [33].

This portion of the gland may be left in situ in a near-total thyroidectomy. If medial retraction limits exposure, the superior pole of the gland should be mobilized (Fig. 17.13e). To properly mobilize the superior pole, the thin anterior suspensory muscle over the larynx should be divided. Branches of the superior thyroid vessels are divided close to the thyroid gland below the external branch of the superior thyroid nerve (Fig. 17.13f). Division of the upper pole pedicle between clamps, en mass, results in a high frequency of injury to this nerve and should be avoided. With the superior pole free, the gland may be retracted medially.

Finally division of the ligament of Berry, the posteromedial attachment of the thyroid, allows the thyroid to be retracted medially and dissected off of the pretracheal fascia to the isthmus. The recurrent laryngeal nerve courses near this posteromedial attachment, so again, proper identification of the nerve is essential. A pyramidal lobe, if present should be resected with the specimen. When performing a lobectomy and isthmusectomy, the junction of the isthmus and opposite lobe is transected with electrocautery (Figs. 17.13f, g). For a total thyroidectomy, mobilize the contralateral lobe as described and remove the entire specimen en bloc. Any suspicious lymph nodes should also be removed.

Blood supply to the parathyroid glands usually comes from the inferior thyroid arteries. If these arteries are not properly ligated, the parathyroid glands risk devascularization. In order to prevent this, individual branches of the inferior thyroid artery should be divided distal to the end branches supplying the parathyroid glands and near the thyroid capsule (Fig. 17.13g). The parathyroid glands should then be gently retracted off of the thyroid capsule. Following division of the inferior thyroid artery, the inferior pole vessels are divided. If parathyroid gland perfusion is compromised during the dissection, then one should immediately autotransplant the gland into the nearby sternocleidomastoid muscle [269, 298, 320]. Some surgeons advocate routine autotransplantation of one or two parathyroid glands into the sternocleidomastoid muscle or forearm muscle to prevent permanent hypoparathyroidism. Any removed parathyroid glands are placed in a specimen cup of sterile saline submerged in sterile ice until the thyroidectomy is completed.

After hemostatis is assured, the strap muscles are approximated with interrupted absorbable sutures. If complete hemostatis is questionable, a small drain may be placed below the strap muscles and brought out through a separate skin incision. The platysma muscle is closed with interrupted absorbable sutures and the skin closed using a running subcuticular stitch. For parathyroid autotransplantation, the excised parathyroid glands are minced into several small pieces. Within the sternocleidomastoid muscle or forearm muscle, small pockets are created by gently spreading with fine forceps. Two or more pieces of parathyroid tissue are placed in each pocket and marked with a silk suture.

Postoperatively, thyroidectomy patients should be treated with exogenous thyroid hormone to suppress TSH-mediated stimulation of the gland. Patients undergoing total parathyroidectomy with reimplantation often require calcium and vitamin D replacement until the autotransplanted tissue functions adequately [268]. To detect distant metastases or residual disease, radioiodine 131I scanning should be performed 6 weeks following surgery and discontinuation of exogenous thyroid replacement. If residual thyroid cancer is detected, then therapeutic doses of 131I should be administered until all disease is eradicated. Diagnostic scans are then repeated yearly. Thyroglobulin levels should also be obtained yearly; an elevated level should raise the suspicion of recurrent thyroid carcinoma [141]. Long-term follow-up in these patients is critical considering

the recurrence rate of thyroid cancer is about 30% after 20 years. The overall progression-free survival of patients with differentiated thyroid cancer is 67% at 10 years and 60% at 20 years after diagnosis. Factors associated with early recurrence are lower age at diagnosis and presence of residual neck disease.

Current management of MTC in children from families having the MEN 2 syndrome relies on the presymptomatic detection of the RET proto-oncogene mutation responsible for the disease, followed by prophylactic total thyroidectomy by about the age of 5 years, before the cancer spreads beyond the thyroid gland [100]. MTC is usually the first tumor to develop in MEN patients and of those children who have a prophylactic thyroidectomy due to presence of a RET mutation, 80% will already have foci of medullary carcinoma within the thyroid gland [268, 321]. Prophylactic thyroidectomy is recommended in infancy for patients with MEN 2B due to the aggressive nature of that subtype of MTC [213, 270, 321]. Unfortunately, external beam radiation and chemotherapy have not been found to be effective in treating MTC, so surgical resection is the only treatment. Patients with MEN 2A have a lifetime risk of hyperparathyroidism of 30%, so at the time of prophylactic thyroidectomy consideration of routine heterotopic autotransplantation should be entertained [28, 128, 321].

17.7 Neuroblastoma

Neuroblastoma is the third most common malignancy in children and the most common cancer in children less then 1 year of age [37, 98]. The annual incidence of neuroblastoma is about 8 per million and is roughly uniform worldwide. In the USA there are more than 600 cases each year. The average age at diagnosis in 17.4 months and 40% are diagnosed before 12 months of age [37, 98]. Neuroblastoma is more common in Caucasians than African-Americans (ratio 1.8:1) in infancy but equivalent after infancy. The male to female ratio is 1.2:1. Primary tumors of the head and neck region occur in 2–4% of afflicted children [42]. When disease is noted in the head and neck, it is most commonly metastatic disease. Infants are more likely to present with tumors in the cervical region.

Environmental factors may play a role in the development of neuroblastoma. Maternal opiate use has been associated with neuroblastoma, while increased folate intake during pregnancy is associated with a lower incidence [62, 90]. Most neuroblastomas appear to be sporadic though increased incidence is found in children with Turner's syndrome, Hirschsprung's disease, central hypoventilation, and neurofibromatosis type 1 [26, 207]. Familial cases of neuroblastoma have also been reported and appear to be transmitted in an autosomal dominant pattern with variable penetrance [152, 153, 179].

17.7.1 Pathology and Genetics

Neuroblastomas are derived from primordial neural crest cells which populate the adrenal medulla and sympathetic ganglia. Based on maturation and differentiation of these neural crest cells, three histologic patterns of these tumors are noted including neuroblastoma, ganglioneuroblastoma, and ganglio-

neuroma. Neuroblastomas consist of mostly neuroblast and few stromal cells and are thus characterized as "stromal-poor" [98]. On histologic examination, small, dense, round cells are seen with hyperchromatic nuclei and scant cytoplasm. Electron microscopy, immunohistochemistry, and cytogenetic studies are currently used to diagnose these tumors. Chromosome 1 deletions, rearrangements, and translocations have been reported in these patients [151, 180, 243]. Deletion of part of chromosome 1p is associated with amplification of N-Myc and is found in up to 25% of neuroblastomas [24, 145, 180, 188, 322]. Deletion of 11q

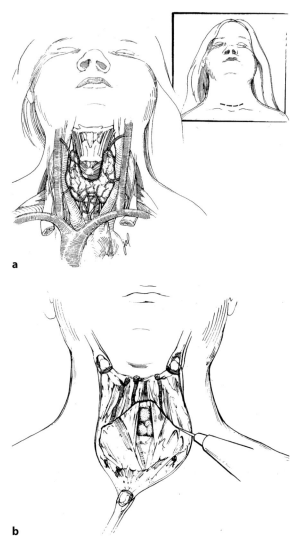

a

b

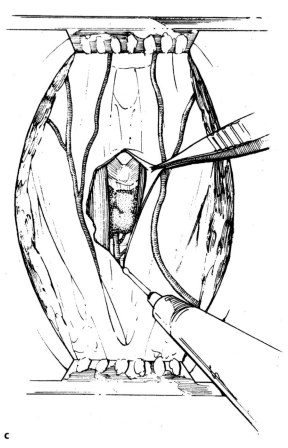

c

Inset illustrates the superior thyroid artery and vein. Superior pole vessels are divided individually, close to the thyroid gland, to avoid injury to the external branch of the superior thyroid nerve. (**e**) Thyroidectomy. Division of the inferior thyroid artery. The relationship between the inferior thyroid artery and recurrent laryngeal nerve (encircled with suture) is defined. The parathyroid glands are identified and preserved by dividing branches of the artery as they enter the thyroid gland. (**f**) Thyroid lobectomy. Transection of thyroid gland. The recurrent laryngeal nerve is identified along its entire course prior to the division of the ligament of Berry. The thyroid is dissected from the pretracheal fascia and divided at the junction of the isthmus and contralateral lobe. (**g**) Thyroid lobectomy. Appearance following right thyroid lobectomy. The recurrent laryngeal nerve and parathyroid glands are preserved.

Fig. 17.13 a–g (**a**) Thyroidectomy. Normal position of the thyroid gland. *Inset* illustrates site for skin incision. (**b**) Thyroidectomy. Elevation of subplatysmal flaps to thyroid notch, superiorly and sternal notch inferiorly. (**c**) Thyroidectomy. The thyroid gland is exposed by separating the strap muscles in the midline. (**d**) Thyroidectomy. Mobilization of the thyroid gland. The middle thyroid vein had been ligated and divided, the recurrent laryngeal nerve identified, and the superior pole mobilized.

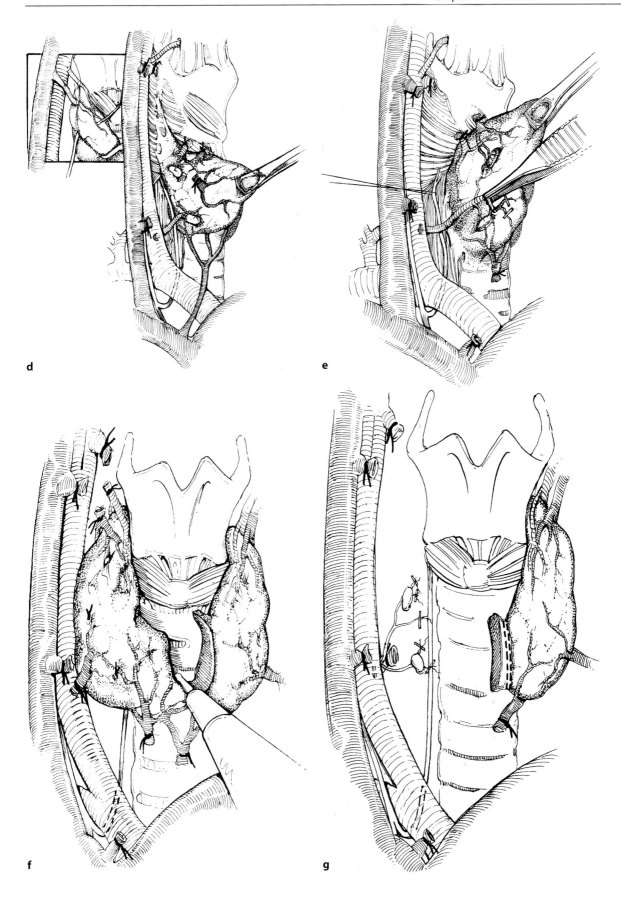

d

e

f

g

and/or 14q is found in 25–50% of neuroblastomas and trisomy 17q is found in half of neuroblastomas [12, 31, 282, 308]. The amplification of the N-myc proto-oncogene in chromosome 1p deletion and trisomy 17q are both associated with poor prognosis [31, 38, 39, 167, 308]. In contrast, expression of the tyrosine kinase receptor gene-A TRK-A is associated with biologically and clinically favorable tumors and good survival [144, 204, 205, 292].

17.7.2 Clinical Presentation

Patients usually present with a nontender, firm mass in the lateral neck [42]. If the tumor extends into the cervical sympathetic chain, Horner's syndrome (ipsilateral ptosis, miosis, and anhidrosis) may be seen [214, 323]. Heterochromia iridis may be present in children who have congenital or acquired Horner's syndrome [96]. Infants with congenital or acquired Horner's syndrome should undergo careful examination and workup for possible neuroblastoma. Metastatic neuroblastoma to the orbits is more common than primary cervical neuroblastoma and may produce proptosis and periorbital ecchymosis. Neuroblastoma may metastasize by lymphatic and/or hematogenous drainage. Cervical neuroblastoma spreads by local invasion of surrounding tissue and shows a high propensity for regional lymph node metastases. Distant disease, including bone and bone marrow involvement, is common at presentation.

Diagnostic evaluation should include routine blood counts, liver and kidney function tests, ferritin levels, and LDH levels. Nearly all neuroblastomas produce catecholamines and their byproducts, homovanillic acid and vanillylmandelic acid, can be measured in the urine. In order to assess for the presence of these products, a 24-h urine collection should be obtained. In order to diagnose neuroblastoma one of the following is needed: a histologic diagnosis of the tumor by microscopy or evidence of metastases to bone marrow on aspirate with elevation in urine or serum catecholamines [40]. In order to stage a neuroblastoma, the following studies are needed: bilateral iliac crest bone marrow biopsy, bone radiography, a radionuclide or MIBG scan, abdominal CT or MRI, chest x-ray and if positive a chest CT, and a MRI/CT of the head and neck for primary tumors of the head and neck.

17.7.3 Staging and Classification

The most common staging system for neuroblastoma is the International Neuroblastoma Staging System (INSS) listed in Table 17.7 [40].

17.7.4 Treatment

Treatment for neuroblastomas arising in the head and neck includes surgery and often chemotherapy. The role of surgery is to establish a tissue diagnosis, stage the tumor, and resect the tumor if possible. For localized cervical neuroblastoma, surgical excision may be curative. When complete surgical excision is possible in stage 1 disease, 5-year survival is 99% [5, 82, 154, 211, 225]. Even if complete surgical resection is possible, children identified as intermediate or high-risk need chemotherapy in addition to surgical resection [183]. Multiagent chemotherapy is used in patients with unresectable disease and advanced disease. Common regimens include cyclophosphamide, carboplatin or cisplatin, etoposide or teniposide, and adriamycin [82, 93, 101, 183, 211, 212, 291]. After chemotherapy, surgical resection may be reconsidered [73, 183]. Radiation is used for unresectable tumors or tumors that are not responsive to chemotherapy including incompletely resected cervical neuroblastoma [50, 93, 134].

Prognosis variables for neuroblastoma include age, stage, MycN status, pathology classification, DNA

Table 17.7 Staging systems for neuroblastoma [40]

International Neuroblastoma Staging System (INSS)	
Stage 1	Localized tumor confined to the area of origin; complete gross excision, with or without microscopic residual disease; identifiable ipsilateral and contralateral lymph nodes negative microscopically
Stage 2A	Unilateral tumor with incomplete gross excision; identifiable ipsilateral and contralateral lymph nodes negative microscopically
Stage 2B	Unilateral tumor with complete or incomplete gross excision; positive ipsilateral regional lymph nodes; identifiable contralateral lymph nodes negative microscopically
Stage 3	Tumor infiltrating across the midline with or without regional lymph node involvement; or unilateral tumor with contralateral regional lymph node involvement; or midline tumor with bilateral lymph node involvement
Stage 4	Dissemination of tumor to distant lymph nodes, bone, bone marrow, liver, or other organs with the exception defined in Stage 4-S
Stage 4-S	Localized primary tumor as defined for Stage 1 or 2 with dissemination limited to liver, skin, or bone marrow

ploidy, location, and metastasis. Infants with primary tumors of the head and neck have a more favorable prognosis. Patients with localized disease that is completely resected have a >90% survival rate. Children with intermediate-risk neuroblastoma treated with surgery and chemotherapy, with or without radiation have long-term survival of 90% [51, 116, 211, 225]. Survival for stage 3 neuroblastoma varies based on age and histologic features [108]. Survival in children with disseminated neuroblastoma (CCG stage IV and POG stage D) is also age dependent but overall survival is ~30% [73, 226]. When recurrence occurs, the disease is usually widely metastatic and the prognosis is poor.

17.8 Germ Cell Tumors

Germ cell tumors account for about 3% of neoplasms in children with an incidence of 4 per million children [119]. Of the germ cells tumors that occur, only 5% occur in the extracranial head and neck region. In general 25–35% of all germ cell tumors are malignant, although malignant germ tumors of the head and neck are rare [15, 74, 294]. Germ cell tumors arise from primitive germ cells and are characterized histologically by the presence of mature tissue from all three germ cell layers. The most common histologic features include skin, and cutaneous appendages, adipose tissue, cystic structures and intestinal epithelium. Mature and immature tissue elements are commonly seen in neonatal cervical teratomas. The majority of cervical germ cell tumors are congenital and present at birth or in early infancy and can be diagnosed by prenatal ultrasound. The anterior lateral neck is the most common site of occurrence though they have also been reported in the pharynx, nasopharynx, paranasal sinuses, skull, and orbit [15, 20, 48, 135, 286, 315]. Large congenital lesions may obstruct the pharynx and produce maternal polyhydramnios or nonimmune fetal hydrops [20, 74, 294]. Following birth, obstructing tumors produce respiratory distress and dysphagia and may require intubation and emergency surgical tracheostomy. Life-threatening airway obstruction has been reported in up to 35% of cases [15]. Prior to surgical excision proper CT/MRI imaging is important to assess the precise anatomy of the tumor and proximity to vital structures. Although rare in the cervical region, pure yolk sac tumors (endodermal sinus tumors) or mixed tumors with yolk sac elements behave as malignant tumors, and metastases, particularly pulmonary metastasis, from congenital teratomas have been reported [19, 267, 286, 300].

Cervical endodermal sinus tumors have been reported. Serum alpha-fetoprotein levels may be elevated in head and neck tumors with endodermal sinus elements [74, 156, 286]. Excision of benign teratomas results in cure. Malignant lesions are treated with surgical resection if possible followed by a multidrug chemotherapy. Patients with unresectable tumors or residual disease may receive irradiation to the primary tumor site. Most patients initially respond to therapy and estimates of long-term disease-free survival in children with unresectable germ cell tumors is around 50% [103].

17.9 Other Soft Tissue Sarcomas

Soft tissue sarcomas other than RMS make up 4% of all tumors in children. These sarcomas are named based on the mature tissue that they resemble, although all of these tumors are derived from primitive mesenchymal cells. Those that occur in infants and small children primarily occur in the head and neck region. Soft tissue sarcomas in infants and younger children often have less aggressive behavior and an excellent prognosis with surgery. Sarcomas which present during adolescence behave more like tumors in the adult population. Most soft tissue sarcomas present as painless, asymptomatic masses in the neck unless there is compression or invasion of adjacent structures. Because of the rarity of these lesions in childhood, most of the available data for treatment come from the adult population. In general, wide local excision is the treatment of choice. Because of the difficulty in obtaining wide negative margins in the head and neck, adjuvant therapy is often used in conjunction with surgical excision.

17.9.1 Fibrosarcoma

Fibrosarcoma is the most common nonrhabdomyomatous soft tissue sarcoma in children younger than 1 year of age and is the most common soft tissue sarcoma after rhabdomyosarcoma in all children, accounting for 11% of the total [194]. Primary head and neck lesions account for approximately 15–20% of fifibrosarcomas [55]. There is a bimodal age distribution with peaks between infancy and to 5 years of age and then again between 10–15 years of age. Histologically, fibrosarcomas tumors consist of spindle cells with a characteristic herringbone pattern. Fibrosarcomas in the first year of life rarely metastasize and can be treated with wide local excision. Radiation is indicated if complete excision is not possible. Fibrosarcoma tumors in adolescents are more aggressive and require multimodality therapy. Survival for nonmetastatic tumors ranges from 83% to 92% in children under 5 years of age and 60% for those older than 5 years [57, 232, 278].

17.9.2 Malignant Peripheral Nerve Sheath Tumor

Malignant peripheral nerve sheath tumors (MPNST) account for 5% of all soft tissue sarcomas in children and 10% occur in the head and neck region. They can arise from the cranial nerves, cervical plexus, or sympathetic chain. In contrast to most of the other head and neck soft tissue sarcomas, MPNSTs commonly present with pain, paresthesias, and muscle weakness. They are associated with neurofibromatosis type I which is characterized by cafe au lait spots, neurofibromas, skeletal dysplasia, and many neoplasms [97]. They are similar in appearance to fibrosarcomas but are far more aggressive. The tumor cells of MPNST, in contrast to fibrosarcoma, are more variable in size and shape and lack a herringbone pattern. Multimodal therapy including wide surgical excision, irradiation, and chemotherapy including vincristine, actinomycin D, cyclophosphamide, and doxorubicin (Adriamycin) are recommended. Survival is generally good for early stage tumors (50–75%) and poor for advanced disease (15–30%) [232].

17.9.3 Synovial Sarcoma

Synovial sarcoma is rare in children but may occur in the head, neck, and trunk in 15–20% of cases [4, 43, 198]. These tumors occur more commonly in older children and young adults and histologically differentiate into a spindle fibrous stroma similar to fibrosarcoma and a glandular component with epithelial differentiation. The tumor is associated with t(x;18) translocation with fusion of SYT-SSX1 and SYT-SSX2 proteins. Those patients with a SYT-SSX2 fusion gene have a better prognosis than those with a SYT-SSX1 fusion gene [4]. In contrast to other nonrhabdomyosarcoma soft tissue sarcomas, synovial sarcomas commonly present with both lymph node and lung metastases. Local disease is treated with local excision. The role of chemotherapy and radiation is unclear, but they are often given in combination with surgery. The 5-year survival rates are greater than 50% [4, 233, 246].

17.9.4 Hemangiopericytoma

Hemangiopericytoma accounts for 3% of all soft tissue sarcomas and occurs most commonly in the lower extremities and retroperitoneum. These tumors occur rarely in the nasal cavity, paranasal sinuses, orbital region, parotid gland, and the neck. It is thought that hemangiopericytomas arise from vascular pericytes or alternatively from mesenchymal cells with pericytic differentiation [148, 215]. Multiple simple and complex genetic translocations have been demonstrated in these tumors [281]. Wide local excision and postoperative chemotherapy is the recommended treatment. Irradiation is added for incompletely resected tumors. Hemangiopericytomas in infants are associated with a better prognosis than those occurring in older children and adults. The reported 5-year survival rate for these tumors is stage-dependent and ranges from 30% to 70% [13, 16, 148].

17.9.5 Malignant Fibrous Histiocytoma

Malignant fibrous histiocytomas (MFH) are rare sarcomas with multiple tissue elements that commonly present in the head and neck region. These tumors rarely occur during the first year of life. Ring chromosomes and 19p+ alterations have been observed in these tumors [4, 178, 248]. Microscopically, MFH has multiple cell types, marked cellular pleomorphism, a storiform pattern, and resembles fibrosarcoma but lacks a herringbone pattern. Treatment is with wide excision and local irradiation for residual tumor with or without chemotherapy. The 3-year survival for head and neck tumors is greater than 50% [58, 235, 265].

17.9.6 Alveolar Soft Part Sarcoma

Alveolar soft part sarcoma is rare in childhood, but when it occurs, it most commonly involves the head and neck. The diagnosis is made based on characteristic light and electron microscopic findings. These tumors possess adenosine triphosphatase and neurosecretory granules suggesting possibly a myogenic and/or neuroepithelial origin [49, 169, 181]. In addition, immunocytochemical studies overwhelmingly support a myogenic origin [245, 293]. These tumors are associated with chromosomal translocations of der(17)t(X;17)(p11.2;q25) leading to ASPL-TFE3 fusion protein [4]. These tumors are slow growing and 80% of children are alive 2 years after diagnosis. Most patients, however, eventually die of the disease. Alveolar soft part sarcomas in younger children and those arising in the head and neck have a better prognosis. Treatment is with wide local excision. Because these sarcomas are very slow growing tumors, radiation and chemotherapy are reserved for recurrent and distant disease.

17.10 Salivary Gland Tumors

Malignant tumors of the salivary glands are rare in children; however, when they do occur, the parotid gland is the most common site, accounting for approximately 90% of the cases. In one series of the 10,000 salivary gland neoplasms reviewed, 430 occurred in children of which only 12% were malignant [150]. Malignant salivary gland tumors are most common in older children and adolescents with a mean age of 13 years [263]. There is a slight female predominance [67, 216, 241, 255]. Histologically, salivary neoplasms in children are similar to those seen in adults. The pleomorphic adenoma is the most common benign neoplasm, and mucoepidermoid carcinoma the most common salivary gland malignancy [241, 311]. Mucoepidermoid carcinoma (MEC) consists of dermoid and mucus-containing cells. Children tend to present with low- or intermediate-grade tumors [216]. Low-grade tumors have a decreased rate of recurrence and nodal metastases. It has been suggested that certain tumor makers, specifically PCNA and KI-67 may be linked to high grade MEC, although other reviews have suggested this is not the case [67, 122]. These tumors have been found in children previously treated for childhood cancer with chemotherapy and radiation. Other types of salivary gland tumors include low-grade acinic cell carcinoma, undifferentiated carcinoma, adenocarcinoma, adenoid cystic carcinoma, peripheral neuroectodermal, and malignant mixed tumors all of which occur less commonly.

The most common presenting sign in children is a firm preauricular mass. Signs particularly concerning for malignancy are rapid growth, facial weakness or pain, and associated lymphadenopathy. Ultrasound, sialogram, and CT scan should investigate a swollen parotid gland not suggestive of acute inflammation [280]. A simple hemangioma or lymphangioma should be treated by surgical excision. A pleomorphic adenoma requires a superficial parotidectomy to avoid recurrence. Mucoepidermoid carcinoma requires a total parotidectomy since even well-differentiated tumors extend beyond the resection margins. For the soft tissue sarcomas, frozen sections allow surface markers, cytogenetic studies, and electronmicroscopy and they are treated appropriately according to the sarcoma or lymphoma protocols as mentioned above.

All firm salivary gland masses should be biopsied [280]. While fine needle aspiration has been used with success in adults, its role in children has not been determined. Incisional biopsy of the parotid gland should be avoided due to the risk of injuring the facial nerve. The only indication for incisional biopsy is for histologic diagnosis of large, unresectable tumors (Figs. 17.14a–d). Superficial or total parotidectomy with preservation of the facial nerve or total excision of the submandibular gland should be the initial procedure. There is controversy over the utility of modified neck dissection in these patients.

In general, superficial or total parotidectomy without facial nerve sacrifice is the recommended surgical treatment for salivary gland tumors [45]. Although adjuvant radiation has not been shown to improve long-term outcomes, adjuvant radiation can be used for local control of high-grade, high stage tumors or for adenoid cystic carcinomas which are difficult to treat with surgery alone [21, 192, 301]. Chemotherapy has been used in cases of high-grade or unresectable lesions, although its long-term benefits are unknown. The prognosis for low-grade mucoepidermoid carcinoma, acinic cell carcinoma and well-differentiated adenocarcinoma is good, whereas high-grade mucoepidermoid carcinoma, poorly differentiated adenocarcinoma, and undifferentiated tumors do poorly. Mucoepidermoid and acinic cell carcinomas have a 5-year survival of greater than 90% [52, 61, 162].

17.11 Nasopharyngeal Carcinoma

Nasopharyngeal carcinoma (NPC) is rare in childhood with an annual incidence of 0.5 per million children. Approximately 10% of the cases in the USA are in children under the age of 16 [161]. It is slightly more common in males and teenagers of African-American descent [14, 229]. Geographically it is more common in China, southeast Asia, the Mediterranean, and Alaska. This geographic variation is thought to be due to both genetic and environmental factors. The two different histopathologic variants are squamous cell and undifferentiated carcinoma. Undifferentiated nasopharyngeal carcinoma, also known as lymphoepithelioma, is most common in children and is associated with EBV exposure [84]. NPC is also known to be associated with certain human leukocyte antigens including HLA A2 Bsin2 haplotype, Aw19, Bw46, and B17 [66, 312]. Cytogenetics has linked NPC with inactivation of p53, retinoblastoma (RB2/p130) tumors suppressor genes, and CYP2E1 [56, 59, 124, 264, 312].

The most common presenting symptom is a painless neck mass although a child may also have earache, tinnitus, deafness, otalgia, nasal obstruction, and epistaxis. At presentation, most children already have metastatic spread to cervical lymph nodes [88]. Auditory symptoms are often the result of a persistent middle ear effusion that may have been present for many months prior to diagnosis of nasopharyngeal cancer. As the cancer invades the base of the skull, cranial nerve palsies and head pain may result. Children may also complain of double vision, eye pain, loss of vision, difficulty swallowing, or hoarseness [66, 217, 312, 324]. Sites of distant metastasis include bone, lung, liver, bone marrow, and mediastinum [66, 260, 312].

Initial laboratory data should include a complete blood count, serum chemistry, liver function tests, and lactic acid dehydrogenase. Elevated LDH levels have been correlated with poor outcomes. Viral capsid an-

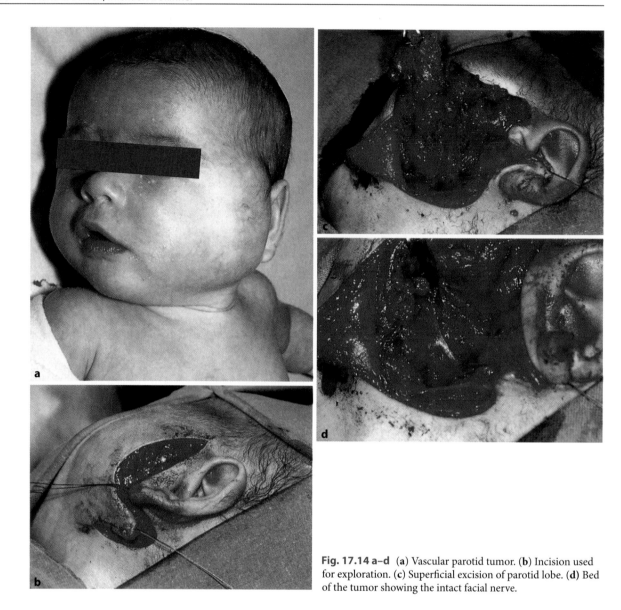

Fig. 17.14 a–d (**a**) Vascular parotid tumor. (**b**) Incision used for exploration. (**c**) Superficial excision of parotid lobe. (**d**) Bed of the tumor showing the intact facial nerve.

tigen IgA and Zebra protein concentration should also be measured for baseline tumor markers. Nasopharyngeal examination and biopsy is performed for diagnosis. For diagnosis and staging, a CT scan and MRI are useful [306]. MRI is considered better for assessing extent of primary tumor and perineural invasion, while CT is better for detecting bone involvement. The role of PET scans is still unclear. In addition, chest x-rays, CT of the chest and abdomen, and radionuclide bone scanning should be performed to evaluate for metastatic disease. Bone marrow biopsy and a lumbar puncture should be performed if there is concern for advanced disease. Undifferentiated nasopharyngeal carcinoma is radiosensitive and responds well to radiotherapy. For metastatic or recurrent NPC, chemotherapy is combined with radiation therapy. Common chemotherapeutic agents include cisplatin, bleomycin, epirubicin, and fluorouracil. The addition of cisplatin-based chemotherapy in addition to radiation has increased the overall 5-year survival of children with nasopharyngeal carcinoma from 20–60% to 70–90% [3, 66, 94, 260, 306, 312].

References

1. Acharya S, Sarafoglou K, LaQuaglia M, et al. (2003) Thyroid neoplasms after therapeutic radiation for malignancies during childhood or adolescence. Cancer 97(10):2397–2403
2. Adde M, Shad A, Venzon D, et al. (1998) Additional chemotherapy agents improve treatment outcome for children and adults with advanced B-cell lymphomas. Semin Oncol 25(Suppl):33–39; discussion 45–48

3. Ahern V, Jenkin D, Banerjee D, et al. (1994) Nasopharyngeal carcinoma in the young. Clin Oncol (R Coll Radiol) 6(1):24–30

4. Albritton KH (2005) Sarcomas in adolescents and young adults. Hematol Oncol Clin North Am 19(3):527–546, vii

5. Alvarado CS, London WB, Look AT, et al. (2000) Natural history and biology of stage A neuroblastoma: A Pediatric Oncology Group Study. J Pediatr Hematol Oncol 22(3):197–205

6. Anderson J, Gordon A, Pritchard-Jones K (1999) Genes, chromosomes, and rhabdomyosarcoma. Genes Chromosomes Cancer 26(4):275–285

7. Anderson JR, Jenkin RD, Wilson JF, et al. (1993) Long-term follow-up of patients treated with COMP or LSA2L2 therapy for childhood non-Hodgkin's lymphoma: A report of CCG-551 from the Children's Cancer Group. J Clin Oncol 11(6):1024–1032

8. Antman K, Crowley J, Balcerzak SP, et al. (1998) A Southwest Oncology Group and Cancer and Leukemia Group B phase II study of doxorubicin, dacarbazine, ifosfamide, and mesna in adults with advanced osteosarcoma, Ewing's sarcoma, and rhabdomyosarcoma. Cancer 82(7):1288–1295

9. ar-Rushdi A, Nishikura K, Erikson J, et al. (1983) Differential expression of the translocated and the untranslocated c-myc oncogene in Burkitt lymphoma. Science 222(4622):390–393

10. Astl J, Dvorakova M, Vlcek P, et al. (2004) Thyroid surgery in children and adolescents. Int J Pediatr Otorhinolaryngol 68(10):1273–1278

11. Atkinson MK, McElwain TJ, Peckham MJ, et al. (1976) Hypertrophic pulmonary osteoarthropathy in Hodgkin's disease: Reversal with chemotherapy. Cancer 38(4):1729–1734

12. Attiyeh EF, London WB, Mosse YP, et al. (2005) Chromosome 1p and 11q deletions and outcome in neuroblastoma. N Engl J Med 353(21):2243–2253

13. Auguste LJ, Razack MS, Sako K (1982) Hemangiopericytoma. J Surg Oncol 20(4):260–264

14. Ayan I, Altun M (1996) Nasopharyngeal carcinoma in children: Retrospective review of 50 patients. Int J Radiat Oncol Biol Phys 35(3):485–492

15. Azizkhan RG, Haase GM, Applebaum H, et al. (1995) Diagnosis, management, and outcome of cervicofacial teratomas in neonates: A Children's Cancer Group study. J Pediatr Surg 30(2):312–316

16. Backwinkel KD, Diddams JA (1970) Hemangiopericytoma. Report of a case and comprehensive review of the literature. Cancer 25(4):896–901

17. Baker LL, Parker BR, Donaldson SS, et al. (1990) Staging of Hodgkin disease in children: Comparison of CT and lymphography with laparotomy. AJR Am J Roentgenol 154(6):1251–1255

18. Bash RO, Crist WM, Shuster JJ, et al. (1993) Clinical features and outcome of T-cell acute lymphoblastic leukemia in childhood with respect to alterations at the TAL1 locus: A Pediatric Oncology Group study. Blood 81(8):2110–2117

19. Batsakis J, Littler, Oberman (1964) Teratomas of the neck: A clinicopathologic appraisal. Arch Orolaryngol (79):619–624

20. Batsakis JG, el-Naggar AK, Luna MA (1995) Teratomas of the head and neck with emphasis on malignancy. Ann Otol Rhinol Laryngol 104(6):496–500

21. Bell RB, Dierks EJ, Homer L, et al. (2005) Management and outcome of patients with malignant salivary gland tumors. J Oral Maxillofac Surg 63(7):917–928

22. Ben-Yehuda D, Polliack A, Okon E, et al. (1996) Image-guided core-needle biopsy in malignant lymphoma: Experience with 100 patients that suggests the technique is reliable. J Clin Oncol 14(9):2431–2434

23. Bernheim A, Berger R, Lenoir G (1981) Cytogenetic studies on African Burkitt's lymphoma cell lines: t(8;14), t(2;8) and t(8;22) translocations. Cancer Genet Cytogenet 3(4):307–315

24. Biegel JA, White PS, Marshall HN, et al. (1993) Constitutional 1p36 deletion in a child with neuroblastoma. Am J Hum Genet 52(1):176–182

25. Birch JM, Hartley AL, Blair V, et al. (1990) Cancer in the families of children with soft tissue sarcoma. Cancer 66(10):2239–2248

26. Blatt J, Olshan AF, Lee PA, et al. (1997) Neuroblastoma and related tumors in Turner's syndrome. J Pediatr 131(5):666–670

27. Boehm T, Foroni L, Kaneko Y, et al. (1991) The rhombotin family of cysteine-rich LIM-domain oncogenes: Distinct members are involved in T-cell translocations to human chromosomes 11p15 and 11p13 Proc Natl Acad Sci U S A 88(10):4367–4371

28. Bongarzone I, Butti MG, Coronelli S, et al. (1994) Frequent activation of ret protooncogene by fusion with a new activating gene in papillary thyroid carcinomas. Cancer Res 54(11):2979–2985

29. Boulad F, Kernan NA, LaQuaglia MP, et al. (1998) High-dose induction chemoradiotherapy followed by autologous bone marrow transplantation as consolidation therapy in rhabdomyosarcoma, extraosseous Ewing's sarcoma, and undifferentiated sarcoma. J Clin Oncol 16(5):1697–1706

30. Bowman WP, Shuster JJ, Cook B, et al. (1996) Improved survival for children with B-cell acute lymphoblastic leukemia and stage IV small noncleaved-cell lymphoma: A pediatric oncology group study. J Clin Oncol 14(4):1252–1261

31. Bown N, Cotterill S, Lastowska M, et al. (1999) Gain of chromosome arm 17q and adverse outcome in patients with neuroblastoma. N Engl J Med 340(25):1954–1961

32. Bradley SJ, Hudson GV, Linch DC (1993) Idiopathic thrombocytopenic purpura in Hodgkin's disease: A report of eight cases. Clin Oncol (R Coll Radiol) 5(6):355–357

33. Brauckhoff M, Gimm O, Thanh PN, et al. (2002) First experiences in intraoperative neurostimulation of the recurrent laryngeal nerve during thyroid surgery of children and adolescents. J Pediatr Surg 37(10):1414–1418

34. Breitfeld PP, Lyden E, Raney RB, et al. (2001) Ifosfamide and etoposide are superior to vincristine and melphalan for pediatric metastatic rhabdomyosarcoma when administered with irradiation and combination chemotherapy: A report from the Intergroup Rhabdomyosarcoma Study Group. J Pediatr Hematol Oncol 23(4):225–233

35. Breneman JC, Lyden E, Pappo AS, et al. (2003) Prognostic factors and clinical outcomes in children and adolescents with metastatic rhabdomyosarcoma—A report from the Intergroup Rhabdomyosarcoma Study IV. J Clin Oncol 21(1):78–84

36. Bridge JA, Liu J, Qualman SJ, et al. (2002) Genomic gains and losses are similar in genetic and histologic subsets of rhabdomyosarcoma, whereas amplification predominates in embryonal with anaplasia and alveolar subtypes. Genes Chromosomes Cancer 33(3):310–321

37. Brodeur G, Maris J (2002) Principles and practice of pediatric oncology. Lippincott, Philadelphia

38. Brodeur GM, Seeger RC, Schwab M, et al. (1984) Amplification of N-myc in untreated human neuroblastomas correlates with advanced disease stage. Science 224(4653):1121–1124

39. Brodeur GM, Azar C, Brother M, et al. (1992) Neuroblastoma. Effect of genetic factors on prognosis and treatment. Cancer 70(6 Suppl):1685–1694

40. Brodeur GM, Pritchard J, Berthold F, et al. (1993) Revisions of the international criteria for neuroblastoma diagnosis, staging, and response to treatment. J Clin Oncol 11(8):1466–1477

41. Brook I (1980) Aerobic and anaerobic bacteriology of cervical adenitis in children. Clin Pediatr (Phila) 19(10):693–696

42. Brown RJ, Szymula NJ, Lore JM Jr (1978) Neuroblastoma of the head and neck. Arch Otolaryngol 104(7):395–398

43. Bukachevsky RP, Pincus RL, Shechtman FG, et al. (1992) Synovial sarcoma of the head and neck. Head Neck 14(1):44–48

44. Burkitt D (1970) Burkitt's lymphoma. Livingstone, Edinburgh

45. Callender DL, Frankenthaler RA, Luna MA, et al. (1992) Salivary gland neoplasms in children. Arch Otolaryngol Head Neck Surg 118(5):472–476

46. Carbone PP, Kaplan HS, Musshoff K, et al. (1971) Report of the committee on Hodgkin's disease staging classification. Cancer Res 31(11):1860–1861

47. Carpenter PA, White L, McCowage GB, et al. (1997) A dose-intensive, cyclophosphamide-based regimen for the treatment of recurrent/progressive or advanced solid tumors of childhood: A report from the Australia and New Zealand Children's Cancer Study Group. Cancer 80(3):489–496

48. Carr MM, Thorner P, Phillips JH (1997) Congenital teratomas of the head and neck. J Otolaryngol 26(4):246–252

49. Carstens HB (1990) Membrane-bound cytoplasmic crystals, similar to those in alveolar soft part sarcoma, in a human muscle spindle. Ultrastruct Pathol 14(5):423–428

50. Castleberry RP, Kun LE, Shuster JJ, et al. (1991) Radiotherapy improves the outlook for patients older than 1 year with Pediatric Oncology Group stage C neuroblastoma. J Clin Oncol 9(5):789–795

51. Castleberry RP, Cantor AB, Green AA, et al. (1994) Phase II investigational window using carboplatin, iproplatin, ifosfamide, and epirubicin in children with untreated disseminated neuroblastoma: A Pediatric Oncology Group study. J Clin Oncol 12(8):1616–1620

52. Castro EB, Huvos AG, Strong EW, et al. (1972) Tumors of the major salivary glands in children. Cancer 29(2):312–317

53. Cavalli F (1998) Rare syndromes in Hodgkin's disease. Ann Oncol 9 Suppl 5:S109–S113

54. Ceccarelli C, Pacini F, Lippi F, et al. (1988) An unusual case of a false-positive iodine-131 whole body scan in a patient with papillary thyroid cancer. Clin Nucl Med 13(3):192–193

55. Chabalko JJ, Creagan ET, Fraumeni JF Jr (1974) Epidemiology of selected sarcomas in children. J Natl Cancer Inst 53(3):675–679

56. Chan AS, To KF, Lo KW, et al. (2000) High frequency of chromosome 3p deletion in histologically normal nasopharyngeal epithelia from southern Chinese. Cancer Res 60(19):5365–5370

57. Chung EB, Enzinger FM (1976) Infantile fibrosarcoma. Cancer 38(2):729–739

58. Clamon GH, Robinson RA, Olberding EB (1984) Prolonged remission of metastatic malignant fibrous histiocytoma induced by combination chemotherapy. J Surg Oncol 26(2):113–114

59. Claudio PP, Howard CM, Fu Y, et al. (2000) Mutations in the retinoblastoma-related gene RB2/p130 in primary nasopharyngeal carcinoma. Cancer Res 60(1):8–12

60. Cleary ML (1991) Oncogenic conversion of transcription factors by chromosomal translocations. Cell 66(4):619–622

61. Conley J, Tinsley PP Jr (1985) Treatment and prognosis of mucoepidermoid carcinoma in the pediatric age group. Arch Otolaryngol 111(5):322–324

62. Cook MN, Olshan AF, Guess HA, et al. (2004) Maternal medication use and neuroblastoma in offspring. Am J Epidemiol 159(8):721–731

63. Correa P, O'Conor GT (1971) Epidemiologic patterns of Hodgkin's disease. Int J Cancer 8(2):192–201

64. Crist W, Gehan EA, Ragab AH, et al. (1995) The Third Intergroup rhabdomyosarcoma study. J Clin Oncol 13(3):610–630

65. Crist WM, Anderson JR, Meza JL, et al. (2001) Intergroup rhabdomyosarcoma study-IV: Results for patients with nonmetastatic disease. J Clin Oncol 19(12):3091–3102

66. Cvitkovic E, Bachouchi M, Armand JP (1991) Nasopharyngeal carcinoma. Biology, natural history, and therapeutic implications. Hematol Oncol Clin North Am 5(4):821–838

67. da Cruz Perez DE, Pires FR, Alves FA, et al. (2004) Salivary gland tumors in children and adolescents: A clinicopathologic and immunohistochemical study of fifty-three cases. Int J Pediatr Otorhinolaryngol 68(7):895–902

68. Dagher R, Helman L (1999) Rhabdomyosarcoma: An overview. Oncologist 4(1):34–44

69. Dahl GV, Rivera G, Pui CH, et al. (1985) A novel treatment of childhood lymphoblastic non-Hodgkin's lymphoma: Early and intermittent use of teniposide plus cytarabine. Blood 66(5):1110–1114

70. Davis RJ, D'Cruz CM, Lovell MA, et al. (1994) Fusion of PAX7 to FKHR by the variant t(1;13)(p36;q14) translocation in alveolar rhabdomyosarcoma. Cancer Res 54(11):2869–2872

71. de Roy van Zuidewijn DB, Songun I, Kievit J, et al. (1995) Complications of thyroid surgery. Ann Surg Oncol 2(1):56–60

72. DeBaun MR, Tucker MA (1998) Risk of cancer during the first four years of life in children from the Beckwith-Wiedemann Syndrome Registry. J Pediatr 132(3 Pt 1):398–400

73. DeCou JM, Bowman LC, Rao BN, et al. (1995) Infants with metastatic neuroblastoma have improved survival with resection of the primary tumor. J Pediatr Surg 30(7):937–940; discussion 940–941

74. Dehner LP, Mills A, Talerman A, et al. (1990) Germ cell neoplasms of head and neck soft tissues: A pathologic spectrum of teratomatous and endodermal sinus tumors. Hum Pathol 21(3):309–318

75. Derias NW, Chong WH, O'Connor AF (1992) Fine needle aspiration cytology of a head and neck swelling in a child: A non-invasive approach to diagnosis. J Laryngol Otol 106(8):755–757

76. Dias P, Parham DM, Shapiro DN, et al. (1990) Myogenic regulatory protein (MyoD1) expression in childhood solid tumors: Diagnostic utility in rhabdomyosarcoma. Am J Pathol 137(6):1283–1291

77. Dias P, Chen B, Dilday B, et al. (2000) Strong immunostaining for myogenin in rhabdomyosarcoma is significantly associated with tumors of the alveolar subclass. Am J Pathol 156(2):399–408

78. Donaldson SS, Hudson MM, Lamborn KR, et al. (2002) VAMP and low-dose, involved-field radiation for children and adolescents with favorable, early-stage Hodgkin's disease: Results of a prospective clinical trial. J Clin Oncol 20(14):3081–3087

79. Douglass EC, Valentine M, Etcubanas E, et al. (1987) A specific chromosomal abnormality in rhabdomyosarcoma. Cytogenet Cell Genet 45(3-4):148–155

80. El-Badry OM, Minniti C, Kohn EC, et al. (1990) Insulin-like growth factor II acts as an autocrine growth and motility factor in human rhabdomyosarcoma tumors. Cell Growth Differ 1(7):325–331

81. Eng C, Smith DP, Mulligan LM, et al. (1994) Point mutation within the tyrosine kinase domain of the RET proto-oncogene in multiple endocrine neoplasia type 2B and related sporadic tumours. Hum Mol Genet 3(2):237–241

82. Evans AE, Silber JH, Shpilsky A, et al. (1996) Successful management of low-stage neuroblastoma without adjuvant therapies: A comparison of two decades, 1972 through 1981 and 1982 through 1992, in a single institution. J Clin Oncol 14(9):2504–2510

83. Exelby PE, Frazell EL (1969) Carcinoma of the thyroid in children. Surg Clin North Am 49(2):249–259

84. Fandi A, Cvitkovic E (1995) Biology and treatment of nasopharyngeal cancer. Curr Opin Oncol 7(3):255–263

85. Favus MJ, Schneider AB, Stachura ME, et al. (1976) Thyroid cancer occurring as a late consequence of head-and-neck irradiation. Evaluation of 1056 patients. N Engl J Med 294(19):1019–1025

86. Feinberg AP (1993) Genomic imprinting and gene activation in cancer. Nat Genet 4(2):110–113

87. Felix CA, Kappel CC, Mitsudomi T, et al. (1992) Frequency and diversity of p53 mutations in childhood rhabdomyosarcoma. Cancer Res 52(8):2243–2247

88. Fernandez CH, Cangir A, Samaan NA, et al. (1976) Nasopharyngeal carcinoma in children. Cancer 37(6):2787–2791

89. Ferraris AM, Racchi O, Rapezzi D, et al. (1997) Familial Hodgkin's disease: A disease of young adulthood? Ann Hematol 74(3):131–134

90. French AE, Grant R, Weitzman S, et al. (2003) Folic acid food fortification is associated with a decline in neuroblastoma. Clin Pharmacol Ther 74(3):288–294

91. Furman WL, Stewart CF, Poquette CA, et al. (1999) Direct translation of a protracted irinotecan schedule from a xenograft model to a phase I trial in children. J Clin Oncol 17(6):1815–1824

92. Galili N, Davis RJ, Fredericks WJ, et al. (1993) Fusion of a fork head domain gene to PAX3 in the solid tumour alveolar rhabdomyosarcoma. Nat Genet 5(3):230–235

93. Garaventa A, De Bernardi B, Pianca C, et al. (1993) Localized but unresectable neuroblastoma: Treatment and outcome of 145 cases. Italian Cooperative Group for Neuroblastoma. J Clin Oncol 11(9):1770–1779

94. Geara FB, Glisson BS, Sanguineti G, et al. (1997) Induction chemotherapy followed by radiotherapy versus radiotherapy alone in patients with advanced nasopharyngeal carcinoma: Results of a matched cohort study. Cancer 79(7):1279–1286

95. Gehan EA, Sullivan MP, Fuller LM, et al. (1990) The intergroup Hodgkin's disease in children. A study of stages I and II. Cancer 65(6):1429–1437

96. George ND, Gonzalez G, Hoyt CS (1998) Does Horner's syndrome in infancy require investigation? Br J Ophthalmol 82(1):51–54

97. Glover TW, Stein CK, Legius E, et al. (1991) Molecular and cytogenetic analysis of tumors in von Recklinghausen neurofibromatosis. Genes Chromosomes Cancer 3(1):62–70

98. Goodman M, Gurney J, Smith M, et al. (1999) Synpathetic nervous system tumors. National Cancer Institute, Bethesda

99. Gordon BG, Warkentin PI, Weisenburger DD, et al. (1992) Bone marrow transplantation for peripheral T-cell lymphoma in children and adolescents. Blood 80(11):2938–2942

100. Gorlin JB, Sallan SE (1990) Thyroid cancer in childhood. Endocrinol Metab Clin North Am 19(3):649–662

101. Green AA, Hayes FA, Hustu HO (1981) Sequential cyclophosphamide and doxorubicin for induction of complete remission in children with disseminated neuroblastoma. Cancer 48(10):2310–2317

102. Gripp KW, Scott CI Jr, Nicholson L, et al. (2002) Five additional Costello syndrome patients with rhabdomyosarcoma: Proposal for a tumor screening protocol. Am J Med Genet 108(1):80–87

103. Grosfeld JL, Billmire DF (1985) Teratomas in infancy and childhood. Curr Probl Cancer 9(9):1–53

104. Grufferman S, Gula M, Olshan A, et al. (1991) In utero X-ray exposure and risk of childhood rhabdomyosarcoma. Paediatr Perinatol Epidemiol (5):A6

105. Grufferman S, Schwartz AG, Ruymann FB, et al. (1993) Parents' use of cocaine and marijuana and increased risk of rhabdomyosarcoma in their children. Cancer Causes Control 4(3):217–224

106. Gu W, Bhatia K, Magrath IT, et al. (1994) Binding and suppression of the Myc transcriptional activation domain by p107. Science 264(5156):251–254

107. Gutierrez MI, Bhatia K, Barriga F, et al. (1992) Molecular epidemiology of Burkitt's lymphoma from South America: Differences in breakpoint location and Epstein-Barr virus association from tumors in other world regions. Blood 79(12):3261–3266

108. Haase GM, Wong KY, deLorimier AA, et al. (1989) Improvement in survival after excision of primary tumor in stage III neuroblastoma. J Pediatr Surg 24(2):194–200

109. Halliday BE, Slagel DD, Elsheikh TE, et al. (1998) Diagnostic utility of MIC-2 immunocytochemical staining in the differential diagnosis of small blue cell tumors. Diagn Cytopathol 19(6):410–416

110. Haluska FG, Brufsky AM, Canellos GP (1994) The cellular biology of the Reed-Sternberg cell. Blood 84(4):1005–1019

111. Hanna SL, Fletcher BD, Boulden TF, et al. (1993) MR imaging of infradiaphragmatic lymphadenopathy in children and adolescents with Hodgkin disease: Comparison with lymphography and CT. J Magn Reson Imaging 3(3):461–470

112. Harness JK, Thompson NW, McLeod MK, et al. (1992) Differentiated thyroid carcinoma in children and adolescents. World J Surg 16(4):547–553; discussion 553–554

113. Hartley AL, Birch JM, Marsden HB, et al. (1988) Neurofibromatosis in children with soft tissue sarcoma. Pediatr Hematol Oncol 5(1):7–16

114. Hartley AL, Birch JM, Blair V, et al. (1993) Patterns of cancer in the families of children with soft tissue sarcoma. Cancer 72(3):923–930

115. Hartley AL, Birch JM, McKinney PA, et al. (1988) The Inter-Regional Epidemiological Study of Childhood Cancer (IRESCC): Past medical history in children with cancer. J Epidemiol Community Health 42(3):235–242

116. Hartmann O, Pinkerton CR, Philip T, et al. (1988) Very-high-dose cisplatin and etoposide in children with untreated advanced neuroblastoma. J Clin Oncol 6(1):44–50

117. Haselkorn T, Bernstein L, Preston-Martin S, et al. (2000) Descriptive epidemiology of thyroid cancer in Los Angeles County, 1972-1995. Cancer Causes Control 11(2):163–170

118. Hatano M, Roberts CW, Minden M, et al. (1991) Deregulation of a homeobox gene, HOX11, by the t(10;14) in T cell leukemia. Science 253(5015):79–82

119. Hawkins EP (1990) pathology of germ cell tumors in children. Crit Rev Oncol Hematol 10(2):165–179

120. Hennekam RC (2003) Costello syndrome: An overview. Am J Med Genet C Semin Med Genet 117(1):42–48

121. Herzog LW (1983) Prevalence of lymphadenopathy of the head and neck in infants and children. Clin Pediatr (Phila) 22(7):485–487

122. Hicks J, Flaitz C (2000) Mucoepidermoid carcinoma of salivary glands in children and adolescents: Assessment of proliferation markers. Oral Oncol 36(5):454–460

123. Hicks J, Flaitz C (2002) Rhabdomyosarcoma of the head and neck in children. Oral Oncol 38(5):450–459

124. Hildesheim A, Anderson LM, Chen CJ, et al. (1997) CYP2E1 genetic polymorphisms and risk of nasopharyngeal carcinoma in Taiwan. J Natl Cancer Inst 89(16):1207–1212

125. Hodgkin T (1823) On some morbid appearances of the absorbent glands and spleen. Med Chir Trans (17):69

126. Hofstra RM, Landsvater RM, Ceccherini I, et al. (1994) A mutation in the RET proto-oncogene associated with multiple endocrine neoplasia type 2B and sporadic medullary thyroid carcinoma. Nature 367(6461):375–376

127. Hostein I, Andraud-Fregeville M, Guillou L, et al. (2004) Rhabdomyosarcoma: Value of myogenin expression analysis and molecular testing in diagnosing the alveolar subtype: An analysis of 109 paraffin-embedded specimens. Cancer 101(12):2817–2824

128. Howe JR, Norton JA, Wells SA Jr (1993) Prevalence of pheochromocytoma and hyperparathyroidism in multiple endocrine neoplasia type 2A: Results of long-term follow-up. Surgery 114(6):1070–1077

129. Hudson M, Donaldson S (2002) Principles and practice of pediatric oncology. Lippincott, Philadelphia

130. Hung W, Anderson KD, Chandra RS, et al. (1992) Solitary thyroid nodules in 71 children and adolescents. J Pediatr Surg 27(11):1407–1409

131. Hutchison RE, Pui CH, Murphy SB, et al. (1988) Non-Hodgkin's lymphoma in children younger than 3 years. Cancer 62(7):1371–1373

132. Hutchison RE, Berard CW, Shuster JJ, et al. (1995) B-cell lineage confers a favorable outcome among children and adolescents with large-cell lymphoma: A Pediatric Oncology Group study. J Clin Oncol 13(8):2023–2032

133. Jackson LA, Perkins BA, Wenger JD (1993) Cat scratch disease in the United States: An analysis of three national databases. Am J Public Health 83(12):1707–1711

134. Jacobson HM, Marcus RB Jr, Thar TL, et al. (1983) Pediatric neuroblastoma: Postoperative radiation therapy using less than 2000 rad. Int J Radiat Oncol Biol Phys 9(4):501–505

135. Jordan RB, Gauderer MW (1988) Cervical teratomas: An analysis. Literature review and proposed classification. J Pediatr Surg 23(6):583–591

136. Kaplan HS (1980) Essentials of staging and management of the malignant lymphomas. Semin Roentgenol 15(3):219–226

137. Kebudi R, Ayan I, Erseven G, et al. (1997) Hypertrophic osteoarthropathy and intrathoracic Hodgkin disease of childhood. Med Pediatr Oncol 29(6):578–581

138. Kelly KM, Womer RB, Sorensen PH, et al. (1997) Common and variant gene fusions predict distinct clinical phenotypes in rhabdomyosarcoma. J Clin Oncol 15(5):1831–1836

139. Khan J, Bittner ML, Saal LH, et al. (1999) cDNA microarrays detect activation of a myogenic transcription program by the PAX3-FKHR fusion oncogene. Proc Natl Acad Sci U S A 96(23):13264–13269

140. King SC, Reiman RJ, Prosnitz LR (1994) Prognostic importance of restaging gallium scans following induction chemotherapy for advanced Hodgkin's disease. J Clin Oncol 12(2):306–311

141. Kirk JM, Mort C, Grant DB, et al. (1992) The usefulness of serum thyroglobulin in the follow-up of differentiated thyroid carcinoma in children. Med Pediatr Oncol 20(3):201–208

142. Knight PJ, Mulne AF, Vassy LE (1982) When is lymph node biopsy indicated in children with enlarged peripheral nodes? Pediatrics 69(4):391–396

143. Kodet R, Newton WA Jr, Hamoudi AB, et al. (1993) Childhood rhabdomyosarcoma with anaplastic (pleomorphic) features. A report of the Intergroup Rhabdomyosarcoma Study. Am J Surg Pathol 17(5):443–453

144. Kogner P, Barbany G, Dominici C, et al. (1993) Coexpression of messenger RNA for TRK protooncogene and low affinity nerve growth factor receptor in neuroblastoma with favorable prognosis. Cancer Res 53(9):2044–2050

145. Komuro H, Valentine MB, Rowe ST, et al. (1998) Fluorescence in situ hybridization analysis of chromosome 1p36 deletions in human MYCN amplified neuroblastoma. J Pediatr Surg 33(11):1695–1698

146. Koscielniak E, Rodary C, Flamant F, et al. (1992) Metastatic rhabdomyosarcoma and histologically similar tumors in childhood: A retrospective European multi-center analysis. Med Pediatr Oncol 20(3):209–214

147. Koscielniak E, Klingebiel TH, Peters C, et al. (1997) Do patients with metastatic and recurrent rhabdomyosarcoma benefit from high-dose therapy with hematopoietic rescue? Report of the German/Austrian Pediatric Bone Marrow Transplantation Group. Bone Marrow Transplant 19(3):227–231

148. Koscielny S, Brauer B, Forster G (2003) Hemangiopericytoma: A rare head and neck tumor. Eur Arch Otorhinolaryngol 260(8):450–453

149. Kramer S, Meadows AT, Jarrett P, et al. (1983) Incidence of childhood cancer: Experience of a decade in a population-based registry. J Natl Cancer Inst 70(1):49–55

150. Krolls SO, Trodahl JN, Boyers RC (1972) Salivary gland lesions in children. A survey of 430 cases. Cancer 30(2):459–469

151. Krona C, Ejeskar K, Abel F, et al. (2003) Screening for gene mutations in a 500 kb neuroblastoma tumor suppressor candidate region in chromosome 1p; mutation and stage-specific expression in UBE4B/UFD2. Oncogene 22(15):2343–2351

152. Kushner BH, Hajdu SI, Helson L (1985) Synchronous neuroblastoma and von Recklinghausen's disease: A review of the literature. J Clin Oncol 3(1):117–120

153. Kushner BH, Gilbert F, Helson L (1986) Familial neuroblastoma. Case reports, literature review, and etiologic considerations. Cancer 57(9):1887–1893

154. Kushner BH, Cheung NK, LaQuaglia MP, et al. (1996) International neuroblastoma staging system stage 1 neuroblastoma: A prospective study and literature review. J Clin Oncol 14(7):2174–2180

155. La Quaglia MP, Corbally MT, Heller G, et al. (1988) Recurrence and morbidity in differentiated thyroid carcinoma in children. Surgery 104(6):1149–1156

156. Lack EE (1985) Extragonadal germ cell tumors of the head and neck region: Review of 16 cases. Hum Pathol 16(1):56–64

157. Lake AM, Oski FA (1978) Peripheral lymphadenopathy in childhood. Ten-year experience with excisional biopsy. Am J Dis Child 132(4):357–359

158. Lawrence W Jr, Anderson JR, Gehan EA, et al. (1997) Pretreatment TNM staging of childhood rhabdomyosarcoma: A report of the Intergroup Rhabdomyosarcoma Study Group. Children's Cancer Study Group. Pediatric Oncology Group. Cancer 80(6):1165–1170

159. Lawrence W Jr, Gehan EA, Hays DM, et al. (1987) Prognostic significance of staging factors of the UICC staging system in childhood rhabdomyosarcoma: A report from the Intergroup Rhabdomyosarcoma Study (IRS-II). J Clin Oncol 5(1):46–54

160. Lawrence W Jr, Hays DM, Heyn R, et al. (1987) Lymphatic metastases with childhood rhabdomyosarcoma. A report from the Intergroup Rhabdomyosarcoma Study. Cancer 60(4):910–915

161. Levine PH, Connelly RR, Easton JM (1980) Demographic patterns for nasopharyngeal carcinoma in the United States. Int J Cancer 26(6):741–748

162. Levine SB, Potsic WP (1986) Acinic cell carcinoma of the parotid gland in children. Int J Pediatr Otorhinolaryngol 11(3):281–286

163. Li FP, Fraumeni JF Jr (1969) Soft-tissue sarcomas, breast cancer, and other neoplasms. A familial syndrome? Ann Intern Med 71(4):747–752

164. Li FP, Fraumeni JF Jr, Mulvihill JJ, et al. (1988) A cancer family syndrome in twenty-four kindreds. Cancer Res 48(18):5358–5362

165. Link MP, Shuster JJ, Donaldson SS, et al. (1997) Treatment of children and young adults with early-stage non-Hodgkin's lymphoma. N Engl J Med 337(18):1259–1266

166. Longo DL, Young RC, Wesley M, et al. (1986) Twenty years of MOPP therapy for Hodgkin's disease. J Clin Oncol 4(9):1295–1306

167. Look AT, Hayes FA, Shuster JJ, et al. (1991) Clinical relevance of tumor cell ploidy and N-myc gene amplification in childhood neuroblastoma: A Pediatric Oncology Group study. J Clin Oncol 9(4):581–591

168. Lukes RJ, Butler JJ (1966) The pathology and nomenclature of Hodgkin's disease. Cancer Res 26(6):1063–1083

169. Machinami R, Kikuchi F (1986) Adenosine triphosphatase activity of crystalline inclusions in alveolar soft part sarcoma. An ultrahistochemical study of a case. Pathol Res Pract 181(3):357–364

170. Mack TM, Cozen W, Shibata DK, et al. (1995) Concordance for Hodgkin's disease in identical twins suggesting genetic susceptibility to the young-adult form of the disease. N Engl J Med 332(7):413–418

171. Magnani C, Pastore G, Luzzatto L, et al. (1989) Risk factors for soft tissue sarcomas in childhood: A case-control study. Tumori 75(4):396–400

172. Magrath I (1990) The pathogenesis of Burkitt's lymphoma. Adv Cancer Res 55:133–270

173. Magrath I. (1993) Principles and practice of pediatric oncology. Lippincott, Philadelphia

174. Magrath I, Bhatia K (1997) The non-Hodgkin lymphomas, 2nd edn Arnold, London

175. Magrath I, Adde M, Shad A, et al. (1996) Adults and children with small non-cleaved-cell lymphoma have a similar excellent outcome when treated with the same chemotherapy regimen. J Clin Oncol 14(3):925–934

176. Magrath IT (1991) African Burkitt's lymphoma. History, biology, clinical features, and treatment. Am J Pediatr Hematol Oncol 13(2):222–246

177. Magrath IT, Ziegler JL (1980) Bone marrow involvement in Burkitt's lymphoma and its relationship to acute B-cell leukemia. Leuk Res 4(1):33–59

178. Mandahl N, Heim S, Willen H, et al. (1989) Characteristic karyotypic anomalies identify subtypes of malignant fibrous histiocytoma. Genes Chromosomes Cancer 1(1):9–14

179. Maris JM, Chatten J, Meadows AT, et al. (1997) Familial neuroblastoma: A three-generation pedigree and a further association with Hirschsprung disease. Med Pediatr Oncol 28(1):1–5

180. Maris JM, Weiss MJ, Guo C, et al. (2000) Loss of heterozygosity at 1p36 independently predicts for disease progression but not decreased overall survival probability in neuroblastoma patients: A Children's Cancer Group study. J Clin Oncol 18(9):1888–1899

181. Mathew T (1982) Evidence supporting neural crest origin of an alveolar soft part sarcoma: An ultra structural study. Cancer 50(3):507–514

182. Matsui I, Tanimura M, Kobayashi N, et al. (1993) Neurofibromatosis type 1 and childhood cancer. Cancer 72(9):2746–2754

183. Matthay KK, Perez C, Seeger RC, et al. (1998) Successful treatment of stage III neuroblastoma based on prospective biologic staging: A Children's Cancer Group study. J Clin Oncol 16(4):1256–1264

184. Maurer HM, Beltangady M, Gehan EA, et al. (1988) The Intergroup Rhabdomyosarcoma Study-I. A final report. Cancer 61(2):209–220

185. Maurer HM, Gehan EA, Beltangady M, et al. (1993) The Intergroup Rhabdomyosarcoma Study-II. Cancer 71(5):1904–1922

186. McClain KL, Joshi VV, Murphy SB (1996) Cancers in children with HIV infection. Hematol Oncol Clin North Am 10(5):1189–1201

187. McGill T (1989) Rhabdomyosarcoma of the head and neck: An update. Otolaryngol Clin North Am 22(3):631–636

188. Mead RS, Cowell JK (1995) Molecular characterization of a (1;10)(p22;q21) constitutional translocation from a patient with neuroblastoma. Cancer Genet Cytogenet 81(2):151–157

189. Meadows AT, Sposto R, Jenkin RD, et al. (1989) Similar efficacy of 6 and 18 months of therapy with four drugs (COMP) for localized non-Hodgkin's lymphoma of children: A report from the Children's Cancer Study Group. J Clin Oncol 7(1):92–99

190. Meazza C, Ferrari A, Casanova M, et al. (2005) Evolving treatment strategies for parameningeal rhabdomyosarcoma: The experience of the Istituto Nazionale Tumori of Milan. Head Neck 27(1):49–57

191. Mellentin JD, Smith SD, Cleary ML (1989) lyl-1, a novel gene altered by chromosomal translocation in T cell leukemia, codes for a protein with a helix-loop-helix DNA binding motif. Cell 58(1):77–83

192. Mendenhall WM, Morris CG, Amdur RJ, et al. (2005) Radiotherapy alone or combined with surgery for salivary gland carcinoma. Cancer 103(12):2544–2550

193. Michalski JM, Meza J, Breneman JC, et al. (2004) Influence of radiation therapy parameters on outcome in children treated with radiation therapy for localized parameningeal rhabdomyosarcoma in Intergroup Rhabdomyosarcoma Study Group trials II through IV. Int J Radiat Oncol Biol Phys 59(4):1027–1038

194. Miser JS, Pizzo PA (1985) Soft tissue sarcomas in childhood. Pediatr Clin North Am 32(3):779–800

195. Miser JS, Kinsella TJ, Triche TJ, et al. (1987) Ifosfamide with mesna uroprotection and etoposide: An effective regimen in the treatment of recurrent sarcomas and other tumors of children and young adults. J Clin Oncol 5(8):1191–1198

196. Mobley DL, Wakely PE Jr, Frable MA (1991) Fine-needle aspiration biopsy: Application to pediatric head and neck masses. Laryngoscope 101(5):469–472

197. Months SR, Raney RB (1986) Rhabdomyosarcoma of the head and neck in children: The experience at the Children's Hospital of Philadelphia. Med Pediatr Oncol 14(5):288–292

198. Moore DM, Berke GS (1987) Synovial sarcoma of the head and neck. Arch Otolaryngol Head Neck Surg 113(3):311–313

199. Morris SW, Kirstein MN, Valentine MB, et al. (1994) Fusion of a kinase gene, ALK, to a nucleolar protein gene, NPM, in non-Hodgkin's lymphoma. Science 263(5151):1281–1284

200. Moussatos GH, Baffes TG (1963) Cervical masses in infants and children. Pediatrics 32:251–256

201. Murphy S, Fairclough D, Hutchison R (1989) Non-Hodgkin's lymphomas of childhood: An analysis of the histology, staging, and response to treatment of 338 cases at a single institution. J Clin Oncol (7):186–193

202. Murphy SB (1980) Classification, staging and end results of treatment of childhood non-Hodgkin's lymphomas: Dissimilarities from lymphomas in adults. Semin Oncol 7(3):332–339

203. Murphy SB, Hustu HO, Rivera G, et al. (1983) End results of treating children with localized non-Hodgkin's lymphomas with a combined modality approach of lessened intensity. J Clin Oncol 1(5):326–330

204. Nakagawara A, Arima M, Azar CG, et al. (1992) Inverse relationship between trk expression and N-myc amplification in human neuroblastomas. Cancer Res 52(5):1364–1368

205. Nakagawara A, Arima-Nakagawara M, Scavarda NJ, et al. (1993) Association between high levels of expression of the TRK gene and favorable outcome in human neuroblastoma. N Engl J Med 328(12):847–854

206. Neglia JP, Friedman DL, Yasui Y, et al. (2001) Second malignant neoplasms in five-year survivors of childhood cancer: Childhood cancer survivor study. J Natl Cancer Inst 93(8):618–629

207. Nemecek ER, Sawin RW, Park J (2003) Treatment of neuroblastoma in patients with neurocristopathy syndromes. J Pediatr Hematol Oncol 25(2):159–162

208. Newman KD (1993) The current management of thyroid tumors in childhood. Semin Pediatr Surg 2(1):69–74

209. Newman KD, Black T, Heller G, et al. (1998) Differentiated thyroid cancer: Determinants of disease progression in patients <21 years of age at diagnosis: A report from the Surgical Discipline Committee of the Children's Cancer Group. Ann Surg 227(4):533–541

210. Nikiforov Y, Gnepp DR (1994) Pediatric thyroid cancer after the Chernobyl disaster. Pathomorphologic study of 84 cases (1991–1992) from the Republic of Belarus. Cancer 74(2):748–766

211. Nitschke R, Smith EI, Shochat S, et al. (1988) Localized neuroblastoma treated by surgery: A Pediatric Oncology Group Study. J Clin Oncol 6(8):1271–1279

212. Nitschke R, Smith EI, Altshuler G, et al. (1991) Postoperative treatment of nonmetastatic visible residual neuroblastoma: A Pediatric Oncology Group study. J Clin Oncol 9(7):1181–1188

213. Norton JA, Froome LC, Farrell RE, et al. (1979) Multiple endocrine neoplasia type IIb: The most aggressive form of medullary thyroid carcinoma. Surg Clin North Am 59(1):109–118

214. Ogita S, Tokiwa K, Takahashi T, et al. (1988) Congenital cervical neuroblastoma associated with Horner syndrome. J Pediatr Surg 23(11):991–992

215. Ordonez NG, Mackay B, el-Naggar AK, et al. (1993) Congenital hemangiopericytoma. An ultrastructural, immunocytochemical, and flow cytometric study. Arch Pathol Lab Med 117(9):934–937

216. Orvidas LJ, Kasperbauer JL, Lewis JE, et al. (2000) Pediatric parotid masses. Arch Otolaryngol Head Neck Surg 126(2):177–184

217. Ozyar E, Atahan IL, Akyol FH, et al. (1994) Cranial nerve involvement in nasopharyngeal carcinoma: Its prognostic role and response to radiotherapy. Radiat Med 12(2):65–68

218. Pacini F, Vorontsova T, Molinaro E, et al. (1999) Thyroid consequences of the Chernobyl nuclear accident. Acta Paediatr Suppl 88(433):23–27

219. Pappa VI, Hussain HK, Reznek RH, et al. (1996) Role of image-guided core-needle biopsy in the management of patients with lymphoma. J Clin Oncol 14(9):2427–2430

220. Pappo AS, Lyden E, Breneman J, et al. (2001) Up-front window trial of topotecan in previously untreated children and adolescents with metastatic rhabdomyosarcoma: An intergroup rhabdomyosarcoma study. J Clin Oncol 19(1):213–219

221. Parham DM, Webber B, Holt H, et al. (1991) Immunohistochemical study of childhood rhabdomyosarcomas and related neoplasms. Results of an Intergroup Rhabdomyosarcoma study project. Cancer 67(12):3072–3080

222. Parkin DM, Stiller CA, Draper GJ, et al. (1988) The international incidence of childhood cancer. Int J Cancer 42(4):511–520

223. Patte C, Auperin A, Michon J, et al. (2001) The Societe Francaise d'Oncologie Pediatrique LMB89 protocol: Highly effective multiagent chemotherapy tailored to the tumor burden and initial response in 561 unselected children with B-cell lymphomas and L3 leukemia. Blood 97(11):3370–3379

224. Percy C, Smith M, Linet M, et al. (1999) Cancer incidence and survival among children and adolescents: United States SEER Program, 1975–1995. National Cancer Institute, Bethesda

225. Perez CA, Matthay KK, Atkinson JB, et al. (2000) Biologic variables in the outcome of stages I and II neuroblastoma treated with surgery as primary therapy: A children's cancer group study. J Clin Oncol 18(1):18–26

226. Philip T, Zucker JM, Bernard JL, et al. (1991) Improved survival at 2 and 5 years in the LMCE1 unselected group of 72 children with stage IV neuroblastoma older than 1 year of age at diagnosis: Is cure possible in a small subgroup? J Clin Oncol 9(6):1037–1044

227. Philip T, Hartmann O, Pinkerton R, et al. (1993) Curability of relapsed childhood B-cell non-Hodgkin's lymphoma after intensive first line therapy: A report from the Societe Francaise d'Oncologie Pediatrique. Blood 81(8):2003–2006

228. Pileri SA, Ascani S, Leoncini L, et al. (2002) Hodgkin's lymphoma: The pathologist's viewpoint. J Clin Pathol 55(3):162–176

229. Plowman P. (1997) Rare tumors. Chapman and Hall, Cambridge

230. Pui CH, Ip SH, Kung P, et al. (1987) High serum interleukin-2 receptor levels are related to advanced disease and a poor outcome in childhood non-Hodgkin's lymphoma. Blood 70(3):624–628

231. Rabes HM, Demidchik EP, Sidorow JD, et al. (2000) Pattern of radiation-induced RET and NTRK1 rearrangements in 191 post-chernobyl papillary thyroid carcinomas: Biological, phenotypic, and clinical implications. Clin Cancer Res 6(3):1093–1103

232. Raney B, Schnaufer L, Ziegler M, et al. (1987) Treatment of children with neurogenic sarcoma. Experience at the Children's Hospital of Philadelphia, 1958–1984. Cancer 59(1):1–5

233. Raney R (1981) Proceedings of the tumor board of The Children's Hospital of Philadelphia: Synovial sarcoma. Med Pediatr Oncol 9(1):41–45

234. Raney RB, Meza J, Anderson JR, et al. (2002) Treatment of children and adolescents with localized parameningeal sarcoma: Experience of the Intergroup Rhabdomyosarcoma Study Group protocols IRS-II through -IV, 1978–1997. Med Pediatr Oncol 38(1):22–32

235. Raney RB Jr, Allen A, O'Neill J, et al. (1986) Malignant fibrous histiocytoma of soft tissue in childhood. Cancer 57(11):2198–2201

236. Raney RB Jr, Tefft M, Maurer HM, et al. (1988) Disease patterns and survival rate in children with metastatic soft-tissue sarcoma. A report from the Intergroup Rhabdomyosarcoma Study (IRS)-I. Cancer 62(7):1257–1266

237. Reed D (1902) On the pathological changes in Hodgkins's disease, with special references to its relation to tuberculosis. Johns Hopkins Hosp Rep (10):133

238. Reiter A, Schrappe M, Parwaresch R, et al. (1995) Non-Hodgkin's lymphomas of childhood and adolescence: Results of a treatment stratified for biologic subtypes and stage—A report of the Berlin-Frankfurt-Munster Group. J Clin Oncol 13(2):359–372

239. Reiter A, Schrappe M, Ludwig WD, et al. (2000) Intensive ALL-type therapy without local radiotherapy provides a 90% event-free survival for children with T-cell lymphoblastic lymphoma: A BFM group report. Blood 95(2):416–421

240. Reiter A, Schrappe M, Tiemann M, et al. (1999) Improved treatment results in childhood B-cell neoplasms with tailored intensification of therapy: A report of the Berlin-Frankfurt-Munster Group Trial NHL-BFM 90. Blood 94(10):3294–3306

241. Ribeiro Kde C, Kowalski LP, Saba LM, et al. (2002) Epithelial salivary glands neoplasms in children and adolescents: A forty-four-year experience. Med Pediatr Oncol 39(6):594–600

242. Ries L, Smith M, Gurney J, et al. (1999) Cancer incidence and survival among children and adolescents. In: United States SEER Program; 1999. National Cancer Institute, SEER Program, NIH. Pub No. 99-4649

243. Roberts T, Chernova O, Cowell JK (1998) NB4S, a member of the TBC1 domain family of genes, is truncated as a result of a constitutional t(1;10)(p22;q21) chromosome translocation in a patient with stage 4S neuroblastoma. Hum Mol Genet 7(7):1169–1178

244. Robertson SJ, Lowman JT, Grufferman S, et al. (1987) Familial Hodgkin's disease. A clinical and laboratory investigation. Cancer 59(7):1314–1319

245. Rosai J, Dias P, Parham DM, et al. (1991) MyoD1 protein expression in alveolar soft part sarcoma as confirmatory evidence of its skeletal muscle nature. Am J Surg Pathol 15(10):974–981

246. Rosen G, Forscher C, Lowenbraun S, et al. (1994) Synovial sarcoma. Uniform response of metastases to high dose ifosfamide. Cancer 73(10):2506–2511

247. Rostock RA, Siegelman SS, Lenhard RE, et al. (1983) Thoracic CT scanning for mediastinal Hodgkin's disease: Results and therapeutic implications. Int J Radiat Oncol Biol Phys 9(10):1451–1457

248. Rydholm A, Mandahl N, Heim S, et al. (1990) Malignant fibrous histiocytomas with a 19p+ marker chromosome have increased relapse rate. Genes Chromosomes Cancer 2(4):296–299

249. Samuel AM, Sharma SM (1991) Differentiated thyroid carcinomas in children and adolescents. Cancer 67(8):2186–2190

250. Sandler E, Lyden E, Ruymann F, et al. (2001) Efficacy of ifosfamide and doxorubicin given as a phase II "window" in children with newly diagnosed metastatic rhabdomyosarcoma: A report from the Intergroup Rhabdomyosarcoma Study Group. Med Pediatr Oncol 37(5):442–448

251. Sandlund JT, Santana V, Abromowitch M, et al. (1994) Large cell non-Hodgkin lymphoma of childhood: Clinical characteristics and outcome. Leukemia 8(1):30–34

252. Santana VM, Abromowitch M, Sandlund JT, et al. (1993) MACOP-B treatment in children and adolescents with advanced diffuse large-cell non-Hodgkin's lymphoma. Leukemia 7(2):187–191

253. Santoro M, Thomas GA, Vecchio G, et al. (2000) Gene rearrangement and Chernobyl related thyroid cancers. Br J Cancer 82(2):315–322

254. Sariban E, Donahue A, Magrath IT (1984) Jaw involvement in American Burkitt's lymphoma. Cancer 53(8):1777–1782

255. Saunders JR Jr, Hirata RM, Jaques DA (1986) Salivary glands. Surg Clin North Am 66(1):59–81

256. Schellong G, Potter R, Bramswig J, et al. (1999) High cure rates and reduced long-term toxicity in pediatric Hodgkin's disease: The German-Austrian multicenter trial DAL-HD-90. The German-Austrian Pediatric Hodgkin's Disease Study Group. J Clin Oncol 17(12):3736–3744

257. Schlumberger M, De Vathaire F, Travagli JP, et al. (1987) Differentiated thyroid carcinoma in childhood: Long term follow-up of 72 patients. J Clin Endocrinol Metab 65(6):1088–1094

258. Scrable H, Witte D, Shimada H, et al. (1989) Molecular differential pathology of rhabdomyosarcoma. Genes Chromosomes Cancer 1(1):23–35

259. Scrable HJ, Witte DP, Lampkin BC, et al. (1987) Chromosomal localization of the human rhabdomyosarcoma locus by mitotic recombination mapping. Nature 329(6140):645–647

260. Serin M, Erkal HS, Elhan AH, et al. (1998) Nasopharyngeal carcinoma in childhood and adolescence. Med Pediatr Oncol 31(6):498–505

261. Seymour JF (1997) Splenomegaly, eosinophilia, and pruritis: Hodgkin's disease, or...? Blood 90(4):1719–20

262. Shapiro DN, Sublett JE, Li B, et al. (1993) Fusion of PAX3 to a member of the forkhead family of transcription factors in human alveolar rhabdomyosarcoma. Cancer Res 53(21):5108–5112

263. Shapiro NL, Bhattacharyya N (2006) Clinical characteristics and survival for major salivary gland malignancies in children. Otolaryngol Head Neck Surg 134(4):631–634

264. Sheu LF, Chen A, Meng CL, et al. (1997) Analysis of bcl-2 expression in normal, inflamed, dysplastic nasopharyngeal epithelia, and nasopharyngeal carcinoma: Association with p53 expression. Hum Pathol 28(5):556–562

265. Shinjo K (1994) Analysis of prognostic factors and chemotherapy of malignant fibrous histiocytoma of soft tissue: A preliminary report. Jpn J Clin Oncol 24(3):154–159

266. Shiramizu B, Barriga F, Neequaye J, et al. (1991) Patterns of chromosomal breakpoint locations in Burkitt's lymphoma: Relevance to geography and Epstein-Barr virus association. Blood 77(7):1516–1526

267. Shoenfeld A, Ovadia J, Edelstein T, et al. (1982) Malignant cervical teratoma of the fetus. Acta Obstet Gynecol Scand 61(1):7–12

268. Skinner MA, DeBenedetti MK, Moley JF, et al. (1996) Medullary thyroid carcinoma in children with multiple endocrine neoplasia types 2A and 2B. J Pediatr Surg 31(1):177–81; discussion 181–182

269. Skinner MA, Norton JA, Moley JF, et al. (1997) Heterotopic autotransplantation of parathyroid tissue in children undergoing total thyroidectomy. J Pediatr Surg 32(3):510–513

270. Skinner MA, Moley JA, Dilley WG, et al. (2005) Prophylactic thyroidectomy in multiple endocrine neoplasia type 2A. N Engl J Med 353(11):1105–1113

271. Slivnick DJ, Ellis TM, Nawrocki JF, et al. (1990) The impact of Hodgkin's disease on the immune system. Semin Oncol 17(6):673–682

272. Smith AC, Squire JA, Thorner P, et al. (2001) Association of alveolar rhabdomyosarcoma with the Beckwith-Wiedemann syndrome. Pediatr Dev Pathol 4(6):550–558

273. Smith LM, Anderson JR, Qualman SJ, et al. (2001) Which patients with microscopic disease and rhabdomyosarcoma experience relapse after therapy? A report from the soft tissue sarcoma committee of the children's oncology group. J Clin Oncol 19(20):4058–4064

274. Smith MB, Xue H, Strong L, et al. (1993) Forty-year experience with second malignancies after treatment of childhood cancer: Analysis of outcome following the development of the second malignancy. J Pediatr Surg 28(10):1342–8; discussion 1348–1349

275. Smith RS, Chen Q, Hudson MM, et al. (2003) Prognostic factors for children with Hodgkin's disease treated with combined-modality therapy. J Clin Oncol 21(10):2026–2033

276. Soldes OS, Younger JG, Hirschl RB (1999) Predictors of malignancy in childhood peripheral lymphadenopathy. J Pediatr Surg 34(10):1447–1452

277. Sonnenblick M, Kramer R, Hershko C (1986) Corticosteroid responsive immune thrombocytopenia in Hodgkin's disease. Oncology 43(6):349–353

278. Soule EH, Pritchard DJ (1977) Fibrosarcoma in infants and children: A review of 110 cases. Cancer 40(4):1711–1721

279. Sozzi G, Bongarzone I, Miozzo M, et al. (1994) A t(10;17) translocation creates the RET/PTC2 chimeric transforming sequence in papillary thyroid carcinoma. Genes Chromosomes Cancer 9(4):244–50

280. Spiro R, Spiro J (1988) Salivary gland tumors. Head and neck cancer. Site-specific problems. Prob gen Surg (5):217

281. Sreekantaiah C, Bridge JA, Rao UN, et al. (1991) Clonal chromosomal abnormalities in hemangiopericytoma. Cancer Genet Cytogenet 54(2):173–181

282. Srivatsan ES, Ying KL, Seeger RC (1993) Deletion of chromosome 11 and of 14q sequences in neuroblastoma. Genes Chromosomes Cancer 7(1):32–37

283. Steel BL, Schwartz MR, Ramzy I (1995) Fine needle aspiration biopsy in the diagnosis of lymphadenopathy in 1,103 patients. Role, limitations and analysis of diagnostic pitfalls. Acta Cytol 39(1):76–81

284. Stefanato CM, Reyes-Mugica M (1996) Masked Hodgkin's disease: The pruriginous disguise. Pediatr Hematol Oncol 13(3):293–294

285. Stein H, Mann R, Delsol G, et al. (2001) World Health Organization classification of tumours. Pathology and genetics of tumours and haematopoietic and lymphoid tissues. Lyon: IARC Press

286. Stephenson JA, Mayland DM, Kun LE, et al. (1989) Malignant germ cell tumors of the head and neck in childhood. Laryngoscope 99(7 Pt 1):732–735

287. Sternberg C (1898) Uber eine Eingenartige unter dem Bilde der Pseudoleukmie verlaufende Tuberculose des lymphatischen. Apparates Z Heilkd (19):21

288. Stiller CA, Parkin DM (1994) International variations in the incidence of childhood soft-tissue sarcomas. Paediatr Perinat Epidemiol 8(1):107–119

289. Stiller CA, McKinney PA, Bunch KJ, et al. (1991) Childhood cancer and ethnic group in Britain: A United Kingdom children's Cancer Study Group (UKCCSG) study. Br J Cancer 64(3):543–548

290. Stratton MR, Fisher C, Gusterson BA, et al. (1989) Detection of point mutations in N-ras and K-ras genes of human embryonal rhabdomyosarcomas using oligonucleotide probes and the polymerase chain reaction. Cancer Res 49(22):6324–6327

291. Strother D, van Hoff J, Rao PV, et al. (1997) Event-free survival of children with biologically favourable neuroblastoma based on the degree of initial tumour resection: Results from the Pediatric Oncology Group. Eur J Cancer 33(12):2121–2125

292. Suzuki T, Bogenmann E, Shimada H, et al. (1993) Lack of high-affinity nerve growth factor receptors in aggressive neuroblastomas. J Natl Cancer Inst 85(5):377–384

293. Tallini G, Parham DM, Dias P, et al. (1994) Myogenic regulatory protein expression in adult soft tissue sarcomas. A sensitive and specific marker of skeletal muscle differentiation. Am J Pathol 144(4):693–701

294. Tapper D, Lack EE (1983) Teratomas in infancy and childhood. A 54-year experience at the Children's Hospital Medical Center. Ann Surg 198(3):398–410

295. Taub R, Kirsch I, Morton C, et al. (1982) Translocation of the c-myc gene into the immunoglobulin heavy chain locus in human Burkitt lymphoma and murine plasmacytoma cells. Proc Natl Acad Sci U S A 79(24):7837–7841

296. Temeck BK, Wexler LH, Steinberg SM, et al. (1995) Metastasectomy for sarcomatous pediatric histologies: Results and prognostic factors. Ann Thorac Surg 59(6):1385–1389; discussion 1390

297. Thomson AB, Wallace WH (2002) Treatment of pediatric Hodgkin's disease. A balance of risks. Eur J Cancer 38(4):468–477

298. Thomusch O, Machens A, Sekulla C, et al. (2003) The impact of surgical technique on postoperative hypoparathyroidism in bilateral thyroid surgery: A multivariate analysis of 5846 consecutive patients. Surgery 133(2):180–185

299. Torsiglieri AJ Jr, Tom LW, Ross AJ, 3rd, et al. (1988) Pediatric neck masses: Guidelines for evaluation. Int J Pediatr Otorhinolaryngol 16(3):199–210

300. Touran T, Applebaum H, Frost DB, et al. (1989) Congenital metastatic cervical teratoma: Diagnostic and management considerations. J Pediatr Surg 24(1):21–23

301. Tran L, Sadeghi A, Hanson D, et al. (1986) Major salivary gland tumors: Treatment results and prognostic factors. Laryngoscope 96(10):1139–1144

302. Tsokos M (1994) The diagnosis and classification of childhood rhabdomyosarcoma. Semin Diagn Pathol 11(1):26–38

303. Tsokos M, Webber BL, Parham DM, et al. (1992) Rhabdomyosarcoma. A new classification scheme related to prognosis. Arch Pathol Lab Med 116(8):847–855

304. Tubergen DG, Krailo MD, Meadows AT, et al. (1995) Comparison of treatment regimens for pediatric lymphoblastic non-Hodgkin's lymphoma: A Childrens Cancer Group study. J Clin Oncol 13(6):1368–1376

305. Turc-Carel C, Lizard-Nacol S, Justrabo E, et al. (1986) Consistent chromosomal translocation in alveolar rhabdomyosarcoma. Cancer Genet Cytogenet 19(3–4):361–362

306. Uzel O, Yoruk SO, Sahinler I, et al. (2001) Nasopharyngeal carcinoma in childhood: Long-term results of 32 patients. Radiother Oncol 58(2):137–141

307. van Krieken JH, Raffeld M, Raghoebier S, et al. (1990) Molecular genetics of gastrointestinal non-Hodgkin's lymphomas: Unusual prevalence and pattern of c-myc rearrangements in aggressive lymphomas. Blood 76(4):797–800

308. Vandesompele J, Baudis M, De Preter K, et al. (2005) Unequivocal delineation of clinicogenetic subgroups and development of a new model for improved outcome prediction in neuroblastoma. J Clin Oncol 23(10):2280–2299

309. Vane D, King DR, Boles ET Jr (1984) Secondary thyroid neoplasms in pediatric cancer patients: Increased risk with improved survival. J Pediatr Surg 19(6):855–860

310. Vassilopoulou-Sellin R, Klein MJ, Smith TH, et al. (1993) Pulmonary metastases in children and young adults with differentiated thyroid cancer. Cancer 71(4):1348–1352

311. Venkateswaran L, Gan YJ, Sixbey JW, et al. (2000) Epstein-Barr virus infection in salivary gland tumors in children and young adults. Cancer 89(2):463–466

312. Vokes EE, Liebowitz DN, Weichselbaum RR (1997) Nasopharyngeal carcinoma. Lancet 350(9084):1087–1091

313. Wagner DK, Kiwanuka J, Edwards BK, et al. (1987) Soluble interleukin-2 receptor levels in patients with undifferentiated and lymphoblastic lymphomas: Correlation with survival. J Clin Oncol 5(8):1262–1274

314. Wakely PE Jr, Kardos TF, Frable WJ (1988) Application of fine needle aspiration biopsy to pediatrics. Hum Pathol 19(12):1383–1386

315. Wakhlu A, Wakhlu AK (2000) Head and neck teratomas in children. Pediatr Surg Int 16(5–6):333–337

316. Walterhouse DO, Hoover ML, Marymont MA, et al. (1999) High-dose chemotherapy followed by peripheral blood stem cell rescue for metastatic rhabdomyosarcoma: The experience at Chicago Children's Memorial Hospital. Med Pediatr Oncol 32(2):88–92

317. Walterhouse DO, Lyden ER, Breitfeld PP, et al. (2004) Efficacy of topotecan and cyclophosphamide given in a phase II window trial in children with newly diagnosed metastatic rhabdomyosarcoma: A Children's Oncology Group study. J Clin Oncol 22(8):1398–1403

318. Weiner M, Leventhal B, Cantor A, et al. (1991) Gallium-67 scans as an adjunct to computed tomography scans for the assessment of a residual mediastinal mass in pediatric patients with Hodgkin's disease. A Pediatric Oncology Group study. Cancer 68(11):2478–2480

319. Weiss LM, Movahed LA, Warnke RA, et al. (1989) Detection of Epstein-Barr viral genomes in Reed-Sternberg cells of Hodgkin's disease. N Engl J Med 320(8):502–506

320. Wells SA Jr, Farndon JR, Dale JK, et al. (1980) Long-term evaluation of patients with primary parathyroid hyperplasia managed by total parathyroidectomy and heterotopic autotransplantation. Ann Surg 192(4):451–458

321. Wells SA Jr, Chi DD, Toshima K, et al. (1994) Predictive DNA testing and prophylactic thyroidectomy in patients at risk for multiple endocrine neoplasia type 2A. Ann Surg 220(3):237–47; discussion 247–250

322. White PS, Maris JM, Beltinger C, et al. (1995) A region of consistent deletion in neuroblastoma maps within human chromosome 1p36.2–36.3. Proc Natl Acad Sci U S A 92(12):5520–5524

323. Woodruff G, Buncic JR, Morin JD (1988) Horner's syndrome in children. J Pediatr Ophthalmol Strabismus 25(1):40–44

324. Woollons AC, Morton RP (1994) When does middle ear effusion signify nasopharyngeal cancer? N Z Med J 107(991):507–509

325. Xia SJ, Pressey JG, Barr FG (2002) Molecular pathogenesis of rhabdomyosarcoma. Cancer Biol Ther 1(2):97–104

326. Xia Y, Brown L, Yang CY, et al. (1991) TAL2, a helix-loop-helix gene activated by the (7;9)(q34;q32) translocation in human T-cell leukemia. Proc Natl Acad Sci U S A 88(24):11416–11420

327. Yamauchi T, Ferrieri P, Anthony BF (1980) The aetiology of acute cervical adenitis in children: Serological and bacteriological studies. J Med Microbiol 13(1):37–43

328. Yip FW, Reeve TS, Poole AG, et al. (1994) Thyroid nodules in childhood and adolescence. Aust N Z J Surg 64(10):676–678

329. Yung L, Smith P, Hancock BW, et al. (2004) Long term outcome in adolescents with Hodgkin's lymphoma: Poor results using regimens designed for adults. Leuk Lymphoma 45(8):1579–1585

330. Zimmerman D, Hay ID, Gough IR, et al. (1988) Papillary thyroid carcinoma in children and adults: Long-term follow-up of 1039 patients conservatively treated at one institution during three decades. Surgery 104(6):1157–1166

Brain Tumors, Intraocular and Orbital Tumors

18

Paul D. Chumas, Susan V. Picton, Harry Willshaw

Contents

18.1 Introduction

In children, brain and spinal cord tumors account for approximately 25% of all cancer (40–50% of all pediatric solid tumors). Overall, they are second only to the leukemias in frequency [1, 2]. There have been reports of an increasing incidence of both adult and pediatric brain tumors which may, in part, be due to "detection bias" although some epidemiology groups suggest that the increases are real [3]. The annual incidence is approximately 2–5 cases per 100,000 (1 in 2,500 children aged 0–16), which translates to approximately 300–400 new cases being diagnosed in the UK per year [4].

A wide variety of tumor types ranging from the highly malignant to the histologically benign is seen in the pediatric age range. However, prognosis depends not only on histological type but also on the location

Table 18.1 Site of tumor by age

Age	% Infratentorial
0–6 months	27
6–12 months	53
12–24 months	74
2–16 years	42

From [14], with permission.

of the tumor with some low-grade tumors (for example, craniopharyngiomas and hypothalamic gliomas) frequently resulting in severe morbidity or sometimes death. Although it is widely taught that infratentorial tumors are more common than supratentorial in the pediatric age-group, it can be clearly seen from Table 18.1 that this ratio varies with age. Overall, there seems to be a slight preference for central nervous system (CNS) tumors in males – in particular in some of the more common tumor types – primitive neuroectodermal tumors (PNET), craniopharyngioma, brain stem glioma, ependymoma, and germ cell tumors arising in the pineal region [5] – the most striking sex preference being seen in relatively rare pituitary adenomas with a 7:1 male:female ratio [5].

For the majority of pediatric brain tumors no specific etiological agent or event can be found. Known risk factors include genetic syndromes (such as Neurofibromatosis I and II, basal cell naevus, tuberous sclerosis, Gorlin, Turcott, Li-Fraumeni, and von Hippel-Lindau), which account for 5% of cases [6], and radiation exposure. Although there has been concern over exposure to low-level electromagnetic radiation (power lines) and from mobile phones, this association remains controversial [7].

The care of children with CNS tumors has probably changed more in the last 25 years than any other pediatric surgical group. This is due to changes at every stage of patient care:

1. Improvement in diagnostic techniques – computerized tomography (CT) in the 1970s, magnetic resonance imaging (MRI) in the 1980s, and functional imaging in the 1990s;
2. Developments in neuroanesthesia (including intra- and perioperative monitoring);
3. Advances in surgery (including use of the operating microscope, the ultrasonic aspirator, stereotaxy, endoscopy, intraoperative functional mapping);
4. Developments in adjuvant therapy (including both chemotherapy and radiotherapy, the use of multicenter trials, the recognition of the detrimental effects of radiotherapy on the developing CNS, the use of fractionated radiotherapy and stereotactic radiosurgery);
5. Improvements in supportive services (physiotherapy; occupational and speech therapy; social, psychological, and educational support; palliative care).

From the surgical perspective, the result has been that a tissue diagnosis can virtually always be achieved regardless of the site and aggressive surgical removal of tumors can usually be attempted. Technology now available aims to use the detail of neuroimaging to help direct the surgeon during the operation. This "neuronavigation" relies on the surgeon registering the patient's head, which is then tracked by infrared cameras. Surgical instruments, fitted with light-emitting diodes, are also tracked as they come into the line of sight of the cameras. The workstation on which the preoperative imaging studies are held will then display where the instrument is within the head and its relationship to the tumor or target. The main drawback of neuronavigation is the fact that the information used is preoperative rather than real time. Intraoperative MRI units (where the patient's head is held within a small MRI magnet or where the operative layout includes a scanner within the operating theatre into which the patient is intermittently placed) are now available but it is yet to be shown that they are cost effective.

Another area of change in the last two decades has been the widespread use of immunohistochemical techniques to further classify poorly differentiated tumors. The World Health Organization (WHO) published a consensus document in 1979, updated in 1993 and again in 2000, giving a standardized reporting system. More recently, it has become clear that in the future CNS tumors may be classified by their molecular genetic profile. Molecular genetics is already important in helping to diagnose rhabdoid tumors/ATRTs (deletions or mutations of the gene hSNF5/INI1) [8], and is of prognostic and therapeutic value in the management of patients with oligodendrogliomas (1p/19q deletion being associated with prolonged survival and chemosensitivity in adults) [9].

Despite these advances, epidemiological data from the UK Childhood Cancer Research Group shows the overall 5- and 10-year survival rates to be approximately 55% and 50%, respectively, and there has been little change in the past 10 years. This is in contrast to the substantial rise in survival rates seen over this period in children with leukemia and non-CNS tumors [10]. This and the recent reporting of improved survival statistics on selected tumor subtypes (e.g., medulloblastoma) have emphasized the need for further collaborative studies. In particular it is hoped that the development of biologically directed therapies and the application of functional imaging to increase the safety and extent of surgical excision will result in significant improvements in outcome. In the last few years, trials in adults have shown significant improvements in survival duration in patients with malignant gliomas (using concomitant Temozolomide [11] or intratumoral chemotherapy [12]) and these results have been the first significant improvement in the management of these patients in the last 40 years. Phase III trials of a number of new agents (including gene therapy) are underway in adult patients – although methods of delivery (for example, convection-enhanced delivery) still need further refinement.

18.2 Phakomatoses

The phakomatoses (or neurocutaneous syndromes) are a group of conditions in which cutaneous stigmata are associated with CNS abnormalities or tumors. Although considered relatively rare, up to 10% of all pediatric astrocytomas are associated with neurocutaneous syndromes [13]. Recognition of these syndromes is important as it may alter the indication and goals of surgery. Likewise, an understanding of the natural history and genetics of the disease is essential for dealing with both patient and family.

18.2.1 Neurofibromatoses

This group comprises by far and away the most common type of phakomatosis and the patients fall broadly into two subtypes – neurofibromatosis types 1 and 2 (NF1 and NF2). Previously, NF1 was known as von Recklinghausen's disease and this, with an incidence of approximately 1/3,000 births, is responsible for more than 90% of cases of neurofibromatosis. It shows an autosomal dominant inheritance with almost 100% penetrance, but up to 50% of cases represent spontaneous somatic mutations [14] with the gene responsible being located on chromosome 17. Optic pathway tumors are the most common type of tumor seen in NF1 but other low-grade gliomas and meningiomas are also seen. The incidence of CNS tumors is approximately 10% [14–16].

Similarly, NF2 is also an autosomal dominant condition with the gene probably being on chromosome 22 [14]. The pathological signature of NF2 is the presence of bilateral acoustic neuromas. Although both NF1 and NF2 may be associated with multiple intradural spinal tumors, these are more common in NF2 than in NF1. Other non-CNS tumors also have an increased frequency in NF2 (including neuroblastoma, sarcoma, leukemia, Wilms' tumor, and ganglioglioma) [14].

The subcutaneous neurofibroma are usually sessile in children but increase in size and in number with puberty and pregnancy and often become pedunculated. These tumors can undergo malignant degeneration in 2–29% of patients (but usually during adult life) [17]. Congenital neurofibromas are often of the plexiform type with a propensity for the periorbital region where they may be progressive and very vascular. A further orbital problem is the characteristic dysplastic lesion seen in NF1 with sphenoid dysplasia leading to pulsatile exophthalmos, and indeed this may be the presenting sign of NF1 in an infant or young child [15].

Other skeletal lesions include congenital bowing of long bones and pseudoarthrosis, vertebral scalloping and scoliosis. Visual problems as a result of an anterior visual pathway tumor may be the first manifestation of NF1 in a young child and may be quite marked by the time medical attention is sought. As a general rule, tumors affecting the optic nerve tend to present at a slightly older age (early 20s) while chiasmatic tumors most often present in the first decade of life often in association with endocrine disturbance and hydrocephalus [18]. In contrast, the defining characteristic of NF2 is the presence of bilateral acoustic tumors, which usually present in adolescence [14, 16].

Another fundamental difference between NF1 and NF2 is the apparent disorganization of the CNS and the presence of hamartomas, heterotopias and low-grade neoplasms in NF1. Macrocephaly may be seen in three-quarters of patients with NF1 [19] and approximately one-third of NF1 patients are intellectually impaired, probably reflecting this widespread intrinsic cerebral disorganization. In addition, MRI scans frequently show areas of abnormal signal intensity but these remain of unknown significance. In contrast, the brains of patients with NF2 do not show this marked disorganization and cognitive function is usually normal.

18.2.2 Tuberous Sclerosis

Tuberous sclerosis (TS), also known as Bourneville's disease, is inherited as an autosomal dominant trait, although many cases are sporadic [16, 20, 21]. The prevalence is approximately 1/10,000 [20] and the disease usually declares itself in childhood with epilepsy and mental retardation. Non-CNS manifestations include "ash leaf spots," facial angiofibromas ("adenoma sebaceum"), café-au-lait spots, shagreen patches (subependymal fibrosis), subungual fibromas, retinal hamartomas, honeycomb lungs, angiomyolipomas of the kidneys, and cardiac rhabdomyomas. In the CNS there are multiple benign hamartomatous lesions which occur in the lining of the lateral and third ventricles (subependymal nodules) and cortical nodules ("tubers").

The characteristic brain tumor in TS is the subependymal giant cell tumor, which is believed to arise from subependymal nodules and nearly always occurs

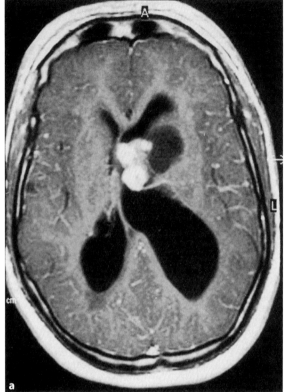

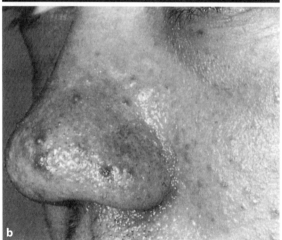

Fig. 18.1 a, b (**a**) Axial T1-weighted MRI with gadolinium showing a giant cell astrocytoma at the Foramen of Monro in an adolescent patient with tuberous sclerosis. (**b**) The classical facial angiofibromas (adenoma sebaceum) of tuberous sclerosis.

at the Foramen of Munro (Fig. 18.1a,b). The sites of these tumors frequently result in obstructive hydrocephalus, which is the usual cause of presentation. The reported incidence of subependymal giant cell tumors ranges from 7 to 23% [22]. Pathologically, these are usually giant cell astrocytomas which are benign and therefore the aim of surgery is to establish free communication of the cerebrospinal fluid (CSF) pathways

rather than necessarily a total resection, which may be difficult to achieve. Surgery may also be considered for intractable epilepsy if it can be shown that one of the tubers or an abnormal area of brain around the tumor is acting as a focus.

18.2.3 Von Hippel-Lindau Disease

This syndrome consists of CNS hemangioblastomas (usually cerebellar but may be spinal and occasionally supratentorial), in association with angiomatosis retinae, cysts/tumors in various organs and polycythemia [16]. This disease usually presents in adulthood and has an autosomal dominant trait with variable penetrance and a positive family history is only seen in approximately 20% of cases. The diagnosis is made by the presence of two or more separate characteristic lesions or a single lesion with a positive family history. The most common associated lesions are pheochromocytomas and renal cysts/tumors (renal cell carcinoma being present in approximately 30% of patients) [16]. Adenomas are also seen in the pancreas, liver, spleen, lung, epididymis and ovaries. The CNS tumors may be multiple and on imaging are usually cystic with a strongly enhancing mural nodule. At surgery, the tumors are highly vascular but usually well demarcated.

18.3 Posterior Fossa Tumors

Tumors in this region fall into two distinct groups – those arising from the cerebellar hemispheres or the fourth ventricle, and those arising from the brain stem itself. These two distinct groups have different clinical presentations and surgical goals and will therefore be discussed separately.

18.3.1 "Cerebellar" Tumors

Within this group of tumors are included cerebellar astrocytomas, medulloblastomas, and ependymomas. Cranial nerve tumors (for example, acoustic neuromas or 5th nerve tumors) will not be discussed due to their relative rarity in children.

As a group, these tumors usually present once they are large enough to cause hydrocephalus by blocking off the outflow of the fourth ventricle. The duration of symptoms rather than type of symptoms correlate with tumor type. Young children, in whom the sutures have not fused, may present with macrocrania, vomiting, and irritability. In older children headache, classically in the morning, and nausea and vomiting are the usual symptoms. It is not infrequent for patients to have been investigated for gastrointestinal problems prior to having a head scan which shows a tumor. If the cerebellar tonsils have been impacted into the foramen magnum, there may be neck pain or head tilt or even opisthotonus. Clinical examination may reveal papilloedema, a 6th nerve palsy (a false localizing sign due to the hydrocephalus) and by the time patient presents there is normally a degree of ataxia and past pointing. If the hydrocephalus is left untreated, the patient will eventually become comatosed.

From a surgical management point of view, there are two main problems: treatment of the hydrocephalus and surgical removal of the tumor. Although historically there was a vogue to insert ventriculoperitoneal shunts into all these patients prior to tumor removal, with the widespread availability of CT and MR scanning these children have tended to present earlier and the usual practice today is to commence dexamethasone and perform early surgery. If required, an external ventricular drain may be inserted either prior to surgery or at the time of surgery. Each tumor type will now be dealt with individually.

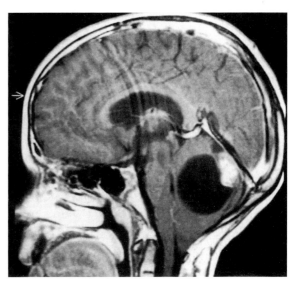

Fig. 18.2 Sagittal T1-weighted MRI with gadolinium showing a large posterior fossa cyst with an enhancing nodule characteristic of a pilocystic astrocytoma. Note that the cerebellar tonsils have herniated through the foramen magnum.

18.3.1.1 Cerebellar Astrocytomas

Cerebellar astrocytomas are virtually always of the low-grade (pilocytic) type in children. This tumor type makes up approximately one-third of childhood posterior fossa tumors [23] with patients being slightly older than those with the malignant posterior fossa tumors. Grossly, these tumors are found to lie either in the cerebellar hemisphere or may involve the midline (vermis). They are either cystic (70%) with a mural nodule or a solid mass (22%) with multiple cystic areas [24]. Although well demarcated, areas where it may be difficult to obtain a complete removal include extension through the cerebellar peduncles into the brain stem (brain stem invasion being reported in 8% of cases) [24], or when tumor is found high in the tentorial notch towards the vein of Galen. The microscopic features of these tumors are characteristic with a biphasic pattern of dense and compact areas with elongated (pilocytic cells) that alternate with loose areas containing stellate astrocytes and microcysts [24]. The cells may contain intracytoplasmic eosinophilic inclusions termed Rosenthal bodies. Vascular proliferation may be seen in cerebellar astrocytomas and unlike other gliomas, this does not indicate a more aggressive behavior of the tumor. Calcification may also be seen in these tumors.

On CT scan, hydrocephalus is often present and in the posterior fossa the classical finding is of a cystic tumor with an enhancing nodule. The tumor is iso- or hypodense on noncontrasted scans. Occasionally, the cyst wall itself enhances and looks thickened and in these cases, surgical excision of the wall is indicated as

it will consist of tumor. However, if the cyst wall does not enhance, then at the time of surgery a thin cyst consisting of gliotic tissue rather than tumor is found. The solid type of tumors can be difficult to differentiate from ependymomas or medulloblastomas. The differential diagnosis of the cystic astrocytoma is with a cystic hemangioblastoma – but the latter are exceptionally rare in the pediatric age group. Today, MRI scanning is usually also obtained as this helps with surgical planning. Cerebellar astrocytomas are usually iso- or hypointense on T1-weighted images and hyperintense on T2-weighted images. Additionally, the MRI will often show on the sagittal plane that the tonsils have herniated through the foramen magnum (Fig. 18.2).

The goal of surgery in these patients is total removal of tumor as this is an important prognostic factor. Additionally, if total surgical excision has been performed then no further adjuvant therapy, specifically radiation, is needed [25]. Garcia et al. reviewed 80 children with cerebellar astrocytoma and the recurrence rate was 2.5% for patients with total removal and 3.5% for patients who had a subtotal removal. Interestingly, radiation did not affect the outcome of patients who had a subtotal excision [25]. Nonetheless, subtotal resection is compatible with long-term survival [26, 27]. From the Garcia study, the 5-, 10-, and 25-year disease-free survival rates were 92%, 88%, and 88% respectively. There are, however, case reports of recurrence after 36 years [28] and occasionally, malignant change is seen in the recurrence. For these reasons these patients require long-term follow-up, with intermittent scanning. Nonsurgical treatment includes radiation or chemotherapy and is only recommended when there is a recurrence and further surgical excision is not feasible, and/or if the recurrent tumor has a malignant histology [29].

18.3.1.2 Medulloblastoma

Medulloblastomas were first described in 1925 by Bailey and Cushing, who suggested that these tumors were derived from a primitive pluripotent cell called the medulloblast. This putative cell has never been found but the name has now become entrenched in the neurosurgical literature. More recently, it has been recognized that the medulloblastoma should be classified under the heading of Primative Neuroectodermal Tumor (PNET). Medulloblastoma is the most common malignant CNS tumor in childhood comprising 15–20% of childhood brain tumors [30] and make up approximately one-third of all posterior fossa tumors in childhood. The peak incidence is between the ages of 3 and 8 years – being slightly younger than the pilocytic astrocytoma age range. However, these tumors may occur in the infancy and are occasionally seen in adults.

Medulloblastomas are most commonly found in the region of the fourth ventricle arising within the vermis. The tumors are reddish in color, friable and frequently vascular. A "desmoplastic" variant has been described which is characterized as being firm and well demarcated but this tends to occur in older children and adults. Recent evidence suggests that this subtype carries a better prognosis compared to classical medulloblastomas [31]. In contrast, large-cell medulloblastoma has been recognized as a distinct subtype which is associated with a poor prognosis [32].

A characteristic of medulloblastoma is the ability to spread via the CSF pathways into the spinal ("drop metastases") or cerebral subarachnoid spaces or within the ventricles. Such dissemination maybe diffuse or nodular and it is reported that 20–30% of patients with medulloblastoma have seeded within the craniospinal axis at the time of diagnosis [30]. Extraneural metastases are seen in 5% of patients [2] and this rate of extraneural deposition does not appear to be altered by the use of a (millipore) filter in association with a ventriculoperitoneal shunt.

Histologically, the classic medulloblastoma is composed of densely packed small cells with hyperchromatic nuclei and very little cytoplasm. There are frequent mitoses and rosettes of the Homer-Wright type are seen in about 20% of cases. Over the last decade cytogenetic and molecular studies have shown that isolated 17p loss and elevated expression of erbB2 and c-myc are associated with a poor prognosis [33].

On CT scanning, medulloblastoma appears as a well-marginated, homogeneously hyperdense mass arising from the vermis and filling the fourth ventricle. The mass typically enhances with contrast and calcification is seen in approximately 15% of cases [30]. Mild to moderate edema is common around the tumor and hydrocephalus is present in 95% of patients [30]. The investigation of choice in all posterior fossa lesions is MRI as it gives far better definition and resolution. The tumors are usually hypodense on T1-weighted images and on T2-weighted images but enhancement is still the rule after gadolinium has been injected (Fig. 18.3a,b); MRI is also superior in picking up subarachnoid seeding and spinal metastases.

The aims of surgery are gross total resection but in approximately one-third of cases a medulloblastoma infiltrates the dorsal brain stem and this precludes total removal [34]. These tumors usually require a long incision in the vermis and this may result in transient truncal ataxia and dysconjugate gaze, which usually resolves over a couple of weeks. In patients in which the tumor has involved the cerebellar peduncle, there may be long-standing ipsilateral dysmetria. Occasionally, patients will suffer with cerebellar mutism, which is poorly understood but tends to resolve over a matter of weeks.

Prognostic Factors

1. Extent of Surgical Resection. Differing definitions and surgical impressions have made this area fraught when trying to undertake comparative studies. It is now generally accepted that a gross total resection is one at which the surgeon feels there is no tumor left and an early CT or MRI examination with and without contrast fails to show any tumor deposit. A subtotal resection is one in which a small amount of tumor is known to have been left by the surgeon or if a postoperative scan shows a small lump of enhancing tissue in the operative bed (<1.5 cm2). Using these strict criteria, there does not appear to be a significant difference in outcome between the two groups [30]. In comparison, patients with a partial excision (>1.5 cm2) or a biopsy alone fare far worse [30].
2. Size/Dissemination. The Chang staging system has been widely employed for many years and characterizes medulloblastoma by tumor size (T stage T1 to T4) and the presence or absence of metastases (M0 to M4). More recently, it has become apparent that preoperative tumor size per se is of no predictive value [30]. However, the presence or absence of dissemination at the time of diagnosis is the most significant factor in predicting the survival of patients with medulloblastoma. It is therefore essen-

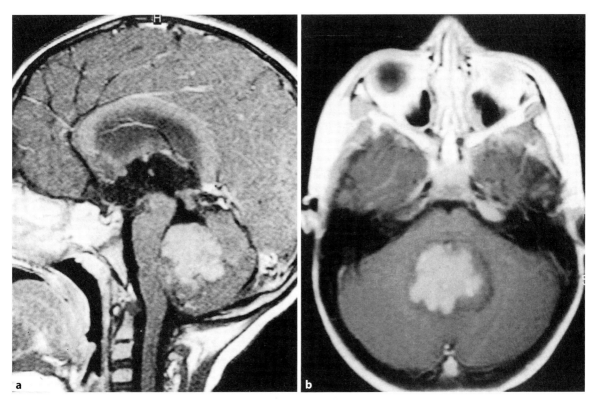

Fig. 18.3 a, b (**a**) Sagittal and (**b**) axial T1-weighted MRI with gadolinium showing a large posterior fossa tumor in the fourth ventricle with variable uptake of contrast. Histologically verified as a medulloblastoma.

tial to arrange a preoperative staging spinal MRI. Furthermore, in order to detect M1 disease (malignant cells identified in the CSF) an LP for cytology should be carried out 10–14 days after the posterior fossa surgery.

3. Age. Probably for multifactorial reasons, younger children fare less well than older children with medulloblastoma (Table 18.1). Younger children are more likely to have disseminated disease at the time of diagnosis and younger patients are less likely to receive aggressive treatment due to the adverse effects of radiotherapy.

Using these three main criteria (gross total/subtotal versus partial/biopsy; < 3 years of age versus >3 years of age; no dissemination versus dissemination) patients with medulloblastoma have been subdivided into "average risk" and "high risk" by the American Children's Oncology Group (COG). It can be estimated that for the poorest group, overall survival is approximately 36% at 5 years with standard postoperative craniospinal axis irradiation, versus 60–80% for children without adverse risk factors [30, 35].

Adjuvant Therapy. It is quite clear from the literature that medulloblastomas are highly radiosensitive. However, follow-up studies have shown that radio-

therapy at a young age may have a devastating effect on final neuro- and cognitive development. These cognitive sequelae are dependent on age at treatment and dose and field of irradiation given [30, 36]. Thus although the "standard" dose of radiation given to patients with medulloblastoma is 5,500 cGy with a dose of 3,600 cGy to the neuraxis [30, 37], it is obvious that these dosages are unacceptable to the immature brain and therefore trials have been undertaken using chemotherapeutic agents to see if it is possible to withhold radiation either temporarily or permanently in very young children [38]. In children older than 3 years the addition of chemotherapy to the standard treatment of surgery and radiotherapy has a resulted in improved survival, even in association with reduced radiotherapy dose to the craniospinal axis [35]. Further clinical trials looking at both survival and quality of survival, while employing lower doses of radiotherapy, are underway. Other areas of research interest include the use of hyperfractionated radiation and of stereotactic radiosurgery for small deposits/recurrences [39].

Endocrine dysfunction is another common problem after radiotherapy [40] with hypothyroidism and growth failure being the most common deficiencies. While the use of growth hormone is beneficial, the final height attained is significantly less than the midparental height [41]. Cushingoid appearance associated with the use of steroids is another common problem during treatment.

Medulloblastoma is clearly a chemosensitive tumor, as demonstrated in numerous phase I and II studies carried out at disease relapse [42, 43]. Chemotherapy has also been used as an adjuvant in medulloblastoma therapy for many years. Studies of chemotherapy given after surgery and before radiotherapy ("sandwich chemotherapy") have shown a survival advantage of 14% at 5 years in patients who received chemotherapy [44]. Standard therapy is, however, to give chemotherapy after completion of radiotherapy as described by Roger Packer and survival is now more than 80% at 5 years [35]. For various reasons – ranging from earlier diagnosis, to better anesthetic and surgical technique and the use of adjuvant therapy – medulloblastomas are one of the few CNS tumors in which there has been a significant improvement in 5-year survival over the last 20–30 years. At present, 5-year survival rates in the range of 70–80% are to be expected [30, 35, 45].

18.3.1.3 Ependymoma

Ependymomas are rare tumors accounting for 6–12% of brain tumors in childhood (30–35 new cases per year in the UK) [46]. Although they may be found throughout the CNS in children, 70% of ependymomas occur in the posterior fossa [47]. Half of these tumors present in pre-school children and the posterior fossa tumors occupy the fourth ventricle and extend through the outlets of the fourth ventricle into the cerebellar pontine angles and down over the cervical medullary junction. On CT, the ependymoma is usually either iso- or hyperdense and may show calcification. Enhancement after contrast is variable. Often MRI with its better definition shows more clearly the spread of the tumor over the cervical canal or out of the Foraminae of Luschka (Fig. 18.4). In the preoperative work-up, it is important that a spinal MRI is performed to look for spinal drop deposits.

Histologically, ependymomas are composed of well-differentiated cells which are often arranged around blood vessels forming perivascular rosettes. These tumors vary from being well differentiated through to having anaplastic features with high cellularity, pleomorphism, necrosis, and high mitotic activity. However, the significance of the histological changes is yet to be verified as there is only a tendency towards worse prognosis with increasing anaplasia [48]. Until recently, reviews in the literature included the highly malignant ependymoblastoma in the anaplastic group and this adversely skewed the survival curve for these children. The ependymoblastoma is now considered to be an embryonal tumor (a variant of the PNET) [49].

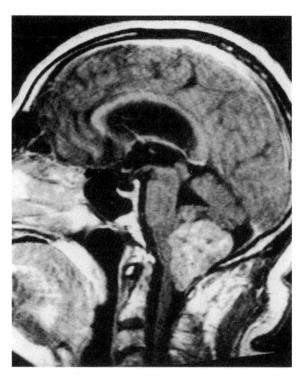

Fig. 18.4 Sagittal T1-weighted MRI with gadolinium showing a large enhancing posterior fossa tumor which has involved the herniated cerebellar tonsils.

With the ependymoblastoma removed from the heading of anaplastic ependymoma, the survival curves are not dramatically different from those showing more low-grade histological features.

At the time of surgery, approximately 10–25% of posterior fossa ependymomas are found to be invading the floor of the fourth ventricle [47, 50]. As with medulloblastomas, the aim of surgery is maximum possible resection without causing neurological deficit. However, due to the frequent extension to the cerebellar pontine (CP) angle, there is a higher incidence of lower cranial nerve palsies after resection. Due to this combination of brain stem invasion and CP angle involvement, the rate of complete resection is relatively low. Recent single institution retrospective studies have emphasized the importance of obtaining gross total removal with 10-year survival rates of over 70% in patients with radiological confirmation of gross surgical removal [51, 52]. This is to be compared with the 30% 5-year survival rate usually quoted for this disease [53]. A multivariate analysis of prognostic factors identified complete resection as the most favorable prognostic factor [54]. This importance of complete resection has led to the concept of second-look surgery, after treatment with chemotherapy, to allow removal of any residual tumor.

Postoperatively, patients should be imaged within 48 h looking for residual tumor. In the absence of dissemination, radiotherapy is given (5,400 cGy to the tumor bed), with spinal radiation only being given to those patients with proven deposits. Results from trials using hyperfractionated and conformal radiotherapy are awaited. In an attempt to avoid radiotherapy in young children various chemotherapeutic trials have been undertaken. There is now evidence that some children can have long-term remission with chemotherapy alone [55] although some children still suffer late recurrences. The approach is still worthwhile in this situation as the chemotherapy can result in very significant delays in the requirement for radiotherapy [56].

18.3.2 Brain Stem Tumors

It is only really since the advent of CT and perhaps even more importantly MRI that the true heterogeneity of this group of tumors has been understood. The classification used here is that based on Abbott et al. [57] and it has allowed for a rational approach to this diverse group of tumors. This has meant that some patients are not subject to any surgical procedures while others are treated aggressively as the underlying tumor may well be benign. The clinical presentation is also somewhat variable and will be discussed with each tumor type.

18.3.2.1 Diffuse Pontine Glioma

Unfortunately, this is the majority of brain stem tumors (comprising 60–70% of the New York series) [57]. It was this tumor group with its dismal prognosis that all patients were assumed to have prior to the advent of modern imaging. The patients present with a short history of ataxia and multiple cranial nerve dysfunction. An MRI scan demonstrates an expanded pons which is hypointense on T1 images (Fig. 18.5a,b). However, the extent of tumor involvement is best appreciated on T2 imaging with the tumor having a hyperintense signal. Enhancement is variable and hydrocephalus is not usually apparent. No treatment has been shown to be effective, with a median survival of 9 months [58]. Radiation has been shown to have a palliative effect and to increase the duration of survival. To date, chemotherapy trials have also failed to demonstrate efficacy but more aggressive regimens and biological "new agents" are currently being evaluated. With the classical MRI picture and clinical history, it is generally agreed that submitting these children to a biopsy is not warranted for diagnosis, although biopsy to obtain tissue for biological studies may be necessary if newer molecular treatments are being considered.

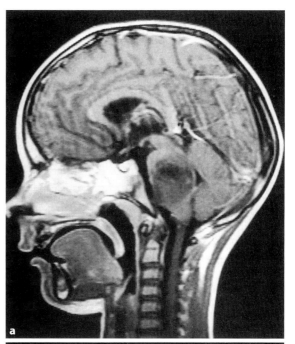
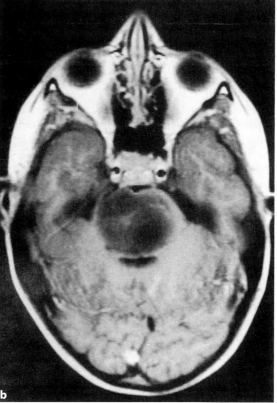

Fig. 18.5 a, b (**a**) Sagittal and (**b**) axial T1-weighted MRI with gadolinium showing massive expansion of the pons by a poorly enhancing tumor – characteristic of a diffuse pontine glioma.

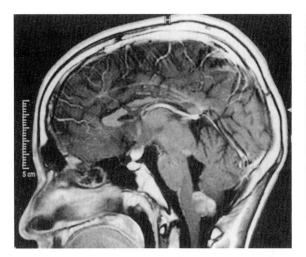

Fig. 18.6 Sagittal T1-weighted MRI with gadolinium showing an exophytic enhancing tumor arising off the medulla. Note also, the tectal plate tumor (with a small area of enhancement) and the enhancing hypothalamic tumor. This 12-year-old boy had presented with hydrocephalus 5 years earlier and on the basis of the CT scan performed at that time, the diagnosis of hydrocephalus secondary to aqueduct stenosis was made. Although asymptomatic, further imaging of the spine revealed another tumor (Fig. 18.10).

18.3.2.2 Focal Tumors

These tumors may arise anywhere within the brain stem and may even be partially exophytic into the CSF spaces. These patients usually have histories going back many months or years, and focal neurological signs. The solid portion of these tumors typically enhances with gadolinium. In the presence of progressive symptoms, surgical debulking of these tumors is a feasible option as the histology is usually of a low-grade astrocytoma. Radiotherapy is not indicated and it is feasible to re-operate on these focal tumors to achieve a complete resection. A subset of these focal tumors is the tectal gliomas, which not infrequently will have been initially "misdiagnosed" as a congenital aqueduct stenosis. These tectal gliomas will frequently show calcification on CT scans [59]. These tumors would seem to have a very benign course and can usually be watched with serial imaging (Fig. 18.6).

18.3.2.3 Exophytic Tumors

These tumors arise from the subependymal glial tissue and fungate into the fourth ventricle [57] with more than 90% of the tumor residing within the ventricular system. The clinical history is long but because of the potential to cause hydrocephalus, patients with these tumors may present with raised intracranial pressure. Additionally, the site of the tumor may result in in-

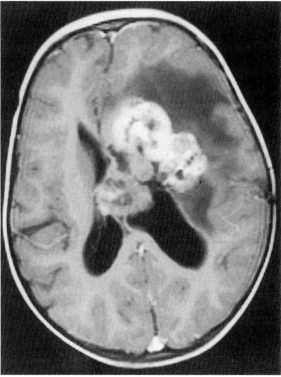

Fig. 18.7 Axial T1-weighted MRI with gadolinium showing a large partially cystic, enhancing tumor involving the parenchyma and with extension into the lateral ventricle. The associated edema is characteristic of a malignant tumor.

tractable vomiting, "failure to thrive" [60], ataxia, and nystagmus. On imaging alone, it can be difficult to differentiate these tumors from medulloblastomas or astrocytomas of the vermis. However, in general, these tumors tend to be isointense and tend to enhance with gadolinium on MRI (Fig. 18.7). The aim of surgery is to shave the tumor flush with the surrounding floor of the fourth ventricle but not to advance ventral to this plain. These tumors are usually benign and surgery followed by surveillance with repeat MRI is required. At the time of tumor recurrence, probably the best form of further therapy is repeat operation.

18.3.2.4 Cervicomedullary Tumor

These glial tumors involve the upper cervical cord/medulla. In effect, they should be treated like spinal cord tumors, the main difference being that as they have "run out of spinal cord" at the level of the decussating white matter tract, they exophytically grow into the cisterna magna [61]. These patients present with long-standing neck pain and gradually develop myelopathy and sensory dysesthesias. These patients also often exhibit torticollis.

Imaging relies on MRI scanning and this shows an enlarged upper cervical cord with distortion of the medulla, usually with an exophytic component going into the cisterna magna. Enhancement with gadolinium is variable. In general, these tumors are low-grade gliomas although very occasionally malignant spinal cord tumors may mimic these findings.

Again, the aim of surgery is to remove as much tumor as possible without damaging normal neural tissues. The cervical tumor is interparenchymal and this requires a midline myelotomy. The exophytic component of the tumor is dealt with in the normal fashion being wary of vascular damage to the posterior inferior cerebellar artery vessels. Some groups find intraoperative electrophysiological monitoring helpful with this group of patients [57]. Postoperatively, these patients are at risk of respiratory failure and problems with protecting their airway and may require tracheostomy and feeding gastrostomies [57].

18.4 Supratentorial Tumors

These tumors usually present clinically with focal neurological signs (e.g., hemiparesis, visual disturbance); or with mass effect either directly due to tumor size or as a result of obstructive hydrocephalus; or with seizures. Supratentorial tumors are a heterogenous group and approximately one-third of these neoplasms involve the cerebral hemisphere [48, 62]. The most common tumor is the low-grade astrocytoma (WHO grade 2), which is composed of fibrillary or protoplasmic neoplastic astrocytes. Other low-grade tumors in this location include juvenile pilocytic astrocytomas (similar to cerebellar astrocytomas), oligodendroglioma, ependymoma, mixed glioma, dysembryoplastic neuroepithelial tumor, and ganglioglioma [48]. During the first 2 years of life, supratentorial tumors are more common than infratentorial and most of these are malignant neoplasms – usually PNETs, choroid plexus carcinomas, or teratomas [48, 63]. Overall, in children, approximately 20% of supratentorial tumors are malignant neoplasms, the most common being the malignant glioma. A brief run through the more common hemispheric tumors will be given prior to discussion of other supratentorial tumor types.

18.4.1 Cerebral Hemispheric Tumors

18.4.1.1 Astrocytomas

This group of tumors comprises one-third of hemisphere neoplasms and shows equal sex distribution with a peak incidence between the ages of 8 and 12 [64, 65]; 10–20% of these tumors will be juvenile pilocys-

tic astrocytomas (having identical histological makeup as those found in the posterior fossa). Malignant gliomas make up a further 20–30% and overall, tumor cysts are found in approximately 40% of children with supratentorial astrocytomas [48].

Once again, it has been shown that gross total/subtotal (>90%) resection confers survival advantage over partial resection/biopsy in both low-grade and high-grade tumors [48]. In spite of the benign histology in the low-grade group, only 60–70% of children will be long-term survivors [48]. This probably reflects the fact that in most series all supratentorial low-grade gliomas are grouped together – including those involving deep vital structure like the hypothalamus and basal ganglia. Nonetheless, the aim of surgery should be to remove as much of the tumor as is safely feasible. The use of radiation postoperatively in these patients with low-grade gliomas is an area of contention. When gross total excision has been accomplished it would seem reasonable to follow these patients with serial imaging. In those patients with partial debulking or biopsy only due to the site of the lesion and in whom clinical progression is occurring, then radiotherapy is indicated. Chemotherapy, using vincristine and carboplatin, is effective and is now used routinely in younger children (less than 8 years of age) and in children with NF1 in whom the use of radiotherapy is to be avoided [66] (Fig. 18.8a–d).

With regard to the malignant tumors, there is clear benefit of adjuvant irradiation and it has been shown that doses of 5,400–6,000 cGy appear to offer longer survival time than does that under 5,000 cGy [67]. Additionally, postirradiation chemotherapy has been shown to significantly increase survival in children with malignant astrocytomas [68] with an increased 5-year survival from 13% in those patients receiving irradiation only to 43% in those also receiving a nitrosourea-based regimen. Recently a newer alkylating agent called Temozolomide has been investigated in both adults and children with high-grade glioma. Although not curative, the use of Temozolomide during and following radiotherapy has been shown to increase duration of survival when compared with radiotherapy alone [69–71]. Further trials of new agents are under way at present.

18.4.1.2 Ependymoma

These tumors make up approximately 10% of all CNS tumors in childhood, and approximately 30% are located supratentorially [48]. Over half of ependymomas occur before 2 years of age [48]. Although the posterior fossa ependymoma is located in relation to the fourth ventricle, the supratentorial ones often lie within the parenchyma and are thought to arise from

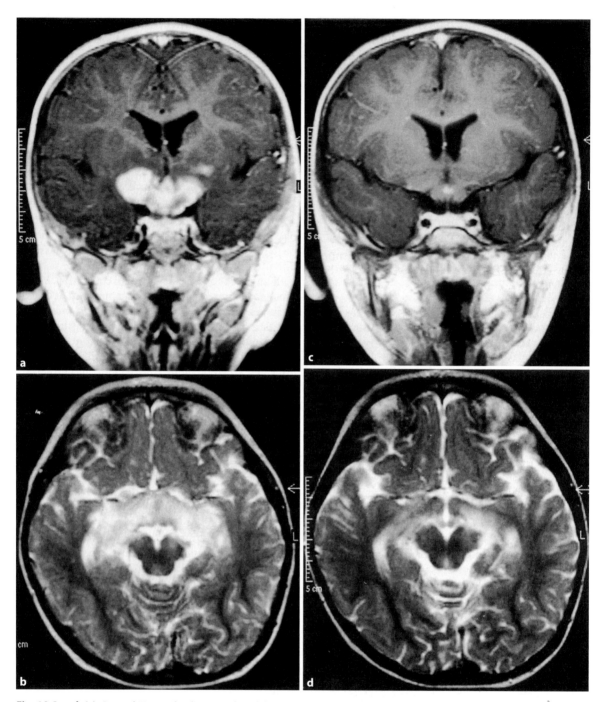

Fig. 18.8 a–d (**a**) Coronal T1-weighted MRI with gadolinium taken at the level of the hypothalamus and third ventricle showing an extensive enhancing tumor – histologically confirmed to be a pilocytic astrocytoma and at surgery found to involve the optic chiasm. (**b**) Axial T2-weighted MRI showing extension of the tumor along the optic radiation. (**c**) and (**d**) are comparable MRI scans from the same 2-year-old patient after chemotherapy with the low grade "Baby Brain" protocol – there being a dramatic reduction in tumor bulk.

ectopic rests of ependymal cells adjacent to the ventricles. Histologically, supratentorial ependymomas are identical to those found in the posterior fossa (see above). Likewise, the aims of surgery are similar to those of the posterior fossa ependymomas. Imaging of the spine is required to exclude drop metastases. Overall, 5-year disease free survival is better than for the infratentorial tumors and ranges between 40% and

60% [72–74], with children with gross total resection faring better and giving recent survival rates of up to 85%. The use and indications for adjuvant therapy are the same as for infratentorial ependymomas.

18.4.1.3 Oligodendrogliomas and Oligoastrocytomas

While pure oligodendrogliomas are rare tumors in the pediatric age group (2–3% of hemispheric tumors) [48], up to 30% of supratentorial gliomas consist of a mixed population of astrocytes and oligodendrocytes – giving them the term "mixed glioma" or "oligoastrocytoma" [48, 64]. Peak incidence is between 6 and 12 years and there is a strong male predominance [48, 75]. These tumors are usually located in the frontal lobe. Histologically, oligoastrocytomas consist of more than 25% astrocytes whereas the oligodendrocytomas are uniform monotonous sheets of cells with perinuclear clear zones or halos producing a "fried egg" appearance [48]. Both tumor types are histologically graded in a similar fashion to astrocytomas. There has been great variation in the incidence of this diagnosis in series of patients with glioma, raising the possibility of international differences in the diagnostic criteria. However, recent advances in our understanding of the cytogenetic changes associated with oligodendrogliomas may help rationalize the diagnostic process. In particular, these tumors often show 1p/19q loss and usually do not show p53 mutations. The 1p/19q loss confers survival advantage and sensitivity to chemotherapy [9].

On CT scan, calcification may be present and there is patchy contrast enhancement with both CT and MRI. Tumor cysts are frequent. The aim of surgery is radical resection and the role of irradiation in these tumors is controversial but probably improves survival in subtotally resected anaplastic tumors. The 5-year survival for pure oligodendrogliomas ranges from 75% to 85% [75, 76]. Malignant mixed tumors fare poorly with similar survival curves to the malignant gliomas.

18.4.1.4 Ganglioglioma

These tumors are also mixed tumors consisting of neoplastic ganglion cells and astrocytes and make up approximately 5% of pediatric brain tumors [48]. Histological grading is based on the astrocytic component of the tumor with regard to features of anaplasia. These tumors have a predilection for the medial temporal lobe and usually present with poorly controlled seizure disorders. Males are more commonly affected and the tumors can occur throughout childhood. Use of MRI demonstrates a well-demarcated cystic temporal lobe mass with no edema.

These are indolent tumors but with often devastating social consequences due to the poorly controlled epilepsy. The aim of surgery is therefore to make the diagnosis, but also to relieve epilepsy. In patients with intractable epilepsy, it is therefore important preoperatively to fully assess the origin of the epileptic focus to confirm that this correlates with the MRI lesion. Long-term survival is seen in 75–90% of patients following radical surgery [76, 77], and radiotherapy is not given in patients who have undergone gross total resection. The role of radiotherapy in patients with a subtotal resection is not yet determined.

18.4.1.5 Primitive Neuroectodermal Tumors (PNET)

These tumors are identical histologically to the infratentorial medulloblastomas. Imaging studies usually demonstrate large, relatively well-demarcated lesions with mixed enhancement patterns and areas of cysts and calcification and possibly hemorrhage [48] (Fig. 18.7). The aim of surgery is to remove as much tumor as possible and preoperatively; these patients require MRI of the spinal axis. Treatment is similar to that for infratentorial medulloblastomas, but the overall prognosis is poor with less than 30% surviving 5 years [32]. Treatment is particularly difficult in young children due to the long-term cognitive consequences of radiotherapy to the supratentorial area.

18.4.1.6 Meningiomas

Although these tumors make up approximately 15% of adult series, they only constitute approximately 2–3% in pediatric series [78]. They are more common in females and in adolescence and may be associated with neurofibromatosis. A far higher percentage of pediatric meningiomas are intraventricular (25%) than in the adult population [48]. As with adult meningiomas, the aim of surgery is total removal including adjacent dura, and long-term survival is expected although recurrence may occur. Occasionally, meningiomas are malignant and may metastasize.

18.4.1.7 Cerebral Metastases

Although common in adults, these tumors only make up approximately 5% of pediatric brain tumors [48] with the most common primary tumors being sarcomas. Patients usually have pulmonary metastases by the time they present with CNS involvement and the prognosis is poor with survival being measured in months.

18.4.2 Midline Tumors

18.4.2.1 Germ Cell Tumors

Intracranial germ cell tumors (GCTs) account for 30% of all GCTs and are histologically identical to extracranial GCTs. Table 18.2 shows the histological classification used for GCTs, which tend to occur in midline sites (suprasellar or pineal), although occasionally they may arise within a ventricle, or within the hemisphere [48]. The management of this group of tumors is covered under Sect. 18.4.3 Pineal Region Tumors.

18.4.2.2 Optic Nerve/Chiasm and Hypothalamic Gliomas

Tumors occurring on the optic pathways make up approximately 5% of all pediatric brain tumors [79] and 75% of these present in the first decade of life. Histologically, these tumors are usually low-grade pilocytic astrocytomas, which very rarely undergo malignant transformation. The tumors may be solid or cystic and are usually fusiform. They may arise primarily in the optic nerve and go on to involve the chiasm or, conversely, they may arise initially in the chiasm and spread to the optic nerves or into the hypothalamus [18]. "Skip" lesions may also be seen along the optic pathways – especially in patients with neurofibromatosis. The symptoms and signs of optic nerve gliomas are dependent upon their anatomical location. The main presenting features are visual failure, squint, proptosis, endocrine dysfunction, and hydrocephalus. Overall,

Table 18.2 Histological classification of intracranial germ cell tumors

Germinoma
Embryonal carcinoma
Yolk sac tumor (endodermal tumor)
Choriocarcinoma
Teratoma
Immature teratoma
Mature teratoma
Teratoma with malignant change
Mixed germ cell tumor

these tumors are associated with good long-term survival but this can be accompanied by slow progressive visual deterioration [18].

The treatment of these tumors remains controversial as their natural history is highly unpredictable – with some tumors progressing despite aggressive treatment while others remain indolent indefinitely [18, 79]. Up to one-third of patients with optic nerve gliomas have neurofibromatosis (NF1) and further evidence for this phakomatosis should be sought at presentation. In general, tumors in patients with NFI behave in a more indolent manner.

Patients with tumors within the orbit or on the intracranial optic nerve tend to present at a slightly later age (6 years) than those with chiasmatic tumors (2–4 years) [18, 79, 80]. Unfortunately, these posteriorly located tumors, which often involve the hypothalamus at presentation, are the most common form of optic nerve glioma making up some 60% [81]. These patients may present with hydrocephalus and/or visual problems and/or pituitary dysfunction and/or hypothalamic dysfunction. The latter classically leading to the diencephalic syndrome (emaciation, pallor, and hyperactivity) seen in up to 20% of patients under 3 years of age [80]. Other symptoms of hypothalamic involvement include diabetes insipidus, anorexia, obesity, and precocious puberty. These tumors also show markedly varying capacity for progression with some remaining indolent while others rapidly increase in size [82].

The imaging investigation of choice is MRI, which usually shows a hypointense tumor on T1-weighted images with enhancement after gadolinium (Fig. 18.8a–c). On T2, high intensity signal may be seen extending to the lateral geniculate bodies, although whether this represents tumor extension or optic tract edema has not yet been determined [80]. Visual evoked responses may be of assistance in monitoring visual function but are of limited value in screening [79].

Management of these tumors remains controversial but in general, patients with reasonable and/or static visual acuity only require surveillance with regular ophthalmic assessment and imaging. Surgery is reserved for problematic proptosis and tumors which are located within the optic nerve but with evidence of spread towards the optic chiasm. Tumors involving the chiasm/hypothalamus may require debulking if there is evidence of tumor progression, although surgery carries an additional risk of further visual impairment. Additionally, histological verification may be important in order to exclude other causes for a suprasellar mass (e.g., germinoma, craniopharyngioma, pituitary adenoma, or a more aggressive astrocytoma). Frequently CSF diversion is required for the treatment of hydrocephalus in patients with posteriorly located tumors (and occasionally this may be complicated by the formation of problematic ascites).

The role of adjuvant therapy in the treatment of optic pathway tumors also remains controversial and is limited to patients with clinical and radiographic evidence of progression. The young age of many of the patients considerably limits the use of radiotherapy; nonetheless, Jenkin et al. [81] have shown that for posterior tumors, irradiation is effective with a 75% 10-year relapse-free survival. Side-effects of irradiation therapy not only include those previously discussed (cognitive impairment, endocrine dysfunction, and secondary malignancy) but also an increased risk of developing Moyamoya phenomenon (cerebral ischemia secondary to spontaneous occlusion of the internal carotid arteries) especially in the setting of NF1 [83]. Of the chemotherapeutic agents available, the nitrosourea-based cytotoxic regimens have been shown to result in symptomatic improvement or stabilization [84]. More recently, carboplatin and vincristine has been reported to be effective in arresting growth in progressive optic gliomas and this is now considered standard treatment for patients with NF1 and young children (less than 8 years) [85] (Fig. 18.8).

18.4.2.3 Craniopharyngiomas

These tumors make up between leukemia is common 5% and 10% of pediatric brain tumors and approximately 15% of all supratentorial tumors [86] and thus are the most common nonglial tumors of childhood. Although 50% of these tumors occur in adults, the peak incidence for the remainder is between the ages of 5 and 10 years [87].

The origin of these unusual tumors has caused much debate over the years but it is generally accepted that they arise from squamous cell rests of an incompletely involuted hypophyseal–pharyngeal duct [88]. Tumors are usually located in the suprasellar region and expand into the hypothalamus and third ventricle. In addition, they grow into the sella and down between the clivus and the brain stem. Approximately one-third of these tumors are purely cystic, while a quarter are purely solid and the remainder mixed – thus overall nearly three-quarters of the tumors are at least partially cystic [88]. The fluid in these cysts is like "engine oil" and contains variable amounts of protein with suspended cholesterol crystals. Calcification is seen in almost all childhood craniopharyngiomas [87].

Histologically, craniopharyngiomas are composed of epithelial cells and form two distinctive variants – the adamantinous and the squamous papillary type. The adamantinous type (48% of all cases) are mainly found in childhood and tend to be cystic tumors, with calcification seen on imaging, and which are prone to recur and have a worse overall outcome. The squamous papillary type (33% of all cases) are usually seen in adults and are generally solid, noncalcified lesions.

Although craniopharyngiomas do not invade neural tissue, they cause an extensive glial reaction – especially around the small finger-like tumor projections which occur within the hypothalamus. Additionally, they frequently are strongly adherent to major arteries and cranial nerves at the base of the brain – in particular the optic chiasm and tracts, the pituitary stalk, and the arteries of the Circle of Willis. It is this unfortunate combination of benign histology and predisposition to form cysts and dense "adhesions" to vital structures that make these tumors such a surgical challenge.

Clinically, these children usually present with signs of raised intracranial pressure secondary to hydrocephalus. Additionally, disturbances of the hypothalamic–pituitary axis may be noted resulting in short stature, diabetes insipidus, obesity, and delayed or precocious puberty. Children of this age may well not complain of visual problems but on presentation over half of them have evidence of visual disturbance (poor acuity, field defect, diplopia or nystagmus) [86]. Plain x-rays show calcification in 85% [87] and may also show an enlarged sella. Calcification is also shown by CT scans and the degree of cystic/solid make up of the tumor and any associated hydrocephalus (Fig. 18.9a,b). Enhancement is intensive but mixed, and coronal scanning may help identify intrasellar extension; MRI is superior to CT for displaying general configuration of the tumor and its relationship to surrounding structures.

The treatment of craniopharyngiomas remains controversial, some proponents advocating aggressive total removal in all children [86, 89], while others consider surgery for craniopharyngiomas as merely palliative and believe that subtotal or partial resection followed by radiation therapy should be the rule [87, 90]. Certainly, if at surgery the hypothalamus is involved, a more conservative approach is warranted to avoid hypothalamic morbidity – as represented by the short, obese, somnolent child. It is becoming more widely accepted that survival and progression-free survival after conservative surgery and radiotherapy are as good as those seen after radical surgery and that there is a lower morbidity associated with the former treatment. However, radiotherapy has its own problems – occasional failure to prevent progression, calcification of the basal ganglia, radiation necrosis (especially of the optic apparatus). Although alternative treatments have been tried (e.g., intracystic injection of radioactive isotopes or bleomycin) these have not been widely adopted [86, 91]. Radiosurgery (single treatment high-dose focused radiotherapy) may have a role in treating small solid tumor remnants situated away from the chiasm [86].

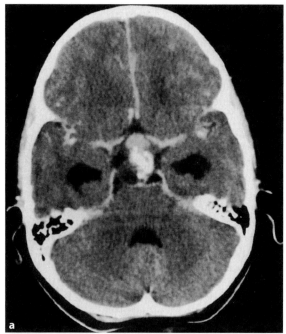

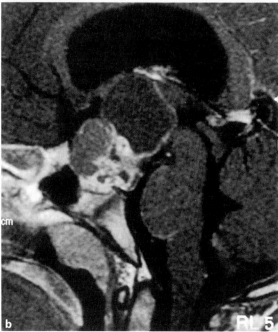

Fig. 18.9 a, b (**a**) Axial CT with contrast showing a partially cystic and partially calcified craniopharyngioma. Note the relationship to the vessels of the Circle of Willis. (**b**) Sagittal T1-weighted MRI shows the extension of the same tumor into the sella turcica, just over the clivus and with a cystic component pushing into the hypothalamus.

18.4.3 Pineal Region Tumors

While making up less than 1% of most adult series [92], pineal tumors are responsible for some 3–8%

Table 18.3 Histological variation of tumors found in the pineal region

Tumors of germ cell origin
(see Table 18.2)
Tumors of pineal parenchyma
Pineocytoma Pineoblastoma Mixed
Tumors of supportive or adjacent tissues
Gliomas Ganglioglioma Meningioma
Non-neoplastic cysts
Pineal cyst Arachnoid cysts
Vascular lesions
Vein of Galen aneurysm Arteriovenous malformations Cavernoma

Adapted from [72].

of childhood brain tumors [93]. Tables 17.2 and 17.3 show the wide variety of tumors that may be found at this location; however, between half and three-quarters of all tumors are either germinomas or of astrocytic origin [92]. Historically, surgical morbidity and mortality rates were high and the standard treatment was shunt insertion for the hydrocephalus and "blind" irradiation of the tumor [94–96]. Improvement in surgical instrumentation and the use of various surgical approaches have resulted in a far more favorable experience in recent years with acceptable mortality rates (0–2%) [92].

Clinically, these children usually present with headache and may have dorsal midbrain syndrome (Parinaud's) consisting of poor upward gaze and difficulty with accommodation. Males are up to four times more likely to develop pineal tumors than females and the average age of presentation is 13 years [92]. Germinomas are particularly prevalent in Japanese adolescent males. Although CT and MRI are useful in delineating the tumor they are not diagnostic (Fig. 18.10). Tumor markers [alpha-fetoprotein (AFP), beta human chorionic gonadatrophin (HCG), and placental alkaline phosphatase (PLAP)] may be raised in both CSF and serum. Preoperative sampling of the CSF is desirable and at the same time cytology can be undertaken. Raised PLAP is classically seen with germinoma, AFP with yolk sac tumors, and raised HCG with choriocarcinoma.

Due to the wide variability in tumor type – not all of which are radiosensitive – it is now generally accepted that tissue diagnosis is required prior to treatment, the only caveat to this being "secretory tumors" which are positive for AFP or HCG. These markers are only positive in malignant germ cell tumors and many trial protocols would recommend up-front chemotherapy with surgery being reserved for postadjuvant residual tumor. Concern has been raised in the literature on the reliability of histological diagnosis from small specimens obtained by stereotactic biopsy [92] – especially as 15% of tumors are of mixed histology [97]. Additionally, the site of pineal tumors with their proximity to the deep venous system has resulted in a higher rate of hemorrhage and morbidity with biopsies in this region than in other areas of the brain. For these reasons, open surgical approaches have gained popularity. However, recent reports of stereotactic biopsy in the management of pineal tumors [98] have shown good diagnostic rates and low morbidity and mortality.

The use of endoscopy in neurosurgery (originally reported in 1923) has increased dramatically over the last two decades, and it is now common practice to treat the hydrocephalus associated with pineal tumors by performing an endoscopic third ventriculostomy (making a small hole through the floor of the third ventricle into the interpeduncular cistern thus bypassing the obstruction at the level of the aqueduct). At the same time, CSF may be obtained for cytology and tumor markers and it may be possible to perform a biopsy of the tumor during the same procedure.

From a surgical perspective, patients with evidence of subependymal seeding or spinal drop metastases require a biopsy (either stereotactic or endoscopic) to obtain a diagnosis. Patients with substantially elevated tumor markers do not require histological confirmation prior to starting treatment. For all other patients, either a biopsy (endoscopic or stereotactic) or an open surgical approach with intraoperative frozen section is required. When the histology is benign, attempt at total removal is undertaken; if the histology is reported as a germinoma, no more than a biopsy is performed; while in those children with malignant pineal region tumors an attempt is made to remove as much tumor as possible.

Postoperative adjuvant therapy is obviously tailored to tumor type with no further treatment being required for benign lesions while radiation and chemotherapy may be required for malignant tumors. The 5-year survival for germinomas treated with radiotherapy is over 90% and therefore many groups recommend radiotherapy alone [92, 97]. Studies are underway to see if it possible to reduce the volume and

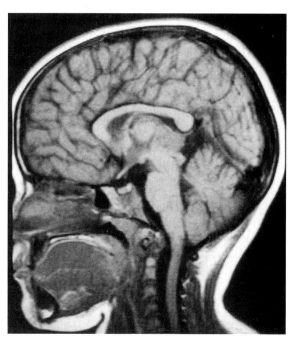

Fig. 18.10 Sagittal T1-weighted MRI showing a pineal tumor compressing the tectal plate. The histology was pineoblastoma.

dose of radiation in patients with germinomas while preserving high cure rates. Secreting tumors have a far poorer prognosis with radiotherapy alone and therefore the use of adjuvant chemotherapy (in particular using etoposide and platinum agents) is now advocated. CSF markers can be used for tumor surveillance and to assess treatment in this group.

18.5 Intraventricular Tumors

As a group, these tumors do not usually present until they have reached sufficient size to obstruct the ventricular system resulting in hydrocephalus. Choroid plexus papillomas may also cause hydrocephalus by overproduction of CSF, although the most likely cause for the hydrocephalus is due to raised protein and cellular debris blocking off CSF absorption. Apart from choroid plexus tumors, the other relatively common tumor types are colloid cysts and the subependymal giant cell astrocytoma. The latter is dealt with under the phakomatoses.

18.5.1 Choroid Plexus Tumors

These relatively rare tumors are histologically divided into choroid plexus papillomas (benign) (Fig. 18.11a) and choroid plexus carcinoma (malignant) (Fig. 18.11b). The latter show focal invasion and dediffer-

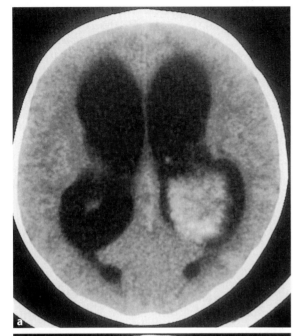

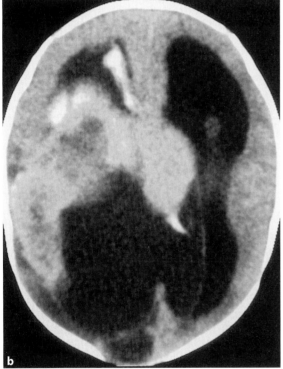

brightly on MRI and CT. In children, they tend to occur in the lateral ventricle [99] while the fourth ventricle is the more typical site in adults [100].

Choroid plexus tumors usually occur in children under 2 years of age in whom there is a small circulating blood volume. This, in combination with the fact that the vascular supply is usually found deep and medial to the tumor, makes these tumors a significant surgical challenge. Complete surgical resection is curative for the papilloma-type and the only long-term survivals reported in the carcinoma-type have occurred after gross total resection and irradiation [101]. The role of presurgical chemotherapy to help devascularize these tumors has been raised by the Toronto group [102] and there are anecdotal reports of success in treating infants with multiagent chemotherapy.

18.5.2 Colloid Cysts

These tumors are rare in childhood but are still occasionally responsible for cases of sudden death. Colloid cysts are benign neuroepithelial cysts whose contents vary from gelatinous to firm in consistency. They are located in the anterior aspect of the third ventricle and may obstruct both Foramen of Munro. It is this site which makes them potentially lethal with their ability to suddenly cause hydrocephalus. Clinically, most patients do not present with acute deterioration or drop attacks but with symptoms of raised intracranial pressure. Various surgical approaches (open via a craniotomy, endoscopic, and stereotactic aspiration) have been advocated for the treatment of these lesions.

18.6 Tumors of the Skull

These "lumps" usually come to light incidentally after minor trauma and 75–90% [103, 104] are benign with the most common being epidermoid or dermoid tumors and with Langerhans' Cell Histiocytosis being the next largest group.

18.6.1 Dermoid and Epidermoid Tumors of the Skull

Fig. 18.11 a, b (**a**) CT scan showing benign choroid plexus papilloma. (**b**) CT scan showing choroid plexus carcinoma.

entiation of cells with marked nuclear pleomorphism [99]. Carcinomas tend to be larger at diagnosis than papillomas and they disseminate along CSF pathways. Both appear as reddish/gray frondular tumors which are highly vascular. For this reason, they enhance

Between them, these tumors probably make up less than 1% of all pediatric brain/skull tumors. Dermoids are usually found around the orbits, around the anterior fontanel and along cranial sutures [104]. These tumors are cysts with stratified keratinizing squamous epithelium forming a capsule of epidermoid and additional dermoid appendages such as hair follicles and sebaceous glands including the walls of dermoids. The tumor usually presents as a painless swelling while those arising around the orbit may present with exophthalmos. Plain x-rays show a rounded erosion of the bone with sclerotic margin while CT scanning shows a lesion which is hypodense. Surgical excision is the treatment of choice.

18.6.2 Fibrous Dysplasia

In this condition, normal bone is replaced by fibrous tissue (fibroblasts and collagen fiber bundles) and the lesion probably represents a developmental defect of mesenchymal tissue [103]. Although occurring in the first few decades of life, lesions are most active during periods of bone growth and during puberty. In nearly 75% of cases only one bone is involved (the cranium being involved in 10–27% of cases) (monostotic form) while in the cases where more than one bone is involved (polyostotic) the cranium is involved in over 50% of cases [103]. If associated with café au lait spots and endocrine dysfunction, the polyostotic form is termed Albright's syndrome. Plain x-ray appearance depends on the amount of bone within the lesion and ranges from radiolucent through to ground-glass or ossified and sclerotic. Growth of the tumor can lead to facial disfigurement or compression of cranial nerves exiting the foramina. Although surgery can be curative, the bones involved often preclude this. These lesions can undergo malignant degeneration to sarcomas (estimated risk of less than 0.5%) but after radiation, this risk may increase up to 44% [103].

18.6.3 Langerhans' Cell Histiocytosis (Histiocytosis X)

This refers to a range of proliferative diseases affecting the reticuloendothelial system which results in the formation of tumor-like lesions. The disease spectrum varies from Letterer-Siwe disease in which there is diffuse systemic involvement and which is progressive and often fatal, through an intermediate stage (Hand-Schüller-Christian disease) in which there is cranial involvement, exophthalmos, and diabetes insipidus; through to eosinophilic granuloma in which solitary lesions are found. The common histological feature is Langerhans' cell histiocytes. In all the conditions, calvarial lesions are the most common and these lesions are usually painful. On plain x-rays they appear punched-out without sclerosis (Fig. 18.12a,b). Diagnosis is obtained at the time of excisional biopsy with curettage. If confirmed, further evaluation (hematological, liver function, chest x-ray and skeletal survey) should be undertaken to determine the extent of active disease. No further treatment is required for single lesions but multiple lesions can be treated with low-dose

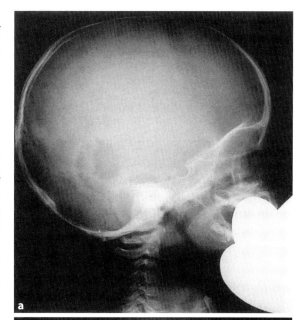
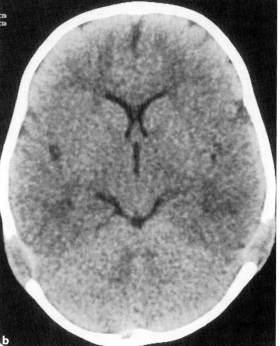

Fig. 18.12 a, b (**a**) Plain x-ray of skull showing punched out lesion of histocytosis on both sides. (**b**) CT scan of the same patient.

radiation (300–1,000 rads); however, multifocal and multisystem disease requires chemotherapy. After surgical excision of a solitary lesion, continuous follow-up is necessary as up to one-third of patients can later develop a new lesion after several years [103].

18.6.4 Hemangioma

Pathologically, these are cavernous hemangiomas growing within the diploe and forming a predominantly lytic lesion on plain x-rays. They have the classic sunburst appearance due to radiating bony spicules. Incision and curettage is usually curative.

18.6.5 Osteoma

These are rare, benign, firm, nontender masses which are dense and well demarcated on plain x-ray. If required they can be easily removed.

18.6.6 Aneurysmal Bone Cyst

Although usually a disease of long bones and spine, approximately 5% occur in the calvarium where they may appear lytic or calcified depending on their age on x-ray. Surgical excision is recommended to prevent hemorrhage after incidental trauma.

18.6.7 Chordomas

These tumors rarely present in childhood but when found in the pediatric population, they are usually located at the skull base involving the clivus and present with lower cranial nerve dysfunction. Metastases to the lung are more frequent in pediatric than in adult chordomas [105]. The investigation of choice to display the tumor extent is MRI. The site makes surgical access difficult but removal has been achieved via far lateral and transoral approaches. Long-term survival for children treated with surgery and radiotherapy approaches 50% [103]. Proton therapy is thought to be more effective than standard radiation for these tumors.

18.6.8 Malignant Primary and Secondary Tumors

Neuroblastoma, because of its relative frequency, is often seen to metastasize to facial bones and the skull. All forms of sarcoma may be located in the cranium although it is rare for the skull bones to be the primary site.

18.7 Spinal Cord Tumors

Spinal cord tumors are divided into extradural and intradural – the latter being further subdivided into

Table 18.4 Types of tumors causing spinal cord compression

Intradural	Extradural
Congenital	Direct spread
Dermoid/epidermoid teratoma	Neural crest tumors (e.g., neuroblastoma) a) Soft tissue tumors (e.g., sarcomas) b) Bony tumors (benign and malignant)
Extramedullary	
Meningioma	
Nerve sheath tumors (schwannoma and neurofibroma)	
	Metastatic
Intramedullary	
Primary (glioma, ependymoma, hemangioblastoma)	
Metastatic (neural „drop" metastases)	

those which are intramedullary (meaning within the parenchyma of the spinal cord) and those that are extramedullary. Table 18.4 shows the types of tumor that may present with spinal cord compression (including extradural compression). Most series include all spinal tumors together and also include developmental anomalies – thus making the true incidence of any type difficult to ascertain. Di Lorenzo et al. [106] found a ratio of intracranial to intraspinal tumors of 6.7 to 1 (making spinal canal tumors some 12–15% of all nervous system tumors). Nearly 70% of these were extramedullary and over 40% of them were extradural. Causes of extradural cord compression include neuroblastomas (Fig. 18.13a–c), tumors of the bony spine and other metastasizing malignancies and these will be discussed in other chapters in this book.

18.7.1 Extramedullary Spinal Tumors

The presenting features depend on the pathology and the age of the child. Delay in diagnosis is the rule rather than the exception. The most common symptom is of pain and motor weakness and in young children the latter may result in regression of ambulatory skills. Sphincter disturbance may also be noticed by delay or regression – although often these symptoms are mistaken as behavioral. Progressive spinal defor-

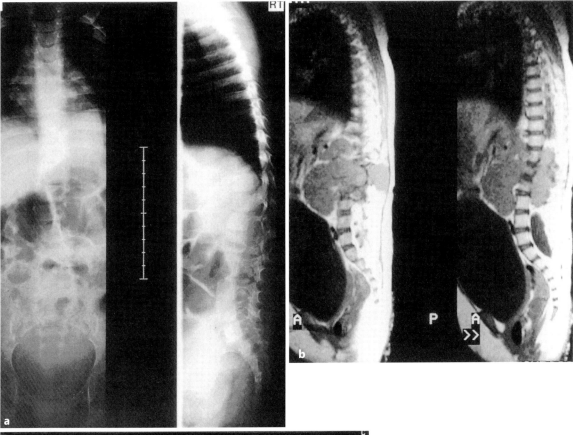

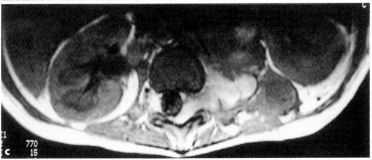

Fig. 18.13 a–c (**a**) Plain anteroposterior and lateral x-rays of a paraplegic 3-year-old child showing gross dilation of the nerve root exit foramina. (**b**) Axial and (**c**) sagittal abdominal MRI with gadolinium from the same patient, showing a large enhancing suprarenal mass entering the spinal canal via the left lumbar nerve root foramen. Histologically, this proved to be a ganglioneuroblastoma.

mity is another method of presentation. Although plain x-rays show abnormalities are present in 50–60% of extramedullary lesions, the investigation of choice today is MRI.

18.7.1.1 Epidermoid and Dermoid Tumors

These lesions are generally believed to result from invagination of skin elements during development. However, occasionally, they may arise after multiple lumbar punctures [107]. Histologically, they are similar to their intracranial counterparts. Dermoids are more common in children and both are usually found in the lumbar region often in association with a cuta-

neous abnormality – hairy patch, port wine, nevus, or dermal sinus. The latter may present with a history of recurrent bouts of meningitis. On MRI scanning, dermoids have the intensity of fat (Fig. 18.14). Complete removal is advocated otherwise recurrence is likely.

18.7.1.2 Teratoma

These tumors either occur within the spinal canal (usually in the lumbar region) or in the sacrococcygeal area. The latter will not be discussed further here. A third of these tumors arise in children less than 5 years of age [108] and the tumors may be cystic or solid and are usually found in the thoracic or lumbar regions.

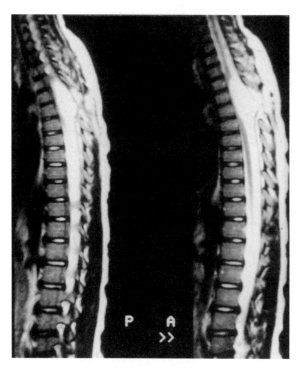

Fig. 18.14 Sagittal T2-weighted MRI of the spine showing a large dermoid (giving the same signal as fat) with marked compression of the spinal cord.

Use of MRI shows multiple tissue signals and surgical excision is the treatment of choice with failure of complete removal resulting in recurrence.

18.7.1.3 Meningioma

Most present in adolescence and usually occur in the thoracic region. Approximately 20% of cases are associated with NF1 [108] and surgical excision is aimed for with good long-term results but with possibly higher rates of recurrence than that seen in adults [108].

18.7.1.4 Nerve Sheath Tumors

Schwannomas are composed of Schwann's cells while neurofibromas are a mixture of Schwann's cells and fibroblasts but with an abundance of collagen fibers. These tumors tend to present around puberty and approximately 25% of them are associated with von Recklinghausen's disease (NF1) [108]. Varying amounts of the tumor may be in the spinal canal with dumb-bell-shaped tumors being seen in 20% of cases. Very occasionally malignant change can occur within them. The investigation of choice is MRI and treatment consists of total removal when feasible.

18.7.1.5 Hemangioblastoma

Hemangioblastomas may occur as part of von Hippel-Lindau disease and approximately 50% of spinal hemangioblastomas occur in conjunction with this syndrome. In general, although hemangioblastoma is rare in children, the spinal lesions are more common than cranial [108]. These tumors may be multiple. Treatment is surgical removal.

18.7.1.6 Metastatic Disease

Extraneural. Involvement of the central nervous system with leukemia is common and may be present at initial diagnosis in up to 30% of patients with acute myelogenous leukemia (AML) [109]. Without prophylactic treatment, patients with acute lymphocytic leukemia (ALL) will develop CNS disease in 50–80% of patients [108] but prophylactic treatment reduces this risk to 2–10%. Leukemia of the CNS presents as either parenchymal or meningeal disease or both and the dural involvement may reach sufficient proportion to produce a mass lesion either within the cranium or within the spinal canal. Hemorrhage can occur from these lesions and infiltration of nerve roots or the spinal cord itself may occur. Diagnosis may be made by CSF cytology and MRI may show meningeal enhancement or masses. Treatment is a combination of radiation and chemotherapy.

Lymphoma can involve the CNS in either primary or secondary fashion. The primary lesions are non-Hodgkins lymphomas and are usually seen in immunocompromised patients [acquired immunodeficiency syndrome (AIDS) or transplant patients], classically being located in the periventricular regions of the cerebral hemispheres. Secondary deposits from both Hodgkin's and non-Hodgkin's lymphomas are seen and are usually extradural – often in the spinal canal. Although generally a medical disease, surgical intervention may be required for acute cord compression not relieved by treatment with chemotherapy.

Neural Origins. The most common causes of drop metastases are PNETs (including the medulloblastomas), anaplastic astrocytomas, ependymomas, and germ cell tumors. Drop metastases are usually seen in the lumbar region. Treatment is generally nonsurgical unless there is a solitary lesion producing acute neurological compression.

18.7.2 Intramedullary Tumors

These relatively uncommon tumors account for only 6% of central nervous system tumors of childhood

[110] and usually occur in adolescence. In the past, these tumors were usually biopsied and given radiotherapy but over the last two decades, it has become apparent that most of these tumors in children should be treated aggressively surgically.

In the pediatric age range, astrocytomas make up approximately 60% of the tumors and ependymomas make up less than 30% (compared with over 50% in

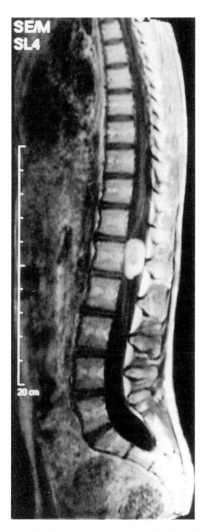

Fig. 18.15 Sagittal T1-weighted MRI of the spine with gadolinium, showing an enhancing tumor arising from the conus.

adults) [110]. Within the pediatric population there is also a predilection for the tumors to occur in the cervical region (nearly 50% versus only 30% in the adult series) [110]. Interestingly, over 10% of patients at presentation will have associated hydrocephalus (the cause of which is still debated) [110].

The imaging of these tumors has been revolutionized by MRI, which has shown them to fall into two types – (a) holocord astrocytomas (these in effect are similar to the cystic variety of cerebral astrocytomas with a small solid component associated with a large rostral and caudal cyst which may extend the whole length of the spinal cord), and (b) focal tumors (Fig. 18.15). With the holocord type of tumor, surgery is restricted to removing the solid component and subsequent follow-up studies will show the rostral and caudal cysts to gradually disappear. Likewise, gross total excision of the focal tumor should be undertaken. For both low-grade astrocytomas and ependymomas, no further adjuvant therapy is required. It should also be noted that the success of surgery is directly related to the preoperative neurological status and therefore an expectant policy while a child gradually deteriorates is not in the long-term interest of the patient. Follow-up is required for these patients and if there is recurrence; further surgery is the first line of treatment.

Surveillance is also required to detect delayed spinal deformity which is more likely to occur the higher up the spinal column the tumor is located. The cause of this deformity (kyphosis or scoliosis) is not clear but probably represents a combination of structural damage (laminectomy) and neuromuscular imbalance. Laminoplasty (the re-insertion and holding down of the laminae in their original position after surgery) is now routinely employed (Fig. 18.16) although there is no evidence to date that this decreases the risk of spinal deformity.

Occasionally, the astrocytomas are malignant (usually with a shorter history) and in these cases radical resection is not indicated as not only is the morbidity associated with aggressive surgery far higher, but also there has been no improvement shown in survival after radical surgery. In this group of patients, total neuroaxis radiation is required but the outlook is dismal.

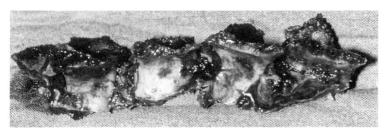

Fig. 18.16 Operative photograph showing four laminae removed en bloc (laminoplasty) which were replaced at the end of the procedure.

18.8 Intraocular Tumors

18.8.1 Retinoblastoma

Retinoblastoma is the most common ocular tumor of childhood, having an incidence world wide of approximately one in every 20,000 live births [111]. The children typically present in the first 2 years of life with either leukocoria or strabismus. Buphthalmos, heterochromia, pseudohypopyon, severe inflammation and raised intracranial pressure are all recognized but rare presentations. Thirty to 40% of the children will have bilateral tumors. All bilaterally affected children, all children with a positive family history, and 8–10% of unilaterally affected children will have a germ line mutation of Rb gene located on chromosome 13.

The retinoblastoma gene, located at the 13q14 site on the long arm of chromosome 13, is a large 2–7 exon 18-kb gene responsible for the production of retinoblastoma protein (pRb). The Rb gene is a ubiquitous oncogene, and both alleles must be lost from a cell for it to undergo malignant transformation. In children with a germ line mutation one allele is missing from all cells and only the "second hit" causing loss of the homologous gene is necessary for retinoblastoma to develop. Loss of that homologue may be triggered by a number of agencies, but oncoviruses and radiation seem to be particularly important.

Gene sequencing enables mutation detection in the vast majority of children with a germ line mutation. This in turn means that family members can be screened and either eliminated from the need for repeated screening, or placed on an intensive screening program to facilitate early tumor detection and treatment. It also provides the information which allows prenatal diagnosis (using amniocentesis or chorionic villus sampling) and even embryo screening.

There is considerable evidence [112] that early detection offers the best chance of successful treatment of retinoblastoma, and one of the major challenges facing clinicians is identification of affected children while the tumors are small enough to allow effective conservative therapy.

In the Western world, where relatively early presentation is the norm, long-term survival can be anticipated in 95% or more of the children. However, in other parts of the world where diagnosis and/or treatment may be delayed until extraocular spread has occurred, 5-year cancer free survival is reduced to less than 20% [113], (Fig. 18.17).

The diagnosis of retinoblastoma is clinical, and requires a detailed fundus examination with the indirect ophthalmoscope. In children of this age a general anesthetic is necessary to allow adequate retinal examination (Figs. 18.17, 18.18).

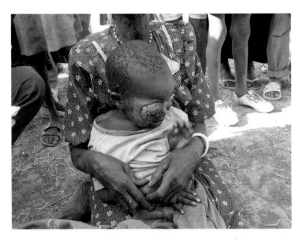

Fig.18.17 Advanced stage retinoblastoma in a child from third world country

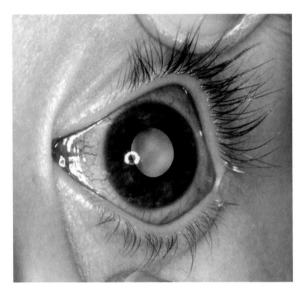

Fig.18.18 Retinoblastoma presenting with leukocoria of the eye

Examination under anesthesia is often combined with ultrasonography to identify calcification within the tumor mass and MRI, looking for evidence of optic nerve involvement. There is no role for diagnostic biopsy and indeed, breaching the corneo-scleral envelope, either spontaneously or iatrogenically, is associated with a substantial increase in orbital and distant dissemination, which in turn carries with it a much poorer prognosis [114].

Differential diagnosis. See Table 18.5.

Retinoblastomas typically consist of masses of basophilic cells arising from the retina interspersed with areas of eosinophilic tumor necrosis and areas of calcifica-

Table 18.5 Table showing a differential diagnostic list of intra-ocular tumours

Primary ocular disease	Coats disease
	Persistent hyperplastic primary vitreous
	Cataract
	Coloboma
	Retinopathy of prematurity
	Myelinated retinal nerve fibers
	Osseous choristoma
Infections	Toxoplasmosis
	Toxocariasis
	CMV retinitis
	Metastatic endophthalmitis
Systemic disorders	Tuberous sclerosis
	Norrie's disease
	Incontinentia pigmenti
	Leukemia
	Metastatic malignancies
Other primary ocular tumors	Retinal astrocytomas
	Medulloepithelioma
	Glioneuroma
	Hemangiomas
	Retinal pigment hamartomas

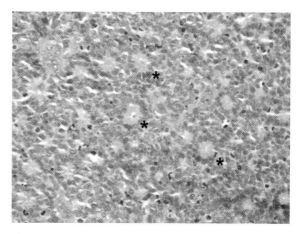

Fig. 18.19 Typical Retinoblastoma with Flexner Wintersteiner rosettes (*asterisks*).

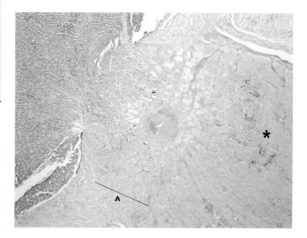

Fig. 18.20 Retinoblastoma with retrolaminar optic nerve invasion.

tion. Well-differentiated tumors show the characteristic Flexner-Wintersteiner rosettes, made up of columnar cells arranged around a clear central lumen (Fig. 18.3). Homer-Wright rosettes are also a common feature but they will also be seen in other small blue cell tumors of childhood such as neuroblastoma and medulloblastoma. Well-differentiated retinoblastomas may also contain fleurettes composed of groups of tumor cells projecting through a fenestrated membrane [115].

Histopathological examination of the enucleated eye also serves to identify adverse features of prognostic significance. Of greatest importance are invasion of the optic nerve (beyond the lamina cribrosa) and invasion of the deeper layers of the choroid (Fig. 18.4). Either of these features will demand postoperative chemotherapy. Invasion into and through the sclera or invasion to the cut end of the optic nerve require more aggressive postoperative chemotherapy and orbital radiotherapy.

For more than 50 years it has been recognized that retinoblastomas are vulnerable to the effects of radiation and for most of that period plaque brachytherapy or external beam radiotherapy have been the mainstays of conservative treatment.

While plaque brachytherapy remains an invaluable treatment modality, external beam radiotherapy has largely been replaced by chemotherapy as the first line conservative management. Recognition of the long-term adverse effects of external beam radiotherapy

on the facial skeleton, the neuro-endocrine system and, particularly, the substantial increase in second tumor formation, has led to this fundamental change in approach. Children with germ line mutations have a fivefold increase in the risk of developing a second malignancy as compared to the general population (with a particularly high relative risk of developing bony or soft tissue sarcomata). That risk of a second malignancy, however, rises to between 18% and 35% by the age of 35 if the children are exposed to external beam irradiation [115, 116].

The most popular chemotherapy regimen employs a combination of vincristine, carboplatin and etoposide given in 3- to 4-week cycles, and most commonly using 6 cycles. The aim of chemotherapy is to reduce the size of the tumor (chemoreduction) and allow complete tumor control with adjunctive focal therapy. Only rarely is complete tumor control, with chemotherapy alone, the objective.

The focal therapies employed include laser therapy (particularly transpupillary thermotherapy) cryotherapy, and plaque brachytherapy. For tumors situated at the macula, complete control with chemotherapy may be attempted to avoid the effect of macula thermotherapy on the child's long-term vision. The results with this approach are variable.

For those children with tumors that cannot be controlled conservatively, or in children with unilateral disease where there is no possibility of preserving a seeing eye, enucleation is recommended.

Enucleation is carried out in such a way that the maximum possible length of optic nerve is obtained, to reduce the possibility of the tumor involving the site of transection of the optic nerve. An orbital implant is placed in the socket at the time of enucleation, and currently the favored implants are those which permit vascular integration. The implant has the extraocular muscles attached to it so that some movement is imparted to the implant during movement of the remaining eye. This in turn ensures a better long-term cosmetic outcome.

Enucleation is usually curative, but families and clinicians must be aware that approximately 1 in 3 enucleated eyes show adverse histological features (optic nerve or deep choroidal invasion by tumor cells) which will necessitate 4 cycles of chemotherapy to reduce the risk of metastatic dissemination. It is also apparent that a proportion of children who have undergone enucleation in childhood develop significant psychological problems related to their enucleation and artificial eye as they grow older. A comprehensive service to the families needs to take account of these later developments.

18.8.2 Medulloepithelioma

Medulloepithelioma is a rare tumor which arises from undifferentiated nonpigmented ciliary epithelium (though there are isolated reports of pigmented medulloepitheliomas in children). A report in 1988 detailed only 16 medulloepitheliomas recorded at the Institute of Ophthalmology in London over a 25-year period [114]. They can be locally invasive with malignant features and orbital invasion, but distant metastases are uncommon.

They most commonly present between 2 and 4 years of age as a pink-colored mass arising from the iris or ciliary body appearing in the anterior chamber of the eye. Secondary changes such as cataract with reduced vision or iris rubeosis and glaucoma may also be presenting features. Histopathological examination has shown that rubeosis iridis is the most common clinicopathological feature.

More than half of all medulloepitheliomas are classified as benign [116] while the remainder show cytological features which may resemble neuroblastoma cells, features of embryonal sarcoma, or astrocytoma cells. When histopathology is difficult, because of poor differentiation, diagnosis may be facilitated by the use of immunohistochemistry to identify the neuro-epithelial origin of the tumor [117].

For some tumors local resection with an iridocyclectomy can be curative. Detailed ultrasonographic examination will serve to indicate the extent of the tumor and is a valuable aid in assessing the feasibility of local resection [118].

Successful conservative treatment with local Iodine 125 brachytherapy has also been described [119], but, in most instances, enucleation of the affected eye is necessary. If examination of the enucleated eye shows evidence of extrascleral extension than surgery needs to be followed by postoperative orbital radiotherapy. Rarely, if there is evidence of orbital recurrence, then orbital exenteration may be required.

18.8.3 Malignant Melanoma of the Iris and Choroid

Malignant melanoma of the choroid is the most common primary ocular tumor but rarely affects children. In a series of 3,706 consecutive ocular melanomas, only 40 affected individuals were less than 20 years of age and 78% were between 15 and 20 [120]. Nonetheless, there are isolated reports of very early onset uveal melanoma [121], and it must be considered in the differential diagnosis of retinoblastoma.

Diagnosis is established by identifying the characteristic ultrasonography findings of high internal reflectivity, and fluorescein angiography shows mottled fluorescence in the early phases.

Treatment depends on the size and location of the melanoma, but options include local resection, plaque brachytherapy, transpupillary thermotherapy with the diode laser or, most commonly, enucleation of the affected eye.

18.8.4 Juvenile Xanthogranuloma (JXG)

JXG is a benign inflammatory lesion of the iris and ciliary body containing histiocytes, lymphocytes, and Touton giant cells. Clinically JXG may take the form of a discrete nodule or a diffuse thickened yellow plaque on the iris, and is often associated with an ipsilateral, yellow papular skin lesion.

JXG is a notorious cause of spontaneous hyphema (bleeding into the anterior chamber of the eye) in children, and if it shows that tendency, treatment with topical or subconjunctival steroids may be necessary.

Occasionally the uveal tract may become diffusely involved in Letterer-Siwe disease, a systemic histiocytic disorder.

18.8.5 Intraocular Vascular Tumors

Vascular intraocular tumors may appear in isolation or as part of a neurocutaneous syndrome (see Sect. 18.8.2 entitled "Phakomatoses).

18.8.6 Choroidal Osteoma

Choroidal osteoma is usually unilateral, and consists of a well-circumscribed, yellow/orange placoid lesion. They show genuine bone formation with osteoblasts, osteocytes, and osteoclasts all present. The bone is laid down in trabeculae and there are intertrabecular marrow spaces.

They require no treatment and are easily identified with CT imaging which shows discrete shield-shaped plaque of calcification in the choroid. It should be considered with differential diagnosis for calcified unilateral retinoblastoma.

18.8.7 Myogenic and Neurogenic Tumors

Myogenic tumors, both leiomyomas and rhabdomyosarcomas, are extremely rare in an intraocular location.

Neurogenic tumors are also extremely rare in this location in childhood. The exceptions are those neurogenic tumors associated with the phakomatoses.

The phakomatoses are a group of disorders in which skin, eye, and central nervous system are involved. Included in this group of disorders are:
– Neurofibromatosis type 1 and 2
– Tuberous sclerosis
– Von Hippell-Lindau syndrome
– Sturge-Weber syndrome
– Klippel-Trenaunay-Weber syndrome
– Wyburn-Mason syndrome

Neurofibromatosis type 1 is a common neurocutaneous condition with an autosomal dominant pattern of inheritance. NF1 has a birth incidence of 1 in 2,500 to 1 in 3,000; the diagnosis is based on clinical assessment and two or more of the features listed in Table 18.6 are required [122]. The causative mutation occurs on the long arm of chromosome 17 at the q11.2 site and results in underproduction of the tumor suppressor protein neurofibrin [123].

Table 18.6 Diagnostic criteria for neurofibromatosis 1

6 or more café au lait macules (>0.5 cm in children or >1.5 cm in adults)
2 or more cutaneous/subcutaneous neurofibromas or one plexiform neurofibroma
Axillary or groin freckling
Optic pathway glioma
2 or more Lisch nodules (iris hamartomas seen on slit lamp examination)
Bony dysplasia (sphenoid wing dysplasia, bowing of long bone +/- pseudarthrosis)
First degree relative with NF1

From [122]

Clinicians should be aware that some individuals with mosaic/segmental NF1 present with six or more café au lait patches and skin fold freckling; however, the skin manifestations are in a restricted segment of the body.

Lisch nodules, a highly characteristic pigmented hamartoma are found in 90–95% of children by the age of 3 years. Histologically they are a variant of neurofibroma and are of value in establishing the diagnosis but need no intervention.

Plexiform neurofibromas, on the other hand, cause significant morbidity because they are diffuse, grow along the length of a nerve, and may involve multiple nerve branches and plexi. The lesions can be nodular, and multiple discrete tumors may develop on nerve trunks. Plexiform neurofibromas infiltrate surrounding soft tissue and bony hypertrophy is evident in some instances.

Facial plexiform neurofibromas causing disfigurement appear during the first 3 years of life and commonly affect the orbits and eyelids. Removal of benign plexiform neurofibromas is difficult due to encroachment of the tumor on surrounding structures and its inherent vascular nature. Life-threatening hemorrhage can occur and expert advice from experienced soft tissue tumor or plastic surgeons is essential before removal. A number of agents (including farnesyl transferase inhibitors, antiangiogenesis drugs, and fibroblast inhibitors) are being used in clinical trials to assess their therapeutic effect on growth of plexiform neurofibromas.

There is an 8–13% lifetime risk of developing malignant peripheral nerve sheath tumors (MPNST) in NF1, but predominantly in individuals aged 20–35 years. These cancers usually but not invariably, arise in pre-existing plexiform neurofibromas.

Optic pathway gliomas (OPG) are grade 1 pilocytic astrocytomas and are found principally in the optic pathways, brainstem, and cerebellum. They occur in about 15% of children with NF1, are often asymptomatic and more indolent than their counterparts in the general population. However, some tumors produce impaired visual acuity, abnormal color vision, visual field loss, squint, pupillary abnormalities, optic atrophy, proptosis, and hypothalamic dysfunction. The risk of symptomatic OPG is greatest in children under 7 years and older individuals rarely develop tumors that require medical intervention [124]. If the integrity of the chiasm is threatened by an optic nerve glioma it is necessary to consider reducing the tumor volume with chemotherapy. Occasionally surgery is warranted to deal with severe proptosis with corneal exposure, or to debulk extensive chiasmal gliomas. Radiotherapy is not advocated in young children because of potential second malignancy [125].

Neurofibromatosis Type 2 (NF2) is an autosomal dominant neurocutaneous disease that is clinically and genetically distinct from NF1 and occurs in approximately 1 in 25,000 individuals. It is caused by inactivating mutations on chromosome 22q11.2 and is characterized by bilateral vestibular schwannomas. Affected individuals also develop schwannomas on other cranial, spinal, peripheral, and cutaneous nerves. Café au lait patches are less numerous than in NF1 and the skin lesions are predominantly schwannomas. Slit lamp examination reveals juvenile subcapsular lens opacities in the majority of patients and multiple retinal astrocytomas are much more likely than in NF1 (Figs. 18.21, 18.22).

Children with Tuberous Sclerosis (TS) show a combination of cutaneous angiofibromas, retinal astrocytic hamartomas, and CNS hamartomas causing developmental delay and epilepsy. The ocular lesions require no treatment and will only cause visual disturbance if they are located at the macula. However, the ophthalmologist may well be the first clinician to recognize the condition, and needs to ensure that a detailed assessment is undertaken, because of the association with renal and cardiac pathology.

Von Hippel-Lindau syndrome is characterized by the formation of retinal capillary angiomas and cerebellar angiomas or hemangioblastomas. The retinal lesion may cause exudation, and since this exudation tends to accumulate at the macula area, it is associated with significant visual loss. In extreme cases the accumulated exudate leads to a retinal detachment, so that treatment at an early stage is desirable.

The aim of treatment is to encourage absorption of the exudate. For lesions between the equator of the globe and the ora serrata, cryotherapy to the base of the hemangioma is most appropriate, using a triple freeze thaw technique. For more posteriorly located

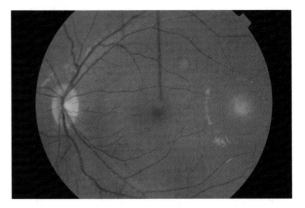

Fig. 18.21 Multiple retinal astrocytomas in neurofibromatosis

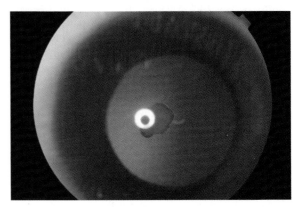

Fig. 18.22 Juvenile subcapsular lens opacities in neurofibromatosis

tumors isolation with argon laser photocoagulation with later sealing of the feeder vessels is the preferred approach.

The major ophthalmic complication of Sturge-Weber syndrome is glaucoma with up to 30% of affected children developing glaucoma [126]. The diffuse choroidal hemangioma, which some affected children show, does not require surgical intervention in the vast majority of cases. If it is associated with sight-threatening retinal exudation, then laser photocoagulation, to promote absorption of the exudate, may be attempted.

18.9 Orbital Tumors

Orbital tumors in childhood may be benign or malignant; they may be derived from any of the structures within the orbit or they may metastasize to the orbit from a distant site. Table 18.7 reflects the nature and origin of the tumors and is a useful template for this discussion.

Table 18.7 Classification of orbital tumors

Primary benign	Derived from orbital structures
Primary malignant	
Secondary benign	Arising from adjacent structures
Secondary malignant	
Orbital cysts	
Metastatic	
Associated with systemic disease	

Table 18.8 Other causes of proptosis in childhood

Lymphoid
Benign reactive lymphoid hyperplasia
Histiocytic
Eosinophilic granuloma
Lacrimal
Ectopic lacrimal gland Lacrimal gland inflammation
Inflammation
Orbital pseudotumor Orbital myositis Wegners Sarcoid Tuberculosis

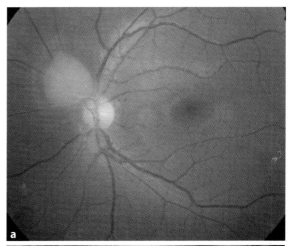

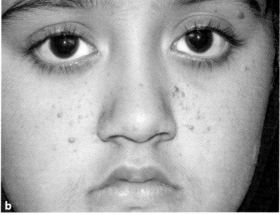

Fig. 18.23 Retinal astrocytoma and adenoma sebaceum in a child with tuberous sclerosis.

18.9.1 Diagnosis

Regardless of their nature, most orbital tumors present with proptosis and limitation of ocular rotations. Pain and inflammation are more variable symptoms and other signs will depend on the tissue of origin. For example, profound visual loss, pupillary abnormality and optic nerve swelling or atrophy are the hallmarks of optic nerve gliomas but are rarely seen with rhabdomyosarcoma.

18.9.2 Primary Benign Orbital Tumors

Neural
– Optic nerve glioma
– Optic nerve meningioma
– Neurofibroma
– Schwannoma

Vascular
– Capillary hemangioma
– Lymphangioma
– Varix
– AV malformation

Adipose and muscular
– Lipoma
– Myofibroma

Fibrous
– Fibroma
– Fibromyxoma
– Fibrous tissue dysplasia

Osseous and cartilaginous
– Osteoma
– Juvenile ossifying fibroma
– Aneurysmal bone cyst

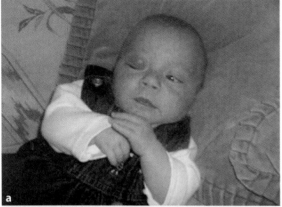

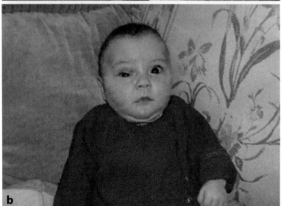

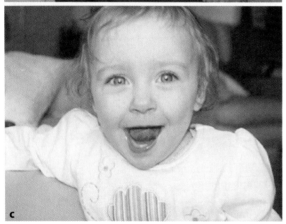

Fig. 18.24 Sequence of clinical photos after intralesional injection of triamcinolone and dexamethasone.

18.9.3 Optic Nerve Glioma

Optic nerve glioma is the commonest intrinsic tumor of the optic nerve. It typically presents around the age of 5 years with loss of vision, painless axial proptosis, and limited ocular movements. Girls are more commonly affected than boys and up to 50% of affected children have NF1 [126].

It is a benign, slow growing, low-grade pilocytic astrocytoma and carries a better prognosis when it is associated with NF1. Occasionally, particularly in younger children, optic nerve glioma shows more aggressive local expansion and these typically are the children likely to need surgical intervention.

The diagnosis is established by imaging which shows a tubular or fusiform swelling of the optic nerve, and characteristic "kinking" of the affected nerve. MRI will show the extent of the tumor, whether there is intracranial extension and any evidence of chiasmal involvement. Visual field testing (in children who are sufficiently cooperative) will identify any involvement of fibers derived from the contralateral optic nerve.

Management consists of observation, including serial visual fields, if the cosmesis is good and there is no threat to the chiasm. Poor vision with severe proptosis, or threatened chiasmal involvement are indication for either chemotherapy (usually with vincristine and carboplatin) or globe sparing optic nerve excision. This surgery can be performed through a lateral orbitotomy if only the orbital portion needs removal, but a craniofacial exposure permits more complete excision of the nerve including the intracranial prechiasmatic portion.

18.9.4 Optic Nerve Meningioma

Optic nerve meningioma is a rare tumor in infants and children. The mean age of presentation is 10 years. It occurs more commonly in males with an increasing incidence with age. The orbit is one of the most common locations. Presentation is of chronic progressive visual loss with mild proptosis associated with diplopia, headache, and ptosis. The tumor is histologically benign but the clinical course tends to be more aggressive in children than in adults. There can be hereditary predisposition and on genetic testing there can be a deletion of part of chromosome 22.

18.9.5 Primary Orbital Cysts

– Dermoid
– Sebaceous
– Hematic
– Hydatid
– Lacrimal duct cyst (Dacryops)
– Microphthalmos with cyst

18.9.6 Malignant Orbital Tumors

Primary Orbital Malignancy
– Rhabdomyosarcoma

– Lacrimal gland adenoid cystic carcinoma
– Sarcoma
– Teratoma

Metastatic orbital malignancy
– Neuroblastoma
– Ewing's sarcoma
– Wilm's tumor

Orbital involvement in systemic malignancy
– Lymphoma
– Leukemia
– Histiocytosis
– Plasmacytosis

18.9.7 Primary Benign Orbital Tumors

– Sinus mucocoele
– Encephalocoele
– Meningocoele

18.9.8 Other Causes of Proptosis in Childhood

Lymphoid
– Benign reactive lymphoid hyperplasia
Histiocytic
– Eosinophilic granuloma

Lacrimal
– Ectopic lacrimal gland
– Lacrimal gland inflammation

Inflammation
– Orbital Pseudotumor
– Orbital myositis
– Wegners
– Sarcoid
– Tuberculosis

Acknowledgements

I would like to thank the following for their help and suggestions with this chapter: Dr. L. Bridges (neuropathology), Dr. J. Livingstone (pediatric neurology), and Dr. R. Taylor (radiotherapy). Special thanks to Mary Walker and Jan Francis for their secretarial help.

References

1. Laurent JP, Cheek WR (1985) Brain tumours in children. J Pediatr Neurosci 1:15–32

2. Allen JC (1985) Childhood brain tumours: Current status of clinical trials in newly diagnosed and recurrent disease. Pediatr Clin North Am 32:633–651

3. McNally RJ, Kelsey AM, Cairns DP, et al. (2001) Temporal increases in the incidence of childhood solid tumours seen in Northwest England (1954–1998) are likely to be real. Cancer 92:1967–1976

4. Parkin DM, Kramarova E, Draper GJ, et al. (1998) International incidence of childhood cancer. IARC Sci Publ, Lyon, p 144

5. Rorke LB (1994) Introductory survey of brain tumours. In: Marlin AE, McLone DG, Reigel DH, Walker ML (eds) Paediatric neurosurgery, 3rd edn. WB Saunders Co, Philadelphia, pp 351–355

6. Bondy ML, Lustbader ED, Buffler PA, et al. (1991) Genetic epidemiology of childhood brain tumours. Genet Epidemiol 8:253–267

7. Draper G, Vincent T, Kroll ME, Swanson J (2005) Childhood cancer in relation to distance from higher voltage power lines in England and Wales: A case-control study. BMJ 330:1290–1293

8. Biegel JA, Tan L, Zhang F, et al. (2002) Alterations of the hSNF5/InI1 gene in central nervous system atypical teratoid/rhabdoid tumours and renal and extrarenal rhabdoid tumours. Clin Cancer Res 8:3461–3467

9. Jenkins RB, Blair H, Ballman KV, et al. (2006) A t(1; 19) (q10; p10) mediates the combined deletions of 1p and 19q and predicts better prognosis of patients with oligodendroglioma. Cancer Res 66:9852–9861

10. Stiller C (1994) Population based survival rates for childhood cancer in Britain 1980–91. BMJ 309:1612–1616

11. Stupp R, et al. (2005) Radiotherapy plus concomitant and adjuvant Temozolomide for glioblastoma. N Engl J Med 352:987–996

12. Wesphal M, Hilt DC, Bortey E, et al. (2003) A phase 3 trial of local chemotherapy with biodegradable carmustine (BCNU) wafers (Gliadel wafers) in patients with primary malignant glioma. Neuro Oncol 5:75–88

13. Kibirige M, Birch J, Campbell R, et al. (1989) A review of astrocytoma in childhood. Pediatr Hematol Oncol 6(4):319–329

14. Greenberg MS (1993) Handbook of neurosurgery, 3rd edn. Greenberg Graphics Inc, Florida, p 686 15. Huson S, Compston D, Harper P (1989) A genetic study of von Recklinghausen neurofibromatosis in South East Wales. II. Guidelines for genetic counseling. J Med Genet 26:712–721

16. Schut L, Duhaime AC, Sutton LN (1994) Phakomatoses: Surgical considerations. In: Marlin AE, McLone DG, Reigel DH, Walker ML (eds) Paediatric neurosurgery, 3rd edn. WB Saunders Co, Philadelphia, pp 473–484

17. Hope DG, Mulvihill JJ (1981) Neurofibromatosis (von Recklinghausen's Disease). Malignancy in neurofibromatosis. In: Riccardi VM, Mulvihill JJ (eds) Advances in neurology, vol 29. Raven Press, New York, pp 35–36

18. Chumas PD (1996) Optic nerve glioma. In: Palmer JD (ed) Neurosurgery 96. Manual of neurosurgery. Churchill Livingstone, Edinburgh, pp 248–251

19. Weichert K, Dire M, Benton C, et al. (1973) Macrocranium and neurofibromatosis. Radiology 107:163–166

20. Sampson J, Scahill S, Stephenson J, et al. (1989) Genetic aspects of tuberous sclerosis in the West of Scotland. J Med Genet 26:28–31

21. Martuza R (1982) Neurofibromatosis and other phakomatoses. In: Wilkins R, Rengachary S (eds) Neurosurgery. McGraw-Hill, New York, pp 511–521

22. Fitz C (1986) Tuberous sclerosis. In: Hoffman HJ, Epstein F (eds) Disorders of the developing nervous system: Diagnosis and treatment. Blackwell Scientific, Boston, pp 625–634

23. Rorke LB, Schut L (1989) Introductory survey of paediatric brain tumours. In: McLaurin RL, et al. (eds) Paediatric neurosurgery: Surgery of the developing nervous system, 2nd edn. WB Saunders Co, Philadelphia, pp 335–337

24. Illgren EB, Stiller CA (1987) Cerebellar astrocytomas. Part I. Macroscopic and microscopic features. Clin Neuropathol 6:185–200

25. Garcia DM, Marks JE, Latifi HR, Kliefoth AB (1990) Childhood cerebellar astrocytomas: Is there a role for postoperative irradiation? Int J Radiat Oncol Biol Phys 18(4):815–818

26. Garcia DM, Latifi HR, Simpson JR, Pickens S (1989) Astrocytoma of the cerebellum in children. J Neurosurg 71:661–664

27. Undjian S, Marinov M, Georgieve K (1989) Long-term follow-up after surgical treatment of cerebellar astrocytomas in 100 children. Childs Nerv Syst 5:99–101

28. Pagni CA, Giordama MT, Canarero S (1991) Benign recurrence of a pilocytic cerebellar astrocytoma 36 years after radical removal: Case report. Neurosurgery 28:606–609

29. O'Brien MS, Krisht A (1994) Cerebellar astrocytomas. In: Marlin AE, McLone DG, Reigel DH, Walker ML (eds) Paediatric neurosurgery. WB Saunders Co, Philadelphia, pp 356–361

30. Sutton LN, Packer RJ (1994) Medulloblastomas. In: Marlin AE, McLone DG, Reigel DH, Walker ML (eds) Paediatric neurosurgery. WB Saunders Co, Philadelphia, pp 362–373

31. Ellison D (2002) Classifying the medulloblastoma: Insights from morphology and molecular genetic. Neuropathol Appl Neurobiol 28:257–282

32. Brown HG, Kepner JL, et al. (2000) Large cell/anaplastic medulloblastoma: A Pediatric Oncology Group study. J Neuropathol Exp Neurol 59:857–865

33. Gajjar A, Hernan R, et al. (2004) Clinical histopatholgic and molecular markers of prognosis: Towards a new disease risk stratification system for medulloblastoma. J Clin Oncol 22:984–993

34. Park T, Hoffman H, Hendrick E, et al. (1983) Medulloblastoma, clinical presentation and management. Experience at the Hospital for Sick Children, Toronto, 1950–1980. J Neurosurg 58:543–552

35. Packer RJ, Gajjar A, et al. (2006) Phase III study of craniospinal radiation therapy followed by adjuvant chemotherapy for newly diagnosed average-risk medulloblastoma. J Clin Oncol 24:4202–4208

36. Roman DD, Sperduto PW (1995) Neuropsychological effects of cranial radiation: Current knowledge and future directions. Int J Radiat Oncol Biol Phys 31:983–998

37. Gerosa M, DiStefano E, Oliva A, et al. (1981) Multidisciplinary treatment of medulloblastoma. A 5-year experience with the SIOP trial. Childs Brain 8:107–118

38. Rutkowski S, Bode U, et al. (2005) Treatment of early childhood medulloblastoma by postoperative chemotherapy alone. N Engl J Med 352:978–986

39. Prados MD, Edwards MS, et al. (1999) Hyperfractionated craniospinal radiation therapy for primitive neuroectodermal tumours: Results of Phase II study. Int J Radiat Oncol Biol Phys 43:279–285

40. Duffner P, Cohen M, Anderson S, et al. (1983) Long-term effects of treatment on endocrine function in children with brain tumours. Ann Neurol 14:528–532

41. Ogilvy-Stuart AL, Shalet SM (1995) Growth and puberty after growth hormone treatment after irradiation for brain tumours. Arch Dis Child 73:141–146

42. Gentet JC, Doz F, et al. (1994) Carboplatin and VP 16 in medulloblastoma: A phase II study of the French Society of Paediatric Oncology (SFOP). Med Pediatr Oncol 23:422–427

43. Lefkowitz IB, Packer RJ, et al. (1990) Results of treatment of children with recurrent medulloblastoma/primitive neuroectodermal tumours with lomustine, cisplatin and vincristine. Cancer 65:412–417

44. Taylor RE, Bailey CC, et al. (2003) Results of a randomisation study of preradiation chemotherapy versus radiotherapy alone for non-metastactic medulloblastoma: The International Society of Paediatric Oncology/United Kingdom Children's Cancer Study Group PNET-2 Study. J Clin Oncol 21:1581–1591

45. Packer R, Sutton L, Goldwein J, et al. (1991) Improved survival with the use of adjuvant chemotherapy in the treatment of medulloblastoma. J Neurosurg 74:433–440

46. Stiller CA, Allen MB, Eatock EM (1995) Childhood cancer in Britain: The national registry of childhood tumours and incidence rates 1978–1987. Eur J Cancer 31A:2028–2034

47. Tomita T, McLone DG, Das L, et al. (1988) Benign ependymomas of the posterior fossa in childhood. Pediatr Neurosci 14:277–285

48. Wisoff JH (1994) Tumours of the cerebral hemispheres. In: Marlin AE, McLone DG, Reigel DH, Walker ML (eds) Paediatric neurosurgery. WB Saunders Co, Philadelphia, pp 392–402

49. Kleihues P, Bueger P, Scheithauer BW (1993) The new WHO classification of brain tumours. Brain Pathol 3:255–268

50. Tomita T (1994) Miscellaneous posterior fossa tumours. In: Marlin AE, McLone DG, Reigel DH, Walker ML (eds) Paediatric neurosurgery. WB Saunders Co, Philadelphia, pp 383–391

51. Pollack IF, Gerszten PC, Martinez AJ, et al. (1995) Intracranial ependymomas of childhood: Long-term outcome and prognostic factors. Neurosurgery 37:655–667

52. Healey EA, Barnes PD, Kupsky WJ, et al. (1991) The prognostic significance of postoperative residual tumor in ependymoma. Neurosurgery 28:666–672

53. Ross GW, Rubinstein LJ (1989) Lack of histopathological correlation of malignant ependymomas with postoperative survival. J Neurosurg 70:31–36

54. Jaing TH, Wang HS, et al. (2004) Multivariate analysis of clinical prognostic factors in children with intracranial ependymomas. J Neurooncol 68:255–261

55. Geyer JR, Sposto R, et al. (2005) Multiagent chemotherapy and deferred radiotherapy in infants with malignant brain tumours: A report from the Children's Cancer Group. J Clin Oncol 23:7621–7631

56. Duffner PK, Horowitz ME, Krischer JP, et al. (1993) Postoperative chemotherapy and delayed radiation in children less than three years of age with malignant brain tumors. New Engl J Med 328:1725–1731

57. Abbott R, Ragheb J, Epstein FJ (1994) Brainstem tumours: Surgical indications. In: Marlin AE, McLone DG, Reigel DH, Walker ML (eds) Paediatric neurosurgery. WB Saunders Co, Philadelphia, pp 374–82

58. Kaplan AM, Albright AL, et al. (1996) Brainstem gliomas in children. A Children's Cancer Group review of 119 cases. Pediatr Neurosurg 24:185–192

59. May PL, Blaser JI, Hoffman HJ, et al. (1991) Benign intrinsic tectal "tumours" in children. J Neurosurg 74:867–871

60. Hoffman HJ, Becker L, Craven MA (1980) A clinically and pathologically distinct group of benign gliomas. Neurosurgery 7:243–248

61. Epstein FJ, Farmer JP (1993) Brainstem glioma growth patterns. J Neurosurg 78:408–412

62. Dohrman GJ, Farwell JR, Flannery JT (1985) Astrocytomas in childhood: A population based study. Surg Neurol 23:64–68

63. Jooma R, Hayward RD, Grant DN (1984) Intracranial neoplasms during the first year of life: Analysis of one hundred consecutive cases. Neurosurgery 14:31–41

64. Duffner PK, Cohen MD, Myers MH, et al. (1986) Survival of children with brain tumours. SEER Programme 1973–1980. Neurology 36:597–601

65. Palma L, Guidetti B (1985) Cystic pilocytic astrocytomas of the cerebral hemispheres. Surgical experience with 51 cases and long-term results. J Neurosurg 62:811–815

66. Packer RJ, Ater J, Allen J, et al. (1997) Carboplatin and vincristine chemotherapy for children with newly diagnosed progressive low grade gliomas. J Neurosurg 86:747–754

67. Marchese MJ, Chang CH (1990) Malignant astrocytic gliomas in children. Cancer 65:2771–2778

68. Sposto R, Ertel IJ, Jenkin RDT, et al. (1989) The effectiveness of chemotherapy for the treatment of high-grade astrocytoma in children. Results of a randomized trial. J Neurooncol 7:165–177

69. Bower M, Newlands ES, et al. (1997) Multicentre CRC phase II trial of temozolomide in recurrent or progressive high-grade glioma. Cancer Chemother Pharmacol 40:484–488

70. Brada M, Hoang ZK, et al. (2001) Multicentre phase II trial of temozolomide in patients with glioblastoma multiforme at first relapse. Ann Oncol 2:259–266

71. Lashford LS, Thiesse P, et al. (2002) Temozolomide in malignant gliomas of childhood: A United Kingdom Children's Cancer Study Group and French Society of Pediatric Oncology Intergroup study. J Clin Oncol 20:4684–4691

72. Kun LE, Kovnar KH, Sanford RA (1988) Ependymomas in children. Pediatr Neurosci 14:57–63

73. Healey EA, Barnes PD, Kupsky WJ, et al. (1991) The prognostic significance of postoperative residual tumour in ependymoma. Neurosurgery 28:666–672

74. Nazar GB, Hoffman HJ, Becker LE, et al. (1990) Infratentorial ependymomas in childhood: Prognostic factors and treatment. J Neurosurg 72:408–417

75. Mork SJ, Lindegaard K-F, Halvorsen TN, et al. (1985) Oligodendroglioma: Incidence and biological behaviour in a defined population. J Neurosurg 63:881–889

76. Warnick RE, Edwards MSB (1991) Paediatric brain tumours. Curr Probl Pediat 21:129–173

77. Sutton LN, Packer J, Rorke LB, et al. (1983) Cerebral gangliogliomas during childhood. Neurosurgery 13:124–128

78. Drake JM, Hendrick EB, Becker LE, et al. (1985–1986) Intracranial meningiomas in children. Pediatr Neurosci 12:134–139

79. Johnson DL, McCullough DC (1994) Optic nerve gliomas and other tumours involving the optic nerve and chiasm. In: Marlin AE, McLone DG, Reigel DH, Walker ML (eds) Paediatric neurosurgery, 3rd edn. WB Saunders Co, Philadelphia, pp 409–417

80. Barkovich AJ, Edwards M (1990) CNS tumours. In: Barkovich AJ (ed) Paediatric neuroimaging. Raven Press, New York, pp 149–204

81. Jenkins D, Angyalfi S, Becker L, Berry M, Runcie R, et al. (1993) Optic glioma in children: Surveillance, resection, or irradiation. Int J Radiat Oncol Biol Phys 25:215–225

82. Hoffman HJ, Humphreys RP, Drake JM, Rutka JT, Becker LE, et al. (1993) Optic pathway/hypothalamic gliomas: A dilemma in management. Pediatr Neurosurg 19:186–195

83. Kestle JR, Hoffman HJ, Mock AR (1993) Moyamoya phenomenon after radiation for optic glioma. J Neurosurg 79:32–35

84. Petronio J, Edwards MS, Prados M, Freyberger S, Rabbitt J, et al. (1991) Management of chiasmal and hypothalamic gliomas of infancy and childhood with chemotherapy. J Neurosurg 74:701–708

85. Moghrabi A, Friedman HS, Burger PC, et al. (1993) Carboplatin treatment of progressive optic pathway gliomas to delay radiotherapy. J Neurosurg 79:223–227

86. Hoffman HJ, Kestle JRW (1994) Craniopharyngiomas. In: Marlin AE, McLone DG, Reigel DH, Walker ML (eds) Paediatric neurosurgery, 3rd edn. WB Saunders Co, Philadelphia, pp 418–428

87. Várady P (1996) Craniopharyngioma. In: Palmer JD (ed) Neurosurgery 96. Manual of neurosurgery. Chuchill Livingstone, Edinburgh, pp 257–263

88. Szeifert GT, Sipos L, Horváth M, Sarker MH, Major O, et al. (1993) Pathological characteristics of surgically removed craniopharyngiomas. Analysis of 131 cases. Acta Neurochir (Wien) 124:139–143

89. Hoffman HJ, da Silva M, Humphreys RP, et al. (1992) Aggressive surgical management of craniopharyngiomas in children. J Neurosurg 76:47–52

90. DeVile CJ, Grant DB, Kendall BE, Neville BGR, Stanhope R, et al. (1996) Management of childhood craniopharyngioma: Can the morbidity of radical surgery be predicted? J Neurosurg 85:73–81

91. Takahashi H, Nakazawa S, Shimura I (1985) Evaluation of postoperative intratumoral injection of bleomycin for craniopharyngioma in children. J Neurosurg 62:120–127

92. Edwards MSB, Baugmartner JE (1994) Pineal region tumours. In: Marlin AE, McLone DG, Reigel DH, Walker ML (eds) Paediatric neurosurgery, 3rd edn. WB Saunders Co, Philadelphia, pp 429–436

93. Hoffman HJ, Yoshida M, Becker LE, et al. (1983) Experience with pineal region tumours in childhood. Experiences at the Hospital for Sick Children. In: Humphreys RP (ed) Concepts in paediatric neurosurgery, vol 4. Karger, Basel, pp 360–386

94. Tien RD, Barkovich AF, Edwards MSB (1990) MR imaging of pineal tumours. Am J Neuroradiol II:557

95. Dearnaly DP, O'Hern RP, Whittaker S, et al. (1990) Pineal and CNS germ cell tumours: Royal Marsden Hospital experience 1962–1987. Int J Radiat Oncol Biol Phys 18:773

96. Abay EO, Laws ER, Grado GL, et al. (1981) Pineal tumours in children and adolescents: Treatment by shunting and radiotherapy. J Neurosurg 55:889–895

97. Edwards MSB, Hudgins RJ, Wilson CB (1988) Pineal region tumours in children. J Neurosurg 68:689–697

98. Regis J, Bouillot P, Rouby-Volot F, et al. (1996) Pineal region tumours and the role of stereotactic biopsy: Review of the mortality, morbidity and diagnostic rates in 370 cases. Neurosurgery 39:907–914

99. Ho DM, Wong T, Liu H (1991) Choroid plexus tumours in childhood: Histopathologic study and clinico-pathological correlation. Childs Nerv Syst 7:437–441

100. Coates TL, Hinshaw DB, Peckman N (1989) Paediatric choroid plexus neoplasm: MR, CT, and pathologic correlation. Radiology 173:81–88

101. Sanford RA, Donahue DJ (1994) Intraventricular tumours. In: Marlin AE, McLone DG, Reigel DH, Walker ML (eds) Paediatric neurosurgery, 3rd edn. WB Saunders Co, Philadelphia, pp 403–408

102. Pillay PK, Humphreys RP, St Clair S, et al. (1992) Choroid plexus carcinomas in children: A role for preresection chemotherapy. AANS Annual Meeting Programme 484 (abstr)

103. Park TS, Kaufman BA (1994) Tumours of the skull and metastatic brain tumours. In: Marlin AE, McLone DG, Reigel DH, Walker ML (eds) Paediatric neurosurgery, 3rd edn. WB Saunders Co, Philadelphia, pp 437–445

104. Ruge JR, Tomita T, Naidich TP, et al. (1988) Scalp and calvarial masses of infants and children. Neurosurgery 22:1037–1042

105. Matsumoto J, Towbin RB, Ball WS (1989) Craniofacial chordomas in infancy and childhood. A report of two cases and review of the literature. Pediatr Radiol 20:28

106. Di Lorenzo N, Giuffre R, Fortuna A (1982) Primary spinal neoplasms in childhood: Analysis by 1234 published cases (including 56 personal cases) by pathology, sex, age and site. Differences from the situation in adults. Neurochirurgia 25:153–164

107. Batnitzky S, Keucher TR, Mealey J Jr, et al. (1977) Iatrogenic intraspinal epidermoid tumours. J Am Med Assoc 237:148–150

108. Coulon RA (1994) Extramedullary spinal tumours. In: Marlin AE, McLone DG, Reigel DH, Walker ML (eds) Paediatric neurosurgery, 3rd edn. WB Saunders Co, Philadelphia, pp 458–472

109. McElwain TJ, Clink HM, Jameson B, et al. (1979) Central nervous system involvement in acute myelogenous leukaemia. In: Whitehouse JMA, Kay HE (eds) Central nervous system complications of malignant disease. Macmillan, London, pp 91–96

110. Epstein FJ, Ragheb J (1994) Intramedullary tumours of the spinal cord. In: Marlin AE, McLone DG, Reigel DH, Walker ML (eds) Paediatric neurosurgery, 3rd edn. WB Saunders Co, Philadelphia, pp 446–57

111. Sanders BM, Draper GJ, Kingston JC (1983) Retinoblastoma in Great Britain 1969–1980: Incidence, treatment and survival. Br J Ophthalmol 72:576–583

112. Antonelli C, Steinhorst F, Ribeiro K, et al. (2003) Extraocular retinoblastoma: A 13-year experience. Cancer 98:1292–1298

113. Stevenson KE, Hungeford JL, Garner A (1989) Local extension of retinoblastoma following intraocular surgery. Br J Ophthalmol 73:739–742

114. Canning R, McCartney ACE, Hungerford JL (1988) Medulloepithelioma (diktyoma). Br J Ophthalmol 72:764–767

115. JA Shields, CL Shields (1992) Intraocular tumours: A text and atlas. WB Saunders Co, Philadelphia, pp 320–332

116. Zimmerman LE, Brougthton WL (1978) A clinicopathologic and follow up study of fifty-six cases of intraocular medulloepithelioms. In: Jakobiec FA (ed) Ocular and adnexal tumours. Aesculapius, Birmingham, pp 181–196

117. Jumper MJ, Char DH, Howes EL, Bitner DG (1999) Neglected malignant medulloepithelioma of the eye. Orbit 18:37–43

118. Ayres B, Brasil OM, Klymberg C, et al. (2006) Ciliary body medulloepithelioma: Clinical, ultrasound biomicroscopic and histopathological correlation. Graefes Arch Clin Exp Ophthalmol 34:695–698

119. Davidorf FH, Craig E, Birnbaum L, Wakely P (2002) Management of medulloepithelioma of the ciliary body with brachytherapy. Am J Ophthalmol 133:841–843

120. Shields CL, Shields JA, Milite J, et al. (1991) Uveal melanomas in teenagers and children. A report of 40 cases. Ophthalmology 98:1662–1666

121. Palazzi MA, Ober MD, Abreu HF (2005) Congenital uveal malignant melanoma: A case report. Can J Ophthalmol 40:611–615

122. Neurofibromatosis. (1998) Conference statement. National Institutes of Health Consensus Development Conference. Arch Neurol Chicago 45:575–578

123. Daston MM, Scrable H, Nordlund M, et al. (1992) The protein product of the neurofibromatosis type 1 gene is expressed at highest abundance in neurons, Schwann cells and oligodendrocytes. Neuron 8:415–428

124. Listernick R, Louis DN, Packer J, et al. (1994) Optic pathway gliomas in children with neurofibromatosis type 1: Consensus statement from the NF1 optic pathway glioma study. J Paediatr Child Health 125:63–66

125. Sharif S, Ferner R, Birch JM, et al. (2006) Second primary tumours in neurofibromatosis 1 patients treated for optic glioma: Substantial risks after radiotherapy. J Clin Oncol 24:2570–2575

126. Listermick R, Darling C, Greenwald M, et al. (1995) Optic pathway tumours in children: The effect of neurofibromatosis type 1 on clinical manifestations and natural history. J Pediatr 127:718–722

Thoracic Tumors

19

Wendy Su, Jean-Martin Laberge

Contents

19.1 Introduction

Pediatric thoracic tumors are diverse and include a wide variety of disease processes. To facilitate the understanding of this subject, thoracic tumors will be discussed in the context of the different regions of the thorax: the chest wall, the lung parenchyma, the mediastinum, and the pleura. The lesions will be further divided according to their malignant potential and their tissue of origin, as the optimal treatment of the individual neoplasm depends on the specific histology.

19.2 Chest Wall Tumors

Chest wall tumors occur rarely in infants and children, accounting for only 1.8% of all solid childhood tumors [1, 2]. Chest wall neoplasms are primarily of mesenchymal origin and comprise a broad spectrum of benign and malignant lesions, arising from the skeletal or soft tissues of the chest wall. The majority are malignant in nature, with distinct behaviors and varying responses to chemotherapy and radiation [2, 3]. Benign tumors are less common in most series, although they may be underreported. Any growing chest wall mass in children should be evaluated promptly because of the high frequency of malignancy. The frequency of malignant tumors identified in nine pediatric series is shown in Table 19.1 [1, 4–11].

19.2.1 Benign Chest Wall Lesions

Pectus carinatum observed in the pubertal adolescent must be distinguished from a neoplasm. In this deformity the protruding costal cartilages can each be pal-

Table 19.1 Relative frequency of malignant chest wall tumors in children, compiled from 9 series[1, 2, 4, 6–11].

Tumor type	n (Total=104)	%
Ewing/PNET	57	54.8
Rhabdomyosarcoma	26	25
Fibrosarcoma	5	4.8
Osteosarcoma	3	2.9
Chondrosarcoma	3	2.9
Synovial sarcoma	2	1.9
Mesenchymal sarcoma	2	1.9
Others [a]	6	5.8

[a] Includes neuroblastoma (2), undifferentiated sarcoma (2), lymphoma and ectomesenchymoma

pated and the chest radiograph is normal. The lesion is often asymmetric and may be confused with a neoplastic growth. Other rib malformations such as bifid rib or focal rib/cartilage protuberance can be diagnosed with physical examination and plain chest radiograph. Usually the cartilage is the site of deformation rather than the bony rib. However, flaring of the anterior calcified part of the rib can usually be appreciated on plain rib radiographs, even though the cartilage deformity itself is not visible. Occasionally imaging with ultrasound is used to confirm the diagnosis and exclude a soft tissue tumor; rarely is CT scan indicated. Referral to a pediatric surgeon in uncertain cases should be done prior to extensive imaging workup.

The chest wall and axillae can be the site of soft tissue lesions encountered elsewhere in the body. Superficial lesions such as pilomatrixomas, dermoid, and epidermoid cysts are common. The latter typically presents in an infant as a pea-size subcutaneous mass below the clavicle with a skin dimple. Excision should be done before the cyst becomes infected or ruptured, which complicates management and results in a bigger scar. Other benign tumors include lymphangiomas and hemangiomas, lipomas and lipoblastomas. These usually are subcutaneous but may be intramuscular, and lymphangiomas can extend intrathoracically. All these lesions may increase dramatically in size. The benign nature can usually be established with imaging or by the presence of characteristic dermal markings in the case of hemangiomas. An incisional or excisional biopsy may be required to exclude soft tissue sarcoma in unclear cases. Lipoblastomas generally present in the first 3 years of life and may be seen at birth. This benign tumor is lobulated and localized; a more infiltrating form is called lipoblastomatosis. Histologically, they may mimic liposarcoma, which is extremely rare under the age of 10, but molecular genetic analysis can be used for definitive distinction [12]. Complete excision is indicated to prevent recurrence, which occurs in 9–22% of lipoblastomatosis.

Mesenchymal harmartoma, (also called vascular hamartoma of infancy or mesenchymoma) is a rare tumor usually noted in infancy, with 40% present at birth. It is a nonneoplastic proliferation of normal skeletal elements, predominantly cartilage [12]. There have not been any reports of malignant degeneration in the literature [13]. The lesion is mostly intrathoracic, but extrapleural, and involves a single or multiple ribs, usually in their posterior or lateral portion. The appearance is typical on chest radiograph (Fig. 19.1), but the intrathoracic component is best evaluated with cross-sectional imaging [14], the easiest to perform in infancy being computed tomography. The most common presentation is respiratory distress due to the mass effect [13, 15]. Several cases now have been diagnosed on prenatal ultrasound as a large thoracic

mass or a fetal pleural effusion [16, 17]. Conservative surgical resection should be performed only to relieve symptoms. Extensive resection of multiple ribs may produce severe scoliosis, thus observation rather than resection is recommended in asymptomatic patients, especially since spontaneous regression may be observed [13, 15–18].

Fibrous hamartoma of infancy is a different entity from chest wall hamartoma. It is a rare, poorly circumscribed, rapidly growing, and superficial soft tissue mass that occurs most frequently in the anterior or posterior axillary fold. There is a marked male predominance. Up to 25% are present at birth and most are diagnosed in the first 2 years of life [12]. Recurrence is rare after excision and usually cured by re-excision.

Other benign tumors can affect the ribs or clavicle. Lesions such as Langerhans cell histiocytosis (the localized form of which was previously referred to as eosinophilic granuloma), aneurysmal bone cyst, and fibrous dysplasia produce intraosseous lesions within the ribs. Radiographically, these lesions typically demonstrate cortical expansion and thinning with a lytic center (Fig.19.2). A chondroma, osteochondroma, or osteoma of the rib will often have characteristic radiographic findings, consisting of a well-defined, ovoid, expansile mass with diffuse or stippled calcification. Unless the imaging is typical, an incisional or excisional biopsy may be necessary to establish the diagnosis for all these lesions. Most are self-limited and follow a benign course, with the exception of the disseminated form of Langerhans cell histiocytosis, which may require chemotherapy to limit the progression of lytic bone lesions and the visceral involvement [19].

Various fibrous tumors can affect the chest wall. Myofibroma and its multicentric counterpart, myofibromatosis, also called congenital generalized fibromatosis, is a benign tumor that is most often detected at birth or in the first 2 years of life. Males are more often affected and familial cases are reported [12]. Some lesions regress spontaneously, and recurrence after excision is uncommon. The prognosis is different when this tumor affects internal organs such as the lungs. Aggressive fibromatosis (or desmoid-type fibromatosis) is locally infiltrative with a tendency for local recurrence, but it does not metastasize. In children this tumor has an equal sex incidence and is usually extra-abdominal, unlike its adult counterpart. Attempts to achieve tumor-free resection margins may result in significant morbidity, and the lesion may ultimately prove fatal, especially if the head and neck are involved [12]. Radiation therapy may be effective but can be associated with significant morbidity [20]. Chemotherapy using vinblastine and methotrexate has been used [21]. A current Children Oncology Group trial is evaluating the safety and efficacy of sulindac, a COX-1 and COX-2 inhibitor, and tamoxifen, an anti-estrogen

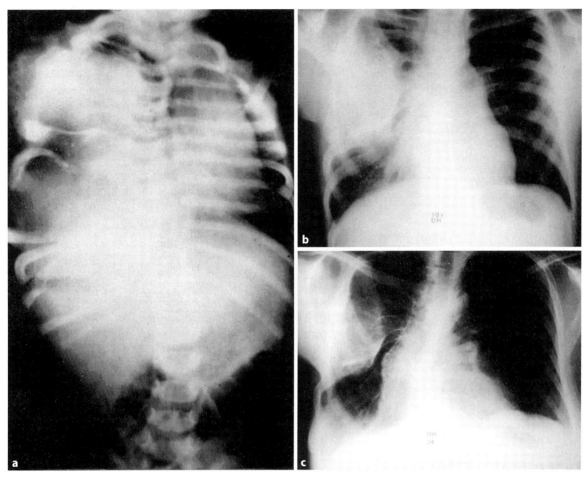

Fig. 19.1a–c (a) Chest radiograph of a 3-month-old girl who presented in 1955 with respiratory distress. Multiple firm masses were palpable in the right axilla. This study demonstrated a large mass nearly filling the right hemithorax. Multiple ribs were involved and calcification was seen within the mass. Extensive bleeding occurred at exploration so only an incisional biopsy was performed. (b) The follow-up radiograph at 10 years of age showed progressive decrease in size of the mass in relation to the hemithorax with functioning lung visible on the right side. (Reproduced with permission from Blumenthal BI, Capitanio MA, Queloz JM, et al. (1972) Intrathoracic mesenchymomas. Radiology 104:107–109). (c) Radiograph at 24 years of age when the patient was admitted for delivery of her first child. The mass has continued to decrease proportionately in size. (Reproduced with permission from John A Kirkpatrick.)

drug, for recurrent tumors or those not amenable to surgery or radiotherapy. Both agents have shown an effect in adult-type desmoid tumors and anecdotally in children [22].

19.2.2 Malignant Chest Wall Lesions

19.2.2.1 Ewing/PNET

This is the most common tumor in all pediatric series of chest wall lesions. It is the second most common sarcoma in bone and soft tissue in children. It occurs primarily in children and young adults with a median age of 13–16 years [23]. In purely pediatric series, the mean age is around 9 years [24]. Up to 6.5% of primary lesions arise in the chest wall. There has been controversy regarding terminology and histogenesis in this entity. Ewing's sarcoma traditionally referred to an undifferentiated small round cell tumor arising in the bone. Tumors exhibiting neuroectodermal differentiation by light microscopy, immunohistochemistry, or electron microscopy were considered distinct and termed primitive neuroectodermal tumors (PNET) [12, 25]. To complicate matters, in 1979, Askin, et al. segregated a group of tumors of soft tissue origin arising in the thoracopulmonary region, with distinct characteristics including a high local recurrence rate, a low risk of systemic spread, and neuroepithelial differentiation [26]. To decrease confusion in this group

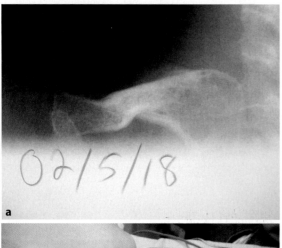

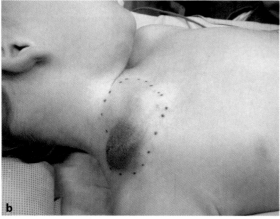

Fig. 19.2 a, b (**a**) Expansile lesion of right clavicle with cortical thinning in a 3-year-old boy. (**b**) The soft tissue mass is outlined. The tumor was eroding through the skin. Ewing's sarcoma/PNET was suspected but biopsy showed Langerhans cell histiocytosis. The patient was treated with prednisone and vinblastine for 6 months and made a full recovery.

of related tumors, Shamberger proposed the term "malignant small round cell tumor" [5]. However, this term has been abandoned in this setting as it is used by pathologists in a broader sense and includes other tumors such as neuroblastoma. Recent immunoperoxidase and cytogenetic studies have confirmed that PNET and Ewing's sarcoma are the same entity and should be considered to be of neuroectodermal derivation [12, 27]. The term Ewing's sarcoma/PNET is now currently used in pathology textbooks, and "Askin tumor" has been gradually abandoned. The typical cytogenetic finding in the Ewing family of tumors is a balanced translocation between chromosomes 11 and 22 [28, 29]. These translocations result in fusion of the EWS gene on chromosome 22 with the FLI1 gene on chromosome 11 or the ERG gene on chromosome 21, both members of the ETS family of transcription factors [30].

Ewing's sarcoma/PNET is an extremely aggressive tumor with frequent metastatic spread and local recurrence, and should be considered as a systemic disease at presentation [23, 31]. The most common presentations are palpable mass, cough, or pain. Respiratory distress from a large malignant pleural effusion or an extensive intrathoracic involvement is less frequent (Fig. 19.3). The most common site of tumor involvement is the rib/intercostal bundle, followed by the clavicle, sternum, scapula, and soft tissues [4, 11]. The evaluation of a suspected chest wall tumor should begin with standard chest radiographs. Both local extension and distant metastasis can be evaluated with computed tomography (CT) scan, to better define the presence of bony involvement, the extent of the soft tissue mass, and the presence of a pleural effusion or pulmonary nodules. A bone scan is appropriate to exclude osseous metastases. The bone scan further defines the extent of primary disease within the rib and the presence of intramedullary "skip" metastasis, which is now preferentially assessed on MRI. Bone marrow aspirate and biopsy are also recommended, and brain scan may be appropriate in selected cases.

The initial intervention is usually an incisional or needle biopsy of the mass. Occasionally a large pleural effusion may yield a sufficient number of malignant cells to establish the diagnosis. When an incisional biopsy is required, proper placement of the incision to avoid compromise of the future resection is of paramount importance. However, adequate diagnostic material for standard histologic, cytogenetic, and biologic studies can usually be obtained with multiple core needle biopsies [32]. In most cases, once the diagnosis is confirmed, chemotherapy is administered prior to definitive surgical resection. Primary resection is limited to the very small lesions, usually those less than 3 cm. Neoadjuvant chemotherapy will generally render the tumor more easily resectable as a result of the decrease in size, vascularity, and sterilizing the margins [4, 33–35], allowing for a more limited resection (Fig. 19.4) [36]. Surgical resection is generally performed after four cycles of chemotherapy, and should be done to achieve local control even if there is no apparent residual tumor. The general approach is to perform a wide excision of all the involved structures, regardless of size [11, 37]. The minimal acceptable margins are 2–5 cm for bone, 5 mm for soft tissues, and 2 mm for periosteum or perichondrium. Whenever possible, an attempt is made to preserve the posterior segment of the rib to minimize the risk or extent of scoliosis [23]. However, Ewing's sarcoma can have "skip lesions" within the marrow cavity [38], and should be investigated prior to resection with either bone scan or magnetic resonance imaging. The adjacent portion of the ribs immediately above and below the involved rib, the attached muscles, and the underlying pleura all should be excised [39]. The resec-

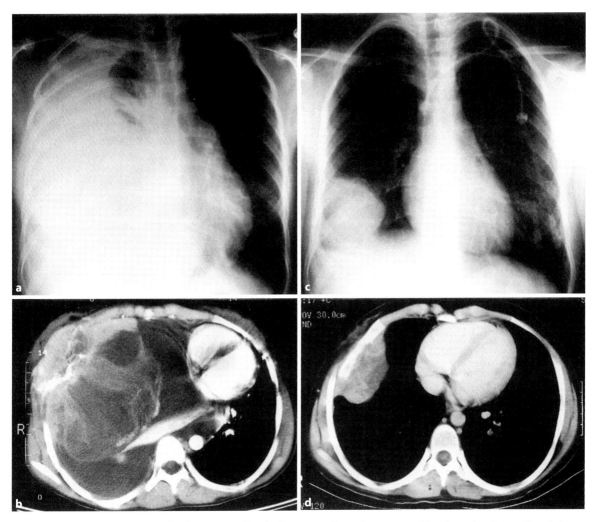

Fig. 19.3 a–d (**a**) Chest radiograph of a 13-year-old girl who presented with a 2-week history of fever, cough, and progressive shortness of breath. Initial chest radiograph showed a large pleural effusion on the right side with erosion of the anterior portion of the 5th rib. (**b**) CT scan subsequently confirmed the effusion as well as a large mass arising from the chest wall and almost filling the hemithorax. Destruction of rib is apparent. Chest radiograph (**c**) and CT scan (**d**) after 3 months of chemotherapy show marked resolution in the size of the tumor.

tion should include any tissue that resembles scarred or residual tumor [31]. The same principles are used for tumors of the sternum and the clavicle, with complete removal of the involved and adjacent structures [39]. The available surgical strategies will be discussed below.

Although the radiosensitivity of this tumor was established by Ewing in his early descriptions, relatively high doses are required [40]. Radiotherapy is used to achieve local control in other sites, but it is associated with significant morbidity for children with chest wall tumors. This includes scoliosis, growth retardation, lung damage, potentiation of the cardiotoxicity of doxorubicin, and a 10–30% risk of secondary malignancy [23, 41–43]. It is usually reserved for tumors that remain unresectable after the 12-week induction

phase, for margins that are microscopically involved after resection, and for patients who have an initial malignant pleural effusion.

Postoperatively, adjuvant chemotherapy is administered to prevent or treat distant metastases and potential pleural seeding [5]. Chemotherapy for Ewing/PNET primarily utilizes a doxorubicin-based regimen, with vincristine, actinomycin-D, and cyclophosphamide (Adria-VAC). Its effectiveness was confirmed in a randomized trial on Ewing tumor at all sites, performed jointly by the Pediatric Oncology Group (POG) and the Children's Cancer Study Group (CCSG) [44]. The response to induction chemotherapy has been shown to correlate with event-free survival [45]. The second intergroup study utilized intermittent high-dose therapy with Adria-VAC and showed an increase

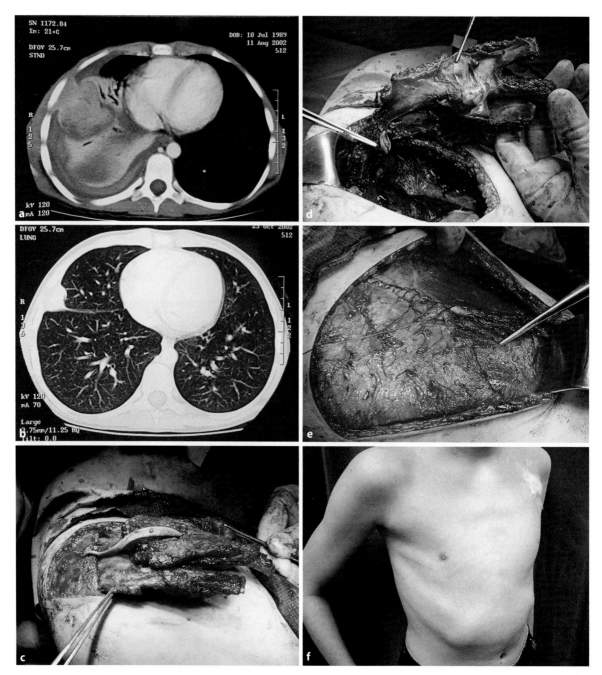

Fig. 19.4 a–f Ewing's sarcoma/PNET in a 12-year-old boy. (**a**) Large pedunculated chest wall tumor with a malignant pleural effusion at presentation. (**b**) Remarkable response after induction chemotherapy with vincristine, doxorubicin, and cyclophosphamide, alternating with ifosfamide and etoposide, for a total of 12 weeks. (**c**) Chest wall resection including 4th, 5th, and 6th ribs and attached muscles and skin (percutaneous biopsy site). Note latissimus dorsi posteriorly. (**d**) Undersurface of ribs showing 2 areas of adherent lung stapled across and resected with the specimen. (**e**) Chest wall reconstructed by detaching the anterior part of the 7th rib from the sternum and resuturing it to the anterior remnant of the 5th rib cartilage. The latissimus dorsi is mobilized and approximated to the pectoralis major and the rectus abdominis to cover the defect without foreign material. (**f**) Result 9 months after surgery. The patient had received postoperative radiotherapy and chemotherapy. He remains disease-free 4 years postoperatively.

in the relapse-free 5-year survival of localized non-pelvic tumors to 73% [46]. The third intergroup study used Adria-VAC alternating with courses of ifosfamide and etoposide and demonstrated additional efficacy in patients with nonmetastatic Ewing's sarcoma [47]. Patients with metastatic disease had an 8-year survival of 32% with standard treatment; this was not improved with the addition of ifosfamide/etoposide [48]. Results of the European Intergroup Cooperative Ewing's Sarcoma Studies showed that patients with primary metastatic disease have an improved outcome after receiving myeloablative megatherapy and stem cell rescue following conventional treatment [49].

The analysis of the third POG/CCSG intergroup study demonstrated no difference in event-free survival between patients with primary chest wall resection and those who were resected after neoadjuvant chemotherapy. However, complete surgical resection is more likely accomplished after neoadjuvant chemotherapy compared to primary resection, and fewer patients require radiation therapy to the chest wall [31].

19.2.2.2 Rhabdomyosarcoma

Rhabdomyosarcoma (RMS) is a malignant tumor of striated muscle origin that commonly occurs in the pediatric age group, accounting for 5% of all pediatric solid tumors (see Chap. 14). It is the second most common malignancy arising from the chest wall. Relatively speaking, RMS in the trunk is rare, comprising only 4–7% of all RMS in the Intergroup Rhabdomyosarcoma Study (IRS)-I, -II, and -III reports, and about half of those originated from the chest wall [50–52]. The IRS is responsible for the development and advances of the multimodal treatment protocols over the last 30 years. The presenting symptoms, initial diagnostic steps, and operative strategy are similar to those discussed for Ewing/PNET, except that chest wall RMS may present in younger children. Treatment is based not only on pretreatment stage, but also on postoperative clinical group. The stage, clinical grouping, histological type, and site of the primary tumor are combined to stratify patients in low-, intermediate-, and high-risk groups. These are discussed in detail in the chapter on soft tissue sarcomas (Chap. 14). Unlike RMS at other sites, the alveolar type is more common than the embryonal type for the chest wall; the alveolar histology is associated with a poorer prognosis in general, but histological type is not of prognostic value for chest wall RMS.

The primary tumor site is an important prognostic determinant for RMS [9], and the chest wall tumors are associated with a poor prognosis [50–53]. Several factors associated with unfavorable outcome after treatment of chest wall RMS have been identified, including tumor size greater than 5 cm, advanced stage

at presentation, local and distant tumor recurrence, but not histologic subtype [9, 11, 50, 54]. The unfavorable outcome of chest wall RMS may be due to a different biology than RMS of more favorable sites. Because these tumors become symptomatic only when large or advanced, they are detected later than tumors at other sites. Involvement of the pleura makes complete surgical resection more difficult, which also may contribute to inferior outcomes [50]. An analysis of 84 children with thoracic sarcomas treated in IRS-II and IRS-III documents the difficulty in achieving a cure for these children [50]. Seventy-six cases were chest wall tumors and the rest were pulmonary (3 cases), pleural (4 cases), and cardiac tumors (1 case). Thirteen patients presented as group I (localized disease, completely resected), 18 as group II (microscopic residual or nodal disease), 31 as group III (gross residual disease or biopsy only), and 22 as group IV (distant metastatic disease). Sixty children (71%) achieved a complete response, seven a partial response, three showed improvement, and 14 had no response or progressed. Of the 60 children with a complete response, 28 had a local recurrence and 11 had a distant recurrence. Only clinical group and recurrence showed statistical significance for overall survival in the multivariate analysis [50]. As expected, outcome was better for patients with totally resected or microscopically residual tumor after resection. Ironically, a higher rate of recurrence occurred in Group I (54%) compared to Group II (27%) suggesting difficulties in accurate pathologic assessment of margin status. As Group I patients were felt to have a complete tumor resection, most did not receive radiation. In contrast, all but two of the Group II patients received 4,000–4,500 cGy to the primary site. These findings suggest that the adequacy of local tumor resection must be very carefully evaluated and may require re-resection for confirmation of margin status and to achieve complete resection. Saenz, et al. reported 15 patients with chest wall primaries (5% of all RMS from Memorial Sloan-Kettering Cancer Center) [55]. Nearly all patients received upfront surgical resection but only 60% had a complete resection; almost all patients received radiation and multiagent chemotherapy, with an overall disease-free survival at 5 years of 66%, the highest reported in the literature [55]. Chui, et al. from St. Jude's Children's Hospital reported 33 patients with truncal RMS among which 20 patients (61%) had a chest wall primary tumor [54]. Tumors 5 cm or smaller were amenable to upfront surgical resection. In patients with tumors larger than 5 cm, either upfront or delayed resection was associated with a 10-year overall survival of 57% compared with 8% in those who had no surgery. Tumor recurrence was local in 44% of cases, and survival after local recurrence was rare (1 of 8). Local treatment failure occurred in 14% of patients treated with gross total resection with or without radiotherapy and in 36% of patients treated with definitive radiotherapy alone. Although this difference was not statistically significant, it underscored the importance of complete tumor resection in the treatment of chest wall RMS [54].

The high local recurrence rate seen in the IRS review and the St. Jude series suggest that there is a need to obtain better local tumor control, incorporating chemotherapy, surgical resection, and radiation. Small chest wall tumors that can be readily resected with adequate margins should have upfront resection followed by appropriate chemotherapy regimen. If the margin is positive after initial diagnostic excisional biopsy, "pretreatment re-excision" should be performed prior to chemotherapy [56]. Frozen section ensuring negative margins is recommended. An arbitrary margin of 0.5 cm circumferentially or an uninvolved fascial margin are considered necessary by the Soft Tissue Sarcoma Committee of the Children's Oncology Group [56]. Large tumors requiring mutilating resection or invading critical structures should receive incisional or core needle biopsy to establish the diagnosis. After 12 weeks of chemotherapy the patient is evaluated by imaging studies as to the potential for complete gross and microscopic excision. Thoracoscopy is sometimes helpful to evaluate the extent of pleural involvement and the presence of any adherence to the lung parenchyma [56]. The excision should include the previous biopsy site and be wide enough to remove the involved chest wall muscles, ribs, and even wedge resection of underlying lung if necessary. It is not necessary to remove the entire length of the rib, or the rib above and below, unless clear margins cannot be obtained otherwise. Wider margins than for other sites are recommended (preferably 2 cm) because of the higher local recurrence rate of chest wall primaries. If the tumor is completely resected with no microscopic or macroscopic residual, no postoperative radiotherapy is required. If the margin is microscopically positive, radiotherapy is required. However, because of the high local recurrence rate, there is a suggestion that additional radiotherapy may benefit all patients with chest wall RMS [50, 55]. Complete or gross total resection, whether upfront or after chemotherapy, will yield superior survival compared with those who never underwent surgical resection based on the St. Jude's series (66% vs. 13% 10-year overall survival) [54]. Assessment of regional lymph node status is also crucial in the management of RMS. Chest wall tumors may drain to the axillary, internal mammary, or infraclavicular nodes, and may require lymphatic mapping to identify the draining lymph node basin unless adenopathy is obvious on physical exam or imaging studies [54, 57].

In general, the 5-year survival for localized RMS is 70%, but it is only 50% for trunk RMS [9, 58]. The analysis of patients with thoracic sarcomas treated in IRS-II and IRS-III showed an estimated 5-year survival at 59% for group I patients, 75% for group II, 44% for group III, and 0 for group IV; the decreased survival in group I compared to group II patients was attributed to a higher local recurrence rate in group I patients as discussed above [50]. The chemotherapy regimen itself is guided by risk assignment. Low-risk group patients receive only vincristine (V) and actinomycin-D (A), plus cyclophosphamide (C) or radiation. Intermediate-risk children receive VAC and dose intensification for those with gross total resection. High-risk patients are those with metastatic disease; they are treated with alternating cycles of VDC (D = doxorubicin) and ifosfamide/etoposide. Additional therapeutic agents using topoisomerase-1 inhibitors such as irinotecan are being evaluated for the high-risk group [58]. Current trials study the effects of irinotecan as an additional agent to the 6 cytotoxic drugs described above, as well as its effect when given as a radiosensitizer during the course of radiotherapy.

In summary, specific considerations for rhabdomyosarcoma of the chest wall are no different from RMS in other locations. Initial detailed metastatic workup is essential to establish the stage of disease [55]. Efforts should be made to remove all visible tumor with an adequate negative margin whenever possible. If initial resection will result in significant morbidity, biopsy is done, followed by chemotherapy and either surgical resection if feasible or preoperative radiotherapy. Surgical resection for residual disease with possible chest wall reconstruction is performed subsequently.

19.2.2.3 Other Chest Wall Tumors

Chondrosarcoma may occur in the pediatric age range in rare occasions, arising usually from the anterior costo-chondral or chondro-sternal junction. As in adults, this is primarily a locally invasive tumor, which responds poorly to chemotherapy or radiotherapy. Aggressive surgical resection following initial biopsy of chondrosarcoma is appropriate. Prognosis is correlated with histologic grade and extent of resection. Wide excision with a 5-cm margin, including a normal rib above and one below the involved rib, together with the underlying pleura, can result in a 96% 10-year survival [59].

Osteosarcoma may rarely arise from the ribs. In contrast to chondrosarcoma, osteosarcomas tend to have earlier hematogenous spread, especially to the lungs, and are responsive to chemotherapy and radiotherapy. As with extremity lesions, initial incisional biopsy followed by neoadjuvant chemotherapy is utilized prior to surgical resection. Local control of osteosarcoma is rarely achieved by chemotherapy and radiotherapy alone. Survival is directly related to the

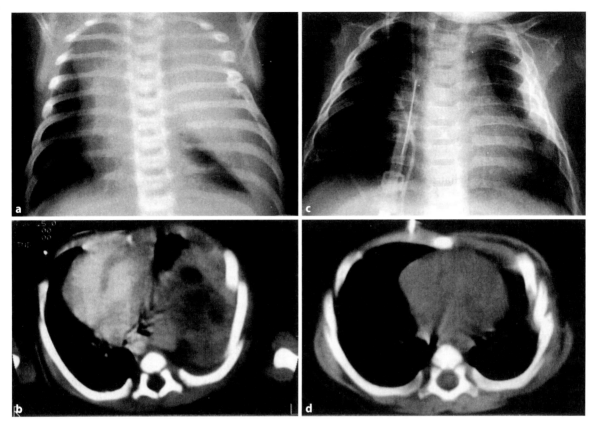

Fig. 19.5 a–d (**a**) Chest radiograph of a newborn child with extensive infantile fibrosarcoma of the left chest. (**b**) CT scan of the same child showing the extensive intrathoracic lesion. (**c**) Follow-up radiograph of the infant after five courses of vincristine, actinomycin, cyclophosphamide (VAC) and doxorubicin and two courses of VAC demonstrating marked tumor regression. (**d**) Follow up CT scan demonstrating the marked tumor regression and small residual lesion. (Reproduced with permission from Shamberger RC, Grier HE, Weinstein HJ, et al. (1989) Chest wall tumors in infancy and childhood. Cancer 63; 774–785.)

presence of metastatic disease as well as the completeness of resection of the primary tumor.

Congenital or infantile fibrosarcoma, (known under several other names, including aggressive infantile fibromatosis) often presents at birth. It accounts for 12% of soft tissue malignancies in infancy, but is more common in the extremities [12]. When it involves the chest wall, it must be distinguished from benign mesenchymal hamartoma. Cytogenetic analysis of the biopsy specimen for the presence of a chromosomal translocation (exchange of material between 12p and 15q, resulting in oncogenic activation of the TRKC receptor tyrosine kinase gene) can be helpful in making the diagnosis [60]. These tumors are responsive to treatment with vincristine, actinomycin-D, and cyclophosphamide (VAC) or doxorubicin in conjunction with VAC [60–62]. In infants with a large congenital fibrosarcoma, initial treatment with chemotherapy can result in significant tumor reduction to allow for a much less extensive resection (Fig. 19.5). Smaller tumors may be treated with resection alone [60].

19.2.2.4 Surgical Resection and Reconstruction

The goals of chest wall resection and reconstruction as defined by Grosfeld include complete removal of the local tumor, restoration of adequate protection of the thoracic viscera, restoration of physiologic function providing for adequate lung and chest wall growth, and an acceptable chest wall appearance [4]. Chest wall resection can be achieved via a standard thoracotomy incision, which should include the initial biopsy site. Serratus anterior or pectoralis muscles may need to be excised with appropriate margins. The extent of rib resection depends on the type of tumor and was already discussed. The importance of surgical resection has been stressed in prior discussions. Incisions must be appropriately placed to allow preservation of overlying skin and, if possible, muscle flaps. In most cases, resection of one or multiple ribs is required. The resulting defect can either be closed primarily or may require chest wall reconstruction.

Reconstruction of a chest wall defect can be difficult. The primary consideration is usually the size and location of the bony and soft tissue defect, although factors such as preoperative pulmonary function, previous chest wall surgery or radiotherapy, and cosmetic considerations can be important. Reconstruction of segments of the chest wall is performed to protect underlying structures, to obtain chest wall rigidity and fixation for effective respiratory effort, to prevent flail segments and reduce paradoxical movements, and prevent herniation. Small defects (those involving fewer than three ribs) can usually be covered primarily with muscle and skin; those greater than 5 cm often require chest wall reconstruction, as a large flail segment would otherwise result. Location is important. Posterior defects of up to 10 cm in diameter can be tolerated as long as the scapula remains to provide stability. Generally, resection of ribs 1 to 4 posteriorly is well tolerated, but if resection also involves the fifth and sixth ribs, additional support is necessary to prevent the scapula from becoming caught below the lower ribs. Resections that include the lower ribs can be reconstructed by reapproximating the diaphragm to the lowest remaining rib. This transforms a thoracic defect into an abdominal defect, which has less physiological consequences. However, this technique cannot be used if the resection extends above the fifth rib. Defects involving the sternum should be reconstructed to protect underlying structures and to prevent the paradoxical motion that occurs with removal of the anterior costal attachments. Defects involving midthoracic segments can be reconstructed with a rib transposition, by disinserting the anterior portion of the rib below the defect from the sternum and fixing it back to the sternum or the remaining extremity of a resected rib in the middle of the defect (Fig. 19.4). We prefer to avoid the use of prosthetic materials whenever possible to decrease the risks of infection and complications related to radiation therapy.

Several materials and techniques have been used to reconstruct large chest wall defects, including fascia lata, omental transplants, contralateral rib grafts, assorted muscle flaps, and numerous prosthetic materials [63, 64]. Prosthetic materials including Marlex (Bard Vascular Systems Division, Billerica, MA), Gore-tex (WL Gore, Co., Flagstaff, AZ) and collagen-coated vinyl mesh have been used to replace missing sections of the chest wall. Gore-tex was the synthetic replacement fabric of choice for chest wall reconstructions in children suggested by Grosfeld, et al. [4]. In larger lesions, a "sandwich" created using two sheets of Marlex mesh and methyl methacrylate can be used. This composite can be shaped to match the contour of the chest wall and produce a solid reconstruction, with the advantages of minimizing paradoxical motion and allowing earlier weaning from the ventilator

[4, 33, 65]. The major deterrence to use of these prosthetic materials in the young infant or growing child is that they do not expand as the child grows and may result in more severe scoliosis than occurs if the defect is closed with living tissue. Prosthetic materials provide a rigid base for reconstructing chest wall defects, but the overlying soft tissue must also be replaced. The pectoralis major, latissimus dorsi, and rectus abdominus myocutaneous flaps, and the greater omentum are all available for use [64]. The latissimus dorsi is particularly useful for pediatric surgeons; it can be based on its superior or inferior pedicle, and can be used in toto or only in part, thus preserving the posterior axillary fold [66]. A pedicled composite osteomuscular flap using the 6th, 8th, and 10th ribs with the latissimus dorsi and serratus anterior has also been described [67]. Free vascularized tissue flaps, created using microsurgical techniques, have recently been used to provide soft tissue coverage of chest wall defects. The tensor fascia lata free flap, which consists of the tensor fascia lata muscle and its overlying fascia and skin, is based on the lateral femoral circumflex vessels. These vessels are anastomosed to either the thoracoacromial or transverse cervical vessels. It is also possible to use vascularized fibular bone grafts to replace missing ribs [68, 69].

19.2.2.5 Long-term Complications

Scoliosis. Scoliosis is a well-established complication of chest wall resection. The severity of the curve is directly related to the number of ribs resected. Resection of the posterior segment of ribs produces more scoliosis than resection of the anterior segments. Similarly, resection of lower ribs produces a greater curve than resection of upper ribs [70]. The convexity of the curve is generally toward the resected side unless there is marked pleural scarring from radiation or empyema (Fig. 19.6). Radiation can also affect growth of the hemivertebrae on the radiated side. Scoliosis is often progressive until the child reaches full stature and therefore requires long-term follow-up. Two of eight long-term survivors in the Indiana series required Harrington rod correction of their severe scoliosis [4].

Restrictive pulmonary function. Pulmonary function has not been extensively evaluated in these patients. Grosfeld performed pulmonary function tests in 13 of his 15 patients undergoing resection [4]. The forced vital capacity (FVC), forced expiratory volume, and functional residual capacities (FRC) studied from 1 month to 10 years after surgery demonstrated minimal early reduction in the FRC and FVC. Progressive worsening over time was noted, with all patients eventually demonstrating pulmonary restrictive disease. This was worsened by the development of scoliosis that was severe enough to warrant surgery in two patients. Further long-term evaluation studies are warranted.

Secondary tumors. The risk of secondary malignancy is estimated at 10–30% following treatment for Ewing's sarcoma/PNET. This is most frequent within the first 5 years but can still occur after 25 years [41–43]. One patient from a recent Italian series developed bronchioloalveolar carcinoma 7 years after treatment of Ewing's sarcoma/PNET of the rib and died of disease a year later [71]. Although no additional patients reported with chest wall sarcoma have developed a secondary sarcoma, their occurrence at other sites from similar treatment is well established [41–43, 71, 72]. The most common secondary malignancies include secondary sarcomas, acute myeloblastic and lymphoblastic leukemias, and bronchioloalveolar carcinoma among others [73]. A sharp increase in risk occurs with doses of radiation greater than 60 Gy. This has stimulated recent efforts to resect the primary tumor and limit the total dose of radiation [72]. Minimizing the dose and area of radiation will decrease the risks for both secondary sarcomas as well as restrictive pulmonary disease. Leukemias have been reported in several series following the use of alkylating agents as well [5, 74, 75].

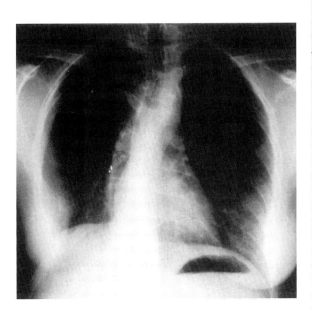

Fig. 19.6 Chest radiograph of a 20-year-old woman who underwent resection at 14 years of age of a histiocytic lymphoma of the chest wall. She had removal of the entire right 7th rib and portions of the 6th and 8th ribs. Reconstruction was with Marlex mesh. This radiograph demonstrates scoliosis which is convex to the side of the resection. (Reproduced with permission from Shamberger RC (1994) Chest wall tumors in infants and children. Semin Pediatr Surg 3: 267–276)

19.3 Pulmonary Parenchymal Tumors

Primary pulmonary tumors are rare in infants and children. The spectrum of pediatric lung tumors is quite different from that occurring in adults [76]. The majority of pulmonary neoplasms in children are malignant in nature, and metastatic lesions are far more common than primary malignancy. In a review by Hartman and Shochat of 230 patients with primary pulmonary tumors, two-thirds were malignant [77]. Hancock, et al. later expanded the review to include 383 primary pulmonary lesions in children, showing that three quarters of all lesions were malignant and one quarter were benign (Table 19.2) [78].

Although children with primary lung tumors represent a heterogeneous group, the evaluation and

Table 19.2 Primary pulmonary tumors in 383 infants and children

Type of tumor	No. (%)*	Mets	Rec	Death	Cyst
Benign	92				
Inflammatory	48 (52.2)		2	4	
Hamartoma	22 (23.9)			4	4
Neurogenic tumor	9 (9.8)				
Leiomyoma	6 (6.5)				
Mucous gland adenoma	3 (3.3)				
Myoblastoma	3 (3.3)				
Benign teratoma	1 (1.1)				
Malignant	291				
Bronchial "adenoma"	118 (40.5)	7	2	1	
Bronchogenic	49 (16.8)	most		44	3
Pulmonary blastoma	45 (15.5)	9	14	19	9
Fibrosarcoma	28 (9.6)		1	9	
Rhabdomyosarcoma	17 (5.8)		3	2	6
Leiomyosarcoma	11 (3.8)		1	5	
Sarcoma	6 (2.1)			2	4
Hemangiopericytoma	4 (1.4)	1		2	
Plasmacytoma	4 (1.4)	2	2	1	
Lymphoma	3 (1.0)				
Teratoma	3 (1.0)			2	
Mesenchymoma	2 (0.7)				2
Myxosarcoma	1 (0.3)			1	

Mets, metastases; Rec, recurrence; Cyst, previous pulmonary cystic malformation

*(%) is percent of benign or percent of malignant tumors.

Reproduced with permission from [78]

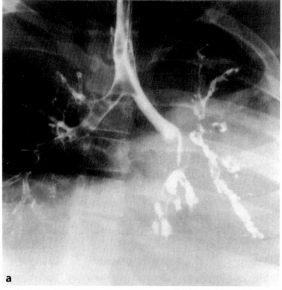

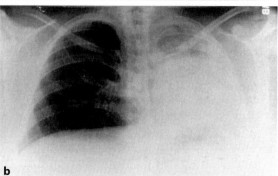

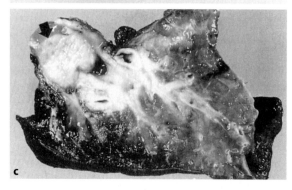

Fig. 19.7 a–c (**a**) A 10-year-old female presented with a 2-month history of left-sided chest pain. A chest radiograph demonstrated collapse of the entire left lung. Attempts at physiotherapy, bronchoscopy, and lavage were unsuccessful at obtaining re-expansion prior to the child's referral for definitive therapy. Bronchoscopy demonstrated a mass obstructing the left main stem bronchus and a bronchogram (**b**) confirmed near complete occlusion of left main stem bronchus with extensive distal bronchiectasis. She was successfully resected with a "sleeve resection" of the main stem bronchus and re-anastomosis of the upper lobe to the carina, but with resection of the lower lobe due to her severe bronchiectasis and extensive parenchymal disease of the lobe. (**c**) Surgical specimen demonstrates the carcinoid tumor (*arrow, top left*) occluding the left bronchus.

treatment are similar in the majority of patients [77, 78]. Most children with benign lesions are asymptomatic, though both benign and malignant tumors can present with cough, fever, hemoptysis, recurrent pneumonitis, and symptoms of partial bronchial obstruction [77–79] (Fig.19.7). Respiratory failure is rare and mostly associated with malignant disease. Computer tomography or magnetic resonance imaging should be performed in children with large space-occupying lesions to determine resectability. Imaging alone may not be able to differentiate benign from malignant lesions; thus excisional, incisional, or in some cases, needle biopsy may be required for definitive diagnosis. Since some of these tumors are endobronchial in origin, a bronchoscopic examination could be performed also for diagnosis but bronchoscopic removal carries a high incidence of recurrence and the risk of severe hemorrhage thus should generally be avoided. Conservative surgical resection is the procedure of choice for benign pulmonary tumors. The principle of resection is to preserve a maximal amount of functioning lung tissue. Thoracoscopic resection is an option in these children in experienced hands. The treatment of malignant lesions varies, depending on location and histology. Sleeve resections should be considered for so-called bronchial adenomas, although this misnomer should not make us forget about their malignant behavior. En bloc resection of draining lymphatics should be done for malignant lesions. In extreme cases, pneumonectomy may be required. Multimodality therapy with adjuvant chemotherapy and possibly radiotherapy may be helpful in children with some of the primary tumors or when metastatic disease is present.

19.3.1 Benign Lung Tumors

19.3.1.1 Inflammatory Myofibroblastic Tumors

Inflammatory myofibroblastic tumor is also known as plasma cell granuloma, inflammatory pseudotumor, fibroxanthoma, and fibrohistiocytoma. Although inflammatory myofibroblastic tumors constitute less than 1% of all lung tumors, they are reported to be the most common cause of solitary lung masses in children, representing as much as 80% of all benign lung tumors and 20% of all primary neoplasms [73, 77, 78, 80]. The pathogenesis is not clearly understood. A history of prior lung infection or trauma in about a third of patients suggests that it may begin as a reactive process. However, recent cytogenetic evidence supports a clonal origin, therefore confirming the lesion as a neoplastic proliferation [81]. Symptoms include fever, cough, dysphagia, hemoptysis, chest pain, and pneumonitis, but 30–70% of children are asymptomatic at the time of presentation [73]. It is more common in teenagers than younger children. The lesion usually appears as a round, well-defined mass on chest radiograph, with calcifications in 25–35% of cases [82]. Although benign in nature, these tumors are occasionally locally aggressive and invade surrounding structures with disregard of tissue planes [83, 84]. Conservative lung resection is recommended for resectable lesions. For unresectable lesions, treatment with nonsteroidal anti-inflammatory agents with antiangiogenic activity via COX2 inhibition have shown promising results in some cases [85].

19.3.2.2 Hamartoma

Pulmonary hamartoma is the second most common benign lung tumor in children. It may present as a solitary or multiple nodules. Up to 25% are calcified with pathognomonic "popcorn" calcification [86]. Some can be quite large and present with fatal respiratory distress in neonates. The lesion may be isolated, or part of Carney's triad, which includes pulmonary hamartoma, extra-adrenal paraganglioma, and gastric leiomyosarcoma, typically occurring in young women [87]. The treatment of choice is conservative pulmonary resection, but lobectomy or pneumonectomy may be required depending on the size and location of the lesion.

19.3.2.3 Other Benign Tumors

A variety of benign lesions may rarely be encountered. Some are mostly endobronchial and present with symptoms related to bronchial obstruction. These include tracheal hemangiomas in infants, granular cell myoblastomas, chondromas, neurofibromas and neurilemmomas, and mucous gland adenomas, the only truly benign "bronchial adenomas" (see below). Other lesions may be endobronchial or pulmonary, such as teratomas, leiomyomas, and lipomas. Rare parenchymal tumors include fibroleiomyomatous hamartoma and lymphangiomyomatosis, which are exclusively seen in females; they may be rarely encountered in the pediatric age group. The latter is sometimes associated with tuberous sclerosis. Sclerosing hemangioma is a solitary parenchymal mass that also occurs occasionally in teenage females [73, 77].

Juvenile papillomatosis is caused by a human papillomavirus, which may be transmitted from mother to child. It usually affects the larynx but extends to the trachea in 5% of patients, and, rarely, to the lung parenchyma [88]. The lesions may produce hoarseness, stridor, and respiratory distress. Resection is often followed by recurrence, although spontaneous regression may be observed in older children [73]. Distal imp-

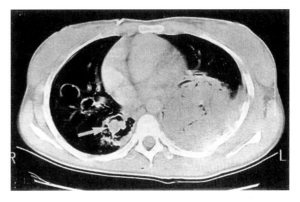

Fig. 19.8 An 18-year-old girl with long-standing respiratory papillomatosis with multiple prior episodes of distal obstruction and multiple laser treatments of the papillomas. She presented with a 6.8-kg (15-lb) weight loss and left chest pain and a mass is shown on this CT. Needle biopsy was consistent with squamous cell carcinoma. Erosion of the ribs can be seen posteriorly. On the right side her airway disease with multiple dilated bronchi and endobronchial papillomas (*arrow, bottom left*) are seen.

lants may be extensive enough to cause pulmonary insufficiency and death, and malignant transformation may occur (Fig.19.8).

19.3.2 Malignant Lung Tumors

19.3.2.1 "Bronchial Adenoma"

Carcinoid tumors, mucoepidermoid carcinomas, and adenoid cystic carcinomas are included under the term "bronchial adenomas," even though they are capable of dissemination, unlike the extremely rare mucous gland adenomas mentioned above. They are the most common primary pulmonary malignancy in children and adolescents, accounting for nearly half of cases [73] (Table 19.2). Most cases are in adolescents [89].

Carcinoid tumors comprise more than 80% of all "bronchial adenomas" in children. They appear to arise from an endobronchial stem cell with neuroendocrine differentiation. Two patterns of growth were described by Andrassy: a polypoid endobronchial lesion or an infiltrating peribronchial mass [90]. The tumor is composed of small, bland-appearing cells in an organoid pattern. Mucoepidermoid carcinoma and adenoid cystic carcinoma occur more frequently in the salivary glands. In the bronchus they appear to arise from the submucosal glands. Symptoms usually result from incomplete bronchial obstruction, such as cough, wheezing, atelectasis, recurrent pneumonia, and hemoptysis. The diagnosis is frequently delayed due to misinterpreting these symptoms as related to asthma. Carcinoid syndrome is extremely rare but Cushing syndrome may occur [89]. Up to 6% will have metastases, and about 2% will recur. In children the mucoepidermoid carcinomas are generally low-grade lesions with a favorable prognosis while the less frequent adenoid cystic carcinoma is more aggressive and frequently fatal [91, 92]. Excellent prognosis is expected for most children with bronchial carcinoids.

The management of these tumors is controversial. They generally occur in a primary or secondary bronchus, thus most lesions are visible by bronchoscopy. Biopsy or endoscopic resection is not recommended because of the high risk of hemorrhage. CT scan and bronchography may be beneficial to determine the degree of bronchiectasis distal to the obstruction, which in turn may affect surgical therapy. Sleeve segmental bronchial resection is the preferred method when feasible [93, 94]. Adjacent lymph nodes should also be removed. When there is significant bronchiectasis distal to the obstruction, lobar resection may be preferred in order to avoid recurrent pulmonary infections (Fig.19.7). When sleeve resection is not possible, there should be no hesitation to proceed with lobectomy, as surgical resection is the primary therapy. Adenoid cystic carcinoma tends to spread submucosally; intraoperative frozen section to confirm the specific nature of the tumor and ensure negative margins will minimize the risk of recurrence or systemic spread. Postoperative monitoring with flexible bronchoscopy may be useful to detect recurrences early.

19.3.2.2 Bronchogenic Carcinoma

Although bronchogenic carcinoma is rare in children, this tumor remains the second most common primary pulmonary malignancy in large reviews [77, 78]. Undifferentiated carcinoma and adenocarcinoma account for 80% of these lesions, with squamous cell carcinoma seen much less frequently (12%), in contrast with adults. These tumors may occur at any age, but are most frequent in adolescence. The majority of children present with disseminated disease; the average survival is only 7 months, and mortality exceeds 90%. Localized lesions can be treated by complete resection, followed by adjuvant therapy.

Bronchioloalveolar carcinoma is a special form of low-grade adenocarcinoma, which has a tendency to spread through the airways. In children, it may occur as a second malignancy after treatment for Ewing's sarcoma, Hodgkin disease and testicular germ cell tumor [73]. It has also been reported in children and young adults with type 1 congenital pulmonary airway malformation (CPAM, formerly called CCAM) of the lung and bronchogenic cysts [95]. Although the topic remains controversial, with just over a dozen case reports, there is pathologic evidence for the carcinogenic potential of the mucous cells found in type 1 CPAM, which speaks in favor of elective resection of these congenital lesions, even when asymptomatic [95–97]. Prognosis is favorable if resection is complete [98].

Squamous cell carcinoma may occur in isolation or can be secondary to recurrent respiratory papillomatosis produced by the human papilloma virus (Fig. 19.8) [99]. These children have laryngeal lesions that seed squamous cells throughout their airways during repeated intubation and endoscopic resection, which leads to distal implants and eventual malignant transformation. Frequent surveillance may be of benefit, although therapeutic options are limited when the disease is diffuse. The tumors are generally moderately to well differentiated and respond poorly to chemotherapy. A few cases have been successfully treated by surgical resection alone.

19.3.2.3 Pleuropulmonary Blastoma

Pleuropulmonary blastoma (PPB) is a rare childhood malignant neoplasm of the lungs, with about 160 pediatric patients reported in the world. The term was defined in 1988 [100] and regroups tumors previously described as pulmonary rhabdomyosarcomas, cystic mesenchymal hamartomas, blastomas, and other types of undifferentiated sarcomas [101, 102]. Recent histologic and immunologic data suggest that PPBs are distinct from the adult type of pulmonary blastoma [100, 103]. The average age of children with PPB is 3–4 years, with a range from the newborn period through 12 years of age, while the "adult" pulmonary blastoma is rarely seen under 10 years of age. PPB is a mesenchymal neoplasm; this is very different from adult-type pulmonary blastoma, which has malignant mesenchymal and epithelial tissue. Adult pulmonary blastoma has not been associated with congenital lung cysts (see below).

Because of the rarity of PPB, a registry has been established to promote research and understanding of this disease [104]. Three types are described based on the morphology and increasing malignant behavior. Type I is purely cystic and mostly seen in younger children. Type I PPB resembles CPAM clinically and radiologically and cannot be differentiated short of histological examination. Type II PPBs are mixed cystic and solid, while type III tumors are predominately solid. Both occur in older children and often arise from pre-existing cystic lesions. Evidence suggests that type I tumors may evolve into the more malignant types II and III if undiagnosed or inadequately treated [105]. Histologically PPBs are thought to arise from pleuropulmonary germ cells [106], and are composed of primitive mesenchymal tissue and disordered epithelial tubules resembling fetal lung tissue, some with variable sarcomatous differentiation [107]. Cytogenetics also identified c-kit expression in solid tumors [103]. Cough, fever, and sometimes pain in the chest suggesting a respiratory infection are often the first symptoms. The chest radiographs may be interpreted as "pneumonia," delaying the diagnosis. Pneumothorax is another common presentation, especially in younger patients [108–110]. Malignant potential increases with the solid component, and more than 20% of patients present with metastatic disease [111]. Frequent sites of metastases are the liver, brain, bone, and spinal cord [112].

The tumor is usually located at the periphery of the lung, but it may also be located in extrapulmonary locations, such as the mediastinum, diaphragm, and/or pleura. Since most of the lung tumors are located peripherally (Fig. 19.9), resection is usually possible by segmental or lobar resection. However, since the limit between the lesion and normal parenchyma may be difficult to determine grossly and because of the high risk of local recurrence and metastatic spread, the surgical procedure of choice for parenchymal PPB is lobectomy. The use of multimodal neoadjuvant chemotherapy and radiation following surgical resection has shown promising results in a few patients with extensive disease and dissemination. Chemotherapeutic agents that have been used include actinomycin D, vincristine, and cyclophosphamide alternating with doxorubicin and cisplatin. Adjuvant chemotherapy is recommended even for type I PPB, in order to decrease the risk of recurrence. Despite aggressive treatment protocols, the prognosis for patients with PPB is not good, with 5-year survival rates of 83% for type 1 and 42% for types 2 and 3. Furthermore, it appears that type II and III lesions have a tendency to recur, even at remote or contralateral sites, despite an apparently complete resection of the primary tumor [78, 103, 105, 112]. PPB has frequently been described in association with cystic lung disease including bronchogenic cysts, CPAM, and air filled cysts [95, 115, 116]. It is not known whether the tumor can develop in pre-existing benign congenital cystic lung disease or whether the cysts in these cases are type I PPB from the outset [117]. The latter opinion has been favored recently, especially since PPB has been identified in fetus and neonates [106, 118]. Being an uncommon tumor, PPB is rarely considered in the differential diagnosis of cystic lung disease in children. Subtle findings in support of a preoperative diagnosis of PPB include the presence of peripherally based lung cysts (Fig.19.9) and multifocal and/or bilateral cystic disease. A history of neoplasia, hyperplasia or dysplasia, and particularly of cystic renal lesions, in the patient, sibling or close relative, should also raise suspicion for PPB since such an association is found in approximately 25% of patients as reported in the International Registry [119, 120]. The difficulty in making a diagnosis of PPB based on

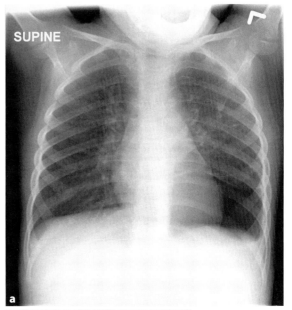

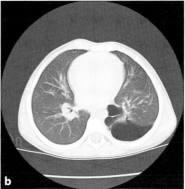

Fig. 19.9 a, b Pleuropulmonary blastoma. A 3-year-old child presented with a 2-month history of low-grade fever and cough. The examination was normal except for decreased breath sounds in the left lower chest. (**a**) Posteroanterior chest radiograph demonstrating a large hyperlucency in the lower left hemithorax with some subsegmental collapse in the upper lobe. (**b**) Computed tomography of the chest confirmed the presence of a multicystic air-filled lesion in the left hemi-thorax. One large and several smaller cysts were identified. Neither calcification nor air-fluid levels were observed within the cysts. At thoracoscopy, the large cystic lesion was attached to the left lower lobe only by a small band of tissue. A margin of normal lung tissue was removed en bloc with the specimen, which was placed in an endobag. A diagnosis of type I pleuropulmonary blastoma was made on microscopic examination, and the case was submitted to the registry (www.ppbregistry.org). (Reproduced with permission from Al-Backer N, Puligandla PS, Su W, Anselmo M, Laberge J-M (2006) Type I pleuropulmonary blastoma in a 3-year-old male with a cystic lung mass. J Pediatr Surg 41:E14.)

imaging alone has led many authors to propose prophylactic removal of all congenital cystic lung lesions, even if asymptomatic [95, 118, 121]. Furthermore, the subsequent development of cystic lung lesions after histological confirmation of PPB should be treated by resection whenever feasible since these lesions invariably demonstrate malignant features. Even with a resected lesion, the diagnosis of type I PPB is not always easy to make, and this tumor may be confused with a type 4 CPAM [117, 122].

19.3.2.4 Rhabdomyosarcoma

Rhabdomyosarcomas of the lung are rare and account for only 0.5% of all childhood rhabdomyosarcomas [123]. Several reported cases appeared to originate in congenital cystic anomalies. Recent reviews by the PPB Registry suggested that most of the reports of "rhabdomyosarcoma in lung cysts" [101, 124–127] are actually PPB. Of 32 cases in these reports, the Registry pathologists reviewed ten and all were rediagnosed as PPB. In four other cases, the reporting institution recategorized their cases as PPB [104]. Thus, most mesenchymal sarcomas in lungs cysts are in fact PPB. It is important to differentiate pulmonary rhabdomyosarcoma from PPB because their clinical behaviors are different. In 25% of PPB cases, there is a familial history of malignancy or dysplasia [119]. This is not true for rhabdomyosarcoma. PPB also has a high incidence of cerebral parenchymal metastases, something not seen in rhabdomyosarcoma. PPB and rhabdomyosarcoma are different malignancies and careful review of pathology to establish the correct diagnosis is essential for optimal patient care. Rhabdomyosarcomas may be pulmonary, endobronchial, or rarely, mediastinal or pleural [130].

19.3.2.5 Other Malignant Pulmonary Tumors

Fibrosarcoma of the lung is a rare low-grade malignancy. It can present in newborns with respiratory distress and may be associated with fatal pulmonary hypoplasia (Fig.19.10). In older children, presenting symptoms include cough, fever, and chest pain. Prognosis with resection is excellent [131].

Malignant fibrous histiocytoma represented 27% of the 26 primary pulmonary sarcomas in Keel's review [132]. Most children were alive with resection alone. Other types of pulmonary sarcomas include synovial sarcoma, leiomyosarcoma, and malignant peripheral nerve sheet tumors [77, 132, 133].

Lymphoma, posttransplant lymphoproliferative disorder, malignant histiocytosis, and Langerhans' cell histiocytosis are other tumors that may have a primary pulmonary manifestation [134].

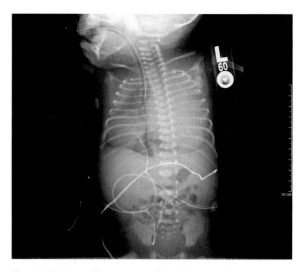

Fig. 19.10 Lung fibrosarcoma. This baby was born prematurely at 34 weeks of gestation because of premature labor, after a prenatal ultrasound examination at 33 weeks showed a large left-sided lung mass causing mediastinal shift but no hydrops. Immediate intubation was required because of respiratory distress, and he failed to stabilized despite high frequency oscillating ventilation. The chest radiograph shows a large solid lung mass filling the entire hemithorax. A total pneumonectomy was required, but the baby failed to improve and died from pulmonary hypoplasia. Microscopic examination showed a fibrosarcoma. (courtesy of Dr. Tom Hui)

19.3.2.6 Lung Metastases

Pulmonary metastases are more frequent than primary tumors in children. The surgical approach depends on the histology of the primary tumor and the response of the primary site to combined-modality therapy [135]. Tumors most frequently considered for pulmonary metastasectomy are osteosarcoma, soft tissue sarcoma, malignant germ cell tumor, and Wilms tumor [136]. The use of CT scan allows for detection of lesions which would not be discovered by routine chest radiographs; however, CT scan can still underestimate the number of nodules, especially in osteosarcoma [137]. Treatment of the pulmonary metastases involves control of the primary tumor and often multimodality therapy – usually chemotherapy in conjunction with metastasectomy – and radiotherapy in some (Wilms tumor). In certain cases resection of isolated pulmonary metastases, especially osteosarcoma, together with chemotherapy has provided cure or long-term survival [138–141]. Not all pulmonary lesions appearing during the course of treatment of a solid tumor are metastatic disease, since 33% of the pulmonary nodules removed in one series of 37 children with known primaries were found to be benign lesions [142]. Thoracoscopic biopsy is an excellent diagnostic tool which can differentiate between benign, infectious, and metastatic lesions in over 90% of cases [143–148]. However, the application of thoracoscopy for tumor resection is still under investigation [148, 149]. Centrally located lesions are less amenable to thoracoscopic excision, and small lesions are difficult to visualize and cannot be palpated when using thoracoscopy.

19.4 Mediastinal Tumors

Tumors of the mediastinum are comprise of a wide spectrum of pathology [150]. Sixty-five to 72% of mediastinal lesions are malignant [151, 152], and about 40% occur in infants and children less than 2 years old. The understanding of the anatomy and tissues present in each compartment is the key to the differential diagnosis of mediastinal tumors. The mediastinum is divided into anterior, middle, and posterior compartments (Fig. 19.11). Anterior mediastinal tumors account for 44% of all mediastinal lesions reported by Grosfeld, et al. [151], and 80% of these are malignant. The major anterior mediastinal tumors can be characterized by the 4 Ts, in the order of frequency: Terrible lymphomas, Teratomas and germ cell tumors, Thymomas, and cysTic hygromas. Twenty percent of mediastinal tumors are found in the middle mediastinal compartment, these are primarily lymphocytic in origin and include Hodgkin's disease and lymphomas. The rare cardiac and pericardial tumors are also found in this compartment. Posterior mediastinal masses account for 36% of all mediastinal tumors, and usually arise from neurogenic structures located at the paravertebral sulcus, including neuroblastoma, ganglioneuroma, and neurofibroma (Table 19.3) [153]. Foregut duplications and extralobar sequestration can be found in both the middle and posterior mediastinum.

These are not neoplasms, but they enter in the differential diagnosis.

Anterior mediastinal tumors may present with respiratory symptoms resulting from tracheal compression and require special anesthetic consideration. Systemic symptoms may be present in patients with lymphoproliferative disease including malaise, fever, weight loss and night sweats. The superior vena cava syndrome is occasionally observed in tumors infiltrating the superior mediastinum. Posterior mediastinal lesions can present as asymptomatic masses or rarely with neurologic symptoms from intraspinal extension or Horner's syndrome from the involvement of the stellate ganglion. Paraneoplastic syndromes such as opsoclonus-myoclonus may be the mode of presentation for neurogenic tumors (Fig. 19.12).

19.4.1 Lymphatic Tumors

Malignant lymphoma of the mediastinum is the most common mediastinal tumor in children, accounting for approximately 60% of all pediatric mediastinal lesions. Two-thirds are non-Hodgkin's lymphomas and one-third are Hodgkin's disease [154, 155]. Lymphoblastic lymphomas are the most common histologic subtype of non-Hodgkin's lymphomas, followed by large cell lymphomas [155, 156]. Patients with Hodgkin's disease or non-Hodgkin's lymphoma require biopsy before initiation of treatment, but resection should not be attempted. The tumor has an excellent response to chemotherapy and radiotherapy and disseminated disease is often present [150]. An open procedure provides the best and safest approach to tissue diagnosis [155]. However, the risk of anesthetic complication from the mass effect of the large mediastinal mass should to be carefully assessed prior to any procedure.

Table 19.3 Tumor histology of posterior mediastinal lesions [153]

Malignant	Number	Benign	Number
Neuroblastoma	32	Ganglioneuroma	14
Malignant schwannoma	1	Neurofibroma	3
Primitive neuroectodermal tumor	2	Benign schwannoma	2
Undifferentiated sarcoma	1	Plasma cell granuloma	1
Liposarcoma	1	Lipoma	1
Malignant paraganglioma (pheochromocytoma)	1	Paraganglioma (pheochromocytoma)	1
		Eosinophilic granuloma	1
		Granulomatous inflammation	1
		Lymphangioma	1

Reproduced with permission from [153]

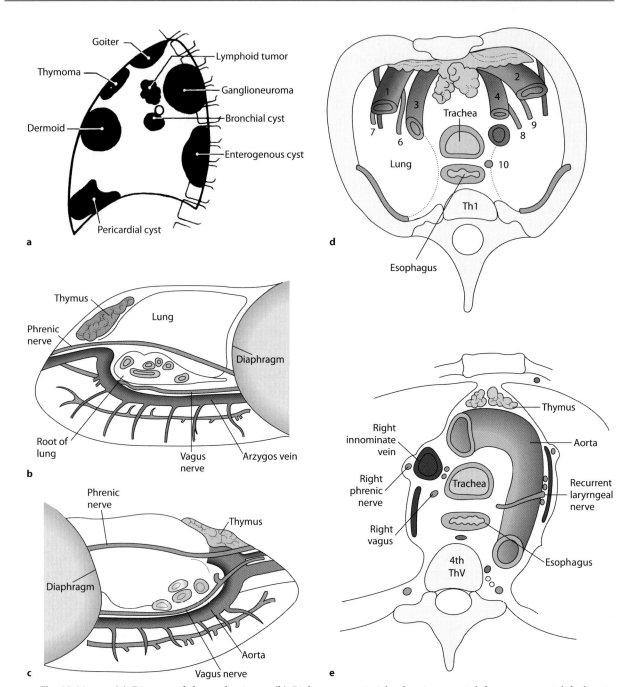

Fig. 19.11 a–e (**a**) Diagram of the mediastinum. (**b**) Right hemi-thorax. (**c**) Left hemi-thorax. (**d**) Structures at the thoracic inlet. 1, 2: Left and right innominate vein; 3: innominate artery; 4: left common carotid; 5: left subclavian artery; 6: right vagus nerve; 7: right phrenic nerve; 8: left vagus nerve; 9: left phrenic nerve; 10: recurrent laryngeal nerve; 11: 1st thoracic nerve. (**e**) Structures at level of 4th thoracic vertebra.

19.4.1.1 Anesthetic Risk Assessment

Tumors in the anterior mediastinum may become large before they produce symptoms. (Figs. 19.13, 19.14). Respiratory collapse during induction of general anesthesia is a recognized risk in children with an anterior mediastinal mass. Anesthetic risks are best assessed using a combination of clinical, functional, and radiological evaluations [154]. Clinical signs and symptoms alone do not correlate well with anesthetic complications [157, 158]. The only symptom that is strongly associated with respiratory collapse is orthop-

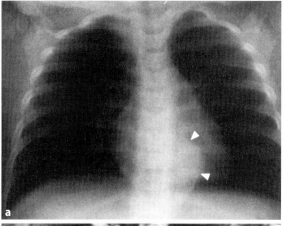

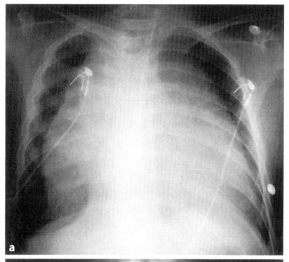

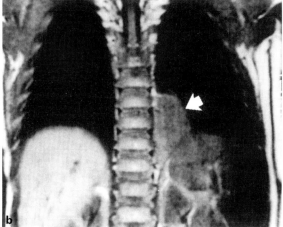

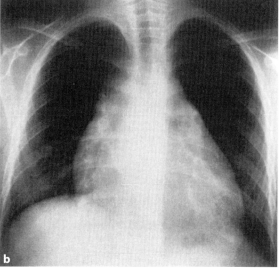

Fig. 19.12 a, b (**a**) An 11-month-old girl presented with op-soclonus. Her neurologist was concerned she might have neu-roblastoma and obtained the chest radiograph shown here and an abdominal ultrasound. The former demonstrated a small paravertebral lesion (*arrows*) and the MRI (**b**) shows a lesion sitting adjacent to the diaphragm, but not extending into the spinal canal (*arrow*). She was successfully resected and followed without any adjuvant therapy. Her opsoclonus slowly resolved over the following year.

Fig. 19.13 a, b (**a**) Chest radiograph of an 8-year-old girl who presented with a 2–3 week history of wheezing, cough, anorexia and weight loss of 2.7 kg (6 lb). The pleural effusion present was tapped to avoid biopsy and the diagnosis of acute lymphoblastic lymphoma was obtained. (**b**) Chest radiograph 1 week after the first course of prednisone, vincristine, doxorubicin, methotrexa-te, and intrathecal cytosine arabinoside (ara-C) demonstrates a dramatic response to therapy.

nea [157–160]. Thus, patients presenting with orthop-nea should avoid general anesthesia for either diagnos-tic or therapeutic procedures as a general rule [154]. As many as 55% of children presenting with Hodgkin's disease have radiographic evidence of tracheal com-pression [161]. Computed tomography was used to define the cross-sectional area of the trachea [162, 163] and applied in two retrospective studies to as-sess the relationship to anesthetic risk [159, 164]. Both Azizkhan, et al. [164] and Shamberger, et al. [159] sug-gested that children with tracheal cross-sectional areas less than 50% of predicted should not receive a general anesthetic. Extensive pulmonary function abnormali-ties were identified in a group of patients with ante-rior mediastinal masses prospectively studied [165].

The peak expiratory flow rate in pulmonary function studies is the best parameter in the prediction of an-esthetic problems. It provides a quantitative reflection of central airway size. It can be easily performed with a hand-held device and compared with the predicted values [154, 165]. A peak expiratory flow rate of less than 50% of predicted is associated with increased anesthetic risks [158, 165]. The measurement of pul-monary function in children with anterior mediastinal masses may add valuable information to the anatomic evaluation obtained by CT scan. In particular, it can

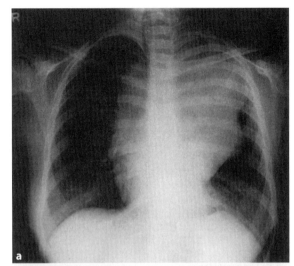

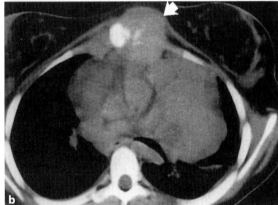

Fig. 19.14 a, b (a) Chest radiograph of a 12-year-old girl obtained because of mild left pleuritic chest pain demonstrates a large anterior mediastinal mass. (b) The CT scan revealed that the mass was eroding through the chest wall and sternum (*arrow*). Because of significant tracheal compression a biopsy was obtained under local anesthesia and Hodgkin's disease was diagnosed.

quantitate the magnitude of pulmonary restriction in relation to the size of the mass and may identify impairment of flow related to compression of airways distal to the carina, which cannot be measured by CT scan. Thus, the clinical, functional, and radiological findings can be incorporated into a simple algorithm to assess anesthetic risk for each individual patient (Figs. 19.15, 19.16) [154].

19.4.1.2 Alternatives to General Anesthesia for Diagnosis

An extrathoracic approach under local anesthesia can be utilized in most patients with anterior mediastinal masses to obtain diagnostic material. This

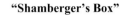

"Shamberger's Box"

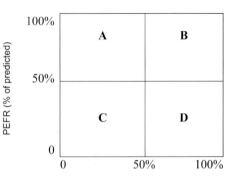

Tracheal Area (% of predicted)

A: Moderate risk (spontaneous ventilation)
B: Low risk (general anesthesia)
C: High risk (local anesthesia)
D: Moderate risk (spontaneous ventilation)

PEFR=peak expiratory flow rate

Fig. 19.15 "Shamberger's box" correlating the peak expiratory flow rate (PEFR) and the tracheal cross-section area. (Reproduced with permission from p. 166 of Ricketts RR (2001) Critical management of anterior mediastinal tumors in children. Semin Pediatr Surg, 10:161–168.)

includes cervical or supraclavicular excision of an enlarged lymph node, thoracentesis for pleural effusion flow cytometry [157], and bone marrow aspirate and biopsy, remembering that leukemias may present as an anterior mediastinal mass (Fig.19.17). Fine needle aspiration of mediastinal masses under CT or ultrasound guidance is generally not acceptable, but multiple passes using core needle biopsies may be a viable alternative [166–170]. Newer techniques utilizing ultrasound-guided endoscopic biopsy have shown improved accuracy in adult patients [171]. The Chamberlain procedure (anterior thoracotomy through the bed of the second rib) can be performed under local anesthesia even in children and should be part of the armamentarium of the pediatric surgeon [172]. Thoracoscopic biopsy requires general anesthesia, and its diagnostic accuracy for lymphoma is still under investigation, despite excellent diagnostic yields for other thoracic lesions using minimally invasive techniques [143, 145, 146, 148]. Careful communication with the pathologist regarding the adequacy of biopsy material is essential when utilizing a minimally invasive technique [173, 174]. For lymphomatous lesions in general, excision of a whole lymph node is preferred over needle or small piecemeal biopsies, in order to assess the nodal architecture.

In patients without extrathoracic disease, pretreatment with steroids or radiation prior to biopsy may reduce tumor size rapidly and allow for safer anesthesia.

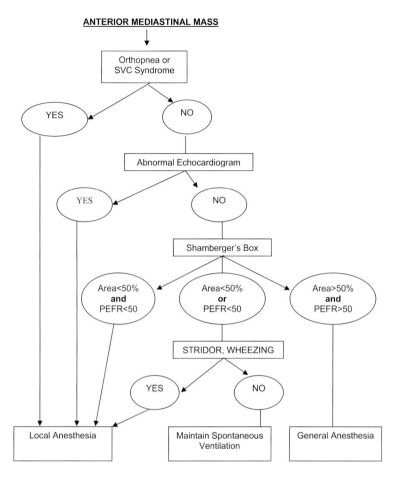

ANTERIOR MEDIASTINAL MASS

Orthopnea or
SVC Syndrome

YES

NO

Abnormal Echocardiogram

YES

NO

Shamberger's Box

Area<50%
and
PEFR<50

Area<50%
or
PEFR<50

Area>50%
and
PEFR>50

STRIDOR, WHEEZING

YES

NO

Local Anesthesia

Maintain Spontaneous
Ventilation

General Anesthesia

Fig. 19.16 An algorithm for the preanesthetic evaluation of children with an anterior mediastinal mass (Reproduced with permission from p. 167 of Ricketts RR (2001) Critical management of anterior mediastinal tumors in children. Semin Pediatr Surg, 10:161–168.)

However, radiation may significantly alter pathology, making the correct diagnosis difficult [175, 176]. In some cases the radiation field can be adjusted to spare an area for biopsy [159]. Pretreatment with steroids may also ablate cytogenetic markers, leading to inaccurate diagnosis [177, 178].

Staging, treatment, and prognosis for lymphoma is discussed in Chap. 15.

Other hematopoietic disorders with mediastinal manifestations include acute myeloblastic leukemia, malignant histiocytosis, and extramedullary hematopoiesis, which can present as paravertebral masses in the posterior-inferior mediastinum of children with chronic hemolytic anemia [134].

Angiofollicular or giant lymph node hyperplasia (also called Castleman's disease) is usually a benign condition, which often affects mediastinal nodes. The grossly enlarged nodes are very vascular on imaging studies. Excisional biopsy is required to differentiate this from lymphoma. The disease sometimes takes a systemic form, in which case the course is complicated with anemia and growth failure. These manifestations sometimes improve with excision of the enlarged node(s) [179].

Langerhans cell histiocytosis in the mediastinum is usually part of a multifocal systemic disease, but rarely may present as an isolated thymic mass. Superior vena cava syndrome has been described. The prognosis for unifocal mediastinal disease is excellent [134].

19.4.2 Teratomas and Germ Cell Tumors

Primary germ cell tumors of the mediastinum account for 6–18% of pediatric mediastinal neoplasms [180]; they are the second most common tumor of the anterior mediastinum. Conversely, 7–10% of all teratomas are mediastinal, making this the third most common site after the sacrococcygeal and gonadal sites [181]. They may present at any age from infancy to adolescence. The majority is benign, but after 15 years of age mediastinal teratomas have a high incidence of malignant behavior, which is usually indicated by elevated levels of tumor markers (see below) [181]. Immature elements are not of prognostic significance in children under 15 years, but they are associated with local aggressiveness and distant metastases above that age [182, 183]. Most mediastinal teratomas are located

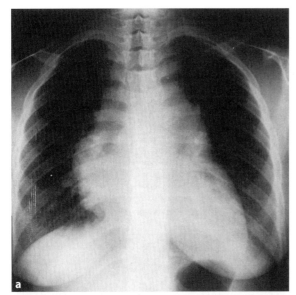

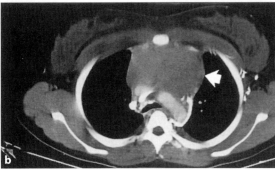

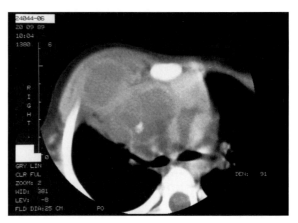

Fig. 19.18 This 2-year-old was referred for a 5-cm by 5-cm hard fixed right chest wall mass that appeared suddenly during an upper respiratory infection. The computed tomography scan shows a bilobed lesion that extends through the chest wall and contains a small area of calcification. An incisional biopsy revealed pus-like material, containing ghost cells and calcified debris. Serum markers were normal. Complete excision of the mass required a right anterior thoracotomy and partial resection of an adherent right middle lobe. Pathologic examination revealed a ruptured mature teratoma with marked inflammatory reaction, containing foci of enteric, respiratory, and squamous mucosa; smooth muscle; salivary glands; pancreas; neuroglial tissue; and bone. (Reproduced with permission from page 983 of Laberge J-M, Nguyen LT, Shaw KS (2005) Teratomas, dermoids and other soft tissue tumors. In Ashcraft KW, Holcomb GW, Murphy JP, (eds) Pediatric surgery, 4th edn. Elsevier Saunders, Philadelphia, Chapter 68, pp 972–996.

Fig. 19.17 a, b (a) Chest radiograph of a 12-year-old girl who presented with facial swelling and plethora. Chest radiograph demonstrated a significant anterior mediastinal mass. Echocardiogram revealed a pericardial effusion and the CT (b) revealed a homogeneous anterior mediastinal mass (*arrow*). Her white cell count was 5.1 with a normal differential count. Fluid aspirated from the pericardium, however, had a white cell count of 724,000 and cytology was diagnostic of lymphoblastic leukemia.

in the anterior mediastinum, but a few have been described in the posterior mediastinum, some with epidural extension; intrapericardial and intracardiac locations are also described, the former presenting in utero or at birth with fetal hydrops or massive pericardial effusion [181]. Infants with an anterior mediastinal teratoma commonly present with respiratory distress, but in older children, the teratoma may be an incidental finding on chest radiograph. It may also present as a chest wall mass with erosion through the soft tissues (Fig. 19.18), with hemoptysis or trichoptysis from bronchial erosion, with rupture into the pleural cavity, or with heart failure [181, 182]. CT scan is the imaging technique of choice in the evaluation of these lesions. It can define the extent of the lesion and possible tra-

cheal compression. A heterogeneous anterior mediastinal mass containing calcification and varying tissue densities is highly suggestive of the diagnosis [184]. Surgical resection via anterior thoracotomy, median sternotomy, or thoracoscopy [185] is usually curative, although malignant elements in the tumor will require further therapy. Thoracoscopic removal is generally not indicated for tumors with elevated markers or other signs suggestive of malignancy.

Approximately 15 to 20% of mediastinal germ cell tumors are malignant. These are complex tumors of varied histology with frequent coexistence of benign elements [186]. Malignant components include seminomas, teratocarcinomas, embryonal carcinomas, germinomas, choriocarcinomas, and yolk sac tumors [187]. They are more common in boys than girls (3:1). A strong association is found in patients with Klinefelter's syndrome, who often present with precocious puberty from the choriocarcinoma elements [181]. Alphafetoprotein and beta-HCG should be obtained preoperatively, as for suspected germ cell tumors in other locations. Diagnostic biopsy should be obtained for large tumors considered difficult to resect either with image-guided needle biopsy or via thoracoscopic or open biopsy [187]. The prognosis for patients with malignant germ cell tumors arising in the mediastinum previously was regarded as dismal with only occasional survivors [153, 188, 189]. The POG/CCSG intergroup study demonstrated successful reduction in tumor bulk with neoadjuvant chemotherapy, facilitating complete resection of tumors with malignant components in 82% of patients [187]. With the combination of multiagent chemotherapy (cisplatin, etoposide, and bleomycin) and aggressive surgical resection, the POG/CCSG intergroup study reported 71% and 69% 4-year overall and event-free survival in patients with malignant mediastinal germ cell tumors [180, 187].

The management of primary mediastinal germ cell tumors should be conservative at diagnosis, with biopsy only for large tumors. Patients with elevated tumor markers or histologic confirmation of malignancy should receive neoadjuvant chemotherapy prior to attempt at resection. Benign tumors and persisting masses after chemotherapy (often due to coexisting elements of benign teratoma) should be resected aggressively, as an excellent outcome can be expected [190].

19.4.3 Thymic Tumors

Tumors or tumor-like lesions arising from the thymus include thymic cysts, thymic hyperplasia, thymomas, and thymolipomas. These lesions represent less than 5% of mediastinal tumors in children. Other lesions such as lymphoma, carcinoid, and lymphangioma may arise in the thymus. When the thymus is primarily involved with lymphomatous disease [191], the diagnosis is usually established only after resection of the mass; additional chemotherapy or radiotherapy is required.

Thymic hyperplasia may take the form of lymphoid follicular hyperplasia, which is often present in myasthenia gravis and associated with a favorable response to thymectomy; it can also present as massive hypertrophy in children. The latter is usually detected incidentally. Two interesting circumstances where massive hypertrophy have been observed are in the recovery phase of a thermal burn, and in association with hyper and hypothyroidism [134].

Thymomas are rare in children as compared to adults, with only 2% presenting in the first two decades of life. They are usually benign and arise in the upper anterior mediastinum or at the base of the neck. Although they may be massive in size, they generally compress adjacent structures rather than invade them. Respiratory distress and superior vena cava syndrome may occur [134]. They are occasionally associated with myasthenia gravis. Surgical resection is curative

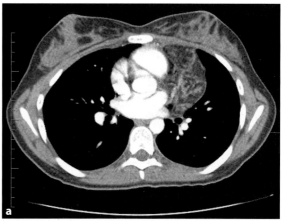

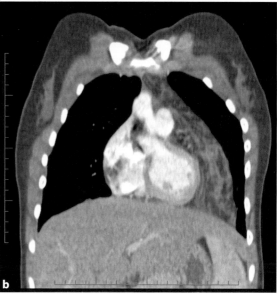

Fig. 19.19 a, b Thymolipoma. This 17-year-old girl had an incidental finding of a heterogenous anterior mediastinal mass during investigation of Crohn's disease. (**a**) This axial cut on CT scan shows the soft tissue mass with fat infiltration, to the left of the aortic arch. (**b**) The extent of the mass to the costo-diaphragmatic angle can be appreciated on this coronal reconstruction. A thoracoscopic resection was performed. (courtesy of Dr. Ken Shaw)

and recurrence is rare (2%) [192]. Malignant thymomas are epithelial in nature and invasive as in adults. Aggressive surgical resection is critical as response to chemotherapy and radiotherapy is limited. Resection of lung, pleura, diaphragm, superior vena cava, and pericardium may be required to achieve complete surgical extirpation.

Thymolipoma is a rare benign tumor of the thymus that often attains huge proportions in clinically asymptomatic patients (Fig. 19.19). Histologically, a thymolipoma is composed of thymic and mature adipose tissue. The tumor usually extends inferiorly to either side of the mediastinum. Associated conditions such as myasthenia gravis [193], aplastic anemia [194], Graves' disease [195], and Hodgkin's disease [196], although possibly coincidental, have been reported in adult patients. One case of erythrocyte hypoplasia and hypogammaglobulinemia has been reported in a child [197]. Surgical resection is necessary for definitive diagnosis and can be accomplished thoracoscopically [197, 198].

19.4.4 Neurogenic Tumors

Tumors of neural crest origin are the most common posterior mediastinal lesions. They arise from the sympathetic chain and range from benign ganglioneuroma to malignant neuroblastoma. Twenty percent of neurogenic tumors are located in the mediastinum. Neuroblastoma is the most common tumor and occurs mostly in infants and young children. (Table 19.3) [153]. Ganglioneuromas present in older children and teenagers as asymptomatic lesions, which are identified incidentally on chest radiographs obtained for unrelated reasons. Radiographically they appear as paraspinal spindle-shaped lesions. Neurogenic tumors may occur anywhere along the paraspinal sulcus from the thoracic inlet to the diaphragm. They are generally well encapsulated and readily resectable. Surgical resection is the treatment of choice and is curative for benign lesions. Several recent series have reported successful thoracoscopic resections [185]. Occasionally they may have extensions along the nerve roots into the spinal canal (Fig. 19.20). Any child with a paraspinal mass requires a CT scan or MRI prior to surgical resection. The optimal treatment for patients presenting with symptomatic spinal cord compression at diagnosis has evolved. Treatment of the so-called dumbbell lesions with extension into the spinal canal must first involve control of the spinal lesion by either laminectomy/laminotomy, radiation, or chemotherapy [199]. Initial resection of the thoracic component entails the risk of potential swelling of the spinal tumor with worsening of neurologic compression and paralysis [153, 200]. Recent studies from France, Italy, and the Pediatric Oncology Group all demonstrated equal efficacy between laminectomy, radiation and chemotherapy to relieve or improve neurologic deficits [201–203]. However, patients treated with chemotherapy usually did not require additional treatment and have less orthopedic sequelae, whereas patients treated either with radiotherapy or laminectomy commonly did [201–203]. Although laminotomy may be a worthwhile alternative with fewer sequelae than laminectomy, the current trend is to use chemotherapy for debulking, now that the fear of inducing tumor necrosis, resulting in edema and increased cord compression, has been

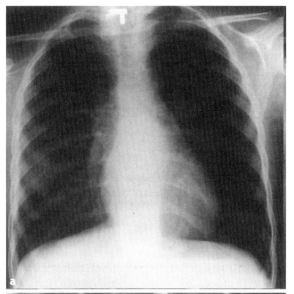

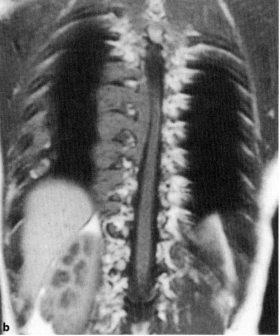

Fig. 19.20a,b (a) Chest radiograph of a 5-year-old girl referred for back pain, which demonstrated a minimal right paraspinal mass, but on the MRI scan (b) a dramatic extension of the tumor was demonstrated through the spinal foramen, and was compressing the spinal cord, although she had no significant neurological symptoms. A percutaneous needle biopsy demonstrated the tumor to be a neuroblastoma.

dispelled. Surgical decompression is reserved for patients who show progressive neurologic deterioration after initiation of chemotherapy [204]. The frequency of complete neurologic recovery in children with intraspinal neuroblastoma inversely correlates with the severity of the presenting neurologic deficits [202], and up to 44% have permanent sequelae [201].

At the time of resection of the primary thoracic mass, the tumor is often closely adherent to the posterior part of the ribs and necessitates removal of part of the periosteum. Often it is impossible to avoid leaving small amounts of residual disease along the sympathetic nerve roots as they emerge from the foramina. These areas are simply marked with small titanium clips for future imaging. A small amount of residual disease results in a stage IIA or IIB, depending on whether the nodes are negative or positive [204]. This has a good prognosis, especially in the chest (see Chap. 11). Ipsilateral nodes are excised if any are visible, but extensive sampling, including contralateral nodes, is not required for thoracic neuroblastomas, unlike for their abdominal counterpart.

Prognosis in neuroblastoma is age dependent, with a better prognosis for infants compared to older children. Intrathoracic neuroblastomas have a more favorable prognosis than abdominal primaries of comparable stage [204, 205]. This is most likely related to the favorable biology of most thoracic neurogenic lesions (see Chap. 11) [206, 207]. In the presence of a maturing ganglioneuroblastoma, it is important to remember that the tumor is as malignant as its most malignant component. A small proportion of older children with thoracic neuroblastoma appear to have a protracted course, with late recurrences and death.

Plexiform neurofibroma may occur in the mediastinum as an isolated lesion or in patients with neurofibromatosis (NF-1 or von Recklinghausen's disease). Resection is required in isolated lesions in order to obtain a histologic diagnosis [208]. In patients with neurofibromatosis, resection is required if the lesions are symptomatic. Rapid growth of these lesions usually occurs if there is malignant transformation to neurofibrosarcoma (Fig. 19.21).

Pheochromocytoma (also called paraganglioma) can also occur along the sympathetic chain in the neck and mediastinum and produce symptoms of compression as well as flushing and hypertension. This tumor has been described in the anterior mediastinum as well. Regional or distant metastases are seen in 15–20% of patients [134]. Other rare neurogenic tumors include neurilemmoma and malignant schwannoma.

19.4.5 Other Mediastinal Tumors

Among the less common mediastinal tumors, there are reports of lipomas and lipoblastomas, and rare instances of liposarcoma. Other sarcomas such as rhabdomyosarcomas, Ewing tumors, mesenchymomas, and other unusual neoplasms may also occur [134]. Rare cases of fibromatosis have also been described.

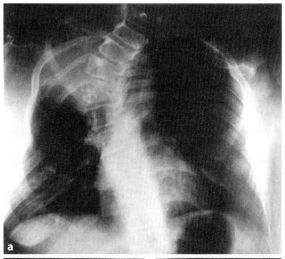
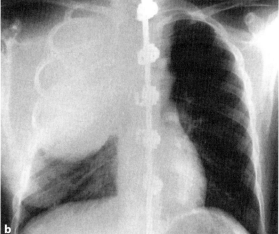
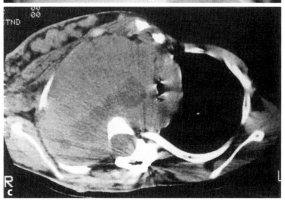

Fig. 19.21 a–c (**a**) Chest radiograph of a 10-year-old boy with neurofibromatosis obtained immediately prior to fusion of his spine. The right apical mass had been stable in size. (**b**) Dramatic increase in the size of the apical mass was noted 9 months later. At resection, malignant degeneration into a neurofibrosarcoma was found. Note thinning of the upper ribs as a result of the long-standing neurofibroma. (**c**) CT scan obtained prior to resection demonstrates the large mass displacing the mediastinum to the left, but not compressing the trachea. Multiple subcutaneous neurofibromas are seen in the subcutaneous tissues of the right chest.

Benign vascular tumors and lymphatic malformations occur as in other parts of the body. When the diagnosis cannot be ascertained by imaging alone, thoracoscopy may be useful [209]. Gorham's disease is worth mentioning; even though it is not a tumor per se, it behaves as one. Gorham's disease or "vanishing bone disorder" is a rare disorder of unknown etiology, characterized by proliferation of vascular channels that results in the destruction and resorption of the osseous matrix [210]. Some consider it as an extreme form of lymphangiomatosis [211]. The shoulder and the pelvis are the most commonly affected sites; however, various locations in all of the other areas of the skeleton have also been reported. The disease may present with pain from lytic bony lesions and pathological fractures, or with chylous pericardial or pleural effusions, which may be life threatening. These effusions may be due to mediastinal extension of the disease process from the involved vertebrae, scapula, ribs, or sternum, or may represent a direct lymphangiomatous involvement of the mediastinum. In general, mediastinal and spinal involvement are associated with a poor prognosis. The treatment is mostly supportive, with isolated trials of radiation therapy, antiosteoclastic and anti-angiogenic medications including pamidronate, zoledronic acid, and alpha-2b interferon [212].

19.5 Pleural-based Tumors

Primary pleural tumors are rare in children. Pleural-based PPB has already been discussed. Pleural rhabdomyosarcomas have been described, but some of these would now be considered as PPB. Rare reports of mesotheliomas in children exist [213]. Pleural fibroma is a lesion that is similar to fibromatoses.

Overall, most pleural lesions encountered will be metastases to the visceral or parietal pleura.

References

1. Kumar AP, et al. (1977) Combined therapy for malignant tumors of the chest wall in children. J Pediatr Surg 12(6):991–999
2. Shamberger RC, Grier HE (1994) Chest wall tumors in infants and children. Semin Pediatr Surg 3(4):267–276
3. Grosfeld JL (1994) Primary tumors of the chest wall and mediastinum in children. Semin Thorac Cardiovasc Surg 6(4):235–239
4. Grosfeld JL, et al. (1998) Chest wall resection and reconstruction for malignant conditions in childhood. J Pediatr Surg 23(7):667–673
5. Shamberger RC, et al. (1994) Malignant small round cell tumor (Ewing's-PNET) of the chest wall in children. J Pediatr Surg 29(2):179–184; discussion 184–185
6. Joseph WL Fonkalsrud EW (1972) Primary rib tumors in children. Am Surg 38(6):338–342
7. Franken EA Jr, Smith JA, Smith WL (1977) Tumors of the chest wall in infants and children. Pediatr Radiol 6(1):13–18
8. Berard J, Jaubert de Beaujeu M, Valla JS (1982) Primary tumors of the ribs in children and adolescents. Apropos of 15 cases. Chir Pediatr 23(6):387–392
9. Raney RB Jr, et al. (1982) Soft-tissue sarcoma of the trunk in childhood. Results of the intergroup rhabdomyosarcoma study. Cancer 49(12):2612–2616
10. Soyer T, et al. (2006) The results of surgical treatment of chest wall tumors in childhood. Pediatr Surg Int 22(2):135–139
11. Dang NC, Siegel SE, Phillips JD (1999) Malignant chest wall tumors in children and young adults. J Pediatr Surg 34(12):1773–1778
12. Fletcher CDM, Unni K, Mertens F (2002) Pathology and genetics of tumors of soft tissue and bone. In: World Health Organization Classification of Tumors. IARC Press, Lyon, France pp. 26–27
13. Ayala AG, et al. (1993) Mesenchymal hamartoma of the chest wall in infants and children: A clinicopathological study of five patients. Skeletal Radiol 22(8):569–576
14. Groom KR, et al. (2002) Mesenchymal hamartoma of the chest wall: Radiologic manifestations with emphasis on cross-sectional imaging and histopathologic comparison. Radiology 222(1):205–211
15. Shimotake T, et al. (2005) Respiratory insufficiency in a newborn with mesenchymal hamartoma of the chest wall occupying the thoracic cavity. J Pediatr Surg 40(4):E13–16
16. Jung AL, et al. (1994) Congenital chest wall mesenchymal hamartoma. J Perinatol 14(6):487–491
17. Odaka A, et al. (2005) Chest wall mesenchymal hamartoma associated with a massive fetal pleural effusion: A case report. J Pediatr Surg 40(5):e5–7
18. Freeburn AM, McAloon J (2001) Infantile chest hamartoma – Case outcome aged 11. Arch Dis Child 85(3):244–245
19. Raney RB Jr, (1991) Chemotherapy for children with aggressive fibromatosis and Langerhans' cell histiocytosis. Clin Orthop Relat Res (262):58–63
20. Merchant TE, et al. (2000) Long-term results with radiation therapy for pediatric desmoid tumors. Int J Radiat Oncol Biol Phys 47(5):1267–1271
21. Skapek SX, et al. (1998) Combination chemotherapy using vinblastine and methotrexate for the treatment of progressive desmoid tumor in children. J Clin Oncol 16(9):3021–3027
22. Lackner H, et al. (2004) Multimodal treatment of children with unresectable or recurrent desmoid tumors: An 11-year longitudinal observational study. J Pediatr Hematol Oncol 26(8):518–522
23. Shamberger RC Grier HE (2001) Ewing's sarcoma/primitive neuroectodermal tumor of the chest wall. Semin Pediatr Surg 10(3):153–160
24. Bourque MD, et al. (1989) Malignant small-cell tumor of the thoracopulmonary region: 'Askin tumor'. J Pediatr Surg 24(10):1079–1083

25. Thomas PR, et al. (1983) Primary Ewing's sarcoma of the ribs. A report from the intergroup Ewing's sarcoma study. Cancer 51(6):1021–1027

26. Askin FB, et al. (1979) Malignant small cell tumor of the thoracopulmonary region in childhood: a distinctive clinicopathologic entity of uncertain histogenesis. Cancer 43(6):2438–2451

27. Dehner LP (1993) Primitive neuroectodermal tumor and Ewing's sarcoma. Am J Surg Pathol 17(1):1–13

28. Lazar A, et al. (2006) Molecular diagnosis of sarcomas: Chromosomal translocations in sarcomas. Arch Pathol Lab Med 130(8):1199–1207

29. Zucman J, et al. (1992) Cloning and characterization of the Ewing's sarcoma and peripheral neuroepithelioma t(11;22) translocation breakpoints. Genes Chromosomes Cancer 5(4):271–277

30. Denny CT (1996) Gene rearrangements in Ewing's sarcoma. Cancer Invest 14(1):83–88

31. Shamberger RC, et al. (2003) Ewing sarcoma/primitive neuroectodermal tumor of the chest wall: Impact of initial versus delayed resection on tumor margins, survival, and use of radiation therapy. Ann Surg 238(4):563–567; discussion 567–568

32. Hoffer FA, Kozakewich H, Shamberger RC (1990) Percutaneous biopsy of thoracic lesions in children. Cardiovasc Intervent Radiol 13(1):32–35

33. Shamberger RC, et al. (1989) Chest wall tumors in infancy and childhood. Cancer 63(4):774–785

34. Rao BN, et al. (1988) Chest wall resection for Ewing's sarcoma of the rib: An unnecessary procedure. Ann Thorac Surg 46(1):40–44

35. Brown AP, Fixsen JA, Plowman PA (1987) Local control of Ewing's sarcoma: An analysis of 67 patients. Br J Radiol 60(711):261–268

36. Hayes FA, et al. (1989) Therapy for localized Ewing's sarcoma of bone. J Clin Oncol 7(2):208–213

37. Ramming KP, et al. (1982) Surgical management and reconstruction of extensive chest wall malignancies. Am J Surg 144(1):146–152

38. Kissane JM, et al. (1981) Sarcomas of bone in childhood: Pathologic aspects. Natl Cancer Inst Monogr (56):29–41

39. Sabanathan S, et al. (1985) Primary chest wall tumors. Ann Thorac Surg 39(1):4–15

40. Ewing J (1972) Classics in oncology. Diffuse endothelioma of bone. James Ewing. Proceedings of the New York Pathological Society, 1921. CA Cancer J Clin 22(2):95–98

41. Tucker MA, et al. (1987) Bone sarcomas linked to radiotherapy and chemotherapy in children. N Engl J Med 317(10):588–593

42. Strong LC, et al. (1979) Risk of radiation-related subsequent malignant tumors in survivors of Ewing's sarcoma. J Natl Cancer Inst 62(6):1401–1406

43. Kuttesch JF Jr, et al. (1996) Second malignancies after Ewing's sarcoma: radiation dose-dependency of secondary sarcomas. J Clin Oncol 14(10):2818–2825

44. Nesbit ME Jr, et al. (1990) Multimodal therapy for the management of primary, nonmetastatic Ewing's sarcoma of bone: A long-term follow-up of the First intergroup study. J Clin Oncol 8(10):1664–1674

45. Arai Y, et al. (1991) Ewing's sarcoma: Local tumor control and patterns of failure following limited-volume radiation therapy. Int J Radiat Oncol Biol Phys 21(6):1501–1508

46. Burgert EO Jr, et al. (1990) Multimodal therapy for the management of nonpelvic, localized Ewing's sarcoma of bone: Intergroup study IESS-II. J Clin Oncol 8(9):1514–1524

47. Grier HE, et al. (2003) Addition of ifosfamide and etoposide to standard chemotherapy for Ewing's sarcoma and primitive neuroectodermal tumor of bone. N Engl J Med 348(8):694–701

48. Miser JS, et al. (2004) Treatment of metastatic Ewing's sarcoma or primitive neuroectodermal tumor of bone: Evaluation of combination ifosfamide and etoposide – A Children's Cancer Group and Pediatric Oncology Group study. J Clin Oncol 22(14):2873–2876

49. Paulussen M, et al. (1993) Results of treatment of primary exclusively pulmonary metastatic Ewing sarcoma. A retrospective analysis of 41 patients. Klin Padiatr 205(4):210–216

50. Andrassy RJ, et al. (1998) Thoracic sarcomas in children. Ann Surg 227(2):170–173

51. Crist W, et al. (1995) The Third Intergroup Rhabdomyosarcoma Study. J Clin Oncol 13(3):610–630

52. Maurer HM, et al. (1988) The Intergroup Rhabdomyosarcoma Study-I. A final report. Cancer 61(2):209–220

53. Maurer HM, et al. (1993) The Intergroup Rhabdomyosarcoma Study-II. Cancer 71(5):1904–1922

54. Chui CH, et al. (2005) Predictors of outcome in children and adolescents with rhabdomyosarcoma of the trunk – The St Jude Children's Research Hospital experience. J Pediatr Surg 40(11):1691–1695

55. Saenz NC, et al. (1997) Chest wall rhabdomyosarcoma. Cancer 80(8):1513–1517

56. Rodeberg DA, et al. (2002) Surgical principles for children/adolescents with newly diagnosed rhabdomyosarcoma: A report from the Soft Tissue Sarcoma Committee of the Children's Oncology Group. Sarcoma 6(4):111–122

57. Neville HL, et al. (2000) Lymphatic mapping with sentinel node biopsy in pediatric patients. J Pediatr Surg 35(6):961–964

58. Rodeberg D, Paidas C (2006) Childhood rhabdomyosarcoma. Semin Pediatr Surg 15(1):57–62

59. Fong YC, et al. (2004) Chondrosarcoma of the chest wall: A retrospective clinical analysis. Clin Orthop Relat Res (427):184–189

60. Loh ML, et al. (2002) Treatment of infantile fibrosarcoma with chemotherapy and surgery: Results from the Dana-Farber Cancer Institute and Children's Hospital, Boston. J Pediatr Hematol Oncol 24(9):722–726

61. Ninane J, et al. (1986) Congenital fibrosarcoma. Preoperative chemotherapy and conservative surgery. Cancer 58(7):1400–1406

62. Grier HE, Perez-Atayde AR, Weinstein HJ, (1985) Chemotherapy for inoperable infantile fibrosarcoma. Cancer 56(7):1507–1510

63. Malangoni MA, et al. (1980) Survival and pulmonary function following chest wall resection and reconstruction in children. J Pediatr Surg 15(6):906–912

64. Mathisen DJ (1990) Surgical techniques for chest wall reconstruction. Ann Thorac Surg 49(1):164–165

65. Weyant MJ, et al. (2006) Results of chest wall resection and reconstruction with and without rigid prosthesis. Ann Thorac Surg 81(1):279–285

66. Lee SL, Poulos ND, Greenholz SK (2002) Staged reconstruction of large congenital diaphragmatic defects with synthetic patch followed by reverse latissimus dorsi muscle. J Pediatr Surg 37(3):367–370

67. Sakaguchi K, et al. (2006) Large chest wall reconstruction using a pedicled osteomuscle composite flap: Report of a case. Surg Today 36(2):180–183

68. Tukiainen E, Popov P, Asko-Seljavaara S (2003) Microvascular reconstructions of full-thickness oncological chest wall defects. Ann Surg 238(6):794–801; discussion 801–802

69. Chang RR, et al. (2004) Reconstruction of complex oncologic chest wall defects: A 10-year experience. Ann Plast Surg 52(5):471–479; discussion 479

70. DeRosa GP (1985) Progressive scoliosis following chest wall resection in children. Spine 10(7):618–622

71. Bacci G, et al. (2005) Second malignancy in 597 patients with Ewing's sarcoma of bone treated at a single institution with adjuvant and neoadjuvant chemotherapy between 1972 and 1999. J Pediatr Hematol Oncol 27(10):517–520

72. Paulussen M, et al. (2001) Second malignancies after Ewing tumor treatment in 690 patients from a cooperative German/Austrian/Dutch study. Ann Oncol 12(11):1619–1630

73. Stocker J (2001) The Respiratory Tract. In: Stocker J, Dehner L (eds) Pediatric Pathology. Lippincot, Williams & Wilkins, Philadelphia, pp. 445–517

74. Young MM, et al. (1989) Treatment of sarcomas of the chest wall using intensive combined modality therapy. Int J Radiat Oncol Biol Phys 16(1):49–57

75. Ozaki T, et al. (1995) Ewing's sarcoma of the ribs. A report from the cooperative Ewing's sarcoma study. Eur J Cancer 31A(13–14):2284–2288

76. Cohen MC Kaschula RO (1992) Primary pulmonary tumors in childhood: A review of 31 years' experience and the literature. Pediatr Pulmonol 14(4):222–232

77. Hartman GE, Shochat SJ (1983) Primary pulmonary neoplasms of childhood: A review. Ann Thorac Surg 36(1):108–119

78. Hancock BJ, et al. (1993) Childhood primary pulmonary neoplasms. J Pediatr Surg 28(9):1133–1136

79. Lal DR, et al. (2005) Primary epithelial lung malignancies in the pediatric population. Pediatr Blood Cancer 45(5):683–686

80. Ayadi-Kaddour A, et al. (2006) Pulmonary inflammatory pseudotumor: Difficulties in diagnosis and prognosis. Tunis Med 84(3):205–208

81. Su LD, et al. (1998) Inflammatory myofibroblastic tumor: Cytogenetic evidence supporting clonal origin. Mod Pathol 11(4):364–368

82. Agrons GA, et al. (1998) Pulmonary inflammatory pseudotumor: Radiologic features. Radiology 206(2):511–518

83. Hedlund GL, et al. (1999) Aggressive manifestations of inflammatory pulmonary pseudotumor in children. Pediatr Radiol 29(2):112–116

84. Shapiro MP, Gale ME, Carter BL (1987) Variable CT appearance of plasma cell granuloma of the lung. J Comput Assist Tomogr 11(1):49–51

85. Applebaum H, et al. (2005) The rationale for nonsteroidal anti-inflammatory drug therapy for inflammatory myofibroblastic tumors: A Children's Oncology Group study. J Pediatr Surg 40(6):999–1003; discussion 1003

86. Eggli KD, Newman B (1993) Nodules, masses, and pseudomasses in the pediatric lung. Radiol Clin North Am 31(3):651–666

87. Carney JA (1999) Gastric stromal sarcoma, pulmonary chondroma, and extra-adrenal paraganglioma (Carney Triad): Natural history, adrenocortical component, and possible familial occurrence. Mayo Clin Proc 74(6):543–552

88. Somers GR, et al. (1997) Juvenile laryngeal papillomatosis in a pediatric population: A clinicopathologic study. Pediatr Pathol Lab Med 17(1):53–64

89. Wang LT, Wilkins EW Jr, Bode HH (1993) Bronchial carcinoid tumors in pediatric patients. Chest 103(5):1426–1428

90. Andrassy RJ, Feldtman RW, Stanford W (1997) Bronchial carcinoid tumors in children and adolescents. J Pediatr Surg 12(4):513–517

91. Seo IS, et al. (1984) Mucoepidermoid carcinoma of the bronchus in a 4-year-old child. A high-grade variant with lymph node metastasis. Cancer 53(7):1600–1604

92. Tsuchiya H, et al. (1997) Childhood bronchial mucoepidermoid tumors. J Pediatr Surg 32(1):106–109

93. Torres AM, Ryckman FC (1988) Childhood tracheobronchial mucoepidermoid carcinoma: A case report and review of the literature. J Pediatr Surg 23(4):367–370

94. Okike N, et al. (1978) Bronchoplastic procedures in the treatment of carcinoid tumors of the tracheobronchial tree. J Thorac Cardiovasc Surg 76(3):281–291

95. Laberge JM, Puligandla P, Flageole H (2005) Asymptomatic congenital lung malformations. Semin Pediatr Surg 14(1):16–33

96. Ota H, et al. (1998) Histochemical analysis of mucous cells of congenital adenomatoid malformation of the lung: Insights into the carcinogenesis of pulmonary adenocarcinoma expressing gastric mucins. Am J Clin Pathol 110(4):450–455

97. Wang NS, Chen MF, Chen FF (1999) The glandular component in congenital cystic adenomatoid malformation of the lung. Respirology 4(2):147–153

98. Ohye RG, et al. (1998) Pediatric bronchioloalveolar carcinoma: A favorable pediatric malignancy? J Pediatr Surg 33(5):730–732

99. Simma B, et al. (1993) Squamous-cell carcinoma arising in a non-irradiated child with recurrent respiratory papillomatosis. Eur J Pediatr 152(9):776–778

100. Manivel JC, et al. (1998) Pleuropulmonary blastoma. The so-called pulmonary blastoma of childhood. Cancer 62(8):1516–1526

101. Pai S, et al. (2006) Correction: Pleuropulmonary blastoma, not rhabdomyosarcoma in a congenital lung cyst. Pediatr Blood Cancer

102. Priest JR, et al. (1997) Pleuropulmonary blastoma: A clinicopathologic study of 50 cases. Cancer 80(1):147–161

103. Boldrini R, et al. (2005) Pulmonary blastomas of childhood: Histologic, immunohistochemical, ultrastructural aspects and therapeutic considerations. Ultrastruct Pathol 29(6):493–501

104. Pleuropulmonary blastoma registry (2006) www.ppbregistry.org/

105. Priest JR, et al. (2006) Type I pleuropulmonary blastoma: A report from the International Pleuropulmonary Blastoma Registry. J Clin Oncol 24(27):4492–4498

106. Miniati DN, et al. (2006) Prenatal presentation and outcome of children with pleuropulmonary blastoma. J Pediatr Surg 41(1):66–71

107 Hachitanda Y, et al. (1993) Pleuropulmonary blastoma in childhood. A tumor of divergent differentiation. Am J Surg Pathol 17(4):382–391

108. Teeratakulpisarn J, et al. (2003) Pleuropulmonary blastoma in a child presenting with spontaneous pneumothorax. J Med Assoc Thai 86(4):385–391

109. Paupe A, et al. (1994) Pneumothorax revealing pneumoblastoma in an infant. Arch Pediatr 1(10):919–922

110. Rubinas TC, et al. (2006) Pneumothorax and pulmonary cyst in a 2-year-old child. Pleuropulmonary blastoma. Arch Pathol Lab Med, 130(4):e47–49

111. Dehner LP (1994) Pleuropulmonary blastoma is THE pulmonary blastoma of childhood. Semin Diagn Pathol 11(2):144–151

112. Priest JR, et al. (2006) Cerebral metastasis and other central nervous system complications of pleuropulmonary blastoma. Pediatr Blood Cancer

113. Parsons SK, et al. (2001) Aggressive multimodal treatment of pleuropulmonary blastoma. Ann Thorac Surg 72(3):939–942

114. Shariff S, et al. (1988) Primary pulmonary rhabdomyosarcoma in a child, with a review of literature. J Surg Oncol 38(4):261–264

115. Federici S, et al. (2001) Pleuropulmonary blastoma in congenital cystic adenomatoid malformation: Report of a case. Eur J Pediatr Surg 11(3):196–199

116. Indolfi P, et al. (2000) Pleuropulmonary blastoma: Management and prognosis of 11 cases. Cancer 89(6):1396–1401

117. Hill DA, Dehner LP (2004) A cautionary note about congenital cystic adenomatoid malformation (CCAM) type 4. Am J Surg Pathol 28(4):554–555; author reply 555

118. Picaud JC, et al. (2000) Bilateral cystic pleuropulmonary blastoma in early infancy. J Pediatr 136(6):834–836

119. Priest JR, et al. (1996) Pleuropulmonary blastoma: A marker for familial disease. J Pediatr 128(2):220–224

120. Boman F, Hill D, Williams G (2006) Familial association of pleuropulmonary blastoma with cystic nephroma other renal tumors: A report from the International Pleuropulmonary Blastoma Registry. J Peds (in press)

121. Tagge EP, et al. (1996) Childhood pleuropulmonary blastoma: Caution against nonoperative management of congenital lung cysts. J Pediatr Surg 31(1):187–189; discussion 190

122. Hill DA, (2005) USCAP Specialty Conference: Case 1-type I pleuropulmonary blastoma. Pediatr Dev Pathol 8(1):77–84

123. Crist WM, et al. (1982) Intrathoracic soft tissue sarcomas in children. Cancer 50(3):598–604

124. Weinberg AG, et al. (1980) Mesenchymal neoplasia and congenital pulmonary cysts. Pediatr Radiol 9(3):179–182

125. Micallef-Eynaud PD, et al. (1993) Intracerebral recurrence of primary intrathoracic rhabdomyosarcoma. Med Pediatr Oncol 21(2):132–136

126. McDermott VG, Mackenzie S, Hendry GM (1993) Case report: Primary intrathoracic rhabdomyosarcoma: A rare childhood malignancy. Br J Radiol 66(790):937–941

127. Iqbal Y, et al. (2003) Lung mass in a child. J Pediatr Hematol Oncol 25(8):677–678

128. Murphy JJ, et al. (1992) Rhabdomyosarcoma arising within congenital pulmonary cysts: Report of three cases. J Pediatr Surg 27(10):1364–1367

129. Allan BT, Day DL, Dehner LP (1987) Primary pulmonary rhabdomyosarcoma of the lung in children. Report of two cases presenting with spontaneous pneumothorax. Cancer 59(5):1005–1011

130. Schiavetti A, et al. (1996) Primary pulmonary rhabdomyosarcoma in childhood: Clinico-biologic features in two cases with review of the literature. Med Pediatr Oncol 26(3):201–7

131. Pettinato G, et al. (1989) Primary bronchopulmonary fibrosarcoma of childhood and adolescence: Reassessment of a low-grade malignancy. Clinicopathologic study of five cases and review of the literature. Hum Pathol 20(5):463–471

132. Keel SB, et al. (1999) Primary pulmonary sarcoma: A clinicopathologic study of 26 cases. Mod Pathol 12(12):1124–1131

133. Daw NC, et al. (2003) Malignant fibrous histiocytoma and other fibrohistiocytic tumors in pediatric patients: The St. Jude Children's Research Hospital experience. Cancer 97(11):2839–2847

134. Dehner L (1987) Mediastinum, lungs, and cardiovascular system. In: Dehner L (ed) Pediatric Surgical Pathology, 2nd edn. Williams & Wilkins, Baltimore, pp. 229–333

135. Kayton ML (2006) Pulmonary metastasectomy in pediatric patients. Thorac Surg Clin 16(2):167–183, vi

136. Karnak I, et al. (2002) Pulmonary metastases in children: An analysis of surgical spectrum. Eur J Pediatr Surg 12(3):151–158

137. Kayton ML, et al. (2006) Computed tomographic scan of the chest underestimates the number of metastatic lesions in osteosarcoma. J Pediatr Surg 41(1):200–206; discussion 200–206

138. Kager L, et al. (2003) Primary metastatic osteosarcoma: Presentation and outcome of patients treated on neoadjuvant Cooperative Osteosarcoma Study Group protocols. J Clin Oncol 21(10):2011–2018

139. Harting MT, et al. (2006) Long-term survival after aggressive resection of pulmonary metastases among children and adolescents with osteosarcoma. J Pediatr Surg 41(1):194–199

140. Harting MT, Blakely ML (2006) Management of osteosarcoma pulmonary metastases. Semin Pediatr Surg 15(1):25–29

141. Su WT, et al. (2004) Surgical management and outcome of osteosarcoma patients with unilateral pulmonary metastases. J Pediatr Surg 39(3):418–423; discussion 418–423

142. Cohen M, et al. (1981) Pulmonary pseudometastases in children with malignant tumors. Radiology 141(2):371–374

143. Rao BN (1997) Present day concepts of thoracoscopy as a modality in pediatric cancer management. Int Surg 82(2):123–126

144. Lima M, et al. (2004) Thoracoscopic management of suspected thoraco-pulmonary malignant diseases in pediatric age. Pediatr Med Chir 26(2):132–135

145. Sailhamer E, et al. (2003) Minimally invasive surgery for pediatric solid neoplasms. Am Surg 69(7):566–568

146. Waldhausen JH, Tapper D, Sawin RS (2000) Minimally invasive surgery and clinical decision-making for pediatric malignancy. Surg Endosc 14(3):250–253

147. Rothenberg SS (1998) Thoracoscopy in infants and children. Semin Pediatr Surg 7(4):194–201

148. Holcomb GW 3rd (1999) Minimally invasive surgery for solid tumors. Semin Surg Oncol 16(2):184–192

149. Spurbeck WW, et al. (2004) Minimally invasive surgery in pediatric cancer patients. Ann Surg Oncol 11(3):340–343

150. King RM, et al. (1982) Primary mediastinal tumors in children. J Pediatr Surg 17(5):512–520

151. Grosfeld JL, et al. (1994) Mediastinal tumors in children: Experience with 196 cases. Ann Surg Oncol 1(2):121–127

152. Zhurilo IP, et al. (2001) Mediastinal tumors and tumor-like formations in children. Klin Khir (9):44–47

153. Saenz NC, et al. (1993) Posterior mediastinal masses. J Pediatr Surg 28(2):172–176

154. Ricketts RR (2001) Clinical management of anterior mediastinal tumors in children. Seminars in Pediatric Surgery 10(3):161–168

155. Glick RD La Quaglia MP (1999) Lymphomas of the anterior mediastinum. Semin Pediatr Surg 8(2):69–77

156. Murphy SB, et al. (1989) Non-Hodgkin's lymphomas of childhood: An analysis of the histology, staging, and response to treatment of 338 cases at a single institution. J Clin Oncol 7(2):186–193

157. Chaignaud BE, et al. (1998) Pleural effusions in lymphoblastic lymphoma: A diagnostic alternative. J Pediatr Surg 33(9):1355–1357

158. Shamberger RC (1999) Preanesthetic evaluation of children with anterior mediastinal masses. Semin Pediatr Surg 8(2):61–68

159. Shamberger RC, et al. (1991) CT quantitation of tracheal cross-sectional area as a guide to the surgical and anesthetic management of children with anterior mediastinal masses. J Pediatr Surg 26(2):138–142

160. King DR, et al. (1997) Pulmonary function is compromised in children with mediastinal lymphoma. J Pediatr Surg 32(2):294–299; discussion 299–300

161. Mandell GA, Lantieri R, Goodman LR (1982) Tracheobronchial compression in Hodgkin lymphoma in children. AJR Am J Roentgenol 139(6):1167–1170

162. Griscom NT (1991) CT measurement of the tracheal lumen in children and adolescents. AJR Am J Roentgenol 156(2):371–372

163. Griscom NT, Wohl ME (1986) Dimensions of the growing trachea related to age and gender. AJR Am J Roentgenol 146(2):233–237

164. Azizkhan RG, et al. (1985) Life-threatening airway obstruction as a complication to the management of mediastinal masses in children. J Pediatr Surg 20(6):816–822

165. Shamberger RC, et al. (1995) Prospective evaluation by computed tomography and pulmonary function tests of children with mediastinal masses. Surgery 118(3):468–471

166. van de Schoot L, et al. (2001) The role of fine-needle aspiration cytology in children with persistent or suspicious lymphadenopathy. J Pediatr Surg 36(1):7–11

167. Shabb NS, et al. (1998) Fine-needle aspiration of the mediastinum: A clinical, radiologic, cytologic, and histologic study of 42 cases. Diagn Cytopathol 19(6):428–436

168. Otani Y, et al. (1996) Use of ultrasound-guided percutaneous needle biopsy in the diagnosis of mediastinal tumors. Surg Today 26(12):990–992

169. Herman SJ, et al. (1991) Anterior mediastinal masses: Utility of transthoracic needle biopsy. Radiology 180(1):167–170

170. Andersson T, Lindgren PG, Elvin A (1992) Ultrasound guided tumour biopsy in the anterior mediastinum. An alternative to thoracotomy and mediastinoscopy. Acta Radiol 33(5):423–426

171. Pugh JL, et al. (2006) Diagnosis of deep-seated lymphoma and leukemia by endoscopic ultrasound-guided fine-needle aspiration biopsy. Am J Clin Pathol 125(5):703–709

172. Olak J (1996) Parasternal mediastinotomy (Chamberlain procedure). Chest Surg Clin N Am 6(1):31–40

173. Ryckman FC, Rodgers BM (1982) Thoracoscopy for intrathoracic neoplasia in children. J Pediatr Surg 17(5):521–524

174. Rodgers BM, et al. (1981) Thoracoscopy for intrathoracic tumors. Ann Thorac Surg 31(5):414–420

175. Ferrari LR, Bedford RF (1990) General anesthesia prior to treatment of anterior mediastinal masses in pediatric cancer patients. Anesthesiology 72(6):991–995

176. Loeffler JS, et al. (1986) Emergency prebiopsy radiation for mediastinal masses: Impact on subsequent pathologic diagnosis and outcome. J Clin Oncol 4(5):716–721

177. Halpern S, et al. (1983) Anterior mediastinal masses: Anesthesia hazards and other problems. J Pediatr 102(3):407–410

178. Frawley G, Low J, Brown TC (1995) Anaesthesia for an anterior mediastinal mass with ketamine and midazolam infusion. Anaesth Intensive Care 23(5):610–612

179. De Paepe M, van der Straeten M, Roels H (1983) Mediastinal angiofollicular lymph node hyperplasia with systemic manifestations. Eur J Respir Dis 64(2):134–140

180. Billmire DF (1999) Germ cell, mesenchymal, and thymic tumors of the mediastinum. Semin Pediatr Surg 8(2):85–91

181. Laberge J, NguyenL, Shaw K (2005) Teratomas, dermoids and other soft tissue tumors. In: Ashcraft K, Holcomb G, Murphy J (eds) Pediatric Surgery. Elsevier Saunders, Philadelphia pp. 972–996

182. Ozergin U, et al. (2003) Benign mature cystic teratoma of the anterior mediastinum leading to heart failure: Report of a case. Surg Today 33(7):518–520

183. Carter D, Bibro MC, Touloukian RJ (1982) Benign clinical behavior of immature mediastinal teratoma in infancy and childhood: Report of two cases and review of the literature. Cancer 49(2):398–402

184. Moeller KH, Rosado-de-Christenson ML, Templeton PA (1997) Mediastinal mature teratoma: Imaging features. AJR Am J Roentgenol 169(4):985–990

185. Partrick DA, Rothenberg SS (2001) Thoracoscopic resection of mediastinal masses in infants and children: An evaluation of technique and results. J Pediatr Surg 36(8):1165–1167

186. Billmire DF (2006) Germ cell tumors. Surg Clin North Am 86(2):489–503, xi

187. Billmire D, et al. (2001) Malignant mediastinal germ cell tumors: An intergroup study. J Pediatr Surg 36(1):18–24

188. Marina N, et al. (2006) Prognostic factors in children with extragonadal malignant germ cell tumors: A pediatric intergroup study. J Clin Oncol 24(16):2544–2548

189. Lack EE, Weinstein HJ, Welch KJ (1985) Mediastinal germ cell tumors in childhood. A clinical and pathological study of 21 cases. J Thorac Cardiovasc Surg 89(6):826–835

190. Billmire DF (2006) Malignant germ cell tumors in childhood. Semin Pediatr Surg 15(1):30–36

191. Nogues A, et al. (1987) Hodgkin's disease of the thymus: A rare mediastinal cystic mass. J Pediatr Surg 22(11):996–997

192. Welch KJ, Tapper D, Vawter GP (1979) Surgical treatment of thymic cysts and neoplasms in children. J Pediatr Surg 14(6):691–698

193. Pan CH, Chiang CY, Chen SS (1988) Thymolipoma in patients with myasthenia gravis: Report of two cases and review. Acta Neurol Scand 78(1):16–21

194. Barnes RD, O'Gorman P (1962) Two cases of aplastic anaemia associated with tumours of the thymus. J Clin Pathol 15:264–268

195. Benton C, Gerard P (1996) Thymolipoma in a patient with Graves' disease. Case report and review of the literature. J Thorac Cardiovasc Surg 51(3):428–433

196. Pillai R, et al. (1985) Thymolipoma in association with Hodgkin's disease. J Thorac Cardiovasc Surg 90(2):306–308

197. Kitano Y, et al. (1993) Giant thymolipoma in a child. J Pediatr Surg 28(12):1622–1625

198. Ferrari G, Paci M, Sgarbi G (2006) Thymolipoma of the anterior mediastinum: videothoracoscopic removal using a bilateral approach. Thorac Cardiovasc Surg 54(6):435–437

199. Shimada Y, et al. (1995) Congenital dumbbell neuroblastoma. Spine 20(11):1295–1300

200. Boglino C, et al. (1999) Spinal cord vascular injuries following surgery of advanced thoracic neuroblastoma: An unusual catastrophic complication. Med Pediatr Oncol 32(5):349–352

201. De Bernardi B, et al. (2001) Neuroblastoma with symptomatic spinal cord compression at diagnosis: Treatment and results with 76 cases. J Clin Oncol 19(1):183–190

202. Katzenstein HM, et al. (2001) Treatment and outcome of 83 children with intraspinal neuroblastoma: The Pediatric Oncology Group experience. J Clin Oncol 19(4):1047–1055

203. Plantaz D, et al. (1996) The treatment of neuroblastoma with intraspinal extension with chemotherapy followed by surgical removal of residual disease. A prospective study of 42 patients – results of the NBL 90 Study of the French Society of Pediatric Oncology. Cancer 78(2):311–319

204. Laberge J (2003) Neuroblastoma. In: O'Neill JJ, et al. (eds) Principles of pediatric surgery. W.B. Saunders, pp. 211–219

205. McLatchie GR, Young DG (1980) Presenting features of thoracic neuroblastoma. Arch Dis Child 55(12):958–962

206. Adams GA, et al. (1993) Thoracic neuroblastoma: A Pediatric Oncology Group study. J Pediatr Surg 28(3):372–377; discussion 377–378

207. Morris JA, et al. (1995) Biological variables in thoracic neuroblastoma: A Pediatric Oncology Group study. J Pediatr Surg 30(2):296–302; discussion 302–303

208. Raffensperger J, Cohen R (1972) Plexiform neurofibromas in childhood. J Pediatr Surg 7(2):144–151

209. Puligandla PS, et al. (2004) Pericardial hemangioma presenting as thoracic mass in utero. Fetal Diagn Ther 19(2):178–181

210. Patel DV (2005) Gorham's disease or massive osteolysis. Clin Med Res 3(2):65–74

211. Aviv RI, McHugh K, Hunt J (2001) Angiomatosis of bone and soft tissue: A spectrum of disease from diffuse lymphangiomatosis to vanishing bone disease in young patients. Clin Radiol 56(3):184–190

212. Mignogna MD, et al. (2005) Treatment of Gorham's disease with zoledronic acid. Oral Oncol 41(7):747–750

213. Fraire AE, et al. (1988) Mesothelioma of childhood. Cancer 62(4):838–847

Rare Tumors

20

Hugo A. Heij

Contents

20.1 Definition

When is a tumor called rare? From a practical point of view we will use the definition in this chapter that a tumor is considered "rare" if there is no treatment protocol available.

One can derive a very long "list of rarities" from the pediatric pathology literature [1–3], which allows the following subdivided definitions:
1. Rare tumors independent of age.
2. Adult-type tumors in children.
3. Rare but typical childhood tumors.
4. Common pediatric tumors with rare histologic features.
5. Common pediatric tumors in rare locations.
6. Seemingly common but in fact rare tumors.
7. Rarely recognized occurrences of common tumors.

In view of the surgical character of this book it seems appropriate to discuss the rare tumors arranged according to their anatomical regions, with special emphasis on the abdominal cavity. The aim of this chapter is not to provide an exhaustive list of all rare tumors, but rather to focus on solid tumors that require surgical treatment. Where possible, guidelines for management will be derived from the available literature. To that purpose, literature searches have been performed in Medline (PubMed) using the type of tumor as MESH term, focusing on reviews. Also, cross references and hand searches of the literature have been done.

20.1.1 IPSO Rare Tumor Registry

Ten years ago, a registry of rare tumors was instituted by the International Society for Pediatric Surgical Oncology (IPSO). The aims of this registry are to collect data and tissue for research, and to provide information and guidance on the management of patients with rare tumors.

The entries provide an impression (but nothing more exact than an impression) of the epidemiology. For the epidemiology and incidence: see also [2]. Table 20.1 provides an overview of the spectrum of tumors registered.

20.2 Inflammatory Myofibroblastic Tumors

These are essentially benign tumors and the reason to present them here is because of the confusion that may arise with malignant tumors.

20.2.1 Terminology

Inflammatory myofibroblastic tumor (IMT) was first described in the lung in 1937, and since then has been reported at various sites. Histopathologically, IMT is a benign solid tumor, mainly composed of spindle-shaped cells, and has a chronic inflammatory component [4]. Synonyms are: inflammatory pseudotumor, pseudosarcomatous myofibroblastic proliferation, plasma cell tumor, xanthomatous pseudotumor, fibroxanthoma, and histiocytoma [4, 5].

The presentation varies according to the location: respiratory symptoms and clubbing in pulmonary IMT; abdominal pain, fever, and weight loss in abdominal IMT [6]. Large fibrous inflammatory pseudotumors may occur in the mesentery, duodenum, jejunum, pancreas, spleen, and liver [4, 5, 7–9].

The most frequent finding is a palpable mass in the abdomen [4, 9–11]. Jaundice was the presenting sign

Table 20.1 Overview of the spectrum of tumors registered with IPSO

Tumor spectrum	
Adrenocortical carcinoma	30
Hamoudi (Frantz) tumor	11
Carcinoid	3
GIST	3
Pancreaticoblastoma	3
Aggressive fibromatosis	3
Pulmonary blastoma	2
Pheochromocytoma	2
Lipoblastoma	2
Chorioncarcinoma liver	2
Desmoplastic tumor abdomen	2
Single entries (n=25)	
Transitional cell carcinoma	
Spindle epithelial tumor with thymus-like differentiation (SETTLE)	
Seminoma	
Renal cell carcinoma	
Mullerian papilloma	
Mucoepidermoid bronchial carcinoma	
Metanephric adenofibroma	
Mesenchymal hamartoma	
Malignant trophoblastic tumor placental site	
Malignant fibrohistiocytoma	
Malignant nonchromaffinic paraganglioma	
Inflamm. myofibroblastic tumor – pt known with neurofibromatosis	
Infantile fibromatosis	
Hemangiopericytoma (infantile type)	
Granulosa-Theca cell tumor	
Gonadoblastoma	
Follicular thyroid ca (lft)	
FNH (focal nodular hyperplasia)	
Embryonic pancreatic tumor	
Ductal adenocarcinoma of pancreas/hepatoblastoma (fetal type)	
Chondroblastoma	
Chemodectoma	
Angiomyolipoma (Tuberous sclerosis)	
Angiomatoid fibrous histiocytoma	
Adenocarcinoma colon	

(with acknowledgement to Dr. D.C. Aronson)

in a 6-year-old boy with IMT in the hilum of the liver [7].

Thoracic IMT has been reported in the heart [12], lung [4], mediastinum, and trachea [5]. A 14-year-old

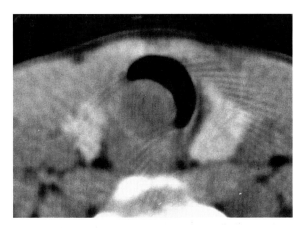

Fig. 20.1 I.M.T. of the trachea. Inflammatory pseudotumor of the trachea. (From [5])

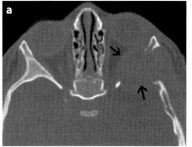

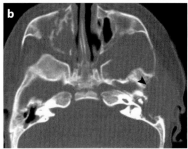

Fig. 20.2 a,b Langerhans cell histiocystosis (**a**) CT scan shows a lytic lesion of the frontal and sphenoid bones (arrows) (**b**) CT scan shows destruction of the temporal bone (arrowhead) (From [20])

boy with IMT of the trachea underwent successful CO_2-laser excision [5] (Fig. 20.1).

The treatment of IMT is complete resection, which may require sacrifice of blood vessels and other vital structures [7, 13]. There are scarce data on recurrence rate, but the available evidence suggests it may be higher than 10%. Tumors that have ill-defined margins and therefore cannot be resected completely have a higher risk of recurrence [8]. Although histologically benign, radiation and cytotoxics have been successfully used in unresectable and recurrent IMT. Corticosteroids have also been advocated under these circumstances [11].

20.2.2   Xanthogranulomatous Pyelonephritis

Xanthogranulomatous pyelonephritis (XPN) is a rare destructive inflammatory process. This condition can be mistaken for a Wilms' tumor; however, the radiographic presence of infection and calculi often help to make a preoperative diagnosis of XPN. Treatment is nephrectomy and antibiotic coverage [14].

20.2.3   Juvenile Xanthogranuloma

Juvenile xanthogranuloma (JXG) is a member of the group of histiocytic proliferative disorders. JXG is a usually benign self-limiting disorder presenting as nodular skin lesions. It occurs mainly in the head and neck region and is present at birth in 5–17% of the cases [15]. In the hand, JXG may arise from the tendon sheath and is called giant cell tumor of the tendon sheath [16].

Disseminated JXG in contrast may involve liver, lungs and CNS, and in young children has a poor prognosis. Various treatments, including surgical re-

section, have been attempted. Dölken, et al. report a 7-month-old girl with life-threatening systemic JXG, including multiple CNS lesions, that responded well to chemotherapy according to the Langerhans cell histiocytosis protocol [17].

20.2.4   Langerhans' Cell Histiocytosis

Histiocytic and dendritic neoplasms in children are rare. They arise from antigen-processing phagocytes (histiocytes) and antigen-presenting dendritic cells, which are derived from the hemopoietic stem cells. The WHO classification distinguishes six entities, of which Langerhans' cell histiocytosis is the most common. Other types are: Langerhans' cell sarcoma and histiocytic sarcoma. These tumors have been described in the vertebral bodies, responding to irradiation, but later metastasizing to the lung [18]; but also as primary pulmonary cystic lesions with fatal outcome despite chemotherapy [19]; as facial swelling [20] (Fig. 20.2); and as cervical lymphadenopathy, with a favorable response to chemotherapy [21].

20.2.5   Association of Malignancy and Langerhans' Cell Histiocytosis

A case of simultaneous occurrence of malignant histocytosis and primary gonadal germ cell tumor was reported in an 18-year-old male by Margolin and Tarweek [22]. The testicular cancer was a stage 1 teratocarcinoma with endodermal sinus tumor elements with malignant histocytosis. The patient died despite treatment with chemotherapy.

Two case reports described the association of histocytosis and germ cell tumors. A 14-year-old boy developed fatal malignant histiocytosis of the spleen during cytotoxic treatment for mediastinal immature teratoma which had been excised 11 months before [23]. A 15-year-old boy presented with chest pain and was diagnosed with a mediastinal germ cell tumor and simultaneous histiocytioc sarcoma of the spleen [24].

20.3 Fibromatosis

Fibromatosis in children comprise a wide spectrum of conditions. A fibroblastic stem cell, called collagenoblast with many oncogenic potentials, has been postulated as the common origin of fibromatoses [25].

Infantile digital fibromatosis (Reye tumor) is a benign condition with a tendency to spontaneous regression. Calcifying aponeurotic fibroma is equally benign and requires conservative excision. In newborns, plantar nodules have been reported, that are classified as precalcaneal congenital fibrolipomatous hamartoma [26, 27]. At the other end of the spectrum are lesions like: low-grade myofibroblastic sarcoma, plexiform fibrohistiocytic tumor, and congenital and infantile fibrosarcoma that require complete (radical) excision [16].

Congenital intestinal fibromatosis has been reported to cause obstruction (Fig. 20.3) [28]. After excision, the prognosis is good [28, 29].

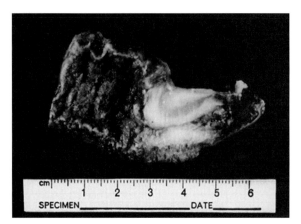

Fig. 20.3 Intestinal fibromatosis. Congenital solitary intestinal fibromatosis. (With kind permission from Numanoglu A, Davies J, Millar AJ, Rode H Congenital solitary intestinal fibromatosis. Eur J Pediatr Surg. 2002 Oct;12(5):337–340. Review)

Aggressive fibromatosis (AF), also called desmoid tumor, arises form the connective tissue of muscles and overlying fascia. The histological features are benign and they do not metastasize, but show local invasiveness and have a tendency to recur. The age distribution peak of pediatric AF is at 8 years (range 0 to 19). The majority occurs sporadically, but they can be associated with Familial Adenomatous Polyposis (FAP) and Gardner syndrome. The recurrence risk after complete excision is significantly lower than in the case of positive surgical margins [30, 31]. If complete excision is not feasible, as in intra-abdominal, mesenteric tumors, NSAIDs and tamoxifen may be effective [32]. The role of cytotoxic agents (a combination of vincristin, actinomycin-D, and cyclophosphamide, VAC) and radiotherapy, although advocated in cases of positive resection margins, is not defined [31].

Mesenteric fibromatosis has been reported in a 13-year-old boy after irradiation for Hodgkin's disease [33].

Fibromatoses in children are difficult to manage for a variety of reasons. They are rare and their clinical behavior is unpredictable. Most cannot be diagnosed without histologic material. Management must therefore be based on an adequate biopsy followed by a detailed discussion between pathologist and surgeon. Although some recur, those that are not malignant are best treated by conservative, nonmutilating excision, with further excision as recurrence occurs. When malignancy is found on biopsy, excision with a margin of normal tissue is necessary. MRI is helpful in planning these procedures. Appropriate staging, including CT-scan of the chest, is indicated [32].

20.4 Vascular Tumors

20.4.1 Malignant Vascular Tumors

Malignant vascular tumors (hemangiosarcoma, malignant hemangioendothelioma, and Kaposi sarcoma) are extremely rare in children.

A case of a 13-year-old girl with malignant hemangioendothelioma has been reported. The tumor was treated by surgical excision of the omentum. However, bloody ascites and multiple peritoneal implants were already present [34].

A series of 18 children were described by the combined Italian and German oncology groups [35]. Surgery is the mainstay of treatment, but even with combined treatment of excision, chemotherapy and radiotherapy the 5-year survival was 30%. A 2-year-old girl with rupture of a angiosarcoma of the spleen and liver metastases came into complete remission after splenectomy, partial liver resection, and treatment with VAI [36].

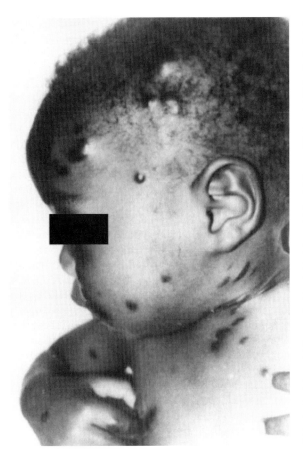

Fig 20.4 Kaposi's sarcoma. (From [38])

Kaposi sarcoma (KS) is associated with HIV in children in Africa (Fig. 20.4), but less frequently in children in industrialized countries [37]. In Africa, it is now one of the most frequent tumors in children [38]. The Human Herpes Virus 8 (HHV 8) is involved in the pathogenesis [39]. Thalidomide appears a promising and affordable inhibitor of angiogenesis [40].

20.4.2 Hemangiopericytomas

Hemangiopericytoma (HPC) is a rare tumor that represents 1% of all vascular tumors and arises not from endothelium but from pericytes, therefore strictly spoken it is not a blood vessel tumor. In children, there are two forms: the infantile (below the age of 12 months) and the adult type.

Although histologically this tumor looks aggressive, it behaves in a benign manner. Spontaneous regression has sometimes been observed. HPC can be localized in the heart, lung, retroperitoneum, or the urinary tract and may present as an abdominal mass causing obstructive symptoms. Subcutaneous tumors may not appear vascular. While the tumor is benign, tumor re-

currence has been recorded more than 10 years later. Imaging studies may show calcification in the soft tissues. The treatment of choice is complete excision of the tumor, which is followed by complete remission in patients with the infantile type. HPC in older children behaves like the adult type. Adjuvant treatment with VAC and IVA [ifosfamide, vincristine, Adriamycin (doxorubicin)] is advised in patients with irresectable lesions or positive margins [41].

20.5   Rare Tumors of the Head

20.5.1 Malignant Mesenchymoma

Malignant mesenchymoma is a rare neoplasm of mesenchymal origin arising in the soft tissues, the extremities, neck, back, sacrum, and occasionally in the mediastinum. See below, the section titled "Ectomesenchymoma."

20.5.2 Brain Metastases in Children

Hematogenous brain metastases are uncommon in children. A literature review revealed an incidence of 4% in over 2,000 reported patients. The incidence varied according to the primary tumor: between 1.3% in Wilms' tumor, 4.4% in neuroblastoma, and 13.5% in germ cell tumor [42]. In the SIOP Wilms' tumor studies between 1971 and 2000, brain metastases were reported in 14 out of 3,040 patients (0.5%). Treatment consisted of multimodal chemotherapy, radiotherapy, and surgery in seven patients. None of the patients survived [43]. In a review of 20 patients reported in the literature, death was recorded in five cases and in the remaining patients survival time of up to 8.5 years was noted [44]. There may be a publication bias in this compiled data since the experience of a single institution with 16 patients with brain metastases from various primary pediatric tumors, reported one survivor at 20 months with alveolar soft part sarcoma [45]. Many of these patients had metastases in multiple organs. In summary, the prognosis of brain metastases from solid tumors in children appears dismal, despite multimodal treatment.

20.5.3 Nasopharyngeal Carcinoma

Epithelial cancers (carcinomas) are the single largest group of rare tumors in children, with an incidence of 2–3% of all childhood malignancies in the Western population. For most sites incidence increases with age, but nasopharyngeal carcinoma (NPC) has a bimodal age distribution, with an early peak in adolescence. The most common presentation is with cervical lymphadenopathy. The role of surgery is therefore limited to biopsy. Chemotherapy (methotrexate, 5-FU, and cisplatinum) and irradiation achieved a high response rate and sustained remission in 91% [2].

In 1997, Srotjan [46] described five children with nasopharyngeal carcinoma with advanced stage IV tumors that were treated with low irradiation dose adjusted to preradiation neoadjuvant chemotherapy. Tumor control was achieved and acute and long-term morbidity reduced.

20.5.4 Salivary Gland Carcinoma

Carcinoma of the salivary gland is very rare in children [47]. Taylor [48] described 15 such children. The primary site was the parotid gland in 11 cases, submandibular gland in three, base of the tongue in one. Six children were treated with complete excision, one required postoperative radiotherapy, five had partial excision, and four tumors were biopsied only. They concluded that complete excision is the treatment of choice.

Mucoepidermoid carcinoma of the parotid has been reported as secondary malignancy in a 17-year-old boy and a 16-year-old girl, who had been treated for osteosarcoma and Ewing's sarcoma, respectively. Subtotal parotidectomy appeared curative. Mucoepidermoid carcinoma has been reported before as secondary tumor after leukemia or lymphoma treatment, but not in sarcoma patients [49].

20.5.5 Synovial Sarcoma of the Larynx in a Child

Morland [50] reported the first case of synovial sarcoma of the larynx in a child. He was treated with combination chemotherapy and radiotherapy, which led to remission for 3 years. Only six cases have been previously reported.

20.6 Rare Tumors of the Chest

20.6.1 Mediastinum

Thymic lesions consist of tumors, cysts, or hyperplasia. Clinical presentation varies from respiratory symptoms to incidental findings on x-rays. About 30 cases in children have been reported in the literature. Benign thymoma, is, unlike in adults, not always associated with myasthenia or other autoimmune diseases. Complete surgical excision is curative. Multiple localizations have been reported. [51]. Malignant thymomas are aggressive and require complete excision.

Stage of the tumor is an independent prognostic factor for survival. Adjuvant chemotherapy and radiotherapy are advocated for invasive tumors [52, 53].

20.6.2 Tracheal and Bronchial Tumors in Children

Primary tumors of the trachea are rare in adults, and even more so in children. Carcinoid represents about one third of the cases, bronchogenic carcinoma one quarter, and mucoepidermoid carcinoma and pleuropulmonary blastoma 9% and 8%, respectively [54–56].

Diagnosis may be delayed because of lack of awareness. Presentation may be with hemoptysis, pneumonia, and other respiratory symptoms. The diagnosis of carcinoid can be improved by octreotide nuclear scan, as these tumors contain somatostatin receptors. Improved imaging will outline the extent of the tumor and hence guide the surgical treatment, which consists of complete excision, if necessary involving lobectomy or pneumonectomy. Endoscopic treatment of carcinoid is discouraged by most authors [57]. Craig, et al. reported on video-assisted thoracoscopic pneumonectomy for bronchial carcinoid affecting the bronchus intermedius in a 14-year-old girl [58].

The outcome of mucoepidermoid carcinoma of the tracheobronchial tree appears good after complete excision [59, 60].

Inflammatory pseudotumor of the trachea has been mentioned above. Cartilaginous neoplasms of the trachea have been described in a child with Mafucci's syndrome, causing obstructive symptoms. Endoscopic laser ablation was successful [61].

20.6.3 Pleuropulmonary Blastoma

Pleuropulmonary blastoma is a rare malignant primary tumor of the lung in children, but 25% of cases are extrapulmonary and metastasize mainly to the CNS. A case of extrapulmonary pleuropulmonary blastoma was reported in a child [62]. This tumor is associated with pre-existing cystic lesions of the lung (congenital cystadenomatoid malformation, CCAM). In fact, the extended classification of CCAM (or Congenital Pulmonary Airway Malformation, CPAM) encompasses 5 types, of which type 4 has a histological picture similar to grade 1 PPB. Table 20.2 [63] presents an overview of this classification.

PPB is also associated with cystic lesions of the kidney: cystic nephroma [64]. Familial cases of this association have been reported [65, 66]. A genetic syndrome has been postulated [67, 68].

The treatment of choice is surgical excision but the prognosis for this type of tumor is poor. Adjuvant che-

Table 20.2 An assessment of the expanded classification of congenital adenomatoid malformations and their relationship to malignant transformation. (From [63])

Type	Proportional incidence	Gross appearance	Microscopy	Other features
0	1–3%	Solid; the lungs are small throughout	Bronchial-type airways that have cartilage, smooth muscle, and glands are separated by abundant mesenchymal tissue	Neonates; other malformations; poor prognosis
1	60–70%	Large cysts (up to 10 cm)	The cysts are lined by pseudostratified ciliated cells that are often interspersed with rows of mucous cells	Presentation may be late; resectable; good prognosis; rare cases show carcinomatous change
2	10–15%	Sponge-like composed of multiple small cysts (up to 2 cm) and solid pale tumor-like tissue	The cysts resemble dilated bronchioles separated by normal alveoli; striated muscle in 5%	Neonates; other malformations; poor prognosis
3	5%	Solid	There is an excess of bronchiolar structures separated by air spaces that are small, have a cuboidal lining, and resemble late fetal lung	Neonates; poor prognosis
4	15%	Large cysts (up to 10 cm)	The cysts are lined by a flattened epithelium resting on loose mesenchymal tissue	Neonates and infants; good prognosis

motherapy has been used successfully in a child with metastatic disease [69]. The registry web site serves as an important resource for physicians and families (http://www.ppbregistry.org).

20.6.4 Cystic Adenomatoid Malformation of the Lung and Malignant Tumors

Apart from PPBs, there are several published cases of other tumors, like mesenchymomas and rhabdomyosarcomas, arising in CCAM [63].

A case of a 22-month-old child with a CCAM who developed rhabdomyosarcoma of the lung was reported by d'Agostino [70]. Among 382 cases of primary pulmonary tumors only 17 had rhabdomyosarcoma, with six of these 17 (35%) arising in a pre-existing pulmonary cystic malformation [71].

20.6.5 Tumors of the Diaphragm

Primary tumors of the diaphragm are rare, even in adults, with fewer than 200 cases reported. In children these tumors are exceptional, with 41 cases published [72]. The majority [32] was malignant; half of these were rhabdomyosarcomas. The presentation may be with chest symptoms or with abdominal symptoms. The diagnosis is often difficult because of the rarity and localization. The treatment depends on the histological diagnosis. Preoperative chemotherapy may shrink the tumor to allow complete excision. [72].

20.6.6 Breast Masses

20.6.6.1 Epidemiology and Etiology

Malignant tumors of the breast are rare in children and adolescents. In this age group, only one-third arise from primary breast tissue; the rest arise from non-breast tissue (rhabdomyosarcoma) or are metastatic tumors. Predisposing factors are: genetic (BRAC-1 and BRAC-2 mutations, Li-Fraumeni syndrome) or exposure to ionizing radiation, as in survivors of Hodgkin's disease [73]. These patients need careful and frequent follow-up according to a detailed schedule [74].

Sixteen patients under the age of 20 years were seen between 1951 and 1990. Four had benign cystosarcoma phyllodes, one osteosarcoma, and metastatic histocytic lymphoma, one had adenocarcinoma, nine had infiltrating ductal carcinoma, and one had an infiltrating lobular carcinoma in addition to an infiltrating ductal carcinoma. The treatment involved a combination of surgery, radiotherapy, and chemotherapy [75].

Eighteen patients with breast cancer were treated over a 25-year period including 16 females and two males. Primary malignancy presented in two of the patients, metastatic disease in 13, and secondary malignancy in three [76].

20.6.6.2 Diagnosis

Mammography in young patients is of limited value; ultrasonography, MRI, and PET-scan are more helpful. Fine needle aspiration cytology has a limited role in children because of pain and fear. Excisional biopsies in prepubertal children involves the risk of damage to the breast bud [77].

20.6.6.3 Treatment

Benign breast masses in adolescent girls are usually fibroadenomas, which may resolve spontaneously. If not excised they should be followed carefully, as ultrasonography cannot distinguish between fibroadenoma and cystosarcoma phyllodes [77]. Phyllodes is malignant in 25% of the cases and should be excised completely with a margin of normal tissue [77].

Two young girls with rhabdomyosarcoma of the breast, one primary and one with metastatic, were treated with surgery and chemotherapy respectively [78].

20.7 Rare Tumors of the Abdomen

20.7.1 Peritoneum, Omentum, and Mesentery

Primary tumors of these structures are often cystic, and benign, with lymphangioma being the most common [79]. Simple surgical excision is the treatment of choice. Peritoneal sarcomas often are very large and pretreatment with neoadjuvant chemotherapy is often necessary to render these tumors operable.

Other extremely rare malignant tumors are discussed below.

20.7.1.1 Peritoneal Mesothelioma

These tumors, although sharing some common histologic features, can vary considerably in biological behavior. Three different types are described: (a) classic, asbestos-related mesothelioma of adults, mainly in the pleural cavity; (b) multicystic mesothelioma, predominantly affecting the pelvic peritoneum of young women and associated with good prognosis [80]; (c) mesothelioma in children, which has an unpredictable behavior [81]. Measuring DNA index by flow cytometry can distinguish the cystic (aneuploid) form from the more malignant (diploid) tumors. In only one case, pathologically proven exposure to asbestos fibers has been reported [82].

The treatment of peritoneal mesothelioma depends on the behavior and appearance. Complete surgical removal is often not possible. There are reports that mesothelioma responds to adriamycin alone or in combination with cisplatinum. Intraperitoneal administration of cisplatinum has also been described [81]. Because of the rarity in children, the diagnosis of mesothelioma is rejected even by pathologists in up to 40% of the cases [83].

20.7.1.2 Desmoplastic Round Cell Tumors

The group of small, blue cell tumors include neuroblastoma, PNET/Ewing's sarcoma and Desmoplastic Small Round Cell Tumor (DSRCT).

These arise from soft tissues with mesothelial linings, are characterized by male predominance, adolescent onset, and aggressive behavior. The tumors are often intraperitoneal, massive, and tend to metastasize early to lymph nodes, liver, and lungs. The immunohistochemical profile of these tumors is often distinctive and reacts to a broad range of antigens. Clinical presentation is usually with a painful mass, but the tumor can also lead to urinary obstruction [84, 85]. Intra-abdominal desmoplastic small round cell tumors may present with retroperitoneal or mesenteric primary with ascites and hepatic metastases. Urogenital involvement has been reported including paratesticular and ovarian localizations [85–87]. Complete surgical excision is usually impossible. Aggressive multidrug chemotherapy can reduce the tumor mass impressively, but the patient remains with residual disease [88].

Kretschmar [89] reported three cases of desmoplastic small cell tumors and reviewed the literature and found 101 cases reported previously which indicated that this tumor is highly malignant and carries a grave prognosis. Only 50% of cases respond to chemotherapy with a median survival of 17 months.

20.7.1.3 Lipoblastoma and Liposarcoma

Lipoblastoma is a benign tumor arising from embryonal fat and therefore only occurs in young children. So far, 85 cases have been described, 12 of them presenting with an abdominal mass. The name lipoblastoma may cause confusion with malignant embryonal tumors, and therefore the term infantile lipoma has been proposed [90]. The treatment of choice is excision [91–93].

Only five cases of liposarcoma in childhood have been documented, with two of them arising from the porta hepatis [94–96]. Three of these five children died, one of them developing a recurrence 12 years after an initial favorable response to surgical excision combined with irradiation and chemotherapy.

20.7.2 Gastrointestinal Tract

20.7.2.1 General

In a recent review, Ladd and Grosfeld [97] presented 58 children and adolescents with gastro-intestinal tumors over a 33-year time frame. The average age was 13.8 years; there were 39 malignant and 19 benign tumors. Over half of the children had lymphomas (Burkitt's in 15, and non-Burkitt's, non-Hodgkin's lymphoma in 15). Six patients had colorectal carcinoma, six had neurogenic tumors, four had inflammatory pseudotumors, three presented with Peutz-Jeghers syndrome; there were two children with carcinoid, two with juvenile colonic polyps, two with hemangioma and one each with leukemic infiltrate and gastric leiomyosarcoma.

In a series of 35 patients reported from Turkey, carcinomas of the large bowel and rectum were the most common, comprising about half of this material [98].

In this chapter, malignant and premalignant tumors of the G-I tract will be discussed.

20.7.2.2 Carcinoma of the Esophagus

Adenocarcinoma of the esophagus has been reported in an 8-year-old boy from India [99]. There was a longstanding history of vomiting, probably due to gastro-esophageal reflux. The patient left the hospital without treatment. The authors quote several other case reports of adenocarcinoma in children with Barrett's esophagus.

20.7.2.3 Smooth Muscle Tumors

In recent years several cases of gastrointestinal smooth muscle tumors, both benign and malignant, have been reported in human immunodeficiency virus (HIV)-infected children [100] Another report mentions similar tumors in the lung of a child with clinical HIV infection [101]. Also, abdominal leiomyosarcomas have been described in very long-term survivors of childhood cancer [102].

Leiomyoma and leiomyoblastoma. These are essentially benign tumors, often occurring at an early age. Symptoms are most commonly caused by complications, such as intestinal obstruction, intussusception, or bleeding. These tumors have been found to occur in the stomach, small intestine, and colon. Usually, excision at the time of treatment of the complication leads to cure [103].

Leiomyosarcoma. Soft tissue sarcoma account for 7% of all childhood malignancies. Sarcomas with intestinal involvement comprise only 2% of this latter group. Leiomyoma often invole the stomach, whereas leiomyosarcoma (LMS) are more often found in the jejunum in children [97]. Over half of LMS occur in newborns. Other risk groups are patients with impaired immunity, e.g., after organ transplantation or due to HIV infection [97, 100–102, 104, 105].

LMS is a highly malignant tumor. The Children's Hospital in Boston reported ten; five (50%) of the children died with metastases. Wide surgical excision is the treatment of choice [106].

Apparently the histological distinction between leiomyosarcoma and leiomyoblastoma is not always easy [107], which could explain why several neonates with "leiomyosarcoma" survived [108, 109].

In total, 27 cases of pediatric intestinal leiomyosarcoma have been reported in the literature. Complete excision and no recurrence after 5 years was achieved. Visceral metastases are atypical [110].

20.7.2.4 GIST

Gastro Intestinal Stroma Tumor has been recognized as a distinct entity by WHO since 1990. Although predominantly a tumor of adulthood, occurrence in children has been reported by several authors and over 50 pediatric cases can be found in the literature [97, 104, 111–114]. Miettinen [115] reported 44 cases of gastric GIST occurring in patients younger than 21 years from the Armed Forces Institute of Pathology.

GIST is a mesenchymal tumor consisting of cells that are very similar to Interstitial Cells of Cajal (ICC), which express the CD 117 antigen, an epitope of the receptor tyrosine kinase KIT, in contrast to smooth muscle tumors like leiomyosarcomas. The great majority of pediatric GIST (88%) is located in the stomach, but small bowel and colon localizations have been reported [104].

The most common symptoms are pain, anemia due to gastro-intestinal bleeding [116], and abdominal masses. The tumor metastasizes to peritoneum, liver, or lymph nodes. Prognostic factors are: mitotic activity, tumor size and tumor site: gastric and colonic tu-

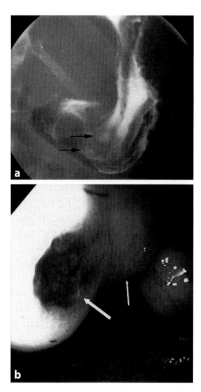

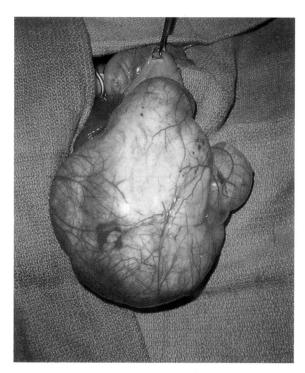

Fig 20.6 Teratoma of the stomach.

Fig 20.5 G.I.S.T. Gastrointestinal stromal tumors arising from the stomach. (From [110])

mors have a better outcome than small bowel or mesenteric primaries [110] (Fig. 20.5).

The association of gastric epithelioid leiomyosarcoma (the older name for a GIST), extra-adrenal paraganglioma, and pulmonary chondroma was described as Carney's Triad. Two of the triad's components are potentially lethal and it is very important that any patient with any of these tumors should be followed long-term. In 1993, Argos [117] reported on 36 cases of Carney's Triad including their own case of a 12-year-old girl. In Miettinen's series [115] only one out of 44 cases had Carney's triad, but Price found two patients with the triad in the five described [113].

Surgical resection is the mainstay of the treatment of GIST. Complete gross resection is recommended and lymphadenectomy is not warranted [104, 110]. Response to chemotherapy is probably low, but imatinib mesylate, a tyrosine kinase inhibitor has been reported to achieve 50% response rate [97, 104, 110].

20.7.2.5 Gastric Teratoma

One hundred and two cases of this usually benign tumor have been reported in the latest review [97]. The majority of the patients are boys, and malignant degeneration has been only rarely described. Abdominal mass, pain,

gastric outlet obstruction, or bleeding are presenting symptoms and signs. After complete resection, no recurrences have been described [118] (Fig. 20.6).

20.7.2.6 Gastric Carcinoma

Fewer than 25 cases of gastric carcinoma in children have been reported [97]. It appears, however, that childhood infection with Helicobacter pylori can play an important causative role in gastric cancer in the adult [119]. Gastric cancer in children has also been described as a secondary tumor after treatment for malignant lymphoma [120]. The most common complaints of stomach cancer in childhood are pain and vomiting, along with symptoms suggesting acid peptic disease. Delay in diagnosis is common and can be avoided by early imaging and endoscopy. Long-term survival is uncommon [121, 122].

The role of chemotherapy and radiation in gastric cancer is still not well defined. Surgery alone may prolong survival. Studies in adults recommend the use of etoposide, doxorubicin (Adriamycin), and cisplatin as primary therapy or combined with surgery and radiation [122].

A 2-year-old boy with pernicious anemia caused by vitamin B12 and iron deficiencies developed atrophic gastritis and gastric carcinoma. This has not been reported previously. Treatment included high subtotal gastrectomy with gastrojejunostomy and re-section of associated lymph nodes and omentectomy and 6 months of chemotherapy. Follow-up after 1 year showed no evidence of recurrent disease [123].

20.7.2.7 Intestinal Polyps and Polyposis Syndromes

Juvenile polyps. Juvenile polyps are hamartomatous in nature and, although benign, considered by some as a premalignant condition [97]. They occur in about 1% of children and are usually detected because of complications. Rectal bleeding is most often the presenting symptom; however, prolapse of the polyp during defecation or straining may also occur. The majority are single (80%) and are located in the rectum, but they have also been reported in colon, stomach, duodenum, and ileum [97]. Colonoscopy is recommended for children with unexplained rectal blood loss and normal proctoscopic examination [124, 125]. Solitary polyps should be excised endoscopically. The finding of a solitary rectal polyp is an indication for colonoscopy to exclude polyposis [126].

Generalized juvenile polyposis. This uncommon disease is characterized by the development of multiple (50 to more than 200) hamartomatous polyps throughout the intestinal tract, mostly in the large bowel; 85% of cases occur in children. In half of the cases, there is a positive family history of polyps or polyposis. The genes involved are SMAD4 on chromosome 18q21.1 or BMPR1A located on the long arm of chromosome 10. The infantile form of this condition is associated with protein-losing enteropathy, anemia, hypoproteinemia, and is often fatal [127]. Eighteen to 35% of patients with juvenile polyposis develop malignant disease by the age of 35. The treatment of choice is colectomy and an anal sphincter-saving procedure. [128].

Peutz-Jeghers syndrome. Peutz-Jeghers Syndrome (PJS) syndrome is autosomal dominantly inherited with an incidence estimated at 1:120,000. It is characterized by abnormal melanin deposits in the skin, lips, and mucous membranes and the formation of multiple hamartomatous polyps throughout the gastrointestinal tract (Fig. 20.7).

The small bowel is involved in 96% of cases, the colon in 27%, the stomach in 24%, and rectum in 24%. Labial pigmentation is a reliable clinical marker in 94% of patients with Peutz-Jeghers syndrome. The causative genetic mutation involves STK11/LKB1 on chromosome 19 [129]. Polyps start to grow in the first decade of life, and 50–60% of patients will develop symptoms by the age of 20 years.

In a large overview of the material removed by polypectomies in children, Peutz-Jeghers syndrome

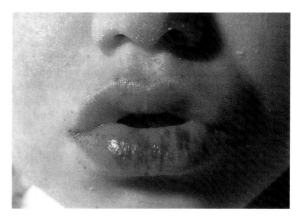

Fig 20.7 Pigmentations of lips in Peutz Jeghers.

accounted for 1.73% of the cases [130]. The complications of bowel obstruction due to intussusception of a polyp and anemia caused by bleeding from these polyps are often noted, sometimes before the typical abnormal pigmentation has developed.

In younger children (below 16 years of age) the gastroduodenal region is frequently the site of the polyps. Apparently these children are at risk for the development of malignant tumors. Two of the 70 patients mentioned earlier developed gastrointestinal adenocarcinoma, perhaps due to degeneration of a polyp, two an ovarian cancer and one a testicular tumor, possibly indicating a genetic disposition. A third case of adenocarcinoma of duodenum and jejunum occuring in an 8-year-old girl with Peutz-Jeghers syndrome was reported later [131]. There is an increased risk of ovarian cancer in relatives of a patient with Peutz-Jeghers syndrome. Whether hamatomatous polyps degenerate into carcinomas (the hamartoma-carcinoma sequence) has been debated. Some investigators consider the polyps as an epiphenomenon to a cancer prone condition [132].

Familial adenomatous polyposis (FAP). This adenomatous autosomal dominant genetic disorder is due to a germline mutation of the APC-gene on chromosome 5q21-22. It is infamous because of its tendency to develop carcinoma of the large bowel, and may cause any significant bowel symptoms during childhood. In families with FAP a colonoscopy is indicated in children before they are 10 years of age [133].

Total colectomy, rectal mucosectomy, and ileoanal anastomosis eliminate the risk for malignant degeneration. Numerous reports have been published on the technical aspects of the ileoanal sphincter-saving operation, which is also applied in patients with ulcerative colitis. Most surgeons prefer the construction of an ileoanal anastomosis, using a "J"-pouch. Early and late complications after these procedures are common and the complication rate can be as high as 41%. Late complications include inflammation ("pouchitis"), diarrhea, or stasis [134]. These complications occur more often in ulcerative colitis patients, whereas the FAP patients as a general rule fare much better [135].

Children in FAP families also have a tendency towards developing liver tumors (hepatoblastoma) more often than in general population [136]. Another interesting link with familial polyposis is Gardner's syndrome and the familial generalized juvenile polyposis, which by and large probably should be managed in a similar fashion as famial polyposis [137].

Although the risk of colon cancer in children under 15 years of age is very low (6%), the youngest patient reported was 9 years. Therefore, the timing of colectomy is under debate as dysplasia can be asymptomatic. Vasudevan, et al. described a group of 11 children who underwent surgery at a mean age of 13 years. Dysplasia was present in 9 patients (82%). The authors advocate early operation to prevent malignant degeneration [138].

20.7.2.8 Colorectal Carcinoma

Uncommon in childhood (less than 1% of all colonic cancers), this tumor has an extremely poor prognosis. This is due to late detection because of ignoring initial symptoms, a high percentage of signet ring or anaplastic lesions present, and often regional lymph node metastases (75% on presentation in the largest published series).

Survival varies from zero to 25%. Even in the event of complete resection it would be advisable to give adjuvant therapy with 5-fluorouracil and leucovorin-based cytotoxics in instances of high-grade lesions or regional lymph node involvement [139–141].

Urinary diversion into the sigmoid colon or use of bowel elsewhere in the urinary tract has also been identified as a risk for the development of adenocarcinoma. Although there usually is a time lag of more than 20 years, and therefore the carcinoma will develop beyond childhood, it is a fact to be kept in mind when constructing urinary conduits in children [142]. Experimental evidence suggests that familial polyposis, ulcerative colitis and ureterosigmoidostomies are conditions with an unstable colonic epithelium, which may become dysplastic, and perhaps deteriorate into malignant degeneration [143].

Brown [140] described seven children aged 10–15 years with carcinoma of the colon and rectum. Distant metastases were present in five and there was no survivors in this series. The youngest patient described was 9 months [97].

20.7.2.9 Carcinoid Tumors

These tumors appear in the gastrointestinal tract, biliary tree, ovaries, bronchi, lungs, and pancreas. The most common sites are the appendix, followed by small inestine and rectum. In one report a case is described of a carcinoid tumor occurring in a rectal duplication [144]. Appendiceal carcinoid is uncommon in infancy but may occur in late childhood and adolescence. Girls are affected three times as often as boys.

In most patients carcinoid is an incidental finding in the appendix removed for acute or recurrent abdominal pain. Usually the tumor is less than 2 cm in diameter and in 75% of the cases it is located near the tip of the appendix. Simple appendectomy is curative in these patients. When the tumor is greater than 2 cm in diameter and occurs at the base, or if there is tumor growth beyond the appendix, a more extensive procedure like partial colectomy is indicated [97]. In the largest reported series of 40 cases, no recurrences, metastases, or tumor related deaths were observed [145].

20.7.3 Bile Ducts

20.7.3.1 Introduction

Two types of tumors occurring in this region deserve mentioning, namely the biliary tract rhabdomyosarcoma and carcinoma arising in the anatomically abnormal bile duct system (Fig. 19.7).

20.7.3.2 Rhabdomyosarcoma

Fewer than 40 cases of rhabdomyosarcoma of the bile ducts have been reported in the literature. The presenting symptom is usually obstructive jaundice [146] (Fig. 20.7).

The diagnosis can be made using abdominal ultrasound, MRI or CT scan. The prognosis for this tumor has been rather poor; 40% of the cases present with metastases, but local growth is a leading cause of death in most instances [147]. The first large series of ten patients was reported in 1985 [148]. At the time of publication there were four survivors following extensive resection and adjuvant radiation and chemotherapy. An interesting development is a recent report in which after an exploratory operation the patient was treated with chemotherapy which caused a dramatic reduction in tumor size. At a second-look operation complete regression of the tumor was observed. The authors claim that with this approach of aggressive surgery can be prevented [149]. Similar experience was reported by Spunt [150], but this has not been confirmed by other authors [151].

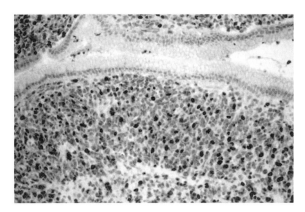

Fig 20.8 Tumor of CBD. Embryonal rhabdomyosarcoma of the common bile duct mimicking choledochal cyst. (From [146])

The role of preoperative imaging is uncertain. ERCP was not found to be helpful in the two cases where it was performed [150]. It is not clear whether MRCP is more accurate than CT-scan [151]. Preoperative (PTC) or intraoperative cholangiography can be useful [151].

20.7.3.3 Carcinoma

The risk of adenocarcinoma developing in a choledochal cyst has been known for many years. A survey of 645 cases of choledochal cyst in Japan treated between 1972 and 1982 disclosed 54 cases (8.4%) of biliary carcinoma. The incidence varied from 0.3% in the pediatric population to 15.6% in the adult cases, indicating that the risk of developing this cancer increases with age [152]. With time, approximately 20–25% of cases will develop malignancy, which carries a poor prognosis since less than 10% are resectable [153]. Patients with an anomalous arrangement of the pancreaticobiliary duct system have an increased cellular proliferative activity in the gallbladder mucosa starting in early childhood [154]. It is presumed that complete cyst excision eliminates the risk of malignant degeneration [153].

Pancreaticobiliary maljunction without dilatation of the common duct is very rare, but nevertheless may be associated with carcinoma in later life. Based on experience in a recent series of seven Japanese children with this anomaly, complete excision of common bile duct and gallbladder followed by hepaticojejunostomy is recommended [155].

20.7.4 Pancreas

20.7.4.1 Introduction

Malignant pancreatic tumors are rare in children. Vossen, et al. quote from a Japanese autopsy statistic, that 0.2% of infant deaths caused by malignant disease are due to pancreatic tumors [156]. A report from Memorial Sloan Kettering describing 17 patients below 21 years in the time period of 33 years between 1967 and 2000, illustrates the spectrum of malignant pancreatic tumors in children. Pancreatoblastoma (5 cases) and solid pseudopapillary or Frantz' tumor (7 cases) were the most frequent. Other tumors were: acinar cell carcinoma (1), nonfunctioning pancreatic endocrine neoplasm (1), malignant VIPoma (1), and PNET (2). The clinical presentation varied: abdominal pain (11), mass (4), anorexia (3). Only three patients were jaundiced. [157]. The pancreas may also be the seat of malignant lymphoma, which may be difficult to diagnose [158].

In this section a more detailed description will be given of four types of pancreatic tumors in children: (a) pancreatoblastoma, (b) solid pseudopapillary or Frantz' tumor, (c) pancreatic ductal Adenocarcinoma, (d) malignant endocrine tumors.

20.7.4.2 Pancreatoblastoma

Pancreatoblastoma (PB) is a malignant epithelial tumor showing mainly acinar differentiation, but occasionally also containing endocrine and ductal cells. These different cellular elements may derive from a pluripotent "blastomatous" cell. This may also explain the fact that a considerable number of PB express alfa-foetoprotein (AFP), and that serum levels are increased in patients with PB. Dhebri, et al. have reviewed the literature on 153 cases [159]. Most of the PB occur in early childhood, but 10% occur in adults. Antenatal diagnosis and successful neonatal management have been reported [160, 161]. The latter patient, and several others in the literature, had the Beckwith-Wiedeman Syndrome (BWS), which is associated with loss of heterozygosity (LOH) on chromosome 11p [162]. The same genetic characteristic has been described in six out of seven patients with PB. Another genetic activation reported in PB is a mutation of the beta-catenin gene [159]. Others have reported multiple chromosomal abnormalities in PB-cells, including MYC-oncogene [163] (Fig. 20.9).

The tumor may arise in any part of the pancreas. The typical mode of presentation is with an abdominal mass, weight loss and pain; jaundice is present in about 10%. Metastases are present at first diagnosis in 17–35% of the patients. The diagnosis should be considered on

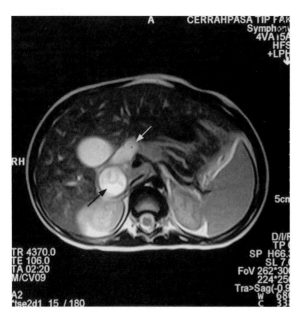

Fig. 20.9 Pancreatoblastoma. A case of pancreatoblastoma prenatally diagnosed as intraperitoneal cyst. (From [160])

the basis of imaging studies and can be confirmed by fine needle aspiration cytology [164]. The treatment consists of complete resection. If this is not possible, neoadjuvant chemotherapy should be given. Various cytotoxic regimes have been advocated: most contain vincristin and cyclophosphamide or ifosfamide, in combination with either actinomycin-D, cisplatinum, doxorubicin, or bleomycin. Postoperative radiotherapy has been advocated for irresectable or incompletely resected cases. See algorithm in Dhebri, et al. [159].

The prognosis in children after complete resection is fairly good, with a reported 5-year survival rate between 50% and 80% [165].

20.7.4.3 Solid Pseudopapillary Tumor; Papillary Cystic Tumor of the Pancreas; Frantz's Tumor

Solid pseudopapillary tumor of the pancreas (SPTP) is known by several names, including the eponym of the author who first described this tumor in 1959 as a separate entity, V.K. Frantz. Since then, more than 700 cases have been reported in the English literature, their ages ranging between 2 and 85 years, with a mean of 22 years. One hundred sixty-five SPTPs have been reported in children below the age of 18 years. Over 90% of the tumors occur in females [166, 167]. It has been suggested that SPTP occurs more often in Asians and Africans than in Caucasians [167].

The cell of origin of SPTP is uncertain. Kosmahl, et al. [168] performed a comprehensive immunocyto-

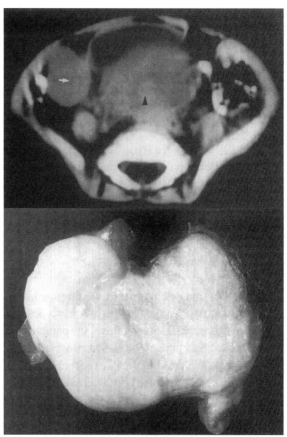

Fig 20.10 Papillary and cystic tumor of the pancreas.

chemical analysis of 59 tumors and concluded that it is difficult to relate the tumor to epithelial cells, even if a mulipotent stem cell origin is considered. On the other hand, SPTP is not a purely endocrine tumor either, both on cytochemical and clinical grounds. The authors postulate that there is a relationship with ovarian rete cells [168]. The tumor may occur in any part of the pancreas, but more often in the tail [168, 169].

The majority of SPTP are localized tumors, particularly in children there are only a few case reports of metastases [170]. Intraperitoneal spread has been observed after abdominal trauma [169]. SPTP is therefore considered as a low-grade malignant tumor.

Most patients present with gastro-intestinal symptoms and a palpable mass. The diagnosis is made by a combination of clinical signs and imaging. Endoscopic ultrasound-guided fine needle aspiration cytology has been advocated, but found conclusive in only a minority of cases [167, 171]. The treatment is complete excision with a margin, but without lymphnode dissection. Intraoperative frozen section is recommended. The prognosis is good in children after complete removal (Fig. 20.10).

20.7.4.4 Pancreatic Ductal Adenocarcinoma

Pancreatic ductal adenocarcinoma (PDAC) is a tumor of the elderly that is exceedingly rare in children. Approximately 37 cases have been reported, although some doubt exists whether these were all adenocarcinomas. In a series of 520 pancreatic neoplasms, 404 were PDACs, two occurred in patients younger than 18 years [172]. The presence of an abdominal mass in the epigastrium, abdominal distension, or obstructive jaundice are the common presenting symptoms.

The diagnosis of a panceatic mass can be made with ultrasonography, MRI, or CT scan. Aggressive surgical procedures are recommended when feasible. In the majority of cases pancreatoduodenectomy or distal pancreatectomy are necessary. Even in instances of anaplastic tumors, survival following extirpative resection has been reported. One author claims that all patients in whom a resection was undertaken were long-term survivors, but others found no better outcome in young patients compared to the elderly [172].

20.7.4.5 Malignant Endocrine Pancreatic Tumors

Whereas in adults, the majority of endocrine pancreatic tumors are insulinomas, which are rarely malignant, in children there is an almost equal distribution of insulinomas and gastrinomas. Unfortunately, most of the insulinomas diagnosed as malignant have already metastasized at diagnosis [156]. Endocrine pancreatic tumors, which are associated with the MEN 1 syndrome, can also be malignant [173]. Malignant endocrine pancreatic tumors have furthermore been reported in children with Tuberous Sclerosis Complex (TSC), an autosomal dominant condition, presenting with epilepsy and mental retardation and known to be associated with benign renal cysts and angiomyolipoma (see also below). TSC1 and TSC2 genes are located on chromosme 9 and 16, respectively. Malignant nonfunctioning islet cell tumors expressing LOH of chromosome 16 (TSC2) were found in two boys [174, 175].

20.8 Rare Tumors of the Genitourinary System

20.8.1 Renal Cell Carcinoma

A retrospective analysis of 22 cases of renal cell carcinoma was reported by Aronson, et al. [176]. Age, tumor size, location, and histology were found not to be predictors of outcome; tumor stage and complete surgical resection were the only significant prognostic determinants. The overall 5-year survival was 30%. The survival rate for tumors that were completely resected was 60% versus 10% for those lesions incompletely resected.

Attempts to treat these tumors by nephron-sparing surgery have also been reported in children. Cook, et al. reported on 15 patients, with a mean age of 7.9 years. Presentation with hematuria, pain, and polycythemia in 75%, whereas 25% were asymptomatic. Treatment consisted of nephrectomy in 10 patients, and partial nephrectomy in five. Excision of metastases was done in 2 patients. Outcome: thirteen are in complete remission, and of the three stage IV patients, 1 died and 1 survived with disease. All of the patients with partial nephrectomy are in complete remission. Two editorial comments warn that the long-term outcome of partial nephrectomy in children is unknown, and that the risk of recurrence has to be established in prospective studies.

20.8.1.1 Renal Cell Carcinoma in Association with Tuberous Sclerosis in Children

Tuberous sclerosis (TS) is an autosomal disorder with incomplete penetrance and variable phenotype (see also under pancreas). Angiomyolipoma and multiple renal cysts are seen in patients with TS. Cases of renal cell carcinoma in patients with TS are usually multiple and may be bilateral [178].

20.8.2 Transitional Cell Carcinoma of the Bladder

Five boys were reported to have transitional cell carcinoma of the bladder [179] Imaging and urine cytology correlated with cystoscopic and biopsy findings. Ultrasound examination was the most sensitive. A special risk category for bladder tumors are patients with bladder augmentation. Transitional cell carcinoma has been reported in three adults who underwent this procedure for neuropathic bladder [180]. In the discussion of this paper, A.B. Retik states the risk starts to rise after a 10-year lag period, in analogy with the experience in the ureterosigmoidostomy patients.

20.8.3 Cystic Partially Differentiated Nephroblastoma

Cystic partially differentiated nephroblastoma (CPDN) is a rare neoplasm. The tumor consists of well-demarcated cystic lesions of the kidney. Blastemal and other embryonic cells are present in the septa of the cysts; MRI can detect the lesions which are highly suggestive of either CPDN or cystic nephroma [181].

Experience in the NWTSG consists of 21 patients, 13 of whom received cytotoxic drugs whereas eight (all stage I) did not. The outcome was 100% survival without recurrences. It is concluded that for stage I patients surgical treatment alone is probably sufficient [182].

20.8.4 B Cell Non-Hodgkin's Lymphoma as a Primary Renal Tumor

Primary renal lymphoma is an extremely rare tumor; only about 35 cases are reported in literature. A 6-year-old boy had a unilateral renal tumor which was thought to be a Wilms' tumor. On review of the histology this proved to be a B cell lymphoma [183].

20.8.5 Prostatic Non-Hodgkin's Lymphoma

A T cell non-Hodgkin's lymphoma of the prostate occurred in a child who presented with actue urinary retention and who responded well to treatment with chemotherapy [184].

20.8.6 Testicular Tumors Before Puberty

Twenty-two neonates less than 1 month of age were found to have testis tumors; seven were diagnosed at birth. Cell types included yolk sac tumors in six, and six had gonadal stromal tumors. Six had juvenile granulosa cell tumors, two gonadoblastoma, one teratoma, and one harmartoma. Serum alpha-fetoprotein was normal in ten tested patients. There were no metastases. Seventeen boys were followed up and there was no evidence of disease. Neonatal tumors are rare but should be considered in the differential diagnosis of scrotal masses in the neonate [185].

Testicular tumors are rare in prepubertal children, and the large majority are germ cell tumors. Serum tumor markers shoud be assessed before operation. If the markers are not elevated and salvageable testis tissue is present on ultrasound, an excisional biopsy with frozen section is advocated. If the tumor is a benign teratoma, the testis can be preserved [186]. Both reports originate from the Prepubertal Testis Tumor Registry (PTTR) created by the Section of Urology of the American Academy of Pediatrics in 1980.

20.9 Ectomesenchymoma

Ectomesenchymoma is a malignant nonepithelial tumor containing two or more cell-types from ectodermal and mesenchymal origin (Figs 20.11). Synonyms are: malignant Triton tumor (MTT) and primary

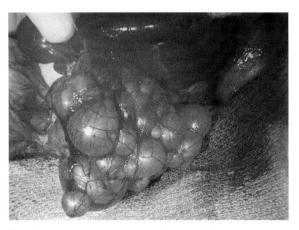

Fig 20.11 Ectomesenchymoma. (From [188])

osteochondrorhabdomyosarcoma. It is considered a variant of the Malignant Peripheral Nerve Sheath Tumor (MPNST) that contains rhabdomyoblasts [187]. This tumor is associated with Neurofibromatosis type 1 (NF1) and usually develops in these patients before the age of 35 years. It is rare in children, with only 24 cases reported, more than half of them in NF1 patients [187]. Predilection sites are: head and neck, trunk, and extremities.

Hajivassiliou, et al. reported a case in a child (gangliorhabdomyosarcoma) with cutaneous nevus syndrome. Review of the literature revealed 35 similar cases [188].

The treatment of MTT consists of wide local excision, the role of chemotherapy is uncertain. The prognosis is grim, with a 5-year survival of 26% [187].

Malignant ectomesenchymoma of the bone is even more rare. Two children were reported: one 10-year-old girl with a tumor of the fibula, and a 15-year-old girl with a tumor of the proximal humerus. A combination therapy of intensive cytotoxics (osteosarcoma protocol) and wide local excision resulted in complete remission in both cases [189–191].

20.10 Malignant Melanoma in Children

Malignant melanoma is rare in children, representing 1–3% of all pediatric malignancies. Two percent of malignant melanomas occur in patients younger than 20 years. Most of pediatric melanomas are seen in adolescents with only 0.3% in prepubertal children. The incidence is 2 per million children (below age 15 years), but is rising [192–194].

Certain (skin) conditions predispose to malignant melanoma. Risk factors in addition to exposure to sunlight [194] are:
1. Giant congenital melanocytic nevi (CMN), 5–15% risk

2. Familial atypical mole/melanoma (FAMM), 100% risk
3. Treatment with chemotherapy for malignant disease
4. Retinoblastoma
5. Xeroderma pigmentosum, (2000 x increased risk)

Malignant melanoma does occur in prepubertal children. Mones and Ackerman [195] describe a group of 11 children between 1 and 10 years of age, (6 younger than 5 years) with melanoma arising de novo. The diagnosis was missed in all cases, both by the clinician and by the pathologist, and all metastasized. One child died. The melanomas were growing fast, and very thick at the time of diagnosis. Confusion with benign Spitz nevus may arise, and the authors point out that the histopathological criteria for melanoma in young children are not different from those in adults.

Approximately half of melanomas in children arise in association with a pre-existing lesion: about 30% within giant CMN and 20% in association with other lesions, like acquired melanocytic nevi or small- or medium-sized CMN [193, 196, 197]. More than half of all melanomas that arise within giant CMNs do so before puberty, whereas melanomas that develop in smaller CMNs often occur after puberty [193]. Prophylactic excision of all giant CMNs, defined as covering 1% body surface in head and neck and 2% elsewhere on the body, is therefore recommended [198]. If a nevus changes in size or aspect, starts bleeding or itching, suspicion should arise. In children where melanoma developed in association with a pre-existing nevus, only 7% of the patients had no signs or symptoms. As the clinical diagnosis is erratic and benign Spitz nevus may be confused with melanoma, the next step is to perform an excisional biopsy of the lesion. If the lesion is smaller than 15 mm, a margin of 1–2 mm is sufficient. It is important to excise the full thickness for adequate staging. Staging depends on the level of penetration (Clarke) or thickness of the lesion (Breslow), and the presence or absence of regional lymphnode and distant metastases. The TNM classification of the American Joint Committee on Cancer is shown in Table 20.3 [199]. For adequate staging of lymphnodes, sentinel node biopsy has been advocated [200].

Treatment guidelines are based on the experience in adults. See American Association of Dermatology online guidelines; National Comprehensive Cancer Network Melanoma Panel. Treatment consists of radical excision, with adequate margins. For lesions less than 1 mm thickness, 1-cm margin is considered adequate; if 1–4 mm thickness: 2-cm margins, and 3-cm margin for lesions with more than 4 mm depth [199]. Enlarged lymphnodes should be removed by formal regional dissection. Elective lymphnode dissection is of no advantage in lesions of <1 mm thickness nor

Table 20.3 Staging of Melanomas [from 199]

Primary Tumor (T)	
pTX	Primary tumor cannot be assessed
pTO	No evidence of primary tumor
pTis	Melanoma in situ
pTl	Tumor 0.75 mm or less in thickness, or Clark Level II
pT2	Tumor greater than 0.75 mm but no more than 1.5 mm in thickness, or Clark Level III
pT3	Tumor greater than 1.5 mm but no more than 4 mm in thickness, or Clark Level IV
pT4	Tumor greater than 4 mm in thickness, or Clark Level V, or satellites present within 2 cm of primary tumor.

Regional Lymph Nodes (N)	
NX	Regional lymph nodes cannot be assessed
NO	No evidence of regional lymph node metastasis
Nl	Metastasis 3 cm or less in greatest dimension in any regional lymph node or nodes
N2	Metastasis greater than 3 cm in greatest dimension in any regional lymph node or nodes and/or in transit metastasis.

Distant Metastasis (M)	
MX	Presence of distant metastasis cannot be assessed
MO	No evidence of distant metastasis
M 1	Distant metastasis present

Stage Grouping			
Stage 1	pTI	NO	MO
	PT2	NO	MO
Stage 2	pT3	NO	MO
Stage 3	pT4	NO	MO
	Any pT	Nl,N2	MO
Stage 4	Any pT	Any N	MO

From Beahrs OH, Henson DE, Hutter RVP, et al (eds): American Joint Committee on Cancer: Manual for Staging of Cancer, 3rd ed. Philadelphia: J. B. Lippincott, 1988, with permission.

in lesions of >4 mm depth. For those between 1 and 4 mm, sentinel node biopsy with routine histopathology and immunohistochemistry is advocated. If the sentinel node is positive, a complete regional node dissection is recommended [193].

Although there is no evidence that chemotherapy is useful in adults, there are some encouraging experiences with a combination of vincristin, cyclophosphamide, and dactinomycin in children [193]. Immunotherapy with Interferon alpha 2b has been found effective. The prognosis is determined by the stage, and there is no evidence that children have a different outlook than adults [193, 196, 197, 199].

References

1. Harms D, Schmidt D (1993) Rare tumors in childhood: Pathological aspects. Experience of the Kiel pediatric tumor registry. Med Pediatr Oncol 21:239–248

2. Walker DA (2005) Rare tumours. In: Voute PA, Barrett A, Stevens MCG, Caron HN (eds) Cancer in children: Clinical management. 5th ed. Oxford University Press, Oxford, pp 396–420

3. Corpron CA, Andrassy RJ (1997) Melanomas and other rare tumors. In: Andrassy RJ (ed) Pediatric surgical oncology. WB Saunders Company, Philadelphia, pp 349–364

4. Karnak I, Senocak ME, Ciftci AO, et al. (2001) Inflammatory myofibroblastic tumor in children: Diagnosis and treatment. J Pediatr Surg 36:906–912

5. Bumber Z, Jurlina M, Manoilovic S, Jakic-Razumovic J (2001) Inflammatory pseudotumor of the trachea. J Pediatr Surg 36:631–634

6. Stringer MP, Ramori P, Yeung K, Capps S, Kieley E, Spitz L (1992) Abdominal inflammatory myofibroblastic tumors in children. Br J Surg 79:1357–1360

7. Kaneko K, Ando H, Watanabe Y, et al. (2001) Aggressive preoperative management and extended surgery for inflammatory pseudotumor involving the hepatic hilum in a child. Surgery 129:757–760

8. Janik JS, Janik JP, Lovell MA, Hendricksonn RJ, Bensard DD, Greffe BS (2003) Recurrent inflammatory pseudotumor in children. J Pediatr Surg 38:1491–1495

9. Sakai M, Ikeda H, Suzuki N, et al. (2001) Inflammatory pseudotumor of the liver: Case report and a review of the literature. J Pediatr Surg 36:663–666

10. DiFiore JW, Goldblum JR (2002) Inflammatory myofibroblastic tumor of the small intestine. J Am Coll Surg 14:502–506

11. Vaughan KG, Aziz A, Meza MP, Hackam DJ (2005) Mesenteric inflammatory pseudotumor as a cause of abdominal pain in a teenager: Presentation and literature review. Pediatr Surg Int 21:497–499

12. Li L, Cerilli LA, Wick MR (2002) Inflammatory pseudotumor (myofibroblastic tumor) of the heart. Ann Diagn Pathol 6:116–121

13. Mergan F, Jaubert F, Sauvat T, et al. (2005) Inflammatory myofibroblastic pseudotumor in children: Clinical review with anaplastic lymphoma kinase, Epstein-Barr virus, and human herpes virus 8 detection analysis. J Pediatric Surg 40:1581–1586

14. Parida SK, Azmy AF, Hollman AS, Wilkinson L, Beattie TJ (1992) Xanthogranulomatous pyelonephritis. Pediatr Rev Commun 6:247–251

15. Hagman C, El-Bahrawy M, Stamp G, Abel RM (2006) Juvenile xanthogranuloma: A case report of a preterm baby. J Pediatr Surg 41:573–575

16. Chinyama CN, Roblin P, Watson SJ, Evans DM (2000) Fibromatosis and related tumours of the hand in children. Hand Clin 16:625–635

17. Dölken R, Weigel S, Schröders H, et al. (2006) Treatment of severe disseminated juvenile systemic xanthogranuloma with multiple lesions in the central nervous system. J Pediatr Hematol Oncol 28:95–97

18. Buonocore S, Valente AL, Nightingale D, et al. (2005) Histiocytic sarcoma in a 3-year old male: A case report. Pediatrics 116(2):e322–325

19. Al-Trabalsi HA, Alshehri M, Al-Shomrani A, et al. (2006) Primary pulmonary Langerhans cell histiocytosis in a two-year-old child. J Pediatr Hematol Oncol 28:79–81

20. Khanna G, Sato Y, Smith RJH, et al. (2006) Causes of facial swelling in pediatric patients: Correlation of clinical and radiologic findings. Radiographics 26:157–171

21. Jain M, Nangia A, Bajaj P (1999) Malignant histiocytosis in childhood. Diagn Cytopathol 1:359–361

22. Margolin K, Traweek T (1992) The unique association of malignant histocytosis and a primary gonadal germ cell tumor. Med Pediatr Oncol 20:162–164

23. Sasou S, Nakamura SI, Habano W, Takano T (1996) True malignant histiocytosis developed during chemotherapy for mediastinal immature teratoma. Hum Pathol 27:1099–1103

24. Song SY, Ko YH, Ahn G (2005) Mediastinal germ cell tumor associated with histiocytic sarcoma of the spleen: Case report of an unusual association. Int J Surg Pathol 13:299–303

25. Hardy JD (1987) The ubiquitous fibroblast. Ann Surg 205:445–455

26. Ortega-Monzo C, Molina-Gallardo I, Monteagudo-Castro C, et al. (2000) Precalcaneal congenital fibrolipomatous hamartoma: A report of four cases. Pediatr Dermatol 17:429–431

27. Jacob CI, Kumm RC (2000) Benign anteromedial plantar nodules of childhood: A distinct form of plantar fibromatosis. Pediatr Dermatol 17:472–474

28. Numanoglu A, Davies J, Millar AJW, Rode H (2002) Congenital solitary intestinal fibromatosis. Eur J Pediatr Surg 12:337–340

29. Choo KL, Borzi PA, Mortimore RJ (2001) Neonatal intestinal obstruction from solitary intestinal fibromatosis. Pediatr Surg Int 17:467–469

30. Abbas AE, Deschamps C, Cassivi SD, ct al. (2004) Chest wall desmoid tumors: Results of surgical intervention. Ann Thorac Surg 78:1219–1223

31. Buitendijk S, van de Ven CP, Dumans TG, et al. (2005) Pediatric aggressive fibromatosis. Cancer 104:1090–1099

32. Knudsen AL, Bulow S (2001) Desmoid tumour in familial adenomatous polyposis. Fam Cancer 1:111–119

33. Bar-Maor JA, Shabshin U (1993) Mesenteric fibromatosis. J Pediatr Surg 28:1618–1619

34. Shih SL, Sheu JC, Chen BF, Ma YC (1995) Malignant hemangioendothelioma presenting as omental masses in a child. J Pediatr Surg 30:118–119

35. Ferrari A, Casanova M, Bisogno G, et al. (2002) Malignant vascular tumors in children and adolescents: A report from the Italian and German Soft Tissue Sarcoma Cooperative Group. Med Pediatr Oncol 39:109–114

36. den Hoed ID, Granzen B, Aronson DC, et al. (2005) Metastasized angiosarcoma of the spleen in a 2-year old girl. Pediatr Hematol Oncol 5:387–390

37. Mueller BU (1999) HIV-associated malignancies in children. AIDS Patient Care STDS 13:527–533

38. Manji KP, Amir H, Maduhu IZ (2000) Aggressive Kaposi's sarcoma in a 6-month African infant: Case report and a review of the literature. Trop Med Int Health 5:85–87

39. Hengge UR, Ruzicka TH, Tyring SK, et al. (2002) Update on Kaposi's sarcoma and other HHV8 associated diseases. Part 2. Lancet Infect Dis 2:344–352

40. Krown SE (2003) Therapy of AIDS-associated Kaposi's sarcoma: Targeting pathogenetic mechanisms. Hematol Oncol Clin North Am 17(3):763–783 (review)

41. Ferrari A, Casanova M, Bisogno G, et al. (2001) Hemangiopericytoma in pediatric ages. A report from the Italian and German Soft Tissue Sarcoma Cooperative Group. Cancer 92:2692–2698

42. Curless RG, Toledano SR, Ragheb J, Cleveland WW, Falcone S (2002) Hematogenous brain metastases in children. Pediatr Neurol 26:219–221

43. van den Heuvel-Eibrink MM, Graf N, Pein F, et al. (2004) Intracranial relapse in Wilms tumor patients. Pediatr Blood Cancer 43:737–741

44. MacRae R, Grimard L, Hsu E, et al. (2002) Brain metastases in Wilms tumor: A case report and literature review. J Pediatr Hematol Oncol 24:149- 153

45. Kebudi R, Ayan I, Görgün O, et al. (2005) Brain metastasis in pediatric extracranial solid tumors: Survey and literature review. J Neurooncol 71:43–48

46. Srotjan P, Benedik MD, Krageli B, et al. (1997) Combined radiation and chemotherapy for advanced undifferentiated nasopharyngeal carcinoma in children. Med Pediatr Oncol 28:366–369

47. Levine DA, Rao BN, Bowman L, et al. (1994) Primary malignancy of the salivary gland in children. J Pediatr Surg 29:44–47

48. Taylor RE, Galtamaneni HR, Spooner D (1993) Salivary gland carcinomas in children: A review of 15 cases. Med Pediatr Oncol 21:429–432

49. Rutigliano D, Wong R, Meyers P, LaQuaglia M (2006) Mucoepidermoid carcinoma as a secondary malignancy in pediatric sarcoma. Presented at BAPS Annual Conference, Stockholm

50. Morland B, Cox G, Randall C, et al. (1994) Synovial sarcoma of the larynx in a child: Case report and histological appearances. Med Pediatr Oncol 23:64–68

51. Lazar CC, Liard A, Lechevallier J, Bachy B, Michot C (2006) Secondary localization of an intra-thoracic benign mesenchymoma in the fossa poplitea: A rare pediatric case. Eur J Pediatr Surg 16:49–51

52. Rothstein DH, Voss SD, Isakoff M, Puder M (2005) Thymoma in a child: Case report and review in the literature. Pediatr Surg Int 21:548–551

53. Dhall G, Ginsburg HB, Bodenstein L, et al. (2004) Thymoma in children. Report of two cases and a review of literature. J Pediatr Hematol Oncol 26:681–685

54. Gaissert HA (2003) Primary tracheal tumors. Chest Surg Clin N Am 13:247–256

55. Curtis JM, Lacey D, Smyth R, Cart H (1998) Endobronchial tumours in childhood. Eur J Radiol 29:11–20

56. Al-Qahtani AR, Di Lorenzo M, Yazbeck S (2003) Endobronchial tumors in children: Institutional experience and literature review. J Pediatr Surg 38:733–736

57. Moraes TJ, Langer JC, Forte V, Shayan K, Sweezey N (2003) Pediatric pulmonary carcinoid. Pediatr Pulmonol 35:318–322

58. Craig ST, Hamzah M, Walker WS (1995) Video assisted thoracoscopic pneumonectomy for bronchial carcinoid tumor in a 14-year-old girl. J Pediatr Surg 30:322–324

59. Welsh JH, Maxson T, Jaksic T, Shahab I, Hicks J (1998) Tracheobronchial mucoepidermoid carcinoma in childhood and adolescence: Case report an review of the literature. Int J Pediatr Otorhinolaryngol 45:265–273

60. Chan EYY, MacCormick JA, Rubin S, Nizalik E (2005) Mucoepidermoid carcinoma of the trachea in a 4-year old boy. J Otolaryngol 34:235–238

61. Moore BA, Rutter MJ, Cotton R, Werkhaven J (2003) Maffucci's syndrome and cartilaginous neoplasms of the trachea. Otolaryngol Head Neck Surg 128:583–586

62. Kelsey AM, McNally K, Birch J, et al. (1997) Case of extrapulmonary, pleuropulmonary blastoma in a child. Pathological and cytogenetic findings. Med Pediatr Oncol 29:61–64

63. MacSweeney F, Papagiannopoulos K, Goldstra P, et al. (2003) An assessment of the expanded classification of congenital adenomatoid malformations and their relationship to malignant transformation. Am J Surg Pathol 27:1139–1146

64. Hill DA (2005) USCAP Specialty Conference, case 1-type I pleuropulmonary blastoma. Pediatr Dev Pathol 8:77–84

65. Bal N, Kayaselcuk F, Polat A, et al. (2005) Familial cystic nephroma in two siblings with pleuropulmonary blastoma. Pathol Oncol Res 11:53–56

66. Delahunt B, Thomson KJ, Ferguson AF, et al. (1993) Familial cystic nephroma and pleuropulmonary blastoma. Cancer 71:1338–1342

67. Knudson AG (2000) Commentary: On a new genetic syndrome. Med Pediatr Oncol 35:428

68. Ishida Y, Kato K, Kigasawa H, et al. (2000) Synchronous occurrence of pleuropulmonary blastoma and cystic nephroma: Possible genetic link in cystic lesions of the lung and kidney. Med Pediatr Oncol 35:85–87

69. DiTullio MT, Indolfi P, Casale F, et al. (1999) Pleuropulmonary blastoma: Survival after intraocular recurrence. Med Pediatr Oncol 33:588–590

70. d'Agostino S, Banoldi E, Dante S, et al. (1997) Embryonal rhabdomyosarcoma of lung arising in cystic adenomatoid malformation. Case report and review of the literature. J Pediatr Surg 32:1381–1383

71. Hancock BS, Di Lorenzo M, Youssef S, et al. (1993) Childhood primary pulmonary neoplasms. J Pediatr Surg 28:1133–1136

72. Cada M, Gertle JT, Traubici J, Ngan BY, Capra ML (2006) Approach to diagnosis and treatment of pediatric primary tumors of the diaphragm. J Pediatr Surg 41:1722–1726

73. van Leeuwen EF, Klokman WJ, van 't Veer MB, et al. (2000) Embryonal rhabdomyosarcoma of lung arising in cystic adenomatoid malformation. Case report and review of the literature. J Clin Oncol 18:487–497

74. Powers A, Cox C, Reintgen DS (2000) Breast cancer screening in childhood cancer survivors. Med Pediatr Oncol 34:210–212

75. Corpron CA, Black CT, Singletary SE, et al. (1995) Breast cancer in adolescent females. J Pediatr Surg 30:322–324

76. Rogers DA, Lobe TE, Rao BN, et al. (1994) Breast malignancy in children. J Pediatr Surg 29:48–51

77. Arca MJ, Caniano DA (2004) Breast disorders in the adolescent patient. Adolesc Med 125:473–485

78. Binokay F, Soyupak SK, Inal M, Celiktas M, et al. (2003) Primary and metastatic rhabdomyosarcoma in the breast: Report of two pediatric cases. Eur J Radiol 48:282–284

79. Gonzalez-Crussi F, Sotelo-Avila C, deMello DE (1986) Primary peritoneal, omental, and mesenteric tumors in childhood. Semin Diagn Pathol 3:122–137

80. Moriwaki Y, Kobayashi S, Harada H, et al. (1996) Cystic mesothelioma of the peritoneum. J Gastroenterol 31:868–874

81. Niggli FK, Gray TJ, Raafat F, Stevens MC (1994) Spectrum of peritoneal mesothelioma in childhood: Clinical and histopathologic features, including DNA cytometry. Pediatr Hematol Oncol 11:399–408

82. Andrion A, Bosia S, Paoletti L, Feyles E, Lanfranco C, et al. (1994) Malignant peritoneal mesothelioma in a 17-year-old boy with evidence of previous exposure to chrysotile and tremolite asbestos. Hum Pathol 25:617–622

83. Kelsey A (1994) Mesothelioma in childhood. Pediatr Hematol Oncol 11:461–462

84. Takekawa Y, Ugajin W, Koide H, Nishio S, et al. (2000) Pathologic, cytologic and immunohistochemical findings of an intra-abdominal desmoplastic small round cell tumor in a 15-year old male. Pathol Int 50:417–420

85. Furman J, Murphy WM, Wajsman Z; Berry AD (1997) Urogenital involvement by desmoplastic small round cell tumor. J Urol 158:1506–1509

86. Roganovich J, Bisogno G, Cecchetto G, D'Amore ESG, Carli M (1999) Paratesticular desmoplastic small round cell tumor: Case report and review of the literature. J Surg Oncol 71:269–272

87. Slomovitz BM, Girotra M, Aledo A, et al. (2000) Desmoplastic small round cell tumor with primary ovarian involvement: Case report and review. Gynecol Oncol 79:124–128

88. Crombleholme TM, Harris BH, Jacir NN, Latchaw LA, Kretschmar CS, et al. (1993) The desmoplastic round cell tumor: A new solid tumor of childhood. J Pediatr Surg 28:1023–1025

89. Kretschmar CS, Colbach C, Bham I, et al. (1996) Desmoplastic small cell tumor. A report of three cases and review of the literature. J Pediatr Hematol Oncol 18:293–299

90. O'Donnell KA, Caty MG, Allen JE, Fisher JE (2000) Lipoblastoma: Better termed infantile lipoma? Pediatr Surg Int 16:458–461

91. McVay M, Keller JE, Wagner CW, et al. (2006) Surgical management of lipoblastoma. J Pediatr Surg 41:1067–1071

92. Arda IS, Senocak ME, Göü S, Büyükpamukçu N (1993) A case of benign intrascrotal lipoblastoma clinically mimicking testicular torsion: A review of the literature. J Pediatr Surg 28:259–261

93. Hicks J, Dilley A, Patel D, et al. (2001) Lipoblastoma and lipoblastomatosis in infancy and childhood: Histopathologic, ultrastructural and cytogenetic features. Ultrastruct Pathol 25:321–333

94. Wright NB, Skinner R, Lee RE, Craft AW (1993) Myxoid liposarcoma of the porta hepatis in childhood. Pediatr Radiol 23:620–621

95. Bouche-Pillon MA, Behar C, Munzer M, Gaillard D, Lefebvre F, et al. (1989) Liposarcoma in children. À propos of 3 cases and a review of the literature. Chir Pediatr 30:181–184

96. Soares FA, Landell GA, Peres LC, Oliveira MA, Vicente YA, Tone LG (1989) Liposarcoma of hepatic hilum in childhood. Med Pediatr Oncol 17:239–249

97. Ladd AP, Grosfeld JL (2006) Gastrointestinal tumors in children and adolescents. Semin Pediatr Surg 15:37–47

98. Büyükpamukçu M, Berbero lu S, Büyükpamukçu N, Sarialio lu F, Kale G, et al. (1996) Nonlymphoid gastrointestinal malignancies in Turkish children. Med Pediatr Oncol 26:28–35

99. Gangopadhyay AN, Mohanty PK, Gopal C, et al. (1997) Adenocarcinoma of the oesophagus in an 8-year-old boy. J Pediatr Surg 32:1259–1260

100. Gould Chadwick E, Connor EJ, Guerra Hanson C, Joshi VV, Abu-Farsakh H, et al. (1990) Tumors of smooth-muscle origin in HIV-infected children. J Am Med Assoc 263:3182–3184

101. Balsam D, Segal S (1992) Two smooth muscle tumors in the airway of an HIV-infected child. Pediatr Radiol 22:552–553

102. Blatt J, Olshan A, Gula MJ, Dickman PS, Zaranek B (1992) Second malignancies in very-long-term survivors of childhood cancer. Am J Med 93:57–60

103. Tamate S, Lee N, Sou H, Nagata N, Takeuchi S, Nakahira M, Kobayashi Y (1994) Leiomyoblastoma causing acute gastric outlet obstruction in an infant. J Pediatr Surg 29:1386–1387

104. Cypriano MS, Jenkins JJ, Pappo AS, Rao BN, Daw NC (2004) Pediatric gastrointestinal stromal tumors and leiomyosarcoma. Cancer 101:39–50

105. Goedert JJ (2000) The epidemiology of the acquired immunodeficiency syndrome. Semin Oncol 27:390–401

106. Lack EE (1986) Leiomyosarcomas in childhood: A clinical and pathologic study of 10 cases. Pediatr Pathol 6:191–197

107. Miser JS, Pizzo PA (1985) Soft tissue sarcomas in childhood. Pediatr Clin North Am 32:779–800

108. Posen JA, Bar-Mao JA (1983) Leiomyosarcoma of the colon in an infant. A case report and review of the literature. Cancer 52:1458–1461

109. Lau WY, Chan CW (1985) Intestinal leiomyosarcoma in childhood. Eur J Pediatr 144:263–265

110. Durham MM, Gow KW, Shehata BM, et al. (2004) Gastrointestinal stromal tumors arising from the stomach: A report of three children. J Pediatr Surg 39:1495–1499

111. Wiechman LS, Tirabassi MV, Tashjian D, et al. GIST: A rare tumor with a novel therapy. Presentation SIOP, Vancouver 2005

112. Hoelwarth ME, personal communication

113. Price VE, Zielenska M, Chilton-McNeill S, et al. Clinical and molecular characteristics of pediatric gastrointestinal stromal tumors (GISTs). Pediatr Blood Cancer 45:20–24

114. Prakash S, Sairan I, Socci N, et al. (2005) Gastrointestinal stromal tumors in children and young adults: A clinicopathologic, molecular and genomic study of 15 cases and review of the literature. J Pediatr Hematol Oncol 27:179–187

115. Miettinen M, Lasota J, Sobin LH (2005) Gastrointestinal stromal tumors of the stomach in children and young adults: A clinicopathologic, immunohistochemical and molecular genetic study of 44 cases with long-term follow-up and review of the literature. Am J Surg Pathol 29:1373–1381

116. Towu E, Stanton M (2006) Gastrointestinal stromal tumour presenting with severe bleeding: A review of molecular biology. Pediatr Surg Int 22:462–464

117. Argos MD, Ruiz A, Sanchez F, Garcia C, Gaztambide J (1993) Gastric leiomyoblastoma associated with extraadrenal paraganglioma and pulmonary chondroma: A new case of Carney's triad. J Pediatr Surg 28:1545–1549

118. Nmadu PT, Mabogunje, Lawrie JH (1993) Gastric teratoma: A case report. Ann Trop Paediatr 13:291–292

119. Blecker U (1996) Heliobacter pylori disease in childhood. Clin Pediatr 35:175–183

120. Brumback RA, Gerber JE, Hicks DG, Strauchen JA (1984) Adenocarcinoma of the stomach following irradiation and chemotherapy for lymphoma in young patients. Cancer 54:994–998

121. McGill TW, Downey EC, Westbrook J, Wade D, de la Garza J (1993) Gastric carcinoma in children. J Pediatr Surg 28:1620–1621

122. Murphy S, Shaw K, Blanchard H (1994) Report of three gastric tumors in children. J Pediatr Surg 29:1202–1204

123. Katz S, Berenheim J, Kaufman Z, et al. (1997) Pernicious anaemia and adenocarcinoma of the stomach in an adolescent. Clinical presentation and histopathology. J Pediatr Surg 32:1384–1385

124. Lowichik A, Jackson WD, Coffin CM (2003) Gastrointestinal polyposis in childhood: Clinicopathologic and genetic features. Pediatr Dev Pathol 6:371–391

125. Mestre JR (1986) The changing pattern of juvenile polyps. Am J Gastroenterol 81:312–314

126. Hyer W (2001) Polyposis syndromes, pediatric implications. Gastrointest Endosc Clin N Am 11:659–682

127. Desi DC, Neale KF, Talbot IC, Hodgson SV, Phillips RK (1995) Juvenile polyposis. Brit J Surg 82:14–17

128. Cameron GS, Lau GYP (1979) Juvenile polyposis coli: A case treated with ileoendorectal pull-through. J Pediatr Surg 14:536–537

129. Doxey BW, Kuwada SK, Burt RW (2005) Inherited polyposis syndromes: Molecular mechanisms, clinicopathology, and genetic testing. Clin Gastroenterol Hepatol 3:633–641

130. Tovar JA, Eizaguirre I, Albert A, Jimenez J (1983) Peutz-Jeghers syndrome in children: Report of two cases and review of the literature. J Pediatr Surg 18:1–6

131. Cordts AE, Chabot JR (1983) Jejunal carcinoma in a child. J Pediatr Surg 18:180–181

132. Jansen M, Leng WWJ de, Bass AF, et al. (2006) Mucosal prolapse in the pathogenesis of Peutz-Jeghers polyposis. Gut 55:10–15

133. Forbes D, Rubin S, Trevenen C, Gall G, Scott B (1987) Familial polyposis coli in childhood. Clin Invest Med 10:5–9

134. Fonkalsrud EW (1996) Long-term results after colectomy and ileoanal pull-through procedure in children. Arch Surg 131:881–886

135. Davis C, Alexander F, Lavery I, Fazio VW (1994) Results of mucosal proctectomy versus extrarectal dissection for ulcerative colitis and familial polyposis in children and young adults. J Pediatr Surg 29:305–309

136. Hughes LJ, Michels VV (1992) Risk of hepatoblastoma in familial adenomatous polyposis. Am J Med Genet 43:1023–1025

137. Naylor EW, Lebenthal E (1979) Early detection of adenomatous polyposis coli in Gardner's syndrome. Pediatrics 63:222–227

138. Vasudevan SA, Patel JC, Wesson DE, et al. (2006) Severe dysplasia in children with familial adenomatous polyposis: Rare or simply overlooked? J Pediatr Surg 41:658–661

139. LaQuaglia MP, Heller G, Filippa DA, Karasakalides A, Vlamis V, et al. (1992) Prognostic factors and outcome in patients 21 years and under with colorectal carcinoma. J Pediatr Surg 27:1085–1090

140. Brown RA, Rode H, Millar AJW, Sinclair-Smith C, Cywes S (1992) Colorectal carcinoma in children. J Pediatr Surg 27:919–921

141. Taguchi T, Suita S, Hirata Y, Ishii E, Ueda K (1991) Carcinoma of the colon in children: A case report and review of 41 Japanese cases. J Pediatr Gastroenterol Nutr 12:394–399

142. Harzmann R, Kopper B, Carl P (1986) Cancer induction by urinary drainage or diversion through intestinal segments? Urologe A 25:198–203

143. Carachi R (1983) Polyposis coli: An experimental animal model. J Pediatr Surg 18:51–57

144. Rubin SZ, Mancer JF, Stephens CA (1981) Carcinoid in a rectal duplication: A unique pediatric surgical problem. Can J Surg 24:351–352

145. Parkes SE, Muir KR, Sheyyab al M, Cameron AH, Pincott JR, et al. (1993) Carcinoid tumors of the appendix in children 1957–1986: Incidence, treatment and outcome. Br J Surg 80:502–504

146. Tireli GA, Sander S, Dervisoglu S, Demirali O, Unal M (2005) Embryonal rhabdomyosarcoma of the common bile duct mimicking choledochal cyst. J Hepatobiliary Pancreat Surg 12:263–265

147. Lack EE, Perez-Atayde AR, Schuster SR (1981) Botryoid rhabdomyosarcoma of the biliary tract. Am J Surg Pathol 5:643–652

148. Ruymann FB, Raney BR, Crist WM, Lawrence W (1985) Rhabdomyosarcoma of the biliary tree in childhood. A report from the Intergroup Rhabdomyosarcoma Study. Cancer 56:575–581

149. Sanz N, Mingo de L, Florez F, Rollan V (1997) Rhabdomyosarcoma of the biliary tree. Pediatr Surg Int 12:200–201

150. Spunt SL, Lobe TE, Pasppo AS, et al. (2000) Aggressive surgery is unwarranted for biliary tract rhabdomyosarcoma. J Pediatr Surg 35:309–315

151. Roebuck DJ, Yang WT, Lam WWM, Stanley P (1998) Hepatobiliary rhabdomyosarcoma in children: Diagnostic radiology. Pediatr Radiol 28:101–108

152. Komi N, Tamura T, Miyoshi Y, Kunitomo K, Udaka H, Takehara H (1984) Nationwide survey of cases of choledochal cyst. Analysis of coexistent anomalies, complications and surgical treatment in 645 cases. Surg Gastroenterol 3:69–73

153. Benjamin IS (2003) Biliary cystic disease: The risk of cancer. J Hepatobiliary Pancreat Surg 10:335–339

154. Tokiwa K, Iwai N (1996) Early mucosal changes of the gallbladder in patients with anomalous arrangement of the pancreaticobiliary duct. Gastroenterology 110:1614–1618

155. Ando H, Ito T, Nagaya M, Watanabe Y, Seo T, Kaneko K (1995) Pancreaticobiliary maljunction without choledochal cysts in infants and children: Clinical features and surgical therapy. J Pediatr Surg 30:1658–1662

156. Vossen S, Goretzki PE, Goebel U, Willnow U (1998) Therapeutic management of rare malignant pancreatic tumors in children. World J Surg 22:879–882

157. Shorter NA, Glick RD, Klimstra DS, et al. (2002) Malignant pancreatic tumors in childhood and adolescence: The Memorial Sloan-Kettering experience 1967 to present. J Pediatr Surg 37:887–892

158. Eisenhuber E, Schoefl R, Wiesbauer P, Bankier AA (2001) Primary pancreatic lymphoma presenting as acute pancreatitis in a child. Med Pediatr Oncol 37:53–54

159. Dhebri AR, Connor S, Campbell F, et al. (2004) Diagnosis, treatment and outcome of pancreatoblastoma. Pancreatology 4:441–451

160. Sugai M, Kimura N, Umehara M, et al. (2006) A case of pancreatoblastoma prenatally diagnosed as intraperitoneal cyst. Pediatr Surg Int e-pub 22:845–847

161. Pelizzo G, Conoscenti G, Kalache KD, et al. (2003) Antenatal manifestation of congenital pancreatoblastoma in a fetus with Beckwith-Wiedeman syndrome. Prenat Diagn 23:292–294

162. Muguerza R, Rodriguez A, Formigo E, et al. (2005) Pancreatoblastoma associated with incomplete Beckwith-Wiedeman syndrome: Case report and review of the literature. J Pediatr Surg 40:1341–1344

163. Barenboim-Stapleton L, Yang X, Tsokos M, et al. (2005) Pediatric pancreatoblastoma: Histopathologic and cytogenetic characterization of tumor and derived cell line. Cancer Genet Cytogenet 157:109–117

164. Montemarano H, Lonergan G, Bulas DI, Selby DM (2000) Pancreatoblastoma: Imaging findings in 10 patients and review of the literature. Radiology 214:476–482

165. Kloeppel G, Kosmahl M, Jaenig U, Luettges J (2004) Pancreatoblastoma: One of the rarest among the rare pancreatic neoplasms. Pancreatology 4:452–453

166. Papavramidis T, Papavramidis S (2005) Solid pseudopapillary tumors of the pancreas: Review of 718 patients reported in the English literature. J Am Coll Surg 200:965–972

167. Zhou H, Cheng W, Lam KY, et al. (2001) Solid-cystic papillary tumor of the pancreas in children. Pediatr Surg Int 17:614–620

168. Kosmahl M, Seada LS, Jaenig U, et al. (2000) Solid-pseudopapillary tumor of the pancreas: Its origin revisited. Virchows Arch 436:473–480

169. Rebhandl W, Felberbauer FX, Puig S, et al. (2001) Solid-pseudopapillary tumor of the pancreas (Frantz tumor) in children: Report of four cases and a review of the literature. J Surg Oncol 76:289–296

170. Andronikou S, Moon A, Ussher R (2003) Peritoneal metastatic disease in a child after excision of a solid pseudopapillary tumour of the pancreas: A unique case. Pediatr Radiol 33:269–271

171. Nadler EP, Novikov A, Landzberg BR, et al. (2002) The use of endoscopic ultrasound in the diagnosis of solid pseudopapillary tumors of the pancreas in children. J Pediatr Surg 37:1370–1373

172. Luettges J, Stigge C, Pacena M, Kloeppel G (2004) Rare ductal adenocarcinoma of the pancreas in patients younger than age 40 years. Cancer 1000:173–183

173. Dotzenrath C, Goretzki PE, Cupisti K, et al. (2001) Malignant endocrine tumors in patients with MEN 1 disease. Surgery 129:91–95

174. Verhoef S, van Diemen-Steenvoorde R, Akkersdijk WL, et al. (1999) Malignant pancreatic tumour within the spectrum of tuberous sclerosis complex in childhood. Eur J Pediatr 158:284–287

175. Francalanci P, Diomedi-Camassei F, Purificato C, et al. (2003) Malignant pancreatic endocrine tumor in a child with tuberous sclerosis. Am J Surg Pathol 27:1386–1389

176. Aronson DC, Medary I, Finlay JL, et al. (1996) Renal cell carcinoma in childhood and adolescents. A retrospective survey for prognostic factor in 22 cases. J Pediatr Surg 31:183–186

177. Cook A, Lorenzo AJ, Pippi Salle J, et al. (2006) Pediatric renal cell carcinoma: Single institution 25-year case series and initial experience with partial nephrectomy. J Urol 175:1456–1460

178. Robertson FM, Cendron M, Klauber GT, et al. (1996) Renal cell carcinoma in association with tuberous sclerosis in children. J Pediatr Surg 31:729–730

179. Hoenig DM, McRae S, Chen SC, et al. (1996) Transitional cell carcinoma of the bladder in the pediatric patient. J Urol 156:203–205

180. Soergel TM, Cain MP, Misseri R, et al. (2004) Transitional cell carcinoma of the bladder following augmentation cystoplasty for the neuropathic bladder. J Urol 172:1649–1652

181. Streif W, Gabner I, Janetschek G, et al. (1997) Partial nephrectomy in a cystic partially differentiated nephroblastoma. Med Pediatr Oncol 28:416–419

182. Blakely ML, Shamberger RC, Norkoo P, et al. (2003) Outcome of children with cystic partially differentiated nephroblastoma treated with or without chemotherapy. J Pediatr Surg 38:897–900

183. Vujanic GM, Webb D, Kelsey A (1995) B cell non-Hodgkin's lymphoma as a primary renal tumour. Med Pediatr Oncol 25:423–426

184. Li CK, Yeung CK, Chow J, et al. (1995) Postatic non-Hodgkin's lymphoma causing acute urinary retention in childhood. Med Pediatr Oncol 25:420–422

185. Levy DA, Kay R, Elder JS (1994) Neonatal testis tumours. A review of the prepubertal testis tumour registry. J Urol 151:715–717

186. Agarwal PK, Palmer JS (2006) Testicular and paratesticular neoplasms in prepubertal males. J Urol 176:875–891

187. Ellison DA, Corredor-Buchmann J, Parham DM, Jackson RJ (2005) Malignant triton tumor presenting as a rectal mass in an 11-month-old. Pediatr Dev Pathol 8:235–239

188. Hajivassiliou CA, Carachi R, Simpson E, et al. (1997) Ectomesenchymoma—One or two tumors? Case report and review of literature. J Pediatr Surg 32:1351–1355

189. Chow LTC, Kumta SM (2004) Primary osteochondrorhabdomyosarcoma (malignant mesenchymoma) of the fibula: A rare tumor in an unusual site—Case report and a review of the literature. APMIS 112:617–623

190. Mrad K, Sassi S, Smida M, et al. (2004) Osteosarcoma with rhabdomyosarcomatous component or so-called malignant mesenchymoma of bone. Pathologica 96:475–478

191. Oppenheimer O, Athanasian E, Meyers P, et al. (2005) Malignant ectomesenchymoma in the wrist of a child: Case report and review of the literature. Int J Surg Pathol 13:113–116

192. Ceballos PI, Ruiz-Maldonado R, Mihm MC (1995) Melanoma in children. New Engl J Med 332:656–662

193. Huynh PM, Grant-Kelsd JM, Grin CM (2005) Childhood melanoma: Update and treatment. Int J Dermatol 44:715–723

194. Oliveria SA, Saraiya M, Geller AC, Heneghan MK, Jorgenson C (2006) Sun exposure and risk of melanoma. Arch Dis Child 91:131–138

195. Mones JM, Ackerman AB (2003) Melanomas in prepubescent children. Review comprehensively, critique historically, criteria diagnostically, and course biologically. Am J Dermatopathol 25:223–238

196. Pensler JM, Hijjawi J, Paller AS (1993) Melanoma in prepubertal children. Int Surg 78:247–249

197. Daryanani D, Plukker JT, Nap RE, et al. (2006) Adolescent melanoma: Risk factors and long-term survival. Eur J Surg Oncol 32:218–223

198. Zaal LH, Mooi WJ, Sillevis Smit JH, van der Horst CMAM (2004) Classification of congenital melanocytic naevi and malignant transformation: A review of the literature. Br J Plast Surg 57:707–719

199. Corpron CA, Andrassy RJ (1997) Melanomas and other rare tumors. In: Andrassy RJ (ed) Pediatric surgical oncology. WB Saunders Co, Philadelphia, pp 349–364

200. Balch CM, Cascinelli N (2006) Sentinel-node biopsy in melanoma. N Engl J Med 355:1370–1371

Reconstructive Surgery

21

Amir F. Azmy

Contents

21.1 Introduction

The outcome of children with primary malignant tumors has improved considerably in recent years due to advanced therapeutic modalities in chemotherapy and radiotherapy. The surgeon plays an important role in improving the quality of life for children who are long-term survivors following multimodal treatment for their malignancies. Any procedure to improve quality of life or cosmetic results should be delayed until a disease-free state is confirmed and recurrence of the tumor is unlikely. The need for reconstructive procedures in the pediatric age group may be related to the long-term sequelae of aggressive treatment of childhood tumors.

Early reconstructive surgery may be required, for example, in patients who have had their bladder removed and reconstruction of the lower urinary tract is fashioned by forming an ileal conduit or continent diversion or, for example, to reconstruct and close a large defect of the chest wall after resection of a large tumor.

Treatment of malignant disease in children may result in loss of part of the body or changes in body function requiring physical restoration. Physical rehabilitation should be considered in initial surgical planning. Consequences of treatment and its possible reconstructive procedures should be discussed with the patient (if he or she is old enough) and the parents. The site of malignancy and its stage dictate the surgical decision.

21.2 Reconstruction After Excision of Head and Neck Cancer

A variety of techniques have been used for closure of surgical defects at the time of primary surgery after complete excision of the primary tumor.
1. Split thickness skin graft. This graft could be used and immobilized by a stent (e.g., maxillary or orbital cavity).

2. Use of local flaps. Small or medium sized defects in the oral cavity or facial defects could be repaired by vascularized local flaps.
3. Regional flaps. The use of a delto-pectoral forehead flap based on the superficial temporal artery.
4. Myocutaneous flaps. For example, the use of the pectoralis major or latissimus dorsi muscles.
5. Microvascular free flaps. Free grafts taken from the groin supplied by the circumflex ileac artery or from the foot supplied by the dorsalis pedis artery, anastomosis between donor veins and superior thyroid or facial arteries and any adjacent veins.

21.3 Mandibular Reconstruction

In reconstructing the mandible, autogenous bone graft is a superior substitute; reconstruction using cancellous bone in trays or struts of cortical bone has also been used. Autogenous bone grafts using a rib or ileac crest show good early results but resorption of bone occurs; improved results may be obtained with the use of a rib attached to a myocutaneous flap.

The use of cancellous rather than cortical bone yields better results. Autogenous marrow and cancellous bone obtained from ileum can be packed into trays fashioned from titanium or stainless steel. The trays serve to stabilize the mandibular fragments and provide a contour for the new bone formed. Aggressive treatment of rhabdomyosarcoma of the mandible in early childhood with chemotherapy, radiotherapy, and surgery may result in severe deformity requiring reconstructive surgery.

Despite achieving a cure, the patient is left with severe deformity of the mandible. Bony osteotomies cannot be performed because of previous irradiation, therefore free tissue transfer of latissimus dorsi muscle and skin, and extraction of the premaxillary nonfunctional teeth along with prosthetic restoration may be necessary to correct the defect. Psychological counseling and appropriate make-up will contribute to improved cosmesis and a satisfying outcome.

21.4 Reconstruction of the Orbit

Children with malignant tumors of the orbit (retinoblastoma) often require excision of the eyeball and receive postoperative irradiation. This results in severe deformity of the orbit and difficulty in achieving reconstruction of the severely contracted socket. Augmentation and formation of an adequate eye socket are required. In 1993 Asato, et al. reported their experience with 25 patients using a free flap transfer with microvascular anastomosis [1]. Various flaps were utilized (groin flap, dorsalis pedis flap, scapular flap,

and others). The design of the donor flap is based on the degree of depression and whether sufficient conjunctiva is present to line the eye socket. Many of the patients may require a minor revision operation such as debulking, dermal fat grafts, canthoplasty, or fascia suspension [1].

Marques, et al. [2] reported their experience with staged reconstruction of the orbit after orbital exenteration and radiotherapy with a follow-up period of between 5 and 18 years. The staged reconstruction includes first orbital filling, second fashioning of the orbital rims and eyelids, and third the cavity is created to receive a static eye prosthesis. Assessment of the results showed that the first stage alone produced a marked improvement in appearance and occluded existing fistulae. The subsequent procedures further improved the aesthetic results; however, some difficulties still exist due to retraction of the tissues and insufficient tissue mobility [2].

21.5 Tissue Expansion

The use of tissue expansion in the treatment of giant melanotic lesions of the scalp allows excision of large tumors and primary closure of the defect with skin created after expansion. The treatment of giant facial congenital melanocytic nevi is advised because of the potential for malignant transformation. The use of tissue expander facilitates excision of giant melanotic lesions of the scalp resulting in excess skin similar in appearance and type to that immediately adjacent to the defect [3].

Two lesions with an increased risk of developing cutaneous malignancy (malignant melanoma) are acquired abdominal nevi (dysplastic nevi) and giant melanocytic nevi [4]. Although the management of these lesions is controversial and the potential for developing malignancy is not well defined [5], resection of all giant congenital melanocytic nevi has been advocated [6] particularly in the scalp where it is difficult to observe changes in the nevus. It is important to carefully establish a plan before attempting soft tissue expansion. Proper placement of the incision and the correct choice of expander size are essential. The incision should be placed where it will not interfere with later skin advancement or compromise the blood supply. The base of the expander should be approximately the same size as the nevus. Expansion is usually begun 3 weeks after the placement and about 10–15% of total expander volume can be injected at one time. Saline is injected at 3- to 4-day intervals if the tissues are responding. When the planned expansion is achieved the expander is removed and the flap is rotated into position.

21.6 Chest Wall Reconstruction After Excision of Large Chest Wall Tumors

Reconstructive procedures after radical resection of a large malignant chest wall tumor are a challenge. Chapelier, et al. [7] described 32 consecutive cases between 1982 and 1993 in which patients underwent radical excision of large chest wall tumors arising from the bone (15 cases) or soft tissue (17 cases) of the chest wall. Nine patients required extensive excision of skin, 12 required sternotomies, and 20 had lateral chest wall resection, 16 of whom required excision of three or more ribs, lung resection with wedge or total resection, and resection of a portion of the diaphragm or abdominal wall. To establish stability of the chest wall various prosthetic materials have been used in 27 patients; marlex mesh was used in 21 cases; polytetrafluoroethylene (PTFE) was used in four patients and polyglactin mesh in two patients.

After sternotomy, methyl methacrylate mesh reinforcement was used in six patients; soft tissue reconstruction using pectoralis major muscle either alone or with skin advancement or myocutaneous flaps was performed. Muscle transposition can be employed to reconstruct defects in the lateral chest wall including latissimus dorsi, pectoralis major muscle, or serratus anterior with advancement of the diaphragm [7]. Pairolero and Arnold [8] reported their experience with 205 consecutive patients over a 9-year period. In 114 with chest wall tumors, a mean of 5.4 ribs were resected.

The skeletal defects were closed with prosthetic material or autologous ribs. Muscle flap procedures used included pectoralis major, latissimus dorsi, rectus abdominus, serratus anterior, external oblique, trapezius, and advancement of the diaphragm or transposition of the omentum. The mean number of operations per patient was 1.9 (range 1–8) and follow-up examination showed excellent results (mean follow-up 32.4 months).

Grosfeld, et al. [9] evaluated the efficacy of extensive chest wall resection and prosthetic reconstruction in 15 children with chest wall malignancies, (mean age 9.6 years). Eleven had primary chest wall malignancies, which included Ewing's sarcoma, rhabdomyosarcoma, chondrosarcoma, primitive neuroectodermal tumor, and mesenchymal sarcoma. Four children had metastatic disease to the chest wall and lungs from Wilms' tumor, osteogenic sarcoma, and neuroblastoma.

Surgical treatment included chest wall resection of two to six ribs and reconstruction with marlex mesh (Devol Inc, Cranston, RI) in seven cases, latissimus dorsi muscle flap in two, prolene mesh in one, and Gortex mesh (Gore Co, Flagstaff, AZ) in five patients. Concomitant en bloc pulmonary resection was also performed including wedge resection in five, lobectomy in two, pneumonectomy in one, and partial resection of the diaphragm in two. Fourteen children received adjunctive treatment with multiagent chemotherapy and irradiation in eight (five preoperatively and three postoperatively) (2,000–4,800 r).

Chest wall resection was done as a delayed primary or second look procedure and adequate skin and subcutaneous tissue coverage was possible. Occasional fluid collection occurred around the gortex patch postoperatively requiring aspiration [9]. In 1991 Gordon, et al. reported a large series of patients with soft tissue sarcoma of the chest wall over a 40-year period. In all, 189 cases had chest wall sarcoma including 32 patients with a desmoid tumor, 23 with liposarcoma, 18 with rhabdomyosarcoma, 17 with fibrosarcoma, 14 instances of embryonal rhabdomyosarcoma, malignant primitive neuroectodermal tumor in 13, malignant fibrous histiocytoma in 11, spindle cell sarcoma in four, synovial sarcoma in three, hemangiopericytoma in three, alveolar sarcoma in three, and other tumor types in 12. Resection was the primary treatment in 94% of cases. Local recurrence occurred in 27% and metastases occurred in 35% of high-grade tumors. The overall 5-year survival rate was 66% for high-grade sarcomas; however, 90% of patients with low-grade tumors survived [10].

21.6.1 Operative Techniques

21.6.1.1 Preoperative Assessment

Patient assessment should include a chest radiograph bronchoscopy and measurement of arterial gases and spirometry, occasionally ventilation perfusion lung scan may be required. Local and extent of the tumor should be precisely identified by performing a computed tomography scan and or magnetic resonance imaging to exclude distant metastasis.

21.6.1.2 Operative Procedure

A single stage procedure of resection and reconstruction is performed using one-lung anesthesia and careful monitoring of pulse, blood pressure, central venous pressure, and arterial blood gas tension. Wide excision with safety margin should be performed including the scar of the previous biopsy site with a 3- to 4-cm normal skin margin. The underlying muscles such as the latissimus dorsi or lateral part of the pectoralis major can often be spared. Complete excision of the tumor and involved tissues may require resection of part or the entire lung, anterior pericardium, subclavian vein, brachiocephalic vein, subclavian artery, or part of the superior vena cava. Partial resection of the diaphragm or abdominal wall may also be necessary.

21.6.1.3 Reconstruction After Lateral Chest Wall Resection

Ipsilateral muscle transposition is used to reconstruct defects of the anteriolateral chest wall. The latissimus dorsi muscle is the most commonly used based on the thoracodorsal vessels. Other coverage may employ the pectoralis major with primary skin closure or a pectoralis major musculocutaneous flap, rectus abdominis musculocutaneous flap, and in cases of local muscles being previously excised or irradiated, a flap based on the internal mammary and superior epigastric vessels with a wide skin island transposed superiorly through a subcutaneous tunnel to cover the lateral defect. The site of the muscle used is closed primarily and reinforced by a sheet of prosthetic mesh to prevent hernia or bulging. Posterior chest wall defects are closed with latissimus dorsi or serratus anterior by muscle transposition with skin advancement.

21.6.1.4 Pectoralis Major Flap

The pectoralis major flap is a myocutaneous flap which can also be used to carry a segment of 5th rib or a portion of sternum. The vascular pedicle is about 1 cm medial to the coracoid process. The artery is the pectoral branch of the thoracoacromial axis; the venous drainage of the flap is the venae comitantes which drain into the axillary vein. The approximate axis of the vascular pedicle is along a line from the coracoid process to the xiphisternum. An island of skin can be raised on a portion of the muscle containing the vascular pedicle. A composite flap can be raised incorporating the 5th rib, which is said to receive its blood supply from the pectoralis muscle in 75% of cases. A segment of the sternum may be used for osteocutaneous transfer relying on the origin of the pectoralis muscle from the sternum; the main use of this flap is in reconstruction of head and neck and chest wall defects. The donor defect can be closed directly or may require a skin graft.

21.6.1.5 Pectoralis Major Muscle

Pectoralis major muscle is frequently used, either unilaterally or bilaterally or transferred on a thoracoacromial vascular pedicle. The muscle is covered with skin advancement or as a musculocutaneous flap. The pectoralis major flap is used for ventral or upper lateral defects in the arc of rotation of the pectoralis major.

The pectoralis major muscle allows an arc of rotation that reaches the entire thoracic wall except the lower sternum (Fig. 21.1). In cases where the sternum has been resected, the muscle could be mobilized from the nondominant side by dividing the humeral attach-

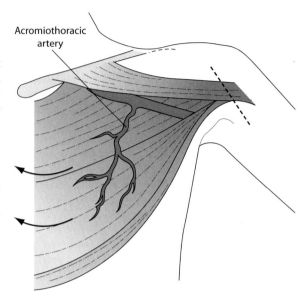

Fig. 21.1 Pectoralis major flap. Division of the humeral attachment allows coverage of the central and upper part of chest wall.

ments and transposing the muscle into the sternal defect to obliterate the space. The contralateral muscle is then transposed without humeral division to cover the deeper muscle. If the sternum is not resected, mobilization of one or both muscles without division of humeral attachment is sufficient for closure of upper sternotomy wounds. To cover defects of lower sternum, the rectus abdominis muscle flaps or omental transposition could be performed.

21.6.1.6 Latissimus Dorsi

Latissimus dorsi muscle is used when the pectoralis major has been previously excised or irradiated and is used for lower or very large defects and the latissimus dorsi is transposed on the thoracodorsal vessels.

The latissimus dorsi is a large flat quadrilateral muscle which arises from the spine of the lower six thoracic vertebrae, the lumber and sacral vertebrae and the posterior crest of the ileum; it has some small slips from the lower four ribs. The muscle is inserted into the intertubercular groove of the humorus. The muscle can be used as a muscle flap or as a myocutaneous flap for island pedicle transfer or free tissue transfer. The muscle is supplied by the thoracodorsal artery (terminal branches of the subscapular artery). The nerve supply is via the thoracodorsal nerve which divides into anterior and posterior divisions; the muscle is large and will support a large amount of skin. The pedicle can be dissected to its origin from the subscapular artery and from the axillary vessels.

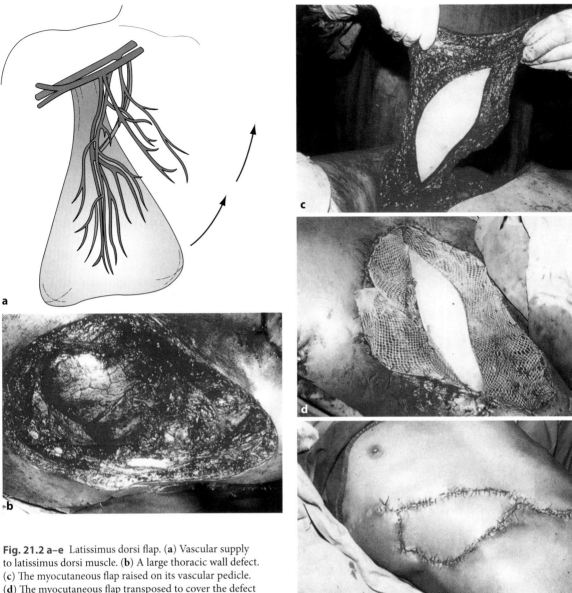

Fig. 21.2 a–e Latissimus dorsi flap. (**a**) Vascular supply to latissimus dorsi muscle. (**b**) A large thoracic wall defect. (**c**) The myocutaneous flap raised on its vascular pedicle. (**d**) The myocutaneous flap transposed to cover the defect supported by an underlying mesh. (**e**) Appearance after completion of repair.

As an island flap, the anterior arc of rotation will allow correction of the lower lateral abdominal wall, chest wall, shoulder, neck, and lower half of the face (Fig. 21.2a–e). The posterior arc of rotation allows the flap to reach the spine, shoulder, and posterior part of the neck. The donor defect can sometimes be closed directly or may require a skin graft. There is no severe disability from the loss of the muscle and the loss of function can be minimized by preserving the posterior division of the thoracodorsal nerve. The major use of the muscle as an island flap is in chest wall reconstruction.

21.6.1.7 Rectus Abdominis Flap

The rectus abdominis muscle is a large flat muscle inserted into the 5th, 6th, and 7th ribs superiorly and into the pubic crest inferiorly. It is commonly used as myocutaneous flap. The muscle has a double arterial supply superiorly from the superior epigastric artery (branch of the internal mammary artery) and inferiorly from the large deep inferior epigastric artery (branch of the external iliac artery). These arteries communicate in a network of vessels within the rectus muscle and communicate with the intercostal arteries and su-

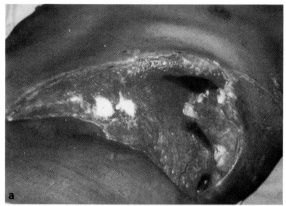

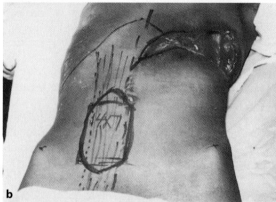

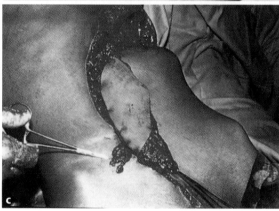

Fig. 21.3 a–c Rectus abdominis flap. (**a**) A large thoracic wall defect. (**b**) Rectus abdominis flap is marked on the skin. (**c**) Rectus abdominis myocutaneous flap is raised.

perficial epigastric vessels. Perforating vessels supply the overlying skin. Venous drainage is via venae comitantes. The rectus abdominis flap can be raised with overlying skin on either superior or inferior pedicle. The superiorly based island myocutaneous flap can be used to cover skin chest wall and lateral trunk defects. It has an arc of rotation which extends to the clavicle on the same side. The donor site can usually be closed directly. The abdominal sheath should be repaired using a locally designed fascial flap or by artificial mesh

to avoid hernia formation. The rectus abdominis flap is very useful in closing large chest wall defects because a large amount of tissue can be raised.

A rectus abdominus musculocutaneous flap is used when latissimus dorsi muscle has been previously excised or irradiated. The procedure requires an experienced plastic surgeon; it is important that the internal mammary artery is patent. The musculocutaneous flap is based superiorly on the superior epigastric vessels and the created abdominal defect is closed. The rectus abdominis muscle flap is preferred because it avoids performing a laparotomy (Fig. 21.3a–c).

The greater omentum is reserved after failure of a musculocutaneous flap. Omental transposition should be reserved as a back-up procedure should muscle transposition fail to cover a soft tissue defect or because of previous irradiation. Omental transposition is suitable for partial thickness resections with sufficient structural stability; omentum can be mobilized to cover a larger area than muscle or musculocutaneous flaps.

21.6.2 Other Flaps

21.6.2.1 The Radial Forearm Flap

The radial forearm flap is a fasciocutaneous flap. The flap is based on the radial artery and venae comitantes. The flap is used primarily in free tissue transfer. The forearm acts as a donor site for a purely facial flap, a fasciocutaneous flap, and an osteocutaneous flap incorporating a segment of the radius. A large amount of tissue can be made available particularly for reconstruction for head and neck on a reliable and constant vascular pedicle [11].

21.6.2.2 Collagen-Coated Vicryl Mesh

A new collagen-coated vicryl mesh bioprosthesis was used in 28 children who needed repair of thoracic and abdominal wall defects. Sixteen children had resection of chest wall for tumors; the others had congenital abdominal wall defects. The new prosthetic material, which has been tested experimentally and used clinically, showed that the material is a perfectly adequate substitute for repair after resection of three or more ribs [12]. The main aim of chest wall resection and reconstruction is complete excision of the tumor with restoration and protection to the thoracic viscera, restoration of physiological function, adequate lung and chest wall growth, and acceptable chest wall appearance.

A major problem after extensive resection and reconstruction is the development of scoliosis, restrictive lung disease, late secondary malignancy in a radiation site, and disseminated metastases.

21.6.3 Pulmonary Function After Chest Wall Resection and Reconstruction

Early and late pulmonary function tests show a reduction in forced vital capacity (FVC) to 31–74% of the predicted value; obstructed lung disease is not present as the ratio of forced expiratory volume (FEV) to FVC is normal and the peak expiratory flow rate is reduced only in proportion to FVC. Restrictive lung disease may be due to in part to the effect of the radiation on the lungs and chest wall deformity. Continued long-term follow-up is essential to determine the true incidence of local recurrence, metastatic disease, or any functional problems [13].

21.6.4 Postoperative Management

Rapid weaning from the ventilator and early physiotherapy are recommended to prevent atelectasis. Adequate pain control and early removal of chest tube drains improve patient comfort. The use of postoperative chemotherapy or radiotherapy may be necessary depending on the type of tumor.

21.6.5 Postoperative Complications

Minor complications may occur including minor skin dehiscence, partial or complete wound dehiscence, hemorrhage, wound infection, and major septic complications. In such cases the prosthetic material will need to be removed with the preservation of the myocutaneous flap and control of infection.

21.6.6 Recommendations for Radical Resection and Reconstruction

1. Wide skin excision in cases of tumor ulcerating through the skin or previous biopsy scar or irradiation.
2. En bloc dissection of the tumor and the involved structures, which may include lung, mediastinal vessels, or pericardium.
3. Prosthetic material must be designed to fit the site of the defect.
4. Chest wall stability must be maintained; marlex mesh is the most commonly used PTFE mesh as it has the advantage of limiting movement of the fluid or air across the chest wall, protects the chest wall, and avoids paradoxical movement.
5. Reconstruction of chest wall using various muscles or musculocutaneous flap should be adjusted to the site and the size of the defect.

21.7 Reconstructive Urology

Surgical extirpation was initially the treatment of choice for children with genitourinary malignancies, especially rhabdomyosarcoma [14]. Michalkiewicz, et al. in 1997 [15] reported on the complications observed following pelvic exenteration at St. Jude Children's Research Hospital from 1963 to 1994. Seventeen children of 43 had pelvic exenteration (median age 3.5 years) for primary neoplasms of the prostate, bladder, or uterus. Early major complications included wound infection (24%), fistula, abscess, and malnourishment (12% each). Late complications included hydronephrosis (35%), bowel obstruction (24%), pyelonephritis, fistulae, lymphedema, and ureteric stenosis (12% each).

The operative management of these tumors has become less aggressive with the evolution of multimodal therapy with preservation and salvage of the affected organ [16]. The improvement and response to chemotherapy and radiotherapy has encouraged avoidance of radical surgery for pelvic organs with rhabdomyosarcoma and limited surgery to partial resection for residual disease after completion of combined chemotherapy and radiotherapy.

Between 1978 and 1991, ten children between 1 and 8 years of age with group III pelvic rhabdomyosarcoma (IRS classification) and considered inoperable at diagnosis were treated primarily with intensive polychemotherapy, complementary radiotherapy and subsequent conservative surgery. Eight of ten children survived free of disease with a functional bladder for (range of follow-up 5.7–18.4 years) [17].

Various reconstructive techniques have been described in cases where limited excision of the bladder could be performed and the remaining bladder could still be functional and its capacity improved with construction of intestinal augmentation. Radical surgery may be required when the tumor involves the base of the bladder or prostate and a urinary reservoir is successfully constructed. Bladder removal with nerve-sparing technique for protection of potency may offer the male patient a satisfactory alternative [18].

In cases of bladder rhabdomyosarcoma arising in the base of the bladder or the prostate and where bladder salvage is not feasible, a total cystectomy will be required and urinary diversion will be necessary to achieve free drainage of urine. The most common procedure for urinary diversion is an ileal conduit. Ureterosigmoidostomy has not been employed in recent years because of recurrent pyelonephritis, metabolic acidosis, and possible risk of malignancy due to urinary excretion of N-nitroso compounds [19, 20]. However, ureterosigmoidoscopy could still be used in selected patients with normal upper tract and renal function in whom long-term outcome is expected to be excellent.

Cutaneous ureteric diversion is suitable in patients where the ureters are obstructed, tortuous and dilated, and easily brought to the skin. This method of diversion may be temporary or permanent; to avoid two cutaneous stomas a transuretero-ureterostomy is therefore performed.

21.7.1 Continent Urinary Diversion

Continent urinary diversion is suitable for children who had radical cystectomy for bladder rhabdomyosarcoma either as a primary procedure at the time of bladder resection or as a secondary procedure after initial ileal loop diversion or cutaneous ureterostomy to achieve a continent stoma. This may also be required in cases with severe bladder fibrosis and contraction due to previous irradiation and not suitable for bladder augmentation. The child should be old enough to look after his own care – particularly intermittent self-catheterization.

21.7.1.1 Evaluation and Preoperative Assessment

1. Evaluation of the upper renal tract and renal function.
2. Mark suitable site for the cutaneous stoma. A stoma therapist should be consulted about the appropriate site and also counseling should be given to the child and his parents about the care of the stoma and the practice of catheterization. The position of catheterizable stoma in the lower abdomen is feasible as there are no external appliances required. The position of the stoma should be checked in various positions (supine, erect, and sitting positions).
3. If the decision is that the continent pouch should be performed at the time of bladder excision, gross tumor excision should be performed and no evidence of spread or metastasis should be insured.
4. Patients undergoing conversion of an ileal loop to a continent pouch diversion, the ureteroileal anastomosis, should be checked – as free reflux or obstruction may be present and should be corrected. The ureteroileal segment could be preserved and incorporated into the pouch.
5. Mechanical and antibacterial bowel preparation should be performed 24 h before operation. Oral laxatives and rectal or colonic washouts should be performed.

A variety of methods to achieve continent urinary diversion have been described and based on providing a large low pressure reservoir, an antireflux procedure and continent cutaneous channel for intermittent catheterization.

21.7.1.2 Kock Pouch

The Kock pouch [21] is fashioned from a small bowel segment away from the ileal cecal valve; the ileal segment is isolated on its vascular pedicle, the central part is detubularized and folded twice to create a large pouch. The segment of the ileum at each end of the pouch (about 6 in) is intussuscepted to provide a nipple valve to prevent leakage of urine or reflux. The ureters are isolated and anastomosed to the afferent loop. To stabilize the nipple, sutures, stable, or cuffs have been used, fixation of the nipple to the pouch wall offers the best result (Fig. 21.4a–c). The purpose of the procedure is to maintain a continent efferent valve and prevent parastomal hernia. Incontinence is due to eversion of the nipple valve when the reservoir is distended. Reoperation is required in more than 20% of cases. Skinner, et al. [22] reported a 15% early and 22% late complication rate; urinary leakage was the most common. A hemi-Kock pouch may be used for bladder augmentation or formation of a neobladder in instances when the ureteral length is not long enough for reimplantation [22].

Skinner, et al., in 1991 [23], reported their experience with 234 consecutive men with invasive bladder cancer who required cystectomy; 119 chose lower urinary tract reconstruction with means of bilateral ureteroileal urethrostomy, six underwent urethrectomy with Kock pouch cutaneous diversion because of involvement of the prostatic urethra, 87 chose a Koch pouch continent urinary diversion, 22 had an ileal conduit; three underwent lower urinary tract reconstruction by conversion of an ileal conduit (2) or as an alternative to revision of an existing Kock cutaneous pouch (1). Four patients underwent lower urinary tract reconstruction at cystoprostatectomy for benign disease (intestinal cystitis, bladder fibrosis). The current method used by Skinner, et al. for lower urinary tract reconstruction after radical cystectomy using a Kock ileal reservoir with bilateral ureteroileal urethrostomy is shown in (Fig. 21.5). The end of the suture line closing the reservoir is anastomosed directly to the urethra because it also is in the antimesenteric portion. That is the most mobile part of the reservoir and will reach without tension. The suture line closing

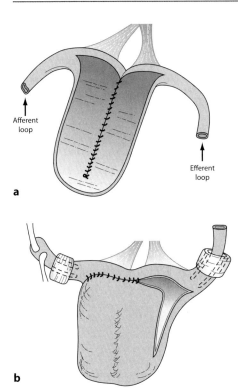

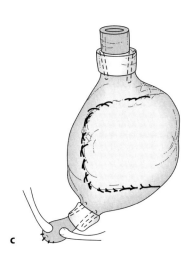

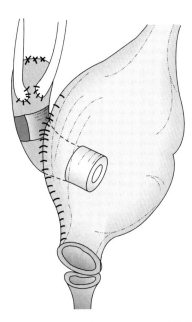

Fig. 21.5 Kock ileal reservoir with bilateral ureteroileal anastomosis and anastomosing of the pouch to the urethra. Reconstructive surgery.

Fig. 21.4 a–c (Opposite) Kock pouch. (**a**) Long segment of ileum doubled to create a large pouch with free ends. (**b**) Afferent and efferent loops are intussuscepted to create a nipple and the ileal loop is constructed into a pouch. (**c**) Kock pouch on afferent and efferent loops to stabilize the nipple.

the reservoir is placed anteriorly under the pubis away from rectal wall.

Bilateral ureteroileal urethrostomy using a Kock ileal reservoir has achieved extraordinary results in terms of patient acceptance, minimal complications, and a low rate of reoperation.

21.7.1.3 Indiana Pouch

The concept of using a continent ileocecal segment is based on the Gilchrist-Merricks procedure [24].

In Gilchrist, et al.'s description of the technique, they use the cecum as a reservoir and the ureters are reimplanted submucosally in an antireflux fashion. Continence is based on the natural antireflux mechanism of the ileocecal valve, antiperistatic action of the terminal ileum and tunneling of the ileum through the abdominal wall in an oblique manner. The technique of Indiana pouch formation started in 1983. The ileocecal segment is marked for pouch reconstruction (Fig. 21.6a,b) using approximately 25 cm of colon and about a 10-cm segment of the ileum from the ileocecal valve. The colon and the ileum are divided and bowel continuity is restored (ileocolostomy). The isolated ileocecal segment on its vascular pedicle is irrigated; the colon is opened on its antimesenteric border down to the cecum; the terminal ileum is tapered and ileocecal valve plicated. Tightening of the ileocecal valve is accomplished around a size 12 French catheter. Tapering is done either with closely inserted silk sutures or with staples [25]. Stapling should be stopped short of the ileocecal valve. Plicating of the terminal ileum is performed at the ileocecal junction. The plication extends to include cecum to tighten the valve to increase the outflow resistance. The ureters are tunneled in the

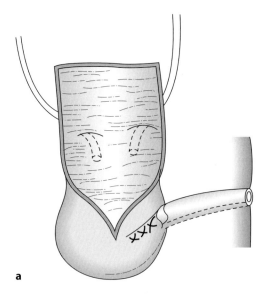

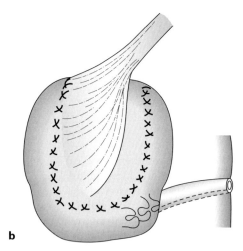

Fig. 21.6 a, b Indiana pouch. (**a**) Ileocecal segment, ureters reimplanted with submucosal tunnel tapering of terminal ileum and plication of ileocecal valve and cecum. (**b**) Indiana pouch completed.

submucosa of the cecum and are stented, before closure of the pouch. The open right colon is folded over and closed transversely; a cecostomy tube is left in situ through the intact cecal wall. The stoma is placed in the lower abdominal wall.

21.7.1.4 Mainz Pouch

The Mainz pouch (mixed augmentation ileum and cecum) for bladder augmentation and continent urinary diversion was described in 1985 [26].

The ileocaecal segments have been used in the Mainz pouch technique for bladder augmentation or orthotopic bladder substitution in the bladder neck or to the urethra. The Mainz pouch provides a low-pressure reservoir with good capacity. The ureters are implanted in the colonic segment in an antireflux fashion. Continence is achieved by intussusception of the nontabularized ileal segment; the intussuscepted part is stabilized by fixing staples and the stoma is situated on the skin (Fig. 21.7a,b).

21.7.1.5 Mitrofanoff Continent Diversion

Mitrofanoff described the use of the appendix as a continent vesicostomy for self-catheterization in 1980 [27]. The Mitrofanoff principle is considered as the best outlet and control mechanism if the urethra is not available regardless of the type of reservoir. Duckett and Schneider described the construction of Pinn's pouch utilizing an ileocecal segment and appendix stoma [28].

The ileocecal segment is selected on its vascular pedicle and detubularized to form a reservoir; ureters are implanted in antireflux fashion. The appendix is mobilized on its artery (a branch of the ileocolic artery), and detached from the cecal wall with a cuff of 3–4 cm which could be used to lengthen the appendix if required.

The appendix is then reversed and the tip is implanted in the cecal wall in a submucosal tunnel and the cecal end of the appendix is sutured to the skin. The appendix conduit is tunneled obliquely through the abdominal wall to make the tract straight and easy to catheterize (Fig. 21.8).

21.7.1.6 Right Colon as a Continent Reservoir

Creating a continent reservoir using the right colon has been used at Lund University Hospital, Sweden, since 1987 [29]. Detubularization of the right colonic segment is performed and the intussuscepted ileal nipple is stapled to maintain continence, anchoring the base of the nipple to the anterior rectus sheath. The ileum is divided 15 cm from the ileocecal valve and transverse colon between the right and middle colic artery. The colonic segment is opened along the anterior tinea down to the ileocecal valve. The distal ileum is intussuscepted into the colon through the ileocecal valve forming a 5-cm-long nipple. A fascial sling is sutured around the end of the ileum and to the anterior rectal sheath; the stoma is situated flush with the skin (Fig. 21.9).

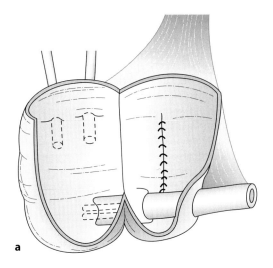

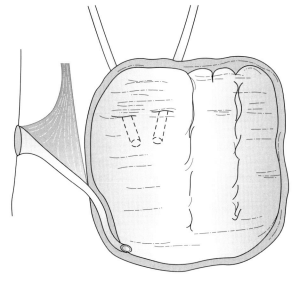

Fig. 21.8 Mitrofanoff diversion (Pinn's pouch with an appendix stoma).

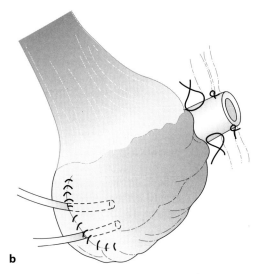

Fig. 21.7 a–b Mainz pouch. (**a**) End to end ileo-ascendostomy is completed. The separated loop of 20-cm ileum is folded into a U-shape and opened along its antimesenteric border. (**b**) The posterior wall of the pouch is completed by side-to-side anastomosis of the colon with the opened ileum.

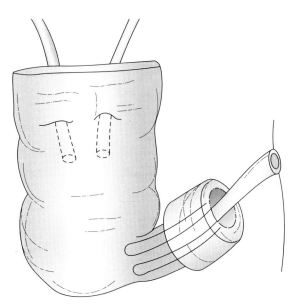

Fig. 21.9 Right colon (Lund reservoir). Intussuscepted ileum through ileocecal valve to form a nipple and a facial sling around end of ileum.

21.7.1.7 The Florida Pouch

A continent reservoir is created using an extended right colon segment isolated with right colic and ileo-colic arteries [30]. The end of the transected transverse colon is folded and shaped as an inverted U and de-tubularization is performed. Both ureters are isolated.

The left ureter is brought behind the mesosigmoid to the right side of the colon segment to prevent ureteric obstruction. A direct mucosa to mucosa anastamosis is performed and both ureters are stented. Bowel plication is performed to achieve continence with interrupted nonabsorbable sutures placed along the ileum, across the ileocecal valve and on to the cecal wall. A second row of plicating sutures are placed 180° from the first row (Fig. 21.10a,b). A flat stoma is sutured to the skin. The advantages of this technique are its simplicity, a decreased incidence of ureteral obstruction, and an acceptable morbidity and complication rate. Postoperative care:

1. Regular 8-hourly irrigation of the pouch is performed to avoid blockage of the catheter with mucous.
2. A "pouchogram" and retrograde "stentogram" is done to check for urine leak on the 8th–10th postoperative day. If there is no leakage the stents are removed.
3. Intermittent catheterization of the reservoir after 2 weeks. Then the cecostomy tube is removed and 3-hourly catheterization is continued.

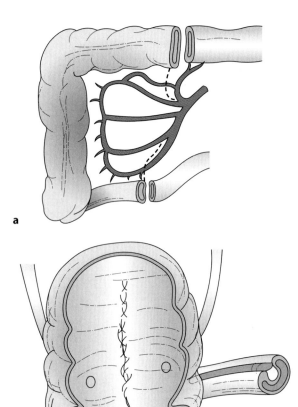

Fig. 21.10 a, b Florida pouch. (**a**) Diagram of extended right colonic segment including cecum, ascending colon and transverse colon based on the right colic and ileocecal arteries. (**b**) The distal end of the bowel is mobilized as an inverted U and the two limbs are detubularized; the posterior wall is sutured, ureteric anastomosis is undertaken without a submocosal tunnel and plication of the ileum.

21.7.2 Bladder Augmentation

Children with rhabdomyosarcoma of the bladder who undergo partial cystectomy sparing the bladder neck and sphincter may require enlargement of the bladder to increase its capacity. At the time of bladder augmentation the child should be free of neoplastic disease locally and systemically. Similarly, children with a fibrosed contracted bladder resulting from treatment (i.e., radiation) will also benefit from bladder augmentation. Following bladder augmentation, intermittent catheterization per urethra may be necessary and the child and his parents should be aware of the risks and complications related to augmentation and taught how to safely catheterize the new bladder.

Various segments of intestinal loops have been used for bladder augmentation (ileum, cecum, ileocecum, sigmoid, etc.). The segment should be long enough to ensure adequate capacity.

In cases where electrolyte absorption may become a problem (particularly in children with irradiated bowel or renal impairment) the stomach may be preferable. The urethra and bladder neck are visualized endoscopically to ensure that the continence mechanism is intact and the rest of the bladder is free from tumor recurrence.

21.7.2.1 Ileocecocystoplasty

Select 20–25 cm of distal ileum starting 10–15 cm from the ileocecal valve. Mark the center and the two free ends of the loop and ensure that the center of the loop will reach the bladder. Divide the ileal loop along its antimesenteric border, suture the medial edges of the divided ileal loop with a continuous 3.0 chronic catgut or vicryl sutures. Fold the open end of the segment over itself and suture each margin to form a cup. Dissect the bladder and elevate it into the wound. Divide the bladder sagittally or coronally, identifying ureteric orifices and insert a feeding tube into each opening. Insert a malecot catheter through the bladder wall and not through the bowel wall. Suture the posterior part of ileal loop to the posterior part of the bladder, using interrupted 3.0 absorbable sutures starting posteriorly through all layers (Fig. 21.11 a–d). An ileocecal segment can be used to provide a large reservoir. The segment is selected on its vascular pedicle and detubularized. The ureters may be reimplanted into the ascending colon with a submucosal tunnel or may be preserved in the trigone. The posterior wall of the ileocolic segment is anastomosed to the posterior wall of the bladder (Fig. 21.12).

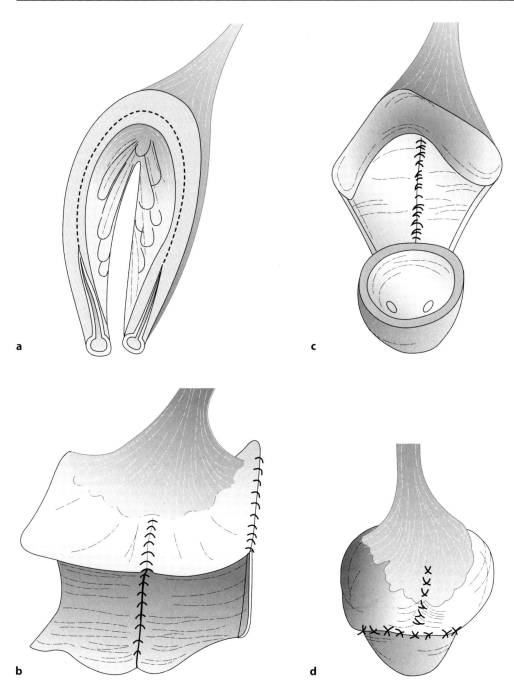

Fig. 21.11 a–d Ileocystoplasty. (**a**) Ileal segment selected on its vascular pedicle. (**b**) Ileal segment completely detubularized. (**c**) Posterior layer of the ileal segment anastomosed to posterior wall of bladder. (**d**) Ileocystoplasty completed.

21.7.2.2 Sigmoidocystoplasty

Sigmoidocystoplasty is an alternative to the use of ascending colon. Select 25 cm of the lower mobile part of the sigmoid colon. Make sure that the segment will reach the bladder without tension then divide the segment and re-establish end-to-end colonic continuity in two layers. Open the chosen sigmoid segment along its antimesenteric border. Leave the proximal few centimeters free for anastomosis of the ureters. Fashion the segment into an S shape and suture the adjacent edges with continuous 3.0 polyglactin sutures. Incise the bladder sagittally as far posteriorly as the trigone and anteriorly to near the bladder neck. Anastomose the sigmoid segment starting posteriorly; all layers are included in the anastomosis using either running or in-

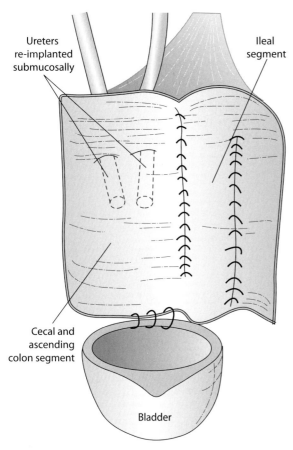

Ureters re-implanted submucosally

Ileal segment

Cecal and ascending colon segment

Bladder

Fig. 21.12 Ileocecocystoplasty. The ileocecal segment is detubularized. The ureters are reimplanted with submucosal tunel. The ileocecal segment is anastomosed to the bladder.

terrupted 3.0 absorbable sutures. Insert ureteric stents and a malecot catheter for urine drainage through the bladder wall (Fig. 21.13a–c).

21.7.2.3 Gastrocystoplasty

The use of gastric segment for bladder augmentation has allowed enlargement of bladder in patients with a short length of bowel due to previous resection – or in children who had pelvic irradiation. The gastric segment will act as a chloride pump and prevent electrolyte disturbances; however, hematuria and dysuria may be complicating symptoms. A wedge gastric cystoplasty is performed using a large wedge of fundus of the stomach based on the right gastroepiploic artery (Fig. 21.14a–c).

The stomach defect is repaired in two layers. The excised wedge graft is brought to the pelvis and is opened to form a flap that is sutured to the bladder. There are some concerns about the development of

malignancy as a potential long-term complication of bowel segment or substitution cystoplasty for bladder augmentation. Colon or small intestine cancer can arise adjacent to the enterovesical anastomosis.

In 1997 Barrington, et al. [31] described four cases of malignancy following augmentation cystoplasty; three were adenocarcinomas of the bladder remnant adjacent to the anastomosis associated with cystitis cystica, dysplasia, and glandular metaplasia. The fourth patient had widespread carcinoma in situ. These observations suggest that all patients with entero or gastrocystoplasties should have regular cystoscopic surveillance.

21.7.2.4 Conversion of an Ileal Conduit to Continent Diversion

In patients who had an ileal conduit diversion at the time of primary excision of bladder tumor and who may wish to achieve urinary continence, a continent diversion can be fashioned [32]. The ileal loop stoma is disconnected from the skin, an intestinal pouch is formed and the ileal loop is anastomosed to it with its attached ureters. A continent stoma is fashioned by using either the appendix or creation of valve mechanism as described (Fig. 21.15).

21.7.2.5 Problems with Bladder Augmentation Using Intestinal Segment

Patient selection is important to ensure that the child will cope with intermittent self-catheterization if necessary. The augmented bladder may take a few months before it stretches. The use of anticholinergic drugs may be required during this period as it may reduce the frequency of catheterization until stretching has occurred. Bladder dysfunction may lead to upper renal tract damage and incontinence. This could be avoided with adequate augmentation and in patients with detrusor muscle instability improvement can be achieved with pharmacologic manipulation. Urinary infection and bacteriuria are commonly observed. Urinary tract infection should be treated promptly and long-term antibiotic therapy may be necessary. Children with vesico-ureteric reflux should have their reflux corrected during the procedure of augmentation. Reflux of infected urine in the augmented bladder will result in recurrent pyelonephritis and back pressure problems

Deterioration of renal function may occur as a result of complication of bladder augmentation using bowel segment. Regular assessment of renal function and treatment of complications are necessary.

Wound infections may occur after use of bowel segment. This is more common when the colon is used

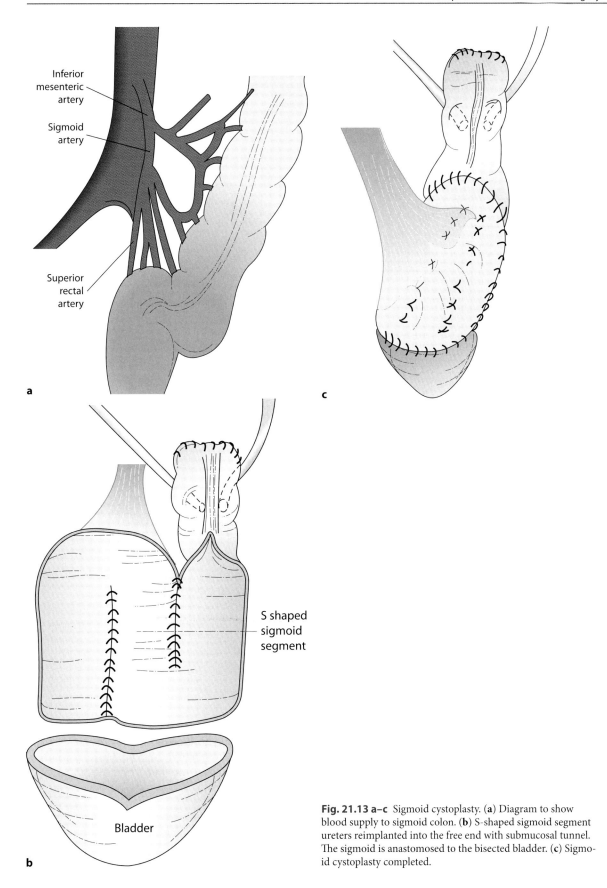

a

b

c

S shaped
sigmoid
segment

Bladder

Fig. 21.13 a–c Sigmoid cystoplasty. (**a**) Diagram to show
blood supply to sigmoid colon. (**b**) S-shaped sigmoid segment
ureters reimplanted into the free end with submucosal tunnel.
The sigmoid is anastomosed to the bisected bladder. (**c**) Sigmoid cystoplasty completed.

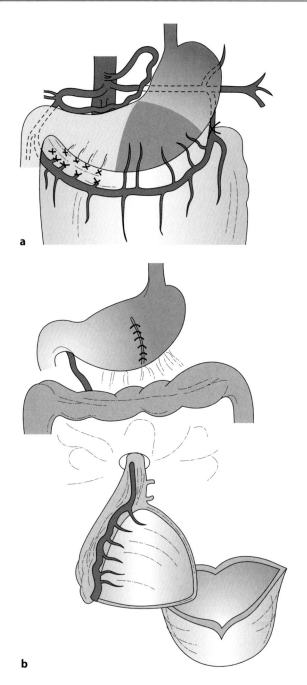

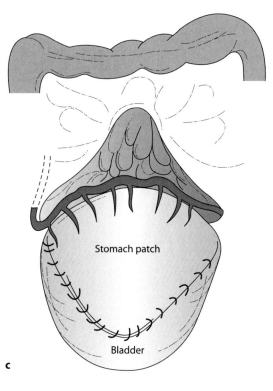

Fig. 21.14 a–c Gastroplasty. (**a**) Blood supply to stomach (wedge is based on right gastroepiploic artery). (**b**) Stomach wedge with its blood supply is drawn through mesocolon to reach the bladder. (**c**) Gastroplasty completed.

as the bowel segment. This complication may be prevented by a good preoperative bowel preparation and perioperative antibiotic administration, insertion of pelvic drains, use of absorbable suture materials and avoidance of tube insertion through the bowel wall. A problem with bladder evacuation is a common complication after augmentation cystoplasty because of unsustained peristaltic contractions during voiding. This can be resolved with intermittent catheterization.

Mucous production could be a problem especially in the early postoperative period. Mucous production decreases with time, but irrigation of the augmented bladder with saline postoperatively may be necessary.

Regarding absorption of electrolytes: an increase in chloride and hydrogen ions may affect the bone buffer and lead to calculus formation.

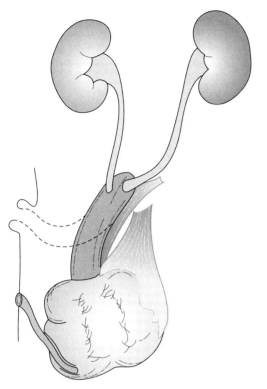

Fig. 21.15 Ileal loop diversion is undone and anastomosed to a Pinn's pouch with an appendix stoma.

21.7.3 Total Bladder Replacement

Total bladder replacement can be performed with one of the common continent intestinal reservoirs (Kock pouch, Indiana pouch, sigmoid colon, detubularized ileum). In cases where the pouch can be anastomosed to the patient's urethra, a hole is made at the bottom of the pouch, a catheter is inserted through the urethra into the pouch, and the base of the pouch is sutured to the posterior urethra (Fig. 21.16 a,b) [33, 34].

Radical cystoprostatectomy represents the most common form of curative treatment for invasive bladder cancer. As a result a urinary reservoir must be created when the urethra can be preserved. Creation of an orthotopic neobladder provides the best functional result. Grosset, et al. in 1998 described the formation of a detubularized sigmoid neobladder with simplified neovesico-urethral anastomosis (Fig. 21.17) [35]. The technique was used in 15 patients with invasive bladder cancer. The urinary reservoir was constructed using the sigmoid colon. Both ureters were reimplanted within a submucosal tunnel and anastomosed to the lowermost part of the pouch anteriorly. The ureters are stented and the pouch drained transurethrally.

The sigmoid neobladder provides good functional results and allows adequate capacity and continence.

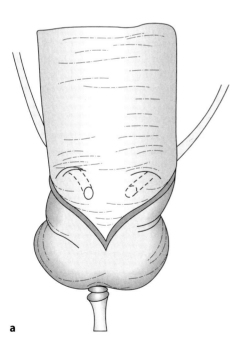

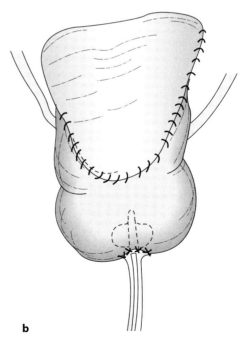

a

b

Fig. 21.16 a, b Total bladder replacement. (**a**) Bladder replacement using right colon. The segment is opened, ileal stump and appendix resected, ureter reimplanted with submucosal tunnel.

A hole is created at the bottom of cecum anastomosing the neobladder to the urethra. (**b**) Right colon bladder replacement completed with indwelling Foley catheter draining the pouch.

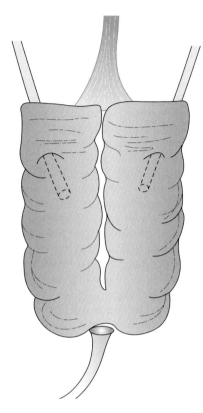

Fig. 21.17 Sigmoid neobladder. Detubularized sigmoid with neobladder urethral anastomosis.

Persistent and occasional nocturnal enuresis in orthotopic urinary diversion: is there a urodynamic difference?

Fifty enuretic men at least 1 year after a radical cystoprostatectomy and ileal neobladder were studied to establish urodynamic criteria differentiating between men with a radical prostatectomy and ileal neobladder who are persistently enuretic and those who are occasionally enuretic. It was concluded that enuretic men had significantly higher residual urine volumes and enterocystometric pressure variables than continent men; also, they had significantly lower flow rates and less urethral resistance.

Pharmacological inhibition of reservoir contraction and/or management of residual urine by clean intermittent catheterization before sleep might cure enuresis [36].

A symptomatic bacteriuria in men with orthotopic ileal neobladders: possible relationship to nocturnal enuresis.

Forty-seven patients with uncomplicated orthotopic ileal neobladders were prospectively studied and it was found that ileal neobladders are associated with a high incidence of a symptomatic bacteriuria during the first year after surgery, spontaneous clearance of bacteriuria with time with no antimicrobial manipula-

tion. There was a significant association between bacteriuria and nocturnal enuresis [37].

21.8 Vaginal Reconstruction

Vaginal reconstruction is required in patients who have had their vagina removed after treatment of pelvic malignancy arising either from the vagina or uterus or bladder infiltrating the vagina.

The use of a bowel segment to replace the vagina has been described. The sigmoid colon has been used but the cecum and ascending colon is favored by some surgeons because of the ease of bringing this segment into the pelvis for anastomosis to the perineum and the reliability of a good blood supply in anastomosing the ileum to the remaining colon to restore bowel continuity. The colocecum is inverted to create a neovagina; lengthening of the inverted segment is achieved by an antimesenteric incision and closure of the mesenteric border. The use of the colocecum produces a good functional result [38].

An abdominoperineal combined approach with a midline or a suprapubic incision is employed. Urethral catheters are inserted. A tunnel is created in the lower portion of the perineum between the bladder and rectum. The greater omentum is mobilized to be utilized later as a pedicle patch to prevent fistula formation and protect the anastomosis. The cecum and ascending colon are mobilized on an ileocolic pedicle. The colon is divided once a segment sufficient to be brought down to the perineum is established. Intestinal continuity is restored by an ileocolic anastomosis. Either the distal or proximal colocecum can be anastomosed to vaginal cuff or perineal skin. The free end is oversewn in two layers, and the appendix removed. The cecum is incised to create an opening of adequate size (Fig. 21.18a–c).

The use of cecum and ascending colon has been advocated for reconstruction of the vagina because of the ease of bringing the cecum down to the perineum and the reliability of the ileocolonic anastomosis that has a lower incidence of vascular compromise or anastomatic leak. The technique gives a good functional and cosmetic result with a lower incidence of late neovaginal orifice stenosis, and mucous production is rarely a problem.

21.8.1 Vaginal Reconstruction Using the Sigmoid Colon

The sigmoid colon segment is selected on its vasculare pedicle (based on the left colic or superior hemorrhoidal artery) close the proximal end of the segment in two layers bringing the distal end to the perineum.

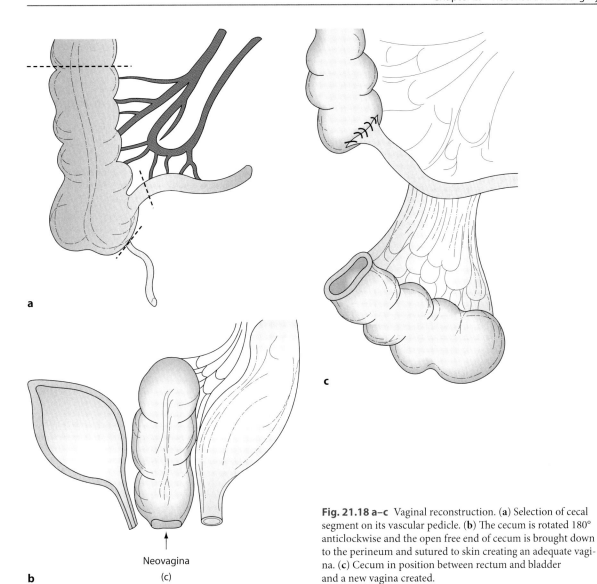

Fig. 21.18 a–c Vaginal reconstruction. (**a**) Selection of cecal segment on its vascular pedicle. (**b**) The cecum is rotated 180° anticlockwise and the open free end of cecum is brought down to the perineum and sutured to skin creating an adequate vagina. (**c**) Cecum in position between rectum and bladder and a new vagina created.

References

1. Asato H, Harii K, Yamada A, et al. (1993) Eye socket reconstruction with free flap. Plast Reconst Surg 92:1061–1067

2. Marques A, Brenda E, Magrin J, et al. (1992) Critical analysis of methods of reconstruction of the exenterated orbits. Brit J Plast Surg 45:523–528

3. Maves MD, Lusk, RP (1987) Tissue expansion in the treatment of giant congenital milanocytic naevi. Arch Otolaryngol Head Neck Surg 133:987–991

4. National Institute of Health Consensus Development Conference Statement, Oct 24–26, 1983 (1984) Precursors to malignant melanoma. J Am Acad Dermatol 10:683–688

5. Rigel DS, Friedman RJ (1985) The management of patients with dysplastic and congenital naevi. Dermatol Clin 3:251–255

6. Maves MD, Rodney P, Lusk MD (1987) Tissue expansion in the treatment of giant congenital melanocytic naevi. Arch Otolaryngol Head Neck Surg 113:987–991

7. Chapelier A, Macchiarini P, Rietjents M, et al. (1994) Chest wall reconstruction following resection of large primary malignant tumors. Eur J Cardio Thoracic Surg 8:351–356

8. Pairolero PC, Arnold PG (1985) Chest wall tumors. J Thorac Cardiovasc Surg 90:367–372

9. Grosfeld JL, Rescorla FJ, West, KNW, et al. (1988) Chest wall resection and reconstruction for malignant conditions in childhood. J Pediatr Surg 23:667–673

10. Gordon MS, Hajdu SI, Bains MS, et al. (1991) Soft tissue sarcoma of the chest wall – Results of surgical resection. J Surg Cardiovasc Surg 101:843–854

11. Soutar DS, Ray AK (1992) The radical arm flap in neck and head reconstruction. In: Jackson IT, Sommerlad BC (eds) Advances in plastic surgery, vol 4. Churchill Livingstone, Edinburgh, pp.77–91

12. Carachi R, Audry G, Ranke A, et al. (1995) Collagen coated vicryl mesh – A new bioprosthesis in pediatric surgical practice. J Pediatr Surg 30:1302–1305

13. Malangoni MA, Offstein, LC, Grosfeld JL, et al. (1980) Survival and pulmonary function following chest wall resection and reconstruction in children. J Pediatr Surg 15:906–912

14. Green GM, Jaffe N (1978) Progress and controversy in the treatment of childhood rhabdomyosarcoma. Cancer Treatment Rev 5:7–27

15. Michalkiewicz EL, Rao BN, Gross E, et al. (1997) Complications of pelvic excentration in children who have genitourinary rhabdomyosarcoma. J Pediatr Surg 32:1277–1282

16. Hayes GM, Lawrence W Jr, Crist WM, et al. (1990) Partial cystectomy in the management of rhabdomyosarcoma of the bladder – A report of the intergroup rhabdomyosarcoma study. J Pediatr Surg 25:719–723

17. Silvan AMA, Gordillo MJO, Lopez AM, et al. (1997) Organ preserving management of rhabdomyosarcoma of the prostate and bladder in children. Med Pediatr Oncol 29:573–575

18. Lepor H, Cregerman M, Crosby R, et al. (1985) Precise localisation of the autonomic nerves from the pelvic plexus to the Corpora Cavernosa – A detailed anatomical study of the adult male pelvis. J Urol 133:207–212

19. Goodwin WE, Harris AP, Kauffmann JJ, et al. (1953) Open transcolonic uretero-intestinal anastomosis – A new approach. Surg Gyn Obstet 97:295–300

20. Miller K, Matsui M, Hautmann R (1990) The augmented functional rectal bladder, first clinical experience. J Urol 143:398A

21. Kock NG, Nilson AE, Nilsson LO, et al. (1982) Urinary diversion via a continent ileal reservoir. Clinical results in 12 cases. J Urol 128:469

22. Skinner DG, Lieskovsky G, Boyd S (1988) Continent urinary diversion, a five and a half year experience. Ann Surg 208:337–344

23. Skinner DG (1991) Lower urinary tract reconstruction following cystectomy: Experience and results in 126 patients using the Kock ilial reservoir with bilateral ureteroileal urethrostomy. J Urol 146:756–760

24. Gilchrist RK, Merricks JW, Hamlin HH, et al. (1950) Construction of a substitute of bladder and urethra. Surg Gyn Obstet 90:752–760

25. Bejany DE, Politano VA (1988) Stapled and non-stapled tapered distal ileum for construction of continent colonic urinary reservoir. J Urol 140:491

26. Thuroff JW, Alken P, Riedmiller H, et al. (2006) The Mainz pouch (mixed augmentation ileum 'n zecum) for bladder augmentation and continent urinary diversion. Eur Urol 50(6):1142–1150

27. Mitroffanof P (1980) Cystostomic continent trans-appendiculaire dans le traitment des vessies neurologiques. Chir Pediatr 21:297–305

28. Duckett JW, Schneider HM (1986) Continent urinary diversion: Variations on the Mitroffanof principle. J Urol 136:58–62

29. Mansson W, Colleen S (1990) Experience with a detubularised right colon segment for bladder replacement canal. J Urol Nephrol 24:53

30. Lockhart JL, Powsang J, Persky L, et al. (1990) A continent colonic urinary reservoir: The Florida Pouch. J Urol 144:864

31. Barrington JW, Fulford S, Griffiths D, Stephenson TP (1997) Tumors in bladder remnant after augmentation enterocystoplasty. J Urol 157:482–485

32. Bihrel R, Foster RS (1991) Continent ileocecal reservoir: the Indiana pouch. In: King LR, Stone AR, Webster GD (eds) Bladder Reconstruction and Continent Urinary Diversion. Mosby, Chicago, pp 308–315

33. Goldwasser B, Webster GD (1985) Continent urinary diversion. J Urol 134:227–236

34. Reddy PK, Lange PH, Fraley EE (1987) Bladder replacement after cystoprostatectomy, efforts to achieve total continence. J Urol 138:495–499

35. Grosset D, Delbos O, Muir GH, et al. (1998) Orthotopic bladder substitution by detubularised sigmoid using a new method of neovesico-urethral anastomosis. Brit J Urol 81:623–627

36. El-Bahnasawy MS, Osman, Y, Gamha MA, et al. (2005) Persistent and occasional nocturnal enuresis in orthotopic urinary diversion: Is there a urodynamic difference? BJU Int 96:137–177

37. Abdel-Latif M, Mosbah A, El-Bahnasaway MS, et al. (2005) Asymptomatic bacteriuria in men with orthotopic ileal neobladders: Possible relationship to nocturnal enuresis. BJU Int 96:391–396

38. Christmas TJ, Hendry WF, Shepherd JH (1991) Anterior pelvic exentration for locally advanced cervical carcinoma with reconstructive of the bladder and vagina using contiguous segment of ileum, caecum and ascending colon. Int Urogynaecol 2:183

Surgical Complications of Childhood Tumors

22

G. Suren Arul, Richard D. Spicer

Contents

22.1 Rare Surgical Presentations of Cancer in Childhood

Most childhood tumors will first present to a physician; some tumors will present in an atypical manner and may mimic a surgical condition. The diagnosis may be missed if the surgeon is not aware of the possibility of cancer. A very great number of rare presentations of childhood cancer have been described in the literature. It is important that the surgeon who is not experienced in the management of childhood cancer is aware that an apparently benign condition could be a manifestation of an underlying malignancy [71, 83] (Table 22.1).

22.2 Soft Tissue Complications

Soft tissue problems are a common cause for surgical consultation on the oncology ward. Immunosuppression, steroid-induced skin changes, and prolonged immobilization all contribute to skin infections. These may start as simple localized infections, which may quickly spread into life-threatening problems. Although the conditions outlined below are all related, they do have significant differences, which are reflected

Table 22.1 Surgical presentation of tumors

Presentation	Neoplastic cause	Ref
Acute abdominal pain	Ruptured Wilms' tumor	[42]
	Ruptured liver tumor	
	Appendicular carcinoid, lymphoma	
Intussusception	Hemangioma	[12, 14]
	Ganglioneurofibroma	[96]
	Lymphoma	[26, 115]
Intestinal obstruction	Leiomyoma	[109]
	Esophageal leiomyoma	[11]
	Intestinal fibromatosis	[17]
	Lymphoma	
Gastrointestinal bleeding	Gastric teratoma	[47]
	Typhlitis	[48]
Perianal abscess	Yolk sac tumors	
	Rhabdomyosarcoma	
Biliary obstruction	Hemangioendothelioma	[106]
	Rhabdomyosarcoma	[16]
Hydronephrosis	Neuroblastoma and other pelvic tumors	[40]
Testicular swelling	Primary tumor	
	Leukemia	[85]
	Lymphoma	
Varicocele	Wilms' tumor	7
Bronchiectasis	Carcinoid	[118]
Priapism and clitoral engorgement	Congenital myeloid leukemia	

in their varying management. Careful clinical diagnosis in conjunction with relevant microbiological, hematological, and biochemical findings is essential.

22.2.1 Cellulitis

Usually soft tissue problems involve no more than simple local infections. However, as these children are often immunosuppressed, a localized infection can quickly spread to a life-threatening cellulitis. Any areas of erythema should be treated suspiciously with swabs of the area and blood cultures being sent. Antibiotics should be employed early in a suspected infection.

Proven cellulitis should be managed by marking the area of erythema so that any progress can be monitored. Intravenous antibiotics are mandatory and should be prescribed after discussion with the infectious disease specialists.

22.2.2 Superficial Abscesses

Conditions such as paronychia and superficial skin abscesses in the groin or axilla are relatively common. In patients with a normal neutrophil count the treatment of choice is incision and drainage of the area of maximum fluctuation. In the cases of neutropenic patients most abscesses will not contain pus but watery fluid containing no neutrophils. These instances are best treated with antibiotics and granulocyte stimulating factor; any areas of fluctuation can be aspirated with a fine needle to provide fluid for culture and sensitivity testing often without the need for incision and drainage.

22.2.3 Radiation Necrosis

Children receiving radiotherapy may develop extensive erythema of the skin and skin necrosis. This was seen more commonly in treatment protocols that advocated large doses of radiation therapy to superficial areas in the body. This is no longer the case with current protocols (Fig. 22.1).

22.2.4 Necrotizing Fasciitis

Established cellulitis may progress to necrotizing fasciitis. The common forms of this disease are either

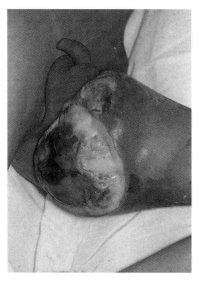

Fig. 22.1 Skin necrosis after chemotherapy and radiotherapy to shrink a rhabdomyosarcoma of the thigh.

caused by group A streptococcus or a mixed flora of anaerobic and aerobic bacteria. This later condition is known as Fournier's gangrene if it occurs around the perineum or Meleney's gangrene if it occurs on the abdominal wall (often associated with a recent operation wound).

In this condition the patient is toxic and complains of severe localized pain. The affected area often has a necrotic appearance from the underlying ischemia. Crepitus may be detected on examination. The diagnosis is made clinically. Once diagnosis is established the treatment is broad spectrum antibiotics (aminoglycoside, penicillin, and metronidazole), intravenous fluid resuscitation, and extensive surgical debridement. Numerous debridements are often required, the defect being closed at a later stage with tissue flaps or skin grafts [94, 99].

Neutropenic patients are at particular risk of developing a pseudomonas fasciitis known as ecthyma gangrenosum (Fig. 22.2) [6, 10, 31, 90]. The patient develops black necrotic ulcers on the buttocks and perineal region. These are initially small but without treatment will spread and coalesce. Unlike necrotizing fasciitis, the treatment is primarily medical with an antibiotic regime including aminoglycoside with an antipseudomonal cephalosporin or penicillin; granulocyte colony stimulating factor (GCSF) may help to revive the neutrophil count [4]. Close observation must be kept on the patient. If large necrotic areas develop then late surgical debridement may be required. Occasionally a diverting colostomy may be necessary.

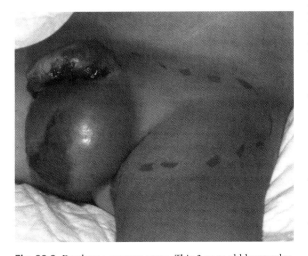

Fig. 22.2 Ecythema gangrenosum. This 3-year-old boy undergoing treatment of acute lymphoblastic leukemia became profoundly neutropenic 10 days after receiving chemotherapy. He developed a pyrexia and a hot erythematous penis and scrotum with areas of necrosis. Blood cultures and swabs of the area grew Pseudomonas aeruginosa. He was treated with antibiotics and G-CSF and recovered fully without the need for surgical intervention.

22.2.5 Compartment Syndrome

Compartment syndrome is a rare problem in childhood and so is often overlooked till a late stage. It can develop in the presence of severe septicemia and shock, particularly after pseudomonas septicemia in the neutropenic patient. In our experience a septic child may complain of lower limb pain; however, as the child is so systematically unwell this can be overlooked. On examination the foot is plantar flexed with tight lower leg muscle compartments. There may be reduced skin sensation over the foot or parasthesia. The pathognomonic sign is extreme pain on the slightest attempt to actively or passively move the foot. Loss of pedal pulses is a late finding. The differential diagnosis is deep vein thrombosis, lower limb cellulitis, or an ischemic arterial problem. The diagnosis is a clinical one; checking compartment pressures and Doppler ultrasound studies can be misleading [78].

Despite the fact that these children are severely ill, surgical decompression under general anesthetic should be performed urgently. All four compartments should be opened right down over the ankle using a medial and lateral incision. The sooner this is done the better the chances of saving the muscles. Though muscle compartments expand markedly after release, use of a loose subdermal tacking suture allows apposition of the wound edge without increasing the compartment pressures. This reduces the need for skin grafting and thus gives a much better cosmetic result. Hemostasis with bipolar diathermy must be done scrupulously as bleeding is a major problem postoperatively. Numerous debridements of dead muscle may be required, although this should be left until demarcation has occurred. Delayed primary closure, tissue flaps, or skin graft may be used subsequently.

22.3 Thoracic Complications

Surgeons may be consulted by oncologists for advice and surgical intervention in children with thoracic complications. The most common request is for biopsying of suspicious lesions on a chest radiograph following treatment – the usual histological finding is of a benign lung scar; however, diffuse fibrosis secondary to chemoradiotherapy, recurrence of tumor, or fungal lesion are other important diagnoses. In addition, surgical consultation may be required to help with management of pleural effusions or severe hemoptysis. Other complications that may arise from thoracic structures involved with tumor, or from iatrogenic procedures, e.g., central lines, biopsy, or thoracoscopy or mediastinoscopy include the following.

22.3.1 Superior Vena Caval Syndrome

The patient is unduly distressed following a procedure on the neck, e.g., after insertion of a central venous catheter or a biopsy. There is venous congestion of the face and neck with distended neck veins and petechial hemorrhage. Color Doppler ultrasound is useful to detect thrombosis in the great veins of the neck. Angiography via the catheter may demonstrate thrombus in the superior vena cava. Assessment at a low-radiation dose, 64-slice CT angiography has been helpful in diagnosing this condition [119]. Rarely, surgical intervention is indicated and most can be managed by supportive measures alone including heparin administration and removal of the central line from this location.

22.3.2 Superior Mediastinal Syndrome

This syndrome results in tracheal compression from trauma, biopsy of tumor (e.g., lymphoma of the mediastinum), or after thoracomediastinoscopy. Rapid intubation and treatment with antibiotics is indicated until the syndrome subsides. Rarely, a tracheostomy is indicated if this syndrome develops rapidly and unsuspected.

22.3.3 Pneumomediastinum, Pneumopericardium, and Surgical Emphysema

The "Michelin man" can be a complication after thoracoscopy from damage to the lung or the airway. This can be treated with antibiotics and a chest drain if a tension pneumothorax results. In rare instances this can occur as a complication of high-pressure ventilation therapy with dissection of air into their interstitial spaces.

22.3.4 Cardiac Tamponade

Cardiac tamponade may result after insertion of a central venous line and needs early recognition. Pericardiac drainage and replacement of a central line is needed.

22.3.5 Pleurodesis

Large malignant pleural effusions may cause respiratory embarrassment. If they do not settle with the treatment of the underlying disease they may require pleurodesis. Very little information has been published concerning children with malignant effusions; most pleurodesis has been undertaken for congenital lymphatic problems (chylothorax) or recurrent spontaneous pneumothorax.

Walker-Renard, et al. reviewed all the literature on pleurodesis of malignant lesions [112]. They found that response rates varied from 93% with talcum powder to 0% for etoposide. Doxycycline, tetracycline, and bleomycin all had success rates around 60–80%. Bacillus Calmette-Guérin (BCG) vacine, quinacrine, and thioptepa were not assessed because of the lack of published data.

Talcum powder may be inserted into the pleural cavity using insufflation; this technique is best done under general anesthetic with thoracoscopy [121], although it can be inserted as a talcum slurry by tube thoracostomy under local anesthetic. Adult respiratory distress syndrome (ARDS), pulmonary edema, and granulomatous pneumonitis have all been described as complications developing postoperatively.

22.3.6 Fungal Lung Lesions

Opportunistic fungal infections are an important cause of morbidity and mortality in the immunosuppressed child. Fungal infections include those caused by Candida albicans, Aspergillus, zygomycetes Cryptococcus, and Mycobacterium avium [100]. The usual presentation of pulmonary fungal infection is fever, malaise, cough, or chest pain. Other problems which may develop include progressive respiratory distress or life-threatening hemoptysis.

Plain chest radiography may show a cavitating lesion, a mass, or pulmonary infiltrates, followed by computed tomography (CT) scan to more accurately identify the lesion (Fig. 22.3 a,b). Bronchoscopy with bronchioalveolar lavage may demonstrate fungal hyphae. Occasionally, either fine needle aspiration or an open biopsy of the lesion is necessary to achieve a definitive diagnosis. The most frequently identified organism is aspergillus. Treatment begins with appropriate antifungal agents, usually amphotericin B. Removal of the bulk of infected lung tissue improves the chances of eradicating the disease [100].

22.3.7 Complications of Long Lines

The development of tunneled silastic central venous catheters by Broviac and Hickman are among the most important milestones in the progress of pediatric oncology. However, as with all surgical procedures they are not without significant complications if they are not performed with care by an experienced operator.

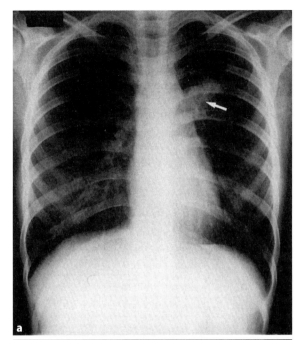

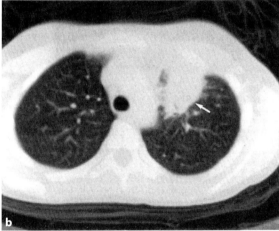

Fig. 22.3 a, b Aspergilloma. This patient, undergoing bone marrow transplantation for a relapsed leukemia, developed an invasive aspergilloma on her left upper lobe bronchus that was gradually eroding into her pulmonary vessels and causing her hemoptysis. Following a lobectomy and removal of the lesion she has made an uneventful recovery. (**a**) Chest x-ray of the patient. (**b**) CT scan of the same patient.

Central venous lines can be placed either percutaneously or at an open operation. Despite the more invasive procedure open placement is required for port insertion and may be actually safer as the vein is carefully identified and hence complications such as accidental puncture of the lung and tearing of the vein are minimized. Most children will require general anesthetic whichever technique is employed. See Chap. 27 [61].

Table 22.2 Complications of central venous catheters

	Complications
Insertion	Hemothorax/hemomediastinum
	– Secondary tearing of the vein
	– Pneumothorax
	– Hematoma secondary to thrombocytopenia
	– Air embolus
	– Cardiac arrhythmias
Usage	Infection
	– Thrombosis of tip/vena cava thrombosis/ atrial thrombus
	– Air embolus
	– Line breakage causing bleeding, introduction of infection and air embolus
	– Dislodgement
Removal	Air embolus
	– Catheter embolus to right side of heart or lungs
	– Dislodgement of septic thrombus

22.3.8 Complications of Catheter Removal

It is important to remember that most operative deaths associated with tunneled catheters occur when they are removed. The reasons for this may be that it is considered a simple procedure often attempted on the ward under local anesthetic or in the anesthetic room by the most junior surgeon. We have heard of three deaths directly attributable to removal of tunneled long lines – in two cases the line was accidentally divided and then embolized, and once a septic thrombus was dislodged; in all three instances a fatal pulmonary embolus resulted. For this reason all our cuffed line removals are done in the operating theater by the following technique. Unless the cuff is readily visible at the exit site a new incision is made proximal to the cuff and the fibrous tissue surrounding the line is dissected free. An incision is made in this fibrous casing in the long axis of the line to reduce the risk of severing the line. The distal part of the line can then be clipped and the line removed while a second person presses firmly over its point of insertion into the vein. The cuff can then be dissected out without risk of damaging the line or causing an air embolus. The incision and exit site are then sutured closed[30].

22.4 Gastrointestinal Complications

22.4.1 Acute Abdominal Pain

22.4.1.1 Overview

The development of the acute abdomen in a child being treated for neoplastic disease often provides the medical and surgical teams caring for that child with a diagnostic and therapeutic dilemma. The cause of the symptoms may be the same as those in a child of similar age without cancer or it may be related to the treatment of cancer. Even simple conditions may be confused by the immunodeficiency, the use of steroids, or cytotoxic drugs and other factors associated with the cancer and/or its treatment. This may lead to localized conditions becoming generalized and the clinical signs of sepsis and inflammation being masked. In addition, the management decisions are complicated by the fact that many of these children are seriously ill at presentation and wound healing may be impaired.

Assessment of the risks of all possible causes is necessary to determine whether a laparotomy is required or if intensive medical treatment is preferable. The present thinking is that both have their place even for the ill child [87], and hence the medical and surgical teams should work closely together in initial assessment and ongoing management.

Table 22.3 shows the likely causes of acute abdominal pain in children with cancer and a suggested structured approach to their treatment. Specific conditions are discussed in detail below.

Table 22.3 Causes of acute abdominal pain in children with cancer

Diagnosis
Neutropenic enterocolitis
Pseudomembranous colitis (Clostridium difficile)
Cytomegalovirus/adenovirus enteritis
Acute graft-versus-host disease
Peptic ulceration (stress or steroids)
Pancreatitis
Hemorrhagic cystitis
Radiation enteritis
Obstruction
Perforation of bowel
Inflammatory cause
Intestinal lymphoma responding to treatment
Rupture of a Wilms' tumor
Hemorrhage into a tumor causing distension
Hepatic tumors
Sudden hepatomegaly stretching liver capsule
Hypercalcemia of malignancy

22.4.1.2 The Role of Diagnostic Imaging

Close cooperation with the radiology department is important for the diagnosis of the acute abdomen in children with cancer. While accurate diagnosis is essential, avoidance of invasive or time-consuming investigations is also important in these seriously ill children. Plain abdominal radiograph may show bowel dilatation, mucosal edema, a space-occupying lesion, free air (outlining the bowel wall), or pneumatosis intestinalis. An erect abdominal radiograph may show free air under the diaphragm though it may be normal in over 10% of bowel perforations; lateral decubitus abdominal radiographs (right side up) may be used in the severely ill patient.

Abdominal ultrasound is an excellent noninvasive method of assessing the bowel for intestinal wall thickness, free fluid, and collections of fluid within the abdomen. Normal colonic wall thickness is ≤2 mm [10]. It can also pick up appendicitis, cholecystitis, and pyelonephritis [39, 76]. Ultrasound examination is relatively inexpensive, avoids ionizing radiation, and can be performed at the bedside. However, it must be remembered that ultrasound is operator-dependent and that excessive bowel gas, especially in the older child, can adversely affect the images; hence a negative scan does not necessarily rule out intra-abdominal pathology.

A CT scan is also noninvasive and requires both intravenous and oral contrast. Restless children will require sedation or general anesthetic for the study. In the immunocompromised patient, CT may demonstrate intra-abdominal abscesses, pseudomembranous colitis, typhlitis, graft-versus-host disease, radiation enteritis, and appendicitis [23, 70].

Contrast studies are beneficial in the relatively well child with chronic symptoms especially for diagnosis of strictures or radiation enteritis [68]. However, care must be taken in patients with colitis because of the risk of bowel perforation [67, 111]; for this reason we prefer to use water-soluble nonionic contrast medium.

22.4.1.3 The Role of Endoscopy

Surgeons are frequently called on to perform either upper or lower gastrointestinal endoscopy on patients with unexplained abdominal symptoms. The number of causes of abdominal pain or bleeding are numerous and, together with judicious use of diagnostic imaging, endoscopy and relevant biopsies may be essential for accurate diagnosis [5, 65, 86, 88].

Obtaining biopsies at endoscopy is not associated with significant sepsis even in severely immunosuppressed patients [49]. Upper gastrointestinal endoscopy can be used to sclerose esophageal varices or inject bleeding ulcers. Careful performance of colonoscopy in patients with viral colitis, typhlitis, and severe graft-versus-host disease is essential in order to avoid overdistension of the colon and reduce the risk of perforation.

22.4.1.4 Assessment of Acute Abdominal Pain in the Child with Malignant Disease

1. Full history with particular reference to the time of onset of pain with regard to other treatments, changes in the neutrophil count and changes in other physiological parameters, i.e., pulse, temperature, blood pressure, respiratory rate.
2. Full examination with special regard to the abdomen looking for focal or generalized tenderness and signs of peritonism. Avoid rectal examination in neutropenic patients if possible.
3. Blood tests to include full blood count, urea, electrolytes, amylase, liver function tests. Clotting studies may reveal disseminated intravascular coagulation. Arterial blood gas sample may show signs of an unexpected metabolic acidosis suggesting ischemia or sepsis. Remember that white cell count, C-reactive protein, and erythrocyte sedimentation rate may all be normal in the presence of immunosuppression.
4. Septic screen to include urine, stool, blood cultures, and sometimes lumbar puncture.
5. Diagnostic imaging – see above.

22.4.1.5 Metabolic Causes of the Acute Abdomen

This usually arises from two main metabolic disorders.
1. Hypercalcemia of malignancy. This can be caused by metastases, osteolytic bone tumors, or humoral factors secreted by endocrine tumors [51], e.g., parathyroid hormone. The symptoms are those of hypercalcemia (weakness, brachycardia, constipation, polyurea, peptic ulceration, and pancreatitis). Fluid resuscitation and pamidonate is of value in the management of acute cancer-related hypercalcemia in children.
2. Tumor lysis syndrome. This was often observed in the treatment of bulky lymphomas following chemotherapy but can occur with any large bulky tumor undergoing necrosis. A rare complication of germ cell tumors and calcium levels should be monitored in all children with solid ovarian masses [62]. The metabolic upset includes hyperuricemia, hyperkalemia, and hyperphosphatemia with hypocalcemia. The patient presents with severe abdominal pain from uric acid crystal crisis, lethargy, and

anuria [1, 9, 123]. Calcification of the gastric mucosa has been reported in association with tumor lysis syndrome in a child with non-Hodgkin lymphoma [8].

The management of such a high-risk patient includes intravenous hydration with at least 2–3 liters/m2 over 24 h using quarter strength saline, 5% dextrose, alkalization of the urine with sodium bicarbonate 100 meq/liter titrating the urine to a ph of 7.0–7.5, drug therapy, allopurinol 300–500 mg/m2 for 3 days to prevent uric acid deposition, and careful monitoring of urine output, ph, urine electrolytes, and urea including calcium and phosphate. Occasionally, dialysis or hemofiltration may be necessary. Recombinant urate oxidase (rasburicase) may be used for prevention and treatment of tumor lysis syndrome in patients with hematological malignancies [114]. Rasburicase is a safe, highly and rapidly effective agent in the treatment and prevention of malignancy-associated acute hyperuricemia and could be considered the treatment of choice to prevent tumor lysis syndrome in children at high risk [79].

22.4.2 Specific Causes of Abdominal Pain

22.4.2.1 Intestinal Obstruction

Vomiting in a child being treated for malignant disease is very common; however, this must be differentiated from the emesis observed in numerous surgical conditions. Obstruction is due to mechanical blockage of the bowel and is common after operation for tumor [84, 98]. Characteristically vomit is bile-stained (green) in mechanical obstruction and in adynamic paralytic ileus. Auscultation is an important denominator. Table 22.4 shows the causes of intestinal obstruction.

It must be noted that sometimes a child presents with obstruction due to abdominal lymphoma. There are two clinical scenarios to be aware of. The first is with localized ileo-cecal disease causing the lead point of an intussusception. In this case localized resection with primary anastomosis is the treatment of choice; biopsy of suspicious mesenteric lymph nodes may also help in staging. If there is diffuse disease then a biopsy alone with intense supportive management is sufficient as the disease will rapidly resolve once chemotherapy is started [14].

22.4.2.2 Radiation Enteritis

Clinical features. Acute systemic upset, with nausea, vomiting, diarrhea, abdominal pain, and gastrointestinal bleeding; commonly complicates radiotherapy to

Table 22.4 Causes of obstruction in relation to the bowel wall

Position of obstructing lesion	Diagnosis
Outside the bowel	Mass effect from large intra-abdominal tumor (compression)
	Postoperative adhesions
In the bowel wall	Primary or secondary tumor within the bowel wall
	Intussusception – after surgery for Wilms' tumor [23], neuroblastoma or other
	Retroperitoneal procedures
	Strictures at an anastomosis, or from radiation enteritis, or enterocolitis
	Paralytic ileus
	Opiate therapy
	Vincristine therapy [Adriamycin (doxorubicin)]
	Anticholinergic effects of medication
	Any of the causes of intestinal inflammation
	Any cause of intraperitoneal sepsis
Within the lumen	Tumor invasion of the lumen

the abdomen and pelvis. Although these acute symptoms usually resolve relatively quickly, about 5% of patients progress to chronic complications after the completion of radiotherapy [35, 68, 117, 120]. Radiation damage to the bowel is dose dependent, although other factors such as previous operations, peritonitis, and concurrent chemotherapy (especially actinomycin-D) may all contribute to worsening the long-term problems [22]. More than one complication may occur and new lesions may develop at later stages; radiation enteritis should, therefore, be considered to be a progressive disease [35]. Complications related to the large bowel include proctocolitis, colorectal and anal strictures, rectal ulcers, spontaneous necrosis, and fistulae to bowel, bladder, or vagina. Small bowel complications include bleeding, adhesions, strictures, malabsorbtion, spontaneous necrosis, fistula, and poor anastomotic healing [117]. Bleeding and fistula or perforation seem to represent the two ends of the spectrum of radiation enteritis suggesting that bleeding represents just mucosal trauma whereas full-thickness bowel wall damage must be present for perforation and fistula formation [35]. Malabsorbtion of fat, vitamin B12, and calcium may also occur [22, 117].

Diagnosis. Diagnosis of the condition can be difficult. A history is important with regard to the time and dosage of radiation. An erect or supine abdominal radiograph may show features of obstruction or perforation. The most important investigations are contrast radiographs, and either small bowel studies or large bowel enemas. Radiological signs of small bowel disease include evidence of submucosal thickening, single or multiple stenoses, adhesions, and sinus or fistula formation [68]. Large bowel strictures usually appear smooth and concentric in outline [117].

Radiation enteritis causes severe villous blunting, distended lymphatics, and replacement of the normal columnar epithelium with cuboidal cells; a pattern consistent with the clinical findings of malabsorption. The submucosal changes include perivascular adventitial fibrosis. Microscopic changes can be found in macroscopically normal bowel [22, 117].

Treatment. Radiation enteritis is a progressive disease [120]. Many patients can be treated conservatively; 5–20% of patients may require surgical intervention [46, 35]. The main indication for surgery is perforation. Patients with strictures are best treated conservatively, initially with bowel rest and decompression followed by low residue diets [22, 120]. If obstruction or fistula makes operative intervention necessary then great care must be taken to handle the bowel gently and avoid resection wherever possible. A high incidence of anastomotic leaks follows bowel resection of irradiated bowel due to a compromised blood supply and poor wound healing. Extensive dissection of adhesions should be avoided and a side-to-side bypass operation considered in some cases. When a resection is inevitable, for instance after perforation or in response to chronic severe blood loss, then more generous resections should be made and the bowel temporarily exteriorized to avoid an anastomosis [35, 120].

Prophylaxis. Many techniques have been used to exclude bowel from the pelvis during radiation therapy for pelvic malignancy using omental slings, tissue expanders, and distension of the bladder or retroversion of the uterus. The use of pelvic vicryl mesh placed at the level of the sacral promontory seems to be the best option in children [69]. In a study of eight children undergoing pelvic irradiation for malignancy who had a pelvic mesh placed before radiotherapy, none suffered from radiation enteritis [69].

Adhesive obstruction. Previous laparotomy, intra-abdominal or pelvic irradiation, and intraperitoneal bleeding or sepsis may lead to adhesion formation. Hence, a child with an intra-abdominal tumor is at significant risk of the late complications of adhesion formation. Operation for adhesions caused by radiotherapy is unrewarding and dangerous; the bowel is often unhealthy, easily damaged, and the adhesions rapidly reform. Adhesions secondary to previous operations are best managed conservatively but failure of the obstruction to resolve after 48 h and signs of ischemia are absolute indications for laparotomy.

22.4.2.3 Treatment of Obstruction in the Terminally Ill Child

Obstruction may occur in the advanced stages of childhood malignancy and although it may be a preterminal event, its management is important for symptom control. Traditional treatment includes stopping oral intake, insertion of a nasogastric tube, decompression, intravenous fluids, and correction of electrolyte abnormalities. Medical management includes anticholinergics, antiemetics, and analgesics. The role of steroids to reduce the degree of perineoplastic inflammation is controversial. Octreotide is a somatostatin analog that stimulates water and electrolyte absorption and inhibits water secretion by the small intestine. It may be useful in the treatment of obstruction and enteric fistulae [113]. Operative intervention with colostomy or bypass procedure may be justified. However, it may be more appropriate to manage these patients with intravenous opiates alone.

22.4.2.4 Neutropenic Enterocolitis

Though this condition may affect any part of the bowel, the most common area to be affected is the distal ileum and cecum and hence the term "typhlitis" is often used. It describes the clinicopathological syndrome of necrotizing inflammation of the cecum occurring in neutropenic patients. Though many cases of appendicitis complicating neutropenia had been described [27]. (usually with fatal results), it was not until 1961 that Amromin first recognized that neutropenic enterocolitis of the cecum was a distinct entity [2, 63].

Incidence. Exact incidence rates are difficult to collect because of the paucity of large studies and the difficulties of defining the relevant population. Several series have suggested an overall incidence of approximately 5% in patients with acute leukemia [29, 72, 91].

Etiology. The condition only develops in the presence of profound neutropenia. This may be disease induced [hematological malignancy, aplastic anemia and immunodeficient diseases such as human immunodeficiency virus (HIV)-induced acquired immunodeficiency syndrome (AIDS)] or secondary to drug treatment (chemotherapy for malignancy and bone marrow transplantation). The condition appears to be more common in acute myelogenous leukemia than in other forms [72, 87].

No definite cause has ever been identified but several hypotheses exist. Damage to the bowel mucosa allows invasion by colonic flora. Septicemia can then develop unchecked by the depleted immune system. Later, shock may increase the ischemia and thus perpetuate the vicious cycle. The initial mucosal insult is probably multifactorial including a direct effect of cytotoxic drugs on the mucosa, profound neutropenia, mucosal hemorrhage due to associated thrombocytopenia, stasis, and by changes in the bacterial flora secondary to prophylactic antibiotics [3, 87, 111, 116]. Why the cecum is most commonly affected is not clear though stasis and a relatively poor blood supply are possible explanations.

The theory that leukemic infiltrates of the bowel wall become necrotic in response to chemotherapeutic regimens causing damage to the mucosal wall and local hemorrhage appears plausible but there is little evidence, on microscopic examination, to support it.

Clinical features. Typically a patient undergoing induction chemotherapy is rendered neutropenic and develops problems between day 4 and 14. Symptoms and signs include diarrhea, vomiting, gastrointestinal bleeding, abdominal distension and sepsis. Examination usually reveals an ill patient with pyrexia, tachycardia, hypotension, and peritoneal irritation which may be diffuse or limited to the right iliac fossa [29, 36, 67, 72, 80, 87, 91].

Pathology. Grossly edematous cecum, mucosal ulceration, congested mesentery, and hemorrhagic mucosa progressing to full thickness necrosis of the bowel wall are seen at laparotomy. Three characteristic anatomical distributions are seen. First, the necrosis is sharply localized to the cecum with relative preservation of the ileum; second, the cecum is involved in extensive disease with other portions of the colon and small intestine; and third the cecum may contain ulcers which also occur sporadically throughout the intestine [111].

The tissues are edematous and blood vessels are dilated and engorged. Tissue structures appear necrotic and frequently masses of organisms are seen within the lesions. Leukemic infiltration is rarely seen but when present is readily identifiable. The usual microscopic pattern is one of hemorrhagic necrosis involving the mucosa and submucosa with a striking lack of acute inflammatory reaction. Occasionally, an exudate resembling a pseudomembrane and consisting of fibrin and cell debris may be found overlying the most severely ulcerated mucosal surfaces. In later stages the process may progress to full thickness involvement of the bowel wall and perforation.

Differential diagnosis. Causes of acute abdominal pain in these patients include acute appendicitis, pseudomembranous colitis, intussusception, pancreatitis, and pelvic abscess [29]. However, studies have shown that the most likely cause of diffuse or localized right iliac fossa abdominal pain in neutropenic patients is typhlitis [70, 72, 87, 111].

The most common organism isolated in septic patients with typhlitis is Pseudomonas aeruginosa [67, 111] though other Gram-negative organisms such as Escherichia coli and Klebsiella are also commonly found [29, 87, 91, 92, 116]. Gram-positive bacteria and fungi are occasionally found [29, 36, 111]. It is important to send multiple stool samples for analysis of C. difficile and its toxins to rule out pseudomembranous colitis.

Investigations. Blood tests are of little help, except to confirm neutropenia (neutrophils <0.5). Other markers of infection and inflammation can be misleading due to the effects of steroids, cytotoxic drugs, and general bone marrow suppression.

Diagnostic imaging studies are essential. Plain radiographs of the abdomen may show a paucity of bowel gas in the right iliac fossa progressing to a right-sided, ill-defined soft tissue mass due to a fluid-filled atonic cecum [111]. Other signs include small bowel ileus, ascites, and occasionally cecal pneumatosis which may not appear until the terminal stages of the disease process. Contrast enema findings include thickened mucosal folds, "thumb-printing" due to edema of the mucosa and cecal contraction [67]. Filling of the appendix rules out acute appendicitis. Contrast enemas may precipitate perforation of the cecum in the debilitated child [70, 111].

The investigation of choice is abdominal ultrasound [76, 92]. Sonographic features of typhlitis include the so-called target sign of a rounded mass with a highly echogenic center and a wide hypoechoic periphery. Remember that this sign is also seen in malignant tumors of the bowel, intussusception, and bowel infarction [67, 76, 92].30,35,61 Appendiceal thickening may indicate an increased risk of serious complications from this disease process [64].

If the ultrasound is not diagnostic or there is a suspicion of a more sinister cause then CT scan should be used. It can detect transmural inflammation, cecal wall thickening, soft tissue mass, and pneumatosis [70, 92].

Having ruled out intussusception, the finding of a soft tissue inflammatory mass in the right iliac fossa by ultrasound or CT in a neutropenic patient with pain and sepsis should be considered diagnostic of typhlitis [39, 70, 92].

Management. Management of these patients remains controversial, and both surgical [29, 72, 91,110, 116] and conservative medical management have been advocated [36, 87]. Recently, large series have shown that aggressive medical treatment with bowel rest, fluid resuscitation, and broad spectrum antibiotics together with selective surgical intervention are associated with good outcomes [87, 92]. Children are treated with intravenous fluids and triple antibiotics (benzylpenicillin, netilmicin, and metronidazole) and closely observed with frequent reassessment by the surgical team, for signs of deterioration. Granulocyte colony stimulating factor (GCSF) has been employed to hasten the return of the neutrophils but thus far its benefits in typhlitis have not been confirmed.

The main indication for surgical intervention is perforation; the other indications for operation include persistent gastrointestinal bleeding despite correction of thrombocytopenia and coagulation defects or clinical deterioration despite maximal supportive therapy. The child will benefit from removal of the source of abdominal sepsis by resection of necrotic bowel and peritoneal lavage [28]. It is important to rule out surgically treatable causes such as intussusception or acute appendicitis. Prognosis is better if the patient is in remission at the time of the operation [29].

Using a combination of aggressive medical and selective surgical management the two largest recent studies have shown a mortality of approximately 8% [87, 92].

22.4.2.5 Pancreatitis

Pancreatitis may rarely develop in some children with cancer following treatment with L-asparaginase, azathioprine, thiazide diuretics, and corticosteroids [60]. In addition it can complicate raised intracranial pressure [25]. or hypercalcemia [60, 104]. After L-asparaginase up to 6.5% of patients will develop pancreatitis [74]. L-asparaginase-induced severe narcotizing pancreatitis has been successfully treated with percutaneous drainage used to flush the infected necrotic parts [103].

Clinical features include severe abdominal pain, vomiting, and shock. Diagnosis is confirmed by a raised serum amylase or lipase level [93]. Full blood count, urea and electrolytes, serum calcium, liver function tests, clotting screen, and an arterial blood gas (ApO2) should be obtained. Chest radiograph can show signs of adult respiratory distress syndrome (ARDS). The abdomen should be assessed by either ultrasound examination or CT scan [76, 93] evaluated for edema, fluid collection, hemorrhage, necrosis, and other complications of pancreatitis.

Treatment is essentially medical, aimed at correction of the shock-like state of the patient with aggressive fluid resuscitation, nasogastric tube insertion, and drainage bowel rest. Intensive care is required if complications such as severe hypocalcemia, disseminated intravascular coagulation or respiratory distress associated with hypoxia develop [93]. Antibiotics may be required particularly in patients who are immunocompromised. Complications of pancreatitis include pancreatic abscess, which often requires urgent debridement and drainage. Pseudocysts may also occur but often will resolve, although in some instances may require drainage either percutaneously or by operative treatment. Octreotide has been used successfully in a child with L-asparaginase induced hemorrhagic pancreatitis [38].

22.4.2.6 Cholecystitis

Though rare, cholecystitis should always be considered in the differential diagnosis of the acute abdomen. In particular acute acalculous cholecystitis is associated with stress, sepsis, and co-existing problems such as leukemia [105]. The usual presentation is with right-upper quadrant pain, pyrexia, and vomiting; jaundice and a palpable mass are sometimes found. Diagnosis is confirmed by ultrasonograph demonstration of gallbladder distension, thickening of the gall bladder wall, pericholecystic fluid collection, and lumen sludge. Patients with cholecystitis usually respond to conservative management with intravenous fluids and antibiotics [105]. Unresponsive cases may require percutaneous drainage or cholecystectomy, either laparoscopically or by open surgery.

22.4.2.7 Ruptured Tumor

Occasionally the cause of the acute abdominal pain is the result of a ruptured tumor. This has been described in patients with Wilms' tumor, hepatoma, neuroblastoma, and B-cell lymphoma. This is often the result of trivial trauma in a child with an unsuspected neoplasm, but can occur spontaneously. Tumor rupture results in a more advanced stage of the disease process and requires more aggressive treatment. Godzinski found that survival after acute nephrectomy for ruptured Wilms' tumor was good but that this was achieved at the expense of long-term morbidity from using doxurubicin (adriamycin) and radiotherapy [42] (Fig. 22.4). An arteriovenous fistula and hemorrhage has been reported as a complication

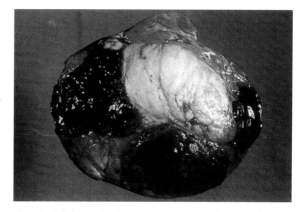

Fig. 22.4 Subcapsular hematoma in a Wilms' tumor. This was about to rupture and had to be removed as an emergency procedure.

following renal biopsy of a suspected bilateral Wilms' tumor [20].

22.4.3 Gastrointestinal Bleeding

Surgeons are occasionally asked to evaluate children on the oncology unit with gastrointestinal bleeding. This can range from small specks of altered blood to frank life-threatening hemorrhage. A list of conditions associated with gastrointestinal hemorrhage is presented in Table 22.5.

Gastric Antral Vascular Ectasia. This is a condition that is being increasingly reported in BMT patients. It was first described by Rider1 back in 1953 but recently has been noted in patients undergoing transplantation [12, 42]. It causes acute and chronic blood loss, at endoscopy the appearance is of red patches within the stomach. Histology shows dilated submucosal capillaries, fibrin thrombi, and fibromuscular hyperplasia. There should be no evidence of GVHD, infection, or ulceration. Ohashi reported five cases all of whom had received conditioning therapy with busulfan and all had a history of microangiopathy.3 Treatment was supportive but did not seem to respond to omeprazole in three of the five patients. Selective angiography had suggested high venous pressures so they were tried on the cardio-selective beta blocker Metoprolol with good results.

22.4.3.1 The Role of Diagnostic Imaging in Acute Gastrointestinal Bleeding

Plain radiographs are rarely useful but may show toxic dilatation of the colon in acute colitis. Contrast studies

Table 22.5 Causes of gastrointestinal bleeding

Site	Cause
Whole bowel	Tumor infiltration of bowel
	Mucosal ulceration from chemoradiotherapy
	Lymphoma
	Acute graft-versus-host disease
	Thrombocytopenia
	Depletion of clotting factors
Liver	Porto-systemic hypertension and varices
	Impaired production of clotting factors
	Veno-occlusive disease
Esophagus	Esophageal varices
	Viral/fungal esophagitis
	Gastroesophageal reflux
	Mallory-Weiss tears
Stomach and duodenum	Peptic ulceration (stress or steroid induced)
	Gastric erosions
	Gastric antral vascular ectasia
Small bowel	Enteritis (see below)
Large bowel	Neutropenic enterocolitis
	Radiation enteritis
	Infective colitis (cytomegalovirus, herpes simplex virus, adenovirus, cryptosporidia, Giardia, Candida)
	Clostridium difficile infection
Non-oncological causes	Ulcerative colitis
	Meckel's diverticulum
	Anal fissure
	Hemorrhoids
	Intestinal duplication
	Hemangioma

should be avoided as they yield little useful information and prevent more useful investigations such as angiography.

Angiography and red cell scans are difficult to set up and time consuming and thus should be held in reserve until upper or lower gastrointestinal endoscopy fail to provide a diagnosis. Angiography has the advantage of accurately detecting the site of the bleeding if the rate exceeds 1.0 cc/min and can be used to embolize a bleeding point. The disadvantage of angiography is that it is an invasive procedure. Radiolabeled red cell scan, on the other hand, can be used in cases with a slower bleeding rate (0.5 cc/min) but provides less precise anatomical location of the bleeding point.

22.4.3.2 The Role of Endoscopy in Acute Gastrointestinal Bleeding

Upper and lower gastrointestinal endoscopy are the most rewarding procedures in detecting the site of bleeding. In a bleeding peptic ulcer endoscopic injection of the ulcer bed with epinephrine and heater probe coagulation may stop the bleeding. In rare instances of liver damage associated with portal hypertension, esophageal varices may be the cause of bleeding and can be injected with sclerosing agents or banded.

22.4.3.3 Algorithm for Management of Gastrointestinal Bleeding

A recommended algorithm for the management of patients with gastrointestinal bleeding is shown in Fig. 22.5.

22.4.3.4 Esophagitis in the Immunosuppressed Patient

The esophagus is a frequent site for infection in the immunosuppressed patient. Patients present with dysphagia, retrosternal chest pain, fever, and upper intestinal bleeding. The patient's symptoms, oropharyngeal cultures and esophageal contrast radiography are not predictive of the cause – therefore, accurate diagnosis depends on endoscopy, mucosal biopsy, and brushings of abnormal-appearing areas and cultures [65].

Endoscopic findings range from discreet vesicles in herpes simplex virus (HSV) esophagitis to erosions and a spectrum of findings from esophagitis to gross ulceration which may complicate any infection and is compounded by gastroesophageal reflux. The most common infecting organism was HSV followed by cytomegalovirus (CMV). Fungal infection also occurs and is usually due to Candida albican [65]. Treatment is supportive with adequate analgesia and appropriate antiviral or antifungal therapy.

22.4.3.5 Infectious Colitis

Immunocompromised patients are at high risk for development of opportunistic infections. Affecting agents include Candida albican, pneumocystitis carnii, C. difficile, cryptosporidia, giardia, CMV, HSV, rotavirus, astrovirus, and adenovirus. Cytomegalovirus infection is particularly associated with colitis and bowel perforation [43]. Investigation of diarrhea includes sending stool culture for anaerobic organisms, C. difficile toxin, and microscopy and culture looking for protozoa, fungi, or viral infestation. Viral infec-

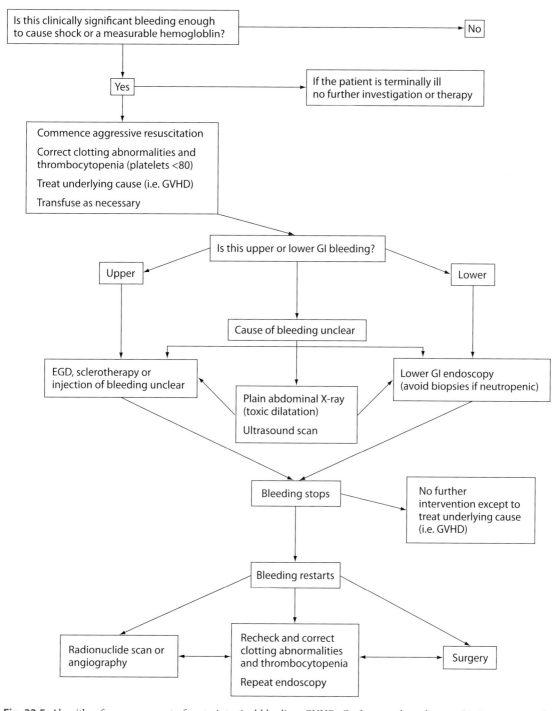

Fig. 22.5 Algorithm for management of gastrointestinal bleeding. GVHD, Graft-versus-host disease; GI, Gastrointestinal; EGD, Esophagogastro-duodenoscopy.

tion is of particular importance in the bone marrow transplant patients as clinically it is difficult to differentiate infection from acute graft-versus-host disease. The consequences of increasing the level of immunosuppression to treat graft-versus-host disease, when the patient is actually suffering from viral colitis, can result in a fatality. Sigmoidoscopy or colonoscopy are useful in making the diagnosis by providing biopsies from affected areas of colon for histology [52, 122]. Histological examination of biopsies may show viral inclusion bodies or fungal colonies. Appropriate

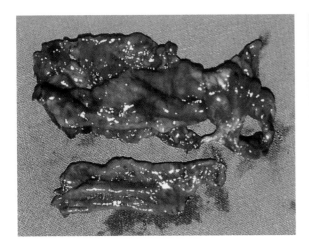

Fig. 22.6 Pseudomembranous colitis.

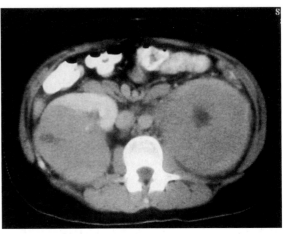

Fig. 22.7 Bilateral infiltration of the kidney in a patient with recurrent T cell lymphoma: CT scan showing both kidneys involved. This patient had to be treated by dialysis for renal failure.

treatment for proven viral infection is with aciclovir or ganciclovir.

Clostridium-difficile-associated diarrhea is now a common problem in hospitals. Changes in the normal bacterial flora of the colon as a result of antibiotic therapy (especially clindamycin and in infants ampicillin) allows overgrowth of C. difficile with subsequent release of toxins that cause mucosal damage and inflammation [50]. Clinical presentation includes mild to moderate diarrhea, antibiotic-associated colitis with or without pseudomembrane formation, and fulminant colitis (Fig. 22.6). Associated symptoms include abdominal cramps and bloody diarrhea. In instances of fulminating colitis the patient presents with an acute abdomen, fever, tachycardia, and lethargy. Toxic dilatation may develop. Diagnosis depends on demonstration of C. difficile toxins in the stool; sigmoidoscopy or proctoscopy and biopsies may be beneficial as most disease is confined to the rectum or sigmoid. However, in 10 % of cases the colitis is limited to the proximal colon. Unfortunately, colonoscopy in these latter cases, in patients with fulminant colitis, may be complicated by perforation.

The treatment of C. difficile associated colitis is cessation of prior antibiotics, and treatment with vancomycin or flagyl preparations is mandatory. Barrier nursing of infected patients is recommended. Though severe colitis can usually be controlled within 48–72 h with antibiotics and appropriate supportive treatment, in some cases this fails and perforation occurs. Emergency celiotomy is mandatory for instances of proven perforation or severe refractory cases unresponsive to nonoperative management [13, 50] colectomy, ileostomy and construction of a Hartman pouch are often required.

22.4.4 Perianal Lesions

Perianal lesions include localized infections, abscesses, and other causes of inflammation such as graft-versus-host disease and radiation proctitis.

Measures to avoid perianal infections include the following points:
1. Avoid rectal examination and the use of suppositories and enemas.
2. Avoid constipation using laxatives/stool softeners.
3. Avoid diarrhea. Clean perianal skin carefully with water (Sitz baths) and soft cloth. Barrier cream may reduce any skin reaction.

Symptomatic perianal infections are a relatively common occurrence in the neutropenic child, complicating 6% of hospitalized leukemic patients [44]. In the case of the profoundly neutropenic patient, no abscess will develop because of the lack of neutrophils to produce pus. The usual findings are of a mixed culture of colonic organisms [4, 41]. Pseudomonas aeruginosa is particularly pathogenic in this region and may quickly progress to necrotizing fasciitis of the anorectal region [4].

Unlike the patient with an intact immune system where surgical incision and drainage of the abscess forms the basis of treatment, the immunocompromised patient should be treated primarily with broad spectrum antibiotics that cover anaerobic and Gram-negative organisms. The regime used includes intravenous benzylpenicillin, netilmicin, and metronidazole. Granulocyte colony stimulating factor may hasten the return of an immunological response though its role is yet to be proven. Constipation should be treated with stool softeners and laxatives. Pain relief may be required. These patients should be observed closely to make sure that no abscess develops when the neutrophil count rises and that the cellulitis does not spread resulting in a necrotizing fasciitis [4, 41, 75]. Indications for surgical intervention are obvious fluctuation, a significant amount of necrotic tissue, or progression to a necrotizing infection [44, 75]. There appears to be no increased morbidity or mortality in those requiring operation [44, 75]. The usual procedure is drainage of the abscess.

22.5 Genitourinary Tract Complications

Renal failure may be a complication seen after many years following treatment with cytotoxic agents and radiotherapy. Patients with neuroblastoma and Wilms' tumor are especially susceptible. Another complication seen in patients receiving therapy for bulky tumor is that of uric acid nephropathy discussed under metabolic causes of the acute abdomen (see "tumor lysis syndrome," above).

22.5.1 Hemorrhagic Cystitis

Hemorrhagic cystitis is a complication resulting from cancer therapy. Several causes have been identified, including alkylating agents, infections, and pelvic irradiation.

The oxazaphosphorine alkylating agents, cyclophosphamide and ifosfamide, are the most important causes. Cyclophosphamide was first introduced as an antineoplastic agent in 1957. Within 2 years Coggins, et al. had reported cases of significant hemorrhagic cystitis (Fig. 22.8) [19]. Acrolein, a liver metabolite of cyclophosphamide produced by microsomal enzymatic hydroxylation, has been identified as the cause of the cystitis. The exact mechanism of action is unknown but contact of acrolein with the urothelium causes sloughing of epithelium, development of inflammatory infiltrates, regeneration of a thinner epithelium, and formation of new blood vessels.

Numerous infectious causes are known. Viral pathogens include BK virus, polyoma virus, adenovirus, and cytomegalovirus. They are thought to be most significant in bone marrow transplant patients who are immunosuppressed and already sensitized by cyclophosphamide. These patients seem to develop a late hemorrhagic cystitis weeks or months after transplantation – there may be a link with graft-versus-host disease. Bacterial causes include E. coli, Klebsiella and Proteus, and fungal causes such as Candida albicans, Aspergillus fumigatus and Cryptococcus neoformans are also implicated in immunosuppressed patients [97].

22.5.1.1 Incidence

The incidence of hemorrhagic cystitis ranges from 2% to 40% in adults; in children this complication seems to be less frequent at around 5–10% [55]. The complication appears to be more frequent during the summer, suggesting that there may be a link with dehydration.

22.5.1.2 Clinical Features

The urological side-effects vary from transient irritative voiding symptoms, including urinary frequency, dysuria, urgency, suprapubic discomfort and stangury with microscopic hematuria, to life-threatening hemorrhagic cystitis [57, 95]. Late complications include bladder fibrosis, necrosis, contracture, and vesicoureteric reflux. The onset of symptoms is variable and may occur during the course of therapy or for several months later [57].

Though the severity of hemorrhagic cystitis does not appear to be dose-related, pediatric patients seem to develop cystitis at lower dosage and shorter duration compared with adults – this may be a consequence of the parenteral route of administration used in most children. There is no correlation with age or sex [55, 95]. However, it is a common complication of allogenic blood and marrow transplantation. In a recent paper they concluded it is more prevalent in matched unrelated donors and unrelated cord blood transplantation than matched related donors [28].

22.5.1.3 Diagnosis

The diagnosis is often made clinically. Urine culture must be obtained to rule out infection. Excretory urograms may show anatomical defects and ultrasound can be diagnostic of hemorrhagic cystitis [53]. Urine cytology is frequently used in adults but has not been useful in children. Urine should be examined by electron microscopy for viral infection. Definitive diagnosis requires cystoscopy and biopsy, and can be useful in ruling out other causes.

22.5.1.4 Prevention

Adequate hydration, diuresis, and frequent bladder voiding all reduce the concentration and the time for which the toxic urine is in contact with the bladder [57, 95]. Care must be taken not to cause overhydration as cyclophosphamide is known to cause damage to renal tubules and inappropriate water retention.

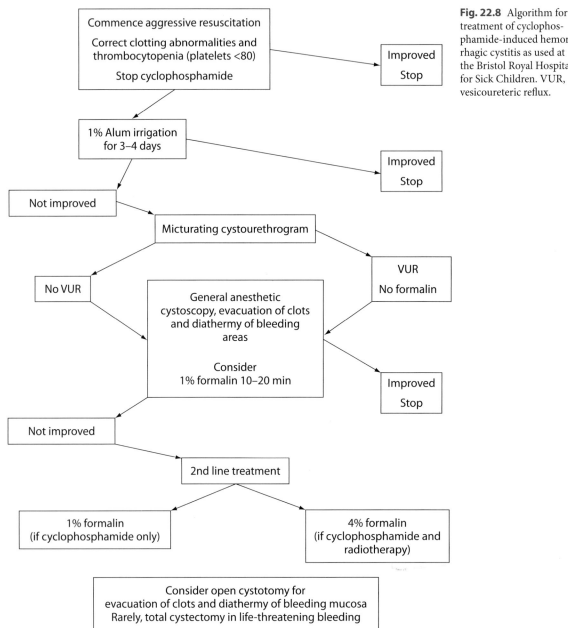

Fig. 22.8 Algorithm for treatment of cyclophosphamide-induced hemorrhagic cystitis as used at the Bristol Royal Hospital for Sick Children. VUR, vesicoureteric reflux.

N-Acetyl cysteine and more recently Mesna (2–mercaptoethane sulfate) have been shown to reduce the incidence of cyclophosphamide-related cystitis [57, 97] by binding and inactivating the toxic acrolein (Table 22.6).

22.5.1.5 Treatment

Many different therapies have been suggested over the last 40 years, few of which have been rigorously tested by randomized controlled trials. Several of the

Table 22.6 Mesna prophylaxis given for cyclophosphamide therapy at the Bristol Royal Hospital for Sick Children

20 mg/kg of intravenous Mesna in 0.9% saline given together with the cyclophosphamide over 1 h
76 mg/kg of intravenous Mesna in maintenance fluids (5% dextrose and 0.225% saline) over the next 23 h
Each urine is checked by dipstix for microscopic hematuria
If hematuria is found then a further 24 h of Mesna is given
Any further doses of cyclophosphamide receive the same regime

management possibilities have only been described in adults (Table 22.7). Fresh frozen plasma, platelets, and blood transfusion should be given as required.

Levine and Richie [57] suggested an algorithm for treatment based on the severity of the disease. Mild acute disease simply requires cessation of cyclophosphamide with good hydration and oral analgesia [55]. More severe disease justifies a more aggressive approach with cystoscopic evacuation of all mucosal clots followed by continuous bladder irrigation with 1–2% alum aluminum potassium sulfate for 2–3 days through a large-bore catheter; alternatively intravesical instillation of prostaglandin F2 followed by cystoscopy, diathermy of any bleeding sites, and instillation of 2.5–4% formalin. In very small children in whom only a very small cystoscope can be passed our experience has been that open cystotomy, clot evacuation, and diathermy of bleeding points can provide excellent control of symptoms and should be considered at an early stage. In unresponsive cases with massive hemorrhage, total cystectomy may be a life-saving procedure.

Though formalin is a well-described treatment, it must be used with extreme caution because of complications of fibrosis, stricture, and renal damage. Before it is used a micturating cystourethrogram must be done to exclude urinary reflux. Formalin should not be used in the presence of reflux.

A review of the presentations and management of children with hemorrhagic cystitis after bone marrow transplantation at The Royal Hospital for Sick Children, Glasgow during the period between 1990 and 1997 showed only six children who developed the disease. During this 8-year period 91 children received a bone marrow transplant. The mean age was 12 years (range 5–15 years); all had prophylaxis with hydration and Mesna. The presentation of hemorrhagic cystitis occurred on average 40 days after chemotherapy (range 26–40 days).

Hemorrhagic cystitis was heralded by a period of microscopic hematuria lasting 4–12 days (mean 9 days). Five patients required continuous irrigation, one with normal saline and his condition settled; the other cases failed due to clot retention and catheter blockage. Irrigation with prostaglandin and alum 1% was tried in two instances but failed to influence the course of the disease. Three children required formal suprapubic vesicostomy with wide stoma; one required temporary urinary diversion and bladder packing and one required emergency cystectomy for massive life-threatening bleeding. Further studies are required to see if earlier intervention during the phase of microscopic hematuria may affect the course of this serious complication. Fibrin glue applied suprapubically while visualizing and insufflating the bladder through a cystoscope achieved hemostasis [81].

22.5.1.6 Outcome

Although hemorrhagic cystitis secondary to cyclophosphamide therapy is usually self-limiting, it can have serious long-term effects especially with regard to bladder fibrosis leading to vesico-ureteric reflux, bladder irritability and incontinence, and ureteric strictures. Renal function may be compromised by the outflow tract obstruction. The long-term problems in some of these patients may require cystectomy or augmentation.

Patients who received more than 50 g of cyclophosphamide probably require long-term surveillance with blood pressure, urinalysis, and assessment of renal function. In addition there is a 4–7% increased risk of bladder malignancy [97]. The risks are greatest in those patients receiving both cyclophosphamide and pelvic irradiation without any uroprotection with Mesna. Urine cytology can be used for early detection of new bladder malignancy [109]. Abnormal cytology or evidence of gross or microscopic hematuria requires further investigation with cystoscopy, bladder biopsy, and excretion urogram.

Table 22.7 Various treatments described for cyclophosphamide induced hemorrhagic

Treatment	Ref.
Cessation of cyclophosphamide	[57]
Hyperhydration	[57]
Frequent or continuous bladder emptying	
Continuous irrigation	[107]
Correction of clotting and platelet abnormalities	
Intravesical therapy with formalin, alum or prostaglandin F2	[21, 37, 54, 56, 73, 82, 89]
Cystoscopy with evacuation of clot and diathermy or laser of hemorrhagic areas	[45]
Open cystotomy, clot evacuation, and diathermy	
Systemic estrogen	[58]
Antiviral therapy if urine cultures are positive	
Cystectomy and neobladder substitution	[77]

22.5.1.7 Other Conditions Affecting the Genitourinary Tract

Renal involvement in non-Hodgkins lymphoma is associated with a poor prognostic factor and renal function should be monitored closely. Renal dysfunction caused by direct tumor involvement may complicate therapy and shorten survival [15]. Ureteral obstruction may be caused by L-asparaginase, an effective antileukemia and antilymphoma agent as it is toxic to many organ systems. This could be managed by a double J stent [18].

Children with leukemia may present with acute testicular swellings which can be mistaken for other acute scrotal conditions, e.g., torsion of the testes, epididymo-orchitis. These children have leukemic infiltration of the testes (Fig. 22.9) and a biopsy usually confirms the presence of leukemic cells in the testes. This

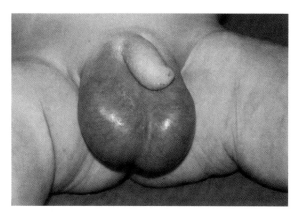

Fig. 22.9 Leukemic infiltration of the testes.

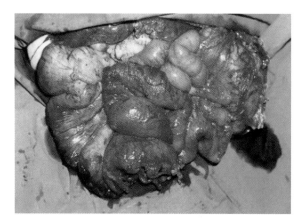

Fig. 22.10 This 4-year-old boy had severe graft-versus-host disease affecting the entire gastrointestinal tract and was managed conservatively for many months. Laparotomy was eventually performed, for persistent intestinal obstruction. Multiple fibrotic strictures were observed and resected. The patient is alive and well 6 years later.

is often a presentation in boys who have had treatment for leukemia and have relapsed after their treatment is finished. The testis is considered a "sanctuary site" for tumor persistence and may require irradiation.

22.6 Intestinal Graft-Versus-Host Disease

Graft-versus-host disease is one of the major complications of bone marrow transplantation. The concept behind transplantation of allograft bone marrow is that new T lymphocyctes will develop which will recognize the host as "self." However, mature T cells may also be transplanted that have already learned what is "not self" and thus may attack host cells that are covered with "foreign" class I and II major histocompatibility antigens.

22.6.1 Clinical Features

Most patients undergoing bone marrow transplantation will develop graft-versus-host disease without specific anti-graft-versus-host disease prophylaxis, at around 2–5 weeks posttransplant. The severity of disease depends on the closeness of the major histocompatibility match, whether the donor marrow has been T cell depleted, the degree of minor histocompatibility match (related to age, sex, race, etc.), and the type of prophylaxis used.

The skin, followed by the gastrointestinal tract (Fig. 22.10) and liver, are the most commonly affected organs. Cutaneous manifestations include pruritus and a fine erythematous or maculopapular rash. In severe cases blistering and desquamation of the skin may occur. A punch biopsy of the skin is required for definitive diagnosis and grading (Table 22.9) of the histological severity of the graft-versus-host disease. In severe disease, the lung can also be affected (though usually in the more chronic form).

Any area of the alimentary tract from the mouth to the anus can be affected. In one study MacGregor, et al. found that up to 70% of patients with graft-versus-host disease had some degree of intestinal involvement [59].

The most common manifestations occur in the small bowel and reflect direct effects on the intestine and secondary infections that develop as a consequence of graft-versus-host disease [24, 32, 66, 101, 108]. Symptoms include nausea, vomiting, abdominal cramps, and diarrhea. The diarrhea may be profuse and cause fluid and electrolyte imbalance. Nutritional problems may occur due to malabsorption and a protein-losing enteropathy. Occasionally mucosal casts are passed per rectum. In severe graft-versus-host disease there can be generalized signs of adynamic ileus,

Table 22.8 Patients at risk of developing acute graft-versus-host disease

1. Bone marrow transplant patients [102]
2. Solid organ transplant patients
3. Transfusion of unirradiated blood products in neonates
4. Transfusion of unirradiated blood products in patients receiving immunosuppressive chemoradiotherapy

Table 22.9 Clinical grading of graft-versus-host disease

Stage	Skin	Bilirubin level (mg/liter)	Intestine
I	Maculopapular rash <25% of BSA	2–3	Diarrhea
		>500 ml/day	
II	Maculopapular rash 25–50% of BSA	3–6	Diarrhea
		>1000 ml/day	
III	Generalized erythroderma	6–15	Diarrhea
		>1500 ml/day	
IV	Generalized erythroderma with bulla formation	>15	Severe abdominal pain, and desquamation with or without ileus

BSA, Body surface area. (From [102])

peritoneal irritation, gastrointestinal bleeding, and perforation: this suggests full thickness inflammation with ulceration.

22.6.2 Investigations

Investigations include blood tests to assess the severity of electrolyte and serum protein levels with complete blood count and a coagulation profile.

Erect and supine abdominal radiographs may show signs of thumb printing, suggesting mucosal edema; pneumatosis may also be observed as erect chest radiographs (or decubitus abdominal radiographs) may show pneumoperitoneum. Contrast barium enema may show typical signs of gastrointestinal graft-versus-host disease but must be used cautiously in very sick patients because of the risks of perforation [33].

Radiological signs include thickened and effaced mucosal folds, thickened bowel wall and rapid transit. In subacute gastrointestinal graft-versus-host disease the contrast studies show a segmental patchy appearance of ulceration with normal and abnormal areas interspersed [33]. Use of CT scan shows fluid-filled, dilated, poorly opacified bowel loops and characteristic abnormally enhanced, thin mucosa.

Histology of intestinal graft-versus-host disease initially shows necrosis of individual intestinal crypt cells (apoptosis). Progression of disease leads to loss of whole crypts with mucosal denudation and ulceration. In extreme circumstances the entire mucosa may be sloughed off [34].

Endoscopic examination can be very useful. The endoscopic appearance of graft-versus-host disease shows edema, erythema, and frank ulceration but these signs are nonspecific [34]. Mucosal biopsy, however, may be characteristic [101] and can help differentiate graft-versus-host disease from opportunistic infections and other causes of colitis [65, 5]. Upper gastrointestinal biopsies have a higher yield than biopsies from the colon or rectum. However, as the disease is patchy the most affected area of bowel should be examined. Invasive procedures such as endoscopy or biopsy should be undertaken because the benefits are often life saving and the actual risks of serious complication are relatively low [5, 49, 101].

22.6.3 Other Problems in Bone Marrow Transplant Patients

In addition to problems with the gastrointestinal tract, the surgeon is occasionally consulted for advice and requests for biopsies to help diagnose problems in patients with liver and respiratory problems. We recently reviewed liver and lung biopsies taken from bone marrow transplant patients at the Bristol Royal Hospital for Sick Children with undiagnosed findings such as worsening liver function and increasing respiratory distress. Of eight liver biopsies (seven by Tru-cut and one by open operation) three were related to graft-versus-host disease, two were due to viral infection, two were related to transfusion siderosis, and one was an aspergilloma. Two open lung biopsies showed one case of cytomegalovirus pneumonitis and one case of radiation fibrosis. Overall we found the complication rate to be low and a number of unsuspected diagnoses were made that altered future management.39

22.6.4 Treatment

Once graft-versus-host disease is documented the treatment is essentially medical with administration of high-dose steroid immunosuppression. The prognosis of graft-versus-host disease is worse if skin, gut, and liver are all involved. The only indication for surgical intervention is perforation of the intestine. Severe hemorrhage is best treated by aggressive medical management with correction of clotting abnormalities, platelet transfusion, and endoscopy. The results of surgical resection in the acute phase are universally poor. Once the disease is quiescent the areas of sloughed intestinal mucosa may heal by forming a stricture that may require bowel resection.

References

1. Alavi S, Arzanian MT, Abbasian MR, Ashena Z (2006) Tumor lysis syndrome in children with non-Hodgkin lymphoma. Pediatr Hematol Oncol 23(1):65–70
2. Amromin GD, Solomon RD (1962) Necrotizing enteropathy. J Am Med Assoc 182:23–29
3. Anderson PE (1993) Neutropenic enterocolitis treated by primary resection with anastomosis in a leukaemic patient receiving chemotherapy. Austr NZ J Surg 63:74–76
4. Angel C, Patrick CC, Lobe T, Rao B, Pui CH (1991) Management of anorectal/perineal infections caused by Pseudomonas aeruginosa in children with malignant diseases. J Pediatr Surg 26:487–492
5. Arul GS, Mullan MH, Cornish J, Oakhill A, Spicer RD (1999) Role of surgical biopsies in the management of bone marrow transplant patients. Medical & Pediatric Oncology 33:95–98
6. Arul GS, RD Spicer (2001) Ecthyma Gangrenosum – A trap for the unwary. The Annals of the Royal College of Surgeons of England 83, pp 47–48
7. Auldist AW (1976) Wilms' tumor presenting as a varicocele. J Pediatr Surg 11:471–472
8. Avci Z, Alioglu B, Canan O, Szcay F, Celasun B, Sarlattoglu F, Ozbek N (2006) Calcification of the gastric mucosa associated with tumor lysis syndrome in a child with non-Hodgkin lymphoma. Pediatr Hematol Oncol 28(5):307–310
9. Baeksgaard L, Sorensen JB (2003) Acute tumor lysis syndrome in solid tumours – A case report and review of the literature. Cancer Chemother Pharmacol 51:187–192
10. Berg A, Armitage JO, Burns CP (1985) Fournier's gangrene complicating aggressive therapy for hematologic malignancy. Cancer 57:2291–2294
11. Bourque MD, Spigland N, et al. (1989) Esophageal leiomyoma in children: Two case reports and review of the literature. J Pediatr Surg 24:1103–1107
12. Bower RJ, Kiesewetter WB (1997) Colo-colic intussusception due to a hemangioma. J Pediatr Surg 12:777–778
13. Bradbury AW, Barrett S (1997) Surgical aspects of Clostridium difficile colitis. Brit J Surg 84:150–159
14. Browne AF, Katz S, Miser J, Boles ET (1983) Blue rubber bleb nevi as a cause of intussusception. J Pediatr Surg 18:7–9
15. Buyukpamukcu M, Caran A, Aydin B, Kale G, Akata D, Yalcin B, Akyuz C, Kutluk T (2005) Renal invovlement in non-Hodgkin's lymphoma and its prognostic effect in childhood. Nephron Clin Pract 100(3):c86–91
16. Caty MG, Oldham KT, Prochownik EV (1990) Embryonal rhabdomyosarcoma of the ampulla of Vater with long term survival following pancreaticoduodenectomy. J Pediatr Surg 25:1256–1260
17. Chang WL, Griffith KM (1991) Solitary intestinal fibromatosis: A rare cause of intestinal obstruction in neonates and infants. J Pediatr Surg 26:1406–1408
18. Chen CH, Lu MY, Lin KH, Peng SF, Jou ST (2004) Ureteral obstruction casued by L-asparaginase-induced pancreatitis in a child with acute lymphoblastic leukemia. J Formos Med Assoc 103(5):380–384
19. Coggins PR, Ravdin RG, Eisman SH (1959) Clinical pharmacology and preliminary evaluation of cytoxan (cyclophosphamide). Cancer Chemo Rep 3:9
20. De Kraker J (1998) Arteriovenous fistula: A complication following renal biopsy of suspected bilateral Wilms' tumor [letter] Med Paediatr Oncol 30:125
21. Donahue LA, Frank IN (1989) Intravesical formalin for haemorrhagic cystitis: Analysis of therapy. J Urol 141:809–812
22. Donaldson SS, Jundt S, Ricour C, Sarrazin D, Lemerle J, Schweisguth O (1975) Radiation enteritis in children. A retrospective review, clinicopathologic correlation, and dietary management. Cancer 35:1167–1178
23. Donnelly LF (1996) CT imaging of immunocompromised children with acute abdominal symptoms. Am J Roentgenol 167:911–913
24. Donnelly LF, Morris CL (1996) Acute graft-versus-host disease in children: Abdominal CT findings. Radiology 199:265–268
25. Eichelberger MR, Chatten J, Bruce DA (1981) Acute pancreatitis and increased intracranial pressure. J Pediatr Surg 16:562–570
26. Ein SH, Stephens CA, Shandling B, Filler RM (1986) Intussusception due to lymphoma. J Pediatr Surg 21:786–788
27. Einhorn M (1961) Temporary remission in acute leukemia after an attack of 'acute appendicitis'. J Am Med Assoc 175:1006–1008
28. El-Zimaity M, Saliba R, Chan K, Shahjahan M, Carrasco A, Khorshid O, Caldera H, Couriel D, Girait S, Khouri I, Ippoliti C, Champlin R, de Lima M (2004) Hemorrhagic cystitis after allogeneic hematoppietic stem cell transplantation; Donor type matters. Blood 103(12):4674–4680
29. Exelby PR, Ghandchi A, Lansigan N, Schwartz I (1975) Management of the acute abdomen in children with leukaemia. Cancer 35:826–829
30. Fasano R, Kent P, Valentino L (2005) Superior vena cava thrombus treated with low-dose, peripherally administered recombinant tissue plasminogen activator in a child: Case report and review of the literature. J Pediatr Hematol Oncol 27(12):637–638
31. Fergie JE, Patrick CC, Lott L (1991) Pseudomonas aeruginosa cellulitis and ecthyma gangrenosum in immunocompromised children. Pediatr Infect Dis J 10:496–499
32. Ferrara UL, Deeg HJ 1991) Graft versus host disease. New Engl J Med 324:667–674
33. Fisk JD, Shulman HM, Greening RR, et al. (1981) Gastrointestinal radiographic features of human graft-versus-host disease. Am J Roentgenol 136:329–336

34. Galati JS, Wisecarver JL, Quigley EMM (1993) Inflammatory polyps as a manifestation of intestinal graft versus host disease. Gastrointest Endosc 39:719–722

35. Galland RB, Spencer J (1985) The natural history of clinically established radiation enteritis. Lancet i:1257–1258

36. Gandy W, Greenberg BR (1983) Successful medical management of neutropaenic enterocolitis. Cancer 51:1551–1555

37. Garat JM, Martinez E, Aragona F (1985) Open instillation of formalin for cyclophosphamide-induced hemorrhagic cystitis in a child. Eur J Urol 11:192–194

38. Garrington T, Ben Sard D, Ingram JD, et al. (1998) Successful management with ocreotide of a child with L-asparaginase induced hemorrhagic pancreatitis. Med Paediatr Oncol 30:106–109

39. Gavan DR, Hendry GM (1994) Colonic complication of acute lymphoblastic leukaemia. Brit J Radiol 67:449–452

40. Gibbons MD, Duckett JW (1979) Neuroblastoma masquerading as congenital ureteropelvic obstruction. J Pediatr Surg 14:420–422

41. Glenn J, Cotton D, Wesley R, Pizzo P (1988) Anorectal infections in patients with malignant diseases. Rev Infect Dis 10:42–52

42. Godzinski J, Weirich A, Tournade MF, et al. (1996) Primary nephrectomy for emergency in SIOP-9 Wilms' tumor patients. Med Pediatr Oncol 27:219

43. Goodman ZD, Boitnott JK, Yardley JH (1979) Perforation of the colon associated with cytomegalovirus infection. Dig Dis Sci 24:376–380

44. Grewal H, Guillem JG, Quan SH, Enker WE, Cohen AM (1994) Anorectal disease in neutropenic leukemic patients. Operative vs. nonoperative management. Dis Colon Rectum 37:1095–1099

45. Gweon P, Shanberg A (1997) Treatment of cyclophosphamide induced hemorrhagic cystitis with neodymium:YAG laser in pediatric patients. J Urol 157:2301–2302

46. Haddad GK, Grodsinsky C, Allen H (1983) The spectrum of radiation enteritis. Surgical considerations. Dis Colon Rectum 26:590–594

47. Haley T, Dimler M, Hollier P (1986) Gastric teratoma with gastrointestinal bleeding. J Pediatr Surg 21:949–950

48. Kaste SC, Flynn PM, Furman WL (1997) Acute lymphoblastic leukemia presenting with typhlitis. Med Pediatr Oncol 28:209–212

49. Kaw M, Przepiorka D, Sekas G (1993) Infectious complications of endoscopic procedures in bone marrow transplant recipients. Digest Dis Sci 38:71–74

50. Kelly CP, Pothoulakis C, La Mont JT (1994) Clostridium difficile colitis. New Engl JMed 330:257–262

51. Kerdudo C, Aerts I, Fattet S, Chevret L, Pacquement H, Doz F, Michon J, Garabedian M, Orback D (2005) Hypercalcemia and childhood cancer: A 7-year experience. Pediatr Hematol Oncol 27(1):23–27

52. Kirchner SG, Horev G (1985) Diagnostic imaging in children with acute chest and abdominal disorders. Pediatr Clin North Am 32:1363–1382

53. Kumar A, Aggarwal S (1990) The sonographic appearance of cyclophosphamide-induced acute haemorrhagic cystitis. Clin Radiol 41:289–290

54. Laszlo D, Bosi A, Guidi S, et al. (1995) Prostaglandin E2 bladder instillation for the treatment of hemorrhagic cystitis after allogeneic bone marrow transplantation. Haematologica 80:421–425

55. Lawrence HJ, Simone J, Aur RJA (1975) Cyclophophamide-induced hemorrhagic cystitis in children with leukemia. Cancer 36:1572–1576

56. Levine LA, Jarrard DF (1993) Treatment of cyclophosphamide-induced hemorrhagic cystitis with intravesical carboprost tromethamine. J Urol 149:719–723

57. Levine LA, Richie JP (1989) Urological complications of cyclophosphamide. J Urol 141:1063–1069

58. Liu YK, Harty JI, Steinbock GS, Holt HA Jr, Goldstein DH, Amin M (1990) Treatment of radiation or cyclophosphamide induced hemorrhagic cystitis using conjugated estrogen. J Urol 144:41–43

59. MacGregor GI, Shepherd JD, Philips GL (1988) Acute graft versus host disease of the intestine. A surgical perspective. Am J Surg 155:680–682

60. Mallory A, Kern F Jr (1980) Drug-induced pancreatitis: A critical review. Gastroenterology 78:813–820

61. Massicotte P, Mitchell L (2006) Thromboprophylaxis of central venous lines in children with cancer: The first steps taken on the long road ahead. Acta Paediatr 95(9):1049–1052

62. Matthew R, Christoper O, Pillippa S (2006) Severe malignancy-associated hypercalcemia in dysgerminoma. Pediatr Blood Cancer 15:621–623

63. McCarville MB, Adelman CS, Li C, Xiong X, Furman WL, Razzouk BI, Pui CH, Sandlund JT (2005) Typhilitis in childhood cancer. Cancer 104(2):380–387

64. McCarville MB, Thompson J, Li C, Adelman CS, Lee MO, Alsammarae D, May MV, Jones SC, Rao BN, Sandlund JT (2004) Significance of appendiceal thickening in association with typhilitis in pediatric oncology patients. Pediatr Radiol 34(3):245–249

65. McDonald GB, Sharma P, Hackman RC, Meyers JD, Thomas ED (1985) Esophageal infections in immunosuppressed patients after marrow transplantation. Gastroenterology 88:1111–1117

66. McDonald GB, Shulman HM, Sullivan KM, Spencer GD (1986) Intestinal and hepatic complications of human bone marrow transplantation. Part II. Gastroenterology 90:770–784

67. McNamara MJ, Chalmers AG, Morgan M, Smith SEW (1986) Typhilitis in acute childhood leukemia: Radiological features. Clin Radiol 37:83–86

68. Mendelson RM, Nolan DJ (1985) The radiological features of chronic radiation enteritis. Clin Radiol 36:141–148

69. Meric F, Hirschl RB, Mahboubi S, et al. (1994) Prevention of radiation enteritis in children, using a pelvic mesh sling. J Pediatr Surg 29:917–922

70. Merine DS, Fishman EK, Jones B, Nussbaum AR, Simmons T (1987) Right lower quadrant pain in the immunocompromised patient: CT findings in 10 cases. Am J Radiol 149:1177–1179

71. Miller SD, Andrassey RJ (2003) Complications in paediatric surgical oncology. J Am Coll Surg 197 (5):832–837

72. Moir CR, Scudamore CH, Benny WB (1986) Typhlitis: Selective surgical management. Am J Surg 151:563–566

73. Mukamel E, Lupu A, deKernion JB (1986) Alum irrigation for severe bladder haemorrhage. J Urol 147:697–699

74. Nguyen DL, Wilson DA, Engelman ED, Sexauer CL, Nitschke R (1987) Serial sonograms to detect pancreatitis in children receiving L-asparaginase. Southern Med J 80:1133–1136

75. North JH Jr, Weber TK, Rodriguez-Bigas MA, Meropol NJ, Petrelli NJ (1996) The management of infectious and noninfectious anorectal complications in patients with leukemia. J Am Coll Surg 183:322–328

76. Ojala AE, Lanning FP, Lanning BM (1997) Abdominal ultrasound findings during and after treatment of childhood acute lymphoblastic leukemia. Med Pediatr Oncol 29:266–271

77. Okaneya T, Kontani K, Komiyama I, Takezaki T (1993) Severe cyclophosphamide-induced hemorrhagic cystitis successfully treated by total cystectomy with ileal neobladder substitution: A case report. J Urol 150:1909–1910

78. Paletta CE, Dehghan K (1994) Compartment syndrome in children. Ann Plast Surg 32:141–144

79. Pession A, Barbieri E (2005) Treatment and prevention of tumor lysis syndrome in children. Experience of Associazione Italiana Ematologia Oncologia Pediatrica Contrib Nephrol 147:80–92

80. Pestalozzi BC, Sotos GA, Choyke PL, Fisherman JS, Cowan KH, O'Shaughnessy JA (1993) Typhlitis resulting from treatment with taxol and doxorubicin in patients with metastatic breast cancer. Cancer 71:1797–1800

81. Purves JT, Graham ML, Ramakumar S (2005) Application of fibrin glue to damaged bladder mucosa in a case of BK viral hemorrhagic systitis. Urology 66(3):641–643

82. Redman JF, Kletzel M (1994) Cutaneous vesicostomy with direct intravesical application of formalin: Management of severe vesical hemorrhage resulting from high dose cyclophosphamide in boys. J Urol 151:1048–1050

83. Riker WL, Goldstein RI (1968) Malignant tumors of childhood masquerading as acute surgical conditions. J Pediatr Surg 3:580–583

84. Ritchey ML, Kelalis PP, Breslow N, et al. (1992) Surgical complications after nephrectomy for Wilms' tumor. Surg Gynec Obstet 175:507–514

85. Roberts JP, Atwell JD (1989) Testicular enlargement as a presenting feature of monocytic leukemia in an infant. J Pediatr Surg 24:1306–1307

86. Roy J, Snover D, Weisdorf S, Mulvahill A, Filipovich A, Weisdorf D (1991) Simultaneous upper and lower endoscopic biopsy in the diagnosis of intestinal graft-versus-host disease. Transplantation 51:642–646

87. Shamberger RC, Weinstein HJ, Delorey MJ, Levey RH (1986) Medical and surgical management of typhlitis in children with acute non-lymphocytic (myelogenous) leukaemia. Cancer 57:603–609

88. Shivshanker K, Chu DZ, Stroehlein JR, Nelson RS (1983) Gastrointestinal hemorrhage in the cancer patient. Gastrointest Endosc 29:273–275

89. Shurafa M, Shumaker E, Cronin S (1987) Prostaglandin F2-alpha bladder irrigation for control of intractable cyclophosphamide-induced hemorrhagic cystitis. J Urol 137:1230–1231

90. Singh TN, Devi KM, Devi KS (2005) Ecthyma gangrenosium: A rare cutaneous maifestation caused by pseudomonas aeruginosa without bacteraemia in a leukaemic patient – A case report. Indian J Med Microbiol 23(4):262–263

91. Skibber JM, Matter GJ, Pizzo PA, Lotze MT (1987) Right lower quadrant pain in young patients with leukaemia. Ann Surg 206:711–715

92. Sloas MM, Flynn PM, Kaste SC, Patrick CC (1993) Typhlitis in children with cancer: A 30–year experience. Clin Infect Dis 17:484–490

93. Spicer RD, Cywes S (1988) Pancreatitis in childhood. Pediatr Surg Int 3:33–36

94. Spirnak JP, Resnick MI, Hampel N, Persky L (1984) Fournier's gangrene: Report of 20 patients. J Urol 131:289–291

95. Stillwell TJ, Benson RC Jr (1988) Cyclophosphamide-induced hemorrhagic cystitis: A review of 100 patients. Cancer 61:451–457

96. Stone MM, Weinberg B, Beck AR, et al. (1986) Colonic obstruction in a child with von Recklinghausen's neurofibromatosis. J Pediatr Surg 21:741–743

97. Strand WR (1996) Haemorrhagic cystitis in children. Dialog Pediatr Urol 19:1–10

98. Surana R, Quinn FM, Guiney EJ (1992) Intussusception as a cause of postoperative intestinal obstruction in children. Brit J Surg 79:1200

99. Sussman SJ, Schiller RP, Shashikumar VL (1978) Fournier's syndrome. Am J Dis Child 132:1189–1191

100. Temeck BK, Venzon DJ, Moskaluk CA, Pass HI (1994) Thoracotomy for pulmonary mycoses in non-HIV-immunosuppressed patients. Ann Thorac Surg 58:333–338

101. Terdiman JP, Linker CA, Ries CA, Damon LE, Rugo HS, Ostroff JW (1996) The role of endoscopic evaluation in patients with suspected intestinal graft-versus-host disease after allogeneic bone-marrow transplantation. Endoscopy 28:680–685

102. Thomas ED, Storb R, Clift RA, et al. (1975) Bone marrow transplantation New Engl J Med 90:895–902

103. Top PC, Tissing WJ, Kuiper JW, Pieters R, van Eijck CH (2005) L-asparaginase-induced severe necrotizing pancreatitis successfully treated with percutaneous drainage. Pediatr Blood Cancer 44(1):95–97

104. Trivedi CD, Pitchumoni CS (2005) Drug-induced pancreatisis; An update. J Clin Gastroenterol 39(8):709–716

105. Tsakayannis DE, Kozakewich HP, Lillehei CW (1996) Acalculous cholecystitis in children. J Pediatr Surg 31:127–131

106. Tunell WP (1976) Haemangioendothelioma of the pancreas obstructing the common bile duct and duodenum. J Pediatr Surg 11:827–830

107. Turkeri LN, Lum LG, Uberti JP, et al. (1995) Prevention of hemorrhagic cystitis following allogeneic bone marrow transplant preparative regimens with cyclophosphamide and busulfan: Role of continuous bladder irrigation. J Urol 153:637–640

108. van Bekkum DW (1991) What is graft versus host disease? Bone Marrow Transpl 7(Suppl 2):110–111

109. Van Dyk OJ, Posso M (1975) Congenital leiomyomatous tumor in a newborn simulating jejunal atresia. J Pediatr Surg 10:139–141

110. Varki AP, Armitage JO, Feagler JR (1978) Typhilitis in acute leukaemia. Cancer 43:695–697

111. Wagner ML, Rosenberg HS, Fernbach DJ, Singleton EB (1970) Typhlitis, a complication of leukemia in childhood. Am J Radiol 109:341–350

112. Walker-Renard PB, Vaughan LM, Sahn SA (1994) Chemical pleurodesis for malignant pleural effusions. Ann Int Med 120:56–64

113. Wallace AM, Newman K (1991) Successful closure of intestinal fistulae in an infant using the somatostatin analogue SMS 201-995. J Pediatr Surg 26:1097–1100

114. Wang LY, Shih LY, Chang H, Jou ST, Lin KH, Yeh TC, Lin SF, Liang DC (2006) Recombinant urate oxidase (rasburicase) for the prevention and treatment of tumor lysis syndrome in patients with hematologic malignancies. Acta Maematol 115(1–2):35–38

115. Wayne ER, Campbell JB, Kosloske AM, Burrington JD (1976) Intussusception in the older child – Suspect lymphosarcoma. J Pediatr Surg 11:789–794

116. Weinberger M, Hollingsworth H, Feuerstein IM, Young NS, Pizzo PA (1993) Successful surgical management of neutropenic enterocolitis in two patients with severe aplastic anemia. Case reports and review of the literature. Arch Int Med 153:107–113

117. Wellwood JM, Jackson BT (1973) The intestinal complications of radiotherapy. Brit J Surg 60:814–818

118. Widburger R, Hollwarth ME (1989) Bronchoadenoma in childhood. Paediatr Surg Int 4:373–380

119. Williams BJ, Mulvihill DM, Pettus BJ, Brothers R, Costello P, Schoepf UJ (2006) Pediatric superior vena cava syndrome: Assessment at low radiation dose 64-slice CT angiography. Thorac Imaging 21(2):71–72

120. Wobbes T, Verschueren RC, Lubbers EJ, Jansen W, Paping RH (1984) Surgical aspects of radiation enteritis of the small bowel. Dis Colon Rectum 27:89–92

121. Yim AP, Low JM, Ng SK, Ho JK, Liu KK (1995) Video-assisted thoracoscopic surgery in the paediatric population. J Paediatr Child Health 31:192–196

122. Yokoyama T, Kondo H, Yokota T, et al. (1997) Colonoscopy for frank bloody stools associated with cancer chemotherapy. Jpn J Clin Oncol 27:111–114

123. Young G, Shende A (1998) Use of pamidronate in the management of acute cancer-related hyercalcemia in children. Med Pediatr Oncol 30:117–122

Supportive Care of Children with Cancer

23

Elspeth Livingston Brewis

Contents

23.1 Introduction

Although cancer is the leading disease cause of death in children, a general practitioner in the UK may only come across a single case in 30 years of general practice [1, 2]. Childhood cancer is a family problem; life for everyone is greatly disrupted and may never be the same again; it is not just the child who suffers [3]. With the observed increase in overall survival of patients with childhood tumors, instead of living with the fear of almost certain death, families experience considerable uncertainty concerning the expectation of long-term survival. In order to support or counsel the families of children with cancer, one needs staff that must have knowledge of the disease and its potential complications and outcome, and how other similar families have coped with the situation [4, 5]. It is then most important to provide parents, children, family members, and caretakers the opportunity to talk about their concerns, fears, hopes, anger, questions, and guilt. The role of support personnel and counselors is to provide the child and parents with time, attention, respect, and information [6].

Parents should be aware that in order to achieve the diagnosis, many essential tests and examinations are required.

23.2 Imparting the Diagnosis

Parents often remember very clearly how they were told that their child had a tumor, that it was cancer, and that it was a life-threatening condition. It is important that undisturbed privacy and adequate time are arranged before disclosing the diagnosis. It is also wise to interview both parents together, or one parent and another trusted person, as one alone may not be able to absorb the details. Discussion between two people given the same information is more helpful than one person trying to explain to others on their own, struggling to remember what was said and not what they thought was said [7]. Some parents will be utterly devastated and shocked at the news ("children don't get cancer"), while others might be "relieved" as the period of doubt and waiting for results has ended. Some might even have prepared themselves for very bad news [8, 9].

Parents should be informed that most children with cancer are involved in clinical trials following specific protocols. Parents need to know the name of the tumor, the prognosis (even if the outlook is poor), that "the best treatment" is available, and who will be looking after their child. It then becomes important to know the likely implications of the disease and any known disfigurement, scars, or disability resulting from treatment. The information should be imparted with full disclosure and honesty. An outline of the treatment program should be presented including the timing of surgery if required, whether adjunctive treatment such as chemotherapy or radiation will be needed, and what routine assessments are planned. They need a careful explanation of what a "clinical trial" means.

At the interview, it is advisable to have a nurse or other support personnel present who stays with the parents offering time for clarification of the information, and answering some of the practical questions, such as what to do about employment, finance, and traveling to and from the hospital. In their initial confusion, parents appreciate advice on how to handle the news, how to manage the lives of the other children in the family, and whether or who will be able to stay with the child in hospital. There are likely to have anxieties about guilt ("I should have taken him to the doctor sooner," "what have I done?"), or anger ("I took him several time to the doctor, I knew there was something wrong"), and fear for the health of the other children in the family. Some parents may even want to know at this early stage that their child will require long-term monitoring for many years to come. Parents need reassurance that they will be kept informed regarding their child's progress.

Parents go through a process of grieving for the loss of their child's health because his/her life is threatened, and they have no control over the situation. Difficult parental behavior might be demonstrated and could be the result of their effort to regain some control of their lives [10]. Often they feel shock and disbelief, along with a feeling of helplessness, failure and guilt [11]. Many parents value a second opportunity to discuss the details with the consultant a day or so later.

23.3 Following Diagnosis

Many treatments are administered as an inpatient, others might be managed at home together with visits to an ambulatory day care facility. However, careful consideration is given to how the family can manage the disruption, the distance from home to hospital, and whether they are likely to be compliant. Home care would ideally be supported be a visiting nurse specialist and social worker [11, 12].

Warning of the expected side-effects of the treatment is essential. Vomiting is a common side-effect although the use of routine antiemetics greatly reduces this problem. A central venous access catheter is used in many patients with cancer and parents must become familiar with catheter care where relevant. Every parent will be shocked and saddened by the loss of their child's hair and need assurance that this is a temporary occurrence and that it will grow back. Although not every child will lose his hair, it can be a devastating psychological problem for children of all ages and of both sexes. Most chemotherapy drugs cause neutropenia resulting in an increased risk of infection. Parents need guidance as to how to reduce the risk, and what steps they should take when pyrexia occurs at home. Contact with other children with viral exanthem or other infectious diseases should be avoided. Other drugs may cause thrombocytopenia. Children with low platelet count should avoid contact sports and other injuries, and are advised to use a soft toothbrush to reduce the risk of bleeding. It may be necessary to administer platelets or even red cell transfusions throughout the treatment period. Other drugs may cause abdominal pain or diarrhea. Sometimes granulocytic growth factor (GCSF) may be required to stimulate the bone marrow to increase production of white blood cells. Any planned immunizations should be delayed until therapy is completed.

23.3.1 What to Tell the Child

Parents need time for discussion about what to tell their child (perhaps with professional assistance), and to compose themselves before returning to him or her. Honesty and simplicity are the first "rules," however; initially it may not be appropriate to give all the details [13]. At the very least the child must have some idea of what is wrong, what to expect with regard to treatment and/or hospital admission, for his lump or pain, etc. The child's ability to understand his illness will vary according to his age, and the degree of communication and trust that already exists within the family; however, he should have an opportunity to ask his own questions [14]. It is wise to ensure that any question is fully understood before being answered, as children often do not use words in the same way used by adults. Even if a parent is not able to answer the child's questions, allowing discussion with a professional is better than denying the subject or telling lies as the child might find out the answer from others. Some parents prefer the consultant to tell the child the diagnosis in person. While being honest may be very difficult at the time, parents need to retain their child's trust. It is also honest to say "I don't know" when that is often the case with difficult questions. If a promise is made to "go and ask doctor" it is important to return with the doctor's response.

Children have the right to know the plan of their care and provided that they understand have their opinion respected [15]. In some countries the child's consent to treatment may be required [16]. Children soon learn about their condition and become very knowledgeable about their treatment, who the people are that care for him, the complex names of the drugs and investigation – and possibly what is happening to other children as well.

With permission from the parents, the outreach nurse liaises with the Primary Health Care Team to keep informed, as the family will need support when the child is out of hospital between treatments [17].

23.4 Implications for Parents and the Family Unit

For most children there will inevitably be short or long periods of hospitalization which mean further disruption to the family and its routines, and usually one or other parent will want to stay in hospital with the sick child most of the time. During these periods the child's physical, emotional, social, cultural, and educational needs must be met if he is to develop and grow through this experience [18]. The employers of either or both parents need to be informed and their cooperation sought. It is often the case that the main wage-earner will want to take special leave for at least a few days. It is vital that parents seek "time out" together to discuss feelings, fears, and problems with each other, offering each mutual support. Indeed they may need to be given the opportunity and encouragement to have occasional diversions at other times. In some instances they may see little of each other, or even avoid talking about such painful matters.

Parents have the task of explaining the situation to the rest of the wider family, including other children. They also have to arrange care for other children in the family, ensuring that they get to school, remain well fed, and are escorted to evening activities (for example sports, visiting friends). Wherever possible it is important for a well sibling to visit the child in the hospital. Children have vivid imaginations and they might think that their sibling is not coming home, or that they look worse than they actually are, that the parents are never coming home again, etc., and "seeing is believing." It is also important for the hospitalized child to see their sibling(s) for reassurance that family life goes on and he or she is not forgotten. The bonds between siblings are usually very strong, despite any age gap or usual rivalry. It is important, however, that if a child (or any visitor) is at all unwell they should not visit until their infection is completely cleared.

While children respond to treatments differently in general, when at home, they handle chemotherapy, ra-diotherapy, and surgery better than adults. A pattern of effect on each child becomes apparent, and parents learn to anticipate the "good days" and "bad days," although they can never be absolutely certain what will occur. Throughout treatment program, which might last for 6 months to a year or more, it is difficult for families to plan activities together. There is always the threat of a sudden return to hospital because of complications, treatment, tumor recurrence, or pyrexia. It is unwise to organize holidays until the treatment program is completed.

Throughout their ordeal the family needs the opportunity to discuss their fears. Many parents may imagine what would happen if their child died, may be convinced that this will happen, and some may even wish to discuss the possibility of death. They need to be encouraged to think positively – a positive and calm attitude in the parent helps the child, yet it is often the attitude of the child itself that helps the parent, especially the young preschool child. Older children have more taxing questions and deeper worries; teenagers may be very silent about their illness or rarely refuse treatment.

Frequently parents experience unjustified personal guilt and question why their child has cancer. It may be difficult for them to accept that there are no answers and that they are not at fault. Parents struggle to handle this difficult situation where they have little control. This situation imposes considerable strain on even the best partnerships. Some might feel like running away, (which occasionally happens, particularly when the parental relationship was somewhat unstable in the first place).

Some men find discussing their feelings very difficult and prefer to remain silent. They may feel responsible for having failed to protect the family. In contrast, women more commonly express their feelings and usually welcome someone to talk to. Parental anger may be manifested by short temper, frustration in handling other healthy children, or even accusations of some imaginary fault.

It is important to recognize the cultural and religious needs of families as a little flexibility with treatment may be required. Recognizing these factors and discussing the issues may address these needs. For example, Muslims may wish privacy next to their child at certain times for prayer. Dietary restriction may be applicable; Jehovah's Witness' may refuse infusion of blood and blood products. There are many aspects of all cultures and religions deserving consideration, and caregivers should be aware of the individual needs [18, 19]. Spiritual support from religious leaders may be helpful.

Ongoing communications with parents is vital in maintaining their trust. It is very frightening to return to one's child to find a blood transfusion in progress, or find that they are absent for a procedure or radiography when the family had not been told. Parents will panic that a complication has occurred, when in fact these measures were "routine" to the staff. The family needs to be updated frequently and hear that the treatment their child is receiving is effective and progressing.

Recognizing parental stress is vital in helping them care for their sick child [23]. In addition, there are often considerable traveling distances between hospital and home. A social worker is invaluable in assisting with advice regarding employment, financial arrangements, or even housing. Not infrequently parents seek additional information about their child's diagnosis independently, and occasionally obtaining information – in libraries or on the internet – may add to their confusion.

The counsel of an outreach nurse or social worker visiting the home to listen, empathize, and guide can provide invaluable support while the child is in hospital. Both the accompanying parent and child need the opportunity to have time to themselves as individuals, even for short periods, especially during long hospital admissions. Other parents in the ward or clinic can be supportive, as they are going through similar experiences. However, one should be sensitive to the additional stress that parents feel when other children in the ward or clinic are very ill, or die, as they and their child cannot be shielded from the realities of life.

23.5 Teenagers

Adolescent patients are a very special group as, in addition to their illness, they are coping with a period of teenage development, multiple body changes, self image, and looking to the future. Any acquired independence from their parents is likely to be reversed in some measure. Their body image might change through cancer treatment at a time when personal appearance and identification with their peer group is vital. They may struggle to carry on as "normal" in seeming silence [21]. Loss of self-esteem and confidence in youngsters facing diagnosis and treatment may be profound. Some may struggle to maintain contact with their friends, and opportunities for communication by telephone and e-mail are essential. Professional care givers should have an understanding of their needs: if a designated teenage orientated unit is unavailable (with appropriately trained staff and support), accommodation with privacy (which is vitally important to teenagers) in a children's facility may be preferable to the isolation of an inappropriate adult unit with elderly patients [21]. As stated, as far as possible family routines and discipline should be maintained [22].

A cancer unit designed for the specific interests of teenagers should have facilities for support from a youth worker, together with advice regarding fertility issues and career advice [23]. Most important is the company of fellow teenagers going through a similar experience. Teenagers have specific "teen-cultural" needs (such as modern music, e-mail, and "texting" communications).

Teenagers may have fears of returning to hospital for appointments, possible admissions, and anything that indicates that they are "different" from other teenagers. The parent of a teenager might want to reside with their child, against the wishes of the youngster. On the other hand, the youngster might be quietly pleased to have one of their parents nearby! These youngsters have more taxing questions and deeper worries, but some teenagers may be very silent about their illness [24, 25].

23.6 Remission and Returning Home

It is important for parents to be aware that a remission is no guarantee of cure. Children should remain out of hospital as much as possible, although this may be difficult with some treatment programs. The hospital discharge should be planned, and the community personnel alerted [26]. It is often not until the child returns home for the first time, be it after a short or long hospitalization, that the full impact of the diagnosis is realized. The parents are suddenly responsible for their child's care. For families who have experienced prolonged inpatient care for their child, returning home can be very daunting, and the confidence of parents might well be somewhat shaken. No longer is there someone easily available to give answers or reassurance therefore providing a contact telephone number at the hospital is essential.

However, the need to get on with family routines is helpful. The child may want to check that nothing has changed in the home during their absence, and often brightens up and eats better and enjoys being in their own environment. Inevitably there will be a lot of visitors, and the experience of this first return home might possibly not be a quiet one.

Immunosuppression due to chemotherapy increases the risk of infection, and the need to avoid direct contact with children or adults with varicella (chicken pox), herpes zoster (shingles), and measles (morbilli) must be stressed. The family is advised that crowded places should be avoided. Both the parents and the child may be anxious about the reaction of others to the child's altered appearance, (such as baldness, disfigurement, or increased/reduced weight, etc.) Adjustments may be necessary because of the use of a wheelchair, or crutches for example – and occasionally a family needs to move their home if access for the child is made impossible by treatment following surgery. Support and advice from occupational and physiotherapists, social worker, and dieticians may be invaluable.

While supporting each other, parents are helping the rest of the family to understand and cope. Parents can feel very isolated within their own community of family and friends, they become frustrated at explaining the circumstances and repeatedly hearing people say that they "understand" when they cannot, or "I don't know how you cope" when there is little choice. Whenever possible it might be wise for the employment of one parent to be re-established, to regain some "normality" for the family, provided that he is able to concentrate. If possible parents should maintain an attitude of calm as children can sense parental stress and become anxious.

The implications and repercussions on family life are considerable, and how each family adjusts will depend upon their normal strategies for living, family dynamics, and the availability of their extended support. The impact is greatest on the immediate family of parents, siblings, and grandparents, but uncles, aunts, cousins, friends, schoolmates, neighbors, etc. will also be affected. Most will have difficulty in knowing how to handle the situation. Sometimes friends withdraw from the family because they do not know what to say, and are apprehensive about facing a possible outburst of emotion (their own or that of the parents). Others may be unexpectedly helpful. Parents (and grandparents) may need encouragement to remember that despite the diagnosis of cancer the child is a normal child and requires appropriate disciplines. There is a temptation to give the sick child everything they want, at the cost of the others, yet this is not in their best interests. Once a child learns that they have control of the parents they could feel insecure through loss of discipline, and treatment compliance could be compromised.

Normal family life as it was has been altered and a new norm develops, even if for a temporary period. It is difficult to give the well children attention when anxieties are focused on the major implications of the diagnosis of cancer. Distance can add to these dilemmas. There are many things to be considered, in maintaining routines, and focusing their efforts in looking after all their children. As a result parents may become tired, not eat or sleep properly, and have no time for personal discussion. If this is not recognized a subsequent rift between parents may occur and can be difficult to heal. Not only does the sick child need care and attention but so do his parents.

During hospital contacts, whether as an inpatient or attending the day unit, both children and parents make contacts with other families. Indeed, many friendships develop as time goes on, some lasting throughout a child's cancer journey, and even beyond. This element of support, found by the parents themselves, plays a vital role in helping families to cope.

23.7 The Other Children

Children over 3 years of age can be involved in a playgroup, nursery, or school. Whenever possible the sick child should continue to attend, or at least interact with his peer group so that the eventual return to group/school will be a smooth transition. Children worry about their appearance (alopecia, disfigurement, body weight changes, etc.) not wanting to be different from their peers. There is also the risk that others may jeer. When a return to school is likely, it is helpful for a professional (e.g., the oncology outreach nurse, and hospital teacher or social worker) to have a meeting at school together with a parent, the child, teachers, and school nurse to provide information and dispel anxieties. This includes information regarding treatment patterns and relevant instructions for specific concerns including anticipated attendance, hair loss, fatigue, levels of concentration, and any special equipment required [27]. Additionally, there is an opportunity to decide what to tell the other school children. If given an opportunity to ask questions the affected child would then know how his anxieties would be handled on returning to school. For a child who has had lengthy hospitalizations or has residual disability, the advice and support of an educational psychologist is important. Sometimes a return to part-time studies initially is relevant and, for a few, home tuition may be appropriate in the short-term. Often contact sports have to be avoided until recovery has reached an adequate stage [28]. The risk of infection and any tendency to bruising require explanations. Whether or not the child will be able to return to his own normal activities will vary greatly.

A single parent may need extra assistance, yet some with family support and their own independence have no additional difficulties. Parents should be encouraged to keep up their own activities and social contacts, especially when treatment activities are based away from home.

Not only do grandparents feel hurt that their grandchild has cancer, but they may feel helpless in assisting their child (the parent of the ill child). Some will be very supportive and help with the other children or domestic duties, and others may be over-bearing and attempts become controlling. They should discuss with the child's parents what is wanted. Some seem totally unable to handle the situation, and may even need looking after themselves, thus adding to the child's parents' dilemma.

Children worry about each other and need the opportunity to play together if at all possible. Sometimes children may think they are to blame for their sibling's illness and reassurance is needed to dispel this fear [29]. Siblings, if not given the opportunity to be informed or involved, will possibly be "attention seeking," demonstrate difficult behavior, or be disruptive [30]. They will feel neglected and isolated if they see little of their parents. However, some will revel in the attention from grandparents or aunts. School or club activities may be the only "normal time" in their lives during this period, yet disruption here may also be demonstrated. It is wise for a sibling's schoolteacher to be aware of the stress that their pupil is experiencing, as sometimes children will confide in a trusted teacher. When the sick child returns home, parents' loyalties become divided, but planning special time with the other children is more valuable than gifts.

Long periods of hospitalization can be very difficult, especially when the sick child comes home and re-establishes his position, and siblings are thrown into a secondary role as the focus of the parents' attention is on the sick child [31]. The sibling's trust in adults can be shaken, particularly if the sick child is suddenly taken to hospital in the middle of the night, with a fever, for example. Good communications within the family is of vital importance in reducing misunderstandings, especially when the sick child has to return to the hospital for further treatment [32].

There are national charitable associations in the UK (for example CancerBACUP), [21, 22] and other countries, that assist families with information and support. Many local groups have been formed for assisting families with moral support and providing practical help [23, 33].

23.8 Surviving Cancer

When the treatment program is complete, parents can experience relief that family life may return to relative normality, yet harbor fear of what the future may hold for their child as active treatment to effect a "cure" has been completed. As parents might worry less about the child and have more time for their own feelings, some can become depressed, or experience the return of confused feelings. This might occur in a parent who apparently handled the situation well initially when in reality they were denied personal time to think of themselves and their own feelings. The continued contact with other families during hospitalization may help lessen the feeling of "isolation" and might last for many months or years.

"It's not over till it's over." No matter how long after the diagnosis and treatment for cancer, when the child experiences pyrexia, an ache, or pain, there will always be anxieties about tumor recurrence. Parents eventually learn to adjust and recognize the common ailments without being overly concerned. They may continue to fear the routine outpatient appointment worrying they may hear some negative news, e.g., a relapse. The older child could also have these anxieties and even the very young can fear returning to hospital [34]. This is a phenomenon that family and friends may not understand.

Once treatment is completed, the child will often regain his former lifestyle, interests, and activities – and should be encouraged to do so. However, problems as a result of the cancer or treatment may continue to exist. The younger the age of the child when receiving aggressive treatment, the greater the potential for problems relating to development. Examples include intelligence changes after brain irradiation, or shortened stature after spinal radiotherapy, etc. [2, 33]. The type of anxieties may change with time – will they be fertile? Will they marry?

It is not uncommon for parents to suspect an episode of relapse before being told. The experience of the disease relapsing is more devastating than when it was first diagnosed, and parents find this very difficult to handle. Having learned to "get back to normal," the significance of the diagnosis at relapse hits harder. This time they already know the implications of treatment – the return to disruption of family life and employment and the actual vulnerability of their child's life [29]. Initially these adjustments all had to be made stage by stage; at relapse they immediately move from ignorance to full realization. The practical readjustments vary depending on possible changes in family circumstances and the new treatment program that is offered.

23.9 Multidisciplinary Team of Social Worker, Play and Occupational Therapists, Play Specialists, Teacher, Dietician, Physiotherapist, Psychologist

There are many professional disciplines involved in the care of a child with cancer, other than the pediatrician and pediatric medical and surgical oncology specialists, and nurses trained in the care of sick children with cancer. These include the social worker, the play or occupational therapist, play leader and assistants, dietician, pharmacist, the hospital school teacher, physiotherapist, psychologist, speech therapist, and others.

Play is an important element of normal development, learning, and expression and is necessary for the sick child, whether in hospital or at home. Additionally, focused play helps the child to understand what is to happen to him. Both parents need to understand the role each plays in the care of their child.

The involvement of teachers in the hospital continuing formal education is important for school-age children. Education is a normal part of life and helps to ensure a smooth transition to school and home life.

Caring for children with cancer is a stressful experience. There should be opportunities for all those professionals involved to interact and discuss needs and changes in the progress of the children in their care. The nature of the treatment means that inevitably children and families become well known, and the effects of relapses and deaths can be considerable and should be recognized. Meetings also provide an opportunity to support each other [36]. Psychological support, whether peer group or professional counseling, should be available for caregivers, with complete confidentiality [6].

23.10 Pediatric Oncology Outreach Nurse

In the UK most centers treating childhood cancer have a pediatric oncology outreach nurse specialist with knowledge of the disease and treatment. The nurse should visit the child and/or parents at home and evaluate how they are coping, listen, advise, teach, and counsel [37, 38]. It is important to become familiar with the parents and child at diagnosis in order for there to be mutual trust to ease the family through the experiences and help with practical nursing skills in the home. In the UK the nurse also administers relevant home treatment [12]. and sets aside time to maintain contact with the family in the ward, in outpatient clinics, at home, and to link with other disciplines needed for the continuing care of the child throughout the months and years ahead. A ward nurse, identified as a named nurse, offers continuity of care and support particularly during admissions [37].

An early visit to the home can provide the opportunity to clarify the understanding of the parents regarding care, medication, and future appointments, etc. How this is done will depend upon the family's specific needs and the local resources available. There is time to discuss feelings and anxieties when the nurse is the visitor [38]. The specialist outreach nurse has a particular role in enabling the child to return to school, and the school to accept the child with their current and potential problems. The Specialist Role is particularly important in palliative and terminal home care, liaising with all the services required in such a situation.

23.11 Palliation, Terminal Care and Bereavement

Palliation is an approach to care which continues from diagnosis, encompassing the whole child, his family, and their needs [41, 42]. It is more commonly thought of as starting when active, curative treatment fails and is no longer appropriate. This does not mean cessation of care, but that the goal treatment is changed aiming for a good quality of life until the time of death [43]. There are Phase II and Phase III trial drugs available, appropriate for consideration in many conditions. Supportive therapy at this stage can sometimes be aggressive, such as radiotherapy given specifically for pain relief, antibiotics in the treatment of infection, or occasionally some other chemotherapeutic or surgical intervention for symptom relief (e.g., in bowel obstruction). All supportive measures as during active treatment – play, school, and all other therapists – continue as before, although changes and adjustments may be necessary.

When death is inevitable, there must be a further discussion between doctor and parents, so that par-

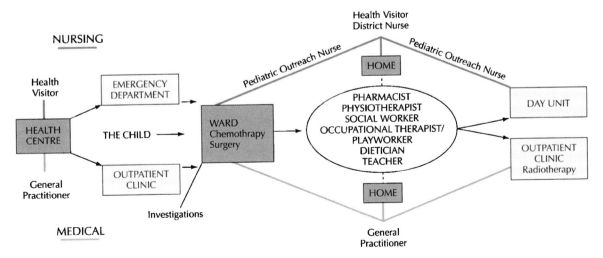

Fig. 23.1 Communications flow chart demonstrating progression from admission, diagnosis and treatment.

ents understand that the end is near. The presence of a nurse during the discussion is useful. If the child is to be nursed at home the presence of the outreach nurse is particularly valuable [37, 40]. It is difficult to explain, and accept, that the child has relapsed and that this time there will be no curative treatment but only that which will hopefully provide a good quality of life for as long as possible. The parent may have suspected that the disease was active again, but probably never thought that nothing more could be done. Absolute honesty is important, giving the parents time for the new information to be understood. Parents have the rest of their lives to live and should feel that everything has been done to try to achieve a cure for their child. There may be hope to have time for some special experiences (there is sometimes "a lot of living to do"), and at the very least hope of comfort [38]. Parents are entering a different period of uncertainty. Even during palliation a Family Bereavement Service can offer support in helping the adjustment to the impending loss.

It does not matter how long the death of a child has been expected, the fact that they are going to die possibly "soon" is something parents never want to hear. However, when death will occur can only be estimated, and only the very broadest guidelines should be offered – each day should be viewed as a good day whether the life-span is expected to last days, weeks, or months.

Whether the child will die at home, in a hospice, or hospital should be discussed [44]; the choice is the parents' and they should be reassured that they can change their minds at any time, and their decision would be respected. It may be appropriate to involve the child or young person in the discussion, depending on their knowledge. After perhaps years of illness working with a particular hospital team, changing supportive caregivers at this time can be very difficult, and it may take a while for parents to feel confident with any change.

23.12 At Home

The general medical practitioner may have had little input due to the hospital attendance of the child during treatment. He can feel vulnerable, as it is rare for a child to die at home [40]. In advance of terminal care at home, a meeting between the general practitioner and other professionals is appropriate. It provides an opportunity for discussion of the child's present status, and the potential progress and problems. It is important to identify a key worker. The link provided by an outreach nurse enables a smooth transition, coordination of care, promoting confidence, and reducing feelings of isolation [45]. This link also facilitates the availability of oncology consultant advice and possibly a combined home visit with the general practitioner and consultant. Parents need the assurance of continued support, to know where it would come from, and who would provide any equipment that may be needed. The parents should become confident in caring for the child at home. They need to know who to contact if they need help or advice. Identifying a key professional, also known to all team members, prevents confusion [39]. This would usually be the outreach nurse.

The visiting nurse's role is to encourage the parents to do as much of the child's care as they wish and are able. Sometimes parents could avoid unnecessary visits to the hospital by developing new skills. Parents need the assurance that they can change the choice of place where their child will die at any time [27]. It is important for parents and children to feel that they have control of their lives, and organize routines for themselves.

Fear of the unknown and isolation can be very difficult to handle. Some children, with adequate symptom control, may have a fairly long palliative phase and continue with normal activities, including school, right up to weeks or even days before dying, when they enter a terminal phase. During this time there can be a number of positive experiences for the family and considerable fun too. With increasing dependence, the mother can become the one the child is likely to constantly seek, which can be difficult for an attentive father. Occasionally an estranged parent returns to the home environment for the sake of the child.

23.12.1 Child's Questions

The questions children ask will depend very much on their development, understanding, and prior experience. They often overhear conversations or sense parental anxieties and become aware that circumstances have changed. They may sense that they are not getting better despite treatments and want to know why. In time they adjust, but may be unaware that they might die [46]. Those who have lost a grandparent or a favorite pet may have some insight into death [48, 49]. Children are often aware that some other children are not around any longer and may have died.

Children need to ask questions with the confidence that they will be given an honest answer, as it takes courage for a child to ask difficult questions. The first person to hear searching questions, or statements, is likely to be one of the parents. It is important to clarify the question, to answer honestly exactly what is asked and no more, taking time to consider the reply. It may be appropriate to ask if the child has thought of an answer.

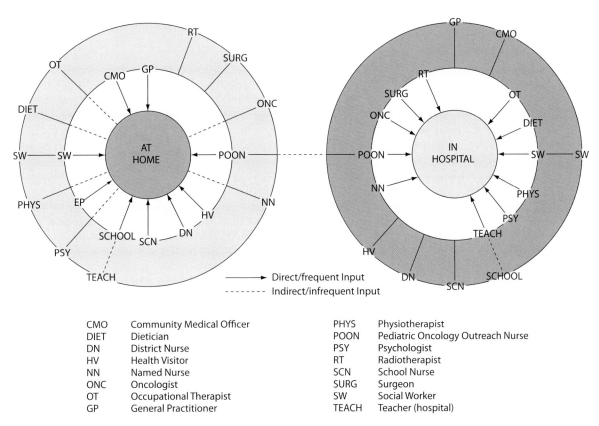

CMO	Community Medical Officer	PHYS	Physiotherapist
DIET	Dietician	POON	Pediatric Oncology Outreach Nurse
DN	District Nurse	PSY	Psychologist
HV	Health Visitor	RT	Radiotherapist
NN	Named Nurse	SCN	School Nurse
ONC	Oncologist	SURG	Surgeon
OT	Occupational Therapist	SW	Social Worker
GP	General Practitioner	TEACH	Teacher (hospital)

Fig. 23.2 This figure illustrates the contacts of the various disciplines involved with the child and the carers

Sometimes children will not ask questions of a parent because they do not want to upset them, or they do not wish to be confronted by an answer they do not want to hear. They might ask a favorite relative, teacher or professional and need assurance that confidentiality will be respected. It is not wrong to say "I don't know," but if one has offered to find out an answer one must return with a reply. It is important not to be shocked at any subject the child chooses, allowing discussion if appropriate, or at least not disallowing the subject. The child will probably change the subject as soon as he has heard enough.

It is important that the subject of death, if asked, is not taboo as this can create other difficulties. Sometimes a child might simply be trying to feel if it is safe to talk about dying. It might be that he just wants the confirmation of love and that he would be missed, or the reassurance that his parents would be alright. The young child could also have feelings of anger, anxiety, fear of separation and being unable to ask questions, so may withdraw feeling insecure [50].

Adolescents may be the most challenging group of patients, as teenagers sometimes appear to consider themselves "immortal" as they often take many risks. They may have feelings of grief (anger, disbelief, anxiety, etc.) manifested by verbal outbursts and body lan-

guage. Some, however, will fully understand the nature of the situation and organize their own funeral [51].

A daily routine is important in any child's life, therefore he should continue attending school whenever possible and maintain contact with friends. Home schooling could be arranged for when it becomes inappropriate to attend the school itself, continuing with education for as long as possible. However, a special activity, trip or event may be considered provided safety is assured, finances are available, and the child is well enough to travel.

Part of the normal routines for children with cancer are hospital visits to the outpatient department or some day facility. Such visits should continue until they cease to be relevant, or the child and parent no longer wish to attend, or traveling becomes too much of an effort for the child.

Siblings of cancer patients need to be involved in caring for their sick sibling if they wish to participate; their companionship is important for the present and their future. At some point the other children should at least be given definite opportunities to ask their own questions; others may need to be told that their sibling might, or will die, as appropriate [46]. Children often overhear conversations, or feel a strained atmosphere, and rather than make it worse may seek to move away from the cause [52], e.g., have a "sleep-over" with a young friend.

As the news that the child will die passes through the family, extended family members will often visit. There may be a need to control this as too many visitors can be stressful for both the child and parents. Allocating one "visitor free" afternoon per week might be one way of permitting some rest. Telephone calls can be redirected to a trusted family member.

23.13 Hospice Care

Often the child could be cared for at home, unless his symptoms cannot be managed by the family and the primary health care team, or the parents wish not to be on their own, or that he would not actually die at home. In the hospice the parents should be as involved with their child as they wish or are able, so that they feel they have done everything that they could for their child. The atmosphere of relaxation and time allows the family to make the best use of their time for all the family and the niceties of life, allowing as much of home life as is possible, with family outings, visits to and from other family members and friends, etc. Accommodation for any sibling is likely to be more readily available in a hospice. In the hospice the staff can take over some of the technical tasks that the child needs, affording the parents real time with their child and their other children. The hospice is also available for respite periods, giving the family a holiday from the total responsibilities and stresses of care – the family too would receive care [53].

It is necessary for an identified nurse to be allocated to look after the child and family for every shift in the 24 hours. As confidence and familiarity grows, it might be possible for the parents to go away to do something else knowing that their child will not be left alone. In this way the parents too can receive care from the staff. Having their own things about them helps parents to make the environment homey, and staff can find ways to help them have some control of their lives and their child's care.

Although the clinical environment of a hospital has the disadvantage of possibly being rushed, the people available to give support would already be familiar.

23.14 Symptom Control

The aim of care, as during active treatment, is to allow the fullest quality of life that symptoms and circumstances will permit. It is pertinent to warn parents of any problems that are likely to occur, and some parents may even ask how their child will die. While it is not possible to be precise, they are probably also

seeking reassurance that every effort will be made to prevent suffering, and to keep their child at home. It is relevant to offer only broad statements at this point. Supporting positive attitudes in the parents will help them to retain some "normality" and the child's confidence. It is important to remember the potential for causing additional problems in an attempt to control symptoms. Some children may hide symptoms from their parents – fearing that if they declare pain or nausea, for example, they will be sent to hospital, or cause their parents extra worry. Some simply lack the words to describe how they feel.

It is not practical to identify every possible symptom that may occur, therefore the commonest problems are noted here. Whenever a symptom occurs it is essential to consider the likely cause as its origin will direct the treatment for control. For example, abdominal pain would not be treated with analgesia if the real cause is unrelieved constipation, a urinary tract infection, spasms, or anxiety. Similarly if a child already receiving morphine had a headache, unrelated to expected complications of the disease, it is reasonable to prescribe paracetamol (US: acetaminophen) for such a common problem. Some unusual symptoms are specific to the diagnosis, for example, some children with brain tumors experience coldness in the limbs. The children themselves may not be particularly aware of this, but the caregivers may express concern. The symptoms come and go, and do not require treatment, other than to increase clothing around the limbs.

Throughout palliation, medications may well increase in number and complexity in an attempt to control unwanted symptoms. However, it is wise to constantly review the medications prescribed and administered, as subsequent prescriptions may be incompatible, or a previous medicine become redundant. Medication can become irksome for the child to take, therefore the minimum dose and frequency necessary for comfort and function should be prescribed. The team looking after the child at home also needs to have confidence in the parents' ability to administer medicines appropriately.

The commonest fear of parents is that the child might suffer pain. Reassurance is needed that every effort will be made to alleviate this symptom [54]. If a child says he has pain, he needs to be believed, and patience applied to discover its cause. Some children behave differently in the presence of pain and caregivers need to recognize body language as the child's energy level diminishes and he becomes quiet and withdrawn, or possibly irritable [55]. Parents are sometimes unable to identify and report pain, especially in those children who have not learned how to describe it. Reassurance, time and an understanding listener or diversion, e.g., play activities, could be opportunities for identifying untreated pain [56]. The cause could also be psychological – worry, anxiety, insecurity, or depression, fear for himself or separation from his parents, or "just not himself" and unable to describe how he feels. Tools for gauging pain, for example a row of four or five faces with expressions varying from very happy to very sad in relation to no pain and the worst pain might be appropriate (careful explanation is needed so that there is no confusion with mood or feelings) [57, 58]. In assessing pain, language appropriate to the child's understanding should be used. The word "pain" may mean little to some small children, and "hurt" or "sore" might be the nearest they can explain – "mild" and "severe" may be better understood if "little" or "big" sore/hurt is used [59, 60]. In the case of children under 2 years of age we need to rely on our own observations and very accurate reporting from the parents.

The pain experienced might depend upon the tumor type, the site of metastases, or any unrelated cause. Some children experience no pain at all, others may only need paracetamol, and yet others need large doses of morphine combined with other analgesic agents. Even a little uncontrolled pain will be bitterly remembered by surviving parents. Further discussion concerning pain management can be found in Chap. 28.

In general, the pain of many procedures can be eliminated or at least reduced to a minimum by simple measures – explanation (to remove fear), a topical anesthetic cream before venepunctures, a respectful approach encouraging trust in the appropriately qualified practitioner [61]. Restraint is never appropriate. Paracetamol is usually very effective in children in the first instance, allowing it time to take effect. The experience of pain is very tiring, and may cause sleepiness.

Morphine-containing drugs cause constipation that can be managed by the administration of prophylactic laxatives or stool softeners. Itchiness of the skin may appear in the first 48 h of morphine administration (a young child might be seen rubbing the end of his nose) and can be resolved by prescribing an antihistamine if it is persistent. Nausea or vomiting may occur in some children and a few develop hypersensitivity to sound and request that the television volume is turned down.

If the oral route is no longer feasible or desirable a subcutaneous infusion can produce good, even pain relief, with little or no disturbance of activities. Most children adapt well and some parents may be able to learn the necessary skills. A variety of ambulatory pumps allow full mobility.

Parents often worry that the child will become addicted to morphine and need reassurance that this is not a major problem when it is required for pain relief. It could be removed in a controlled way if it were no longer needed. For example, morphine might be required for severe bone pain due to metastases; once

the desired effect of a radiotherapy course is evident, the morphine can be reduced or even stopped.

It may be appropriate for neuropathic pain in a clearly defined area to be relieved by a minute transdermal electrical impulse. Their diverting action by counter stimulation can be invaluable for focused pain relief.

Steroids have many benefits, not least of which is the relief of bone pain, its anti-inflammatory effect, or reduction of cerebral edema. However, if high doses are required there is a risk of Cushing's syndrome, associated with a change in body image (obesity, and possibly diabetes mellitus). This problem could be unacceptable to parents especially if the benefits are short-lived. Steroids also reduce immunity, and infection problems could result. Steroids are often used in "short sharp" doses in patients with a brain tumor.

Nonsteroidal anti-inflammatory drugs may be used for musculoskeletal pain, spasm, or inflammation. In addition to relieving general aches and pains, paracetamol is very useful as an antipyretic agent.

Vomiting can be a very distressing symptom and on occasions a difficult one to control. Simple measures to achieve control should be considered including altering the timing of drugs, or food, the types of food, the positioning of the child during a meal and avoidance of unpleasant smells. Dramatic or persistent vomiting or nausea requires treatment. It is important to identify the cause of vomiting (which could be anxiety, pain, treatment, constipation, metastases, etc.) A child who has suffered vomiting during chemotherapy may have become used to a particular antiemetic. Some drugs cause sleepiness or thirst, and others may result in anxiety and hyperactivity. (An antiemetic can be added to the subcutaneous preparations but may not be tolerated locally). Any increased drowsiness caused by the antiemetics may be preferable to nausea or vomiting. Abdominal spasm may occur and require administration of an antispasmodic.

The child's nutrition should be maintained, with supplements if necessary, throughout the period of palliation, but tube feeding avoided. There could come a point when it no longer remains appropriate to encourage a child to eat more than he wishes, but fluid intake should always be encouraged – thirst can be distressing. As the child's activity decreases, the daily calories required becomes reduced; however, this is an area that parents find most distressing, and needs careful explanation.

Breathing can become a problem in patients with lung metastases, for example. The respiratory distress may be associated with cough and is best soothed by using morphine, which also reduces the anxiety level. The benefits of oxygen are usually short-lived, and therefore rarely appropriate. Often the dyspnoea is more distressing to the observer than to the patient himself, but the draught caused by the oxygen may be comforting. Occasionally a bronchodilator could be useful in relieving bronchospasm. In the presence of a significant pleural effusion, a pleural tap may give effective relief.

Bladder retention maybe painful and if so should be relived by catheterization. An indwelling catheter may be necessary in some instances. An indwelling catheter would not mean that the child would be either bed- or housebound, although it would mean some readjustment. Urinary infections are painful and distressing and the administration of an appropriate antibiotic is very justified.

Patients with brain tumors may experience seizures. The events may appear for the first time as the child's condition deteriorates. Controlling seizure activity may be difficult, but an initial benefit for some can be achieved by giving a rectal preparation of diazepam. Medication might be appropriate if there were general agitation, or anxiety; it might be reasonable to prescribe another appropriate drug.

Some children may develop severe anemia as a result of chemotherapy or tumor infiltration of the bone marrow. A blood transfusion could be justified in the interest of allowing activity and improving the quality of life.

23.15 Support Networks

All those professions who helped in the active treatment phase will continue to have a role whether care is given at home, hospice, or hospital, although their approach will change as care needs change. Play, education, and schooling are essential elements to the life of a child, no matter the age, and the contribution of these specialists will help to uphold a degree of normality and help to continue normal routines. Periodically dietary intake can vary with treatment and morbidity, and the nutritionist has a vital role, the advice changing accordingly. The physiotherapist can encourage activity, and help remove fear of bodily changes and restrictions in limbs, etc. Skin care becomes especially important as mobility decreases. Scratching an itchy skin, sweating dryness, sores, etc., cause additional problems. Although not needed by all individuals, a clinical psychologist should be available for support and advice to alleviate emotional difficulties in child and/or parents.

23.16 Spiritual and Religious Support

All individuals have the right to respect, privacy, and dignity irrespective of religion (or none), cultural or ethnic considerations. Children should be allowed the freedom to ask questions on present issues, and express their fears and thoughts for the future. The spiritual needs of the patient and family should not be neglected and access to the appropriate leaders may be needed for support. The child may not be able to discuss such fears with his parents, therefore another person (possibly a professional) should be available to be entrusted with his confidence [56]. The child needs the reassurance of such company, love and an atmosphere of confidence and trust.

23.17 Terminal Care

Terminal care is defined as the phase of a patient's care in which death is imminent. During this phase therapies can be reduced as they become "redundant" – "heroic" interventions become inappropriate, and the major goal is to create an atmosphere promoting the comfort of the patient [60]. Ongoing opportunities to discuss progress and changes with doctors are invaluable. These help build a planned approach for the parents who are caring for their child, whether they are at home, in the hospice, or hospital. As the child's condition deteriorates, parental care responsibilities may become more difficult and the professional caregiver may assume a greater role in the nursing care, perhaps relieving the parents of some of the responsibilities they had assumed, albeit with guidance during earlier stages. Indicating the assistance available to them enables them to have more time with their child, and it may help to prevent any additional guilt feelings. However, parents become exhausted, and the idea of relinquishing responsibility may be difficult for them to accept.

23.17.1 Children's Fears

Even a young child can be aware of a change in their body image, actual or potential, or a decreasing ability to do things and may get frustrated and angry and not wish people to see the changes. The older child may discuss such things. As the terminal state progresses the child may have an increased wish for privacy. There are times when a child's privacy may need to be specifically respected, yet they may fear going to sleep, or being left alone. Following long months of more and more treatment, children realize they are not getting better, and some children come to know that they are dying; the very young may make statements of facts in their play (e.g., "heaven is a nice place of snow and flowers," others might ask "what is heaven like?") [47]. The older child might even want to arrange their own funeral, or decide who will have his belongings. As long as the child discovers that it is safe to talk about these things, he will decide how much is discussed. The child's progress to understand what is happening will vary according to age and development, life experience, and overheard conversations. The very young may fear separation and demand a parent (usually the mother) to be present all the time [47]. The teenager may be fully aware, and even assume a degree of control – he or she may or may not discuss feelings, fears, etc.

23.17.2 Parents Preparing for the Child's Death

Many parents of children who die may never have attended a funeral before. They might seek information from the doctor, spiritual adviser, nurse, or social worker as to what will happen and how to handle it. It may be helpful to indicate that they might have difficult questions to ask, and that someone is always available to answer them at any time. Some parents only want to face such questions after the child has died, while others may arrange the funeral in detail well in advance.

During the final phase, when a simple enquiry "how is the child?," seems inappropriate, it is important to remain in contact with the family. Professionals should remember that their feelings can be seen through their own body language and communicated to the dying child, resulting in him withdrawing his trust and causing a feeling of insecurity. Even though conversations may not be relevant, listening will help, and neither parent nor child should be ignored, as they already feel isolated in their own unique situation. The need for a professional presence may change; some parents will be confident enough to have less of a presence, others might wish for more and it is important for the professional to be sensitive to the subtle changes. The next home visit or communication should be arranged on leaving the house, with the understanding that it can be cancelled or rearranged according to the family needs.

As time slips away, being with their child becomes very precious for parents, and they may forget to look after themselves and fail to eat properly. As parents see that life is ebbing away, they may ask "How long?," "How will I know?," "How will I cope?," "Who will I call?" This last question is perhaps the easiest, and one should have the knowledge to give relevant guidance, and reassurance that they need not be alone However, most parents wish to be present when their child dies if at all possible, and some parents may even wish to be on their own if possible. Occasionally some may start to "back away" emotionally from their child through fear of the unknown. Professionals should not remove all hope, but guide the change to hope for realistic goals of comfort and support [63].

Professionals involved in care can provide opportunities for parents to physically relax (even if they cannot sleep), and not feel guilty for taking short breaks from the bedside. A Family Bereavement Service can provide support even before a child dies. Professionals also have their feelings – opportunities should be identified for mutual support. A means of reporting progress of the child and family back to the base team members can prove supportive.

23.18 After the Child Dies

No matter for how long the child's death has been expected, there is shock at the time of death and behavior will vary from normality or quiet numbness to hysteria and anything in between. Most parents manage to cope and function. Each parent will probably respond differently at the time of the child's death (and perhaps throughout the bereavement). There is no rush and the parents should have as much time with their dead child as they wish, before they are washed and dressed [38]. Even in a hospital setting parents should be given the opportunity to do this themselves, this last act could help them feel that they did everything they possibly could. Parents need time and privacy to say goodbye to their loved one.

Support and guidance should be available to the parents from doctors, nurses, religious leaders, or funeral director. It is important for the funeral to be arranged according to the parents' wishes, considering religious or cultural rites and feasibility. Parents should make as many of the arrangements themselves as they wish, rather than have another family member take over the task.

It is easy to think that siblings should be shielded from such experiences, but they could benefit from being given the choice of being involved, with a simple, honest explanation of what has happened, and what will happen. It is important for the sibling not to feel left out of these events. It is sensible to allow siblings the choice of seeing the child who has just died, as this can help them understand about death. A straightforward explanation of how their dead sibling looks and feels should be offered before the child makes his decision to see the body or not. If this experience is denied it is possible that the sibling might have worse ideas about death, or later accuse a parent because he was not given the choice. Siblings can also have a role in helping to choose clothes and flowers, and maybe what to put in the coffin to accompany the child. However, one can only guide parents, they are the ones who will live with their decisions, and the professional can only offer advice and present options.

Although the interval before the funeral may seem long, this is a valuable adjusting period for the parents, siblings, and the rest of the family. The funeral itself is a ceremony that gives the opportunity to openly grieve and say goodbye. At this stage some parents may not "feel anything at all" and function almost as normal (which can be disturbing to other family members), while other bereaved parents may only be able to function with assistance or encouragement.

Many of the feelings that parents experience at diagnosis return – anger, disbelief, anxiety, guilt, as well as sadness. For some there might be a feeling of relief if the last illness was protracted and had unpleasant aspects. Parents who have been able to participate in their child's care can at least have the feeling of knowing that they did their best. The question "why" returns causing anguish – "Why did he die, why did he get cancer, why did the cancer come back when 'it had been put away?'" Some parents might feel bitterness. There can be many expressions of anger especially when the loss is sudden. Some parents, even at this time, can express gratitude to professionals for all that has been done in trying to treat the cancer, or for helping to ease the passage to death, for the treatment, the support, etc., which can be difficult for professionals to accept – "they only did their job."

Losing a child is the worst experience in life. The parent has lost part of himself and some feel physically empty [64, 65]. Grieving is a very tiring exercise. The day no longer has the intense activity and anxiety of caring for the dying child. It takes a lot of effort performing even the simplest tasks, such as making tea, getting out of bed, etc. Life seems to have lost its purpose; however, caring for the other children can provide some purpose to each day.

Parental self-esteem becomes low, and the feeling of worthlessness is compounded by the fact that despite their efforts their child died [49]. Parents can feel guilt that they have failed, or survived, and become short tempered over even minor events. For example, they may feel irritation at another child, because that child is well, doing normal things, and the child who has died cannot. Yet parents may become over protective of surviving children, and fear that they too could come to harm or even, irrationally, fear they too might die, while giving parents a reason for living [29].

Tiredness continues as the parents find sleeping difficult, have no interest in eating, and certainly no interest in going to find diversion with friends. Some people avoid going to the usual shops for fear of meeting someone who does not know that their child has died. One parent might make frequent (even daily) visits to the grave over many months, and another hardly visits at all. In time parents pretend that life is "fine" because everyone around them seems to expect that they are getting "better" and will "get over it." Other people get on with their lives, and the initial support and attention lessens. It can seem to the parents that others have

forgotten their child, as friends and family perhaps become wearied of having to listen to the bereaved. The situation becomes very isolating. However, gradually better days appear between the sad ones.

For some, particularly mothers, the need to talk is very strong; for others, usually fathers, it is too painful to talk about their deceased child. Because of this a father might feel accused that he cares less than the mother. Parents often have a fear of forgetting, and talking about their child is one way to keep memories alive. They need frequent reassurance that they will not forget. For some there can be happy dreams, and for others no dreams or maybe disturbing ones. With patient listening and reassurance things will probably improve. There can be feelings of the child being near them, as they "search" for him. Photographs, clothes (which might still have the child's smell), toys, etc. become very precious reminders. Indeed a parent may not allow the other children to play with his toys, while others may be pleased to see toys still being actively used. It is not uncommon for other people to try to persuade parents to clear out the now unwanted toys and clothes, frightened that a bedroom might become a shrine to the dead child. Parents agreeing together need to sort these items out in their own time. Most parents would probably have made some adjustments by the first anniversary, even if very small.

For each parent the experience is unique and different no matter how close the relationship. They first need to adjust to the strange situation and feelings they have within themselves and probably find it difficult to share with their partner, for fear of making things worse for the other. A solution needs to be found, and a trusted friend may be able to help by listening to the anguish, perhaps being a "catalyst" [66].

Some parents manage to return to the routine of work quite quickly as often there is a need for financial income. Work may become simply a way to fill in the day, yet concentration is likely to be poor, as the bereaved have difficulty in thinking of anything other than their child. For those who have no employment the days are very long. A Family Bereavement Service facility could help all family members, including children.

The feelings of anger, guilt, disbelief, loss, and sadness come and go in any order and at any time. There are no rules as to how long a phase may last, or the order in which they come or go or return [64]. Many parents find the return of disbelief hard to understand, especially if it is experienced 6 or 9 months after their child's death, at a time when they feel that "it's getting worse." Indeed during this period some parents can experience extreme tiredness and despair at missing their child, as it is a long time since they saw them, and they yearn for touch, smell, and sound of him. A parental wish to have their child back just for one more day, or to die just to be with their child, can be strong even if brief. Writing about (or a letter to) their child might be helpful.

Together with the loss of the child goes the loss of future expectations that the child would never fulfill. Over the next months and years there are anniversaries of what the child did "this time last year," or "he should have been doing…this year." The loss of their child is felt daily, but the most difficult of all is the birthday. The first anniversary of the death might also be hard, as well as family holidays (such as Christmas or an equivalent). The second year can sometimes be worse than the first. It is not uncommon for a spell of depression to occur at 18 months or even later – and friends might well not understand.

It is not uncommon for parents to have physical symptoms, although these may not manifest immediately. These include headaches, abdominal, chest or back pain, stomach ulcers, depression, sleep disturbance, nervous rashes, anorexia, etc. Some of these symptoms may require medical attention.

An unmarked grave has its own anguish, and sometimes there is a degree of comfort in the headstone being in place, although it is a very "final" act to have it erected. There can be happy times again, although parents may experience guilt [65]. Parents fear not being able to love a subsequent baby (yet this does not happen) or that it too might be taken away [67]. Time is not "a healer" but provides space to learn to readjust. For a few a professional counselor may be needed to assist the adjustment phase.

23.18.1 Siblings

During the illness, siblings have adjusted to a preoccupied atmosphere. When the sick child dies, the sibling suddenly becomes the only focus for the attention of parents (and grandparents, etc.) who may be too wrapped up in their own grief to notice his. Children do not like to see their parents sad and crying, and might avoid talking of the dead sibling, yet need to know that crying is allowed. The sibling gets upset and angry too; he might be reluctant to go to bed, might not sleep at night and have nightmares. His behavior may become difficult and demanding one minute, and happy and playful the next. A surviving child might try to be the child who has died in an effort to be noticed. He may withdraw himself from people in order to avoid getting hurt again [68]. A young child might cling to his parents, and an older one choose to visit friends (where there is not the sadness of home). A special toy or some item of clothing of the dead sibling can be comforting.

Meanwhile the sibling has to adjust to the lack of a playmate. After advising school or play group of the bereavement, a sibling will benefit from the normality of that school or group. Some children may seem to adjust quickly, but months later they may lose interest in schoolwork, or become uncommunicative with difficult behavior patterns, as the child gets wearied of "being good." Siblings too need time, patience, trust, and the opportunity to express how they feel. It may be that at play or in the back of the car, where parental faces cannot easily be seen, that questions will be asked or statements made. Words used in play in the past – "I wish you were dead" – could be a problem, as some children think their siblings' death was their fault. The exercise of composing a special photograph album, or scrap book about his dead brother or sister would encourage discussion and allow memories [69]. Children who are allowed to talk about their dead sibling should adjust well in time to their new lives without them. If parents find this particularly difficult, then perhaps a professional counselor could assist [66]. It is important that their normal routines are disrupted as little as possible. Family Bereavement Services are also available to children.

Grandparents find the death of a grandchild very difficult to bear. They hurt because they are unable to prevent the pain that their child (the parent) is suffering, and they have their own loss. They wish that they, who have lived a full life, could have died instead.

People do not know what to say to those who are bereaved of a child, they cannot risk the tears of the bereaved or possibly their own and may change the subject even when the bereaved themselves mentions the child's name. As a result people can say unhelpful things such as – "I know how you feel" (they cannot unless they too have been bereaved of a child), "you'll get over it" (one *never* does but gets used to living without the child and adjusting to the new life), "you can have another child" (no subsequent child or surviving sibling can *replace* the child who has died, but can provide a different focus) [71]. Worse still is when a friend avoids the bereaved not knowing how to approach, for fear of causing upset.

23.18.2 The Professional

It is important for the physician and oncology nurse to be available with time, attentiveness, and empathy to listen. One should not be judgmental but respect silence and appear relaxed and unshocked. When a child has just died it is probably most helpful to say little but listen; whatever is said is likely to be remembered. Being available for company when the bereaved wishes it, is valuable, as is knowing when to come and when to go. Support from a professional involved with their child's illness may be welcomed intermittently over many months, or declined due to the association with painful times.

After some weeks or months many parents feel the need to understand more of their child's illness and accept an opportunity of an interview with the consultant. Some may seek an opportunity to revisit the hospital while many others may find the idea of even seeing the establishment frightening and to be avoided. Some parents may take advantage of meeting with others bereaved of a child through cancer, perhaps in the form of a support group [40].

It is stressful being in the company of those whose child is dying or has died, but unless one has lost a child under similar circumstances one does *not* know what it is like, but with the experience of being with other families, one could have a element of understanding. Professionals cannot support a family in this situation without some emotional involvement themselves. However, in order to be helpful the professional needs to maintain some personal control, concentrating on the positive aspects of the experience. One can deal with the intensity of one's own emotions at a different time, perhaps sharing with a colleague.

23.19 Conclusion

The diagnosis of cancer in a child is devastating news and, no matter the age of the child, the family and its individuals will never be the same again. It is not in the natural order of life events that a child should die before parents or grandparents and the diagnosis threatens the expectations of life and the future. The social impact touches those who have known the child since birth – family, other relatives, friends, teachers, school mates, general practitioner, and many others. Others involved in the treatment will probably be affected on a personal level as well. Throughout care, communication is vitally important – between professional and child, professional and parent, parent and child, parent and siblings, and between professionals. Multidisciplinary support, understanding the implications of the diagnosis, anticipating problems and alleviating them where possible are important adjuvants to care [72]. These things will help families develop and hopefully strengthen through the experience of the child's survival.

It is important to remember throughout a child's cancer journey the value and importance of school, play, and play therapy. The inclusion of siblings along with maintaining normal family routines wherever possible is vital to the function of the family unit, and the success with emotional survival, no matter the outcome. Listening, empathy, and support will sustain.

References

1. Ekert H (1989) Incidence of childhood cancers. In: Childhood cancer – Understand and coping. Gordon and Breach, Melbourne, p 13
2. Hollis R (1997) Childhood cancers into the 21st century. Paediatr Nurs 9:12–15
3. Shone N (1995) Introduction. In: Cancer – A family affair. Sheldon, London, pp 1–4
4. Tomlinson D (2004) Paediatric oncology nurse education: The development of a national framework. J Clin Nurs 13(5):646–654
5. Adams DW (1979) The nature of helpful intervention. In: Childhood malignancy – The psychological care of the child and family. CC Thomas, Springfield, p 78
6. Potter F (1996) Counseling in cancer care. Prof Nurse 12:191–192
7. Wooley H, Stein A, Forrest GC, Baum JD (1989) Imparting the diagnosis of life threatening illness in children. Br Med J 298:1623–1626
8. Taylor J, Muller D (1995) Nursing adolescents – Research and psychological perspectives. Blackwell Science Ltd, Oxford; B6:78 (Action for Sick Children policy paper 3: Adolescents in hospital)
9. Buckman R (1990) I don't know what to say. Macmillan, London, 5:43–45
10. Williams HA (1992) Comparing the perception of support by parents of children with cancer and by professionals. J Pediatr Oncol Nurs 9:184
11. Kelly KP, Porock D (2005) A survey of pediatric oncology nurses' perceptions of parental educational needs. J Pediatr Oncol Nurs 22(1):58–66
12. Brewis, EL (2004) Oncology outreach: History in the making. Paediatr Nurs 16(9):24–27
13. Bluebond-Langner M (1978) What terminally ill children know about their world. The private lives of dying children. University Press, Princeton, pp 135–165
14. Ekert H (1989) Responses and emotions. In: Childhood cancer – Understanding and coping. Gordon and Breach, Melbourne, pp 135–165
15. Scotland Commissioner for Children: Article 24. www.sccyp.org.uk
16 Fulton Y (1996) Children's rights and the role of the nurse. Paediatr Nurs 8:29–31
17. Goldman A, Beardsmore S, Hunt J (1990) Palliative care for children with cancer: Home, hospital or hospice? Arch Dis Child 65:641–643
18. Harrison J (1992) Spirituality needs more attention. Nurs Times 88:58
19. Green J (1991) Death with dignity. Macmillan, London, pp 1–2
20. Wright PS (1993) Parents' perceptions of their quality of life. J Pediatr Oncol Nurs 10:139–145
21. Rechner M (1990) Adolescents with cancer: Getting on with life. J Pediatr Oncol Nurs 7:139–144
22. www.cancerbacup.org.uk
23. www.click4tic.org.uk
24. Ritchie MA (2001) Psychosocial nursing care for adolescents with cancer. Compr Pediatr Nurs 24(3):165–175

25. www.canteen.org.uk

26. Wong DL (1991) Transition from hospital to home for children with complex medical care. J Pediatr Oncol Nurs 8:6

27. Larcombe I, Walker J (1989) General comments. In: Return to school after treatment for cancer. Cancer Research Campaign, Christie Hospital, Manchester, pp 89–91

28. Jossi KL (2000) Kids growing up with cancer: Pediatric oncology nurses care for their patients and help with families cope with the realities of having a child with cancer. Nurs Spectr (Wash D C) 10(2):6–7

29. Adams DW, Deveau EJ (1984) Early treatment, relapse, after death. In: Coping with childhood cancer, where do we go from here? Reston, Virginia, pp 79–82, 109

30. Hewitt J (1990) The sibling response to hospitalization. Paediatr Nurs 2:12–13

31. Miller S (1996) Living with a disabled sibling – A review. Paediatr Nurs 8:21–23

32. Murray, JS (1999) Methodological triangulation in a study of social support for siblings of children with cancer. J Pediatr Oncol Nurs 16(4):194–200

33. www.CLICSargent.org.uk

34. Adams DW (1979) Helping the child and family toward normal living, parent reactions (after the death of a child). In: Childhood malignancy – The psychological care of the child and family. CC Thomas, Springfield, 125:pp 156–158

35. Kun LE, Milheron RK, Crisco JJ (1983) Quality of life in children treated for brain tumours: Intellectual, emotional and academic function. J Neurosurg 58:1–6

36. Harding J (1996) Children with cancer: Managing stress in staff. Paediatr Nurs 8:28–31

37. Hunt J (1995) The paediatric oncology community nurse specialist: The influence of employment location and funders on models of practice. J Adv Nurs 22:126–133

38. Brewis EL (1990) Care of the terminally ill child. In: Thompson J (ed) The child with cancer – Nursing care. Scutari Press, London, pp 155–166

39. Leenders F (1996) An overview of policies guiding health care for children. Nurs Stand 10:33–38

40. Baum JD, Dominica Sister Frances, Woodward RN (1990) Listen – My child has a lot of living to do. Oxford University Press, Oxford, pp 23–24

41. Dominica F (1987) Reflections of death in childhood. Br Med J 294:108–110

42. Scottish Partnership Agency for Palliative and Cancer Care. Palliative cancer care guidelines. SHHD, Edinburgh, 10(2,1)

43. Beardsmore S, Alder S (1994) Terminal care at home – The practical issues. In: Hill L (ed) Caring for dying children and their families. Chapman and Hall, London, pp 162–166

44. Goldman A, Beardsmore S, Hunt J (1990) Palliative care for children with cancer: Home, hospital or hospice? Arch Dis Child 65:641–643

45. Gould D (1996) Multiple partnerships in the community. Paediatr Nurs 8:27–31

46. Stickney D (1987) Water bugs and dragonflies – Explaining death to children. Mowbray, London

47. Bluebond-Langner M (1978) How terminally ill children come to know themselves and their world. The private worlds of dying children. Princeton University Press, New Jersey, pp 166–197

48. Goodall J (1994) Thinking like a child about death and dying. In: Hill L (ed) Caring for dying children and their families. Chapman and Hall, London, pp 16–32

49. Adams DW, Deveau EJ (1984) Helping children understand death. In: Coping with childhood cancer, where do we go from here? Reston, Virginia, pp 141–152

50. Williams M (1995) The velveteen rabbit. Heinemann, London

51. Edwards J (2001) A model of palliative care for the adolescent with cancer. Int J Palliat Nurs 7(10):485–488

52. Sheldon F (1995) Children and bereavement – What are the issues? Eur J Palliative Care 1:42–44

53. www.helpthehospices.org.uk/education/content/children_understanding.pdf

54. Ahmedzai S, Brooks D (1994) Pain control in palliative care. Hosp Update 2:549

55. Goldman A (1993) Pain management. Arch Dis Child 68:423–425

56. May L (1992) Reducing pain and anxiety in children. Nurs Stand 4:25–28

57. Buckingham S (1993) Pain scales for toddlers. Nurs Stand 7:12–13

58. Morton N (1993) Balanced analgesia for children. Nurs Stand 7:8–10

59. Devine T (1990) Pain management in paediatric oncology. Paediatr Nurs 2:11–13

60. McGrath PJ, Beyer J, Cleeland D, Eland J, McGrath PA, Portenoy R (1990) Report of the sub-committee on assessment and methodological issues in the management of pain in cancer. Pediatrics 86:814–817

61. Kelter LK, Altman A, Cohen D, et al. (1990) Report of the subcommittee on the management of pain associated with procedures in children with cancer. Pediatrics 86:826–831

62. O'Brien T (1992) Terminal care/palliative care – What do we mean? Palliative care today. CCT Healthcare Communications, London, 5:26

63. Gear P (1991) The terminally ill child. Paediatr Nurs 3:22–23

64. Brewis EL (1990) Care of the terminally ill child. In: Thompson J (ed) The child with cancer – Nursing care. Scutari Press, London, pp 19–22

65. Schiff HS (1979) Bereavement and pleasure. In: The bereaved parent. Souvenir Press, London, pp 126–127, 143–144

66. Buckman R (1990) I don't know what to say. Macmillan, London, p 194

67. Davey N (1995) Paediatric bereavement care. Paediatr Nurs 7:24

68. Hitcham M (1995) Direct work techniques with the siblings of children dying from cancer. In: Smith SC, Pennels M (eds) Interventions with bereaved children. Jessica Kingsley Publications, London, p 38

69. Neville R (1995) Making memory stores with children and families. In: Smith S, Pennels M (eds) Interventions with bereaved children. Jessica Kingsley Publications, London, p 267

70. Hemmings P (1995) Communicating with children through play. In: Smith S, Pennels M (eds) Interventions with bereaved children. Jessica Kingsley Publications, London, p 19

71. Sawley L (1988) What will I say? Nurs Times 8:57

72. Brady N (1994) Symptom control in dying children. In: Hill L (ed) Caring for dying children and their families. Chapman and Hall, London, p 138

Long-term Effects of Childhood Cancer Therapy on Growth and Fertility

24.1

Michelle Reece-Mills, Louise E. Bath,
Christopher J. Kelnar, W. Hamish B. Wallace

Second Tumors

24.2

Charles Keys, Robert Carachi

Contents

24.1 Long-term Effects of Childhood Cancer Therapy on Growth and Fertility

24.1.1 Introduction

Survival rates for most childhood malignancies have improved remarkably over the past decade with an overall survival rate for England and Wales for children less than 15 years of age quoted as 75% (1993 and 1997) [1]. This improvement has been attributed to advances in treatment, better supportive care, and centralizing treatment in specialized centers with entry of patients into clinical trials [2, 3]. Approximately 1 in every 640 individuals in the US between the ages of 20 and 39 years is a survivor of childhood cancer [4]. Long-term survival rates vary with cancer type, demographic characteristics such as age, gender and race, tumor characteristics such as location and extent of disease, morphology, and genetic alterations.

Attempts to improve survival in poor prognosis groups have led to therapeutic protocols that use more intensive therapy increasing the probability of treatment complications and long-term adverse outcomes in survivors.

With the improvement in survival rates, focus has shifted to minimizing the late effects associated with intense cancer therapy. For example, in the treatment of Wilms' tumor and Hodgkin's lymphoma, survival rates have been maintained despite a reduction in the overall intensity of treatment used for most patients. Reports concerning the frequency and severity of late effects of treatment vary widely and accurate estimates of the incidence and severity are difficult to define. Previous cohort studies have estimated that between 33% and 75% of adult survivors experience problems [5, 6].

The Childhood Cancer Survivor Study (CCSS) – a large cohort study in the US – found that more than 40% of survivors of childhood cancer report long-term adverse effects in specific areas of health. Patients treated for soft-tissue sarcomas were identified as among those with the highest risk of such problems [7]. The cohort demonstrated a 10.8-fold excess in overall mortality. Recurrence of the original cancer was the leading cause of death among 5-year survivors, accounting for 67% of deaths [8]. Nevertheless, the overall proportion of survivors affected is currently relatively small [9].

A recent study looking at the barriers to follow-up care of survivors in the US and the UK found that the majority of survivors are not receiving recommended health care. Key barriers identified included a general lack of awareness of late effects by survivors, a lack of capacity for survivor care within cancer institutions, primary care physicians being unfamiliar with the health care needs of survivors, and a general lack of communication between survivors, cancer centers, and primary care physicians. Strategies to overcome these barriers are being investigated [10].

The late effects of cancer therapy may be subdivided into:

1. Impairment of endocrine function
2. Abnormal growth
3. Sub-fertility
4. Cardiac and renal complications
5. Pulmonary fibrosis and restrictive lung disease
6. Secondary malignancies
7. Neurological impairment
8. Cognitive decline and psychological effects
9. Reduced quality of life
10. Early death

The risk of late effects are directly related to the treatment received rather than the underlying pathological diagnosis. Their anticipation and detection are essential as they may be amenable to prevention and treatment [11]. The following chapter focuses on impaired endocrine function, abnormal gonadal sub-fertility, and secondary malignancy.

24.1.2 Endocrine Late Effects

Endocrine disturbances have been documented in 20–50% of childhood cancer survivors resulting from the underlying condition, the nature, and cumulative dosage of cytotoxic chemotherapy, and the dose and schedule of irradiation [12].

Patients with central nervous system tumors are at increased risk with the prevalence of an endocrinopathy documented in more than 70%. This is often as a result of radiation injury to the hypothalamus, thyroid, or gonads [13].

Endocrine abnormalities often impose a negative impact on growth, body image, sexual function, and quality of life.

The range of endocrine complications includes gonadal damage, thyroid disorders, and dysfunction of the hypothalamic-pituitary axis. Neuroendocrine abnormalities may occur following external radiation for a number of tumors when the hypothalamic-pituitary axis falls within the fields of radiation. Deficiency of one or more anterior pituitary hormones, most commonly growth hormone, has been demonstrated after therapeutic cranial irradiation for primary brain tumors, prophylactic cranial irradiation for acute lymphoblastic lymphoma (ALL), and total body irradiation (TBI) as conditional treatment before bone marrow transplant (BMT).

24.1.2.1 Direct Radiation Damage to the Hypothalamic Pituitary Axis (HPA)

Following cranial radiotherapy patients are at risk of: growth hormone deficiency, an attenuated pubertal growth spurt, early or delayed puberty, and multiple pituitary hormone deficiencies.

The impact of radiation is dependent on the total dose, fraction size, number of fractions, and the duration of therapy (see Chap. 8). Lower radiation doses are associated with isolated growth hormone deficiency while higher doses may cause panhypopituitarism. A tissue's radiosensitivity is directly proportional to its mitotic activity and inversely proportional to its cellular differentiation. Radiation effects on slowly proliferating tissues such as the brain only become obvious with time.

The pathophysiology of radiation-induced damage has not been completely elucidated. Direct neuronal injury has been proposed to be the main mechanism rather than reduced cerebral blood flow.

The hypothalamus has been shown to be more radiosensitive than the pituitary and is damaged by lower doses of cranial radiation. This is suggested by suppression of insulin-mediated and spontaneous growth hormone secretion following cranial irradiation but preservation of the growth hormone response to hypothalamic-releasing factors [14–16]. Doses of less than 50 Gray (Gy) affect the hypothalamus with subsequent growth hormone deficiency. Higher doses used in the treatment of nasopharyngeal carcinomas and tumors of the base of the skull may cause direct anterior pituitary damage leading to early and multiple pituitary hormone deficits [17–20]. The pituitary hormones are generally lost in the following order: growth hormone, leutenizing hormone/follicle stimulating hormone, ACTH, and thyroid stimulating hormone [21].

Hypothalamic-pituitary dysfunction secondary to radiation is also time dependent [22, 23]. The progressive nature of the hormonal deficits following radiation damage to the hypothalamic–pituitary axis can be attributed to the delayed effects of radiotherapy on the axis or the development of secondary pituitary atrophy following a lack of hypothalamic releasing factors [24–26].

An additional risk factor is the age of the child at the time of radiotherapy. Younger children have been shown to be more sensitive than older children and adults to radiation-induced damage of the hypothalamic-pituitary axis [27].

24.1.2.2 Growth Hormone Deficiency

Growth hormone deficiency is usually the first and frequently the only manifestation of neuroendocrine dysfunction following cranial irradiation. It is classically characterized by diminished spontaneous (physiological) growth hormone secretion in the presence of preserved peak responses to provocative tests although the latter will also become abnormal [28].

Growth hormone is usually secreted in an intermittent pulsatile pattern with the majority of secretory bursts during sleep. Spontaneous growth hormone secretion is determined by the number of pulses, pulse amplitude, and the total 24-h integrated GH concentration derived from sampling every twenty minutes over a 24-h period. The reported frequency of radiation-induced growth hormone deficiency reported will be influenced by the physiological or pharmacological test used. Most prospective studies have used provocative testing and so the true extent of growth hormone deficiency may be underestimated.

The severity and onset of GH deficiency are dose dependent and the incidence increases with time elapsed after irradiation. Virtually all children treated with cranial irradiation doses in excess of 30 Gy will be growth hormone deficient 2 years after treatment. Low-dose cranial irradiation (18–24 Gy) used as CNS-directed therapy in ALL may lead to isolated growth hormone deficiency [29–33]. Isolated growth hormone deficiency has also been documented following total body irradiation with doses as low as 10 Gy [32, 34].

Short stature after cancer treatment has been well documented, particularly following cranial and craniospinal irradiation [35].

The effect of final height is more profound with treatment at a younger age [36].

Outcome in adult height and sitting height is poor in children surviving medulloblastoma due to craniospinal irradiation (CSRT) and chemotherapy. A study at the Children's Hospital of Philadelphia evaluated adult height and sitting height in 51 medulloblastoma patients stratified into four groups: G1, GH-deficient (GHD) patients treated with 23–39 Gy craniospinal radiation but not treated with GH [recombinant human (rh)GH]; G2, patients treated with rhGH; G3, patients who were not GHD; and G4, patients treated with 18 Gy CSRT and rhGH [37].

Sitting height. The sitting heights were available for 35 patients (two in group G1, 26 in group G2, two in group G3, and five in group G4), and the results are shown in Fig. 24.1. Compared with the general popu-

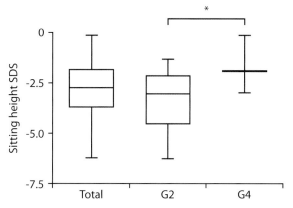

Fig. 24.1 Sitting height outcome. Sitting height SDS in total patients (n = 35), in group G2 (n = 26), and in group G4 (n = 5). The *box and whiskers plot* represents +2 SD and -2 SD (*error bars*), the 25 and 75% (*box*), and the mean (*horizontal bar*). *, P = 0.021.

lation, the sitting heights were impaired in all of the children (total group mean SDS, -2.96; P <0.0001). In groups G2 and G4, the mean sitting height SDS were -3.3 ± 1.43 and -1.62 ± 1.16, respectively. Similar to the comparison of standing adult height outcome, the sitting height of group G4 was significantly taller than that of group G2 (P = 0.021). Therefore, higher dosing of rhGH and reduced CSRT doses improved sitting height, although sitting height SDS was still short in comparison to the normal population. Although limited to two patients, the sitting height SDS for group G3 (non-GHD patients) was -2.0. The adult stature in the entire group G3 was shorter than midparental height and not different from group G2, whose spinal growth was impaired despite rhGH treatment. These observations suggest that despite GH sufficiency in group G3, the loss of stature in comparison to midparental height is due to CSRT injury to spinal growth.

Early diagnosis and treatment is important as response to growth hormone is poorer than in idiopathic growth hormone deficiency especially in children who have received spinal radiotherapy [38].

Growth hormone deficiency is also believed to cause a reduced lean body mass and increased fat mass, metabolic abnormalities including an adverse lipid profile and glucose intolerance, reduction in bone mineral density and impaired quality of life [39–42]. Insulin resistance, impaired glucose tolerance or even type 2 diabetes mellitus have been recently reported in children who have received total body irradiation [43].

It is well accepted to treat documented growth hormone deficiency in childhood with replacement doses of recombinant human growth hormone. Diagnosis of GH insufficiency can sometimes be problematic at times, however, especially in the early postirradiation period [44]. Measurements of peak growth hormone secretion will miss deficits confined to qualitative, subtle differences in pulsality (neurosecretory dysfunction) [45] and those in whom there is an inability to augment pubertal growth hormone adequately [46, 47]. Measurements of insulin-like growth factors and their binding proteins are unreliable indicators of growth hormone secretion in this situation [48]. A high index of suspicion for growth hormone deficiency is therefore needed following irradiation.

Growth in children is a sensitive marker of growth hormone status. The presence of significant growth deviation over a 1-year period (growth velocity below the 25th percentile) or a drop in height of greater than or equal to one standard deviation is highly suggestive of clinically significant growth hormone deficiency. However, obesity can result in preservation of a normal height velocity with a worsening height prognosis, as can precocious puberty, another common consequence of cranial irradiation in young girls.

Growth monitoring is an essential part of follow-up of children who have received cranial irradiation as part of treatment. Sitting and standing heights should be measured every 3–6 months. The sitting height is obtained by using a sitting height stadiometer and is particularly important in those who received spinal irradiation. The impact of spinal irradiation on spinal growth is such that greater auxological emphasis must be placed on the leg length changes rather than the total height. Spinal irradiation will particularly impair late pubertal growth.

With biochemical or clinical evidence of growth hormone deficiency (height velocity <5 cm/year) treatment is usually commenced with recombinant growth hormone as a daily subcutaneous injection. Due to the evolving nature of growth hormone insufficiency it is important that treatment begin as soon as possible.

Growth hormone is potentially mitogenic and concerns have been raised about its use in cancer survivors. However, long-term studies of patients treated with physiological replacement doses of recombinant growth hormone have failed to demonstrate any increased risk of tumor recurrence or increased frequency of second tumors although continued surveillance is needed [49–51].

However, most centers do not advocate introducing therapy within the first 2 years after cancer treatment as this is the time of highest relapse.

24.1.2.3 Abnormalities of Gonadotrophin Secretion

Gonadotrophin deficiency. Disruption of gonadotrophin secretion generally occurs at radiation doses above 40 Gy [52, 53]. Deficiencies of both follicle-stimulating hormone (FSH) and leutenizing hormone

(LH) have been documented. The clinical picture shows considerable variability from subclinical abnormalities detectable only by gonadotrophin releasing hormone (GnRH) testing to a significant reduction in circulating sex hormones levels and delayed puberty. Gonadotrophin deficiency is generally a reflection of hypothalamic dysfunction [54]. It is therefore possible to restore gonadal function and fertility by use of exogenous GnRH replacement therapy. Because of differential sensitivities of testicular and ovarian cell types to cytotoxic chemotherapy or radiotherapy, spontaneous progression through puberty is no guarantee of subsequent fertility.

Precocious puberty. The effect of cerebral irradiation on the hypothalamic-pituitary-gonadal axis (HPGA) is dose dependent. Whereas higher doses cause a deficiency, lower doses can cause premature activation leading to early or precocious puberty. The mechanism for early puberty following irradiation is believed to be secondary to disinhibition of cortical influences on the hypothalamus.

The definition of precocious puberty is the onset of puberty before the age of 8 years in girls and 9 years in boys. This can be distinguished from early puberty, which means onset between 8 and 10 years in girls and 9 and 11 years in boys.

Low-dose cranial irradiation (18–24 Gy) used in central nervous system prophylaxis for ALL has been associated with a higher incidence of early or precocious puberty, an effect seen mainly in girls. No increased frequency of precocious puberty over the normal population has been documented in male ALL survivors [55, 56]. This may reflect sex differences in the control of the onset of puberty (Fig. 24.2).

Ogilvy-Stuart et al. demonstrated that in 46 GHD children previously irradiated for brain tumors (25–47.5 Gy) the onset of puberty occurred at an early age in both sexes and there was a significant linear association between age at irradiation and age at onset of puberty, i.e., the younger the age at irradiation the earlier the onset of puberty [57].

The consequence of early puberty is that of a premature pubertal growth spurt followed by early epiphyseal fusion and a reduction in final adult height.

Children with precocious puberty are also usually growth hormone deficient. Both problems contribute to a poorer prognosis with respect to final height potential by reducing peak height velocity [58], and the time over which childhood growth can take place.

Height loss after radiation has also been shown to be disproportionate with a significant portion being a loss of sitting height [59]. Direct radiation to the spine further disrupts spinal growth with only a partial response to growth hormone therapy, which mainly stimulates long bone growth. Thus, the younger the

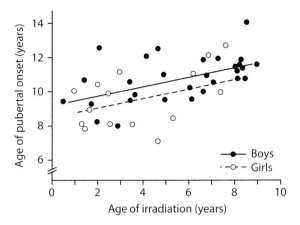

Fig. 24.2 Age at onset of puberty compared with age at irradiation in children treated for brain tumors [57].

child at the time of irradiation, the greater the risk of subsequent skeletal disproportion [60].

Close monitoring of these patients is essential after treatment with respect to growth and puberty. Six-monthly clinical assessment of pubertal status is needed as well as auxology measurements. Growth hormone and gonadotrophin secretion and bone age should be done as indicated.

Suppressing pubertal progression and delaying skeletal fusion with GnRH analogues and treatment with growth hormone gives the best prognosis in terms of height potential although the final height achieved is still lower than target [61, 62].

Hypothyroidism. The risk of hypothyroidism following treatment for childhood cancer is related to radiation field, dose, and adjuvant chemotherapy. Chemotherapy alone has not been shown to cause hypothyroidism [63]. Thyroid dysfunction may occur due to central thyroid stimulating hormone (TSH) deficiency following cranial irradiation, primary end organ damage due to direct irradiation to the gland or a combination of both, for example following craniospinal irradiation or TBI.

TSH deficiency. The hypothalamic pituitary axis and production of TSH appears least vulnerable to radiation damage. The risk of TSH deficiency from cranial irradiation is dose [64] and time related [65] as for other pituitary hormone deficiencies. However, the risk is low. In a survey of 71 children who had been treated with cranial irradiation, 6% showed evidence of TSH deficiency at a median of 12 years follow up [65]. The risk of TSH deficiency occurs at doses >50 Gy.

End organ damage. The thyroid gland is sensitive to direct irradiation. Hypothyroidism, thyroid nodules,

and hyperthyroidism have all been described. Primary hypothyroidism is the most common consequence of direct radiation injury and occurs frequently at doses that exceed 26 Gy. In a population of 1,787 adults and children who received neck irradiation for Hodgkin's disease the risk for developing hypothyroidism was 47% at 27 years [66] and approximately half the patients with thyroid dysfunction were diagnosed in the first 5 years. The presence of thyroid nodules after radiation is very common. The percentage reported with thyroid cancer varies from 14% to 40%, the risk increasing with time since treatment, and those treated at a young age most at risk [67, 68].

Combined central and primary hypothyroidism. The commonest cause for thyroid dysfunction now seen by the pediatric endocrinologist is due to a combined effect of primary and central dysfunction due to cranial and direct irradiation. The patients most at risk are those who have received craniospinal irradiation for brain tumors. In one study [69] of 119 patients who had been treated as children with craniospinal irradiation, raised TSH levels were seen in 22% who had received craniospinal irradiation alone and 69% who had received craniospinal irradiation and chemotherapy. The overall prevalence of primary dysfunction was 28% compared to 3% for central dysfunction. In a more recent study evaluating thyroid function in children treated with craniospinal irradiation (36 vs. 23 Gy) with or without chemotherapy, those treated with the lower dose of radiotherapy who also received chemotherapy, and those treated at a younger age, had the highest incidence of hypothyroidism (100% for those aged <5 years) [70]. There is a risk of primary hypothyroidism after TBI, which may be compounded by a central decline in TSH production. After fractionated TBI the risk is reduced – only 16% in one study had features of thyroid dysfunction at long-term follow-up [71].

Evaluation of thyroid dysfunction. Biochemical diagnosis of thyroid dysfunction is based on basal thyroid function tests – TSH and free thyroxine (FT4) level. Detection of primary hypothyroidism is relatively easy with rising TSH levels and declining FT4 levels. If there is evidence of increasing TSH levels with persisting normal FT4 levels (compensated primary hypothyroidism), treatment should be started prior to overt hypothyroidism as persistently elevated TSH levels are thought to increase the risk of thyroid cancer.

The diagnosis of central or combined hypothyroidism can be notoriously difficult. Treatment should be considered for individuals at risk who have a low normal or subnormal FT4 level, especially if declining over time, with low, normal, or mildly raised TSH levels, with or without symptoms [72].

24.1.3 Fertility

Direct damage to the gonads may occur due to radio-therapy involving the spine or pelvis or by systemic chemotherapy. This may lead to subfertility or infertility in both males and females.

24.1.3.1 The Effects of Chemotherapy

The extent of cytotoxic damage to the gonads is dependent on the agent used, the age and sex of the patient, and the dose received. Toxic chemotherapeutic agents include alkylating agents such as the nitrogen mustard compounds (cyclophosphamide, ifosfamide, and melphalan); nitrosoureas (carmustine, CCNU), busulphan, thiotepa, and cisplatin; procarbazine, and etoposide. Alkylating agents act as inhibitors of DNA synthesis and damage those cells with rapid mitotic activity such as the germinal cells of the testicular tubules leading to severe germinal aplasia and oligospermia/azoospermia in adulthood [73].

The germinal epithelium is more sensitive to the detrimental effects of chemotherapy than the somatic cells. This means that following gonadotoxic chemotherapy, male patients may become oligospermic or azoospermic but testosterone production by the Leydig cells is unaffected so secondary sexual characteristics develop normally [74, 75]. However, with higher doses of chemotherapy, Leydig cell dysfunction also occurs [76].

Treatment of Hodgkin's lymphoma has traditionally been associated with a high rate of azoospermia due to the use of procarbazine and alkylating agents such as chlorambucil and cyclophosphamide. Newer hybrid regimens have been designed with the above agents being alternated with anthracycline agents resulting in significantly less gonadotoxicity [77].

Ovarian dysfunction has also been documented after chemotherapy with a significant number seen following treatment of Hodgkin's lymphoma [65–68]. Causative agents include procarbazine and the alkylating agents. These effects are age and dose related [78–82].

24.1.3.2 The Effects of Radiotherapy

The degree of radiation damage depends on the field of treatment, total dose, and fractionation schedule [83–86]. In males, doses as low as 0.1–1.2 Gy can cause Sertoli cell damage with impaired spermatogenesis and with doses greater than 4 Gy leading to permanent infertility [83–85]. Germ cells are more susceptible to radiation damage than somatic cells. Leydig cells responsible for testosterone production in males,

are relatively radio-resistant, and are damaged at doses of around 20 Gy in prepubertal boys and up to 30 Gy in sexually mature males [87, 88].

In females, total body, abdominal, or pelvic irradiation may lead to ovarian and uterine damage, the extent being dependent on the radiation dose, fractionation schedule, and age at time of treatment.

The human ovary contains a fixed pool of primordial oocytes maximal at 5 months of gestation, which declines with increasing age in a biexponential manner, eventually leading to menopause at an average of 50–51 years. At this age, approximately 1,000 oocytes remain. The number of primordial oocytes present at the time of treatment, together with the dose of radiotherapy received by the ovaries, determines the fertile "window" and the age at which premature ovarian failure occurs [89].

The radiosensitivity of the human oocyte has recently been estimated to be less than 2 Gy [90]. The Faddy-Gosden equation

$$dy/\text{day } x = - y \left[0.0595 + 3{,}716 / (11{,}780 + y) \right]$$

where x denotes age, $y(x)$ is population at age x, with initial value $y(0) = 701{,}200$; the initial value denotes population at birth provides a mathematical model for calculating the rate of natural follicular decline in women.

A recent study has looked at predicting the age of ovarian failure after radiation based on data obtained from young women who developed ovarian failure after total body irradiation.

It is not possible to diagnose ovarian failure clinically, biochemically, or radiologically before the onset of puberty. The above mathematical model may be useful in predicting the onset of ovarian failure in women receiving radiotherapy [89] (Table 24.1).

Acute ovarian failure, defined as the loss of ovarian function within 5 years of diagnosis, is known to develop in a subset of survivors of pediatric and adolescent cancers. A cohort study with female participants >18 years from the CCSS was conducted looking at incidence and risk factors. Acute ovarian failure developed in small subset (6.3% of cases) especially in those treated with at least 1,000-cGy radiation to the ovaries [91].

Abdominal and pelvic irradiation are used in the treatment of a variety of malignancies such as Wilms' tumor, pelvic rhabdomyosarcoma, and Ewing's sarcoma of the pelvis or spine with dose and volume dependent upon the diagnosis and tumor size. The prevalence of ovarian failure following whole abdominal radiotherapy has been unacceptably high with the majority of patients failing to complete pubertal development without hormone replacement therapy. The introduction of flank irradiation in 1972 has resulted in

Table 24.1 Predicted age at ovarian failure with 95% confidence limits for ages at treatment from 0 to 30 years and for doses 3, 6, 9, and 12 Gy

Age	3 Gy			6 Gy			9 Gy			12 Gy		
	Low	Mean	High	Low	Mean	High	Low	Mean	High	Low	Mean	High
0	31.2	35.1	39.0	18.7	22.6	26.5	9.8	13.7	17.6	4.0	7.9	11.8
1	31.3	35.2	39.1	19.0	22.9	26.8	10.4	14.3	18.2	4.8	8.7	12.6
2	31.5	35.4	39.3	19.3	23.2	27.1	10.9	14.8	18.7	5.5	9.4	13.3
3	31.6	35.5	39.4	19.7	23.6	27.5	11.5	15.4	19.3	6.2	10.1	14.0
4	31.7	35.6	39.5	20.1	24.0	27.9	12.1	16.0	19.9	6.9	10.8	14.7
5	31.9	35.8	39.7	20.5	24.4	28.3	12.7	16.6	20.5	7.7	11.6	15.5
6	32.1	36.0	39.9	20.9	24.8	28.7	13.3	17.2	21.1	8.4	12.3	16.2
7	32.2	36.1	40.0	21.3	25.2	29.1	13.9	17.8	21.7	9.1	13.0	16.9
8	32.4	36.3	40.2	21.7	25.6	29.5	14.6	18.5	22.4	9.9	13.8	17.7
9	32.6	36.5	40.4	22.1	26.0	29.9	15.2	19.1	23.0	10.6	14.5	18.4
10	32.8	36.7	40.6	22.6	26.5	30.4	15.8	19.7	23.6	11.4	15.3	19.2
11	33.0	36.9	40.8	23.0	26.9	30.8	16.5	20.4	24.3	12.1	16.0	19.9
12	33.2	37.1	41.0	23.5	27.4	31.3	17.1	21.0	24.9	12.9	16.8	20.7
13	33.4	37.3	41.2	23.9	27.8	31.7	17.8	21.7	25.6	13.6	17.5	21.4
14	33.6	37.5	41.4	24.4	28.3	32.2	18.5	22.4	26.3	14.4	18.3	22.2
15	33.9	37.8	41.7	24.9	28.8	32.7	19.1	23.0	26.9	15.1	19.0	22.9
16	34.1	38.0	41.9	25.4	29.3	33.2	19.8	23.7	27.6	15.9	19.8	23.7
17	34.3	38.2	42.1	25.9	29.8	33.7	20.5	24.4	28.3	17.0	20.5	24.4
18	34.6	38.5	42.4	26.4	30.3	34.2	21.2	25.1	29.0	18.0	21.3	25.2
19	34.9	38.8	42.7	27.0	30.9	34.8	21.8	25.7	29.6	19.0	22.0	25.9
20	35.1	39.0	42.9	27.5	31.4	35.3	22.5	26.4	30.3	20.0	22.8	26.7
21	35.4	39.3	43.2	28.0	31.9	35.8	23.2	27.1	31.0	21.0	23.5	27.4
22	35.7	39.6	43.5	28.6	32.5	36.4	23.9	27.8	31.7	22.0	24.3	28.2
23	36.0	39.9	43.8	29.1	33.0	36.9	24.6	28.5	32.4	23.0	25.0	28.9
24	36.3	40.2	44.1	29.7	33.6	37.5	25.3	29.2	33.1	24.0	25.7	29.6
25	36.7	40.6	44.5	30.3	34.2	38.1	25.9	29.8	33.7	25.0	26.5	30.4
26	37.0	40.9	44.8	30.8	34.7	38.6	26.6	30.5	34.4	26.0	27.2	31.1
27	37.3	41.2	45.1	31.4	35.3	39.2	27.3	31.2	35.1	27.0	27.9	31.8
28	37.7	41.6	45.5	32.0	35.9	39.8	28.0	31.9	35.8	28.0	28.7	32.6
29	38.0	41.9	45.8	32.5	36.4	40.3	29.0	32.6	36.5	29.0	29.4	33.3
30	38.3	42.2	46.1	33.1	37.0	40.9	30.0	33.2	37.1	30.0	30.1	34.0

significantly less pubertal failure but the onset of a premature menopause may occur with time. Irradiation involving the uterus in childhood is associated with an increased incidence of nulliparity. Even if a pregnancy is achieved there is a high incidence of early miscarriage or intrauterine growth retardation with small-for-gestational-age offspring due to problems with uterine blood flow and distensibility [92–94].

Permanent menopause may be induced in women over 40 years of age following gonadal radiotherapy treatment with 6 Gy, while significantly higher doses are required to completely destroy the oocyte pool and induce ovarian failure in younger women and children [95]. This reflects the smaller follicle reserve in older patients and hence increased susceptibility to smaller doses of irradiation.

Determination of the impact of chemotherapy and radiotherapy on gonadal function currently involves regular clinical assessment of pubertal status, biochemical assessment of gonadotrophins and sex steroids, menstrual history in females, and semen analysis in males. It has not been possible to detect early gonadal damage in a prepubertal child due to a lack of a sensitive marker of gonadal function.

Inhibin B is a potential marker of gonadotoxicity in this age group. It is secreted primarily from Sertoli cells in males and developing small antral follicles in females. It plays a key role in spermatogenesis and folliculogenesis in adult males and females, respectively. Gonadotoxic chemotherapy has been shown to be associated with a reduction in inhibin B levels [86]. A pilot study assessing inhibin B in relation to sensitive measurements of gonadotrophins as markers of the early gonadotoxic effects of chemotherapy in prepubertal children treated for cancer found that in prepubertal girls with cancer, chemotherapy is associated with suppression of inhibin B. Sustained suppression following treatment may indicate permanent ovarian damage. In prepubertal boys, chemotherapy had little immediate effect on Sertoli cell production of inhibin B. Inhibin B, together with sensitive measurements of FSH, may be a potential marker of the gonadotoxic effects of chemotherapy in prepubertal children with cancer [87].

24.1.3.3 Fertility Protection and Preservation

Infertility is functionally defined as the inability to conceive after 1 year of intercourse without contraception. Rates of permanent infertility and compromised fertility after cancer therapy vary and depend on many factors. The effects of chemotherapy and radiation therapy depend on the drug or location of the radiation field, dose, dose intensity, method of administration, disease, age, gender, and pretreatment fertility of the patient. Male infertility can result from the disease itself as seen in patients with testicular cancer and Hodgkin's lymphoma or more frequently from damage or depletion of germinal stem cells (Table 24.2). Measurable effects of chemotherapy or radiotherapy include compromised sperm number, motility, morphology, and DNA integrity. In females, fertility is affected by any treatment that decreases the number of primordial follicles, affects hormonal balance, or interferes with the functioning of the ovaries, fallopian tubes, uterus, or cervix.

Male and female fertility may be transiently or permanently affected by cancer treatment or only manifest in women later through premature ovarian failure. Female fertility may be compromised despite maintenance or resumption of cyclic menses. Even if women are initially fertile after cancer treatment, the duration of their fertility may be shortened with a premature menopause.

There is a paucity of data regarding rates of male and female infertility following most current cancer treatments and oncologists have difficulty providing precise guidance to patients about their risks for infertility.

A review of current literature by the American Society of Clinical Oncologists assessed cancer patients' interest in fertility preservation, quality of evidence supporting current and forthcoming options for preservation of fertility in men and women, and the role of the oncologist in advising patients.

Available evidence suggests that fertility preservation is very important to many people diagnosed with cancer. Infertility from cancer treatment may be associated with psychosocial distress. Even though cancer survivors can become parents through routes such as adoption and third party reproduction (using gamete donation or a gestational carrier) most prefer to have a biological offspring even if they have concerns about birth defects that could result if the parent had cancer treatment before conception or anxiety about their own longevity or their child's lifetime cancer risk [98–101].

Parents may also be interested in fertility preservation on behalf of their children with cancer. Impaired future fertility is difficult for children to understand but potentially traumatic for them as adults. The use of established methods of fertility – semen cryopreservation and embryo freezing – in postpubertal minor children requires parental consent. However, the modalities available to prepubertal children to preserve fertility are limited by their sexual immaturity and are essentially experimental.

Advances in assisted reproductive technologies have focused attention on the possibility of preserving gonadal tissue for future use [102–104]. Such technique does raise a number of important legal and ethical is-

Table 24.2 Best assessment of risk of subfertility following current treatment for childhood cancer by disease

Low risk of subfertility (<20% risk)
1. Acute lymphoblastic leukemia
2. Wilms' tumor
3. Soft tissue sarcoma stage 1
4. Germ cell tumors (with gonadal preservation and no radiotherapy)
5. Retinoblastoma
6. Brain tumor
– Surgery only
– Cranial irradiation <24 Gy
Medium risk of subfertility
1. Acute myeloblastic leukemia
2. Hepatoblastoma
3. Osteosarcoma
4. Ewing's sarcoma
5. Soft tissue sarcoma
6. Neuroblastoma
7. Hodgkin's disease – "hybrid therapy"
8. Brain tumor
– Craniospinal radiotherapy
– Cranial irradiation >24 Gy
High risk of subfertility (>80% risk)
1. Total body irradiation
2. Localized radiotherapy; pelvic/testicular
3. Chemotherapy conditioning for bone marrow transplant
4. Hodgkin's disease – alkylating agent-based therapy
5. Soft tissue sarcoma – metastatic
Low risk <20%, High risk >80%

sues. Concerns include protection of children's reproductive rights and obtaining valid informed consent both for storage and for future use of cryopreserved material. Given the absence of proven therapeutic benefit and potential risk associated with these procedures, together with the uncertainty of predicting infertility from new chemotherapeutic and reproductive strategies, it is questionable whether such treatment is justified or ethical in children without scientific trials. The technique of autotransplantation in patients following cancer treatment raises the theoretical possibility of reintroduction of malignant cells.

Current recommendations from the American Society of Clinical Oncology suggest that the two methods of fertility preservation with the highest likelihood of success are sperm cryopreservation for postpubertal males and embryo freezing for females. Conservative surgical approaches and transposition of ovaries or gonads or gonadal shielding before radiotherapy may also preserve fertility in selected cases. Other available

fertility preservation methods should be considered experimental and be performed in centers with the necessary expertise after due ethical process [105].

Although data are limited, there appears to be no detectable increased risk of disease recurrence associated with most fertility preservation methods and pregnancy even in hormonally sensitive tumors [106, 107].

Aside from hereditary genetic syndromes, there is no evidence that a history of cancer, cancer therapy, or fertility interventions increase the risk of cancer or congenital abnormalities in progeny. Available studies, including large registry studies, have shown no increased risk of genetic abnormalities, birth defects, or cancers in children of cancer survivors [108–113].

24.1.4 Conclusion

Endocrine disturbances are common in childhood cancer survivors with an increased prevalence in patients with central nervous system tumors.

Growth hormone deficiency is the commonest endocrine abnormality following cranial radiotherapy occurring between 2 and 5 years from treatment depending on the dose. Multiple pituitary hormone deficiencies also occur at higher doses. Serial monitoring of height, sitting height, weight, and pubertal staging with calculation and interpretation of height velocity and body mass index are essential to enable anticipation and prompt management of growth and puberty problems.

Fertility in both males and females can be affected by cancer treatment given prepubertally. The two methods of fertility preservation with the highest likelihood of success are sperm cryopreservation for postpubertal males and embryo freezing for females. Oncologists should discuss with families how cancer treatment can affect fertility prior to the commencement of therapy and fertility preservation offered where appropriate and available.

A major challenge for the future remains to maintain a high cure rate for childhood cancers while further reducing endocrine and other late effects associated with therapy.

References

1. National Registry of Childhood Tumours
2. Stiller CA, Draper GJ (1998) The epidemiology of cancer in children. In: Voute PA, Kalifa C, Barrett A (eds) Cancer in children: Clinical management, 4th edn. Oxford University Press, Oxford p 3s
3. Stiller CA (1994) Centralized treatment, entry to trials and survival. Br J Cancer 70:352–362

4. National Cancer Policy Board: Weiner SI, Simone IV, Hewitt M (eds) (2003) Childhood cancer survivorship: Improving care and quality of life. National Academy of Sciences, Washington, DC 32

5. Stevens MCG, Mahler H, Parkes S (1998) The health status of adult survivors of childhood cancer. Eur J Cancer 34:694–698

6. Lackner H, Benesch M, Schagerl S, et al. (2000) Prospective evaluation of late effects after childhood cancer therapy with a follow up of over 9 years. Eur J Pediatr 159:750–758

7. Hudson MM, Mertens AC, Yasui Y, et al. (2003) Health status of adult long term survivors of childhood cancer: A report from the Childhood Cancer Survivors Study. JAMA 290:1583–1592

8. Mertens AC, Yasui Y, Neglia JP, et al. (2001) Late mortality experience in five-year survivors of childhood and adolescent cancer: The Childhood Cancer Survivor Study. J Clin Oncol 19(13):3163–3172

9. Robison LL, Green D, Hudson M, et al. (2005) Long-term outcomes of adult survivors of childhood cancer: Results from the childhood cancer survivor study. Cancer 104(11):2557–2564

10. Oeffinger K, Wallace WHB (2006) Barriers to follow-up care of survivors in the United States and the United Kingdom. Pediatr Blood Cancer 46:135–142

11. Kissen GDN, Wallace WHB (1995) Long-term follow up therapy based guidelines. United Kingdom Children's Cancer Study group (UKCCSG), Pharmacia, Leicester

12. Sklar CA (2001) Endocrine complications of the successful treatment of neoplastic diseases in childhood. Growth Genet Horm 17:37–42

13. Sklar CA (2002) Childhood Brain Tumours. J Pediatr Endocrinol 15(2):669–673

14. Jorgensen EV, Schwartz ID, Hvizdala E, et al. (1993) Neurotransmitter control of growth hormone secretion in children after cranial radiation therapy. J Pediatr Endocrinol 6:131–142

15. Schmiegelow M, Lassen S, Poulsen HS, et al. (2000) Growth hormone response to a growth hormone-releasing hormone stimulation test in a population-based study following cranial irradiation of childhood brain tumors. Horm Res 54:53–59

16. Lustig RH, Schriock EA, Kaplan SL, Grumbach MM (1985) Effect of growth hormone-releasing factor on growth hormone release in children with radiation-induced growth hormone deficiency. Pediatrics 76:274–279

17. Saaman NA, Bakdash MM, Caderao JB, et al. (1975) Hypopituitarism after external irradiation. Evidence for both hypothalamic and pituitary origin. Ann Intern Med 83:771–777

18. Blacklay A, Grossman A, Ross RJ, et al. (1986) Cranial irradiation for cerebral and nasopharyngeal tumours in children: Evidence for the production of a hypothalamic defect in growth hormone release. J Endocrinol 108:25–29

19. Lam KS, Wang C, Yeung RT, et al. (1986) Hypothalamic hypopituitarism following cranial irradiation for nasopharyngeal carcinoma. Clin Endocrinol (Oxf) 24:643–651

20. Pai HH, Thornton A, Katznelson L, et al. (2001) Hypothalamic/ pituitary function following high-dose conformal radiotherapy to the base of skull: Demonstration of a dose-effect relationship using dose-volume histogram analysis. Int J Radiat Oncol Biol Phys 49:1079–1092

21. United Kingdom Children's Cancer Study Group Late Effects Group. Therapy based long term follow-practice statement: Hypothalamic pituitary axis. United Kingdom Children's Cancer Study group (UKCCSG), Pharmacia, Leicester, p 19

22. Lam KS, Tse VK, Wang C, et al. (1991) Effects of cranial irradiation on hypothalamic-pituitary function- A five year longitudinal study in patients with nasopharyngeal carcinoma. Q J Med 78(286):165–176

23. Littley MD, Shalet SM, Beardwell CG, et al. (1989) Hypopituitarism following external radiotherapy for pituitary tumours in adults. Q J Med 70(262):104–107

24. Clayton PE, Shalet SM (1991) Dose dependency of time of onset of radiation-induced growth hormone deficiency. J Pediatr 118:226–228

25. Schmiegelow M, Lassen S, Poulsen HS, et al. (2000) Growth hormone response to a growth hormone-releasing hormone stimulation test in a population-based study following cranial irradiation of childhood brain tumors. Horm Res 54:53–59

26. Spoudeas HA, Hindmarsh PC, Matthews DR, et al. (1996) Evolution of growth hormone neurosecretory disturbance after cranial irradiation for childhood brain tumours: A prospective study. J Endocrinol 150:329–342

27. Shalet SM, Price DA, Gibson B, et al. (1976) The effect of varying doses of cerebral irradiation on growth hormone production in childhood. Clin Endocrinol (Oxf) 5:287–290

28. Bercu BB, Diamond FB Jr (1986) Growth hormone neurosecretory dysfunction. Clin Endocrinol Metab 15:537–590

29. Shalet SM, Price DA, Beardwell CG, et al. (1979) Normal growth despite abnormalities of growth hormone secretion in children treated for acute leukemia. J Pediatr 94:719–722

30. Costin G (1988) Effects of low-dose cranial radiation on growth hormone secretory dynamics and hypothalamic-pituitary function. Am J Dis Child 142:847–852

31. Shalet SM, Beardwell CG, Jones PH, et al. (1976) Growth hormone deficiency after treatment of acute leukemia in children. Arch Dis Child 51:489–493

32. Brennan BM, Rahim A, Mackie EM, et al. (1998) Growth hormone status in adults treated for acute lymphoblastic leukemia in childhood. Clin Endocrinol (Oxf) 48:777–783

33. Kirk JA, Raghupathy P, Stevens MM, et al. (1987) Growth failure and growth-hormone deficiency after treatment for acute lymphoblastic leukemia. Lancet 1(8526):190–193

34. Ogilvy-Stuart AL, Clark DJ, Wallace WH, et al. (1992) Endocrine deficit after fractionated total body irradiation. Arch Dis Child 67:1107–1110

35. Muller HL, Klinkhammer-Schalke M, Kühl J, et al. (1998) Final height and weight of long-term survivors of childhood malignancies. Exp Clin Endocrinol Diabetes 106:135–139

36. Ogilvy-Stuart AL, Shalet SM (1995) Growth and puberty after growth hormone treatment after irradiation for brain tumours. Arch Dis Child 73:141–146

37. Xu Weizhen, Janss A, Moshang T (2003) Adult height and adult sitting height in childhood medulloblastoma survivors. J Clin Endocrinol Metab 88(10):4677–4681

38. Sulmont V, Brauner R, Fontoura M, Rappaport R (1990) Response to growth hormone treatment and final height after cranial or craniospinal irradiation. Acta Paediatr Scand Suppl 79:542–549

39. de Boer H, Blok GJ, Van der Veen EA (1995) Clinical aspects of growth hormone deficiency in adults. Endocr Rev 16:63–86

40. Talvensaari K, Knip M (1997) Childhood cancer and later development of the metabolic syndrome. Ann Med 29:353–355

41. Kaufman JM, Taelman P, Vermeulen A, Vandeweghe M (1992) Bone mineral status in growth hormone-deficient males with isolated and multiple pituitary deficiencies of childhood onset. J Clin Endocrinol Metab 74:118–123

42. Stabler B (2001) Impact of growth hormone (GH) therapy on quality of life along the life-span of GH-treated patients. Horm Res 56(1) 55–58

43. Gorska, et al. (2006) Eur Soc Ped Endocrin (abstract)

44. Spoudeas HA, Hindmarsh PC, Matthews DR, Brook CG (1996) Evolution of growth hormone neurosecretory disturbance after cranial irradiation for childhood brain tumours: A prospective study. J Endocrinol 150:392–42

45. Spiliotis BE, August GP, Hung W, et al. (1984) Growth hormone neurosecretory dysfunction. A treatable cause of short stature. JAMA 251:2223–2230

46. Moell C, Garwicz S, Westgren U, et al. (1989) Suppressed spontaneous secretion of growth hormone in girls after treatment for acute lymphoblastic lymphoma. Arch Dis Child 64:252–258

47. Crowne EC, Moore C, Wallace WH, et al. (1992) A novel variant of growth hormone (GH) following low dose cranial irradiation Clin Endocrinol (Oxf) 36:59–68

48. Achermann JC, Hindmarsh PC, Brook CG (1998) The relationship between the growth hormone and insulin-like growth factor axis in long-term survivors of childhood brain tumours. Clin Endocinol (Oxf) 49:639–645

49. Ogilvy-Stuart AL, Ryder WD, Gattamaneni HR, et al. (1992) Growth hormone and tumour recurrence. Br Med J 304:1601–1605

50. Swerdlow AJ, Reddingius RE, Higgins CD, et al. (2000) Growth hormone treatment of children with brain tumors and risk of tumor recurrence. J Clin Endocrinol Metab 85:4444–4449

51. Sklar CA, Mertens AC, Mitby P, et al. (2002) Risk of disease recurrence and second neoplasms in survivors of childhood cancer treated with growth hormone: A report from the Childhood Cancer survivor Study. J Clin Endocrinol Metab 87:3136–3141

52. Sanders JE, Buckner CD, Leonard JM, et al. (1983) Late effects on gonadal function of cyclophosphamide, total-body irradiation, and marrow transplantation. Transplantation 36:252–255

53. Pasqualini T, Escobar ME, Domene H, et al. (1987) Evaluation of gonadal function following long-term treatment for acute lymphoblastic leukemia in girls. Am J Pediatr Hematol Oncol 9:15–22

54. Hall JE, Martin KA, Whitney HA, et al. (1994) Potential for fertility with replacement of hypothalamic gonadotrophin-releasing hormone in long term female survivors of cranial tumors. J Clin Endocrinol Metab 79:1166–1172

55. Leiper AD, Stanhope R, Kitching P, et al. (1984) Precocious puberty after hypothalamic and pituitary irradiation in young children. N Engl J Med 311:920

56. Quigley C, Cowell C, Jimenez M, et al. (1989) Normal or early development of puberty despite gonadal damage in children treated for acute lymphoblastic leukemia. N Engl J Med 321:143–151

57. Ogilvy-Stuart AL, Clayton PE, Shalet SM (1994) Cranial irradiation and early puberty. J Clin Endocrinol Metab 78:1282–1286

58. Didock E, Davies HA, Didi M, et al. (1995) Pubertal growth in young adult survivors of childhood leukemia. J Clin Oncol 13:2503–2507

59. Davies HA, Didock E, Didi M et al. (1994) Disproportionate short stature after cranial irradiation and combination chemotherapy for leukemia. Arch Dis Child 70:472–475

60. Shalet SM, Gibson B, Swindell R, Pearson D (1987) Effect of spinal irradiation on growth. Arch Dis Child 62:461–464

61. Cara JF, Kreiter ML, Rosenfield RL (1992) Height prognosis of children with true precocious puberty and growth hormone deficiency: Effect of combination therapy with gonadotrophin releasing hormone agonist and growth hormone. J Pediatr 120:709–715

62. Adan L, Souberbielle JC, Zucker JM, et al. (1997) Adult height in 24 patients treated for growth hormone deficiency and early puberty. J Clin Endocrinol Metab 82:229–233

63. Van Santen HM, Vulsma T, Dijkgraaf MG, et al. (2003) No damaging effect of chemotherapy in addition to radiotherapy on the thyroid axis in young adult survivors of childhood cancer. J Clin Endocrinol Metab 88:3657–3663

64. Constine LS, Woolf PD, Cann D, et al. (1993) Hypothalamic-pituitary dysfunction after radiation for brain tumors. N Engl J Med 328:87–94

65. Schmiegelow M, Feldt-Rasmussen U, Rasmussen AK, et al. (2003) Assessment of the hypothalamo-pituitary-adrenal axis in patients treated with radiotherapy and chemotherapy for childhood brain tumor. J Clin Endocrinol Metab 88:3149–3154

66. Hancock SL, Cox RS, McDougall IR (1991) Thyroid diseases after treatment of Hodgkin's disease. N Engl J Med 325:599–605

67. Crom DB, Kaste SC, Tubergen DG, et al. (1997) Ultrasonography for thyroid screening after head and neck irradiation in childhood cancer survivors. Med Pediatr Oncol 28:15–21

68. Acharya S, Sarafoglou K, LaQuaglia M, et al. (2003)Thyroid neoplasms after therapeutic radiation for malignancies during childhood or adolescence. Cancer 97:2397–2403

69. Livesey EA, Brook CG (1989) Thyroid dysfunction after radiotherapy and chemotherapy of brain tumours. Arch Dis Child 64:593–595

70. Paulino AC (2002) Hypothyroidism in children with medulloblastoma: A comparison of 3600 and 2340 cGy craniospinal radiotherapy. Int J Radiat Oncol Biol Phys 53:543–547

71. Sanders JE, Pritchard S, Mahoney S, et al. (1986) Growth and development following marrow transplantation for leukemia. Blood 68:1129–1135

72. Gleeson HK, Shalet SM (2004) The impact of cancer therapy on the endocrine system in survivors of childhood brain tumours. Endocr Relat Cancer 11:589–602

73. Cicognani A, Pasini A, Pession A, et al: (2003) Gonadal function and pubertal development after treatment of a childhood malignancy. J Pediatr Endocrinol Metab 16: S321–326

74. Kreuser ED, Xiros N, Hetzel WD, Heimpel H (1987) Reproductive and endocrine gonadal capacity in patients treated with COPP chemotherapy for Hodgkin's disease. J Cancer Res Clin Oncol 113:260–266

75. Thomson AB, Campbell AJ, Irvine DS, et al. (2002) Semen quality and spermatozoal DNA integrity in survivors of childhood cancer: A case-control study. Lancet 360:361–367

76. Gerl A, Muhlbayer D, Hansmann G, et al. (2001) The impact of chemotherapy on Leydig cell function in long term survivors of germ cell tumors. Cancer 91:1297–1303

77. Viviani S, Santoro A, Ragni G, et al. (1985) Gonadal toxicity after combination chemotherapy for Hodgkin's disease. Comparative results of MOPP vs ABVD. Eur J Cancer Clin Oncol 21:601–605

78. Waxman JH, Terry YA, Wrigley PF, et al. (1982) Gonadal function in Hodgkin's disease: Long-term follow-up of chemotherapy. Br Med J (Clin Res Ed) 285:1612–1613

79. Clark ST, Radford JA, Crowther D, et al. (1995) Gonadal function following chemotherapy for Hodgkin's disease: A comparative study of MVPP and a seven-drug hybrid regimen. J Clin Oncol 13:134–139

80. Mackie EJ, Radford M, Shalet SM (1996) Gonadal function following chemotherapy for childhood Hodgkin's disease. Med Pediatr Oncol 27:74–78

81. Chiarelli AM, Marrett LD, Darlington G (1999) Early menopause and infertility in females after treatment for childhood cancer diagnosed in 1964-1988 in Ontario, Canada. Am J Epidemiol 150:245–254

82. Whitehead E, Shalet SM, Blackledge G, et al. (1983) The effect of combination chemotherapy on ovarian function in women treated for Hodgkin's disease. Cancer 52:988–993

83. Speiser B, Rubin P, Cassarett G (1973) Aspermia following lower truncal irradiation in Hodgkin's disease. Cancer 32:692–698

84. Centola GM, Keller JW, Henzler M, Rubin P (1994) Effect of low-dose testicular irradiation on sperm count and fertility in patients with testicular seminoma. J Androl 15:608–613

85. Clifton DK, Bremner WJ (1983) The effect of testicular x-irradiation on spermatogenesis in man. A comparison with the mouse. J Androl 4:387–392

86. Rowley MJ, Leach DR, Warner GA, Heller CG (1974) Effect of graded doses of ionizing radiation on the human testis. Radiat Res 59:665–678

87. Shalet SM, Tsatsoulis A, Whitehead E, Read G (1989) Vulnerability of the human Leydig cell to radiation damage is dependent upon age. J Endocrinol 120:161–165

88. Castillo LA, Craft AW, Kernahan J, et al. (1990) Gonadal function after 12-Gy testicular irradiation in childhood acute lymphoblastic leukemia. Med Pediatr Oncol 18:185–189

89. Wallace WH, Thomson AB, Saran F, et al. (2005) Predicting age of ovarian failure after radiation to a field that includes the ovaries. Int J Radiat Oncol Biol Phys 62:738–744

90. Wallace WHB, Thomson AB, Kelsey TW (2003) The radiosensitivity of the human oocyte. Hum Reprod 18:117–121

91. Chemaitilly W, Mertens AC, Mitby P, et al. (2006) Acute ovarian failure in the childhood cancer survivor study. J Clin Endocrinol Metab 91:1723–1728

92. Sanders JE, Hawley J, Levy W, et al. (1996) Pregnancies following high-dose cyclophosphamide with or without high-dose busulfan or total-body irradiation and bone marrow transplantation. Blood 87:3045–3052

93. Bath LE, Critchley HO, Chambers SE, et al. (1999) Ovarian and uterine characteristics after total body irradiation in childhood and adolescence: Response to sex steroid replacement. Br J Obstet Gynaecol 106:1265–1272

94. Critchley HO, Wallace WH, Shalet SM, et al. (1992) Abdominal irradiation in childhood: The potential for pregnancy. Br J Obstet Gynaecol 99:392–394

95. Lushbaugh CC, Casarett GW (1976) The effects of gonadal irradiation in clinical radiation in therapy: A review. Cancer 37:1111–1125

96. Wallace EM, Groome NP, Riley SC, et el. (1997) Effects of chemotherapy-induced testicular damage on inhibin, gonadotrophin, and testicular secretion: A prospective longitudinal study. J Clin Endocrinol Metab 82:3111–3115

97. Crofton PM, Thomson AB, Evans AE, et al. (2003) Is inhibin B a potential marker of gonadotoxicity in prepubertal children treated for cancer? Clin Endocrinol (Oxf) 58(3):296–301

98. Rosen A (2005) Third-party reproduction and adoption in cancer patients. J Natl Cancer Inst Monogr: 34:91–93

99. Fossa SD, Aass N, Molne K (1989) Is routine pre-treatment cryopreservation of semen worthwhile in the management of patients with testicular cancer? Br J Urol 64:524–529

100. Schover LR, Brey K, Litchin A, et al. (2002) Knowledge and experience regarding cancer, infertility, and sperm banking in younger male survivors. J Clin Oncol 20:1880–1889

101. Schover LR, Rybicki LA, Martin BA, et al. (1999) Having children after cancer. A pilot survey of survivors' attitudes and experiences. Cancer 86: 697–709

102. Brinster RL, Zimmerman JW (1994) Spermatogenesis following male germ-cell transplantation. Proc Natl Acad Sci U S A 91:11298–11302

103. Schlatt S, von Schonfeldt V, Schepers AG (2000) Male germ cell transplantation: An experimental approach with a clinical perspective. Br Med Bull 56:824–836

104. Newton H (1998) The cryopreservation of ovarian tissue as a strategy for preserving the fertility of cancer patients. Hum Reprod Update 4:237–247

105. Lee SJ, Schover LR, Partridge AH, et al. (2006) American Society of Clinical Oncology recommendations on fertility preservation in cancer patients. J Clin Oncol 24:2917–2931

106. Oktay K (2005) Further evidence on the safety and success of ovarian stimulation with letrozole and tamoxifen in breast cancer patients undergoing in vitro fertilization to cryopreserve their embryos for fertility preservation. J Clin Oncol 23:3858–3859

107. Oktay K, Buyuk E, Libertella N, et al. (2005) Fertility preservation in breast cancer patients: A prospective controlled comparison of ovarian stimulation with tamoxifen and letrozole for embryo cryopreservation. J Clin Oncol 23(19):4347–4353

108. Thomson AB, Campbell AJ, Irvine DC, et al. (2002) Semen quality and spermatozoal DNA integrity in survivors of childhood cancer: A case-control study. Lancet 360:361–367

109. Green DM, Whittton JA, Stovall M, et al. (2002) Pregnancy outcome of female survivors of childhood cancer: A report from the Childhood Cancer Survivor Study. Am J Obstet Gynecol 187:1070–1080

110. Sankila R, Olsen JH, Anderson H, et al. (1998) Risk of cancer among offspring of childhood-cancer survivors. Association of Nordic Cancer Registries and the Nordic Society of Paediatric Haematology and Oncology. N Engl J Med 338:1339–1344

111. Stovall M, Donaldson SS, Weathers RE, et al. (2004) Genetic effects of radiotherapy for childhood cancer: Gonadal dose reconstruction. Int J Radiat Oncol Biol Phys 60:542–552

112. Green DM, Whitton JA, Stovall M, et al. (2003) Pregnancy outcomes of partners of male survivors of childhood cancer: A report from the Childhood Cancer Survivor Study. J Clin Oncol 21:716–721

113. Boice JD Jr, Tawn EJ, Winther JF, et al. (2003) Genetic effects of radiotherapy for childhood cancer. Health Phys 85:65–80

24.2 Second Tumors

The survival of childhood cancers has improved greatly in the last 30 years. With better diagnostic and therapeutic regimens most children who are now diagnosed with cancer will have a survival rate at 5 years of approximately 70% [1]. This improved survival is achieved at the expense of the long-term effects of having a childhood malignancy and their irradiation and chemotherapeutic treatments. These late effects include reduced fertility, cardiovascular morbidity, adverse endocrine function, and psychological effects. The development of a second malignant neoplasm (SMN) is also a well-recognized late outcome.

As more children survive into adulthood the extent of SMNs is becoming more apparent. However, such malignancies are difficult to study for several reasons. They take a long time to develop, which requires long follow-up and retrospective data collection. Furthermore, small cohorts of patients make results difficult to interpret. However, large cancer groups have published data from large cohorts of children with cancer and have identified prevalence rates and general patterns of associated tumors. Also certain risk factors have been found such as genetic susceptibilities, effects of treatment regimens, lifestyle, and environmental factors.

24.2.1 Incidence and Associations

Overall in the US, SMNs in survivors of cancer account for 6–10% of all cancers [1]. A European cohort study showed an overall incidence of 3% of developing an SMN after a childhood cancer [2]. More recently a cohort study of over 16,000 patients identified an overall risk of developing an SMN by 25 years as 4.2% [3] (Table 24.3).

Various patterns of associations between primary and SNMs have been noted.

The association between retinoblastoma and developing an SMN, especially sarcomas, has long been known [5]. The proposed mechanism is a combination of genetic susceptibility and radiotherapy exposure. One study showed a 30-year cumulative incidence of SMN of 35% in patients who received radiotherapy and 5.8% in those who did not [6].

Wilms' tumor patients are also known to develop SMNs. One study showed an incidence of 0.4% [7]. These SNMs tend to be bone and soft tissue sarcomas, and are often in the field of previous irradiation. Acute myeloid leukemia, lymphoma, and brain tumors have also been reported (Figs. 24.3a–b).

Table 24.3 First and second tumors associated with risk factors. (Adapted from [4])

First tumor	Second tumor	Risk factors
Retinoblastoma	Bone and soft tissue sarcoma, pineal, melanoma	Genetic disease, radiation
Wilms' tumor	Bone and soft tissue sarcoma, leukemia, brain	Radiation
Neuroblastoma	Thyroid, bone and soft tissue sarcoma	Radiation
Sarcomas	Other sarcomas of bone and soft tissues	Radiation; neurofibromatosis
Lymphoma	Leukemia, other lymphoma, sarcoma	Alkylating agents, epipodophyllotoxins; radiation

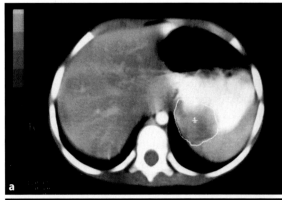

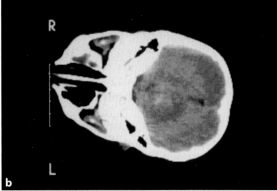

Fig. 24.3 a, b (**a**) This is a CT scan of a two-year-old boy who presented with a large abdominal mass. He had a large Wilms' tumor on the left side invading the liver. He subsequently was found to have chromosome breakage syndrome when he became unwell following chemo- and radiotherapy. (**b**) Two years later after his treatment was completed, he developed signs of raised intracranial pressure. This CT scan of the brain shows a separate brain tumor. He succumbed shortly after treatment was instituted. His brother also died after treatment for a rhabdomyosarcoma of the head and had a second tumor, a ganglioneuroblastoma of the abdomen discovered at post mortem.

Sarcomas have been the subject of many studies occurring either as the primary tumor, which then develop an SMN, or as the SMN following a different primary tumor. Following the treatment of soft tissue sarcomas several SMNs have been recognized including a second sarcoma, brain tumors, leukemias, neuroblastomas, and lymphomas [8].

The risk of SMN following a Ewing sarcoma has been the subject of debate. One recent study reported a relative risk of 12.7% of developing an SMN at 20 years [9]. A second sarcoma following irradiation accounted for most of these.

Brain tumors are the most common solid tumor of childhood, and SMNs following them are well recognized [10]. The incidence is variable and there can be a wide variety of neoplasms including non-Hodgkins

lymphoma, basal cell carcinoma, malignant melanoma, and Kaposi sarcoma.

SMN following lymphoma is also becoming more prevalent. Most patients with Hodgkin's lymphoma can now be cured, making this more common. The risk of lung cancer is significantly increased in patients with previous Hodgkin's disease [11]. Other SMNs include leukemia and cancers of the esophagus, stomach, colon, and breast [12]. Patients with non-Hodgkin's lymphoma have also been shown to have an increased risk of all malignancies, especially leukemia and lung cancer [13]. Hodgkin's disease has also been reported as an SMN following leukemia, but in general this is very rare for reasons that are still unknown [14].

Thyroid neoplasms following radiotherapy for childhood malignancy is a well-established late outcome. Primary malignancies include lymphomas, leukemias, Wilms' tumor, and neuroblastomas. These thyroid neoplasms can be either benign or malignant [15].

24.2.2 Risk Factors/Etiology

The risk of developing an SMN is a balance of genetic predisposition, exposure to previous therapy, lifestyle, and environmental factors.

Much has been written about the genetic susceptibility of SMN in children. The risk of developing an SMN is increased in two common pediatric conditions; neurofibromatosis type I, and the genetic form of retinoblastoma [4]. Neurofibromatosis type I is carried by a mutation on chromosome 17 and accounts for 0.5% of childhood cancers. This gene is associated with an increased risk of developing an SMN.

The genetic form of retinoblastoma involves a constitutional alteration of chromosome 13. These patients have been reported to have a 50% risk of developing an SMN by 50 years of age [16]. Li-Fraumeni syndrome is a known indicator of cancer manifesting as sarcomas and subsequent risk of SMNs. A germline p53 gene mutation is accountable for this [17].

Other inherited cancer syndromes include multiple endocrine neoplasias and familial adenomatous polyposis. Beckwith-Wiederman syndrome is associated with primary Wilms' tumor and SMN hepatoblastoma (Fig. 24.4a,b). Recent evidence has shown increased RET gene expression in patients who develop thyroid SMN following radiotherapy [18].

Exposure to radiotherapy has long been linked to an increased risk of developing a subsequent neoplasm. Factors that may influence this include age of the child, field of radiation, and dose of irradiation, in addition to the type of primary neoplasm. In general the younger the age at which radiotherapy is received, the greater the risk. Low doses of radiation are asso-

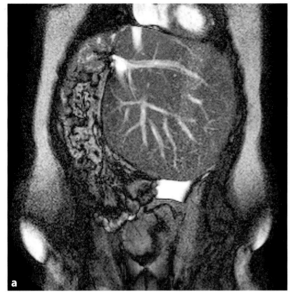

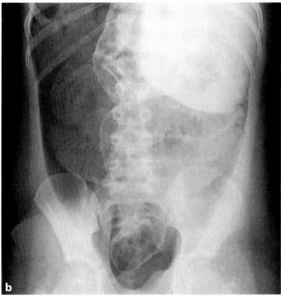

Fig. 24.4 a, b (**a**) This is a scan of a child with a familial right-sided hepatoblastoma that has been successfully resected and following treatment was cured. Genetic studies on the family revealed he had the APC gene mutation. On follow-up 3 years later he developed rectal bleeding. This scan shows compensatory growth of the residual normal left lobe of liver. (**b**) This x-ray demonstrates a complication of a pneumoperitoneum after an attempted biopsy of polyps in the colon. Multiple polyps were encountered. The patient had a total colectomy, and is well.

ciated with thyroid neoplasms [15] and higher doses with sarcomas, although no definite dose threshold has been found [19]. The development of breast tumors following radiation is not thought to be dose related but may be due to a specific susceptibility [20].

Chemotherapy agents are also known to be associated with the development of SMNs. Alkylating agents and epipodophyllotoxins are the most well known and are associated with secondary leukemia [4].

Evidence suggests that the risk of SMN development is further increased with combined radiotherapy and chemotherapy [21, 22].

24.2.3 Summary

As patients with childhood tumors achieve longer survival more SMNs are being seen. These can occur in some well-established patterns that may follow genetic predisposition. They may result as a late effect of exposure to irradiation and some chemotherapeutic agents.

All patients with childhood malignancies require long-term follow-up. Long-term prospective surveillance of all children with malignancies will afford improved understanding of incidence and possible etiology of these SMNs. This may provide the opportunity to prevent and treat these malignancies.

References

1. Bhatia S, Sklar C (2002) Second cancers in survivors of childhood cancer. Nat Rev Cancer 2(2):124–132
2. De Vathaire F (1994) Incidence of second malignant neoplasms (SMN) after a cancer in childhood: A European cohort study of 4111 children. Med Pediatr Oncol 23:174–175
3. Jenkinson HC, Hawkins MM, Stiller CA, Winter DL, Marsden HB, Stevens MCG (2004) Long-term population-based risks of second malignant neoplasms after childhood cancer in Britain. Br J Cancer 91(11):1905–1910
4. Meadows AT (2001) Second tumours. Eur J Cancer 37(16):2074–2081
5. Draper GJ, Sanders BM, Kingston JE (1986) Second primary neoplasms in patients with retinoblastoma. Br J Cancer 53(5):661–671
6. Wenzel CT, Halperin EC, Fisher SR (2001) Second malignant neoplasms of the head and neck in survivors of retinoblastoma. Ear Nose Throat J 80:108–112
7. Carli M, Frascella E, Tournadde MF, et al. (1997) Second malignant neoplasms in patients treated on SIOP Wilms' tumour studies and trials1,2,5 and 6. Med Pediatr Oncol 29(4):239–244
8. Rich DC, Corporan CA, Smith MB, et al. (1997) Second malignant neoplasms in children after treatment of soft tissue sarcoma. J Pediatr Surg 32(2):369–372
9. Bacci G, Longhi A, Barbieri E, Ferrari S, et al. (2005) Second malignancy in 597 patients with Ewing sarcoma of bone treated at a single institution with adjuvant and neoadjuvant chemotherapy between 1972 and 1999. J Pediatr Hematol Oncol 27(10):517–520

10. Buyukpamukcu M, Varan A, Yazici N, et al. (2006) Second malignant neoplasms following the treatment of brain tumors in children. J Child Neurol 21(5):433–436

11. Lorigan P, Radford J, Howell A, Thatcher N (2005) Lung cancer after treatment for Hodgkin's lymphoma: A systematic review. Lancet Oncol 6(10):773–779

12. Dores G, Metayer C, Curtis R, et al. (2002) Second malignant neoplasms among long-term survivors of Hodgkin's disease: A population-based evaluation over 25 years. J Clin Oncol 20(16):3484–3494

13. Mudie NY, Swerdlow AJ, Higgins CD, et al. (2006) Risk of second malignancy after non-Hodgkin's lymphoma: A British Cohort Study. J Clin Oncol 24(10):1568–1574

14. Ragusa R, Russo S, Villari L, Schiliro G (2001) Hodgkin's disease as a second malignant neoplasm in childhood: Report of a case and review of the literature. Pediatr Hematol Oncol 18(6):407–414

15. Acharya S, Sarafoglou K, LaQuaglia M, et al. (2003) Thyroid neoplasms after therapeutic radiation for malignancies during childhood or adolescence. Cancer 97(10):2397–2403

16. Wong FL, Boice JD, Abramson DH (1997) Cancer incidence after retinoblastoma. Radiation dose and sarcoma risk. JAMA 278(15):1262–1267

17. Yonemoto T, Tatezaki S, Ishii T (2004) Multiple primary cancers in patients with osteosarcoma: Influence of anticancer drugs and genetic factors. Am J Clin Oncol 27(3):220–224

18. Collins BJ, Chiappetta G, Schneider AB (2002) RET expression in papillary thyroid cancer from patients irradiated in childhood for benign conditions. J Clin Endocrinol Metab 87(8):3941–3946

19. Caglar K, Varan A, Akyuz C (2006) Second neoplasms in pediatric patients treated for cancer: A center's 30-year experience. J Pediatr Hematol Oncol 28(6):374–378

20. Guibout C, Adjadj E, Rubino C (2005) Malignant breast tumors after radiotherapy for a first cancer during childhood. J Clin Oncol 23(1):197–204

21. Cohen RJ, Curtis RE, Inskip PD (2005) The risk of developing second cancers among survivors of childhood soft tissue sarcoma. Cancer 103(11):2391–2396

22. Bassal M, Mertens AC, Taylor L (2006) Risk of selected subsequent carcinomas in survivors of childhood d cancer: A report from the Childhood Cancer Survivor Study. J Clin Oncol 24(3):476–483

Minimally Invasive Surgery in the Diagnosis and Treatment of Childhood Cancer

25

George W. Holcomb, Benno M. Ure

25.1 Introduction

Two of the early pioneers in minimally invasive surgery (MIS) were Drs. Stephen Gans and Bradley Rodgers. In the early 1970s, Dr. Gans described the use of laparoscopy for a variety of indications in 16 infants and children. In addition, in collaboration with Storz Endoscopy America (Los Angeles, CA), he helped design the first set of laparoscopic instruments for pediatric patients [1]. Dr. Rodgers authored two papers in the late 1970s and early 1980s describing the use of thoracoscopy for evaluation and biopsy of intrathoracic conditions. In a series of patients between 1975 and 1978, he and his colleagues described 65 thoracoscopic procedures in 57 children [1]. Thirty-four operations were performed in immunosuppressed patients to rule out Pneumocystis carinii pneumonia. Twenty of these were proven to have Pneumocystis pneumonia for a diagnostic accuracy of 100%. Fifteen operations were performed for the diagnosis of intrathoracic tumors. Four years later, Drs. Rodgers and Ryckman described over 150 thoracoscopic procedures for evaluation of intrathoracic pathology [2]. Twenty-five of these operations were undertaken for the diagnosis or staging of intrathoracic tumors in patients from 8 months to 18 years of age. Forty-eight percent were performed for parenchymal tumors, 44% for mediastinal masses, and 8% for pleural disease. In this series, general anesthesia with endotracheal intubation and spontaneous ventilation was used in children under 3 years of age.

In children older than 3 years, a four-rib intercostal nerve block in the region where the thoracic cannulas were inserted afforded localized parietal pleural anesthesia. Intravenous ketamine anesthesia was also used. All of these methods employed spontaneous ventilation allowing maintenance of a sufficient pneumothorax to aid in a complete examination. There were minimal complications in this extremely early series.

Except for these two publications, there were very few reports in the literature describing the use of laparoscopy or thoracoscopy for the treatment of benign or malignant disease until 1988. Soon thereafter, an exponential increase in the use of MIS for all conditions occurred. By the mid-1990s, there were a number of papers describing utility of laparoscopy in adults for pancreatic, ovarian, gastric, and colon cancers [3–11]. Moreover, a number of adult surgeons reported their experience using thoracoscopy for lung and esophageal cancers [12–17]. As the use of MIS in children for benign disease was slow to evolve, so too was its utilization for malignant conditions. The primary reason for this gradual evolution in children with cancer centered on the limited experience among most pediatric surgeons with MIS for benign conditions. Thus, the decade of the 1990s was largely spent training pediatric surgeons in this evolving technology. In the USA in 1996, the National Cancer Institute (NCI) funded a number of studies involving the use of MIS in the treatment of various malignancies in adults and children to evaluate the potential impact of this novel approach on the quality of life for cancer patients. As with new chemotherapeutic agents, the NCI felt that it was important to evaluate these new endoscopic approaches by funding randomized clinical trials. Along with a number of adult studies, the NCI funded the surgical sections of the Children's Cancer Group (CCG) and the Pediatric Oncology Group (POG) to conduct two prospective randomized controlled, surgeon-directed studies to evaluate the role of MIS in children with cancer. Unfortunately, these studies closed in 1998 due to a lack of patient accrual. An attempt was made to evaluate why a randomized controlled trial looking at cancer in children had failed

[18]. Interestingly, in this review, family preference for either the open or MIS approach was not considered to be a major limitation for patient enrollment. However, there appeared to be a strong bias of individual surgeons favoring one approach over the other that was probably directly correlated with one's experience with MIS. This lack of surgical expertise with MIS was likely the single most important reason for failure of this study. Thus, the study may have been conceived and funded ahead of the development of MIS expertise among pediatric surgeons.

Over the past 5 years, experience with MIS in children with cancer has grown substantially to the point that this modality can now be considered an acceptable approach for many tumors. In the abdomen, laparoscopy is used primarily for biopsy of new lesions or for second look procedures. Moreover, in a number of institutions, laparoscopic resection of certain malignancies is employed. The use of thoracoscopy is maturing faster due to the fact that biopsy of mediastinal masses or wedge resection of pulmonary lesions lends itself quite nicely to the thoracoscopic approach. In addition, for many reasons, resection of posterior mediastinal masses can be accomplished thoracoscopically. This chapter will describe the impact of MIS on tumor cell behavior, the use of laparoscopy and thoracoscopy for children with cancer and, finally, a review of the available literature describing these minimally invasive approaches in children with cancer.

25.2 Impact of Minimally Invasive Techniques on Tumor Cell Behavior

The benefits of minimally invasive surgery have been attributed to several mechanisms, including a specific impact on the immune system. Numerous experimental studies have confirmed that minimally invasive surgery interferes less with the function of various cell populations that play a key role in the host's defense. These cell populations include monocytes-macrophages, polymorphnuclear leucocytes (PMN), and lymphocytes [19]. These specific immunological effects have been attributed to less trauma associated with the minimally invasive technique, and to the metabolic properties of the gas used to create the pneumoperitoneum or pneumothorax.

These beneficial effects have been confirmed by recent experimental work. When compared to laparotomy, laparoscopy had advantages such as lower migration of PMNs to the abdominal cavity and reduced abdominal macrophage cytokine release [20]. Similar effects were seen when CO_2 was compared to air insufflation. Moreover, the use of CO_2 during laparoscopy compared to minilaparotomy with a similar length of abdominal incision was associated with

reduced circulatory cytokine release, prevention of hepatic macrophages from expansion, and preservation of normal intra-abdominal cell distribution [21]. The effects of the CO_2 used for pneumoperitoneum have not only been identified in the peritoneal cavity and the circulatory system, but in distant organs as well. The pulmonary macrophage reactive oxygen species release was reduced after pneumoperitoneum with CO_2 when compared to air [20]. Besides the impact on macrophage function, a lack of increase in the number of leucocytes, a reduction in their phagocytic activity, and other parameters of cellular activation, such as surface expression of CD11b and concentration of elastase, are associated with CO_2 pneumoperitoneum [22]. Numerous controlled clinical trials have confirmed that pneumoperitoneum-based surgery results in reduced levels of circulatory cytokines and a better preserved cell-mediated immunity in patients [22–27].

It has been postulated that local acidification, which occurs during CO_2 pneumoperitoneum, represents the major factor in the above-mentioned alteration of cell behavior [28, 29]. The release of cytokines and free oxygen radicals, as well as the mitochondrial activity of macrophages and polymorphonuclear cells, are down regulated by CO_2-associated pH-modulation in vitro [29–31]. A recent randomized clinical trial suggested that CO_2 laparoscopy preserves the production of cytokines by lowering the abdominal pH, interestingly without affecting macrophage phagocytosis [32].

Currently, controversy exists about the role of such direct and indirect effects of CO_2 in patients with malignant disease. It has been postulated that the alteration of host defense mechanisms may interfere with the clearing of tumor cells that have been spread during the operation. In addition, a direct impact on the behavior of tumor cells has been suggested. However, the results of experimental studies using adult tumor cells, such as colon or breast adenocarcinoma, were not conclusive [33]. In numerous animal studies, pneumoperitoneum, in comparison to an open procedure, enhanced wound implants and increased the growth, weight, and invasiveness of tumors [34–39]. Other authors have found opposite effects, including a decrease in tumor growth, wound implants, cell proliferation, and an increase in cell necrosis [40–42]. However, such effects have not been confirmed by clinical studies on adults with cancer. Several prospective and randomized trials on colon cancer resected by laparoscopy versus conventional surgery have shown similar recurrence rates and overall survival [43–45].

Little is known about the impact of CO_2 pneumoperitoneum on the behavior of pediatric tumor cells. Schmidt, et al., investigated several pediatric tumor cell lines in vitro and found a potentially beneficial effect [46]. The proliferation rate of neuroblastoma, hepatoblastoma, hepatocellular carcinoma, and lymphoma cells was significantly reduced for up to 4 days after exposure to CO_2 versus air or helium. CO_2, but not helium, exposure reduced the activity of several cell lines, which makes hypoxic effects unlikely. There was no impact on rhabdomyosarcoma cells. However, it remains unclear whether CO_2 interferes with the activation of oncogenes that are involved in stimulating progression of the cell cycle regulation or with the inactivation of tumor suppressor genes in pediatric tumors.

The in-vivo behavior of neuroblastoma cells after pneumoperitoneum was recently investigated by Iwanaka, et al. [47]. The authors used a small animal retroperitoneal neuroblastoma model. There was no significant difference in survival, tumor growth, or distant metastases in animals with CO_2 pneumoperitoneum versus laparotomy. In this study, the tumor remained untouched. In subsequent experiments, the authors showed that port-site recurrences were similar when biopsies were performed during CO_2 versus gasless pneumoperitoneum [48]. Fondrinier and colleagues found no significant differences in carcinomatosis between CO_2 laparoscopy, laparotomy, and controls 2 weeks after peritoneal implantation of an aneuploid tumor cell line [49]. However, similar studies on other types of pediatric tumors, such as lymphoma, hepatoblastoma, and rhabdomyosarcoma are lacking.

To date, clinical studies have not confirmed an alteration in the behavior of tumor cells by minimally invasive techniques in children. A recent survey of the Japanese Society of Pediatric Surgery showed no port-site recurrence in 85 children undergoing laparoscopic and 44 undergoing thoracoscopic procedures for neuroblastoma, hepatoblastoma, nephroblastoma, and other tumors [50]. However, it is well recognized that further work is needed to demonstrate that long-term survival and recurrence rates are not compromised by the beneficial immunological effects of minimally invasive techniques.

25.3 Laparoscopy in Pediatric Oncology

The laparoscopic approach has been widely used in children with suspected cancer to establish the diagnosis, for staging purposes, for evaluation of recurrent or metastatic disease, and for tumor resection. The spectrum of malignancies in children undergoing laparoscopic biopsy include the whole range of pediatric abdominal and retroperitoneal tumors, such as neuroblastoma, nephroblastoma, hepatoblastoma, rhabdomyosarcoma, teratoma, lymphoma, and numerous others [51–58]. In these reports, the conversion rate was less than 5%. The diagnostic accuracy of laparoscopic biopsies for various malignant conditions has been reported to be up to 100% [51–54]. No major complications associated with the laparoscopic approach were reported. Spurbeck and his coinvestigators did not observe any port-site recurrences in 27 children [55], nor did Iwanaka, et al., in 24 children [59], but the duration of follow-up may not be long enough to draw final conclusions.

A limited number of reports have confirmed that laparoscopy may be a valid tool for resection of solid pediatric malignancies in selected patients. However, the feasibility of laparoscopic tumor resection is somewhat limited in most reported series. Warmann, et al., had to convert in 5 out of 9 procedures [51], and Iwanaka, et al., converted in 2 out of 19 [59]. Most reports concerning laparoscopic resection of specific tumors deal with neuroblastoma. Iwanaka, et al., operated on 5 patients with 1 conversion due to poor visualization around the large vessels [60]. De Lagausie, et al., resected 9 adrenal neuroblastomas and converted 1 case due to adhesions [61]. There were neither intraoperative complications nor evidence of recurrence or port-site metastases observed during a mean follow-up of 15 months. The feasibility of laparoscopic resection for various other types of tumors can only be derived from case reports. Pancreatic tumors including insulinoma [62, 63], renal tumors such as nephroblastoma [64] and numerous other rare conditions have been successfully resected using laparoscopy in a limited number of children with defined disease. These initial data are encouraging, but long-term follow-up data are not yet available.

Several authors from Japan have recommended laparoscopic resection of neuroblastoma identified by mass screening [65–67]. The applicability of laparoscopy for resection was excellent due to the limited extent of the disease and to well-encapsulated tumors with a size of less than 5 cm in diameter. However, the appropriate indication for laparoscopic resection of neuroblastomas identified by mass screening has been a matter of debate. Komuro, et al., suggested resecting tumors which do not regress for several months or increase in size to more than 5 cm [68]. Other authors advocate resection of smaller neuroblastomas with a size of less than 2 cm [65, 67].

Most authors prefer the transabdominal approach as the optimal route for laparoscopic tumor exposure [51–58]. In general, even for children with retroperitoneal tumors, the transperitoneal route has been recommended [69–71]. However, Steyaert, et al., successfully used a retroperitoneoscopic approach in 10 cases [72]. Pampaloni, et al., have suggested performing transabdominal laparoscopic surgery for right sided masses and preferred the retroperitoneoscopic approach for left-sided tumors [73].

Technical aspects of laparoscopic surgery in children with suspected malignancy include using low pressure pneumoperitoneum to preserve the integrity of the peritoneal cell layers, and minimizing the spread of tumor cells by using endobags. Iwanaka, et al., showed experimentally that local or intravenous chemotherapeutic agents, such as cyclophosphamide, reduced the incidence of port-site metastasis of neuroblastoma [47]. The authors therefore recommended administration of chemotherapy as soon as possible after laparoscopic biopsies were taken in children with chemotherapy-sensitive tumors. However, clinical evidence of the advantages of this concept is currently unavailable.

In conclusion, laparoscopic techniques can be recommended as a first choice in children with a suspected abdominal or retroperitoneal malignancy requiring biopsy. With meticulous selection of patients, the feasibility of laparoscopic resection in children with neuroblastoma or several other types of malignant tumors is excellent. The known short-term benefits of minimally invasive surgery such as less pain and faster recovery are applicable in these patients, but data on long-term results in larger series of children are lacking.

25.3.1 Patient and Personnel Positioning

There are not nearly as many preoperative considerations for the child undergoing laparoscopic biopsy, assessment of resectability, or even tumor resection when compared to a thoracoscopic procedure. An enema the night before the operation may be helpful in evacuating the colon for a mid to lower abdominal lesion. An orogastric tube should be inserted and the bladder should be emptied following induction of anesthesia. The bladder can be emptied with a Credé maneuver or a urinary catheter can be introduced if a long procedure is anticipated. For a midline upper abdominal lesion, the patient is positioned supine on the operating table. The surgeon and assistants can stand at the foot of the table, much like would occur for a laparoscopic fundoplication. For a right-upper or left-upper abdominal procedure, the patient positioning and location of the personnel should be similar to a laparoscopic cholecystectomy or a laparoscopic splenectomy, respectively. One or two monitors can be used for upper abdominal operations.

For pelvic operations, often a single monitor is acceptable and should be placed at the foot of the bed. The surgeon and assistant stand opposite each other on each side of the table. In general, if the lesion is a left-lower abdominal or left pelvic mass, the surgeon should stand on the patient's right side and vice versa for a right-lower abdominal or pelvic mass. For a pelvic lesion, it is important to evacuate the bladder completely so a temporary urinary catheter may be advisable.

Cannulas or "stab incisions" can be used for introduction of the instruments. If a biopsy or second look procedure is planned, stab incisions afford a very cosmetically pleasing means to introduce the instruments and obtain the biopsy with minimal scarring and discomfort. An endoscopic retrieval bag should be used to extract the specimen to prevent port-site recurrences. In general, biopsy of masses, assessment of resectability, and second look procedures constitute the majority of indications for the use of laparoscopy in children with abdominal masses (Fig. 25.1). Large tumors such as Wilms' tumor or dense fibrotic le-

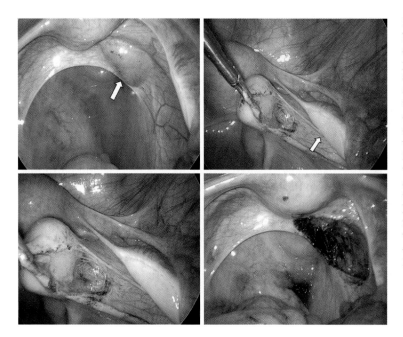

Fig. 25.1 Second-look laparoscopy can be useful after adjuvant therapy in certain circumstances. In this teenage patient who previously had undergone laparotomy and resection of a large germ cell tumor, second-look laparoscopy was performed to determine whether evidence of residual disease existed. *Upper left*, Residual disease is seen along the right pelvic side wall (*white arrow*). *Upper right*, this mass is being resected from the pelvic side wall. Note the normal right ovary (*white arrow*). *Lower left*, further dissection of the mass is achieved. *Lower right*, the mass has been completely excised with hemostasis controlled by cautery. (Reprinted with permission from Pediatric Surgery, 4th edn, Ashcraft, Holcomb, Murphy, eds, Elsevier, 2005, p 676.)

sions such as neuroblastoma are probably not good candidates for minimally invasive resection. Although rarely performed currently, staging laparotomy for Hodgkin's disease is also a good indication for laparoscopy in children with cancer.

25.4 Thoracoscopy in Pediatric Oncology

In a patient undergoing a thoracoscopic operation, a number of considerations need to be addressed preoperatively. One is the location of the lesion to be either biopsied or resected. For lesions in the lung parenchyma in which a wedge excision or biopsy is indicated, the issue of whether the lesion should be localized preoperatively is important. Most surface lesions can be visualized at thoracoscopy and do not need localization. However, if the lesion is small, consideration should be made for preoperative localization as sometimes it can be difficult to visualize a small lesion on the surface of the lung when the lung is collapsed. Preoperative localization is important for the thoracoscopic procedure when compared with the open operation because of the loss of tactile sensation resulting in the inability to palpate the lesion with one's hands. If the lesion is deeper in the parenchyma, preoperative localization should be strongly considered. A number of techniques are possible for preoperative localization. One is percutaneous placement of a wire into the lesion using CT guidance (Fig. 25.2) [74]. Also, in combination with wire localization, either methylene blue or a drop of the patient's own blood may be instilled in the area to be resected in case the wire is dislodged [75]. At some institutions, methylene blue has been banned so the use of a blood patch from the patient can also be efficacious. All of these techniques are effective in experienced hands. However, if the wire localization is utilized and the surgeon plans to use insufflation to partially collapse the ipsilateral lung for creation of an adequate working space for thora-coscopy, one should not collapse the lung too quickly following patient positioning and draping. Otherwise the wire may become dislodged from the lesion as the lung is pulled away from the chest wall with positive pressure insufflation.

Another important component of the thoracoscopic approach is the use of double lumen endotracheal intubation. The smallest double lumen tube is a 26 French. Thus, the smallest patient in whom such a tube can be utilized is usually around 6 to 8 years of age. Therefore, if a thoracoscopic operation is planned for a younger patient and collapse of the ipsilateral lung is important, other modalities should be considered to effect collapse of the ipsilateral lung. If the patient is undergoing a left thoracoscopic operation, a relatively easy technique is to place an uncuffed endotracheal tube in the right mainstem bronchus, which usually allows minimal ventilation to the left lung. If a right thoracoscopy is needed, it is sometimes possible to position an uncuffed endotracheal tube down the left mainstem bronchus, although this is not as easy as on the right side. Another useful technique is positioning the endotracheal tube in the trachea and inserting a Fogarty catheter down the right mainstem bronchus. With the Fogarty catheter being used as a bronchial blocker, there should be minimal ventilation to the right side.

Another method that evolved over the past decade is the use of positive pressure insufflation in the thoracic cavity. Early in the 1990s, insufflation was not considered helpful and nonvalved cannulas were routinely utilized. It was felt that collapse of the lung through endotracheal blockade was more helpful than using positive pressure insufflation inside the rigid thoracic cavity. However, most surgeons who perform a large number of thoracic operations, whether for benign or malignant processes, now use valved cannulas and positive pressure CO_2 insufflation to effect lung collapse. An insufflation pressure of 6–8 torr usually will result in good collapse in most patients.

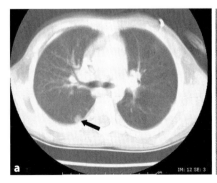
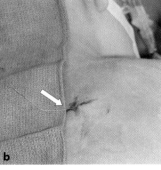

Fig. 25.2 a, b Preoperative localization is important for thoracoscopic operations when compared to the open operation because of the lack of tactile sensation with one's hands. Preoperatively, the patient was noted to have a posterior lung nodule (*black arrow*) (**a**). This lesion was localized preoperatively and the wire is seen exiting the patient's skin (*white arrow*) (**b**).

Certainly, positive pressure helps augment the initial lung collapse if endobronchial blockade is also being employed. Therefore, if cannulas are being used, they should have valves and stopcocks so that the positive pressure insufflation can be retained in the chest to partially collapse the ipsilateral lung.

25.4.1 Patient and Personnel Positioning

Another important consideration is patient positioning. By positioning the patient on the operating room table in different positions, the surgeon can take advantage of gravity to improve visualization. For instance, for an anterior mediastinal lesion, the patient should be placed in about a 30° supine position with a roll under the ipsilateral side. With the use of insufflation and/or endobronchial blockade, the lung should fall more posterior and improve visualization of the anterior mediastinum. Conversely, for a posterior mediastinal lesion, the patient should be placed in an approximately 30° prone position, which allows the lung to fall anterior and improve exposure in the posterior mediastinum (Fig. 25.3). For parenchymal nodules, the patient can be placed more or less in a 90° decubitus position although the patient can be tilted anterior or posterior if the lesion is more posterior or anterior. For lesions on the diaphragm which require assessment and possible biopsy, the patient should be placed more in a reverse Trendelenburg position to allow the lung to fall away from the diaphragm. Conversely, for a lesion in the apex of the thoracic cavity, the table can be placed more in a head-up position to promote the lung falling more caudal away from the area of concern.

For lesions in the upper part of the thoracic cavity, one or two monitors should be placed at the head of the operating table. In general, the surgeon should stand to the patient's back if the lesion is more anterior and the monitor should be over the patient's shoulder so that the lesion is located between the surgeon and the monitor. Conversely, if the lesion is more posterior, then the surgeon should work from the patient's front and the monitor should be over the patient's shoulder as well, keeping the lesion between the monitor and the surgeon. Ideally, the scrub nurse should stand next to the surgeon and the assistant should stand opposite the surgeon. If an additional assistant is available to hold the camera, that person should be on the same side as the surgeon. Similarly, these principles should remain the same for lesions in the lower aspect of the thoracic cavity. However, the monitor(s) should be toward the foot of the bed so that the lesion is between the surgeon and the monitor. This "in-line" arrangement allows an ergonomically facile procedure to be performed.

Finally, a comment should be made about concern for port-site metastases. There is no doubt that port-site metastases are an area of significant concern and diligence should be sought to avoid this complication. In adults, this incidence of port-site metastases was initially thought to be as high as 20%. Now, it appears closer to the incidence of wound metastases after open surgery [76]. In a survey from the Japanese Society of Pediatric Endosurgeons, 29 institutions were queried [50]. There was a total of 129 endosurgical procedures reported for pediatric malignancies. There were no port-site metastases observed in any patient in this survey. In a recent review of the literature, there was only one case of port-site metastases reported. This was a child who underwent thoracoscopic surgery for osteogenic sarcoma [77]. In summary, this problem does not occur as often as initially feared, although it is important to place all specimens into an endoscopic retrieval bag for exteriorization of the specimen (Fig. 25.4).

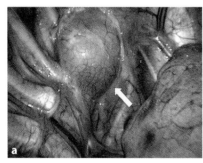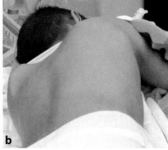

Fig. 25.3 a, b Patient positioning is an important preoperative consideration for a thoracoscopic (or laparoscopic) operation. This teenager had a posterior mediastinal mass (*white arrow*) which turned out to be a ganglioneuroma (**a**). For access to this posterior mediastinal lesion, the patient was placed in a 30° prone position to allow the lung to fall away from the posterior mediastinum (**b**).

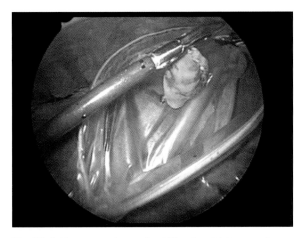

Fig. 25.4 Cancer specimens should be placed into an endoscopic retrieval bag prior to removal from the patient.

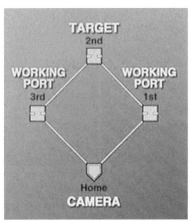

Fig. 25.5 A good analogy to remember where to position the cannulas for a laparoscopic or thoracoscopic operation is the concept of a baseball diamond. If home base represents the cannula through which the telescope/camera is inserted, first and third base represent the working ports for the surgeon. The targeted lesion is at second base and the viewing monitors are in right center and left centerfield if two monitors are used. If only one monitor is utilized, it is placed in centerfield.

25.4.2 Operative Technique

Following endotracheal anesthesia and patient positioning (as discussed previously), the patient is widely prepped and draped. The prep and drape should extend from the sternum anteriorly to the vertebral column posteriorly and from the axilla superiorly to the iliac crest inferiorly. It is important to widely prep and drape for several reasons. First, conversion to a thoracotomy may be needed. Second, one never knows where one will exteriorize the chest tube/chest drain so it is important to have the lower costal margin prepped for options about selecting the position of the drain. Third, the surgeon cannot be completely certain where he/she will place the cannulas as port placement should be individualized according to the operation. As a general statement, the cannula through which the telescope attached to the camera is inserted should be in the center of a triangle with the two working ports. A good analogy to always remember is the concept of a baseball diamond (Fig. 25.5). If home base represents the cannula through which the telescope/camera is inserted, first and third base represent the working ports for the surgeon. The lesion is at second base and the monitors are either in right center and left center field or in center field (if only one monitor is used). If this concept is used for all thoracoscopic operations, whether for benign or malignant lesions, an ergonomically efficient setup is provided. In addition, one should always remember that space, or lack of space, can be a problem in operating in the chest of children. This is especially true in the younger child. Therefore, it is often helpful to try to place the telescope/camera port as far away from the lesion as possible so that this port is out of the way of the operating ports for the surgeon. In addition, as an endoscopic stapler is used for most excisional biopsies of parenchymal nod-

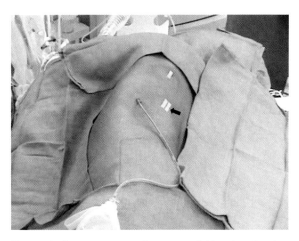

Fig. 25.6 The port positions for a young child undergoing thoracoscopic wedge excision of a metastatic lesion are seen. The largest incision (*arrow*) was positioned as far away from the lesion as possible so that the stapler could be opened within the chest cavity. A small silastic drain was exteriorized through a stab incision.

ules, it is important to remember that 4–5 cm of the stapler must be within the thoracic cavity before the stapler will open. Therefore, when selecting a site for insertion of the stapler, it is again important to position the stapler port away from the lesion so that adequate intrathoracic space is available to open the stapler (Fig. 25.6). Angulated staplers are now available and, as a general statement, the angulated staplers are easier to ligate and divide the lung parenchyma

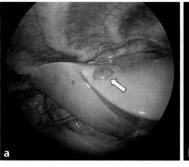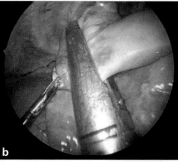

Fig. 25.7 a, b Staplers are the easiest and safest means to extract a pulmonary parenchymal lesion. In this patient with a suspected metastatic Wilms' tumor, the lesion (*arrow*) is seen on the edge of the right upper lobe (**a**). The stapler has been placed across the parenchyma and the lesion has been incorporated in the wedge resection (**b**).

for pulmonary wedge resection (Fig. 25.7). The other working port can often be a "stab incision" through which a 3-mm instrument is directly introduced into the thoracic cavity (Fig. 25.6). The advantage of using a stab incision is that there is greater mobility with an instrument placed directly through the thoracic interspace rather than working through a previously placed interface cannula as angulation and movement of the cannula can often be limited by the ribs. Second, there is a cost advantage of using as few cannulas as possible [78]. In addition, there is rarely a problem with CO2 leak through the stab incision if an adequate insufflation flow is achieved. Finally, as previously mentioned, an endoscopic retrieval bag is mandatory for all biopsy or wedge resection specimens to prevent port-site recurrences. In general, morcellation of cancer specimens is not advisable. Available bags are now 10 mm or 15 mm in size. For most cancer operations, the 10-mm bag is sufficient and can be introduced through the port in which the stapler is also inserted. It is vitally important not to extract a specimen that is too large through a small port-site as there is concern that tearing the bag will result in spillage of the specimen which might lead to implantation around the parietal surface of the thoracic cavity or to port-site recurrence. Therefore, enlarge the site through which the bag is exteriorized if the specimen is large.

25.5 Literature Review

There have been several series which have reviewed the use of laparoscopy and thoracoscopy in children with cancer. The first one was published in 1995 and described 85 children from 15 CCG (now Children's Oncology Group) institutions who underwent 88 minimally invasive procedures [57]. Twenty-five patients underwent a laparoscopic operation and 60 patients had a total of 63 thoracoscopic procedures. At this early stage in the use of minimally invasive surgery, both modalities were considered useful for assessment of resectability, for staging purposes, and for evaluation of recurrent or metastatic disease. In 2000,

another review described 59 children undergoing 15 laparoscopic and 47 thoracoscopic operations [54]. Diagnostic accuracy again was 100% in all cases and no patient was found retrospectively to have been inadequately treated based on decisions made from tissue obtained through the minimally invasive approach. These data confirmed the previous data from the CCG review. Another report in 2003 describing 28 children undergoing the minimally invasive approach for diagnostic purposes confirmed these data as well [79]. The largest review to date is a retrospective review from St. Jude in which 101 patients undergoing 113 minimally invasive operations were described [55]. Interestingly, 64 patients underwent a laparoscopic operation and 49 had a thoracoscopic procedure. In most series, thoracoscopic operations are more common. In this review, seven abdominal tumors were excised. Thirty patients underwent their laparoscopic operation due to complications of the malignancy or its treatment. In the patients who underwent a thoracoscopic procedure, most of them required wedge resection of a lung nodule. In this series, fourteen cases (29%) had to be converted to an open thoracotomy because of the inability to localize the suspected lesion. In those situations in which conversion was required due to inability to localize the lesion at operation, none of the patients had undergone an attempted preoperative needle localization. A recent paper has described 24 biopsies and 24 excisions that were performed laparoscopically or thoracoscopically for neuroblastoma, ovarian solid tumors, and other solid tumors [56]. The authors related that the length of the hospitalization and the time to initiation of postoperative feeding was significantly shorter in the group who underwent an endosurgical approach when compared to an open operation. However, the time to initiation of postoperative chemotherapy was shorter only in those with an abdominal neuroblastoma.

A number of papers have described the use of thoracoscopy alone in patients with cancer. In 2002, Rothenberg and his colleagues described 52 patients undergoing 63 thoracoscopic operations over a 7-year period [80]. Eight patients required conversion in this series. Two recent reports have also described the utility of thoracoscopy for resection of neurogenic tumors. In one series, 17 children underwent resection of mediastinal neurogenic tumors over a 6-year period [81]. In this series, 10 patients underwent a thoracoscopic approach and 7 had an open operation. There was no difference between operative time or blood loss between the two groups, but postoperative hospitalization was shorter following thoracoscopic resection (p <0.05). There were no regional recurrences in either group. In a report from France, 21 patients underwent thoracoscopic resection of neurogenic tumors over a 5-year period [82]. One patient required conversion to an open operation. The diagnosis was neuroblastoma or ganglioneuroblastoma in 16 cases and ganglioneuroma in five cases. In this series, two patients developed a postoperative chylothorax which required postoperative chest drainage. No other complications developed.

A final mention should be made of the use of image-guided techniques for children with pulmonary nodules [83, 84]. In a recent report from Toronto, a series of 28 patients undergoing a thoracoscopic lung biopsy was compared with 35 patients having a percutaneous image-guided biopsy [83]. Adequate tissue for pathologic diagnosis was obtained in 100% of the patients with a thoracoscopic biopsy versus 80% of those patients who underwent an image-guided biopsy. However, due to the fact that 18% of the patients in the thoracoscopy group suffered a persistent air leak which required temporary chest tube drainage, the authors concluded that the percutaneous technique should be considered as the initial approach for children with pulmonary nodules. Most pediatric surgeons would disagree with this conclusion because a persistent air leak following wedge resection of a pulmonary nodule should be an extremely unusual complication.

In the early stages in the use of laparoscopy and thoracoscopy for children with cancer, most of the indications centered on biopsy or evaluation of resectability or as a second look procedure to see if there was any residual disease. Gradually, primary minimally invasive resections have evolved such that resection of an amenable abdominal tumor and of many posterior mediastinal lesions can now be considered fairly standard. This evolution from straight-forward biopsy/evaluation operations to more complex procedures is representative of the evolution that has happened for not only adults with cancer, but for most minimally invasive procedures in children. As a number of articles have been published over the last 10 years detailing the efficacy of the minimally invasive approach and the paucity of complications, now would be the optimal time to reinstitute the concept of a prospective, randomized trial looking at the open versus the minimally invasive approach in children with cancer.

Although this trial was funded 10 years ago, the trial was ahead of the MIS learning curve for most pediatric surgeons. Such a trial would likely be embraced now as most pediatric surgeons are comfortable with these minimally invasive approaches.

References

1. Rodgers BM, Moazam F, Talbert JL (1979) Thoracoscopy in children. Ann Surg 189:176–180
2. Ryckman FC, Rodgers BM (1982) Thoracoscopy for intrathoracic neoplasia in children. J Pediatr Surg 17:521–524
3. Warshaw AL, Gu ZY, Wittenberg J, et al. (1990) Preoperative staging and assessment of resectability of pancreatic cancer. Arch Surg 125:230–233
4. Cuschieri A (1988) Laparoscopy for pancreatic cancer: Does it benefit the patient? Eur J Surg Oncol 14:41–44
5. Fockens P, Huibretse K (1993) Staging of pancreatic and ampullary cancer by endoscopy Endoscopy 25:52–57 (review)
6. Spinelli P, DiFelice G (1991) Laparoscopy in abdominal malignancies. Probl Gen Surg 8:329–347
7. Watt I, Stewart I, Anderson D, et al. (1989) Laparoscopy, ultrasound and computer tomography in cancer of the esophagus and gastric cardia: A prospective comparison for detecting intra–abdominal metastases. Br J Surg 76:1036–1039
8. Colin-Jones DG, Rosch T, Dittler HJ (1989) Staging of gastric cancer by endoscopy Endoscopy 25:34–38 (review)
9. Phillips EH, Franklin M, Carroll BJ, et al. (1992) Laparoscopic colectomy. Ann Surg 216:703–707
10. 10 Bleday R, Babineau T, Forse RA (1993) Laparoscopic surgery for colon and rectal cancer Semin Surg Oncol 9:59–64 (review)
11. Buschbaum HJ, Lifshitz S (1984) Staging and surgical evaluation of ovarian cancer Semin Oncol 11:227–237 (review)
12. Sisler GE (1993) Malignant tumors of the lung: Role of video assisted thoracic surgery. Chest Surg Clin N Am 3:307–317
13. Kirby TJ, Rice TW (1993) Thoracoscopic lobectomy. Ann Thorac Surg 56:784–786
14. Naruke T, Asamura H, Kondo H, et al. (1993) Thoracoscopy for staging of lung cancer. Ann Thorac Surg 56:661–663
15. Shennib HA, Landreneau R, Mulder DS, et al. (1993) Video-assisted thoracoscopic wedge resection of the T1 lung cancer in high-risk patients. Ann Surg 218:555–560
16. Krasna MJ, McLaughlin JS (1993) Thoracoscopic lymph node staging for esophageal cancer. Ann Thorac Surg 56:671–674
17. Dowling RD, Ferson PF, Landreneau RJ (1992) Thoracoscopic resection of pulmonary metastases. Chest 102:1450–1454
18. Ehrlich PF, Newman KD, Haase HM, et al. (2002) Lessons learned from a failed multi-institutional randomized control study. J Pediatr Surg 37:431–436

19. 19 Neuhaus SJ, Watson DI (2004) Pneumoperitoneum and peritoneal surface changes: A review. Surg Endosc 18:1316–1322

20. Ure BM, Niewold TA, Bax NMA, et al. (2002) Peritoneal, systemic, and distant organ immune responses are reduced by a laparoscopic approach and carbon dioxide versus air. Surg Endosc 16:836–842

21. Jesch NK, Vieten G, Tschernig T, et al. (2005) Mini-laparotomy and full laparotomy, but not laparoscopy, alter hepatic macrophage populations in a rat model. Surg Endosc 19:804–810

22. Gupta A, Watson DI (2001) Effect of laparoscopy on immune function. Br J Surg 88:1296–1306

23. Jacobi CA, Wenger F, Opitz I, et al. (2002) Immunologic changes during minimally invasive surgery. Dig Surg 19:459–463

24. Karayiannakis AJ, Makri GG, Mantzioka A, et al. (1997) Systemic stress response after laparoscopic or open cholecystectomy: A randomized trial. Br J Surg 84:467–471

25. Le Blanc-Louvry I, Coquerel A, Koning E, et al. (2000) Operative stress response is reduced after laparoscopic compared to open cholecystectomy: The relationship with postoperative pain and ileus. Dig Dis Sci 45:1703–1713

26. Hendolin HI, Paakonen ME, Alhava EM, et al. (2000) Laparoscopic or open cholecystectomy: A prospective randomised trail to compare postoperative pain, pulmonary function, and stress response. Eur J Surg 166:394–399

27. Neudecker J, Sauerland S, Neugebauer E, et al. (2002) The European Association for Endoscopic Surgery clinical practice guideline on the pneumoperitoneum for laparoscopic surgery. Surg Endosc 16:1121–1143

28. West MA, Baker J, Bellingham J (1996) Kinetics of decreased LPS-stimulated cytokine release by macrophages exposed to CO2. J Surg Res 63:269–274

29. West MA, Hackman DJ, Baker J, et al. (1997) Mechanism of decreased in vitro murine macrophage cytokine release after exposure to carbon dioxide. Ann Surg 226:179–190

30. Kos M, Kuebler JF, Jesch NK, et al. (2006) Carbon dioxide differentially affects the cytokine release of macrophage subpopulations exclusively via alteration of extracellular pH. Surg Endosc 20:570–576

31. Kuebler JF, Kos M, Jesch NK, et al. (2007) Carbon dioxide suppresses macrophage superoxide anion production independent of extracellular pH and mitchondrial activity. J Pediatr Surg 42:244–248

32. Neuhaus SJ, Watson DI, Ellis T, et al. (2001) Metabolic and immunologic consequences of laparoscopy with helium or carbon dioxide insufflation: A randomized clinical study. ANZ J Surg 71:447–452

33. Are C, Talamini MA (2005) Laparoscopy and malignancy. J Laparoendosc Adv Surg Tech A 15:38–47

34. Ishida H, Murata N, Yamada H, et al. (2000) Pneumoperitoneum with carbon dioxide enhances liver metastases of cancer cells implanted into the portal vein in rabbits. Surg Endosc 14:239–242

35. Hopkins MA, Dulai RM, Occhino A, et al. (1999) The effects of carbon dioxide pneumoperitoneum on seeding of tumor in port sites in a rat model. Am J Obstet Gynecol 181:1329–1333

36. LeMoine MC, Navarro F, Burgel JS, et al. (1998) Experimental assessment of risk of tumor recurrence after laparoscopic surgery. Surgery 123:427–431

37. Wu JS, Brasfield EB, Guo LW, et al. (1997) Implantation of colon cancer at trocar sites is increased by low pressure pneumoperitoneum. Surgery 122:1–7

38. Jacobi CA, Orderman J, Bohm B, et al. (1997) The influence of laparotomy and laparoscopy on tumor growth in a rat model. Surg Endosc 11:618–621

39. Jones DB, Guo LW, Reinhard MK, et al. (1995) Impact of pneumoperitoneum on trocar site implantation of colon cancer in hamster model. Dis Colon Rectum 38:1182–1188

40. Gutt CN, Riemer V, Kim ZG, et al. (1999) Impact of laparoscopic colonic resection on tumour growth and spread in an experimental model. Br J Surg 86:1180–1184

41. Bouvy ND, Marquet RL, Jeekel J, et al. (1997) Laparoscopic surgery is associated with less tumour growth stimulation than conventional surgery: An experimental study. Br J Surg 84:358–361

42. Bouvy ND, Marquet RL, Jeekel H, et al. (1996) Impact of gasless laparoscopy and laparotomy on peritoneal tumor growth and abdominal wall metastases. Ann Surg 224:694–700

43. Korolija D, Tadic S, Simic D (2003) Extent of oncological resection in laparoscopic versus open colorectal surgery: Meta-analysis. Langenbecks Arch Surg 387:366–371

44. Schwenk W, Haase O, Neudecker J, et al. (2005) Short term benefits for laparoscopic colorectal resection. Cochrane Database Syst Rev 20:CD003145

45. Tilney HS, Lovegrove RE, Purkayastha S, et al. (2006) Laparoscopic versus open subtotal colectomy for benign and malignant disease. Colorectal Dis 8:441–450

46. Schmidt AI, Reismann M, Kübler JF, et al. (2006) Exposure to carbon dioxide and helium alters in vitro proliferation of pediatric tumor cells. Pediatr Surg Int 22:72–77

47. Iwanaka T, Arya G, Ziegler MM (1998) Minimally invasive surgery does not improve the outcome in a model of retroperitoneal murine neuroblastoma. Pediatr Surg Int 13:149–153

48. Iwanaka T, Arya G, Ziegler MM (1998) Mechanism and prevention of port-site tumor recurrence after laparoscopy in a murine model. J Pediatr Surg 33:457–461

49. Fondrinier E, Boisdron-Celle M, Chassevent A, et al. (2001) Experimental assessment of tumor growth and dissemination of a microscopic peritoneal carcinomatosis after CO2 peritoneal insufflation or laparotomy. Surg Endosc 15:843–848

50. Iwanaka T, Arai M, Yamamoto H, Fukuzawa M, et al. (2003) No incidence of port-site recurrence after endosurgical procedure for pediatric malignancies. Pediatr Surg Int 19:200–203

51. Warmann S, Fuchs J, Jesch NK (2003) A prospective study of minimally invasive techniques in pediatric surgical oncology: Preliminary report. Med Pediatr Oncol 40:155–157

52. Saenz NC, Conlon KC, Aronson DC, et al. (1997) The application of minimal access procedures in infants, children, and young adults with pediatric malignancies. J Laparoendosc Adv Surg Tech A 7:289–294

53. Sandoval C, Strom K, Stringel G (2004) Laparoscopy in the management of pediatric intra-abdominal tumors. JSLS 8:115–118

54. Waldhausen JH, Tapper D, Sawin RS (2000) Minimally invasive surgery and clinical decision-making for pediatric malignancy. Surg Endosc 14:250–253

55. Spurbeck WW, Davidoff AM, Lobe TE, et al. (2004) Minimally invasive surgery in pediatric cancer patients. Ann Surg Oncol 11:340–343

56. Iwanaka T, Arai M, Kawashima H, et al. (2004) Endosurgical procedures for pediatric solid tumors. Pediatr Surg Int 20:39–42

57. Holcomb GW 3rd, Tomita SS, Haase GM, et al. (1995) Minimally invasive surgery in children with cancer. Cancer 76:121–128

58. Silecchia G, Fantini A, Raparelli L, et al. (1999) Management of abdominal lymphoproliferative diseases in the era of laparoscopy. Am J Surg 177:325–330

59. Iwanaka T, Arai M, Ito M, et al. (2001) Surgical treatment for abdominal neuroblastoma in the laparoscopic era. Surg Endosc 15:751–754

60. Iwanaka T, Arai M, Ito M, et al. (2001) Challenges of laparoscopic resection of abdominal neuroblastoma with lymphadenectomy. A preliminary report. Surg Endosc 15:489–492

61. de Lagausie P, Berrebi D, Michon J, et al. (2003) Laparoscopic adrenal surgery for neuroblastomas in children. J Urol 170:932–935

62. Lo CY, Tam PK (2003) Laparoscopic pancreatic resection of an insulinoma in a child. Asian J Surg 26:43–45

63. Carricaburu E, Enezian G, Bonnard A, et al. (2003) Laparoscopic distal pancreatectomy for Frantz's tumor in a child. Surg Endosc 17:2028–2031

64. Duarte RJ, Denes FT, Cristofani LM, et al. (2004) Laparoscopic nephrectomy for Wilms tumor after chemotherapy: Initial experience. J Urol 172:1438–1440

65. Yamamoto H, Yoshida M, Sera Y (1996) Laparoscopic surgery for neuroblastoma identified by mass screening. J Pediatr Surg 31:385–388

66. Nakajima K, Fukuzawa M, Fukui Y, et al. (1997) Laparoscopic resection of mass-screened adrenal neuroblastoma in an 8-month-old infant. Surg Laparosc Endosc 7:498–500

67. Kouch K, Yoshida H, Matsunaga T, et al. (2003) Extirpation of mass-screened adrenal neuroblastomas by retroperitoneoscopy. Surg Endosc 17:1769–1772

68. Komuro H, Makino S, Tahara K (2000) Laparoscopic resection of an adrenal neuroblastoma detected by mass screening that grew in size during the observation period. Surg Endosc 14:297

69. Skarsgard ED, Albanese CT (2005) The safety and efficacy of laparoscopic adrenalectomy in children. Arch Surg 140:905–908

70. Mirallie E, Leclair MD, de Lagausie P, et al. (2001) Laparoscopic adrenalectomy in children. Surg Endosc 15:156–160

71. Castilho LN, Castillo OA, Denes FT, et al. (2002) Laparoscopic adrenal surgery in children. J Urol 168:221–224

72. Steyaert H, Juricic M, Hendrice C, et al. (2003) Retroperitoneoscopic approach to the adrenal glands and retroperitoneal tumours in children: Where do we stand? Eur J Pediatr Surg 13:112–115

73. Pampaloni EL, Valeri A, Mattei R, et al. (2004) Initial experience with laparoscopic adrenal surgery in children: Is endoscopic surgery recommended and safe for the treatment of adrenocortical neoplasms? Pediatr Med Chir 26:450–459

74. Waldhausen JHT, Shaw DWW, Hall DG, et al. (1997) Needle localization for thoracoscopic resection of small pulmonary nodules in children. J Pediatr Surg 32:1624–1625

75. Pursnani SK, Rausen AR, Contractor S, et al. (2006) Combined use of preoperative methylene blue dye and microcoil localization facilitates thoracoscopic wedge resection of indeterminate pulmonary nodules in children. J Laparoendosc Adv Surg Tech A 16:184–187

76. Curet MJ (2004) Port site metastases. Am J Surg 187:705–712

77. Sartoreli KH, Patrick D, Meagher DP (1996) Port-site recurrence after thoracoscopic resection of pulmonary metastasis owing to osteogenic sarcoma. J Pediatr Surg 31:1443–1444

78. Ostlie DJ, Holcomb GW III (2003) The use of stab incisions for instrument access in laparoscopic operations. J Pediatr Surg 38:1837–1840

79. Sailhamer E, Jackson CA, Vogel AM, et al. (2003) Minimally invasive surgery in pediatric solid neoplasms. Am Surg 69:566–568

80. Smith TJ, Rothenberg SS, Brooks M, et al. (2002) Thoracoscopic surgery in childhood cancer. J Pediatr Hematol Oncol 24:429–435

81. Petty JK, Bensard DD, Patrick DA, et al. (2006) Resection of neurogenic tumors in children: Is thoracoscopy superior to thoracotomy? J Am Coll Surg 196(3):484–488

82. Lacreuse I, Becmeur F, Valla JF Thoracoscopic resection of neurogenic tumours in children. Submitted, J Laparoendosc Adv Surg Tech A

83. Hayes-Jordan A, Connolly BL, Temple M, et al. (2003) Image-guided percutaneous approach is super to the thoracoscopic approach in the diagnosis of pulmonary nodules in children. J Pediatr Surg 38:745–748

84. Connolly BL, Chait PG, Duncan DS, et al. (1999) CT-guided percutaneous needle biopsy of small lung nodules in children. Pediatr Radiol 29:342–346

New Treatments and New Strategies

26

Edward M. Barksdale, Jr.

Contents

26.1 Introduction

Recent advances in molecular and cell biology have opened new avenues for the understanding of the genetic nature of cancer. Emergence of novel treatment approaches over the last 50 years has resulted in significant improvement in the prognosis of childhood cancer. The long-term survival rate for pediatric cancer patients in the 1960s was approximately 20% and currently is in the range of greater than 75% [1]. Specifically, the survival in patients with Wilm's tumor has dramatically increased from 30% to 90% during this period [2]. Despite these impressive trends in survival, little progress has been made in the therapy of many pediatric brain tumors, neuroblastoma, and soft-tissue sarcomas. Furthermore, the focus of mainstream cancer therapies to target the proliferating cells has led to significant side-effects in normal developing tissues, organs, and bone marrow predisposing children to growth delay, cognitive impairments, and secondary malignancies [3]. Clearly, strategies that are both more targeted and effective are mandated in these patients.

Enhanced understanding of cancer biology further reinforces the complex and dynamic nature of the genomic events surrounding tumor development, progression, and metastasis. Despite this complexity there appear to be subset of molecular, biochemical, cellular, and immunologic traits or fingerprints that characterize all the events in the cell's neoplastic transformation from the normal to the premalignant and then to the malignant phenotype. Hanahan and Weinberg (2000) postulated that cancer was a "manifestation of six essential alterations in cell physiology that collectively dictate malignant growth." These six "hallmarks of cancer" include: (1) autonomous provision of growth signals; (2) resistance to growth inhibitory signals; (3) evasion of apoptosis; (4) replication without limits; (5) sustained angiogenesis; and (6) local tissue invasion and distant metastasis [4]. Recent work over the last two decades gives credence to a possible seventh trait: evasion of host tumor immune detection or immunosurveillance [5]. In this context the inherent genomic instability of cancers frequently render them rapidly moving targets for therapies directed at only one component of their behavior.

The classic paradigm for cancer therapy consists of radical surgery, multiagent chemotherapy, and external beam radiation all directed primarily at limiting the proliferative potential of the cancer cell. This chapter will focus on the emerging therapies and strategies that are in late preclinical phases of development or currently being utilized in early clinical trials, usually in adults. Some of these promising therapies may have applications in the treatment of pediatric solid tumors, while others may remain preclinical yet provide a limited forecast of the possibilities that lie on the horizon of pediatric cancer care. This chapter will specifically focus on immune-based (cellular, vaccine, and monoclonal), antiangiogenesis, and gene and antisense therapies to provide a conceptual foundation of understanding of these novel and emerging cancer strategies. Although these therapies are presented as different subcategories, they are often complementary and overlapping in their application. This is a dynamic and evolving area of combined medical and scientific interest; more detailed reviews of these topics may be obtained in the references.

26.2 Immunotherapy

Increased understanding of the molecular, cellular, and immunologic mechanisms of tumor-host interactions has led to greater insights regarding the potential for therapeutic manipulation to enhance the rejection of invasive and metastatic cancer. Even as early as the late 19th century William Coley, an American surgeon, observed that tumor regression could be mediated by bacterial toxins [6]. Although Burnet hypothesized that cancer occurred due to an impairment in immunosurveillance in the mid-20th century, the role of the immune system in the pathogenesis of cancer did not gain acceptance until the late 20th century [7]. A preponderance of evidence now exists that the immune system plays a significant role in cancer biology. This includes the spontaneous regression of certain tumors like neuroblastoma, the presence of antitumor antibodies and immune effector cells in patients with treated tumors, the correlation of lymphocytic infiltration in cancer tissue specimens with survival, the 200-fold increased rate of malignancy patients with congenital or acquired immunodeficiencies and the fivefold increase in cancer posttransplantation [8–10].

The immune response may be broadly categorized into two interrelated components: innate and adaptive immunity. Innate immunity consists of nonspecific, antigen-independent killing that is mediated by neutrophils, macrophages, monocytes, dendritic cells, natural killer cells, eosinophils, and complement activation pathways. This is the first line of immunologic defense against bacterial or parasitic infection. Innate immunity does not induce immunologic memory directly but may critically orchestrate the development of the adaptive immune response. Adaptive immunity involves antigen-specific immune recognition by T and B cells and subsequent clonal expansion of immuneffector and memory cells. This complex network forms the biologic defense against viral infection and likely malignant transformation by directly targeting pathogens or autologous cells expressing foreign or altered proteins for destruction. Concurrently, this system has evolved to both recognize self-antigens to avoid their destruction and to delete autoreactive immuneffector cells known as clonal deletion. Many tumors express altered self-antigens that may either evoke an immune response, or due to homology with the native or wild-type protein, induce tolerance. This capacity to discriminate self versus non-self is one of the hallmarks of the immune system and a critical concept in understanding the design, limitations, and side effects of immune based therapies [11]. Enhancing immunoreactivity to malignantly transformed cells while limiting the induction of autoimmunity is the principal goal of cancer immunotherapy.

Although many preclinical studies have demonstrated tumor eradication in mice, progress toward the development of effective antitumor strategies in humans has been limited [12, 13]. The principle barrier to the development of more effective immunotherapies is related to the cancer cell's ability to escape detection or immunosurveillance and the development of tumor-specific immune tolerance. Tumors have evolved numerous mechanisms to induce a state of anergy. Some of these mechanisms include the downregulation of MHC/HLA Class I molecule expression, the loss of tumor antigens, defective death receptor signaling (FAS-L and others), expression of immunosuppressive cytokines (TGF-, IL10), migration of immunosuppressive T regulatory or suppressor cells to the tumor microenvironment, and the lack of costimulatory molecule expression. Another important tolerogenic mechanism is immunoediting or the selection tumor cell clones that are not recognized by the antitumor immune response [14–16]. Two broad categories of immunotherapies have emerged to disrupt the tolerogenic state induced by cancers: antibody-based therapies (monoclonal antibodies) and T cell-based therapies (adoptive/cell transfer and vaccine based).

26.2.1 Monoclonal Antibody Therapy

Three decades ago the technique of monoclonal antibodies (mAbs) was developed and shortly thereafter much enthusiasm emerged about their potential as an anticancer immunotherapy [17]. Despite the initial interest the early therapeutic agents were marginally effective due to: (1) the immunogenicity of the vaccines; (2) the direction against ineffective cell targets. These therapies utilized unmodified murine mAbs, which were unable to kill targets due to their inability to fix complement, elicit antibody-dependent cellular cytotoxicity (ADCC) with host mononuclear cells and their limited *in vivo* survival. Furthermore, these antibodies did not target appropriate surface molecules critical to tumor survival, which limited their effectiveness [18–20]. Present modifications utilizing fully human or humanized antibodies and mAbs directed against cell surface targets like cytokines, growth factors, and death signal receptors have significantly improved the overall effectiveness of these antibodies making them the most rapidly growing class of immunotherapeutic agents in clinical use [21].

Based on the early lessons, various therapeutic strategies have emerged in the current design of monoclonal antibodies against cancer. Targets for monoclonal antibodies include the tumor cell (direct specificity), the host tissue (indirect specificity), or the negative immunoregulatory checkpoints in the antitumor inflammatory cascade (indirect specificity). Several approaches directed against the tumor cells include activation of the death pathways, activation of antibody dependent cellular cytotoxicity (ADCC), blockade of growth factor stimulated cell proliferation, and antibody mediated delivery of cytotoxic agents. Examples of these include CD30-directed mAbs which activate the tumor necrosis factor alpha (TNF-α), tumor cell death-signaling pathway, promoting apoptotic death in the target tumor cell. Monoclonal antibodies have also been utilized against host tissue targets like angiogenic molecules or basement membrane proteins. Avastatin, a humanized antibody approved for the treatment of metastatic colon cancer, is a potent angiogenesis inhibitor that targets vascular endothelial growth factor. Alternative targets for monoclonal antibodies include the host cells that regulate immune response. Examples of these agents include anti-CTLA-4, which eliminates a negative T-cell receptor signaling pathway, and mAbs that eliminate CD4+CD 25+ T reg cells [20].

Several mAbs have been approved for clinical use and well over 100 antibodies are presently being evaluated in therapeutic clinical trials [21]. Some of the mAbs currently approved for therapy of solid tumors include Trastuzumab (Hercecptin), a mAb directed against HER-2/neu; the epidermal growth factor receptor (EGFR), important in some breast and gastrointestinal tumors; and Bevacizumab (Avistatin) which targets vascular endothelial growth factor (VEGF). Pediatric solid tumors like sarcomas, neuroblastomas, and gliomas may express these same molecules and be candidates for treatment with these mAbs. The human mouse chimeric antidisialoganglioside (GD2) antibody-cytokine fusion protein ch14.18-IL-2 and the anti-GD2 murine IgG3 antibody 3F8 are two mAbs currently being studied in neuroblastoma. They target the disialoganglioside, GD2, the most highly expressed antigen on the surface of neuroblastoma and activate the complement cascade and antibody directed cellular cytotoxicity. Favorable outcomes have been reported in patients who have minimal residual disease following conventional therapies [22–26]. The effectiveness of monoclonal antibodies in therapy against solid tumors is limited by the impaired exposure and incomplete penetration to all the tumor cells [27].

26.2.2 T Cell-Based Therapies

The work pioneered by Rosenberg and others has demonstrated that cells in the immune system can be therapeutically exploited as anticancer agents. Tumor reactive C8+ cytotoxic T lymphocytes (CTLs), CD4+ helper cells, natural killer cells, and antigen presenting cells (dendritic cells, macrophages, etc.) are among the most promising candidates for cell-directed therapies.

These therapies are based on the fundamental concept that tumors selectively express different protein antigens (Ag) relative to normal tissue that may function as specific targets of the immune response by cytotoxic T cells. T-cell-based immunotherapies may utilize the adoptive transfer of autologous ex vivo stimulated T cells or vaccine strategies directed at the in vivo activation of tumor reactive T cells [28, 29]. T-cell activation is a multistage process that first involves antigen-specific engagement of the T cell receptor complex (TCR), which is triggered by the recognition of peptides complexed with MHC Class I or II molelcules. The TCR-Ag interaction is facilitated by the engagement of adjacent adhesion molecules like intercellular adhesion molecule 1 (ICAM-1) expressed by the antigen presenting cell and its specific ligand leukocyte function antigen 1 (LFA-1) on the T cell to form a supermolecular activation complex (SMAC) (Fig. 26.1). Costimulation, the binding of other APC surface molecules with their T cell ligands, is required in order to achieve further T cell activation and expansion. The most important of these APC costimulatory signaling molecules are B7.1 and B7.2 which bind CD28 on T cells. Absent or inadequate CD28 signaling/costimulation results in the induction of a tolerogenic response to the specific antigen [30].

26.2.3 Adoptive Cell Transfer

Adoptive cell transfer techniques involve three principal steps in order to produce potent antitumor responses: (1) isolation of antitumor T cells from patients with cancer; (2) ex vivo expansion and activation of these CTL; (3) autologous reinfusion of CTL with ap-

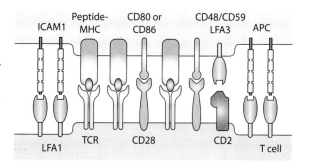

Fig. 26.1 Supermolecular activation complex (SMAC). T cell receptor-antigen-major histocompatibility complex (TCR-Ag(Peptide)-MHC) binding is facilitated by the engagement of adjacent adhesion molecules like intracellular adhesion molecule 1 (ICAM-1), CD 80/CD86, and CD48/CD59 (LFA-3) expressed by the antigen-presenting cell to their specific ligands leukocyte function antigen 1 (LFA-1), CD2, and CD28 on the T cells respectively to form the supermolecular activation complex (SMAC) or "immunologic synapse." [102]

propriate growth factors [31]. CTLs recognize antigens secreted by tumors that consist of 8–10 amino acid peptide fragments or epitopes derived from cytoplasmic proteins that have undergone proteosomic degradation. These epitopes are then covalently bound in the cleft of the Class I Human Leukocyte Antigen (HLA), also known as the Major Histocompatibility Complex (MHC) located within the T cell receptor (TCR) [32]. Expression cloning techniques, which involve the identification of these peptide fragments by transfecting complementary DNA (cDNA) libraries from tumors into target cells expressing the appropriate MHC molecule, have led to the identification of numerous tumor antigens and the genes that encode them [33]. Adoptive therapies utilizing the immunodominant peptide epitopes isolated from these tumors coadministered with an immunoadjuvant like IL-2 have demonstrated that high levels of tumor-reactive T cells may be generated. These overexpressed target peptides usually fall into one of three categories: oncogenes, tumor unique antigens, and tissue differentiation antigens [31, 34] (Table 26.1). Despite the propagation of numerous preclinical and clinical studies, most T-cell-based immunotherapies fail to generate a sustained antitumor response. In fact a recent review of the multiple clinical trials utilizing these therapies only demonstrated a 3%

clinical response rate [13]. The failure of these strategies may be secondary to insufficient CTL activation, aberrant activation of the antitumor cell, or the endogenous immune response or failure of proliferation of the antitumor lymphocytes in the host or tumor microenvironment.

26.2.4 Vaccine Therapy

The holy grail of tumor immunotherapy is the development of a preventive vaccine that will eradicate cancers in a manner analogous to the smallpox vaccine. Although 10–20% of all human tumors may be caused by viruses and other microorganisms, the vast majority of human malignancies are the result of either exogenous carcinogens or endogenous genomic events that result in malignant transformation [35]. Hepatitis B and Human Papilloma virus vaccines will undoubtedly markedly diminish the worldwide incidence of hepatic and cervical malignancies respectively [36, 37]. The goal of the ideal vaccine for cancer prevention would provide a sustained response against oncogenesis over the entire life of the individual (Fig. 26.2). These preventive therapies would likely require periodic boosters to both stimulate and maintain immune memory. These

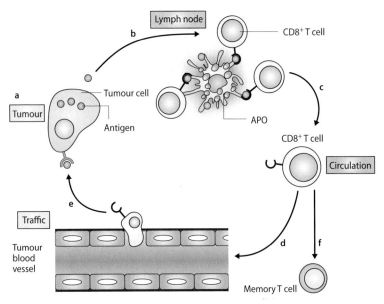

Fig. 26.2 a–f The six steps necessary for an effective antitumor CD8+ T-cell response. Tumor lysis mediated by antigen specific CD8+ T cells is a multistep process. Each of the six steps is an immunoregulatory checkpoint that may be modulated by a host of factors. These steps include: (**a**) expression of peptide antigen by the tumor; (**b**) antigen uptake and processing by antigen-presenting cells (APC) and subsequent antigen presentation by the APC to T cells in the lymph node; (**c**) T-cell proliferation by tumor antigen specific T cells; (**d**) access to and entry into the tumor; (**e**) evasion by CD8+ cytotoxic T cells by immuno-suppressive and immunoregulatory factors in the tumor microenvironment to recognize and lyse their tumor targets; (**f**) generation of memory T cells. Tumor immunotherapy utilizing T-cell-based strategies may fail at each of these critical steps. Advances in the development of immunoassays and immunodiagnostic techniques have not only improved the understanding of antitumor response but have facilitated the development of strategies to overcome the specific factors that may impair the immunotherapeutic response at each of these steps [103].

Table 26.1 Categories T-cell defined antigens

Vaccine setting	Antigen targeted by the vaccine	Time for the induction of the immune reaction	Status of the immune system to be activated	Foremost effector mechanism to be activated	Lesion targeted by the immune reaction	Required duration of the induced reaction
Therapeutic	Tumor-associated T-cell epitopes from mutated proteins, differentiation antigens, embryo/testis antigens, overexpressed antigens, or oncoantigens	Short because of the threat posed by tumor growth	Negatively imprinted by a growing tumor with expanded immature suppressor myeloid cells and regulatory T cells; debilitated by previous therapies	CTLs; antibody production is often seen as detrimental	Large, actively proliferating and genetically unstable	Short (months)
Preventive	Mostly oncoantigens	Long, which gives plenty of time to induce an optimal immune reaction; repeated booster and recall vaccinations are required	A normal immune system that has not yet perceived a possible incipient tumor	A coordinate induction of T-helper cells, antibodies, and CTLs; antibody-mediated down modulation of oncoantigens might prevent tumor development	Not yet existing, or small; localized; endowed with an indolent proliferative activity; not sheltered from the immune attack by an abundant stroma	Persistent, potentially lifelong

From [38]

vaccines would also need to simultaneously thwart the development of self-reactive clones that would lead to the development of autoimmune disease. The efficacy of this type of vaccine appears to require the coadministration of other immunoadjuvants like cytokines, allogeneic MHC glycoproteins, costimulatory molecules, and microbial CpG. Furthermore, the data support that in order for these preventive vaccines to be effective they must be initiated early in the process of tumorigenesis [38].

In contrast to preventive vaccines, therapeutic vaccines are more readily applicable to current cancer therapy. Various categories of vaccines exist including tumor cells (autologous or allogeneic), tumor cell lysates (membrane and heat shock proteins), gene-modified tumor cells (encoding cytokine genes or costimulatory molecules), and tumor-dendritic cell fusion products. Vaccines may also be based on purified antigenic peptides, synthetic peptides, naked DNA, recombinant viruses, and recombinant bacteria [38] (Table 26.2). Both autologous and allogeneic tumor cell vaccines have been trialed for several decades but are labor intensive and only marginally

effective because they fail to evoke sustained antitumor immune responses. Many of these trials have utilized melanomas or allogeneic melanoma cell lines [39]. Genetic modification of tumor cells with cytokine genes have demonstrated modest effects in several phase I and II clinical trials. These vaccines constructed to express, GM-CSF, IL-2, B&-1, and CD40L have serologic and pathologic evidence of an immune response; however, clinical responses have been marginal [40]. Peptide-based vaccines that contain the appropriate HLA-restricted amino acid sequences can be designed and constructed to improve the binding affinity to T cells. These sequences based on tumor-specific, tumor-unique, and tissue-differentiation antigens can be engineered by markedly enhancing the binding affinity and stability of the TCR-MHC tumor peptide complex, resulting in enhanced antitumor immunity. This involves minimal changes in the amino acids of a specific epitope (peptide sequence). These vaccines are quite labor intensive and require exact HLA typing and matching with the precise tumor peptide epitope. Examples of these tumor antigens include: [41, 42].

Table 26.2 Key differences between anti-tumor vaccines in cancer therapy and prevention

Antigen	Tissue Expression	
	Tumors	Normal Tissue
Differentiation antigens (overexpressed)		
Tyrosinase	Melanoma	Melanocytes
MART1/Melan-A	Melanoma	Melanocytes
GP100	Melanoma	Melanocytes
Differentiation antigens (normally expressed)		
Prostate-specific antigens	Prostate cancer	Prostate
CD20, idiotype	B-cell malignancies	B cells
Cancer-testis antigens		
MAGE1, MAGE3	Melanoma, others	Testis, placenta
GAGE and others	Melanoma, others	Testis, placenta
Oncofetal antigens		
CEA	Colon cancer, others	Liver, others
AFP	Liver cancer	-
Mutated antigens		
CASP8	Head and neck cancer	-
CDK4, MUM3	Melanoma	-
Beta-catenin	Melanoma, lung, others	-

Classification of T-cell-defined antigens with a partial list of examples. (Note overexpressed or mutated oncogenic proteins – such as RAS, BCR-ABL, and p53 – are additional potential target antigens and T cells that recognize such antigens can be generated in vitro. However, as such antigens have not previously been identified as targets of endogenous tumor-reactive T cells in humans, they are not considered to be "T-cell-defined" antigens.)

AFP, alpha fetoprotein; CASP8, caspase-8; CDK4, cyclin-dependent kinase 4; CEA, carcinoembryonic antigen; MAGE, melanoma antigen; MART1, melanoma-associated antigen recognized by T cells 1

(From Yee C, Greenberg P (2002) Modulating T-cell immunity to tumours: New strategies for monitoring T-cell responses. Nat Rev Cancer 2:409-419)

Recent understanding of the role of T-cell activation by "professional" antigen presenting cells (monocytes, macrophages, and dendritic cells), the regulation of T-cell activation by regulatory T (suppressor) cells, and the role of T-cell trafficking and costimulation may lead to further advances in the effectiveness of cellular therapies. Dendritic cells (DC), the most potent antigen presenting cells, hold great promise as an adjuvant immunotherapy or cancer vaccine (Fig. 26.3). Primarily due to the marginal efficacy of other vaccine strategies, DC-based vaccines have emerged as a viable alternative to conventional vaccine strategies. DC, a population of bone-marrow-derived cells, reside in an immature state at peripheral sites where they monitor for environmental alterations such as viral infection or malignant transformation. These changes stimulate antigen uptake via phagocytosis that initiates DC differentiation and proliferation. These APC subsequently migrate to regional lymphoid organs where they present high concentrations of tumor antigens to naive T cells that are then activated. This stimulation of T-cell-activation, also known as priming, results in numerous CTLs directed against the tumor [43]. DC-based therapies offer several sites for therapeutic manipulation of the cellular immune response. DC may be activated ex vivo with agents like GM-CSF, Interleukin-4 (IL-4), or CD-40L, or DC may be loaded with antigen. Alternatively, DC may be activated in vivo by simultaneous injection of tumor peptides with an immunoadjuvant like CD-40 antibodies, chemokines, and immunoglobulin G Fc fragment. Ex vivo engineering of DC has gained the greatest favor and allows manipulation of CD 34+ hematopoetic DC progenitors or monocytes that are naive and unexposed to the tolerogenic effects of the tumor microenvironment [44] (Fig. 26.4).

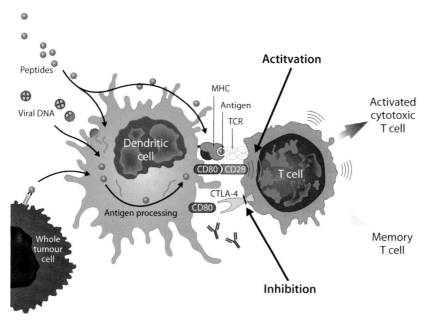

Fig. 26.3 Dendritic cell (antigen-presenting cell)-T cell stimulation. Dendritic cells and other antigen-presenting cells can process antigens such as peptides or whole-tumor cells, can become infected by viral vectors that then express tumor-associated antigens for presentation, or can be ex vivo pulsed with peptides then injected. These antigen-presenting cells present to the T cell, causing activation of the T cell. Upon activation, CTLA-4 is upregulated and inhibits prolonged activation of the T cell. Antibodies to CTLA-4 can block the inhibitory signals and cause prolonged activation. CTLA-4, cytotoxic T-lymphocyte-associated protein 4; MHC, major histocompatibility complex; TCR, T-cell receptor [104].

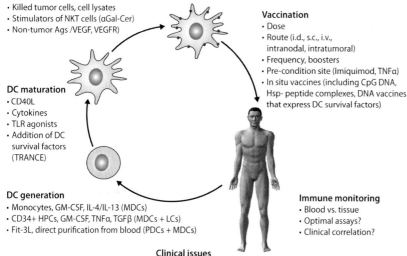

Antigen loading
- Peptides (MHC I-restricted, MHC II-restricted)
- Proteins
- Ag-Ab complexes, receptor targeting, Hsp-peptide complexes (cross-presentation)
- RNA, DNA (single gene or whole tumor-derived, lysosomal targeting sequences, genes encoding cytokines, chemokines, co-stimulatory molecules or survival factors)
- Viral vectors
- Killed tumor cells, cell lysates
- Stimulators of NKT cells (αGal-Cer)
- Non-tumor Ags /VEGF, VEGFR

Vaccination
- Dose
- Route (i.d., s.c., i.v., intranodal, intratumoral)
- Frequency, boosters
- Pre-condition site (Imiquimod, TNFα)
- In situ vaccines (including CpG DNA, Hsp- peptide complexes, DNA vaccines that express DC survival factors)

DC maturation
- CD40L
- Cytokines
- TLR agonists
- Addition of DC survival factors (TRANCE)

DC generation
- Monocytes, GM-CSF, IL-4/IL-13 (MDCs)
- CD34+ HPCs, GM-CSF, TNFα, TGFβ (MDCs + LCs)
- Fit-3L, direct purification from blood (PDCs + MDCs)

Immune monitoring
- Blood vs. tissue
- Optimal assays?
- Clinical correlation?

Clinical issues
- Standardized response criteria (WHO, RECIST)
- Clinical setting (metastatic disease, minimal residual disease, adjuvat therapy, maintenace, prophylaxis)
- Combination therapies

Fig. 26.4 Clinical dendritic cell (DC) vaccines. A variety of strategies have been devised to use DC vaccines in the immunotherapy of cancer. DC may be generated (isolated/purified), matured, and antigen loaded ex vivo. Generation strategies may result in heterogeneous DC populations that may have varying numbers of macrophages, monocytes, and other immune-effector cells. DC maturation strategies employ the use of various cytokines and other agonist and survival factors. DC are then loaded with peptides proteins (antigen), cytokines, chemokines, DC survival factors, factors that stimulate other immune-effector cells or other nontumor antigens. Following preparation of the DC they may be delivered via a variety of routes and the immune response to therapy may be assessed by various monitoring techniques. The correlation of these monitoring immunologic assays with clinical outcome will determine the true efficacy of these therapies. Adapted from [105].

Table 26.3 Vaccine approaches to cancer treatment

Vaccines can be based either on cancer cells or on the genetic identification of cancer antigens.
Many of these materials can be used to pulse, transfect, or tranduce APCs or can be administered with a variety of adjuvants or cytokines.

Vaccines based on cancer cells are derived from: whole cancer cells (both autologous and allogeneic preparations); gene-modified cancer cells (genes encoding cytokines or co-stimulatory molecules); cancer cell extracts (lysates, membranes, and heat-shock proteins); and cancer cells fused to APCs

Vaccines based on the genetic identification of cancer antigens include:
purified cancer antigens (natural or recombinant); synthetic peptides; „naked" DNA (for example, plasmids); recombinant viruses (adenovirus, vaccinia, or avipox); and recombinant bacteria (Bacille Calmete-Guerin and listeria).

Adapted from [31]

Table 26.4 Blockade of negative immunoregulatory checkpoints that impair immunotherapy

Host negative immunoregulatory mechanism	Potential intervention to release checkpoint on the immune response
Signals mediated by negative T cell costimulatory molecule CTLA-4 after interaction with CD80, 86 family on APCs deliver signals that terminate T cell activation	Antibody-mediated blockade of CTLA-4 to enhance antitumor immunity induced by vaccine
PD1 interaction with PDL1 or PDL2 inhibits T cell receptor-mediated proliferation and activation of CD4+ T cells	Anti-PDL1 antibody
CD4+ CD25+ negative regulatory Tregs (supressor T cells) inhibit antitumor immune responses	Oncotoxin (IL-2 diphtheria toxin ONTAK), anti-IL-2Rα *Pseudomonas* toxin (LMB-2), or CD25-directed antibody (PC61) therapy to deplete Tregs
IL-2-mediated self-tolerance that leads to apoptosis of tumor-specific T cells	IL-15 to facilitate the survival of NK and memory phenotype CD8 T cells in lieu of IL-2
CD4+ NK T cell generation of IL-13 that indirectly (through the action of TGFβ) inhibits CD8+ cell-mediated antitumor responses. TGFβ is also synthesized directly by tumor cells or by host cells via other mechanisms	IL-13Rα IgFc or anti-TGFβ monoclonal antibody

APCs, antigen-presenting cells; PD1, programmed cell death-1; PDL1, PD1, Ligand 1; NK, natural killer; TGF, transforming growth factor; CTLA-4, cytotoxic T-lymphocytic antigen-4

Geiger, et al. demonstrated that tumor lysate-pulsed DC could be used to safely treat patients with advanced recurrent neuroblastoma that had failed conventional therapy, generate specific antitumor T cell responses, and yield regression of metastatic disease [45]. Other investigators have shown in preclinical models that DC transduced with cytokine genes or coadministered with cytokines may provide potentially effective therapies in neuroblastoma [46–48]. Few studies have been initiated in the immunotherapy of pediatric sarcomas; however, advances are being made relative to the understanding of the immunobiology of these tumors and potential strategic targets for cellular therapies [49].

Research on the role of cellular immunity has also led to improved understanding of the immunoregulatory checkpoints in the immune response. (Table 26.4)

These "brakes on the immune system" include the downregulation of MHC Class I expression by tumor cells, the absence of expression of the B7 family of costimulatory molecules (CD80, CD86), secretion of immunosuppressive factors like TGF-β, the expression of the negative regulatory T cells (Treg) that inhibit the antitumor response, and the immuno-inhibitory signaling receptor molecules cytotoxic T lymphocyte antigen-4 (CTLA-4, CD152) and programmed cell death-1 (PD-1) [50]. Regulatory or suppressor T (Treg) cells are a functionally distinct population of thymic-derived CD4+CD25+ immunoeffector cells that maintain the state of self tolerance and eliminate autoreactive CTL, including those that may be directed against tumor antigens. Large numbers of these cells have been found in breast, ovarian, pancreatic, and lung cancer. The expression of the transcriptional repressor

FOXP3, a forkhead protein, and chemokine-mediated migration by CCL2 supports the assumption that T-reg cells may create a microenvironment that favors tumor proliferation through direct effects on CTL and antigen presenting cell trafficking [51, 52].

26.3 Angiogenesis

The principle approach of classic anticancer chemotherapy has focused on the cancer cell. However, the inherent genetic instability of the malignantly transformed cell may render this a "moving target" for cell-directed therapies due to the propensity of malignancies to acquire drug resistance [53]. In contrast, the endothelial cell in the tumor microenvironment has greater genomic stability and this trait may render it a more stable and susceptible target for therapeutic manipulation [54].

Over the last 30 years a large body of work has demonstrated that the development of new capillaries from existing blood vessels or angiogenesis plays a critical role in the tumor formation and metastasis in a variety of malignancies including the pediatric cancers neuroblastoma and nephroblastoma [55]. This complex, highly regulated process stimulated locally by tissue hypoxia, the secretion of high levels of proangiogenic molecules like VEGF, PDGF, NOS, oncogene activation, and tumor suppressor mutation appears to be a distinct component of the repertoire that every tumor must acquire to survive. Laboratory evidence suggests that this occurs early in the premalignant stages of tumor development and may in fact be the "second hit" or signal that is felt to be necessary for transformation [56].

Angiogenesis is a multistep process that consists of local membrane degradation of the endothelial cell tube, invasion of the surrounding stroma, endothelial cell proliferation, migration and differentiation, capillary tube or "sprout" formation, tubular fusion and coalescence to form vascular loops which will allow blood to circulate into the region [57]. Each tumor appears to have its own distinct threshold or "angiogenic switch," when it progresses from the nonangiogenic to angiogenic phenotype. This angiogenic switch is felt to be a necessary step in malignant transformation and local tissue invasion [58] (Fig. 26.5). Furthermore, this phenotype increases the potential for metastasis by both enhanced tumor shedding into the general circulation and by the secretion of factors such as proteases that disrupt the basement membrane at distinct sites to allow metastatic growth [59, 60]. This process appears to be driven in some tissue sites by proangiogenic oncogenes, like EGFR, N-myc, and bcl-2 which are also important oncogenes in pediatric tumors. Other studies have identified an increasing number of angiogenic

inducers, the foremost of which appear to be VEGF and bFGF; however, others include placental growth factor, pleiotrophin, platelet-derived growth factor-BB, and transforming growth factor-β [61].

A number of studies utilizing advanced techniques of immunohistochemistry to evaluate primary tumors have demonstrated that vessel number and density within the primary tumor may correlate with both the metastatic potential and the long-term prognosis for many malignancies [62, 63]. There may also be tissue and tumor-specific angiogenic factors yet to be identified. There are also a number of naturally secreted endogenous angiogenesis inhibitors like angiostatin, endostatin, thrombospondin-1, and tumstatin which physiologically oppose the process [64]. It is hypothesized that under normal conditions in all tissues there is a dynamic balance between proangiogenic factors and angiogenic inhibitors that maintains a homeostatic block on the angiogenic switch [58]. Much scientific and clinical interest has recently focused on these categories of molecules as potential therapeutic anticancer adjuvants. In fact, a number of clinical trials in adult patients with advanced cancer have been initiated with drugs like Bevacizumab (Avastin), endostatin, angiostatin, VEGF-Trap, and TNP-470, which appear to have exclusively antiangiogenic inhibitory effects. While drugs like celecoxib (Celebrex), a cyclooxegenase-2 (COX-2) inhibitor, a potent anti-inflammatory drug and bortezomib (Velcade), a proteosome inhibitor used in multiple myeloma both have strong antiangiogenic activity in addition to their other effects [65].

The antiangiogenesis drugs may have direct or indirect inhibitory effects on tumor growth. An "indirect" angiogenesis inhibitor blocks angiogenic protein synthesis, neutralizes angiogenic protein, or blocks the endothelial receptor for the protein. Resistance to these indirect inhibitors may emerge through the selection of mutated malignant clones that have bypassed the blockade or survive through alternative angiogenic pathways [66]. A "direct" angiogenesis inhibitor prevents endothelial cells from responding to multiple angiogenic proteins. These inhibitors function through a mechanism that is independent of the more genetically unstable tumor cell and targets the more stable endothelial cell.

An understanding of tumor angiogenesis and the role of the endothelial cell in tumor progression has led to another potential modification of the current approach to the administration of cytotoxic chemotherapy. The classic "drug holiday" or period off chemotherapy, which is used to allow recovery of the bone marrow from the myeloablative effects of chemotherapy, has been found experimentally to allow the growth of the endothelial cell. Dose reduction with increased frequency of dosing or so-called metronomic

a Dormant

b Perivascular detachment and vessel dilation

c Onset of angiogenic sprouting

d Continuous sprouting; new vessel formation and maturation; recruitment of perivascular cells

e Tumour vasculature

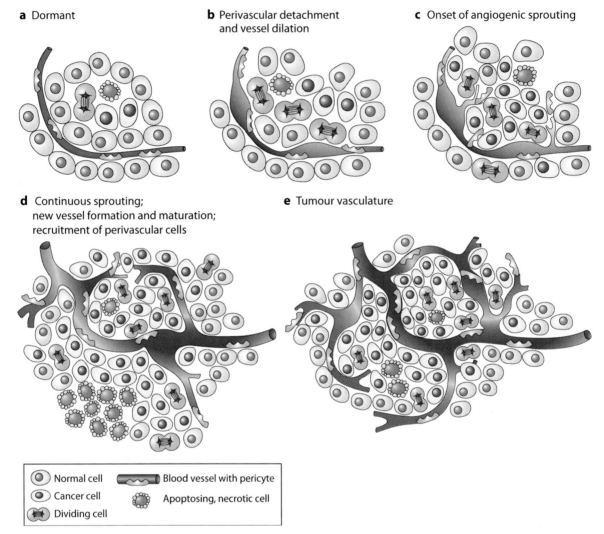

◉ Normal cell	▬▬ Blood vessel with pericyte
◉ Cancer cell	✺ Apoptosing, necrotic cell
✹ Dividing cell	

Fig. 26.5 a–e The angiogenic switch. (**a**) Most tumors begin as autonomously dividing cells that reach a steady state between replication and apoptosis and remain as dormant avascular nodules. The angiogenic switch is a critical event in tumor development and progression allowing for exponential tumor growth. This switch begins with (**b**) perivascular detachment and vascular dilatation, followed by the (**c**) onset of angiogenic sprouting, (**d**) neovascular development and growth with associated migration of perivascular cells. A (**e**) neovascular network engulfs the tumor providing critical metabolic substrates to hypoxic and necrotic areas of tissue to further potentiate tumor cell proliferation. Adapted from [106].

chemotherapy has been found to decrease the risk of drug resistance in these tumors and induce the expression of endogenous angiogenesis inhibitors [67].

Numerous endogenous and synthetic angiogenesis inhibitors have recently been developed that offer great promise in their therapeutic efficacy against a variety of tumors in preclinical trials. Some of these drugs have also been entered into clinical trials in adult malignancy; however, no published data exist for the clinical use of these drugs in pediatric solid tumors. In several murine tumor models of hepatoblastoma, nephroblastoma, and neuroblastoma, a number of angiogenesis inhibitors have demon-

strated efficacy but remain to be formally investigated in clinical trials [54]. In contrast, many trials are currently underway that are looking at the utility of these agents as components of the repertoire of anticancer therapy.

Endostatin, a 20-kD fragment of the basement membrane protein collagen XVIII with potent angiogenic inhibitory effects, is the prototypic inhibitor. It is a highly evolutionary conserved protein found in C. elegans. It has the broadest spectrum of antineoplastic spectrum of any endogenously occurring angiogenesis inhibitor, targeting more than 12% of the human genome, and is the most studied endogenous angiogenesis inhibitor [64]. Its mechanism of activity is based on its inhibition of VEGF binding to its receptor (KDR/Flk-1); blockade of tyrosine kinase phosphorylation of this receptor; inhibited blockade of intracellular signaling pathway; blockade of extracellular signaling kinase, p38 mitogen activated protein kinase (MAPK), as well as other yet-to-be determined signaling pathways. It has minimal toxicity and may reach its designated targets in some tissues through oral administration. Endostatin plasma levels may be induced by some oral drugs such as prednisolone, slazosulfapyridine, and celecoxcib [68].

26.4 Gene Therapy

Gene therapy, the introduction of genetic material into cells for therapeutic indications, may be an important treatment strategy for a variety of malignancies. Gene therapy encompasses a broad spectrum of experimental strategies extending from the direct delivery of "suicide genes" to the transduction of specific antigen or cytokine genes into the tumor cell that will elicit a vigorous antitumor response. Other potential targets for anticancer gene therapy may be immunoeffector cells, such as T cells, macrophages, and dendritic cells or the extracellular matrix. Three major categories of anticancer gene therapy exist: (1) immune enhancement, (2) direct tumor killing, (3) bone marrow pro-

tection [69]. Although clinical trials have been performed in adults with marginal success, the number of studies in children remain limited due to significant safety considerations [70].

The successful introduction of genetic material into eukaryotic cells requires a transduction method that will both successfully insert the genetic material in the particular cell of interest with adequate efficiency and will promote sufficient expression of the gene in the cell type. Transduction methods may result in permanent or transient alteration of the host genetic material. Alternatively, expression of the transgene may be constituitive or regulated. Although numerous techniques of gene transfer exist, they fall into two major categories, viral and nonviral techniques. The principle viral techniques involve retroviruses, adenoviruses, adeno-associated viruses, pox viruses, and herpes simplex viruses. The viral techniques offer ease of in vivo delivery and sustained high level transgene expression but may interfere with normal cell function or evoke an immune response. Nonviral techniques utilize DNA encapsulated in cationic lipids (liposomes) or physical methods like gene gun or hydrodynamic gene transfer techniques to introduce genetic material into the cell. Although nonviral methods of gene delivery offer advantages of ease of production and diminished toxicity, the efficiency of in vivo delivery is diminished and lacks sustained high-level expression [69] (Table 26.5),

Table 26.5 Characteristics of vectors used for gene therapy

Vector	Packaging capacity	Ease of production	Integration into host genome	Duration of expression	Transduction of postmitotic cells	Pre-existing host immunity	Safety concerns	Germline transmission
Non-viral	Unlimited	+++	Rarely	Usually transient	++	None	–	–
Retroviral	a 8.0 kb	Producer cell lines for onco-retroviral but not lentiviral vectors	Yes	Long-term	Lentiviral vectors ++ Onco-retroviral vectors	None	Insertional mutagenesis	–/+
Adenoviral	a 30.0 kb	+/–	No	Transient	Very efficient	+++	Inflammatory response	–
AAV	4.6 kb	Cumbersome	Rarely	Long-term in postmitotic cells	Efficient	++	–	+/–
Herpes	a 150 kb	+/–	No	Transient	++	+++	Inflammatory response	–

Viral vectors have been favored in the cancer gene therapy due to their ability to facilitate in vivo delivery to a variety of sites and the capacity to maintain prolonged transgene expression. Two categories of viral vectors are recognized: integrating and nonintegrating. One of the most common viral methods of gene transfer is through the use of retroviruses. Following cellular entry the viral DNA undergoes reverse transcription to DNA by viral reverse transcriptase. Subsequently, the DNA molecules undergo nuclear translocation, nuclear entry via the nucleopore and stable genomic integration. The virally integrated DNA or provirus is then translated into protein [7]. Retroviral vectors are constructed by substituting the gene of interest in the viral protein coding regions. Packaging of these particles using helper or packaging cell lines that contain structural viral proteins facilitate genomic incorporation [70]. Adenovirus, adeno-associated virus, and herpes virus vectors are incorporated into episomes that are not integrated into the host DNA and are subsequently lost over time. These offer distinct advantages in clinical situations when transient transgene expression is desired.

The most efficient viral vectors for transgene expression are the adenoviruses [69]. These viruses do not require cell division for transduction, may be produced in high titers, transduce with high levels of efficiency without host genomic incorporation (episome), and have high level early transgene expression. Principle limitations of this vector are based on its capacity to provoke a potent antiviral immune response and its hepatic tropism which may augment its toxicity [70]. Furthermore, their episomal location make them useful only for transient gene expression. Recent modifications in their structure to eliminate wild-type genes may render these "designer" adenovirus vectors less immunogenic and allow for their longer in vivo life and function [69]. Recombinant adeno-associated viruses (rAAV), members of the parvovirus family, are another category of viruses that may be used as vectors. These nonenveloped, single-standed, replication-incompetent DNA viruses easily integrate into the host genome but require the coadministration of a helper virus (adenovirus or herpes virus) for replication. The enhanced safety profile, low immunogenicity, ability to transfect nondividing cells, and the ability to achieve long-term expression make these viruses a nearly ideal vector. The production of neutralizing antibodies by some individuals, high titer transduction requirement, limited packaging capacity for genetic material, and lack of reliable packaging cells are some of the significant limitations to the utility of this gene therapy vector. Pox viruses, a family of DNA viruses, have a large genomic capacity that permits significant amounts of foreign DNA incorporation. These viruses incorporate into the cytoplasm and are independent of host transcription regulation. These viruses may be engineered to produce large amounts of gene product. These viruses are limited by their limited expression of the transgene and host cytolytic properties. Recombinant herpes simplex virus vectors have also been utilized as vectors but are hampered by their induction of a robust inflammatory response. Modifications of the virus and delivery systems may improve this vector strategy [70].

Cancer gene therapy encompasses a broad range of approaches from direct tumoricidal effects to indirect immune responses that lead to cell death. Current applications of gene therapy fall into four major categories of approaches: immunotherapy, tumor suppressor therapy, suicidal therapy, and chemoprotection. A more detailed discussion of the application of gene therapies as a component of immunotherapy has been discussed above.

Tumor suppressor genes are a category of naturally occurring genes like p53, APC (adenomatosis polyposis coli), RB (retinoblastoma). p16INK4a, PTEN, and p14ARF that prevent malignant transformation of the host cell. Many cancers result from the loss of function or expression of these genes and theoretically the restoration of this single gene will reverse the complex process of tumorigenesis. The delivery of these genes to malignant cells in which their expression is defective or absent results in cell growth arrest, apoptosis, and genomic stability [70]. Two major principles guide this form of gene therapy: (1) delivery of a single gene will induce growth inhibition and/or death in the cancer cell; (2) transgene delivery to adjacent normal tissue will have minimal effects. The effectiveness of this type of therapy is also critically dependent on the delivery of the viral vector to other adjacent tumor cells not directly exposed to the vector to invoke a "bystander effect." This process may also induce indirect effects on the adjacent normal tissues by impacting the expression of growth factors like IGF-I and VEGF. The inhibition of these substances has negative paracrine effects on growth and survival of normal cells within the tumor microenvironment. This is the critical component of the effective gene therapy utilizing tumor suppressors (Fig. 26.6). The prototype for this form of gene therapy is p53 gene therapy for nonsmall cell cancer of the lung which provided the proof of principle that delivery of the tumor suppressor gene was tumoricidal in vivo [71]. This study demonstrated the safety and efficacy of this approach with one-third of the patients showing a clinical response to treatment. Currently modifications of viral factor delivery systems are being utilized to refine this therapy. Alternatively blocking oncogenes expression via techniques of antisense oligonucleotides or ribozyme delivery of suicide genes to cancer cells may be an effective strategy (Fig. 26.6). Several malignancies depend on onco-

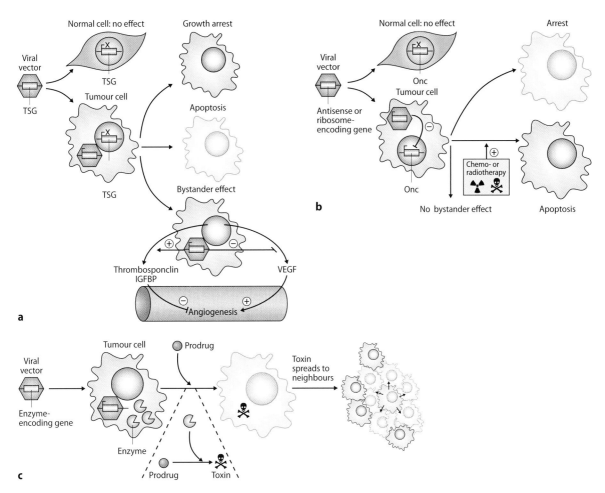

Fig. 26.6 a–c Cancer gene therapy: (**a**) Tumor suppressor gene (TSG) therapy or (**b**) inhibition of oncogene expression. (**a**) Viral vectors encoding tumor suppressor genes are delivered to the tumor microenvironment and will infect normal and tumor cells. They will typically have no effect in normal cells but will induce growth arrest or apoptosis in tumor cells. These TSG may exert innocent bystander effects, e.g., p53 gene therapy which abrogates endothelial vascular endothelial growth factor (VEGF) secretion and induces thrombospondin and insulin-like growth factor 1 production (antiangiogenic factors). (**b**) Alternatively, transgene delivery of oncogene inhibitors like antisensene oligonucleotides which directly inhibit oncogene expression or ribozymes which cleave oncogene transcripts. These may lead to growth arrest, apoptosis or increase chemo- and radiosensitivity of the tumor cells. Adapted from [69]. (**c**) Transgene delivery of a suicide gene like a prodrug concerting enzyme may activate toxic metabolites in the infected cell that is cytotoxic to this and nearby cells inducing a „potent bystander effect". Adapted from [69]

gene induction for the maintenance of the malignantly transformed state. Disrupting the expression of these genes in select tumors results in the restoration of the nonmalignant phenotype.

The delivery of suicide genes to cancer cells is a second category of emerging gene therapy for cancer. This technique involves the delivery of enzymes encoding genes that allow the cancer to metabolize a nontoxic prodrug administered separately into a potent cytotoxic agent (Fig. 26.6c). The most broadly studied enzyme-prodrug combination is herpes simplex virus thymidine kinase (HSV-tk)-gancicolvir, enzyme-prodrug combination. The HSV-tk phosphorylated ganciclovir, which results in its incorporation into the host DNA inhibiting DNA synthesis [72]. Other enzyme-prodrug combinations are listed above (Table 26.6).

Although the techniques of suicide gene therapy have demonstrated in vitro responses, the clinical efficacy of this therapy has been marginal. This may in large part be secondary to inadequate in vivo delivery mechanisms to target all malignant cells, especially in the setting of widespread metastatic disease.

The third category of gene therapy involves techniques of chemoprotection to decrease the myeloablative toxicities of chemotherapy. Expression of the multidrug resistance gene (MDR) makes tumor cells resistant to the effects of chemotherapy by encoding for a transmembrane pump that actively eliminates

Table 26.6 Enzyme-prodrug combinations for suicide gene therapy

Enzyme	Prodrug	Product	Mechanism
HSV-tk	Ganciclovir	Ganciclovir triphosphate	Blocks DNA synthesis
Cytosine deaminase	5-Fluorocytosine	5-Fluorouracil (5-FU)	Pyrimidine antagonist: blocks DNA and RNA synthesis
Carboxylesterase	CPT-11	SN38	Topoisomerase inhibitor
Cytochrome P450	Cyclophosphamide	Phosphoramide mustard	DNA alkylating agent: blocks DNA synthesis
Purine nucleoside phosphorylase	6-Mercaptopurine-DR	6-Mercaptopurine	Purine antagonist: blocks DNA synthesis

From [69]

cytotoxic agents. MDR gene-transduced hematopoietic bone marrow progenitor cells have been shown to have decreased toxic effects [72, 73]. This strategy is still in its early stages of evolution but may hold great promise, particularly in the pediatric population.

Another emerging category of gene therapy for cancer is the use of therapeutic viral infection to treat the cancer. Reports in the mid to late 20th century utilizing viruses to treat conditions such as cervical cancer emerged as a theoretical approach to care but lacked the molecular or genomic foundation to be advanced into a sound treatment paradigm. Currently the construction of replication-competent viruses that replicate only in rapidly dividing cells and also lack virulence genes are being safely exploited for anticancer gene therapies. Among these agents are a group of herpes virus mutants G207 and HSV-1716 used in clinical trials to treat malignant glial cell tumors and metastatic melanoma, respectively. Replication of the attenuated adenovirus mutant, ONYX-015, relies on inhibition of p53 function and may be used to eliminate malignant cells with loss of p53. Normal cells expressing this tumor suppressor prevent replication of this virus [74]. Adenovirus defective in E1A proteins, which typically bind and neutralize RB and its analogues, have also been shown in preclinical trials to selectively kill cells with defective RB [75, 76]. Other viral constructs like the adenovirus Calydon CN706 and others have been designed to exploit tissue-specific regulatory elements in the replication process in areas like the prostate or colon as a means of cancer cell killing [77].

26.5 Antisense Strategies

One of the major spin-offs of the human genome project has been the improved understanding of the molecular basis for cancer development, progression, and

metastasis. Numerous molecular targets have been identified through a variety of genomic and proteomic technologies. Antisense oligonucleotide (ASO) strategies are an emerging novel anticancer therapy based on the specificity of the Watson-Crick base pair interactions [78]. These antisense oligonucleotides are single-stranded, chemically modified, DNA-like molecules that are typically 17–22 nucleotides in length and designed to be complementary to the selected gene's mRNA based on Watson-Crick base pair binding specificity. The native targeted mRNA sequence is termed the "sense" sequence, while the complementary oligodeoxyribonucleotide (oligonucleotide) is the "antisense" sequence. Watson-Crick-specific complementary binding of the mRNA (sense)-DNA (antisensense) complex leads to activation of RNase-H, a ubiquitous intranuclear enzyme, mediated cleavage of the target mRNA. RNase H cleaves the mRNA strand of the mRNA-ASO hybrid allowing the ASO to bind to another identical mRNA, while the cleaved mRNA undergoes rapid degradation. This technique targets the messenger RNA that encodes the nucleotide sequence that will undergo translation to a specific protein normally upregulated during oncogenesis by the ribosome. Selective partial inhibition or deactivation of this protein then dysregulates growth, differentiation, and apoptosis of the targeted cell [79, 80]. Techniques have been developed to specifically target tumor cells with a safe pattern of side effects. Recent studies have demonstrated that this form of therapy may inhibit translation inducing alterations in mRNA transport, modulating or inhibiting mRNA splicing, and arresting translation by triple helix formation [81]. Some of these antisense sequences may contain motifs that possess nonspecific or "off target" effects that are different from its specific target. An example of this is the CpG motif found in some ASOs that have an immunostimulatory activity in addition to its translation inhibitory effect [82].

Double-stranded siRNA (small interfering) also inhibits gene expression by direct Watson-Crick-specific hybridization to a target RNA that leads to posttranscriptional gene silencing. These siRNAs are incorporated into a multiprotein RNA-inducing silencing complex leaving the antisense strand to guide this complex to its homologous RNA targets by endonucleolytic cleavage. Theoretically siRNAs offer superior potency and specificity; however, few biologically active molecules have been identified. Utility of this approach has also been limited by production costs and toxicities [83].

Numerous major barriers currently exist to the clinical applicability of this technique. These include the identification of sites on the mRNA of the particular gene that are accessible antisense hybridization techniques, methods of delivery to the tissue of origin, in vivo stabilization and resistance to degradation, limitation of toxicities, and increasing the affinity to the specific mRNA sequence [78]. Chemical modification of the ASO backbone may lead to improved tissue distribution and bioavailability through increased resistance to nuclease digestion while retaining potent hybridization and RNase-H activity.

26.5.1 Antisense Targets

The elucidation of the role of target genes associated with neoplastic progression produces a growing list of antisense gene candidates. The most promising candidates are the targets that are upregulated during or as a consequence of cancer progression and therapeutic resistance and are not otherwise amenable to inhibition with antibodies or small molecules. Although a number of ASOs have been identified in preclinical models of tumor, only a select group of protein targets have been clinically applicable. Some of these targets include members of the BCL2 family, protein kinase C (PKC) family, the inhibitors of apoptosis family (IAP), and the heat shock protein family. Among the most studied antisense targets are the BCL2 family members (BCL2 and BCL-XL). This class of oncogenes promotes tumor progression by inhibiting apoptosis or programmed cell death through BCL-2, a mitochondrial-membrane protein that functions to heterodimerize with BAX and the other proapoptotic regulators, thereby inhibiting the release of cytochrome c from the mitochondria and the subsequent steps of the apoptotic cascade [84]. The selective and competitive dimerization between pairs of these antagonists and agonists of the BCL2 family of proteins determines how a cell responds to an apoptotic signal. BCL-2 overexpression has often been implicated in treatment resistance by tumors. BCL-XL is another antiapoptotic BCL-2 family member that may be coexpressed in some tumors and some may switch between the two pathways [85–89].

Protein Kinase C (PKC) belongs to a class of serine/threonine kinases that regulate numerous intracellular "arising from G-protein-coupled receptors, receptors with tyrosine kinase activity and nonreceptor tyrosine kinases" [90]. Enhanced PKC expression is associated with oncogenesis and multidrug resistance phenotype. PKCα inhibitors block proliferation, affect the growth and survival of tumors, promote apoptosis, and sensitize tumor cells to chemotherapy [91–93].

Survivin, an inhibitor of apoptosis (IAP) gene family, encodes proteins that protect cells from undergoing apoptosis through the inhibition of caspases, the key effector proteins of the apoptotic cell death cascade [94]. This protein is highly expressed in many adult malignancies including breast, lung, pancreas, colon, and prostate cancers but is largely unexpressed in normal tissue [95, 96]. Survivin is also present in many pediatric brain tumors, soft tissue sarcomas, and neuroblastomas. Overexpression in tumor cells inhibits chemotherapy induced, BAX-induced, and FAS-induced apoptosis. High-level expression is correlated with poor prognosis in solid tumors. Survivin is the fourth most common gene expressed in cancer cells but not in normal tissue. This selectivity of Survivin in addition to its physiologic functions make it an ideal target for therapeutic antisense interventions [97].

Survivin has been identified in primary pediatric central nervous system tumors, soft tissue sarcomas, and neuroblastoma; however, detailed analysis of these tumors remains quite limited at present. Studies have shown that 10–50% of medulloblastomas in children may express Survivin and that the level of expression may correlate with both histology and prognosis. Diagnostic and therapeutic implications are emerging from these observations. Over 80% of rhabdomyosarcoma, the most common pediatric soft tissue sarcoma, may overexpress this molecule. Studies also indicate that Survivin in these tissues may serve as an excellent target for antisense and other RNA silencing technologies. Survivin expression appears to be correlated with unfavorable histology, advanced disease, and poor prognosis in neuroblastoma [98]. Promising results of preclinical data implicate Survivin-targeted strategies utilizing antisense techniques as a feasible approach to therapy in the future [99].

The heat shock proteins (HSP) are a family of highly conserved molecular chaperones that are induced by signals such as hypertension, oxidative stress, activation of Fas death receptor, and cytotoxic drugs that directly interfere with apoptosis. Antisense strategies to target these important molecular chaperones are currently being studied and hold promise in the therapy of some malignancies [100].

Success of antisense therapies will be predicated upon the improved understanding of the relative importance of the identified target, dose optimization and scheduling, successful clinical trial data from sensitive tumors, and rational use of combination regimens.

Future antisense techniques are being designed to prolong in vivo half life, improve tissue distribution, increase potency, and decrease toxicity.

26.6 Conclusion

The progress made in the last three decades in the understanding of the molecular, genetic, cell signaling, and immunologic foundations has led to significant advances in our efforts to either cure cancer or make it a chronic disease. Many of these novel strategies that have been introduced to adult oncology have only recently begun to be used in the treatment of pediatric malignancies. It becomes increasingly clear from the adult experience that Ehrlich's "magic bullet" or therapy that will cure all cancer does not yet exist but that the optimal approach to treating malignancy must employ a strategy based on the use of multiple modalities [101]. As our understanding of cancer cell biology and the host response continues to proliferate, these novel and emerging therapeutic strategies will become conventional and new therapies will emerge. Our focus must remain on the close collaboration of scientist and clinician to achieve this goal of a cure.

References

1. Pearson HA (2002) History of pediatric hematology oncology. Pediatr Res 52:979–992
2. Poplack DG (2002) Principles and practice of pediatric oncology. In: Pizzo PA, Poplack DG (eds) Principles and practice of pediatric oncology. Lippincott Williams & Wilkins, Philadelphia
3. Feig SA (2001) Second malignant neoplasms after successful treatment of childhood cancers. Blood Cells Mol Dis 27:662–666
4. Hanahan D, Weinberg RA (2000) The hallmarks of cancer. Cell 100(1):57–70
5. Zitvogel L, Tesniere A, Kroemer G (2006) Cancer despite immunosurveillance: Immunoselection and immunosubversion. Nat Rev Immunol 6(10):715–727
6. Nauts HC (1989) Bacteria and cancer: Antagonisms and benefits. Cancer Surv 8:713–723
7. Burnet FM (1970) The concept of immunological surveillance. Prog Exp Tumor Res 13:1–27
8. Everson TC, Cole WH (1966) Spontaneous regression of cancer. Saunders, Philadelphia, pp 88–163
9. Penn I (1988) Tumors of the immunocompromised patient. Annu Rev Med 39:63–73
10. Penn I (1994) De novo malignancy in pediatric organ transplant recipients. J Pediatr Surg 29:221–226
11. Matzinger P (1994) Tolerance, danger and the extended family. Annu Rev Immunol 12:991–1045
12. Offringa R (2006) Cancer. Cancer immunotherapy is more than a numbers game. Science 314:68–69
13. Rosenberg SA, Yang JC, Restifo NP (2004) Cancer immunotherapy: Moving beyond current vaccines. Nat Med 10(9):909–915
14. Dunn GP, Bruce AT, Ikeda H, Old LJ, Schreiber RD (2002) Cancer immunoediting: From immunosurveillance to tumor escape. Nat Immunol 3:991–998
15. Kim R, Emi M, Tanabe K, Arihiro K (2006) Tumor-driven evolution of immunosuppressive networks during malignant progression Cancer Res 66:5527–5536
16. Drake CG, Jaffee EE, Pardoll DM (2006) Mechanisms of immune evasion by tumors. Adv Immunol 90:51–81
17. Köhler G, Milstein C (1975) Continuous cultures of fused cells secreting antibody of predefined specificity. Nature 256:495–497
18. Carter P (2001) Improving the efficacy of antibody-based cancer therapies. Nat Rev Cancer 1:118–129
19. von Mehren M, Adams GP, Weiner LM, et al. (2003) Monoclonal antibody therapy for cancer. Annu Rev Med 54:343–369
20. Waldmann TA (2006) Effective cancer therapy through immunomodulation. Annu Rev Med 57:65–81
21. Kohzoh I, Akinori T, (2006) Comparing antibody and small-molecule therapies for cancer. Nat Rev Cancer 6:714–727
22. Hank JA, Surfus J, Gan J, et al. (1994) Treatment of neuroblastoma patients with antiganglioside GD2 antibody plus interleukin-2 induces antibody-dependent cellular cytotoxicity against neuroblastoma detected in vitro. J Immunother 15:29–37
23. Mujoo K, Kipps TJ, Yang HM, et al. (1989) Functional properties and effect on growth suppression of human neuroblastoma tumors by isotype switch variants of monoclonal antiganglioside GD2 antibody 14.18. Cancer Res 49:2857–2861
24. Kushner BH, Kramer K, Cheung NK (2001) Phase II trial of the anti-G(D2) monoclonal antibody 3F8 and granulocyte-macrophage colony-stimulating factor for neuroblastoma. J Clin Oncol 19(22):4189–4194
25. Sondel PM, Hank JA (2001) Antibody-directed, effector cell-mediated tumor destruction. Hematol Oncol Clin North Am 15(4):703–721
26. Cheung NK, Kushner BH, Kramer K (2001) Monoclonal antibody-based therapy of neuroblastoma. Hematol Oncol Clin North Am. 15:853–866
27. Stacy KM (2005) Therapeutic mabs: Saving lives and making billions. Scientist 19:17–19.
28. Boon T, Coulie PG, Van den Eynde B (1997) Tumor antigens recognized by T cells. Immunol Today 18:267–268
29. Rosenberg SA (1999) A new era for cancer immunotherapy based on the genes that encode cancer antigens. Immunity 10:281–287
30. Shastri N, Schwab S, Serwold T (2002), Producing natures gene–chips: The generation of peptides for display by MHC Class I molecules. Annu Rev Immunol 20:463–493

31. Rosenberg SA (2001) Progress in human tumour immunology and immunotherapy. Nature 411:380–384

32. Pardoll DM (2002) Spinning molecular immunology into successful immunotherapy. Nat Rev Immunol 2:227–238

33. Wang RF, Rosenberg SA (1996) Human tumor antigens recognized by T lymphocytes: Implications for cancer therapy. J Leukoc Biol 60:296–309

34. Dudley ME, Wunderlich JR, Yang JC, et al. (2002) A phase I study of non-myeloablative chemotherapy and adoptive transfer of autologous tumor antigen-specific T lymphocytes in patients with metastatic melanoma. J Immunother 25:243–251

35. Stewart BW, Kleihues P (eds) (2003) World cancer report. IARC Press, Lyon

36. Chang MH, Shau WY, Chen CJ, et al. (2000) Hepatitis B vaccination and hepatocellular carcinoma rates in boys and girls. JAMA 284:3040–3042

37. Villa LL, Costa RL, Petta CA,et al. (2005) Prophylactic quadrivalent human papillomavirus (types 6, 11, 16 and 18) L1 virus-like particle vaccine in young women: A randomized double-blind placebo-controlled multicentre phase II efficacy trial. Lancet Oncol 6:271–278

38. Lollini PL, Cavallo F, Nanni P, Forni G (2006) Vaccines for tumour prevention. Nat Rev Cancer 206–214

39. Palena C, Abrams SI, Schlom J, Hodge JW (2006) Cancer vaccines: Preclinical studies and novel strategies. Adv Cancer Res 95:115–145

40. Pietersz GA, Pouniotis DS, Apostolopoulos V (2006) Design of peptide-based vaccines. Curr Med Chem 13:1591–1607

41. Reilly RT, Machiels JP, Emens LA, Jaffee EM (2002) Cytokine gene-modified cell-based cancer vaccines. Methods Mol Med 69:233–257

42. Gilboa E (2004) The promise of cancer vaccines. Nat Rev Cancer 4:401–411

43. Saito H, Frieta D, Dubsky P, Palucka AK (2006) Dendritic cell-based vaccination against cancer. Hematol Oncol Clin North Am 20:689–710

44. Fong L, Engelman EG (2000) Dendritic cells in cancer immunotherapy. Annu Rev Immunol 18:245–273

45. Geiger JD, Hutchinson RJ, Hohenkirk LF, et al. (2001) Vaccination of pediatric solid tumor with tumor lysate-pulsed dendritic cells can expand specific T cells and mediate tumor regression. Cancer Res 61(23):8513–8519

46. Iinuma H, Okinaga K, Fukushima R, et al. (2006) Superior protective and therapeutic effects of IL-12 and IL-18 gene transduced dendritic neuroblastoma fusion cells on liver metastasis of murine neuroblastoma. J Immunol 176(6):3461–3469

47. Redlinger RE Jr, Mailliard RB, Lotze MT, et al. (2003) Synergistic interleukin-18 and low-dose interleukin 2-promote regression of established murine neuroblastoma in vivo. J Pediatr Surg 38(3):301–307

48. Redlinger RE Jr, Shimizu T, Remy T, et al. (2003) Cellular mechanisms of interleukin-12 mediated neuroblastoma regression. J Pediatr Surg 38(2):199–204

49. Maki RG (2006) Future directions for immunotherapeutic intervention against sarcomas. Curr Opin Oncol 18(4):363–368

50. Alegre ML, Frauwirth KA, Thompson CB (2001) T-cell regulation by CD28 and CTLA-4. Nat Rev Immunol 1:220–228.

51. Salomon B, Bluestone JA (2001) Complexities of CD28/B7: CTLA-4 costimulatory pathways in autoimmunity and transplantation. Annu Rev Immunol 19 2225–2252

52. Chambers CA, Kuhns MS, Egen JG, Allison JP (2001) CTLA-4 mediated inhibition in regulation of T cell responses: Mechanisms and manipulation in tumor immunotherapy. Annu Rev Immunol 19:565–594

53. Lengauer C, Krinzler KW, Vogelstein B (1998) Genetic instabilities in human cancers. Nature 396:642–649

54. Kerbel RS (1991) Inhibition of tumor angiogenesis as a strategy to circumvent acquired resistance to anti-cancer therapeutic agents. Bioessays 13:31–36

55. Davidoff AM, Kandel JJ (2004) Antiangiogenic therapy for the treatment of pediatric solid malignancies. Semin Pediatr Surg 13(1):53–60

56. Knudson AG (1971) Mutation and cancer: Statistical study of retinoblastoma. Proc Natl Acad Sci U S A 68:820–823

57. Carmeliet P (2000) Mechanisms of angiogenesis and arteriogenesis. Nat Med 6:389–395

58. Hanahan D, Folkman J (1996) Patterns and emerging mechanisms of the angiogenic switch during tumorigenesis. Cell 86:353–364

59. Brooks PC, Silletti S, von Schalscha TL, et al. (1998) Disruption of angiogenesis by PEX, a noncatalytic metalloproteinase fragment with integrin binding activity. Cell 92:391–400

60. Ruegg C, Yilmaz A, Bieler G, et al. (1998) Evidence for the involvement of endothelial cell integrin alpha Vbeta 3 in the disruption of tumor vasculature induced by TNF and IFN-gamma. Nat Med 4:408–414

61. Relf M, LeJeune S, Fox S, Smith K, Leek R, Moghaddam A, Whitehouse R, Bicknell R, Harris AL(1997) Expression of the angiogenic factors vascular endothelial growth factor, acidic and basic fibroblast growth factor, tumor growth factor beta-1, platelet-derived endothelial growth factor, placenta growth factor and pleiotrophin in human primary breast cancer and its relation to angiogenesis. Cancer Res 57:963–969

62. Meitar D, Crawford SE, Rademaker AW, et al. (1996) Tumor angiogenesis correlates with metastatic disease, N-myc amplification, and poor outcome in human neuroblastoma. J Clin Oncol 14:405–414

63. Abrahamson LP, Grundy PE, Rademaker AW, et al. (2003) Increased microvascular density predicts relapse in Wilm's tumor. J Pediatr Surg 38:325–330

64. Folkman J (2006) Antiangiogenesis in cancer therapy-endostatin and its mechanisms of action. Exp Cell Res 312:594–607

65. Folkman J (2006) Angiogenesis. Annu Rev Med 57:1–18

66. Kerbel R, Folkman J (2002) Clinical translation of angiogenesis inhibitors. Nat Rev Cancer 2:727–739

67. Hanahan D, Bergers G, Bergsland E (2000) Less is more, regularly: Metronomic dosing of cytotoxic drugs can target tumor angiogenesis in mice. J Clin Invest 105:1045–1047

68. Abdollahi A, Hahnfeldt P, Maercker C, Grone HJ, Debus J, Ansorge W, Folkman J, Hlatky L, Huer PE (2004) Endostatin's antiangiogenic signaling network. Mol Cell 13:649–663

69. McCormick F (2001) Cancer gene therapy: Fringe or cutting edge? Nat Rev Cancer 1:130–141

70. Nathwani AC, Benjamin R, Nienhuis AW, Davidoff AM (2004) Current status and prospects for gene therapy. Vox Sang 87:73–81

71. Roth JA, Nhuyen D, Lawrence DD, et al. (1996) Retrovirus-Mediated wild-type of p53 gene transfer to tumors of patients with lung cancer. Nat Med 2:985–991

72. Cowan KH, Moscow JA, Huang H, et al. (1999) Paclitaxel chemotherapy after autologous stem cell transplantation and engraftment of hematopoietic cells transduced with a retrovirus containing the multidrug resistance complementary DNA (MDR1) in metastatic breast cancer patients. Clin Cancer Res 5:1619–1628

73. Hanania EG, Giles RE, Kavanagh J, et al. (1997) Results of MDR-1 vector modification trial indicate that granulocyte/macrophage colony-forming unit cells do not contribute to post-transplant hematopoietic recovery following intensive systemic therapy. Proc Natl Acad Sci USA 93:15346–15351

74. Kim DH, McCormick F (1996) Replicating viruses as selective cancer therapeutics. Mol Med Today 2:519–527

75. Barker DD, Berk A (1987) Adenovirus proteins from both E1B reading frames are required for transformation of rodent cells by viral infection and DNA transfection. Virology 156:107–120

76. Fueyo J, Gomez-Manzano C, Alemany R, et al. (2000) A mutant oncolytic adenovirus targeting the RB pathway produces anti-glioma effect in vivo. Oncogene 19:2–12

77. Rodriguez R, Schuur ER, Lim HY, et al. (1997) Prostate attenuated replication competent adenovirus (ARCA) CN706: A selective cytotoxic prostate specific antigen-positive prostate cancer cells. Cancer Res 57:2559–2563

78. Moolten FL (1986) Tumor chemosensitivity conferred by inserted herpes thymidine kinase genes: Paradigm for a prospective cancer control strategy. Cancer Res. 46:5276–5281

79. Gleave ME, Monia BP (2005) Antisense therapy of cancer. Nat Rev Cancer 5:468–479

79. Orr RM, Monica BP (1998) Antisense therapy for cancer. Curr Opin Investig Drugs 1:199–205

80. Crooke ST (1998) Molecular mechanisms of antisense drugs: RNase H. Antisense Nucleic Acid Drug Dev 8:33–134

81. Monia BP, et al. (1993) Evaluation of 2'-modified oligonucleotides containing 2'-deoxy gaps as antisense inhibitors of gene expression. J Biol Chem 269:4514–4522

82. Carpentier AF, Chen L, Maltonti F, et al. (1999) Oligodeoxynucleotides containing CpG motifs can induce rejection of a neuroblastoma in mice. Cancer Res 59:5429–5432

83. Ameyar-Zazoua M, Guasconi V, Ait–Si–Ali S (2005) siRNA as a route to new cancer therapies. Expert Opin Biol Ther 5:221–224

84. Reed JC (1994) Bcl-2 and the regulation of programmed cell death. J Cell Biol 124:1–6

85. Zangemeister-Wittke U, Leech SH, Olie RA, et al. (2000) A novel bispecific antisense oligonucleotide inhibiting both bcl-2 and bcl-xl expression efficiently induces apoptosis in tumor cells. Clin Cancer Res 6:2547–2555

86. Gleave ME, Tolcher A, Miyake H, et al. (1999) Progression to androgen independence is delayed by adjuvant treatment with antisense Bcl-2 oligodeoxynucleotides after castration in the LNCaP prostate tumor model. Clin Cancer Res 6:2891–2898

87. Webb A, Cunningham D, Cotter F, et al. (1997) BCL-2 antisense therapy in patients with non-Hodgkin lymphoma. Lancet 349:1137–1141

88. Miyake H, Monia BP, Gleave ME (2000) Inhibition of progression to androgen-independence by antisense bcl-2 oligonucleotides plus taxol after castration in the Shionogi tumor model. Int J Cancer 86:855–862

89. Gautschi O, Tschopp S, Olie RA, et al. (2001) Activity of a novel bcl-2/bcl-xl bispecific antisense oligonucleotide against tumors of diverse histologic origins. J Natl Cancer Inst 93:463–471

90. Newton AC (1997) Regulation of protein kinase C. Curr Opin Cell Biol 9:161–167

91. Swannie HC, Kaye SB (2002) Protein kinase C inhibitors. Curr Oncol Rep 4:47–46

92. Wang XY, Repasky E, Liu HT (1999) Antisense inhibition of protein kinase Cα reverses the transformed phenotype in human lung carcinoma cells. Exp Cell Res 250:253–263

93. Geiger T, Muller M, Dean NM, et al.(1998) Antitumor activity of PKC-α antisense oligonucleotide in combination with standard chemotherapeutic agents against various human tumors transplanted intonude mice. Anticancer Drug Des 13:35–45

94. Altieri DC (2003) Survivin versatile modulation of cell division and apoptosis in cancer. Oncogene 22:8581–8589

95. Ambrosini G, Adida C, Altieri DC (1997) A novel anti-apoptosis gene, survivin, expressed in cancer and lymphoma. Nat Med 3:917–921

96. Fukuda S, Pelus L (2006) Survivin, a cancer target with an emerging role in normal adult tissues. Mol Cancer Ther 5:1087–1098

97. LaCasse EC, Baird S, Korneluk RG, et al. (1998) The inhibitors of apoptosis (IAPS) and their emerging role in cancer. Oncogene 17:3247–3259

98. Fangusaro JR, Caldas H, Jiang Y, Altura R (2006) Survivin: An inhibitor of apoptosis in pediatric cancer. Pediatr Blood Cancer 47:4–13

99. Chen J, Wu W, Tahir SK, et al. (2000) Down-regulation of survivin by antisense oligonucleotides increases apoptosis, inhibits cyokinesis and anchorage-independent growth. Neoplasia 2:235–241

100. Ciocca DR, Oesterreich S, Chamness GC, et al. (1993) Biological and clinical implications of heat shock protein 27,000 (Hsp27): A review. J Natl Cancer Inst 85:1558–1570

101. Ehrlich P (1956). On immunity with special reference to cell life: Croonian lecture. In: B Himmelweir (ed) The collected papers of Paul Ehrlich: Immunology and cancer research. 148–192

102. Friedl P, den Boer A, Gunzer M (2005) Tuning immune responses: Diversity and adaptation of the immunological synapse. Nat Rev Immunol 5:532–545

103. Lake RA, Robinson BWS (2005) Immunotherapy and chemotherapy-A practical partnership. Nat Rev Cancer 5:397–405

104. Tarassoff CP, Arlen PM, Gulley JL (2006) Therapeutic vaccines for prostate cancer. Oncologist 11:451–462

105. O'Neill DW, Adams S, Bhardwaj N (2004) Manipulating dendritic cell biology for the active immunotherapy of cancer. Blood 104:2235–2246

106. Bergers G, Benjamin LE (2003) Tumorigenesis and the angiogenic switch. Nat Rev Cancer 3:401–410

Central Venous Access

27

Gregor Walker, Constantinos A. Hajivassiliou

Contents

27.1 Introduction

Approximately 200,000 central venous lines (CVLs) are inserted in the UK annually and a significant proportion are indwelling lines inserted for the administration of chemotherapy or to serve the other needs of patients with oncological problems.

The advances in cancer care have been paralleled by similar advances in central line design and construction. The history of central access and treatment through indwelling catheters is relatively short: in 1968 Dudrick [1] inserted a catheter in the superior vena cava of beagle puppies that was maintained in situ for a long period. Broviac, et al. introduced a catheter suitable for long-term use in 1973 [2], and Hickman modified this in 1975 [3] by increasing catheter wall thickness and lumen diameter. The evolution of materials used to construct these catheters has also been revolutionized by the replacement of thrombogenic, relatively noncompliant, and variably antigenic rubber, nylon, polyvinyl, or polyurethane catheters with those made of silicone, associated with a concomitant decrease in the complication rate and duration of indwelling catheter time.

Multiple lumen catheters have been designed for use in patients requiring long-term simultaneous administration of two or more parenteral solutions, e.g., chemotherapy, antibiotics, antifungal agents, and parenteral nutrition. Since the introduction of intravenous therapy teams, there have been dramatic improvements in catheter and catheter site care, bringing about a reduction in complications [4]. Furthermore, the introduction of fully implantable central access systems (Figs. 27.1, 27.2) has afforded further benefits, especially freedom of lifestyle, to these patients [5, 6].

27.2 Indications for the Insertion of Central Lines

Patients with oncological problems will almost always require treatment with chemotherapy. Administration of chemotherapy is the most important specific indication for the insertion of a central venous line. However, the needs of cancer patients are often quite complex; therefore, a CVL may be required for other uses besides chemotherapy.

27.2.1 Administration of Chemotherapeutic Agents

The use of multiple lumen catheters has been of particular value in patients requiring multimodal treatments. Patients undergoing bone marrow transplantation require vascular access during preparation for transplant, high-dose chemotherapy, and total body irradiation.

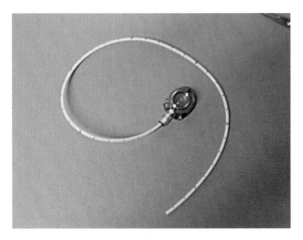

Fig. 27.1 Fully implantable device (port-a-cath) allowing patients a much less restricted lifestyle

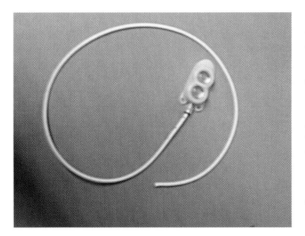

Fig. 27.2 Dual lumen port affording the advantages of double lumen lines in a totally implantable device

Supportive therapy is also required during preparation for engraftment and following transplantation.

27.2.2 Administration of Intravenous Alimentation

Intestinal complications of chemotherapy requiring bowel rest (e.g., typhlitis) or effectively leading to a malabsorption type syndrome occur relatively frequently in neutropenic patients with leukemia during aggressive treatment with chemotherapy [7]. Many children with cancer are malnourished during their induction of chemotherapy, manifesting in weight loss. Their nutritional requirements can be met by parental feeding despite inadequate absorption from the gastrointestinal tract. Nutritional support can also be maintained without the need for long hospital stays through home parenteral nutrition programs.

27.2.3 Resuscitation

Central access is also invaluable in the intensive care unit and monitoring of these patients, pre- and post-transplantation, during and after major oncological surgery, and in the management of complications such as tumor lysis syndrome.

27.2.4 Monitoring and Repeat Blood Sampling

Monitoring central venous pressure is important in monitoring patients in the intensive care facility or during major surgical procedures. Frequent blood sampling, from the catheter during courses of chemotherapy, avoids the need for frequent venepuncture in the pediatric patient.

27.2.5 Administration of Antibiotics

As many of these patients are immunocompromised, they may require frequent courses of intravenous antibiotics for prolonged periods to manage episodes of systemic sepsis.

27.2.6 Repeated Transfusion of Blood and Blood Products

CVLs are used for the administration of whole blood, packed cells, white cells, platelets, and plasma factors, and plasma may be required in patients with granulocytopenia, immune suppression, and patients with recurrent or chronic blood loss. Central lines are also useful for patients requiring exchange blood transfusions and apheresis.

27.2.7 Hemodialysis

This may be necessary for various reasons [8] and a specially modified large caliber line (semi-rigid dual lumen catheter) can be inserted to allow hemodialysis to be performed. It is possible to use the same tract of an existing central line and sequentially dilate it with special venous dilators to permit insertion of the hemodialysis catheter. This preserves a valuable entry point to the central circulation as oncology patients are likely to require multiple line insertions.

27.3 Methods of Venous Access

27.3.1 General Principles Applying to Gaining Intravenous Access: "The 5A's"

– Asepsis
– Antisepsis
– Adequate access
– Anatomical placement
– Avoidance of complications

All the above are self explanatory: aseptic technique should be employed with appropriate antisepsis of the surrounding skin/tissues. Chlorhexidine is superior to betadine as it is associated with a lower incidence of line infection [9]. The line inserted should be adequate for the purpose intended (single/multiple lumen, appropriate diameter, etc.) and should be inserted in the appropriate central location. The operator's experience and appropriate choice of the technique for insertion are also important factors in avoidance of complications.

27.3.1.1 Peripheral Venous Access

Peripheral venous access is indicated for short-term administration of fluids and drugs. There are a number of advantages over central venous access. There is evidence that drugs administered peripherally reach effective levels as quickly as those given centrally as long as they are flushed with a bolus of saline [10].

The basilic and cephalic veins in the ante cubital fossa and the dorsal veins of the hands and feet are usually easily accessible in most patients. The origin of the cephalic vein in the "anatomical snuff box" is a site favored by medical staff, earning it a reputation as the "house-man's vein." Occasionally cannulae may need to be inserted blindly, where no vein is visible or palpable. In this situation veins which are relatively fixed in their position such as the medial cubital vein or the long saphenous vein at the ankle are useful. Different peripheral cannulation sites are more appropriate in different age groups. In neonate and infants, the scalp is a useful alternative site for peripheral access, although it is necessary to shave the hair around the site of insertion.

Some agents when given peripherally can contribute to the development of vasculitis (e.g., calcium, dopamine, chemotherapy agents); however, parenteral nutrition can be successfully administered into peripheral veins. Patients who require only short-term nutritional support are ideal candidates for this peripheral parenteral nutrition. Advantages of using peripheral access include the avoidance of the complications associated with the insertion and the care of central venous cannulae. However, administration of chemotherapy commonly leads to complications if given in the periphery. Other means to reduce the incidence of thrombophlebitis and prolong the life-span of peripheral lines include the simultaneous administration of fat emulsion (intralipid) and the use of a topical vasodilator such as transdermal glycerin trinitrate [11].

Peripheral lines are available in a variety of diameters, each color-coded in a universal manner, regardless of manufacturer. The smallest cannulae have the highest gauge.

27.3.1.2 Peripherally Sited Central Venous Access

The risks involved in central line insertion can be avoided by using specifically designed silicone catheters that can be placed in a peripheral vein and advanced into a more central position (PIC-line). This allows the administration of solutions that may be venotoxic when given peripherally, but avoids some of the complications associated with central line insertion [12].

Most commercially available long-lines come with an introducing kit. Ideal sites for insertion include the antecubital fossa veins, the femoral vein, or in small children the long saphenous vein at the ankle. To reduce the incidence of complications, if an upper limb vein is used the catheter should be advanced into the superior vena cava, and if a lower limb vein is used it should lie in the external/common iliac vein [13].

There have been recent reports of this type of cannula being associated with cardiac tamponade, after the tip of the line migrated through the wall of the right atrium [14, 15] leading to the recommendation that the tip of the line should rest in the central veins rather than the right atrium. The less compliant polyurethane lines of extremely fine caliber (e.g., <2FG) are most likely to cause this problem, partially due to the high pressure "jetting" effect at the tip of the line [16].

27.3.1.3 Central Venous Access

Central venous access is indicated if venous access is required for a prolonged period of time, if peripheral access is unsuccessful, or when hypertonic or venotoxic solutions are to be used. Central lines are available in two major forms – polyethylene catheters that are more rigid and suitable for short-term access/monitoring, and silicone catheters that are more suited for long-term use. The complications of central line insertion are listed in Table 27.1. The site chosen, underly-

Table 27.1 Commonest complications of Central Line Insertion

Complication	Incidence [reference]
Infection	1–20% [19]
Hemorrhage	1–3% [45]
Dislodgement	7% [46]
Phlebitis	4% [45]
Thrombosis	1.5–3% [45, 46]
Thromboembolism	1% [45]
Air embolism	Rare (<0.1%) [47]
Pneumothorax	2% [29]
Hemothorax	0.2% [29]

Table 27.2 A selection of central line manufacturers

Name	Address	Device
Vygon Corporation	East Rutherford NJ	Various
Gesco International	San Antonio TX	Per-Q-Catheter, various
Dow Corning	Ithaca, NY	Various
Pharmacia Inc.	St. Paul MN	Port-a-cath, various
Bard Corp	Murray Hill, NJ	Various
Cook Inc.	Bloomington, IN	Broviac, various

ing condition of the patient, and the experience of the clinician determine the incidence of these complications [17]. Junior trainees should be supervised until they feel comfortable and demonstrate competency in carrying out this procedure.

As the list of complications is long, the clinician may be tempted to advise repeated peripheral cannulae. In a large review of 585 children who required venous access, Ziegler, et al. found that in 385 with peripheral lines there was a complication rate of 9%, and in 200 children with central access, the rate was 20% [18]. However, as the central lines were in place for a longer period than the peripheral lines, the complication rate per patient per day was actually lower in the central line group.

The reported risk of developing a catheter-related infection ranges between 1% and 20% [19], but this should also be expressed as "per 100 intravascular device days." Infection can be reduced by meticulous aseptic technique at the time of insertion and each time the line is accessed or the dressing damaged at the exit site. A 2% chlorhexidine solution is an appropriate choice of agent and appears to be superior to betadine [9]. A collagen subcutaneous cuff as found on some central lines can reduce the risk of infection if the patient is nonseptic at the time of insertion [20]. The cuff can also add to the security of the line if inserted to a distance of greater than 2 cm from the exit site [21].

Manufacturers of commercially available central lines are listed in Table 27.2. A recent modification popularized in the USA is the Groshong valve [22]. This patented system allows the tip of the catheter to be rounded and closed. The valve opens inwards when blood is aspirated and outwards during infusions. It remains closed when the line is not in use so clamping of the line is not necessary. Lines only require flushing once weekly.

There are three main sites commonly used for central lines – the subclavian vein, the femoral vein, and the neck veins (internal and external jugular veins). Each of these sites will be discussed.

27.3.2 Catheterization of the Subclavian Vein

The subclavian vein may be percutaneously catheterized using the Seldinger technique [23]. The apex of the lung lies higher on the left so pneumothorax is a more common complication using this side (Fig. 27.3).

Unless there is a suspected cervical spine injury, this technique is facilitated by placing a roll under the thoracic spine, thereby extending it, a head down position to engorge the great veins, and the patient facing towards the contralateral side.

27.3.2.1 Technique

1. Scrub hands and observe strict aseptic technique.
2. Cleanse the patient's skin with an antiseptic solution and drape appropriately. The wider the sterile field, the better.
3. Infiltrate local anesthetic (e.g., 0.5% bupivacaine) to an area 0.5 cm below the clavicle just lateral to the mid-clavicular line.
4. Attach a 2.5-ml syringe onto the needle and flush with heparinized saline.
5. Puncture the skin just below the clavicle lateral to the mid-clavicular line and advance the needle superiorly until the clavicle is met. Manipulate the needle to pass under the clavicle and point the tip medially.

Fig. 27.3 Anatomical specimen of the neck and thoracic inlet showing the protrusion of the apex of the lung/pleura (arrows) in close proximity to the sites of percutaneous puncture for accessing the subclavian veins

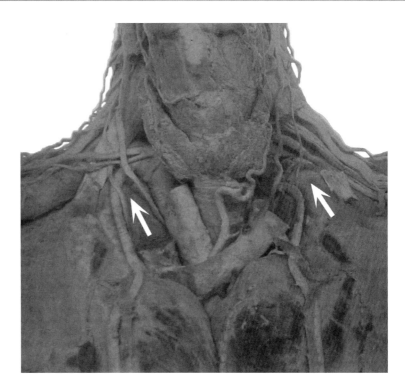

6. At this point flush a very small amount of saline through the needle to evacuate any plugs of skin or tissue in the needle.
7. Place a finger of the other hand in the sternal notch, and direct the needle towards this target, gently aspirating the syringe as the needle is advanced.
8. Visualize the needle passing under the clavicle towards the tip of the finger in the sternal notch.
9. Free aspiration of blood indicates the correct position. If this is not achieved, withdraw slowly, while aspirating. Flashback of blood almost invariably occurs as the needle is withdrawn.
10. Once the vein has been accessed, firmly secure the end of the needle with one hand, and with the other remove the syringe. There should be free flow of blood from the end of the needle at this time.
11. Pass the guidewire through the needle until the tip is in the vena cava (Fig. 27.4). This should pass easily; if this is not the case, this indicates incorrect placement. This part of the procedure should be done with image intensifier help.
12. Remove the needle over the guidewire and make a small skin incision to allow the exit of the tunneling device and catheter and also subsequently the passage of the tissue/venous dilator and split sheath introducer.
13. Tunnel the line from a position lateral to the areola of the breast to the guidewire entry point and

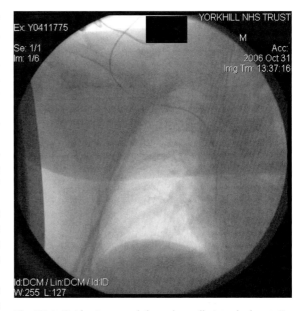

Fig. 27.4 Guidewire passed through needle into the heart. On this occasion it traversed the right atrium and terminated into the IVC and was withdrawn prior to the procedure continuing

cut to size (ideally with the help of the image intensifier).
14. Pass the dilator over the guidewire and with a gentle but firm advancing and rotating force, advance the venous dilator/split sheath introducer into the SVC/RA.

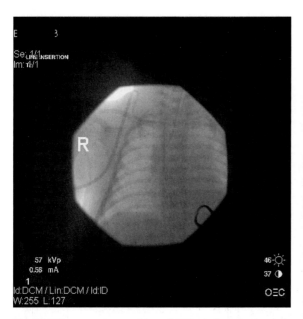

Fig. 27.5 Inappropriate position of CVL tip into the innominate vein

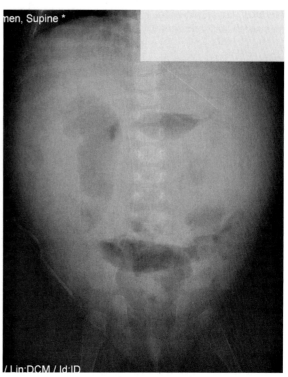

Fig. 27.6 A femoral line placed into the IVC

15. When the correct position is radiographically confirmed, the guidewire and venous dilator are removed leaving the outside thin split sheath introducer in situ. This allows the tip of the previously tunneled catheter to be advanced to the correct position (SVC/RA junction) and the sheath split and removed while holding the catheter in place.
16. Advance the catheter over the guidewire until it reaches the desired position, then remove the guidewire.
17. Flush all lumina of the line and secure it in place using one of several methods to reduce the chance of displacement and migration [24–26].
18. Confirm that bilateral breath sounds are present.
19. Proper catheter position should be documented in all cases with a chest radiograph as inappropriately positioned lines should be remanipulated (Fig. 27.5).

27.3.3 Catheterization of the Femoral Vein

Percutaneous femoral vein catheterization has been used for long-term venous access (it is also the site of access for many invasive vascular techniques, e.g., cardiac catheterization, embolization, etc.). In the absence of significant abdominal distension the central venous pressure recorded through a femoral line is also an accurate reflection of supradiaphragmatic venous pressure [27]. Although it would seem that femoral lines are more likely to be complicated by infection there is

no evidence of this [28]; indeed there is a lower rate of insertion-related complications compared to other sites [29]. Thrombotic complications, however, are more common.

For long-term access, the femoral vein is cannulated by a long saphenous vein cut down at the groin. A subcutaneous tunnel is fashioned to the anterior abdominal wall after the vein is exposed. A cuffed catheter can then be inserted through the tunnel and into the vein and can be advanced to the desired level up to the right atrium (Fig. 27.6).

27.3.4 Catheterization of the Jugular Veins

The external and internal jugular veins can be used for central access. Both can be accessed percutaneously or by an open technique. The external jugular vein is an appropriate site for venous cut down in children under general anesthetic and the number of complications related to insertion is low. Indeed, it is the site of choice for the insertion of the first central line in this institution.

Percutaneous access of the internal jugular vein is preferably performed on the right. The pathway to the right atrium is straight, and there is virtually no chance of thoracic duct injury. Again, it is best if the patient is placed head down with a roll under the shoulders to extend the neck, with the patient facing the contralateral side. If there is suspected cervical spine trauma this position will not be possible. Recently published guidelines (2002) from the National Institute for Clinical Excellence have recommended the use of 2-dimensional ultrasound to locate the vein prior to percutaneous insertion. This policy increases the success rate of internal jugular venous access in children although the avoidance of arterial injury is not as marked as in adult practice [30]. This technique has also been described with subclavian access [31].

27.3.4.1 Totally Implantable Devices

These consist of central venous lines that are inserted as documented above but instead of being tunneled to an exit site, a port is buried in a subcutaneous pocket, usually on the lateral chest wall, and secured through small fixing holes in its periphery. The port is a chamber with a self-sealing injection port (Figs. 27.1, 27.2). A recent addition to the choice of ports is a dual lumen device, with the obvious advantages it affords (Fig. 27.2). The ports are made of stainless steel, titanium alloy or synthetic plastic materials and have a silicone dome on the anterior surface to allow access. The silicone compound has "bleeding" properties such that after the needle is withdrawn, the access hole seals spontaneously. Access to the port is achieved via a specially designed "non-coring" Huber needle through the skin (Fig. 27.7).

Advantages of implantable devices include decreased infection rate with appropriate care [32], decreased dislodgement rate [21], minimal maintenance [33], and freedom of activities [34]. The most pleasing aspect of these devices to our patients is the ability to continue with normal activities such as swimming and other sports. Although access to the port involves puncturing the overlying skin, this is initially sensitized by using local anesthetic cream (EMLA, Ametop) until the area eventually becomes insensitive as time progresses. The skin, however, may break down over the patch and lead to complications, e.g., infection.

27.4 Complications of CVLS and Their Treatment

A central line, however carefully and expertly inserted, is still a foreign body in direct contact with the circulation. Most of the potential complications have already been reported and studied (Table 27.1), but the clinician should remain vigilant to identify and treat any potential permutation or new complication that may

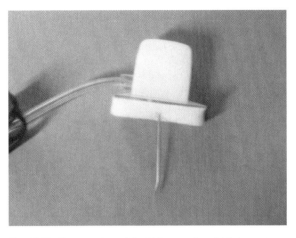

Fig. 27.7 Close up view of the Huber needle, which is constructed in such a way to penetrate the silicone dome of the port reservoir by pushing away the layer of silicone instead of "coring" through its thickness

arise. Infection is a serious complication, especially in immunocompromised patients and can be treated aggressively with antibiotics with reasonable success [35], although in the setting of sepsis, 20–60% of catheters will be removed [32]. Some organisms (e.g., staphylococcus epidermidis [36], *pseudomonas* species, and *candida albicans* [37], etc.) are virtually impossible to eradicate and will require line removal and a new line to be inserted. Although some success is reported by replacing the line through the same tract [38], in severely immunocompromised patients the commonest protocol involves removal of the line, antibiotic administration, and line replacement several days later once the infection is controlled. There is a paucity of published evidence regarding an optimal delay before line reinsertion. Published articles pertain predominantly to the use of short-term central venous lines in the intensive care setting and extrapolation of this evidence to cuffed tunneled lines is tenuous. One controversy with short-term central lines is the practice of routine replacement to prevent catheter-related sepsis. In a telephone survey in 1997, 52% of intensive care units in the UK had a policy of replacing lines before 7 days [39]. Recommendations from the USA do not support a practice of routine replacement [40].

Another relatively recent advance is the introduction of antibiotic-impregnated lines [41], which are reportedly associated with lower rates of bacterial colonization [42]. Techniques used include bonding minocycline and rifampicin to both internal and external surfaces or chlorhexidine and silver sulfadiazine to the external surface [43]. This technology is widely available with percutaneously inserted central lines rather than tunneled long-term central lines. However, these lines are less compliant as a result of the manufacturing process of impregnation and careful consideration should be made prior to their use.

Hemorrhage can be caused by damage to the vein, inadvertent puncture of an artery or the heart [44], and exacerbated by thrombocytopenia/impaired clotting in pancytopenic patients. While in most cases general measures (mainly local pressure application) suffice, in some, vascular reconstruction/emergency cardiac surgery may be necessary to correct the problem. Mortality is indeed associated with this thankfully rare complication. Phlebitis is rarely observed with correctly positioned central lines and is more commonly the result of peripheral administration (mainly through necessity) of venotoxic solutions or due to displacement of the tip of the central line from the correct position. Thrombosis is also a sequel of the presence of the line in the circulation as such and this may lead to vein stricture and/or thrombosis. Pulmonary embolus is a rare complication usually resulting from the dislodgement of a thrombus from the right atrium (RA). Keeping the catheter tip proximal to the RA avoids this complication.

Prior to each use, the line should be checked for free flow of blood both ways. If in doubt, a chest radiograph and possibly an echocardiogram should be performed to assess the position and presence of thrombus around the line. Early detection and treatment will reduce the chances of thromboembolic complications. Air embolism can occur during insertion of the line or through a breach of the integrity of the line. The former can be avoided if the patient remains in head down position until the line is inserted, flushed, and sealed and the latter by regular careful inspection of the integrity of the line and all obturator parts.

Pneumothorax is a well-recognized, although rare, complication of percutaneous subclavian vein access and all patients/families should be warned about this possibility. If recognized early, it is successfully treated by the insertion of a chest drain. Chylothorax is a very rare complication of central venous access, almost exclusively after left-sided approach due to the proximity of the thoracic duct to the confluence of the internal jugular vein with the left subclavian. It can be avoided by ensuring open approaches remain above the confluence of the two great veins.

If the line is advanced too far (i.e., into the RA), it can cause atrial arrhythmias by interfering with the SA or AV node or ventricular arrhythmias by interfering directly with the ventricular myocardial wall. In such cases, the line should be remanipulated in the correct position as soon as possible. Fracture of the catheter, if complete, can result in the distal segment embolizing into the pulmonary vasculature. This can be successfully retrieved through a transfemoral minimally invasive technique best done in the cardiac catheter suite.

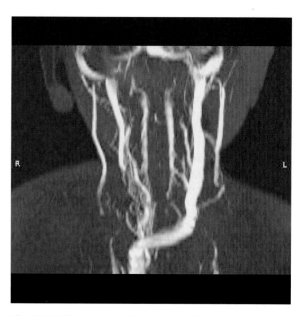

Fig. 27.8 MR venogram showing complete occlusion of the right internal jugular and subclavian veins with the development of tortuous collateral circulation. CVL cannulation was achieved by percutaneous subclavian access of the innominate vein

Many unfortunate patients require repeated insertions of central lines over long periods of time and this eventually results in obliteration/thrombosis of the available veins. In order to avoid fruitless invasive explorations, an angiogram would be indicated if a new attempt at central access is required in such a patient. Until recently, the investigation of choice was a formal angiogram, which is associated with a high level of radiation and the possibility of allergic reaction to intravenous contrast, or B-mode ultrasound, but these investigations have now been virtually superseded by detailed MR angiography which can effectively guide the surgeon to the appropriate vessel while at the same time being safer and much less invasive for the patient (Fig. 27.8).

27.5 Summary

Technological advances in material manufacture and design have revolutionized the safety of implantable central lines, by reducing their antigenicity and thrombogenic potential, while at the same time augmenting their longevity in the circulation. Surgical technique has evolved in parallel to allow for safe and minimally invasive placement of these lines that afford a more successful and comfortable method of administering the necessary chemotherapeutic and supportive agents to oncology patients.

References

1. Dudrick SJ, Wilmore DW, Vars HM, Rhoads JE (1968) Long-term total parenteral nutrition with growth, development, and positive nitrogen balance. Surgery 64(1):134–142

2. Broviac JW, Cole JJ, Scribner BH (1973) A silicone rubber atrial catheter for prolonged parenteral alimentation. Surg Gynecol Obstet 136(4):602–606

3. Hickman RO, Buckner CD, Clift RA, Sanders JE, Stewart P, Thomas ED (1979) A modified right atrial catheter for access to the venous system in marrow transplant recipients. Surg Gynecol Obstet 148(6):871–875

4. Johnson A, Oppenheim BA (1992) Vascular catheter-related sepsis: Diagnosis and prevention. J Hosp Infect 20(2):67–78

5. De Backer BA, Vanhulle A, Otten J, Deconinck P (1993) Totally implantable central venous access devices in pediatric oncology-our experience in 46 patients. Eur J Pediatr Surg 3(2):101–106

6. Bland KI, Woodcock T (1984) Totally implantable venous access system for cyclic administration of cytotoxic chemotherapy. Am J Surg 147(6):815–816

7. Sala A, Pencharz P, Barr RD (2004) Children, cancer, and nutrition-A dynamic triangle in review. Cancer 100(4):677–687

8. Rossi R, Kleta R, Ehrich JH (1999) Renal involvement in children with malignancies. Pediatr Nephrol 13(2):153–162

9. Maki DG, Ringer M, Alvarado CJ (1991) Prospective randomised trial of povidone-iodine, alcohol, and chlorhexidine for prevention of infection associated with central venous and arterial catheters. Lancet 338(8763):339–343

10. Barsan WG, Hedges JR, Nishiyama H, Lukes ST (1986) Differences in drug delivery with peripheral and central venous injections: Normal perfusion. Am J Emerg Med 4(1):1–3

11. Khawaja HT, Williams JD, Weaver PC (1991) Transdermal glyceryl trinitrate to allow peripheral total parenteral nutrition: A double-blind placebo controlled feasibility study. J R Soc Med 84(2):69–72

12. Thiagarajan RR, Ramamoorthy C, Gettmann T, Bratton SL (1997) Survey of the use of peripherally inserted central venous catheters in children. Pediatrics 99(2):E4

13. Racadio JM, Doellman DA, Johnson ND, Bean Jacobs BR (2001) Pediatric peripherally inserted JA, central catheters: Complication rates related to catheter tip location. Pediatrics 107(2):E28

14. Pezzati M, Filippi L, Chiti G, Dani C, Rossi S, Bertini G, Rubaltelli FF (2004) Central venous catheters and cardiac tamponade in preterm infants. Intensive Care Med 30(12):2253–2256

15. Nowlen TT, Rosenthal GL, Johnson GL, Tom DJ, Vargo TA (2002) Pericardial effusion and tamponade in infants with central catheters. Pediatrics 110(1):137–142

16. Angle JF, Matsumoto AH, Skalak TC, O'Brien RF, Hartwell GD, Tegtmeyer CJ (1997) Flow characteristics of peripherally inserted central catheters. J Vasc Interv Radiol 8(4):569–577

17. Waitt C, Waitt P, Pirmohamed M (2004) Intravenous therapy. Postgrad Med J 80(939):1–6

18. Ziegler M, Jakobowski D, Hoelzer D, Eichelberger M, Koop CE (1980) Route of pediatric parenteral nutrition: Proposed criteria revision. J Pediatr Surg 15(4):472–476

19. Maki DG, Kluger DM, Crnich CJ (2006) The risk of bloodstream infection in adults with different intravascular devices: A systematic review of 200 published prospective studies. Mayo Clin Proc 81(9):1159–1171

20. Maki DG, Cobb L, Garman JK, Shapiro JM, Ringer M, Helgerson RB (1988) An attachable silver-impregnated cuff for prevention of infection with central venous catheters: A prospective randomized multicenter trial. Am J Med 85(3):307–314

21. Wiener ES, McGuire P, Stolar CJ, Rich RH, Albo VC, Ablin AR, Betcher DL, Sitarz AL, Buckley JD, Krailo MD (1992) The CCSG prospective study of venous access devices: An analysis of insertions and causes for removal. J Pediatr Surg 27(2):155–163

22. Delmore JE, Horbelt DV, Jack BL, Roberts DK (1989) Experience with the Groshong long-term central venous catheter. Gynecol Oncol 34(2):216–218

23. Kirkemo A, Johnston MR (1982) Percutaneous subclavian vein placement of the Hickman catheter. Surgery 91(3):349–351

24. Reardon PR, McKinney GP, Craig ES, Reardon MJ (2003) A loop technique for the safe, secure, and convenient fixation of subclavian central venous catheters to the chest wall. Am J Surg 185(6):536–537

25. Sri PT, Corbally M, Fitzgerald RI (2003) New technique for fixation of Broviac catheters. J Pediatr Surg 38(1):51–52

26. Babu R, Spicer RD (2001) "Cuff-stitch" to prevent inadvertent dislodgement of central venous catheters. Pediatr Surg Int 17(2–3):245–246

27. Desmond J, Megahed M (2003) Is the central venous pressure reading equally reliable if the central line is inserted via the femoral vein. Emerg Med J 20(5):467–469

28. Deshpande KS, Hatem C, Ulrich HL, Currie BP, Aldrich TK, Bryan-Brown CW, Kvetan V (2005) The incidence of infectious complications of central venous catheters at the subclavian, internal jugular, and femoral sites in an intensive care unit population. Crit Care Med 33(1):13–20

29. Eisen LA, Narasimhan M, Berger JS, Mayo PH, Rosen MJ, Schneider RF (2006) Mechanical complications of central venous catheters. J Intensive Care Med 21(1):40–46

30. Grebenik CR, Boyce A, Sinclair ME, Evans RD, Mason DG, Martin B (2004) NICE guidelines for central venous catheterization in children. Is the evidence base sufficient? Br J Anaesth 92(6):827–830

31. Brooks AJ, Alfredson M, Pettigrew B, Morris DL (2005) Ultrasound-guided insertion of subclavian venous access ports. Ann R Coll Surg Engl 87(1):25–27

32. Adler A, Yaniv I, Steinberg R, Solter E, Samra Z, Stein J, Levy I (2006) Infectious complications of implantable ports and Hickman catheters in paediatric haematology-oncology patients. J Hosp Infect 62(3):358–365

33. Goossens GA, Vrebos M, Stas M, De Wever I, Frederickx L (2005) Central vascular access devices in oncology and hematology considered from a different point of view: How do patients experience their vascular access ports? J Infus Nurs 28(1):61–67

34. Borst CG, de Kruif AT, van Dam FS, de Graaf PW (1992) Totally implantable venous access ports-the patients' point of view. A quality control study. Cancer Nurs 15(5):378–381

35. Capdevila JA (1998). Catheter-related infection: An update on diagnosis, treatment, and prevention. Int J Infect Dis 2(4):230–236

36. Erbay A, Ergonul O, Stoddard GJ, Samore MH (2006) Recurrent catheter-related bloodstream infections: Risk factors and outcome. Int J Infect Dis 10(5):396–400

37. Nahata MC, King DR, Powell DA, Marx SM, Ginn-Pease ME (1988) Management of catheter-related infections in pediatric patients. J Parenter Enteral Nutr 12(1):58–59

38. Somme S, Gedalia U, Caceres M, Hill CB, Liu DC (2001) Wireless replacement of the "lost" central venous line in children. Am Surg 67(9):817–819

39. Cyna AM, Hovenden JL, Lehmann A, Rajaseker K, Kalia P (1998) Routine replacement of central venous catheters: Telephone survey of intensive care units in mainland Britain. Br Med J 316(7149):1944–1945

40. Cook D, Randolph A, Kernerman P, Cupido C, King D, Soukup C, Brun-Buisson C (1997) Central venous catheter replacement strategies: A systematic review of the literature. Crit Care Med 25(8):1417–1424

41. Hachem R, Raad I (2002) Prevention and management of long-term catheter related infections in cancer patients. Cancer Invest 20(7–8):1105–1113

42. Darouiche RO, Raad II, Heard SO, Thornby JI, Wenker OC, Gabrielli A, Berg J, Khardori N, Hanna H, Hachem R, Harris RL, Mayhall G (1999) A comparison of two anti-microbial-impregnated central venous catheters. Catheter Study Group. N Engl J Med 340(1):1–8

43. O'Grady NP (2002) Applying the science to the prevention of catheter-related infections. J Crit Care 17(2):114–121

44. Bagwell CE, Salzberg AM, Sonnino RE, Haynes JH (2000) Potentially lethal complications of central venous catheter placement. J Pediatr Surg 35(5):709–713

45. Cortelezzi A, Moia M, Falanga A, Pogliani EM, Agnelli G, Bonizzoni E, Gussoni G, Barbui T, Mannucci PM (2005) Incidence of thrombotic complications in patients with haematological malignancies with central venous catheters: A prospective multicentre study. Br J Haematol 129(6):811–817

46. Schwarz RE, Coit DG, Groeger JS (2000) Transcutaneously tunnelled central venous lines in cancer patients: An analysis of device related morbidity factors based on prospective data collection. Ann Surg Oncol 7(6):441–449

47. Heckmann JG, Lang CJ, Kindler K, Huk W, Erbguth FJ, Neundorfer B (2000) Neurologic manifestations of cerebral air embolism as a complication of central venous catheterization. Crit Care Med 28(5):1621–1625

Palliative Care and Pain Management

28

John Currie

Contents

28.1 Introduction

It is one of the "Rights of the Child" not to have to endure pain [1, 2]. In the past there was little knowledge or understanding of pain in children [3]. Many of us were taught that babies do not feel pain. Minor operations such as circumcision were often performed on neonates with no analgesia. We now know this to be a cruel misconception and in fact neonates have an enhanced, more global response to pain. Sensitization of the nervous system by trauma at such an early age can lead to different pain behavior in later life [4]. This global response in neonates is due in part to the poor hyalinization of nerves at this early stage of life, and also to the inability to localize pain until the brain develops a proper body image in the first few months of life.

This better understanding of pediatric pain has led to a revolution in pain management for acute and peri-operative pain in children. Most children's hospitals now have a well established "pain team" who ensure protocols are followed and that pain is adequately assessed and treated. It is from this initiative that the problem of chronic pain in children came to be recognized. These principles have been applied to chronic pain due to terminal disease.

Pain is an adaptive mechanism. Pain is a sensation and a reaction to that sensation. It helps us to avoid noxious stimuli in our environment and protect any injury while healing takes place. Pain is incorporated in our body image, localized and then changes our behavior. Our body image and pain behavior develop throughout childhood. For instance, a child under 5 years of age may describe any pain as "tummy ache" [5]. The pain may be somatic, visceral, or both, each type of pain having a different effect on the child. Somatic pain is easier to incorporate into the body image; a cut or broken arm can be seen. It is part of the body, outside of "self." Visceral pain, on the other hand, is more difficult to visualize. It is mediated mainly by C fiber pathways with anatomical connections into the limbic system. This is more frightening and has a greater emotional response. It is also harder to localize. We do not have a well-developed internal body image. A good example of this is appendicitis, which presents as a central abdominal pain until our nervous system works it all out.

Pain may be useful and protective, and this is easier to tolerate, and usually time limited. Chronic pain can be thought of as "useless" pain. This can lead to more suffering. Suffering is a global concept, associated with negative feeling, and impairs quality of life. This type of pain needs a different approach and this is what is provided by pain clinics in their pain management programs.

If the pain is associated with neoplasia then these negative feelings are enhanced. Any worsening of the pain will be interpreted by the patient and their family as progression of the disease. The final stage is palliative care. Here pain and symptom management is the goal, realizing that a cure is impossible and the outcome hopeless. This situation is obviously very psychologically demanding on staff as well as devastating for the family. The more closely staff are involved with the care of these children then the more difficult this situation will be. Nurses in particular will be in need of psychological support when caring for a dying child.

A palliative care team is extremely valuable for providing objective advice regarding difficult decisions and support to the primary care team. This team should meet regularly in an environment conducive to open discussion, rather than on the ward itself. In our own institution the team consists of our lead oncologist, pain management consultant, liaison psychiatrist, pediatrician, surgeon, and the nurses who coordinate care in the child's home as well as during ward admissions. We find that this approach works well. It is also useful to maintain close contact with the hospital ethics committee for help with end of life decisions and "do not resuscitate" orders.

Pain from childhood tumors is chronic "useless" pain which may develop as the disease progresses to become terminal pain needing palliative care. There may be acute events related to the progression of the disease, such as fractures related to bone metastases, pleuritic pain due to infection, or pain due to lymphoedema, for example.

What do we mean by "chronic pain?" The most widely accepted definition is that of Bonica [6]. He defined chronic pain as:

Pain which persists a month beyond the usual course of an acute disease or reasonable time for an injury to heal or is associated with a chronological pathological process which causes continuous pain or pain which recurs at intervals for months or years.

In palliative care the ongoing disease process leads to a chronic pain picture which is progressive. The last few years have seen a considerable development in our understanding of pain mechanisms [7]. Laboratory and clinical studies have demonstrated increased spontaneous activity involving both mechanosensitivity and chemosensitivity in damaged peripheral nerves [8]. The consequent increased neural activity effects changes in both the dorsal root ganglion and the dorsal horn of the spinal cord (Fig. 28.1). This is a well-known phenomenon of dorsal horn windup. Abolition of spontaneous activity from damaged nociceptors or nerves may allow remodeling of the dorsal horn, and other areas of the central nervous system, resulting in prolonged pain relief.

This is an example of how the nervous system adapts to a chronic stimulus. The nervous system "learns" and tends to facilitate chronic stimulation. This has led to the concept of the plasticity of the nervous system which is now well established [9–11]. Understanding of the way in which the nervous system adapts to chronic pain inputs has lead to a range of techniques and specific drug treatments for the control of chronic pain [12].

This "learning" takes place throughout the nervous system all the way through to how the body image is mapped into higher centers and hence to consciousness [13] (Fig. 28.2).

Thus the pain may become "neuropathic" (from the Greek "neuro," meaning nerves, and "pathy," meaning abnormality). This is pain either originating from abnormal firing of nerve cells, or abnormal propagation of sensory input so that nonnoxious sensations are perceived as painful. This type of pain relies on dif-

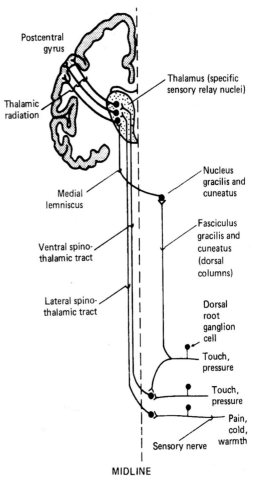

Fig. 28.2 Mapping of the body image through the thalamus to the post central gyrus. The post central gyrus is the area of the sensory cortex where the body is mapped as the homunculus (little man).

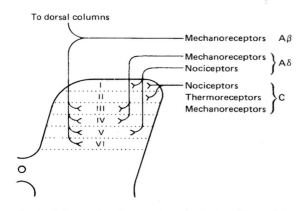

Fig. 28.1 Integration of sensory input in the dorsal horn of the spinal cord.

ferent transmitters within the nervous system, notably the n-methyl d-aspartate (NMDA), gamma amino butyric acid (GABA), and alpha-amino-3-hydroxy-5-methyl-4-isoxazolepropionate (AMPA) systems [14–16]. Neuropathic pain does not usually respond to conventional analgesic regimes and is opiate resistant.

28.2 Management of Pain in the Child with Advanced Malignancy

The effects of a tumor are complex and debilitating. As the tumor grows it may compress local tissues or nerves causing pain. Compression of nerves is a classic way in which neuropathic pain in produced. Indeed, compression by ligature is the most common way of producing an experimental neuropathic pain model. The tumor may also infiltrate into a nerve bundle or plexus causing pain. Infiltration into bone will initially cause painful pressure on the periosteum and may progress to cause pathological fractures. The same is true of bone metastases. Tumors also produce secretions which can act locally or systemically. Locally acting secretions include kallikreins [17, 18] and bradykinin [19, 20], which cause pain in nerve endings adjacent to the tumor. Recent research has focused on the purine pain pathway, mediated by adenosine triphosphate [21–23]. This is particularly interesting with relation to pain caused by tumors due to the very high levels of adenosine triphosphate in cancer cells. Systemically cancers produce substances that alter metabolism and the immune response. This leads to systemic pain, which is not well understood. Pain can also result from recumbence and pressure on thinned and weakened tissues.

Successful management of pain and other symptoms of pediatric tumors demands a team approach. Nurse pain specialists will liaise with the ward teams on a day-to-day basis, and in particular with the home support nurses. This latter group is key to managing pain at home. Most children are better nursed at home with their families where possible. This is particularly true at the end stages of life. The ideal is for the child to die comfortably at home. Other members of the team will include a psychologist and perhaps also a psychiatrist to try to help with the inevitable depression and anxiety. Where a family has a strong religious faith then close involvement with their church and hospital chaplain, etc., is extremely helpful. The physiotherapists can help with stiffness and pain due to recumbence as well as breathing exercises and helping to clear secretions. Any acute exacerbations of pain can be assessed with the help of the diagnostic imaging department to diagnose fractures, effusions, etc.

When assessing a patient with pain due to malignancy, adequate enquiry to obtain information is essential. We use a detailed questionnaire that the child fills in with the help of the family. This can identify the different types of pain the child has, as well as how it changes during each day. A pain diary can help with how the pain is responding to treatment or progressing.

The first step is to try to gain control and break the cycle of pain. Patient-controlled methods are preferably as they give some control to the child. They have something they can do. This can also help allay the fear that the pain may crescendo and become completely uncontrollable. Children often fear what the pain may be like rather than deal with what it is. Anyone who has performed a venipuncture on a child will know this well! A transcutaneous nerve stimulation device is extremely useful and is often our first line of approach. For visceral pain we have found a TSE (Transcutaneous Spinal Electro-analgesia) machine extremely useful. This is coupled with explanation and reassuring the patient and family, i.e., explanation as to why the child has pain, due to the mechanisms we have described, and reassurance that pain does not necessarily mean progression of the disease.

Sometimes more of an intervention event is necessary to break the cycle of pain. This may be a local anesthetic injection or an infusion of medication. It is important to get control of the pain in order to gain the confidence of the child and family.

Then a systematic approach is followed, developing a plan to deal with the pain. This is where the team approach is essential to monitor progress and avoid over treatment. Careful enquiry must be made as to the effect of the pain on the child's sleep pattern. If the child is kept awake or woken by pain, the whole family will be woken and lose sleep. This has a detrimental effect on everyone's mood and ability to cope. Pain relief must be first directed to give the child a good night's sleep. Melatonin is extremely useful for re-establishing normal sleep patterns. After that, pain control at rest is the goal, followed by pain control for whatever activity the child may be capable of. Pain control during all activity may not be possible, but some degree of mobility can usually be achieved, even if only from bed to chair.

28.3 Medical Treatment

There is still a place for conventional analgesia regimes. Many children will respond and not progress to the more intractable pain picture. Care must be taken to give adequate analgesic doses of these drugs and to make full use of the synergism between different drug groups. A good example of this is to combine paracetamol with nonsteroidal anti-inflammatory drugs (NSAIDs).

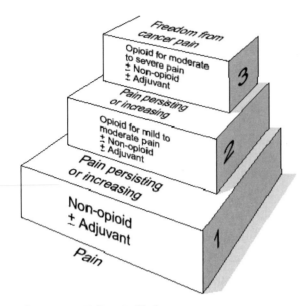

Fig. 28.3 WHO "Pain Ladder."

This represents the first stage of the World Health Organization analgesic ladder (Fig. 28.3). Most units would progress from this first stage to stage three, strong opiates. This bypasses stage two, weak opiates. Stage two is unlikely to control the pain for long, and the side effects of the weak opiates are out of proportion with their efficacy in controlling pain.

Morphine is the standard opiate used and will initially be given intravenously to determine the required dose. This can then be converted to oral morphine given as a long-lasting (continuous) preparation twice daily. Breakthrough pain can be controlled by oral morphine given as the standard preparation. As long as oral intake is possible this is the ideal regime as is effective in most cases. Diamorphine can be used if morphine becomes ineffective, as it is a more powerful analgesic with the added benefit of a more profound anxiolytic action. It is extremely soluble making it the ideal agent for subcutaneous administration usually as an infusion. Fentanyl patches allow opiate absorption without a cannula. Patches are available in different strengths allowing titration of the dose. Each patch will give a steady dose of opiate through the skin for 72 h. Oral morphine can be used for breakthrough effect.

Nerve blocking techniques are useful, and may be peripheral or central. Laboratory and clinical studies have demonstrated increased spontaneous activity involving both mechanosensitivity and chemosensitivity in damaged peripheral nerves. The consequent increased neural activity effects changes in both the dorsal root ganglion and the dorsal horn of the spinal cord [8]. Abolition of spontaneous activity from damaged nociceptors or nerves may allow remodeling of the dorsal horn, and other areas of the central nervous system, resulting in prolonged pain relief. Local anesthetic administered by subcutaneous infiltration or directly to specific nerves can produce long-lasting pain relief for a variety of chronic painful conditions [10, 12]. Pain relief will often last for months [17]. Intrapleural blocks can be very useful for upper abdominal pain as well as pain in the thorax. A catheter can be used and an infusion given. This can be a very useful "event" to gain control of pain that has become intractable.

Many treatments despite involving short-term modification of the neural pathways nevertheless have long-term effects, for example, injecting local anesthetic drugs. We are manipulating the plasticity of the nervous system. I like to think of this as rebooting the system so that the normal program can run. In this computer age children relate well to this analogy.

Some pain may be mediated by the sympathetic nervous system and be helped by sympathetic blockade [24]. A good example is coeliac plexus block for pain mediated by upper abdominal tumors, particularly those affecting the pancreas. We have, in our unit, a particular interest in coeliac plexus block for upper abdominal pain [25, 26] (Figs. 28.4–28.7).

Stellate ganglion block can be very effective in controlling pain mediated by the sympathetic nervous system in the upper quadrants. A block using local anesthetic such as levo-bupivacaine gives long-term relief and seldom needs to be repeated (Fig. 28.8).

In chronic pain epidural block is often a technique of last resort. The catheter can be tunneled to allow for long-term use. There are difficulties involved in managing a patient with a long-term epidural catheter, but these can be overcome with careful monitoring. These epidural infusions can be successfully managed at home. There are more drug preparations now available for administration by the epidural or caudal route as well as techniques for modification of neuronal function at this level [27, 28]. Catheters can also be placed intrathecally and this is an extremely effective method of achieving pain control [29]. The high risk of infection limits its usefulness [30]. Reservoirs of medication can be implanted under the skin, but this technique is limited by cost not just of the system itself but also in terms of resources to manage it effectively. The most common drugs used in these central blocks are local anesthetics such as levo-bupivacaine and opiates such as morphine or diamorphine. Adjuvant drugs such as clonidine can enhance the effect of local anesthetic.

The position of the tip of the epidural catheter can be confirmed by radiography or ultrasound to ensure accurate delivery of the medication (Fig. 28.9).

Other more invasive techniques may include nerve destruction, but this is seldom employed in children. An exception is ablation of the coeliac plexus after successful block with local anesthetic. A single localized lesion may be the major source of pain, for example,

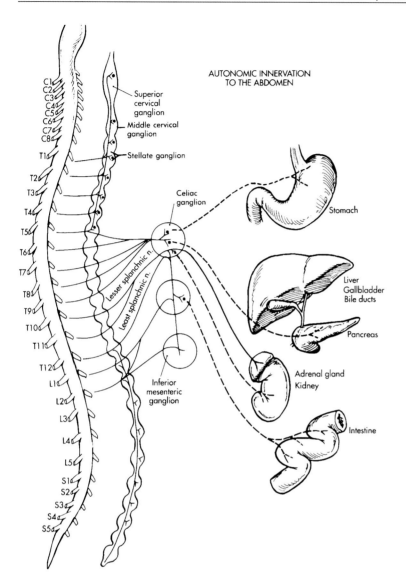

Fig. 28.4 The autonomic innervation of abdominal viscera.

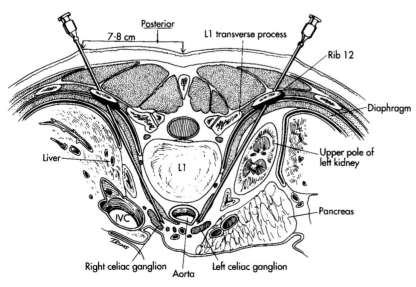

Fig. 28.5 Showing the positioning of the two needles for coeliac plexus (ganglion) block.

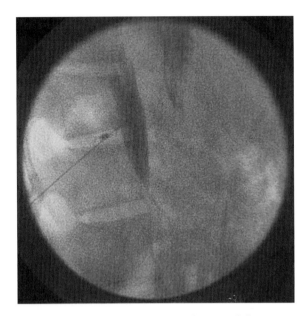

Fig. 28.6 Lateral radiograph showing dye around the aorta at the level of the coeliac ganglion.

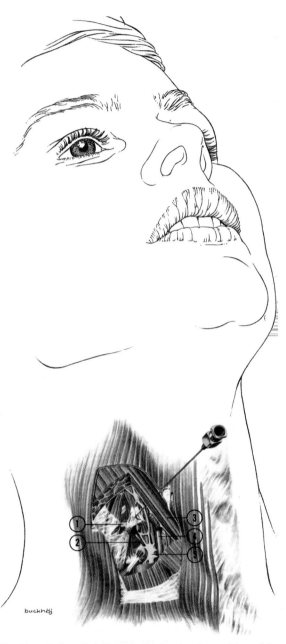

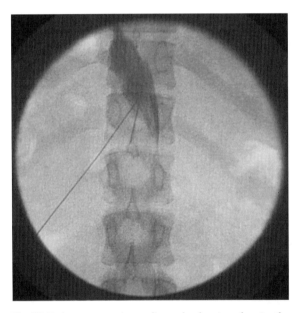

Fig. 28.7 Antero-posterior radiograph showing dye in the midline at T12

Fig. 28.8 Stellate Ganglion Block, showing the position of the ganglion in the neck and enlarged to show position of the needle adjacent to the ganglion. (1) Tranverse process of C6, (2) Vertebral artery, (3) Sternocleidomastoid muscle, (4) Common carotid artery, (5) Stellate ganglion

collapse of a vertebra due to tumor infiltration causing pain by nerve compression. This may be treated by injecting polymethyl methacrylate into the vertebra, which hardens and supports the damaged spine. Although obviously rarely used this is an extremely effective technique for controlling this type of very localized pain. We have ourselves used this successfully in a case of vertebral collapse due to hemo-lymphangioma.

The use of other techniques such as acupuncture and aromatherapy can be very effective [27]. Careful patient selection is important, particularly for acupuncture. Aromatherapy has the major advantage of allowing parental involvement. Modern treatment regimes can lead to excessive "medicalization" of the child. The ability to be involved in care is very valuable to parents.

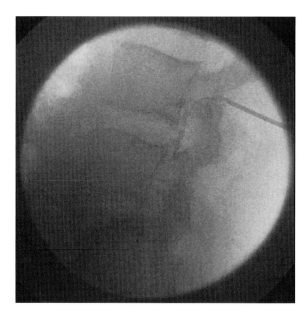

Fig. 28.9 Radiograph of the epidural catheter passing caudad in the epidural space

28.4 When the Drugs Don't Work

Most pain related to cancer will be controlled with opiates as the final stage of the analgesic ladder. The palliative team really comes into its own when these standard techniques fail and "the drugs don't work." This is when these more invasive techniques will be employed. Morphine may not control the pain. The pain may be mediated by different pathways particularly if the pain becomes neuropathic. The main pathway in this process is the N-methyl D-aspartate (NMDA) system.

More specific agents are now available for this neuropathic pain and their mechanisms of action are better understood. [16, 17]. Our first line treatment for somatic neuropathic pain is gabapentin, lamotrigine being preferred for visceral pain. Ketamine is an excellent NMDA blocker and can be used intravenously or as part of an epidural infusion. Psychological side effects limit its use intrathecally. Methadone is also a very effective NMDA blocking agent, but its usefulness is limited by its narrow therapeutic index and significant side effects.

28.5 Other Symptoms

Nausea is a common symptom of cancer pain associated with renal or hepatic dysfunction, chemotherapy, and of course opiates. In children, however, we find that if the dose of opiates is appropriate for the pain then side effects do not present a significant problem.

It is only when the dose is escalated in a futile attempt to control pain that has become opiate resistant, that the unwanted effects emerge. Nausea can be as distressing as the pain itself and should be treated aggressively [36]. The cause should be determined, whether it be due to chemotherapy or metabolic dysfunction. Hypercalcemia, which may occur particularly in metastatic tumors, must always be excluded, as it is a potent cause of vomiting. The antiemetic will be chosen with regard to the cause of vomiting in each particular patient.

Excess secretions can be a major problem in the end stages of palliative care. The child may be too weak to cough and clear normal secretions or infection may lead to increased secretions. This may lead to noisy breathing or indeed choking which is very distressing to relatives and staff caring for the child. Hyoscine usually applied as a patch is very effective in relieving this symptom.

In a pain management program the input of other health care professionals is essential. This is particularly important in palliative care especially at the end of life. Depression and anxiety are features of terminal care in even the youngest of patients. This must be recognized particularly as many of the drugs to help with this can take days to work. A particular feature of palliative care is terminal agitation. The cause of this is multifactorial. Factors include poor metabolism of drugs at the end of life as well as increased anxiety. Nozinan (levomepromazine) is the most effective treatment, and has the added advantage of being an excellent antiemetic.

New drugs on the horizon which may be useful for neuropathic pain are levetiracetam an antiepileptic with a novel mode of action [31], and the AMPA blocking agent Anandamide.

Many of these new techniques and methods have resulted in some ethical dilemmas. For instance, most of the drugs used are not licensed for use in children or are being prescribed for conditions that are "off-license" for that drug.

28.6 The Future

There are many promising new developments in the study of chronic pain. We have several new drugs which can be used to modify the method of transmission of chronic pain and research continues in this area. New developments in functional MRI give us a better understanding of the central changes associated with chronic pain and its treatment. Remapping sensory input into consciousness is an exciting possibility [32, 13]. There is also increasing evidence of a genetic basis or predisposition to chronic pain syndromes opening up further avenues of treatment [33, 34, 36].

These advances will help us in our understanding of the effects of our therapies on the pain pathways and central pain perception, and may also provide guidence in the choice of appropriate treatment.

The drugs and dosages that we use in our clinic are listed in Table 28.1 [37].

Table 28.1 Drugs and dosages used in author's clinic

Neuropathic pain drugs
These drugs should be titrated slowly up to the effective dose. This will help to avoid unwanted effects. They should not be stopped suddenly, but weaned off gradually. Doses for pain management are generally lower than those used to control epilepsy.
Gabapentin: >60 kg max dose up to 3600 mg/24 h <45 kg max dose up to 2400 mg/24 h <30 kg max dose up to 1200 mg/24 h <20 kg not recommended Preparations available: capsules: 100 mg, 300 mg (can be opened & mixed with food, e.g., jam, etc.) Tablets: 600 mg, 800 mg
Amitryptilline: requires ECG before commencement. >50 kg 25 mg PM - aim for 25 mg BD <50 kg 10 mg PM - aim for 10 mg BD <30 kg not recommended Preparations available: oral solution: 25 mg/ml, 50 mg/5ml Tablets: 10 mg, 50 mg
Carbamazepine: >40 kg 100 mg PM should be effective at this dose <40 kg not recommended Preparations available: tablets: 100 mg, 200 mg, 400 mg Chewtabs (tegretol): 100 mg, 200 mg Oral solution (tegretol): 100 mg/5ml Suppositories (tegretol): 125 mg, 250 mg Slow release (tegretol retard): 200 mg, 400 mg
Lamotrigine: >50 kg START 10 mg BD (max 40 mg.BD) >30 kg START 5 mg BD (Max 25 mg BD) <30 kg not recommended Titrate to effect. We start this with child as in-patient as adverse reactions, particularly a rash may be a problem. Preparations available: tablets: 25 mg, 50 mg, 100 mg, 200 mg Soluble: 5 mg, 25 mg, 100 mg
Topiramate >30 kg 2–6 mg/kg per day in two divided doses. Initiate 25 mg nightly with weekly increments of 1–3 mg/kg withdraw very slowly.
NSAIDs (Non Steroidal Anti Inflammatory Drugs)
Caution if bleeding risk, asthma, atopy, renal dysfunction, GI ulceration/bleeding, on anticoagulants, (avoid if <6 months or weight <10 kg).
Diclofenac: 1 mg/kg up to 8 hourly Preparations available: tablets: 25 mg, 50 mg Suppositories: 100 mg Modified release (diclomax SR): 75 mg Modified release (voltarol retard): 100 mg

Table 28.1 *(Continued)* Drugs and dosages used in author's clinic

Ibuprofen: 10 mg/kg up to 6 hourly   Preparations available: tablets: 200 mg, 600 mg   Oral suspension: 100 mg/5mls   Effervescent granules: 600 mg/sachet
Naproxen: <5 years not recommended   >5 years 10 mg/kg in 2 divided doses   Preparations available: tablets: 250 mg, 500 mg   Oral solution: 125 mg/ml   Suppositories: 500 mg
Piroxicam: <15 kg 5 mg stat   16–25 kg 10 mg daily   26–45 kg 15 mg daily   >46 kg 20 mg daily   Preparations available: capsules: 10 mg, 20 mg   Melts (Feldene): 20 mg   Suppositories: 20 mg
Antiemetics should be chosen in relation to the cause of the vomiting.   Ondansetron: is a specific 5HT three serotonin antagonist.   Dose: 0.1 mg/kg (100 micrograms) 8 hourly   Preparations available: tablets: 4 mg, 8 mg   Oral lyophilisates (zofran melt): 4 mg, 8 mg   Domperidone: does not readily cross the blood-brain barrier, so causes less central effects. It acts at the chemoreceptor trigger zone.   Dose: 200–400mcg/kg 4–8 hourly   <20 kg not recommended   Preparations available: tablets: 10 mg   Oral solution: 5 mg/5mls   Suppositories: 30 mg   Hyoscine: Topical hyoscine preferred (Scopoderm TTS):   Dose: >35 kg 1 mg patch   Not recommended <10 years   Preparations available: 1 mg/72 h when in contact with skin.   Metoclopramide   500 micrograms/kg/24 h   Oral or IV   Methotrimeprazine   Excellent for intractable nausea/vomiting. Sedative and useful for „terminal agitation" in palliative care.   Initial dose 0.25 mg/kg daily given in 2 or 3 divided doses. This dosage may be increased gradually until an effective level is reached which should not surpass 40 mg/day for a child less than 12 years of age.
Opioids
Minimum monitoring standard for in-patients. Do not mix opioids or routes of administration.
Loading dose   >3 months old 0.1–0.2 mg/kg (100–200micrograms/kg).   Switch to oral as soon as possible.

Table 28.1 *(Continued)* Drugs and dosages used in author's clinic

Oral opiods
MST: opioid naïve child: <15 kg expert use only
15–25 kg: 5 mg BD
25–50 kg: 10 mg BD >50 kg: 15-20 mg BD Preparations available: tablets: 5 mg, 10 mg, 30 mg, 100 mg Sachets: 20 mg, 30 mg, 60 mg, 100 mg, 200 mg
Oramorph: opioid naïve child: one fifth of total MST dose for breakthrough 4/6 hourly. Preparations available: oral solution: 10 mg/5mls If more than 3 doses of oromorph per day add to MST dose by adding total dose of drug to MST dose and divide to 2 equal doses. Always titrate to effect. Doses may be considerably higher in children who are not opiate naïve.
Diamorphine: Extremely soluble and so is useful in small volumes for subcutaneous administration. When converting from morphine start with 1/4 to 1/3 of combined oral MST and oromorph dose Sevredol: As oromorph, one fifth of total MST dose for breakthrough 4/6 hourly. Preparations available: oral solution: tablets: 10 mg, 20 mg Conversion to MST as per oromorph recommendations.
Oxycontin and oxycodone are alternatives to MST and ORAMORPH
Tramadol: >12 years 50 mg 6 hourly >60 kg 100 mg 6 hourly Preparations available: capsules: 50 mg Soluble: 50 mg Slow release: 100 mg, 150 mg, 200 mg Effectiveness limited by high incidence of nausea.
Dihydrocodeine: 0.5–1 mg/kg 6 hourly Preparations available: tablets: 30 mg Oral solution: 10 mg/5mls Slow release: 60 mg

Topical opioids
Fentanyl: opioid naïve child: 25mcg/hr patch Under 30 kg: half patch Under 15 kg: quarter patch Patch should not be cut but placed over nonporous dressing such as Tegederm to give desired surface area of patch next to the skin. Preparation available: patch 25 = 25mcg/hr for 72 h Patch 50 = 50mcg/hr for 72 h Patch 75 = 75mcg/hr for 72 h Patch 100 = 100mcg/hr for 72 h When starting evaluation of the analgesic effect should not be made before the system has been worn for 24 h to allow the gradual increase in plasma-fentanyl concentration. It also may take 17 h or longer for the plasma-fentanyl concentration to decrease by 50%. Patches should be changed every 72 h.

NMDA (N-methyl-D-aspartic acid) antagonist
These drugs should only be used by specialists for severe intractable pain. Ketamine: Binds to specifically to phencyclidine site (PCP site) of the NMDA receptor-gated channel and blocks NMDA receptors. It can be associated with general disturbances of sensory perception. This is an anesthetic and adequate training before use is essential. Sublingual: may be used to test efficacy 1 mg/kg diluted in 5 mls water: spit out after 2 min or if feeling dizzy. Intravenous: start at 15 mg/kg in 24-h period diluted in normal saline to give dose of 2–4ml/hr. May need up to 25 mg/kg/24hours, Epidurally: Epidural agents must be preservative free. Start with bolus of 0.6 mg/kg and then 0.8– 1 mg/kg in 24-h period. Methadone: Epidurally: as per epidural ketamine doses

References

1. Southall DP et al. (2000) The Child-Friendly Healthcare Initiative (CFHI): Healthcare Provision in Accordance With the UN Convention on the Rights of the Child. Pediatrics 106(5):1054–1064

2. http://www.childfriendlyhealthcare.org/publications/pediatrics.htm

3. Bonica JJ (1990) Evolution and current status of pain programs. J Pain Sympt Manage 5(6):368–374 (review)

4. Taddio A, Katz J (2005) The effects of early pain experience in neonates on pain responses in infancy and childhood. Paediatric Drugs 7(4):245–257 (review)

5. Franck LS, Greenberg CS, Stevens B (2000) Pain assessment in infants and children. In: Yaster M (ed) The pediatric clinics of North America. Lippincott, Philadelphia, pp 487–512

6. Bonica JJ (1990) The management of pain, 2nd edn, vol 1. Lea and Febiger, Pennsylvania

7. Fitzgerald M, Howard RF (2003) The neurobiologic basis of pediatric pain. In: Schecter NL, Berde CB, Yaster M (eds) Pain in infants, children and adolescents, 2nd edn. Lippincott, Philadelphia, pp 19–42

8. Hu P, McLachlan EM (2001) Long-term changes in the distribution of galanin in dorsal root ganglia after sciatic or spinal nerve transection in rats. Neuroscience 103(4):1059–1071

9. Bago M, Dean C (2001) Sympathoinhibition from ventrolateral periaqueductal gray mediated by 5-HT(1A) receptors in the RVLM. Am J Physiol Regul Integr Comp Physiol 280(4):R976–R984

10. Holmberg K, Shi TJ, Albers KM, Davis BM, Hokfelt T (2001) Effect of peripheral nerve lesion and lumbar sympathectomy on peptide regulation in dorsal root ganglia in the NGF-overexpressing mouse. Exp Neurol 167(2):290–303

11. Scislo TJ, Kitchen AM, Augustyniak RA, O'Leary DS (2001) Differential patterns of sympathetic responses to selective stimulation of nucleus tractus solitarius purinergic receptor subtypes. Clin Exp Pharmacol Physiol 28(1-2):120–124 (review)

12. Chabal C (1994) Membrane stabilizing agents and experimental neuromas. In: Fields HL, Liebeskind JC (eds) Pharmacological approaches to the treatment of chronic pain: New concepts and critical issues. Progress in pain research and management, vol 1. IASP Press, Seattle, pp 205–210

13. Halligan PW, Zeman A, Berger A (1999) Phantoms in the brain. Question the assumption that the adult brain is "hard wired." BMJ 319(7210):587–588

14. Centre for Synaptic Plasticity. http://www.bris.ac.uk/Depts/Synaptic/info/glutamate.html

15. Dev KK, Henley JM (1998) The regulation of AMPA receptor-binding sites. Mol Neurobiol 17(1-3):33–58

16. Parpura V, Basarsky TA, Liu F, Jeftinija K, Jeftinija S, Haydon PG (1994) Glutamate-mediated astrocyte-neuron signalling. Nature 369(6483):707–708

17. Dendorfer A, Wolfrum S, Dominiak P (1999) Pharmacology and cardiovascular implications of the kinin-kallikrein system. Jpn J Pharmacol 79:403–426

18. Skidgel RA, Alhenc-Gelas F, Campbell WB (2003) Relation of cardiovascular signaling by kinins and products of similar converting enzyme systems; prologue: Kinins and related systems. New life for old discoveries. Am J Physiol Heart Circ Physiol 284:H1886–891

19. Dendorfer A, Wolfrum S, Wagemann M, Qadri F, Dominiak P (2001) Pathways of bradykinin degradation in blood and plasma of normotensive and hypertensive rats. Am J Physiol Heart Circ Physiol 280:H2182–H2188

20. Kuoppala A, Lindstedt KA, Saarinen J, Kovanen PT, Kokkonen JO (2000) Inactivation of bradykinin by angiotensin-converting enzyme and by carboxypeptidase N in human plasma. Am J Physiol Heart Circ Physiol 278(4): H1069–H1074

21. Kozlowska M, Smolenski RT, Makarewicz W, Hoffmann C, Jastorff B, Swierczynski J (1999) ATP depletion, purine riboside triphosphate accumulation and rat thymocyte death induced by purine riboside. Toxicol Lett 104(3):171–181

22. Kondo M, Yamaoka T, Honda S, et al. (2000) The rate of cell growth is regulated by purine biosynthesis via ATP production and G1 to S phase transition1. J Biochem 128(1):57–64

23. Yegutkin GG, Samburski SS, Jalkanen S (2003) Soluble purine-converting enzymes circulate in human blood and regulate extracellular ATP level via counteracting pyrophosphatase and phosphotransfer reactions. FASEB J 17(10):1328–1330. Epub 2003 May 20

24. Schurmann M, Gradl G, Wizgal I, Tutic M, Moser C, Azad S, Beyer A (2001) Clinical and physiologic evaluation of stellate ganglion blockade for complex regional pain syndrome type I. Clin J Pain 17(1):94–100

25. Cleary AG, Sills JA, Davidson JE, Cohen AM (2001) Reflex sympathetic dystrophy. Rheumatology (Oxford) 40(5):590–591

26. Ceballos A, Cabezudo L, Bovaira M, Fenollosa P, Moro B (2000) Spinal cord stimulation: A possible therapeutic alternative for chronic mesenteric ischaemia. Pain 87(1):99–101

27. McCleane G (2004) Pharmacological strategies in relieving neuropathic pain. Expert Opin Pharmacother 5(6):1299–1312

28. Manning DC (2004) New and emerging pharmacological targets for neuropathic pain. Curr Pain Headache Reports 8(3):192–198

29. Cousins MJ, Mather LE (1984) Intrathecal and extradural administration of opioids. Anesthesiol 61:276–310

30. Chaney MA (1995) Side effects of intrathecal and extradural opiates. Can J Anaesth 42:891–903

31. Lynch BA, Lambeng N, Nocka K et al. (2004) The synaptic vesicle protein SV2A is the binding site for the antiepileptic drug levetiracetam. Proc Natl Acad Sci 101(26):9861–9866

32. Maihofner C, Handwerker HO, Neundorfer B, Birklein F (2003) Patterns of cortical reorganisation in complex regional pain syndrome. Neurology 61(12):1707–1715

33. Buskila D, Neumann L, Press J (2005) Genetic factors in neuromuscular pain. Cns Spectr 10(4):281–284

34. Finegold AA, Mannes AJ, Iadarola MJ (1999) A paracrine paradigm for in vivo gene therapy in the central nervous system: Treatment of chronic pain. Hum Gene Ther 10(7):1251–1257

35. Kaye P (1994) Pocket book of symptom control. EPL Publications, Northampton, p 72

36. Smith O (1999) Pain-killer genes. Science 284(5420):1634

37. Currie JM (2006) Management of chronic pain in children. Arch Dis Childhood 91:111–114

Parents' Associations and Support Groups

29

Marianne C. Naafs-Wilstra

Parent Organizations – Partners in the Care for Children with Cancer

The International Confederation of Childhood Cancer Parent Organizations (ICCCPO) is an international network representing organizations of parents of children with cancer worldwide. Since its founding in 1994, ICCCPO has increased its membership in 2006 from the initial 9 members to 97 member organizations representing parents and children from 61 countries. ICCCPO works closely with other childhood cancer organizations, in particular with the International Society of Paediatric Oncology (SIOP).

ICCCPO's mission is to share information and experiences in order improve access to the best possible treatment and care for children with cancer everywhere in the world.

ICCCPO Has Several Core Goals

- *Education* of parents, survivors, doctors, nurses, psychologists, teachers, etc. Parent organizations can share their special experiential expertise in order to increase each others' knowledge and to help direct services more appropriately.
- *Public awareness* of the general public with regard to childhood cancer, the needs of children with cancer and their families, the increased chances of cure, and the continuing need for medical and psychosocial monitoring and support.
- *Development* of parent organizations where they don't yet exist. This can be at a local and national level. ICCCPO supports and trains parents to create and lead parent organizations and to strengthen this worldwide movement. Parent organizations are encouraged to act as advocates for their children regarding medical and psychosocial care, school and education, health insurance, etc.
- *Advocacy* for adequate medical and psychosocial care, for advance of the cure rates of children with cancer throughout the world, and for equal access to health insurance and employment of survivors.

In practice, the needs of families and their children differ immensely in various countries. In the industrialized countries effectively all children get diagnosed and treated. Treatment is provided to similar standards, with more than 70% of children surviving. Parent organizations can focus on psychosocial care, eg. welfare, education, emotional, and long-term survivor support.

In lower income countries, most children do not get diagnosed and even if they do, treatment is inadequate or – in the best cases – palliative. Eighty percent of children with cancer in the world fall into this category. Parent organizations in these countries are striving to educate doctors and families about early diagnosis, giving support to help families travel to a center, and providing the drugs that are essential for treatment.

ICCCPO helps parent organizations develop against this varied background of needs.

ICCCPO Activities to Help Parent Organizations Worldwide to Achieve Their Mission

Information and Sharing

Annual conference. Each year ICCCPO holds an international conference, usually at the occasion of the annual SIOP conference. This enables parent organizations, survivor organizations, support organizations, and professionals to meet and take part in lectures and workshops and to informally network.

Regional conferences. ICCCPO also organizes a regional conference wherever the continental SIOPs have their biannual meeting. These meetings provide an excellent forum to discuss the needs of children with cancer and their families from a certain part of the world and to tailor informational sessions and workshops to the wishes of parent organizations and health care professionals in that specific region, to share best practices and thus try to jointly find the best strategy. Next to these joint meetings with the medical professionals,

ICCCPO organizes other regional conferences in areas where, for instance, a common culture or language guarantees the best communication.

Information. ICCCPO provides a range of information through a number of channels. The ICCCPO Newsletter is published two times a year in a digital version, and the ICCCPO website is a major resource for parent organizations and individual parents throughout the world. It brings together information about parent organizations around the world, and provides links to sites which contain information of value for parents and their families.

Public Awareness

International Childhood Cancer Day. This annual event on February 15th helps ICCCPO member organizations to raise awareness and funds for use at a local level.

Development

Twinning. There are many examples of parent organizations twinning to provide development support. For example, a resource-rich member providing support to a resource-poor member, or a member with a long experience of an issue supporting another, to avoid "re-inventing the wheel." Often these twinning programs are jointly run with hospitals in the two different countries.

Local visits. ICCCPO officers visit local parent organizations, often in combination with regional conferences.

Advocacy

ICCCPO works with SIOP in developing guidelines for professionals and parent organizations to help provide holistic treatment and care.

ICCCPO sits at the table with specialists and reviews ethical and informational aspects of innovative treatment studies.

ICCPO believes that every child deserves the chance to live and therefore helps to improve diagnosis and access to treatment and palliative care in resource-poor countries.

ICCCPO strives to improve support for survivors and their families to avoid these families being disadvantaged as a result of cancer.

With ever-competing demands on governments, it falls to those affected, and those working in this field

to advocate the case for children with cancer. No one is better placed than those who have experienced the trauma of life-threatening illness to a child, or who have had to endure inequality as a result of it.

Local Parent Organizations and Their Activities

Local parent organizations are often linked to a certain treatment center. Their activities differ according to the needs of parents in different places, and the resources available to them, but in general organizations work in the following areas.

They provide parents with *information* about the disease and the treatment, about psychosocial issues and coping strategies, and about the hospital and the treatment team. They also give information about financial and insurance issues. They do this through arranging presentations, discussion groups, newsletters, brochures, books, resource lists, and a website.

Parent organizations provide *financial assistance*, home-from-homes, respite care, and information about practical issues such as home care, school programs, and funeral arrangements. They raise funds to help pay for treatment or to improve the children's ward in the hospital. This kind of practical support is especially seen in less wealthy countries where basic medical treatment and funds to travel to the hospital are lacking.

Most parent organizations offer *social support* through recreational programmes for children, like day trips or camps. Often siblings are involved, and sometimes the entire family. They sometimes fund computer links between ill children and their schoolmates to reduce social isolation.

Parent organizations offer *emotional support* in the form of peer-to-peer counseling. Parents who went through the same are only half a word away. There can be special sessions for mothers and fathers separately, for teenage patients or siblings, and for bereaved parents.

Parent organizations often work with the medical team to improve medical and psychosocial care and create change that will benefit them and their children.

National Parent Organizations and Their Activities

National parent organizations generally coordinate and share information and resources among various local groups via meetings, conferences, newsletters, and electronic media. They sometimes support local parent organizations by offering a training program for current and future leaders and volunteers. Often national organizations provide services that would be difficult and costly to organize at each local site, like books, a national newsletter, and camps. Many national organizations sponsor an annual conference for all parents or for group representatives.

National organizations often have access to health care policy-makers. They have the ear of national cancer societies and governmental bodies concerned with cancer policy, health benefits, special educational programs for sick children, funding of childhood cancer research and treatment, etc. They act as advocates, represent parent and survivor concerns, and work with national pediatric oncology organizations, nurses, social workers, and psychologists. Some are active lobbyists in the legislative arena and with employers and insurance companies.

The size of national organizations varies considerably. They count between 5 and 200 local chapters; some only have one chapter, e.g., the national organization. They also vary in their annual budget: organizations in many nations, especially those in the less affluent countries, have very minimal funds.

ICCCPO members and their contact details can be found on the ICCCPO website: www.icccpo.org.

Contact
Marianne C. Naafs-Wilstra
ICCCPO Secretariat
Schouwstede 2B
3431 JB Nieuwegein
The Netherlands
Tel + 31 30 2422944
Email: icccpo@vokk.nl
www.icccpo.nl

Subject Index